Introduction to Clinical Medicine

Editorial Board

Introduction to Clinical Medicine

Edited by

Harry L. Greene, MD

Associate Professor of Medicine
University of Arizona College of Medicine
Chief, Section of General Medicine
University of Arizona Health Sciences Center
Tucson, Arizona

Associate Editors

Richard J. Glassock, MD

Professor of Medicine
UCLA School of Medicine, Los Angeles
Chairman, Department of Medicine
Harbor-UCLA Medical Center
Torrance, California

Mark A. Kelley, MD

Vice Dean for Clinical Affairs
Associate Professor of Medicine
University of Pennsylvania School of Medicine
Philadelphia, Pennsylvania

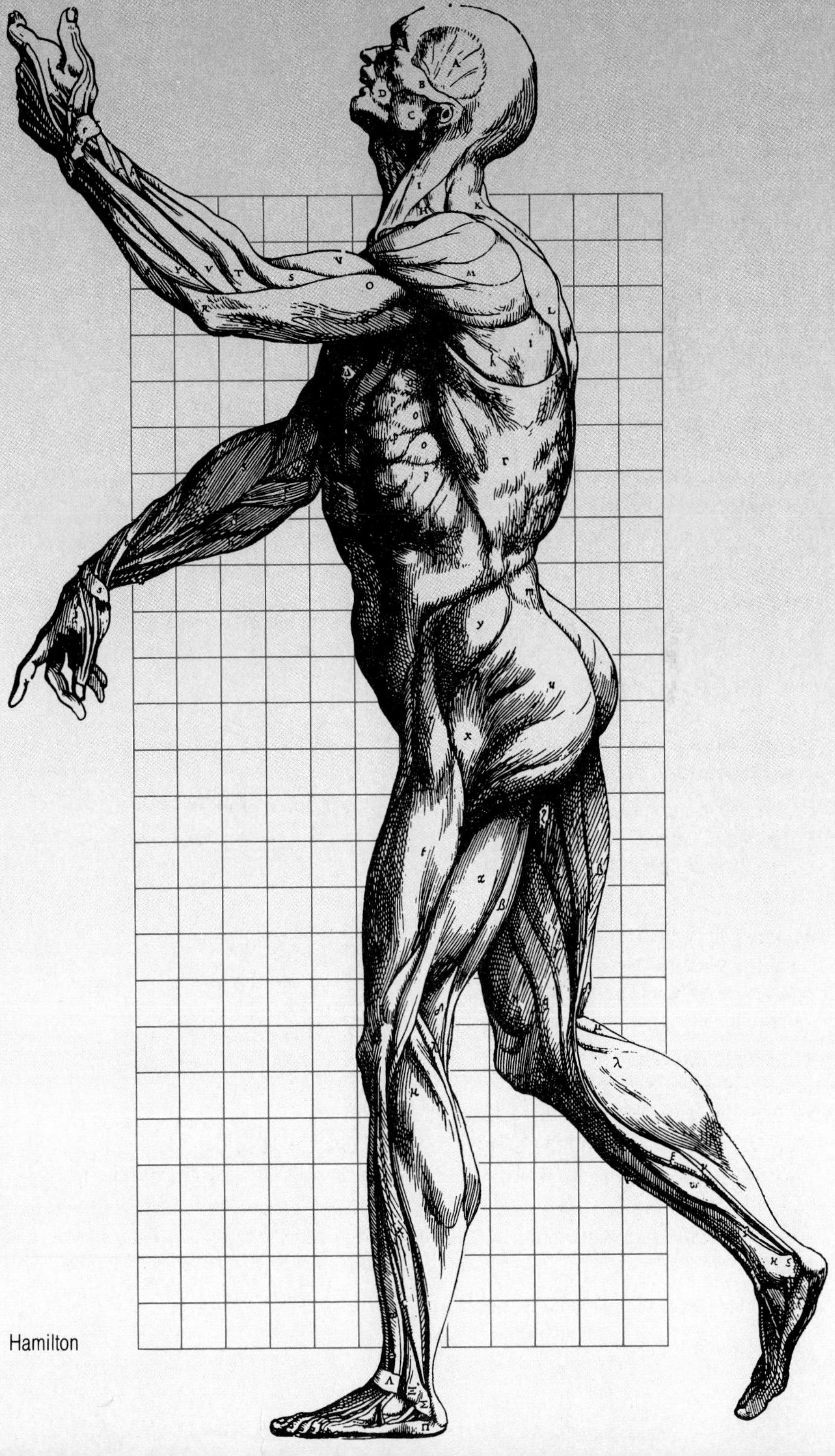

B. C. Decker Inc. Philadelphia Hamilton

Publisher

B.C. Decker Inc
One James Street South
11th Floor
Hamilton, Ontario L8P 4R5

B.C. Decker Inc
320 Walnut Street
Suite 400
Philadelphia, Pennsylvania 19106

Sales and Distribution

United States and Puerto Rico
Mosby–Year Book Inc.
11830 Westline Industrial Drive
Saint Louis, Missouri 63146

Canada
Mosby–Year Book Ltd.
5240 Finch Ave. E., Unit 1
Scarborough, Ontario M1S 5A2

Australia
McGraw-Hill Book Company Australia
Pty. Ltd.
4 Barcoo Street
Roseville East 2069
New South Wales, Australia

Brazil
Editora McGraw-Hill do Brasil, Ltda.
rua Tabapua, 1.105, Itaim-Bibi
Sao Paulo, S.P. Brasil

Colombia
Interamericana/McGraw-Hill de Colombia, S.A.
Carrera 17, No. 33-71
(Apartado Postal, A.A., 6131)
Bogota, D.E., Colombia

Europe, United Kingdom, Middle East, and Africa
Wolfe Publishing Limited
Brook House
2-16 Torrington Place
London WC1E 7LT
England

Hong Kong and China
McGraw-Hill Book Company
Suite 618, Ocean Centre
5 Canton Road
Tsimshatsui, Kowloon
Hong Kong

India
Tata McGraw-Hill Publishing Company, Ltd.
12/4 Asaf Ali Road, 3rd Floor
New Delhi 110002, India

Indonesia
Mr. Wong Fin Fah
P.O. Box 122/JAT
Jakarta, 1300 Indonesia

Japan
Igaku-Shoin Ltd.
Tokyo International P.O. Box 5063
1-28-36 Hongo, Bunkyo-ku,
Tokyo 113, Japan

Korea
Mr. Don-Gap Choi
C.P.O. Box 10583
Seoul, Korea

Malaysia
Mr. Lim Tao Slong
No. 8 Jalan SS 7/6B
Kelana Jaya
47301 Petaling Jaya
Selangor, Malaysia

Mexico
Interamericana/McGraw-Hill de Mexico,
S.A. de C.V.
Cedro 512, Colonia Atlampa
(Apartado Postal 26370)
06450 Mexico, D.F., Mexico

New Zealand
McGraw-Hill Book Co. New Zealand Ltd.
5 Joval Place, Wiri
Manukau City, New Zealand

Portugal
Editora McGraw-Hill de Portugal, Ltda.
Rua Rosa Damasceno 11A-B
1900 Lisboa, Portugal

South Africa
Libriger Book Distributors
Warehouse Number 8
"Die Ou Looiery"
Tannery Road
Hamilton, Bloemfontein 9300

Singapore and Southeast Asia
McGraw-Hill Book Co.
21 Neythal Road
Jurong, Singapore 2262

Spain
McGraw-Hill/Interamericana de Espana, S.A.
Manuel Ferrero, 13
28020 Madrid, Spain

Taiwan
Mr. George Lim
P.O. Box 87-601
Taipei, Taiwan

Thailand
Mr. Vitit Lim
632/5 Phaholyothin Road
Sapan Kwai
Bangkok 10400
Thailand

Venezuela
Editorial Interamericana de Venezuela, C.A.
2da. calle Bello Monte
Local G-2
Caracas, Venezuela

Introduction to Clinical Medicine

Library of Congress catalog card number: 90-82202

ISBN 1-55664-233-4

Notice

The authors and publisher have made every effort to ensure that the diagnosis and care recommended herein, including choice of drugs and drug dosages, is in accord with the accepted standards and practice at the time of publication. However, since research and regulation constantly change clinical standards, the reader is urged to check the product information sheet included in the package of each drug, which includes recommended doses, warnings, and contraindications. This is particularly important with new or infrequently used drugs.

Contributors

Abigail Adams, MD, Assistant Professor of Medicine, University of Massachusetts Medical School; Internist, University of Massachusetts Medical Center, Worcester, Massachusetts

Steven A. Adelman, MD, Assistant Professor of Psychiatry, University of Massachusetts Medical School; Director, Ambulatory Psychiatry Services, University of Massachusetts Medical Center, Worcester, Massachusetts

Cheryl L. Albright, MD, Research Associate, Stanford University; Research Staff, Department of Medicine, Stanford University School of Medicine, Stanford, California

Scott R. Allen, MD, Fellow, General Medicine, University of Massachusetts Medical Center, Worcester, Massachusetts

Joseph S. Alpert, MD, Edward Budnitz Professor of Cardiovascular Medicine, and Director, Department of Medicine, University of Massachusetts Medical School, Worcester, Massachusetts

Jack E. Ansell, MD, Professor of Medicine and Pathology, University of Massachusetts Medical School; Staff Physician, University of Massachusetts Medical Center, Worcester, Massachusetts

Jonathan S. Appelbaum, MD, Instructor in Medicine, University of Massachusetts Medical School, Worcester; Staff Physician, Day Kimball Hospital, Putnam, Massachusetts

Neil Aronin, MD, Associate Professor of Medicine and Physiology, University of Massachusetts Medical School; Endocrinologist, University of Massachusetts Medical Center, Worcester, Massachusetts

Canan A. Avunduk, MD, PhD, Assistant Professor of Medicine, University of Masssachusetts Medical School, Worcester, Massachusetts

Helen Beattie, MPH, EdD, Director of Primary Care Services, Northern County Health Care, Inc., East Hardwick, Vermont

Rita S. Berman, MD, MPH, Assistant Professor, Harvard Medical School and University of Massachusetts Medical School; Private Dermatology Practice, Brighton, Massachusetts

Joseph R. Benotti, MD, Associate Professor of Medicine, University of Massachusetts Medical School; Director, Invasive and Interventional Cardiology, St. Vincent's Hospital, Worcester, Massachusetts

Sandra L. Bertman, PhD, Professor of Humanities in Medicine, University of Massachusetts Medical School; Director, Program of Medical Humanities, University of Massachusetts Medical Center, Worcester, Massachusetts

Gregory Bishop, MD, Assistant Professor of Medicine, University of Massachusetts Medical Center; Dermatologist, Fallon Clinic, Worcester, Massachusetts

Robert M. Black, MD, Associate Professor of Medicine, University of Massachusetts Medical School; Director, Renal Division, St. Vincent's Hospital, Worcester, Massachusetts

Brian D. Blackbourne, MD, Chief Medical Examiner, County of San Diego, San Diego, California

Neil R. Blacklow, MD, Chairman, Department of Medicine, and Richard M. Haidach Distinguished Professor in Medicine, University of Massachusetts Medical School, Worcester, Massachusetts

Robert D. Blute, Jr., MD, Assistant Professor of Urology, University of Massachusetts Medical School; Staff Urologist, University of Massachusetts Medical Center, and Chief of Urology, St. Vincent's Hospital, Worcester, Massachusetts

Jean Boucher, RNC, MS, ET, Enterostomal Clinical Nurse Specialist, University of Massachusetts Medical Center, Worcester, Massachusetts

Andrew I. Cederbaum, MD, Associate Professor of Medicine, University of Massachusetts Medical School; Chief, Hematology/Oncology, The Medical Center of Central Massachusetts–Memorial, Worcester, Massachusetts

David A. Chad, MD, Associate Professor of Neurology, University of Massachusetts Medical School; Attending Physician, University of Massachusetts Medical Center, Worcester, Massachusetts

Sarah H. Cheeseman, MD, Associate Professor of Medicine, Pediatrics, and Molecular Genetics and Microbiology, University of Massachusetts Medical School, Worcester, Massachusetts

David M. Clive, MD, Associate Professor of Medicine, University of Massachusetts Medical School; Staff Nephrologist and Director of Medical Residency Training, University of Massachusetts Medical Center, Worcester, Massachusetts

Carolyn C. Compton, MD, PhD, Associate Professor of Pathology, Harvard Medical School; Director, Gastrointestinal Pathology, Massachusetts General Hospital, Boston, Massachusetts

Susan Connor, RN, Formerly Nurse Coordinator of Gynecology, University of Massachusetts Medical Center, Worcester, Massachusetts

R. William Corwin, MD, Pulmonary Specialist, and Assistant Clinical Professor of Medicine, Brown University Program in Medicine; Staff Pulmonary Physician, Rhode Island Health Association, Providence, Rhode Island

James E. Dalen, MD, MPH, Vice Provost for Medical Affairs, Dean, College of Medicine, and Professor, Department of Internal Medicine, University of Arizona College of Medicine, Tucson, Arizona

Julie A. D'Andrea, RN, MA, MSN, Staff Nurse and Risk Manager, University of Massachusetts Medical Center, Worcester, Massachusetts

Dennis Davidson, MD, Director, Preventive Cardiology Clinic, Stanford University School of Medicine, Stanford, California

Diana DeCosimo, MD, Assistant Professor and Assistant Director of General Medicine, University of Massachusetts Medical School; Associate Medical Director, Center for Health and Fitness, University of Massachusetts Medical Center, Worcester, Massachusetts

Don P. Deprez, MD, Associate Medical Staff, University of Massachusetts Medical Center, and Physician, Department of Obstetrics and Gynecology, The Medical Center of Central Massachusetts, Worcester, Massachusetts

Lewis Dexter, MD, Professor of Medicine, Emeritus, Harvard Medical School, Boston, and Visiting Professor of Medicine, Emeritus, University of Massachusetts Medical School, Worcester; Senior Physician, Emeritus, Brigham and Women's Hospital, Boston, Massachusetts

Gary V. Doern, PhD, Professor of Medicine and Molecular Genetics and Microbiology, University of Massachusetts School of Medicine; Director, Department of Clinical Microbiology, University of Massachusetts Medical Center, Worcester, Massachusetts

Paul W. Doherty, MD, Former Assistant Chief of Nuclear Medicine, Veterans Administration Medical Center, West Roxbury, Massachusetts

Carl J. D'Orsi, MD, Professor and Vice-Chairman, Department of Radiology, University of Massachusetts Medical School, Worcester, Massachusetts

Deborah M. Dufresne, MS, OTR/L, Instructor, Occupational Therapy, Worcester State College, Worcester; Private Practice Therapist, Leicester, Massachusetts

Gregory L. Eastwood, MD, Dean, School of Medicine, Medical College of Georgia, Augusta, Georgia

Judith Eaton, MD, Formerly Assistant Professor of Psychiatry and Obstetrics and Gynecology, University of Massachusetts Medical School; Currently Active Staff, The Medical Center of Central Massachusetts, Worcester, Massachusetts

Thomas H. Ebert, MD, Associate Professor of Medicine, University of Massachusetts Medical School; Chief, Nephrology, The Medical Center of Central Massachusetts–Memorial, Worcester, Massachusetts

W. Thomas Edwards, PhD, MD, Associate Professor and Vice-Chair, Department of Anesthesiology, University of Massachusetts Medical School; Director of Pain Management Services, University of Massachusetts Medical Center, Worcester, Massachusetts

R. Curtis Ellison, MD, Professor of Medicine, and Chief, Section of Preventive Medicine and Epidemiology, Evans Department of Medicine, Boston University School of Medicine, Boston, Massachusetts

Charles H. Emerson, MD, Professor of Medicine, University of Massachusetts Medical School, Worcester, Massachusetts

Kathleen F. Erickson, PT, MS, Director of Physical Therapy, University of Massachusetts Medical Center, Worcester, Massachusetts

John F. Erkkinen, MD, Physician, Maine Medical Center, Portland, Maine

George H. Eypper, MD, Assistant Professor of Medicine, University of Massachusetts Medical School, Worcester, Massachusetts

Patrick G. Fairchild, MD, Assistant Professor of Medicine, University of Massachusetts Medical School; Director, HIV Clinical Center, University of Massachusetts Medical Center, Worcester, Massachusetts

John W. Farquhar, MD, C. F. Rehnborg Professor of Disease Prevention, Stanford University School of Medicine, Stanford; Director, Stanford Center for Research in Disease Prevention, Palo Alto, California

Steven A. Franks, MD, Assistant Professor, University of Massachusetts Medical School; Chief of Dermatology, The Medical Center of Central Massachusetts, Worcester, Massachusetts

Patricia Gamble-Hovey, MSW, LICSW, Coordinator, Oncology Social Services and Psychosocial Services, Division of Hematology-Oncology, Primary Children's Medical Center, Salt Lake City, Utah

Nelson M. Gantz, MD, Professor of Medicine, and Professor of Molecular Genetics and Microbiology, University of Massachusetts Medical School; Hospital Epidemiologist, University of Massachusetts Medical Center, Worcester, Massachusetts

Ann Gateley, MD, Associate Professor of Medicine, University of New Mexico Medical School; Associate Program Director, Internal Medicine, Veterans Affairs Medical Center, Albuquerque, New Mexico

David F. Giansiracusa, MD, Associate Professor and Associate Chairman, Department of Medicine, and Director, Division of Rheumatology and Immunology, University of Massachusetts Medical School, Worcester, Massachusetts

Francis J. Gilroy, MD, Associate in Medicine, University of Massachusetts Medical School, Worcester; Staff Physician, Tri River Family Health Center, Uxbridge, Massachusetts

Barry Ginsberg, MD, Formerly Assistant Professor, Department of Psychiatry, University of Massachusetts Medical School, Worcester, Massachusetts

Richard H. Glew, MD, Professor of Medicine, Molecular Genetics and Microbiology, University of Massachusetts Medical School; Chief of Medicine, The Medical Center of Central Massachusetts, Worcester, Massachusetts

Edward L. Goldberg, MD, Staff Physician, Veterans Affairs Hospital, Providence, Rhode Island

Robert J. Goldberg, MD, Associate Professor of Medicine and Epidemiology, University of Massachusetts Medical School, Worcester, Massachusetts

Perry A. Gotsis, MD, Formerly Assistant Professor of Medicine, University of Massachusetts Medical School, Worcester, Massachusetts; Currently Staff, Naples Community Hospital, Naples, Florida

Harry L. Greene, MD, Associate Professor of Medicine, University of Arizona College of Medicine; Chief, Section of General Medicine, Arizona Health Sciences Center, Tucson, Arizona

Linda C. Greene, RN, BSN, Pre-Authorization Nurse Manager, FHP Corporation, Tucson, Arizona

Thomas W. Griffin, MD, Associate Professor of Medicine, University of Massachusetts Medical School; Director, Clinical Research, Division of Oncology, University of Massachusetts Medical Center, Worcester, Massachusetts

Paul T. Gross, MD, Assistant Clinical Professor of Neurology, Harvard Medical School, Boston; Staff Neurologist, Lahey Clinic Medical Center, Burlington, Massachusetts

Sandra A. Hall, RN, MSN, Assistant Professor of Nursing, Worcester State College, Worcester, Massachusetts

David S. Hatem, MD, Instructor of Medicine, University of Massachusetts Medical School; General Medicine Staff, University of Massachusetts Medical Center, Worcester, Massachusetts

Roger B. Hickler, MD, Lamar Soutter Distinguished Professor of Medicine, University of Massachusetts Medical School; Staff Physician, University of Massachusetts Medical Center, Worcester, Massachusetts

Janice C. Hitzhusen, MD, Assistant Professor of Medicine, University of Massachusetts Medical School; Staff, St. Vincent's Hospital, Worcester, Massachusetts

Timothy B. Hopkins, MD, Assistant Professor of Urology, University of Massachusetts Medical School; Urologist, The Medical Center of Central Massachusetts and University of Massachusetts Medical Center, Worcester, Massachusetts

Sandra L. Horowitz, MD, Assistant Professor of Neurology, University of Massachusetts Medical School; Director, EEG Sleep Clinic, St. Vincent's Hospital, Worcester, Massachusetts

Rolf D. Hubmayr, MD, Associate Professor of Medicine, Thoracic Diseases Section, Mayo Medical School; Consultant, Division of Thoracic Diseases and Internal Medicine, Mayo Clinic, Rochester, Minnesota

James P. Hughes, MD, Assistant Professor, University of Massachusetts Medical School, Worcester, Massachusetts

Todd W. Hunter, MD, Assistant Professor, University of Massachusetts Medical School, Worcester, Massachusetts

Merle R. Ingraham, MD, Senior Associate in Psychiatry, University of Massachusetts Medical School; Consultant, The Medical Center of Central Massachusetts, Worcester, Massachusetts

Richard S. Irwin, MD, Professor of Medicine, University of Massachusetts Medical School; Director, Division of Pulmonary and Critical Care Medicine, University of Massachusetts Medical Center, Worcester, Massachusetts

Irving Jacoby, MD, Associate Clinical Professor of Medicine and Surgery, University of California, San Diego, School of Medicine; Assistant Director, Department of Emergency Medicine, and Associate Director, Hyperbaric Medicine Center, UCSD Medical Center, San Diego, California

Elise Jacques, MD, Associate Professor of Medicine, University of Massachusetts Medical School; Chief of Gastroenterology, Worcester City Hospital, Worcester, Massachusetts

Brian F. Johnson, MD, Professor of Medicine and Pharmacology, University of Massachusetts Medical School; Director, Division of Clinical Pharmacology, University of Massachusetts Medical Center, Worcester, Massachusetts

Thomas A. Johnson, MD, Associate Professor, Vice-Chair, and Director of Education, Department of Obstetrics and Gynecology, and Associate Professor of Family and Community Medicine, University of Massachusetts Medical School, Worcester, Massachusetts

William P. Johnson, MD, Clinical Assistant Professor of Medicine, University of Arizona College of Medicine; Physician, University Medical Center, Tucson, Arizona

Katherine L. Kahn, MD, Assistant Professor, University of California, Los Angeles, School of Medicine, Los Angeles, California

Barbara F. Katz, JD, General Counsel, Massachusetts Eye and Ear Infirmary, Boston, Massachusetts

Edward L. Kazarian, MD, Assistant Professor of Surgery, Division of Ophthalmology, University of Massachusetts Medical School, Worcester, Massachusetts

Joseph M. Kelly, DDS, Associate Professor of Surgery, University of Massachusetts Medical School; Chief, Dental Service, University of Massachusetts Medical Center, Worcester, Massachusetts

Brian J. Keroack, MD, Rheumatology Fellow, University of Michigan Medical School; Fellow, Division of Rheumatology, University of Michigan Medical Center, Ann Arbor, Michigan

Howard Kirshenbaum, MD, Assistant Professor of Medicine, University of Massachusetts Medical School, Worcester, Massachusetts

Harvey J. Kowaloff, MD, Associate Professor of Medicine, University of Massachusetts Medical School, Worcester, Massachusetts

Jean L. Kristeller, PhD, Assistant Professor of Medicine, University of Massachusetts Medical School, Worcester, Massachusetts

F. John Krolikowski, MD, Assistant Professor of Pathology, University of Massachusetts Medical School; Director of Laboratories, Genica Pharmaceutical Corporation, Worcester, Massachusetts

Lawrence M. Kulla, MD, Clinical Neurologist, South Shore Neurology Associates, South Weymouth, Massachusetts

Laszlo Leb, MD, Associate Professor of Medicine, University of Massachusetts Medical School; Hematologist and Senior Attending Physician, St. Vincent's Hospital, Worcester, Massachusetts

Peter H. Levine, MD, Professor of Medicine, University of Massachusetts Medical School; Director, Blood Research Laboratory, The Medical Center of Central Massachusetts, Worcester, Massachusetts

Lynn Li, MD, Assistant Professor, University of Massachusetts Medical School; Medical Director, Geriatrics, and Staff Physician, Department of Medicine/Primary Care, University of Massachusetts Medical Center, Worcester, Massachusetts

Marcia K. Liepman, MD, Associate Professor of Medicine, University of Massachusetts Medical School; Staff Physician, Worcester Memorial Hospital, Worcester, Massachusetts

Christopher Longcope, MD, Professor of Medicine and Obstetrics and Gynecology, University of Massachusetts Medical School, Worcester, Massachusetts

John C. Love, MD, Assistant Clinical Professor, University of Vermont College of Medicine, Burlington, Vermont; Cardiologist in Private Practice, Portland, Maine

Gertrude W. Manchester, MD, Assistant Professor of Medicine, University of Massachusetts Medical School; Associate Director, Primary Care Clinic, University of Massachusetts Medical Center, Worcester, Massachusetts

James L. McGuire, MD, Associate Professor of Medicine, and Director of Rheumatology Clinic and Fellowship, Stanford University School of Medicine, Stanford; Chief of Rheumatology, Palo Alto Veterans Administration Hospital, Palo Alto, California

William J. McLaughlin, MD, Assistant Professor of Obstetrics and Gynecology, University of Massachusetts Medical School, Worcester, Massachusetts

John A. Merritt, MD, Associate Professor of Medicine, Yale University School of Medicine; Physician, Hospital of St. Raphael, New Haven, Connecticut

James A. Michaels, PT, MS, Associate in Orthopedics, University of Massachusetts Medical School; Director of Acute Rehabilitation Services, University of Massachusetts Medical Center, Worcester, Massachusetts

Sherri F. Murkland, RD, MEd, Nutrition Support Dietitian, University of Massachusetts Medical Center, Worcester, Massachusetts

Judith K. Ockene, PhD, Professor of Medicine, and Director, Division of Preventive and Behavioral Medicine, University of Massachusetts Medical School, Worcester, Massachusetts

Judith Freiman Olson, MSW, LICSW, Administrative Director, Human and Community Services, St. Vincent's Hospital, Worcester, Massachusetts

Morris Ostroff, MD, MPH, MBA, FACEP, Associate Clinical Professor of Surgery and Emergency Medicine, University of Connecticut School of Medicine, Farmington; Chief of Emergency Medicine and Assistant Vice-President, Mount Sinai Hospital, Hartford, Connecticut

Cynthia B. Passarelli, MD, Associate in Neurology, University of Massachusetts Medical School; Neurologist, Fallon Clinic, Worcester, Massachusetts

Linda A. Pape, MD, Associate Professor of Medicine, University of Massachusetts Medical School; Director of Noninvasive Cardiology, University of Massachusetts Medical Center, Worcester, Massachusetts

Dennis D. Patton, MD, Professor of Radiology and Optical Sciences, and Director, Division of Nuclear Medicine, University of Arizona College of Medicine, Tucson, Arizona

Rashmi V. Patwardhan, MD, Associate Professor of Medicine, University of Massachusetts Medical School; Educational Coordinator, St. Vincent's Hospital, Worcester, Massachusetts

Liberto Pechet, MD, Professor of Medicine and Pathology, and Chief, Division of Hematology and Hematology Laboratory, University of Massachusetts Medical School, Worcester, Massachusetts

John R. Person, MD, Associate in Medicine/Dermatology, University of Massachusetts Medical School, Worcester; Staff Dermatologist, Fallon Clinic, Auburn, Massachusetts

Linda G. Peterson, MD, Associate Professor of Psychiatry, University of Massachusetts Medical School; Director, Consultation/Liaison Service, University of Massachusetts Medical Center, Worcester, Massachusetts

Daniel E. Pritchard, BS, RRT, Formerly Director of Respiratory Therapy, University of Massachusetts Medical Center, Worcester, Massachusetts

Ardath Quinlan, BS, Director of Quality Assurance, University of Massachusetts Medical Center, Worcester, Massachusetts

Steven D. Reich, MD, Associate Professor of Medicine and Pharmacology, University of Massachusetts Medical School, Worcester; Vice President of Medical Affairs, Parexel International Corporation, Cambridge, Massachusetts

James M. Rippe, MD, Associate Professor of Medicine, University of Massachusetts Medical School; Director, Exercise Physiology and Nutrition Laboratory, University of Massachusetts Medical Center, Worcester, Massachusetts

Mai-Lan Rogoff, MD, Associate Professor, Psychiatry and Pediatrics, University of Massachusetts Medical School, Worcester, Massachusetts

Jonathan S. Rothman, MD, Senior Associate, Department of Psychiatry, University of Massachusetts Medical School; Active Staff, The Medical Center of Central Massachusetts, Worcester, Massachusetts

Richard I. Rothstein, MD, Assistant Professor of Medicine, Dartmouth Medical School; Director, Gastrointestinal Motility Laboratory, Dartmouth-Hitchcock Medical Center, Hanover, New Hampshire

James A. Russell, DO, Associate in Neurology, Guthrie Clinic, Sayre, Pennsylvania

Arthur R. Russo, MD, Assistant Professor of Medicine, University of Massachusetts Medical School; Director of General Medicine, University of Massachusetts Medical Center, Worcester, Massachusetts

Mary Ellen M. Rybak, MD, Associate Professor of Medicine, University of Massachusetts Medical School, Worcester, Massachusetts

Marjorie Safran, MD, Associate Professor of Medicine, University of Massachusetts Medical School, Worcester, Massachusetts

Mark J. Scharf, MD, Assistant Professor of Medicine, Division of Dermatology, University of Massachusetts Medical School, Worcester, Massachusetts

Joel H. Schwartz, MD, Associate Professor of Medicine, University of Massachusetts Medical School, Worcester; Medical Oncologist, Salem Hospital, Salem, and Former Director of Oncology, St. Vincent's Hospital, Worcester, Massachusetts

Joel M. Seidman, MD, Associate Professor of Medicine and Physiology, University of Massachusetts Medical School; Chief of Pulmonary Medicine, The Medical Center of Central Massachusetts–Memorial, Worcester, Massachusetts

Wayne E. Silva, MD, Professor of Surgery, University of Massachusetts Medical School; Staff Surgeon, University of Massachusetts Medical Center, Worcester, Massachusetts

L. Michael Snyder, MD, Professor of Internal Medicine, University of Massachusetts Medical School; Chief of Laboratory Medicine, St. Vincent's Hospital, Worcester, Massachusetts

John L. Stock, MD, Associate Professor of Medicine, University of Massachusetts Medical School; Chief of Endocrinology, The Medical Center of Central Massachusetts, Worcester, Massachusetts

Judith P. Stone, MSW, LICSW, Associate in Psychiatry and Pediatrics, University of Massachusetts Medical School; Administrative Director, Patient Placement, University of Massachusetts Medical Center, Worcester, Massachusetts

Sarah L. Stone, MD, Assistant Professor of Medicine, University of Massachusetts Medical School, Worcester, Massachusetts

Gary M. Strauss, MD, Formerly Associate Professor of Medicine, University of Massachusetts Medical School, Worcester; Currently Medical Oncologist, Harvard Community Health Plan, Boston, Massachusetts

Steven L. Strongwater, MD, Associate Professor of Medicine, University of Massachusetts Medical School; Staff Rheumatologist, and Director of Medical Specialties Clinics, University of Massachusetts Medical Center, Worcester, Massachusetts

Helen K. Sumpter, BA, Coordinator of Bereavement, Division of Oncology, University of Massachusetts Medical Center, Worcester, Massachusetts

Kenneth J. Tabor, PharmD, Assistant Director, Drug Surveillance and Epidemiology Department, Glaxo Inc., Research Triangle Park, North Carolina

Catherine S. Thompson, MD, Associate Professor of Medicine, Division of Nephrology, University of Texas Medical School at Houston, Houston, Texas

Thomas E. Ukena, MD, PhD, Associate Professor of Pathology, University of Massachusetts Medical Center; Assistant Chief of Pathology, The Medical Center of Central Massachusetts, Worcester, Massachusetts

Katherine S. Upchurch, MD, Assistant Professor of Medicine, University of Massachusetts Medical School; Staff Rheumatologist, The Medical Center of Central Massachusetts, Worcester, Massachusetts

Carol A. Waksmonski, MD, Instructor in Medicine, Harvard Medical School; Associate Director, Echocardiography Laboratory, Beth Israel Hospital, Boston, Massachusetts

Allen D. Ward, MD, Assistant Professor of Medicine, University of Massachusetts Medical School; Chief of Oncology, Worcester Hahnemann Hospital and Worcester City Hospital, Worcester, Massachusetts

Earle B. Weiss, MD, Professor of Medicine, University of Massachusetts Medical School, Worcester; Senior Pulmonary Research Scientist, Department of Anesthesia Research Laboratories, Brigham and Women's Hospital, Boston, Massachusetts

Michael D. Wertheimer, MD, Associate Professor of Surgery, and Director, Breast Clinic, University of Massachusetts Medical School, Worcester, Massachusetts

Deborah Wexler, MSW, Social Services, Division of Oncology, University of Massachusetts Medical Center, Worcester, Massachusetts

Harold A. Wilkinson, MD, PhD, Professor and Chairman, Division of Neurosurgery, University of Massachusetts Medical School; Chief of Neurosurgery, University of Massachusetts Medical Center, Worcester, Massachusetts

William F. Winchell, MD, Staff Rheumatologist, Newton-Wellesley Hospital, Newton, Massachusetts

Thomas H. Winters, MD, Associate Clinical Professor of Medicine, Boston University School of Medicine; Medical Director, Medsite Occupational Health Center, Boston, Massachusetts

Rosalie S. Wolf, PhD, Professor, University of Massachusetts Medical School; Associate Director, Center on Aging, University of Massachusetts Medical Center, Worcester, Massachusetts

Robert A. Yood, MD, Assistant Professor of Medicine, University of Massachusetts Medical School; Director of Rheumatology, St. Vincent's Hospital, and Chief of Rheumatology, Fallon Clinic, Worcester, Massachusetts

Bruce S. Zaret, MD, Physician in Private Practice, Hollywood, Florida

John K. Zawacki, MD, Associate Professor of Medicine, University of Massachusetts Medical School; Interim Chair, Department of Gastroenterology, University of Massachusetts Medical Center, Worcester, Massachusetts

Justin A. Zivin, MD, PhD, Professor of Neurosciences, University of California School of Medicine, San Diego, California

Preface

Introduction to Clinical Medicine is a work stimulated by and intended for medical students. It is primarily designed to help bridge the chasm between the basic sciences and the wards. The format identifies the problems (e.g., pruritus, cough) that the patient will describe and helps the student move through the history, physical examination, and laboratory data to arrive at a diagnosis. In many chapters, we have included decision-making algorithms to aid in visualizing the process and thinking through clinical issues. For students interested in more information, brief reference lists are provided at the end of each chapter.

The problems discussed were generated by the General Medicine/Primary Care faculty at the University of Massachusetts Medical School and at the University of Arizona Health Sciences Center based on their own experience and perceived student need. They are the result of years of ward teaching and general medicine practice. Section I, "Principles of Clinical Medicine," covers mundane but crucial issues, such as working with other health care members on the team, what to do with the mass of literature that confronts the new physician, how to get maximum value from the laboratories, how to begin saving money for patients and society, and how to write orders and prescriptions. Chapters on high-technology diagnostics (Nuclear Medicine, Radiology and Magnetic Resonance Imaging) are presented to give the student an appreciation of these fields. Section II, "Internal Medicine: A Signs and Symptoms Approach," uses a problem-oriented approach to delineate patient problems. In this way, the book is a logical extension of the history and physical examination, leading directly to clinical decisions. Diseases and diagnostic entities are heavily indexed and cross-referenced as a complement to the signs and symptoms approach. Section II and Section III, "Adolescent Medicine, Geriatric Medicine, Behavioral Medicine," are divided into subsections (e.g. "Endocrinology," "Behavioral Medicine") with each individual complaint (e.g. amenorrhea, anxiety) given a full chapter's discussion. In some cases, tasks that must be undertaken by the physician, such as delivering bad news, what to do when a patient dies, and handling the issue of patients who leave against medical advice, are addressed. Sections IV and V cover general medical problems (e.g., otolaryngology, gynecology) and medical-legal issues. Issues about which many physicians have lacked knowledge as a result of inadequate teaching in medical schools (e.g., ostomy, informed consent) are mentioned to stimulate student thought. Post-hospital care issues such as the importance of discharge planning, home care, and health maintenance responsibilities are also discussed. Finally, four appendices provide valuable information for patient care in an easily used format.

The book has been designed to make information easily accessible to the reader. Color has been used purposefully in the algorithms to indicate diagnostic procedures and medications. The numerous summary tables are highlighted with color screens to enhance readability. In addition, full-color illustrations appear throughout the book. Students should find that all of these features increase the usefulness of the text and facilitate their understanding of the material presented.

Harry L. Greene, M.D.

Acknowledgments

This book is a reality because of the encouragement of James E. Dalen, M.D., Vice Provost for Medical Affairs and Dean, College of Medicine, University of Arizona. He has established an environment wherein teaching is important and is provided in an unthreatening manner, in which all may learn. Special thanks go to Rubin Bressler, M.D., Neil Blacklow, M.D., Peter H. Levine, M.D., Gilbert E. Levinson, M.D., John A. Merritt, Jr., M.D., Alan L. Michelson, M.D., and Francis X. Dufault, M.D., who have encouraged faculty participation and support of this work since its inception. Through the years I have been fortunate to have a number of excellent teachers who have helped stimulate my interest in doing an introductory clinical book. They include Eugene Braunwald, Lewis Dexter, Kelley Skeff, Daniel Federman, Oglesby Paul, Marshall Wolf, Charles Mengel, George Thorn, Louis Weinstein, Patrick Henry, Douglas Griggs, and John Lukens. A deep debt of gratitude must go to Sheila Putnam, Kathleen Tedesco, Joyce McKenna, Suzanne Howatt, Marcia Atchue, Joanne Scott, Sheri Schober, and Luz Palomarez who tirelessly assisted with the preparation of the manuscript. Thanks are also due to Nora Provost Radcliffe, Art Director for the book, and Dimitri Karetnikov, who prepared the beautiful full-color illustrations. Special thanks go to Arnold Relman, Marcia Angell, Marlene Thayer, and the staff at the *New England Journal of Medicine*, all of whom helped and supported me during my sabbatical in Boston when much of this book was completed. Dana Dreibelbis, Lynne Gery, Brian Decker, and the entire staff of B.C. Decker have been remarkable in their support and production of this book.

Finally, thanks to my parents, Harry and Helen Greene, my wife, Linda, and our children, Harry III, Michele, and Jennifer, who were constantly there with support and encouragement.

Harry L. Greene, M.D.

Contents

Constitutional

Dermatology

Endocrinology

Gastroenterology

Genitourinary

Hematology

Infectious Diseases

Musculoskeletal

Neurology

Oncology

Ophthalmology

Pulmonary

Renal

III Adolescent Medicine, Geriatric Medicine, Behavioral Medicine 533

Adolescent Medicine

Geriatric Medicine

Behavioral Medicine

IV Oral Cavity; Ears, Nose, and Throat; Gynecology 603

Principles of Clinical Medicine I

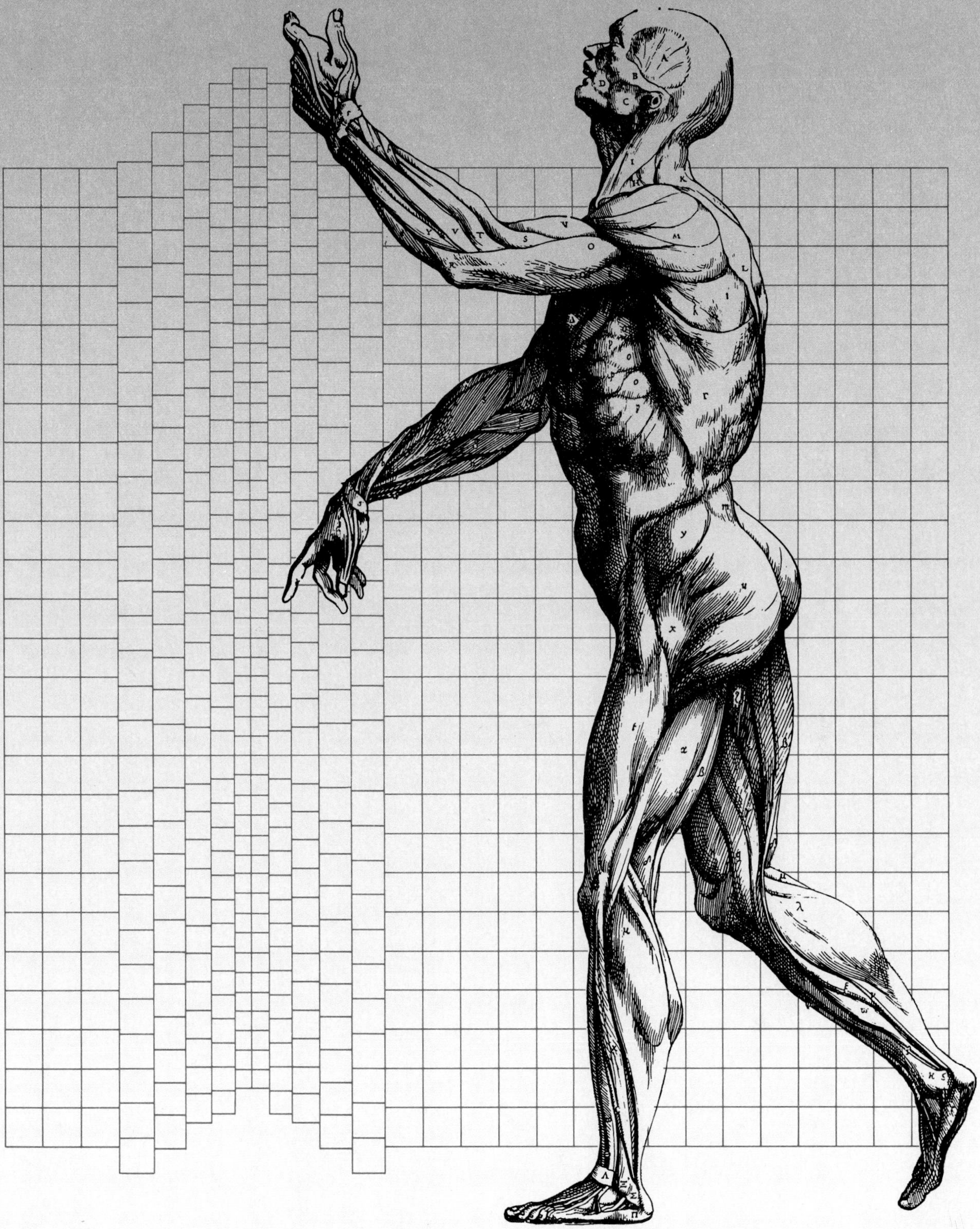

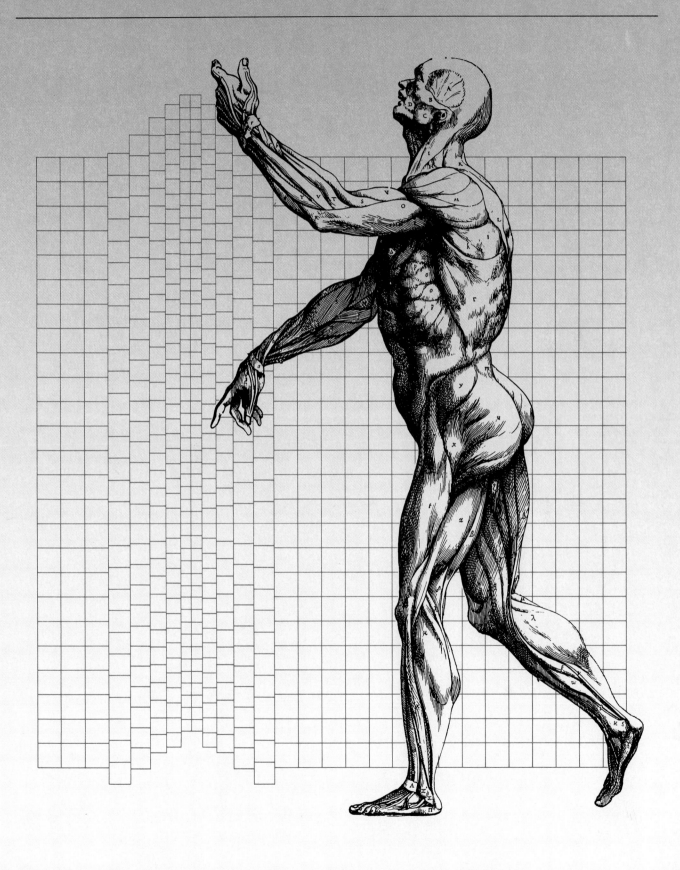

Approach to the Medical Clerkship

Carol A. Waksmonski, MD

Harry L. Greene, MD

For most of us, the third-year clerkship in medicine is one of the most exciting and stimulating times of our lives. It is a time when much of basic science becomes relevant, as it seldom could in the lecture theater. It is a period when physical diagnosis and history taking are for "keeps," and the most thorough patient evaluation on the chart may be yours. Because of the weight of your first real clinical responsibility, you will feel some apprehension and anxiety. These feelings can help prepare you for one of the most rapid growth and learning periods you will have experienced between birth and internship. Many of the conditions for learning will be right; you will be highly motivated and well prepared, have a high need to know, and will learn in small groups or one on one. There will also be a few impediments to learning: fatigue; interruptions; anxiety, if too stressed; and a certain number of menial tasks that historically have been delegated to the student. There will be ample feedback as you develop your clinical skills.

One important aspect of this experience will be your approach to the patient. The patients you have seen up to now have often been selected especially for you because of their ability to tell their stories, their classic physical findings, their stability, or their affability. Now you will have to learn to master patients who are anxious, depressed, hostile, angry, or frightened. Some of your patients may be poor autobiographers or, indeed, may not be able to give you a history. You must develop speed and facility in history taking and physical examinations and establish good relationships with family members. You will confront the challenges of dealing with the terminally ill or an unanticipated death. It will be necessary to work closely with other health care professionals, each with his or her own agenda and personality.

So let us begin. As soon as you know that you are getting a patient to work up, start your preparation. Dress professionally and have your instruments, database or history-taking forms, and writing materials with you. It is important for a patient to have confidence in you, and that confidence starts with being prepared. Much of the apprehension about new admissions is experienced before one actually meets the patient ("How sick is the person?" "Will he die on me?" "Can I manage his problem?" "Will he let me examine him?" "How can I, as a student, offer him anything?"). Try to see the patient as soon as possible to dissipate this fear and anxiety, and start to initiate more constructive problem-solving behavior. Introduce yourself properly. The patient will be more anxious than you, and through your self-confidence, patience, courtesy, gentleness, and consideration, you will begin to establish yourself as your patient's student physician and friend and provide therapy for his or her anxiety. Be systematic and thorough in your history (see Chapter 2, "The Medical Interview") and physical examination. It is not uncommon for a careful student to discover an early melanoma or breast cancer on a patient who is admitted for another problem. If aspects of the history or laboratory data are lacking, do whatever is necessary to complete the database on your patient.

Write up your patient as quickly, concisely, and legibly as possible, leaving most of the available time to synthesize the data gathered thus far and to consider any laboratory studies that may be needed. Construct a list of problems (Fig. 1-1) and provide a reasonable differential diagnosis for each problem. It takes practice to master the synthesis process. Gleaning pertinent facts from the history, physical examination, and laboratory tests and then formulating a differential diagnosis list and a therapeutic plan is a challenge. A good foundation of pathophysiology will be helpful in this regard. Also, feel free to consult the more experienced members of your team. To the student the medical literature appears vast, so a useful first step is to read about each item in your problem or differential diagnosis list under the appropriate heading in this text. This material may be supplemented by any one of the excellent current medicine texts (see Chapter 7, "Critically Reviewing the Medical Literature").

Try to get an idea of the incidence of each illness so that you can use the odds in developing your differential diagnosis. Begin by reading in a standard medicine textbook. When you feel you have narrowed the prospects to two or three, consult the current literature for reviews of these subjects in peer-reviewed journals. Your residents should be able to guide you to the appropriate references, or you can get them from a computerized literature search (see Chapter 6, "Computer Applications in Internal Medicine"). As you work up each disease problem, try to think of ways in which the disease could have been prevented (e.g., vaccination, prophylactic antibiotics). Think of ways to lessen its effects (e.g., seat belts in auto accidents) or ways in which health care teaching could have eliminated the disease in your patient (e.g., smoking and chronic obstructive pulmonary disease or lung cancer). Think about the implications for other

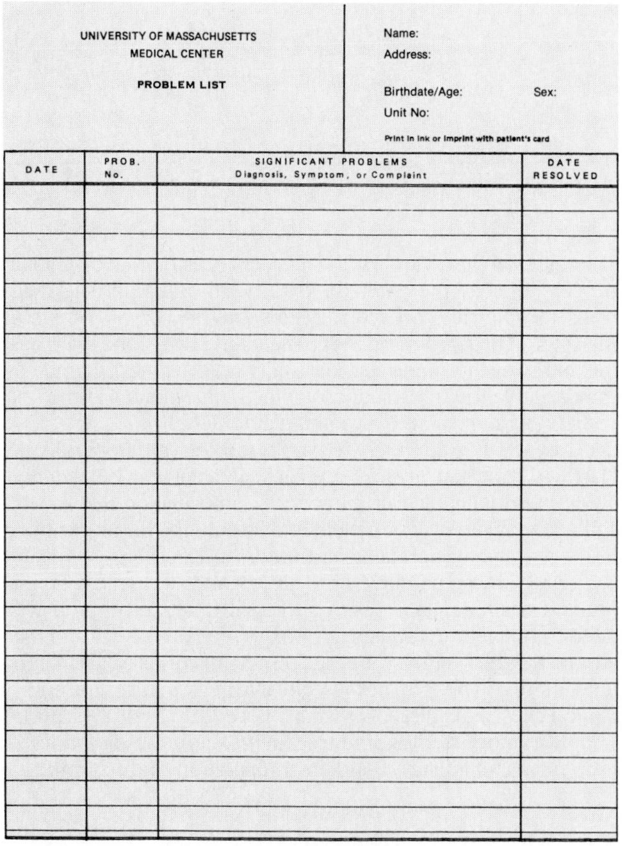
UNIVERSITY OF MASSACHUSETTS
MEDICAL CENTER
PROBLEM LIST

Name:
Address:
Birthdate/Age: Sex:
Unit No:
Print in ink or imprint with patient's card

DATE	PROB. No.	SIGNIFICANT PROBLEMS Diagnosis, Symptom, or Complaint	DATE RESOLVED

Figure 1-1 A sample problem list from the University of Massachusetts Medical Center.

family members, and intervene or arrange evaluations for them (e.g., inform daughters of premenopausal women with breast cancer of their own risk of breast cancer and encourage them to learn self-examination techniques and undergo mammography).

During this process you will be expected to write orders for the patient's diet, activity level, vital signs, medications, and special studies or tests (see Chapter 12, "Writing Orders on Hospitalized Patients"). Try to learn how the tests you order are performed and what they cost (see Chapter 11, "Cost Containment"). Recording pertinent information in a small notebook will come in handy when you encounter a similar work-up. You will have to request the appropriate blood work. Whenever possible, perform the phlebotomy yourself so that you will become a true expert. Get to know your laboratories; examine your patient's peripheral smears, urine sediments, and Gram and acid-fast bacillus stains, and become adept at these procedures. In the modern era many hospitals do not facilitate this type of learning, but it is crucial to your ability to become the complete physician and lessens your dependence on others. You will have to familiarize yourself with the radiology department so that you can readily review your patient's studies and mentally commit yourself before the "official reading" comes (see Chapter 17, "Nuclear Medicine Studies," and Chapter 18, "Radiology and Magnetic Resonance Imaging"). Likewise, you should know the pathology and cytology laboratories and review studies there as well. Chapter 9, "Optimal Utilization of the Laboratory," gives you a useful overview of each lab and how it can help you. The more you know about what happens to your patient's specimens and tests, the better you can interpret the results. Establish rapport with one person in each lab who can help you when a value seems abnormal or when you have a technical question.

Much of your guidance will be provided by residents and by the attending staff. Good interpersonal relationships at this level are critical to a valuable experience. Remember that students are welcomed by busy and often overburdened residents. You will have a well-defined role on the ward team and will be an important functioning member. You should ask questions and anticipate problems, and be available, affable, and, above all, *honest*. If you don't know, say so. Ask for help. You are here to learn, not to create an illusion of knowledge. You will learn to work with other health care professionals, especially nursing staff, pharmacists, dietitians, and various therapists. Review who they are and what they do. See Chapter 8, "Interacting with Other Health Care Professionals," so that you can optimize and enhance your learning from these specially trained groups.

The goal of our book is to provide practical information to help you with the medical clerkship experience, to present a foundation for dealing with common problems, and to ease the metamorphosis from student to physician. You will find your clerkship a most rewarding and enjoyable experience.

Good luck! These are the first days of your life as a doctor.

Reference

Huth EJ. A library for internists VI. Recommendations from the American College of Physicians. Ann Intern Med 1988; 108:497.

The Medical Interview

William P. Johnson, MD

2

The medical interview is the cornerstone of the diagnostic process. Despite the emphasis on biotechnical aspects of diagnosis, the clinical process still begins with the person-to-person interview. The process by which the interview is conducted and the interviewer's interpersonal skills and mannerisms are as important as the information obtained. Questionnaires can be mailed to patients before an ambulatory visit to save time (Fig. 2-1) or used as guidelines for data recording (see Appendix IV, "Defined Data Base Form"). A great deal of data can be obtained from questionnaires, but much of the information that can be gained by observing the patient and listening to his or her story is lost if only questionnaires are used.

Interviewing patients, although not always easy, is interesting and challenging. To be a successful interviewer, you will need to call on the assets that have gotten you this far and that you share with others—honesty, respectful curiosity, and a genuine interest in people. Because the interview initiates the entire clinical process, it influences what follows: the physical examination, laboratory studies, and treatment. Mastering the basics is important, and it takes discipline, preparation, and practice.

The Interviewing Process

The medical interview has four functions: (1) determining the nature of the problem; (2) developing and maintaining a therapeutic relationship; (3) communicating information, educating the patient, and implementing a treatment plan; and (4) coaching to see that the treatment plan is followed or modified so that it can be accepted and implemented.

Approaching the Patient

Establishing rapport with the patient leads to a relationship based on shared respect and trust and forms the basis for optimal, satisfying health care. The clinical setting is unique in that this rapport can be developed relatively quickly with effective communication. The right attitude empowers the patient to communicate with you. A characteristic of the right attitude is active listening. The interview is not an interrogation. Listening conveys a sense of respect, openness, and tolerance. Illness may threaten a patient's sense of connection to other people and to the world in general. If patients feel that the physician is really listening to and understanding them, their sense of isolation and despair is reduced. Rapport and empathy must be sincere; the "I know just how you're feeling" refrain will be interpreted as phony unless it's clear that you mean it. You must also recognize that in the clinical setting, the physician is in a position to shame a patient. For some people, the illness experience in itself is humiliating. The physician can avoid compounding this by accepting people as they are and being careful to avoid censure, fault finding, and moralizing.

HEALTH HISTORY QUESTIONNAIRE

DATE:
NAME:
ADDRESS:

BIRTHDATE/AGE: SEX:
UNIT NUMBER:

PRINT IN INK OR STAMP WITH PATIENT CARD

IDENTIFICATION DATA: Please fill in the following information. PLEASE PRINT.

> Name ______________ > Date ________ MR # ________

> Address ______________ > City ________ > State ____ > Zip ______

> Date of Birth ___ / ___ / ___ Home Phone ( ) ________ Work Phone ( ) ________

> SEX:
1 ☐ Male
2 ☐ Female

> CURRENT MARITAL STATUS:
1 ☐ Single
2 ☐ Married
3 ☐ Separated
4 ☐ Divorced
5 ☐ Widowed

> RACE:
1 ☐ White
2 ☐ Black
3 ☐ Hispanic
4 ☐ Asian
5 ☐ Other ________

> HEALTH INSURANCE:
1 ☐ Blue Cross
2 ☐ Blue Shield
3 ☐ Private Insurance Company
4 ☐ Preferred Provider Organization
5 ☐ Health Maintenance Organization
6 ☐ Medicare
7 ☐ Medicaid
8 ☐ Other ________
9 ☐ None

Specify (HMO) ________

> Who referred you to UMC Primary Care Clinic? ________
1 ☐ Self
2 ☐ Friend or relative
3 ☐ Other physician outside UMC
4 ☐ UMC Emergency Room
5 ☐ Another UMC physician
6 ☐ Other ________

HOSPITALIZATIONS: List all your hospitalizations as best as you can.
Type of illness/surgery/hospitalization (please be specific - you may use an additional blank sheet of paper if necessary) — Year

1 ________ ____
2 ________ ____
3 ________ ____
4 ________ ____
5 ________ ____
6 ________ ____

MEDICATIONS:
What prescribed medicines do you presently take? (List name, dosage, and how often you take it).

________ ________
________ ________
________ ________
________ ________
________ ________

Do you take any non-prescription medicines (over the counter) or tonics?
For example: laxatives, diet pills, vitamins, antacids, or cold remedies?

☐ YES ☐ NO If yes, please list any non-prescription drugs.

________ ________
________ ________
________ ________
________ ________

ALLERGIES: Are you allergic to or have you had a "bad reaction" to any medicines or other substances?

☐ YES ☐ NO If yes, list the medicine and reactions.

________ ________
________ ________

SOCIAL HISTORY:

Live with: ☐ Spouse ☐ Parents ☐ Relatives ☐ Friend ☐ Alone ☐ Other

> How many years of formal education have you completed?
1 ☐ No high school
2 ☐ Some high school
3 ☐ High school diploma
4 ☐ Some college
5 ☐ College degree
6 ☐ Graduate school
7 ☐ Special Education

> Present employment status:
1 ☐ Working part-time
2 ☐ Working full-time
3 ☐ Unemployed
4 ☐ Retired
5 ☐ Disabled

> What is your usual occupation? ________

What are your (or your household's) sources of income?
☐ Salary ☐ Pension ☐ Social Security ☐ Disability Comp. ☐ Other

Are you now involved in any of the following organizations?
☐ Community group ☐ School group ☐ Church ☐ Veterans' group ☐ Other

Do you receive any community services?
☐ Home health aide ☐ VNA ☐ Homemaker ☐ Meals on Wheels ☐ Visiting friend

HEALTH MAINTENANCE:

> 1. Do you exercise at least 3 times a week? ☐ Yes ☐ No
2. Do you brush your teeth at least once a day? ☐ Yes ☐ No
3. Do you floss to clean between your teeth at least once a day? ☐ Yes ☐ No
4. Do you see a dentist on a regular basis? ☐ Yes ☐ No
Name ________
5. Do you see an eye doctor on a regular basis? ☐ Yes ☐ No
Name ________
6. WOMEN ONLY - How often do you perform breast self-examination?
☐ Never ☐ Every 6 months ☐ Every three months ☐ Every month
7. Do you have a home evacuation plan (fire drill) in case of fire? ☐ Yes ☐ No
8. Do you know what to do in case of accidental poisoning or drug overdose and how to get help for this? ☐ Yes ☐ No
9. How often do you use seat belts?
☐ Never ☐ 25% of the time ☐ 50% of the time ☐ Almost always
10. Are you often exposed at work to excessive or loud noises without ear plugs or protectors? ☐ Yes ☐ No
11. Do you think you are exposed at work to any of the following:
1. unsafe conditions ☐ Yes ☐ No
2. hazardous chemicals, solvents, or dust ☐ Yes ☐ No
3. other conditions you wish to discuss ☐ Yes ☐ No
12. Do you think that at work
1. you lift too much weight ☐ Yes ☐ No
2. you do jobs that result in bone or muscle aches ☐ Yes ☐ No

> HEALTH HABITS:

1. Do you currently smoke cigarettes? ☐ Yes ☐ No
2. If you do not currently smoke cigarettes, have you ever smoked cigarettes? ☐ Yes ☐ No
3. If you currently smoke or have ever smoked:

How many packs per day?	AND	For how many years?
1 ☐ ½ pack or less		1 ☐ 5 years or less
2 ☐ ½ to 1 pack		2 ☐ 5 to 10 years
3 ☐ 1 to 1½ packs		3 ☐ 10 to 15 years
4 ☐ 1½ to 2 packs		4 ☐ 15 to 20 years
5 ☐ More than 2 packs		5 ☐ More than 20 years

4. If you are an ex-smoker, how long ago did you stop smoking?
1 ☐ 6 months or less
2 ☐ 6 to 12 months ago
3 ☐ 1 to 2 years ago
4 ☐ 2 to 10 years ago
5 ☐ More than 10 years ago
5. On the average, how many drinks do you have per day?

	Weekdays	AND	Weekends
(One drink = One 12 oz. beer	1 ☐ None		1 ☐ None
= One 4 oz. glass of wine	2 ☐ 0-2		2 ☐ 0-2
= One 1 oz. shot of whiskey)	3 ☐ 3-5		3 ☐ 3-5
	4 ☐ 6-10		4 ☐ 6-10
	5 ☐ More than 10		5 ☐ More than 10

6. Have you ever tried to cut down on drinking? ☐ Yes ☐ No
7. Have you ever been annoyed by criticism of your drinking? ☐ Yes ☐ No
8. On the average, how much of the following beverages do you consume?

Tea	Coffee	Colas
1 ☐ None	1 ☐ None	1 ☐ None
2 ☐ 0-2 cups/day	2 ☐ 0-2 cups/day	2 ☐ 0-2 cans/day
3 ☐ 3-6 cups/day	3 ☐ 3-6 cups/day	3 ☐ 3-6 cans per day
4 ☐ More than 6 cups/day	4 ☐ More than 6 cups/day	4 ☐ More than 6 cans/day

9. Have you ever been advised by a physician to modify your diet? ☐ Yes ☐ No
10. Do you purposely restrict any of the following in your diet?
Fats/cholesterol ☐ Yes ☐ No
Sugar/carbohydrates ☐ Yes ☐ No

> PREVENTION/SCREENING TESTS:

Please give the approximate date of the last time you had any of the following examinations, tests or immunizations. (If you are unsure of a date, please mark a ? next to the date.)

	DATE		DATE
1 ☐ Glaucoma screening/eye exam	____	6 ☐ Tetanus immunization	____
2 ☐ Chest X-ray	____	7 ☐ Influenza immunization	____
3 ☐ Sigmoidoscopy	____	8 ☐ Pneumococcus immunization	____
4 ☐ Rectal exam	____	9 ☐ Hepatitis immunization	____
5 ☐ Tuberculin (TB) skin test	____	39 ☐ Rubella test/immunization	____
20 ☐ Guaiac stool cards	____	45 ☐ Cholesterol level	____
WOMEN ONLY		MEN ONLY	
10 ☐ Mammogram	____	13 ☐ Testicular exam	____
11 ☐ Breast exam	____		
12 ☐ PAP smear	____		

> FAMILY HISTORY: Has any **BLOOD RELATIVE** had any of the following?
Please indicate by X's which of the following health problems you, your parents, your grandparents, or your siblings have had (include blood relatives only).

	SELF (1)	PARENT (2)	GRAND-PARENT (3)	BROTHER OR SISTER (4)		SELF (1)	PARENT (2)	GRAND-PARENT (3)	BROTHER OR SISTER (4)
(1) Allergies	☐	☐	☐	☐	(14) Tuberculosis	☐	☐	☐	☐
(2) Asthma	☐	☐	☐	☐	(15) Kidney disease	☐	☐	☐	☐
(3) Anemia	☐	☐	☐	☐	(16) Stomach/duodenal ulcer	☐	☐	☐	☐
(4) Diabetes	☐	☐	☐	☐	(17) Hepatitis	☐	☐	☐	☐
(5) Alcoholism	☐	☐	☐	☐	(18) Arthritis	☐	☐	☐	☐
(6) Psychiatric illness	☐	☐	☐	☐	(25) Hypercholesterolemia	☐	☐	☐	☐
(7) Glaucoma	☐	☐	☐	☐	(26) Colon polyp(s)	☐	☐	☐	☐
(8) Epilepsy	☐	☐	☐	☐	(19) Lung cancer	☐	☐	☐	☐
(9) Stroke	☐	☐	☐	☐	(20) Breast cancer	☐	☐	☐	☐
(10) Heart Disease	☐	☐	☐	☐	(21) Colon/rectal cancer	☐	☐	☐	☐
(11) Hypertension (high blood pressure)	☐	☐	☐	☐	(22) Prostate cancer	☐	☐	☐	☐
(12) Chronic bronchitis	☐	☐	☐	☐	(23) Skin cancer	☐	☐	☐	☐
(13) Emphysema	☐	☐	☐	☐	(24) Other cancers (Specify) ________				

REVIEW OF SYMPTOMS AND PROBLEMS BY SYSTEMS

1. ENDOCRINE:

In the past year, have you had:
1. An unexplained weight gain of 10 lbs. or more ☐ Yes ☐ No
2. An unexplained weight loss of 10 lbs. or more ☐ Yes ☐ No
3. Heat intolerance ☐ Yes ☐ No
4. Cold intolerance ☐ Yes ☐ No
5. Excessive appetite ☐ Yes ☐ No
6. Unusual thirst ☐ Yes ☐ No
7. Abnormal hair growth ☐ Yes ☐ No

Have you ever had:
> 8. Sugar diabetes ☐ Yes ☐ No
9. X-ray treatments of your face, tonsils, neck or face ☐ Yes ☐ No
10. Treatment for thyroid problems ☐ Yes ☐ No
> 11. Surgery: 1. thyroid gland operation ☐ Yes ☐ No
2. parathyroid gland operation ☐ Yes ☐ No

Figure 2-1 A sample health history questionnaire.

Figure continues on following page

2. EYES, EARS, NOSE, THROAT:

In the past year, have you had:

1. Recurrent or frequent eye pain ☐ Yes ☐ No
2. Failing vision not corrected with glasses ☐ Yes ☐ No
3. Trouble with your hearing ☐ Yes ☐ No
4. Frequent or recurrent ear pain or discharge ☐ Yes ☐ No
5. Severe nosebleeds ☐ Yes ☐ No
6. Troublesome nasal discharge or stuffy nose ☐ Yes ☐ No
7. Bad or painful teeth ☐ Yes ☐ No
8. Persistent or troublesome sores on the lips or tongue ☐ Yes ☐ No
9. Persistent hoarseness ☐ Yes ☐ No

Have you ever had:

10. A temporary loss of vision in one or both eyes ☐ Yes ☐ No
> 11. Glaucoma ☐ Yes ☐ No
12. Retinal detachment ☐ Yes ☐ No
> 13. Cataract ☐ Yes ☐ No
14. Allergy testing ☐ Yes ☐ No
> 15. Surgery 1. eye operation ☐ Yes ☐ No
2. ear operation ☐ Yes ☐ No
3. nose/sinus operation ☐ Yes ☐ No
4. mouth or throat ☐ Yes ☐ No

3. RESPIRATORY:

In the past year, have you:

1. Had a chronic (daily) cough ☐ Yes ☐ No
2. Coughed up blood ☐ Yes ☐ No
3. Had shortness of breath which interfered with your normal functions ☐ Yes ☐ No

Have you ever had:

> 4. Tuberculosis ☐ Yes ☐ No
> 5. A positive (abnormal) skin test for TB ☐ Yes ☐ No
> 6. Asthma ☐ Yes ☐ No

4. CARDIOVASCULAR:

In the past year, have you had:

1. Frequent skipped or irregular heartbeats ☐ Yes ☐ No
2. Repeated bothersome chest pain on exertion ☐ Yes ☐ No
3. Shortness of breath if you lie flat ☐ Yes ☐ No
4. Swollen (not just puffy) ankles or feet ☐ Yes ☐ No
5. Painful leg cramps brought on by walking ☐ Yes ☐ No

Have you ever had:

> 6. Rheumatic fever ☐ Yes ☐ No
> 7. High blood pressure ☐ Yes ☐ No
> 8. A heart attack or coronary ☐ Yes ☐ No
> 9. Angina ☐ Yes ☐ No
10. Heart murmur ☐ Yes ☐ No
> 11. Surgery 1. a heart operation ☐ Yes ☐ No
2. artery surgery ☐ Yes ☐ No

5. GASTROINTESTINAL:

In the past year, have you had:

1. Persistent difficulty or pain in swallowing ☐ Yes ☐ No
2. Frequent episodes of vomiting ☐ Yes ☐ No
3. Persistent troubles with gas, heartburn, or indigestion ☐ Yes ☐ No
4. Frequent abdominal pains ☐ Yes ☐ No
5. Persistent constipation requiring laxatives ☐ Yes ☐ No
6. Recent change in bowel habits ☐ Yes ☐ No
7. Blood in or around the stool ☐ Yes ☐ No
8. Blood in the toilet bowl ☐ Yes ☐ No
9. Blood on the toilet paper ☐ Yes ☐ No
10. Black or tarry stools ☐ Yes ☐ No
11. A recent loss of appetite ☐ Yes ☐ No

Have you ever had:

12. Ulcer problems ☐ Yes ☐ No
13. Jaundice, hepatitis or other liver disease ☐ Yes ☐ No
> 14. Ulcerative colitis or regional enteritis ☐ Yes ☐ No
15. Diverticulitis ☐ Yes ☐ No
16. Gall stones ☐ Yes ☐ No
17. Polyp or tumor of the bowel or rectum ☐ Yes ☐ No
> 18. Surgery 1. hernia repaired ☐ Yes ☐ No
2. appendix removed ☐ Yes ☐ No
3. gall bladder removed ☐ Yes ☐ No
4. stomach operation ☐ Yes ☐ No
5. intestinal or rectal operation ☐ Yes ☐ No
6. other type of abdominal surgery ☐ Yes ☐ No

6. GENITOURINARY:

In the past year, have you had:

1. Persistent trouble passing urine ☐ Yes ☐ No
2. Bloody urine ☐ Yes ☐ No
3. To get up more often than once at night to urinate ☐ Yes ☐ No

Have you ever had:

4. An infection of the kidney or bladder ☐ Yes ☐ No
> 5. Kidney or bladder stones ☐ Yes ☐ No
6. Treatment for VD ☐ Yes ☐ No
> 7. Surgery 1. kidney operation ☐ Yes ☐ No
2. bladder operation ☐ Yes ☐ No

7. GENITOURINARY - MEN ONLY:

In the past year, have you had:

1. A discharge from your penis ☐ Yes ☐ No
2. A lump or swelling of your testicle ☐ Yes ☐ No
3. A decrease of your sex drive or potency more than you think is normal ☐ Yes ☐ No

Have you ever had:

> 4. Surgery 1. Prostate operation ☐ Yes ☐ No
2. Penis operation ☐ Yes ☐ No
3. Testicle operation ☐ Yes ☐ No
4. Sterilizing operation ☐ Yes ☐ No

MEN . . . GO TO HEMATOLOGY SECTION

8. OBSTETRICS-GYNECOLOGY - WOMEN ONLY:

1. Are you pregnant or think you are pregnant ☐ Yes ☐ No
If no, is inability to get pregnant a problem ☐ Yes ☐ No

> 2. When was your last period DATE ______________

In the past year, have you had:

3. A troublesome vaginal discharge ☐ Yes ☐ No
4. Repeated pain with intercourse ☐ Yes ☐ No
5. A decreased sex drive more than you think is normal ☐ Yes ☐ No

If you are no longer having periods, go on to Question 12

6. Gone six or more months without a period ☐ Yes ☐ No
7. Trouble with irregular periods ☐ Yes ☐ No
8. Severe cramps or backaches with period that limit activity ☐ Yes ☐ No
9. Excessive bleeding or flow with your periods ☐ Yes ☐ No
10. Vaginal spotting or bleeding in-between your periods ☐ Yes ☐ No
11. Been achieving birth control by:
☐ pills ☐ loop, coil, IUD ☐ diaphragm ☐ other ☐ none
12. Vaginal bleeding or spotting after menopause ☐ Yes ☐ No

Have you ever had:

13. An abnormal Pap smear ☐ Yes ☐ No
14. Been told your mother was given Stilbesterol (DES) or hormones during her pregnancy with you ☐ Yes ☐ No
> 15. Surgery 1. tubes or ovaries operated on or removed ☐ Yes ☐ No
2. uterus removed (hysterectomy) ☐ Yes ☐ No
3. ectopic pregnancy (pregnancy in the tubes) ☐ Yes ☐ No
4. other female operation ☐ Yes ☐ No

9. HEMATOLOGY:

In the past year, have you had:

1. Prolonged bleeding (more than is normal for you) from a cut, injury or tooth removal ☐ Yes ☐ No

Have you ever had:

2. Anemia ☐ Yes ☐ No
> 3. Hemophilia or some other bleeding disease ☐ Yes ☐ No
> 4. Leukemia or other cancer of the blood ☐ Yes ☐ No
> 5. Surgery 1. spleen removed ☐ Yes ☐ No
2. biopsy or removal of lymph gland ☐ Yes ☐ No

10. SKIN/BREAST:

In the past year, have you had:

1. A persistent skin rash or problem ☐ Yes ☐ No
2. Moles or skin lumps that have changed either in size or color ☐ Yes ☐ No
3. Lumps or soreness in the breast or nipple ☐ Yes ☐ No
4. A bloody discharge from the nipple(s) ☐ Yes ☐ No

Have you ever had:

> 5. Psoriasis ☐ Yes ☐ No
> 6. Surgery 1. Skin cancer removed ☐ Yes ☐ No
2. Breast operation or biopsy ☐ Yes ☐ No

11. MUSCULOSKELETAL:

Since your 18th birthday, have you:

> 1. Had any fractures or dislocations to your bones or joints ☐ Yes ☐ No
> 2. Been injured in a road traffic accident ☐ Yes ☐ No
> 3. Injured your head ☐ Yes ☐ No
> 4. Been injured in an assault or fight (excluding injuries during sports) ☐ Yes ☐ No
> 5. Been injured after drinking ☐ Yes ☐ No

MUSCULOSKELETAL (continued):

In the past year, have you had:

6. Back pain which interfered with your normal activity for more than 2 or 3 days ☐ Yes ☐ No
7. Troublesome joint stiffness or pain ☐ Yes ☐ No
8. Recurrent aches, pains or cramps in the muscles ☐ Yes ☐ No
9. To use a cane, crutch/walker ☐ Yes ☐ No

Have you ever had:

> 10. Gout ☐ Yes ☐ No
> 11. Surgery 1. amputation of an arm, hand, or other body parts ☐ Yes ☐ No
2. operation of the neck, back or other joints ☐ Yes ☐ No

12. NEUROLOGY:

In the past year, have you had:

1. Recurring severe headaches ☐ Yes ☐ No
2. Troublesome double vision ☐ Yes ☐ No
3. Troublesome dizzy spells ☐ Yes ☐ No
4. Lost your ability to speak for a few minutes ☐ Yes ☐ No
5. Blackout spells ☐ Yes ☐ No
6. Serious trouble with memory or coordination ☐ Yes ☐ No

Have you ever had:

> 7. A stroke ☐ Yes ☐ No
8. Paralysis ☐ Yes ☐ No
> 9. Multiple sclerosis ☐ Yes ☐ No
10. Seizures in the past 5 years ☐ Yes ☐ No

13. PSYCHOSOCIAL:

In the past few months, have you:

1. Often had difficulty sleeping (trouble falling asleep or frequent awakening) ☐ Yes ☐ No
2. Often felt tiredness which lasts more than two hours after arising ☐ Yes ☐ No
3. Found that you sleep more than is usual for you ☐ Yes ☐ No
4. Felt depressed or blue most of the time ☐ Yes ☐ No
5. Felt lonely much of the time ☐ Yes ☐ No
6. Repeated spells when you can't stop crying ☐ Yes ☐ No
7. Often wished you were dead ☐ Yes ☐ No
8. Felt a strong need to take your life ☐ Yes ☐ No
9. Often had troublesome panicky feelings for no apparent reason ☐ Yes ☐ No

Have you ever had:

10. A nervous breakdown ☐ Yes ☐ No
11. Shock treatment ☐ Yes ☐ No
12. Attempted suicide ☐ Yes ☐ No
13. Been hospitalized for problems with your nerves ☐ Yes ☐ No
14. Been seen by a psychiatrist, psychologist, or counselor for personal problems ☐ Yes ☐ No

PATIENT'S CONCERNS/NEEDS:

In your opinion, what are your most important health problems?

1. ____________ 2. ____________ 3. ____________
4. ____________ 5. ____________ 6. ____________

What health problems do you want to talk about today?

1. ____________ 2. ____________ 3. ____________ 4. ____________

Would you like to talk to a social worker about any of the following:

☐ Living situation ☐ Financial situation ☐ Transportation ☐ Other ____________

Figure 2-1 *Continued*

People who come to a university medical center for care expect that students will participate in their care. There is no reason to apologize about your status as a student. Introduce yourself in a straightforward fashion. The title of doctor carries with it knowledge, obligations, and expectations that you cannot yet fulfill. Rapport and professionalism do not depend upon familiarity, so use the patient's surname unless instructed to do otherwise. Inquire about the patient's comfort and do whatever you can to put the patient and yourself at ease. Also do whatever you can to ensure privacy, although this can be a nearly impossible task in the university hospital. Be equipped with note paper, writing instruments, and a checklist to guide the interview. Sitting during the interview is recommended, but don't sit on the patient's bed without his or her permission; it is best to sit in your own chair at the bedside, where the patient can easily see you.

Within a few minutes of meeting the patient, assess his or her reliability. If you question the patient's reliability, perform a mini mental status examination (Table 2-1). Evidence of cognitive impairment does not mean there is no value in talking further with the patient, but you will have to make certain allowances for this.

Conducting the Interview

There is no one right way to record information obtained in the interview. Some clinicians can record information as it is given without distracting from the interview, but others prefer to use intermittent summary notes and other techniques. Feel free to experiment; with time and practice, you will find a method that works for you.

Questioning is the main technique for eliciting information. There are primary and secondary types of questions. Primary questions include open-ended (How can I help you?), limited-choice (What medicines are you taking?), and yes/no (Did you vomit?) questions. Secondary questions include clarification (How often do you take that medicine?) and elaboration (In addition to that medicine what else do you take?).

Most medical interviews include the history of the present illness, the previous medical history, a review of systems, the family history, and a social history. The interview sequence is not fixed. It is often a good idea to begin with the social history (inquire about the patient's background and so forth) in order to put the patient's illness complaints in perspective. Although flexibility in the interview allows the patient's history to develop in a natural order, following a routine is insurance against omission and can help keep you on track when you are tired or distracted.

Social History. As stated, this is a good place to begin. Two important and often revealing questions are "Who are the important people in your life?" and "Where are they now?"

History of Present Illness. Begin with the patient's view of the current problem. Good starting points include asking the patient to tell you about his or her problem(s) and asking the patient when he or she last felt 100 percent well. Get a clear description of the major symptom or symptom cluster and characterize it as outlined in the next section.

Review of Systems. The review of systems enables you to examine organ systems with words. Commit the sequence to memory (use a 3 × 5 card initially) and begin each category with broad questions (Any trouble with your lungs?) before asking specifics (Any history of asthma?). Many physicians do the review of systems while they are doing the physical examination, e.g., asking about eye problems while examining the eyes.

Previous Medical History. Organizing this section in a problem-oriented fashion can be very useful.

Family History. The family history often gives you insight into the patient's problem. Don't discount this part of the history.

Learn to make transitional statements between the preceding categories, or your patient will become confused; e.g., "I am going to ask you a series of questions now that may seem unrelated, but your answers will help me understand more about your problem."

It will take time and experience to learn to focus and regulate the interview tactfully. Review of your own recorded interviews with an experienced interviewer can be invaluable in this regard.

Table 2-1 The Short Portable Mental Status Questionnaire

1. What is the date today?
2. What day of the week is it?
3. What is the name of this place?
4. What is your telephone number?
   (If the patient does not have a phone: What is your street address?)
5. How old are you?
6. When were you born?
7. Who is the president of the United States now?
8. Who was the president just before that?
9. What was your mother's maiden name?
10. Subtract 3 from 20 and keep subtracting 3 from each new number you get, all the way down.

When this test is administered to community-dwelling elders, the specificity is found to be better than 90%. The sensitivity (the ability of the test to detect impairment) is not as great and may be as low as 50%. This means that although 90% of normal elders are identified correctly as not impaired, as few as half of the demented patients are detected. Thus there are few false-positive results but many false-negative results.

Scoring: 0– 2 errors: Intact
3– 4 errors: Mild impairment
5– 7 errors: Moderate impairment
8–10 errors: Severe impairment

Symptom Analysis

During the interview, you don't deal directly with the disease but with the illness. Recall that illness is the patient's perception of the injury and his or her reaction to it. The illness is manifested by signs and symptoms; therefore, symptom analysis is the major focus of the interview. The interpretation of illness and its translation into a formal disease process is a challenging experience.

Symptom analysis starts with the patient's description and is refined to a set of precise dimensions. Use the following parameters to help dictate the symptom into a defined organ system:

1. Location
2. Radiation
3. Chronology or timing
4. Quality
5. Security
6. Setting or onset
7. Modifying factors
8. Associated symptoms

Unfortunately, there is usually not one clear-cut symptom but rather multiple ones. Persevere and look for the predominant symptom, which is often characterized by chronology and pattern.

Concluding the Interview

The final minutes of the interview may be very revealing. Most patients have agenda items that they keep until the end of the interview. These items are often the most important for them. It is crucial to allow adequate time for these questions. Try closing with final questions like these: "Are there other issues you wanted to talk about?" "Do you have any questions?" "What are your own ideas about what is wrong?" "What do you think caused or is causing the problem?"

Follow-Up

Usually, you will need to return to the bedside to expand on the database after the initial interview. Let the patient know that you will probably return with more questions after you have had a chance to review and digest the information already obtained. The return visit can often be pleasantly surprising, as the patient reveals or recalls important new information.

Immediately after seeing a patient is an excellent time to study that patient's complaint or disease. Reading almost always broadens the differential diagnosis and supports new avenues to explore with the patient.

Illness Behavior

The process that takes a patient's symptoms and reduces them to a disease entity is artificial; one cannot simply reduce a complex human problem to a narrow biologic issue with satisfactory results. It is also not realistic to think that, in a single interview, the busy clinician can understand fully the psychosocial variables that are active in each patient. However, if you understand a few psychosocial concepts of illness behavior, the ultimate outcome of your interview will be more satisfying to you and your patient.

Explanatory Models. All patients come to the medical interview with explanatory models for their symptom complex. The patient's explanatory model contains the patient's understanding of the cause of his or her illness, its pathophysiology and expected course and prognosis, and the treatment he or she believes should be administered. This can be assessed if the patient trusts you.

Illness Meaning. After assessing the explanatory model, inquire about illness meaning. Generally, patients try to understand their experiences and perceptions by attributing or assigning causes to them. For the patient distressed by physical complaints, a causal explanation provides some control for them. Illness attributions are important to the clinician because they reveal the meanings patients attach to their symptoms. This meaning of illness determines the patient's illness behaviors, coping responses, and emotional reactions. Patients are more likely to feel genuinely supported when they sense that the clinician's behavior expresses a concern based on a personal understanding. This psychosocial concern can and has been devalued and replaced with a sterile scientific quest for the control of symptoms; however, such a value transformation disables the clinician and disempowers the patient.

Illness Problems. Illness problems consist of the experiential, family, economic, interpersonal, occupational, and daily-life problems that arise secondary to the disease and its treatment. For example, the onset of back pain in a construction worker may require him to curtail his work activities or even change careers, lead to significant economic problems, decrease his sexual relations, interfere with lifestyle and recreation, result in marital discord, disrupt his social network, and lead to disability lawsuits and serious personal distress—all while he is seeking medical care. Awareness of illness problems may help you understand the patient's illness behavior.

Major illness problems frequently encountered include the following:

1. Family problems created or worsened by sickness
2. Financial problems created or worsened by sickness
3. Changes in the patient's personal identity and social role in the context of permanent disability or disease
4. Maladaptive coping responses that patients and families use to manage sickness, such as denial, passive-aggressive behavior, and doctor shopping
5. Conflict in personal beliefs between patients (and family) and clinicians concerning the cause or nature of the sickness, the expected course, and the objectives for treatment
6. Inappropriate adoption of sick role and illness behavior for psychological, social, or financial gain
7. Conflict in cultural values concerning treatment between patients and clinicians due to substantial differences in social class, lifestyle, and ethnic norms
8. Inappropriate use of alternative or indigenous health care providers

Clinical Negotiation. Clinical negotiation involves the development of a therapeutic alliance between the clinician and the patient. Elements of this alliance involve trust, establishment of expertise, patient education, and acceptance (on the part of both parties). If conceptual differences arise between the clinician and the patient regarding explanatory models, illness meanings, and the like, these will need to be recognized and negotiated. This clinical negotiation is necessary if one wishes to change patient behavior and motivate the patient to accept therapy (discussed in more detail in Chapter 149, "Principles of Behavioral Change").

Remember that it is not the purpose of the clinical interview to ferret out the innermost secrets of the illness experience. The interview assists the clinician in establishing his or her role in helping patients and those around them come to terms with (accept, master, or change) their symptoms and the implication of illness. This is the essence of empowering patients!

References

Kleinman A, et al. Culture, illness and cure: Clinical lessons from anthropologic and cross cultural research. Ann Intern Med 1978; 88:251.

Lazare A. Shame and humiliation in the medical encounter. Arch Intern Med 1987; 147:1653.

Lepowski ZJ. Psychosocial aspects of disease. Ann Intern Med 1969; 71:1197.

Levinson D. A guide to the clinical interview. Philadelphia: WB Saunders, 1987.

Lipkin M Jr, et al. The medical interview: A core curriculum for residencies in internal medicine. Ann Intern Med 1984; 100:277.

Suchman AL, et al. What makes the patient-doctor relationship therapeutic? Exploring the connexional dimension of medical care. Ann Intern Med 1988; 108:125.

Health Maintenance and Preventive Care

Katherine L. Kahn, MD

Harry L. Greene, MD

3

During recent decades, patients, physicians, and policy makers have shown strong interest in preventive care. However, what once seemed to be a straightforward issue has evolved into a complex look at the goals and limitations of health care. Table 3-1 contrasts the purpose of a *diagnostic evaluation* in a patient with a problem, the *periodic health examination* in a basically well individual, and *screening* in a generally well population. This chapter describes the basic principles of health maintenance, particularly with respect to the periodic health examination.

Assets and Debits of Screening

When a patient presents without a specific complaint, the physician's task is to ask the patient to identify a problem, to ascertain that there is no hidden agenda, and finally to approach the patient who truly appears well. Although it is common for the physician and patient to recognize and take risks in the evaluation of the sick patient (e.g., risk of diagnostic needle aspiration), the use of tests and the introduction of uncertainty into the risk–benefit equation for the well person are more difficult. In order to use the preventive medicine approach most effectively, it is helpful to acknowledge the potential problems and assets associated with screening. A false-negative test is one that describes a normal result despite the patient's having an abnormality. The unfortunate consequence is false reassurance. For example, a patient who smokes might be inappropriately reassured by a normal chest film, when in fact he or she has severe smoking-induced obstructive lung disease that was not documented by the radiograph. The false-positive test is also a problem in screening the well patient, for it may cause anxiety or lead to inappropriate further testing and diagnoses in the truly well individual. A classic example is the VDRL test for syphilis, which, in 10 percent of elderly persons, is a biologically false-positive test. Imagine the anxiety and frustration that might be suffered by an elderly patient told she had syphilis when in fact the problem was a false-positive test.

Cost is another factor to be considered when the well person is evaluated. Cost evaluations must include cost of the test and cost of the follow-up evaluation for an abnormal screening test, particularly when the test result is false-positive. Consider, for example, the false-positive stool test for occult blood. Ingestion of red meat decreases the predictive value of the fecal test for occult blood by increasing the false-positive rate. The well person whose stool tests positive for occult blood must be followed with further tests to confirm that the blood in the stool is secondary to the ingested meat and not to a lesion bleeding in the bowel. Cost evaluations must also include cost of any follow-up sigmoidoscopy or other test used to evaluate the blood. Similarly, if a patient with asymptomatic hyperuricemia is treated to control the elevated level of uric acid in the blood and then develops a drug rash (as 15 percent of patients treated with allopurinol do), the occurrence of that rash must also be considered a "cost" of screening.

Labeling is a phenomenon that describes a change in the patient's behavior as a consequence of knowing a new diagnosis. For example, a group of workers showed increased absenteeism after they were told of their diagnosis of hypertension. Discrimination is also a potential problem associated with screening. Patients may be stigmatized by the diagnosis of hypertension, an abnormal electrocardiogram, proteinuria, or HIV positivity and then be denied a job promotion or, in the case of HIV positivity, an insurance policy.

Well persons may be resistant to screening because they may not want the attention of a physician and the discomfort associated with tests and procedures. Patients are often dubious about a physician's ability to detect occult disease, particularly given stories of a "well patient's" sudden death soon after a check-up. Historically, patient groups with the highest prevalence of a disease, and thus the most to gain from screening, sometimes have been most resistant to screening. For example, women of lower socioeconomic status are more likely to develop cervical cancer and, ironically, are less likely to participate in opportunities for a Papanicolaou smear screening.

Two biases inherent in screening should be considered. As shown in Figure 3-1, lead-time bias represents an illusion of prolongation of the patient's life span, although in fact it is unchanged; only the time from detection to death has been prolonged. Length bias describes the possibility that screening tests will preferentially detect cases with longer preclinical stages. Because less aggressive diseases (i.e., cancers with slower growth rates) have a longer presymptomatic period than aggressive diseases, the slower-growing cancers are more likely to be detected by screening. The bias occurs because screening trials have a greater opportunity to detect cancers that are slow growing and thus associated with a more prolonged survival. Both the lead time and the length bias emphasize the need for screening tests to be evaluated after consideration of these potential biases.

Table 3-1 Approaches to the Patient

	Type of evaluation		
Purpose of evaluation	*Diagnostic evaluation*	*Periodic health examination*	*Screening*
Subjects to be studied	Patient with a problem	Well individual	Well population
Objective	Diagnosis	Identify unrecognized disease	Identify unrecognized disease
	Resolution of a problem	Identify unrecognized risk of disease	Identify unrecognized risk of disease

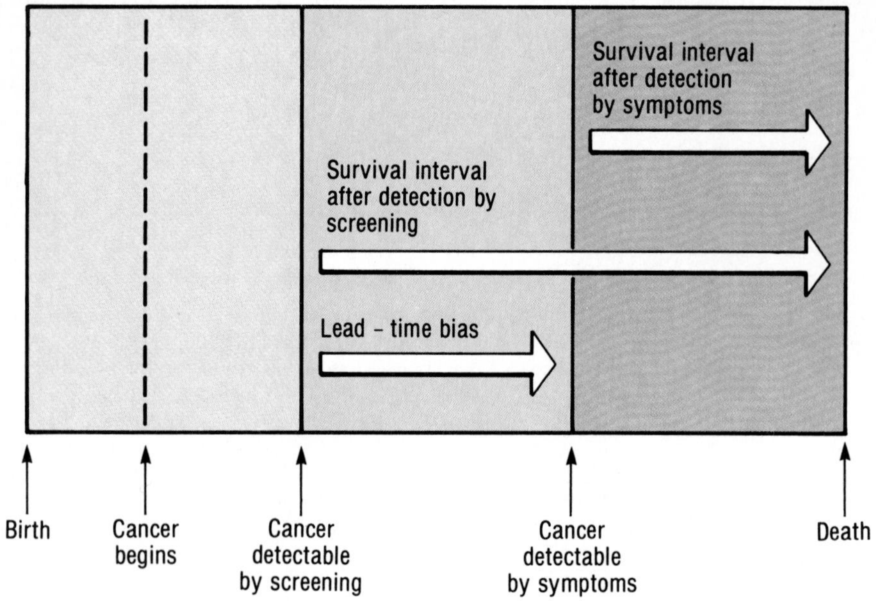

Figure 3-1 Lead-time bias.

Approach to the Patient

The benefits of appropriately used screening evaluations are decreased morbidity, decreased mortality, and improved quality of life. Although often difficult, each of these outcomes should be considered in relation to cost. Evaluation of a test or procedure for screening should include assessment of the *disease* being screened, assessment of the *test* itself, and assessment of the proposed *intervention*. The ideal disease for screening is one with a high prevalence, because such a disease is associated with improved predictive value and cost-effectiveness. If the disease being studied has identifiable risk factors, the detection rates can be improved by directing screening efforts toward individuals with appropriate risk factors. For example, although it is not appropriate to screen all persons for colorectal cancer, it is appropriate to screen those whose age, family history, or previously known conditions place them at increased risk for cancer of the colon. For screening to be most effective, the disease should have a latency period during which its detection would actually result in decreased morbidity and mortality. The *test* must have a reasonable cost and reasonable acceptability to the individual being tested. The screening test and follow-up diagnostic capabilities must be available. The *intervention* must truly decrease morbidity and mortality, not simply by advancing the time of diagnosis but by improving survival or function. Treatment methods must be available and acceptable.

Identifying Patients at High Risk

A fundamental principle of screening or health maintenance is that the greater the prevalence of the condition in the studied population, the more successful the attempts at screening. This is where the clinician's skill at identifying significant risk factors becomes critical. Patient history, family history, social habits, occupational exposures, and physical examination can provide clues that individualize the approach to patient care and allow for optimizing the preventive approach. Tables 3-2 to 3-9 illustrate the 10 leading causes of death in the United States by decade and so illuminate the kind of screening that might be emphasized for patients of various age groups.

Age is certainly an important factor in identifying patients at high risk. Health maintenance care, however, may be individualized even beyond considerations of age. Family history is a relevant risk factor when a family member has coronary heart disease at an early age (50 years old), hypertension, obesity, thyroid disease, colorectal cancer, breast cancer, or malignant melanoma. Cigarette smoking is a risk factor for chronic obstructive lung disease, coronary heart disease, and cancer of the oropharynx, esophagus, bladder, and lung. Exposure to radiation during childhood increases the risk of subsequent development of thyroid disease, including thyroid cancers. High-dose therapeutic radiation, particularly in combination with chemotherapy, increases the likelihood of subsequent leukemia. Fair-skinned individuals, particularly those who are exposed to the sun a great deal, are at risk for melanoma.

Blacks have a higher incidence of hypertension, obesity, alcoholism, and sickle cell disease than whites, as well as a greater likelihood of cancer of the uterine cervix, oral cavity, lung, and prostate. Native-born Japanese have a high incidence of gastric cancer. Chinese have an increased incidence of nasopharyngeal carcinoma. Ashkenazi Jews are at risk for Tay-Sachs disease.

The role of occupational exposure in the etiology of disease has increased annually and should be carefully noted: Asbestos exposure has been associated with lung cancer and mesothelioma; polyvinyl chloride exposure is associated with the development of hepatic angiocarcinoma; exposure to hydrocarbons, rubber, and dye is associated with an increase in bladder carcinoma; and petrolatum exposure increases the risk for development of cancer of the skin and scrotum.

Physical Examination

The identification of persons at high risk is only part of the approach to health maintenance. The other criteria noted previously regarding the disease, the test, and the patient must also be considered. The physical examination provides a useful set of screening modalities, which are noted in the next section. Figure 3-2 summarizes the physical examination as it relates to health maintenance and preventive care.

Evaluation of blood pressure and weight is an important part of the screening physical examination because the chronic conditions of hypertension and obesity are associated with improved outcomes when interventions are conducted appropriately. Ask the patient about persistent sores of the skin or in the mouth and lumps anywhere in the body. Examine the skin with the patient undressed, looking for melanoma and basal and squamous cell carcinomas. Search carefully for abnormal lymph

Table 3-2 Leading Causes of Death from Birth to 18 Months and Preventive Services

Schedule of visits

Schedule at 2, 4, 6, 15, and 18 mo. Five visits are required for immunizations. Because of lack of data and differing patient risk profiles, the scheduling of additional visits and the frequency of the individual preventive services listed in this table are left to clinical discretion (except as indicated in footnotes).

	Preventive services*		
Leading causes of death	*Screening*	*Parent counseling*	*Immunizations and chemoprophylaxis*
Conditions originating in perinatal period Congenital anomalies Heart disease Injuries (non–motor vehicle) Pneumonia/influenza	Height and weight Hemoglobin and hematocrit[†] *High-risk groups* Hearing[‡] (HR1) Erythrocyte protoporphyrin (HR2)	**Diet** Breastfeeding Nutrient intake, especially iron-rich foods **Injury Prevention** Child safety seats Smoke detector Hot-water-heater temperature Stairway gates, window guards, pool fence Storage of drugs and toxic chemicals Syrup of ipecac, poison-control telephone number **Dental Health** Baby bottle tooth decay **Other Primary Preventive Measures** Effects of passive smoking	Diphtheria-tetanus-pertussis (DTP) vaccine[§] Oral poliovirus vaccine (OPV)[¶] Measles-mumps-rubella (MMR) vaccine[**] *Haemophilus influenzae* type b (Hib) conjugate vaccine[††] *High-risk groups* Fluoride supplements (HR3) **First Week** Ophthalmic antibiotics[‡‡] Hemoglobin electrophoresis (HR4)[‡‡] T_4/TSH[§§] Phenylalanine[§§] Hearing (HR1) **Remain Alert for:** Ocular misalignment Tooth decay Signs of child abuse or neglect

High-risk categories

HR1: Infants with a family history of childhood hearing impairment or a personal history of congenital perinatal infection with herpes, syphilis, rubella, cytomegalovirus, or toxoplasmosis; malformations involving the head or neck (e.g., dysmorphic and syndromal abnormalities, cleft palate, abnormal pinna); birth weight below 1,500 g; bacterial meningitis; hyperbilirubinemia requiring exchange transfusion; or severe perinatal asphyxia (Apgar scores of 0–3, absence of spontaneous respirations for 10 min, or hypotonia at 2 hr of age).

HR2: Infants who live in or frequently visit housing built before 1950 that is dilapidated or undergoing renovation; who come in contact with other children with known lead toxicity; who live near lead-processing plants or whose parents or household members work in a lead-related occupation; or who live near busy highways or hazardous-waste sites.

HR3: Infants living in areas with inadequate water fluoridation (less than 0.7 ppm).

HR4: Newborns of Caribbean, Latin American, Asian, Mediterranean, or African descent.

* This list of preventive services is not exhaustive. It reflects only those topics reviewed by the US Preventive Services Task Force. Clinicians may wish to add other preventive services after considering the patient's medical history and other individual circumstances.
† Once during infancy.
‡ At age 18-mo visit, if not tested earlier.
§ At ages, 2, 4, 6, and 15 mo.
¶ At ages 2, 4, and 15 mo.
** At age 15 mo.
†† At age 18 mo.
‡‡ At birth.
§§ Days 3 to 6 preferred for testing.
Data in Tables 3-2 to 3-9 are from the U.S. Preventive Services Task Force Guide to Clinical Preventive Services.

nodes, because Hodgkin's disease is a potentially curable disease with higher survival rates when it is localized. Evaluate the oral cavity for lumps, leukoplakia, redness, ulcerations, or roughened areas, which may be associated with carcinoma of the oral cavity, particularly in the smoking or drinking patient who is more than 50 years old. Examine the thyroid gland for nodules, taking particular care in the patient with a history of radiation exposure to the head and neck.

In the heart examination one should seek a normal, regular rhythm and crisp sounds, with careful focus on a normally split second heart sound. Recognition and subsequent closure of an atrial septal defect in a young adult is one of the vivid success stories in medicine today. Patients with valvular heart disease, history of rheumatic fever, mitral valve prolapse, bicuspid aortic valve, or valvular prosthesis should be identified and appropriate prophylaxis or suppressive therapy administered.

Women should be assessed for their risk of breast cancer by noting the presence of any of the following risk factors: age more than 40, nulliparity after age 30, family history of breast cancer in first-degree relatives, early menarche, late menopause, or previous breast malignancy. Ask the patient about her own performance of breast self-examination, and teach or reiterate the proper technique for doing so. The breast must be examined carefully because cancerous lumps are sometimes only subtly palpable and are often difficult to distinguish from the lumpiness and asymmetries of normal breast tissue. Pay attention to the axilla, which contains both the tail end of normal breast tissue and lymph nodes. Examine the nipple region for irregularity and discharge. The pelvic examination is essential to a screening evaluation and should include a Papanicolaou smear on a regular basis in women who are sexually active or more than 18 years old. The incidence of cervical car-

Text continues on page 20

Table 3-3 Leading Causes of Death from Ages 2 to 6 Years and Preventive Services

Schedule of visits

One visit is required for immunizations. Because of lack of data and differing patient risk profiles, the scheduling of additional visits and the frequency of the individual preventive services listed in this table are left to clinical discretion (except as indicated in footnotes).

	Preventive services*		
Leading causes of death	*Screening*	*Patient and parent counseling*	*Immunizations and chemoprophylaxis*
Injuries (non–motor vehicle) Motor vehicle crashes Congenital anomalies Homicide Heart disease	Height and weight Blood pressure Eye exam for amblyopia and strabismus[†] Urinalysis for bacteriuria *High-risk groups* Erythrocyte protoporphyrin[‡] (HR1) Tuberculin skin test (PPD) (HR2) Hearing[§] (HR3)	**Diet and Exercise** Sweets and between-meal snacks, iron-enriched foods, sodium Caloric balance Selection of exercise program **Injury Prevention** Safety belts Smoke detector Hot-water-heater temperature Window guards and pool fence Bicycle safety helmets Storage of drugs, toxic chemicals, matches, and firearms Syrup of ipecac, poison-control telephone number **Dental Health** Tooth brushing and dental visits **Other Primary Preventive Measures** Effects of passive smoking *High-risk groups* Skin protection from ultraviolet light (HR4)	Diphtheria-tetanus-pertussis (DTP) vaccine[¶] Oral poliovirus vaccine (OPV)[¶] *High-risk groups* Fluoride supplements (HR5) **Remain Alert for:** Vision disorders Dental decay, malalignment, premature loss of teeth, mouth breathing Signs of child abuse or neglect Abnormal bereavement

High-risk categories

HR1: Children who live in or frequently visit housing built before 1950 that is dilapidated or undergoing renovation; who come in contact with other children with known lead toxicity; who live near lead-processing plants or whose parents or household members work in a lead-related occupation; or who live near busy highways or hazardous-waste sites.

HR2: Household members of persons with tuberculosis or others at risk for close contact with the disease; recent immigrants or refugees from countries in which tuberculosis is common (e.g., Asia, Africa, Central and South America, Pacific Islands); family members of migrant workers; residents of homeless shelters; or persons with certain underlying medical disorders.

HR3: Children with a family history of childhood hearing impairment or a personal history of congenital perinatal infection with herpes, syphilis, rubella, cytomegalovirus, or toxoplasmosis; malformations involving the head or neck (e.g., dysmorphic and syndromal abnormalities, cleft palate, abnormal pinna); birth weight below 1,500 g; bacterial meningitis; hyperbilirubinemia requiring exchange transfusion; or severe perinatal asphyxia (Apgar scores of 0–3, absence of spontaneous respirations for 10 min, or hypotonia at 2 hr of age).

HR4: Children with increased exposure to sunlight.

HR5: Children living in areas with inadequate water fluoridation (less than 0.7 ppm).

* This list of preventive services is not exhaustive. It reflects only those topics reviewed by the US Preventive Services Task Force. Clinicians may wish to add other preventive services after considering the patient's medical history and other individual circumstances.

† Ages 3–4.

‡ Annually.

§ Before age 3, if not tested earlier.

¶ Once between ages 4 and 6.

Table 3-4 Leading Causes of Death from Ages 7 to 12 Years and Preventive Services

Schedule of visits

Because of lack of data and differing patient risk profiles, the scheduling of additional visits and the frequency of the individual preventive services listed in this table are left to clinical discretion (except as indicated in footnotes).

Leading causes of death	Preventive services* *Screening*	 *Patient and parent counseling*	 *Chemoprophylaxis*
Motor vehicle crashes Injuries (non–motor vehicle) Congenital anomalies Leukemia Homicide Heart disease	Height and weight Blood pressure *High-risk groups* Tuberculin skin test (PPD) (HR1)	**Diet and Exercise** Fat (especially saturated fat), cholesterol, sweets and between-meal snacks, sodium Caloric balance Selection of exercise program **Injury Prevention** Safety belts Smoke detector Storage of firearms, drugs, toxic chemicals, matches Bicycle safety helmets **Dental Health** Regular tooth brushing and dental visits **Other Primary Preventive Measures** *High-risk groups* Skin protection from ultraviolet light (HR2)	*High-risk groups* Fluoride supplements (HR3) **Remain Alert for:** Vision disorders Diminished hearing Dental decay, malalignment, mouth breathing Signs of child abuse or neglect Abnormal bereavement

High-risk categories

HR1: Household members of persons with tuberculosis or others at risk for close contact with the disease; recent immigrants or refugees from countries in which tuberculosis is common (e.g., Asia, Africa, Central and South America, Pacific Islands); family members of migrant workers; residents of homeless shelters; or persons with certain underlying medical disorders.

HR2: Children with increased exposure to sunlight.

HR3: Children living in areas with inadequate water fluoridation (less than 0.7 ppm).

* This list of preventive services is not exhaustive. It reflects only those topics reviewed by the US Preventive Services Task Force. Clinicians may wish to add other preventive services after considering the patient's medical history and other individual circumstances.

Table 3-5 Leading Causes of Death from Ages 13 to 18 Years and Preventive Services

Schedule of visits

One visit is required for immunizations. Because of lack of data and differing patient risk profiles, the scheduling of additional visits and the frequency of the individual preventive services listed in this table are left to clinical discretion (except as indicated in footnotes).

Leading causes of death	Preventive services* *Screening*	 *Counseling*	 *Immunizations and chemoprophylaxis*
Motor vehicle crashes Homicide Suicide Injuries (non–motor vehicle) Heart disease	**History** Dietary intake Physical activity Tobacco/alcohol/drug use Sexual practices **Physical Exam** Height and weight Blood pressure *High-risk groups* Complete skin exam (HR1) Clinical testicular exam (HR2)	**Diet and Exercise** Fat (especially saturated fat), cholesterol, sodium, iron,‡ calcium‡ Caloric balance Selection of exercise program **Substance Use** Tobacco: cessation/primary prevention Alcohol and other drugs: Driving/other dangerous activities while under the influence Treatment for abuse *High-risk groups* Sharing/using unsterilized needles and syringes (HR12)	Tetanus-diphtheria (Td) booster** *High-risk groups* Fluoride supplements (HR15) **Remain Alert for:** Depressive symptoms Suicide risk factors (HR11) Abnormal bereavement Tooth decay, malalignment, gingivitis Signs of child abuse and neglect

Table continues on following page

Table 3-5 *(Continued)*

Leading causes of death	Preventive services*: *Screening*	Preventive services*: *Counseling*
	Laboratory/Diagnostic Procedures *High-risk groups* Rubella antibodies (HR3) VDRL (HR4) Chlamydial testing (HR5) Gonorrhea culture (HR6) Counseling and testing for HIV (HR7) Tuberculin skin test (PPD) (HR8) Hearing (HR9) Papanicolaou smear (HR10)†	**Sexual Practices** Sexual development and behavior§ Sexually transmitted diseases: partner selection, condoms Unintended pregnancy and contraceptive options **Injury Prevention** Safety belts Safety helmets Violent behavior¶ Firearms¶ Smoke detector **Dental Health** Regular tooth brushing, flossing, dental visits **Other Primary Preventive Measures** *High-risk groups* Discussion of hemoglobin testing (HR13) Skin protection from ultraviolet light (HR14)

High-risk categories

HR1: Persons with increased recreational or occupational exposure to sunlight, a family or personal history of skin cancer, or clinical evidence of precursor lesions (e.g., dysplastic nevi, certain congenital nevi).

HR2: Males with a history of cryptorchidism, orchiopexy, or testicular atrophy.

HR3: Females of child-bearing age lacking evidence of immunity.

HR4: Persons who engage in sex with multiple partners in areas in which syphilis is prevalent, prostitutes, or contacts of persons with active syphilis.

HR5: Persons who attend clinics for sexually transmitted diseases, attend other high-risk health care facilities (e.g., adolescent and family-planning clinics), or have other risk factors for chlamydial infection (e.g., multiple sexual partners or a sexual partner with multiple sexual contacts).

HR6: Persons with multiple sexual partners or a sexual partner with multiple contacts, sexual contacts of persons with culture-proven gonorrhea, or persons with a history of repeated episodes of gonorrhea.

HR7: Persons seeking treatment for sexually transmitted diseases; homosexual and bisexual men; past or present intravenous (IV) drug users; persons with a history of prostitution or multiple sexual partners; women whose past or present sexual partners were HIV infected, bisexual, or IV drug users; persons with long-term residence or birth in an area with high prevalence of HIV infection; or persons with a history of transfusion between 1978 and 1985.

HR8: Household members of persons with tuberculosis or others at risk for close contact with the disease; recent immigrants or refugees from countries in which tuberculosis is common (e.g., Asia, Africa, Central and South America, Pacific Islands); migrant workers; residents of correctional institutions or homeless shelters; or persons with certain underlying medical disorders.

HR9: Persons exposed regularly to excessive noise in recreational or other settings.

HR10: Females who are sexually active or (if the sexual history is thought to be unreliable) aged 18 or older.

HR11: Recent divorce, separation, unemployment, depression, alcohol or other drug abuse, serious medical illnesses, living alone, or recent bereavement.

HR12: Intravenous drug users.

HR13: Persons of Caribbean, Latin American, Asian, Mediterranean, or African descent.

HR14: Persons with increased exposure to sunlight.

HR15: Persons living in areas with inadequate water fluoridation (less than 0.7 ppm).

* This list of preventive services is not exhaustive. It reflects only those topics reviewed by the US Preventive Services Task Force. Clinicians may wish to add other preventive services after considering the patient's medical history and other individual circumstances.

† Every 1–3 yr.

‡ For females.

§ Often best performed early in adolescence and with the involvement of parents.

¶ For males.

** Once between ages 14 and 16.

Table 3-6 Leading Causes of Death from Ages 19 to 39 Years and Preventive Services

Schedule of visits

Schedule every 1 to 3 yr. The recommended schedule applies only to the periodic visit itself. The frequency of the individual preventive services listed in this table is left to clinical discretion, except as indicated in footnotes.

	Preventive services*		
Leading causes of death	*Screening*	*Counseling*	*Immunizations*
Motor vehicle crashes Homicide Suicide Injuries (non–motor vehicle) Heart disease	**History** Dietary intake Physical activity Tobacco/alcohol/drug use Sexual practices **Physical Exam** Height and weight Blood pressure *High-risk groups* Complete oral cavity exam (HR1) Palpation for thyroid nodules (HR2) Clinical breast exam (HR3) Clinical testicular exam (HR4) Complete skin exam (HR5) **Laboratory/Diagnostic Procedures** Nonfasting total blood cholesterol Papanicolaou smear[†] *High-risk groups* Fasting plasma glucose (HR6) Rubella antibodies (HR7) VDRL (HR8) Urinalysis for bacteriuria (HR9) Chlamydial testing (HR10) Gonorrhea culture (HR11) Counseling and testing for HIV (HR12) Hearing (HR13) Tuberculin skin test (PPD) (HR14) Electrocardiogram (HR15) Mammogram (HR3) Colonoscopy (HR16)	**Diet and Exercise** Fat (especially saturated fat), cholesterol, complex carbohydrates, fiber, sodium, iron,[‡] calcium[‡] Caloric balance Selection of exercise program **Substance Use** Tobacco: cessation/primary prevention Alcohol and other drugs: Limiting alcohol consumption Driving/other dangerous activities while under the influence Treatment for abuse *High-risk groups* Sharing/using unsterilized needles and syringes (HR18) **Sexual Practices** Sexually transmitted diseases: partner selection, condoms, anal intercourse Unintended pregnancy and contraceptive options **Injury Prevention** Safety belts Safety helmets Violent behavior[§] Firearms[§] Smoke detector Smoking near bedding or upholstery *High-risk groups* Back-conditioning exercises (HR19) Prevention of childhood injuries (HR20) Falls in the elderly (HR21) **Dental Health** Regular tooth brushing, flossing, dental visits **Other Primary Preventive Measures** *High-risk groups* Discussion of hemoglobin testing (HR22) Skin protection from ultraviolet light (HR23)	Tetanus-diphtheria (Td) booster[¶] *High-risk groups* Hepatitis B vaccine (HR24) Pneumococcal vaccine (HR25) Influenza vaccine** (HR26) Measles-mumps-rubella vaccine (HR27) **Remain Alert for:** Depressive symptoms Suicide risk factors (HR17) Abnormal bereavement Malignant skin lesions Tooth decay, gingivitis Signs of physical abuse

High-risk categories

HR1: Persons with exposure to tobacco or excessive amounts of alcohol, or those with suspicious symptoms or lesions detected through self-examination.

HR2: Persons with a history of upper-body irradiation.

HR3: Women aged 35 and older with a family history of premenopausally diagnosed breast cancer in a first-degree relative.

HR4: Men with a history of cryptorchidism, orchiopexy, or testicular atrophy.

HR5: Persons with family or personal history of skin cancer, increased occupational or recreational exposure to sunlight, or clinical evidence of precursor lesions (e.g., dysplastic nevi, certain congenital nevi).

HR6: The markedly obese, persons with a family history of diabetes, or women with a history of gestational diabetes.

HR7: Women lacking evidence of immunity.

HR8: Prostitutes, persons who engage in sex with multiple partners in areas in which syphilis is prevalent, or contacts of persons with active syphilis.

HR9: Persons with diabetes.

Table continues on following page

Table 3-6 (*Continued*)

High-risk categories (*continued*)

HR10: Persons who attend clinics for sexually transmitted diseases, attend other high-risk health care facilities (e.g., adolescent and family planning clinics), or have other risk factors for chlamydial infection (e.g., multiple sexual partners or a sexual partner with multiple sexual contacts, age less than 20).

HR11: Prostitutes, persons with multiple sexual partners or a sexual partner with multiple contacts, sexual contacts of persons with culture-proven gonorrhea, or persons with a history of repeated episodes of gonorrhea.

HR12: Persons seeking treatment for sexually transmitted diseases; homosexual and bisexual men; past or present intravenous (IV) drug users; persons with a history of prostitution or multiple sexual partners; women whose past or present sexual partners were HIV infected, bisexual, or IV drug users; persons with long-term residence or birth in an area with high prevalence of HIV infection; or persons with a history of transfusion between 1978 and 1985.

HR13: Persons exposed regularly to excessive noise.

HR14: Household members of persons with tuberculosis or others at risk for close contact with the disease (e.g., staff of tuberculosis clinics, shelters for the homeless, nursing homes, substance abuse treatment facilities, dialysis units, correctional institutions); recent immigrants or refugees from countries in which tuberculosis is common, migrant workers; residents of nursing homes, correctional institutions, or homeless shelters; or persons with certain underlying medical disorders (e.g., HIV infection).

HR15: Men who would endanger public safety were they to experience sudden cardiac events (e.g., commercial airline pilots).

HR16: Persons with a family history of familial polyposis coli or cancer family syndrome.

HR17: Recent divorce, separation, unemployment, depression, alcohol or other drug abuse, serious medical illnesses, living alone, or recent bereavement.

HR18: Intravenous drug users.

HR19: Persons at increased risk for lower-back injury because of past history, body configuration, or type of activities.

HR20: Persons with children in the home or automobile.

HR21: Persons with older adults in the home.

HR22: Young adults of Caribbean, Latin American, Asian, Mediterranean, or African descent.

HR23: Persons with increased exposure to sunlight.

HR24: Homosexually active men, IV drug users, recipients of some blood products, or persons in health-related jobs with frequent exposure to blood or blood products.

HR25: Persons with medical conditions that increase the risk of pneumococcal infection (e.g., chronic cardiac or pulmonary disease, sickle cell disease, nephrotic syndrome, Hodgkin's disease, asplenia, diabetes mellitus, alcoholism, cirrhosis, multiple myeloma, renal disease, or conditions associated with immunosuppression).

HR26: Residents of chronic care facilities or persons suffering from chronic cardiopulmonary disorders, metabolic diseases (including diabetes mellitus), hemoglobinopathies, immunosuppression, or renal dysfunction.

HR27: Persons born after 1956 who lack evidence of immunity to measles (receipt of live vaccine on or after first birthday, laboratory evidence of immunity, or a history of physician-diagnosed measles).

[*] This list of preventive services is not exhaustive. It reflects only those topics reviewed by the US Preventive Services Task Force. Clinicians may wish to add other preventive services after considering the patient's medical history and other individual circumstances.
[†] Every 1–3 yr.
[‡] For women.
[§] For young males.
[¶] Every 10 yr.
[**] Annually.

Table 3-7 Leading Causes of Death from Ages 40 to 64 Years and Preventive Services

Schedule of visits

Schedule every 1 to 3 yr. The recommended schedule applies only to the periodic visit itself. The frequency of the individual preventive services listed in this table is left to clinical discretion, except as indicated in footnotes.

	Preventive services[*]		
Leading causes of death	*Screening*	*Counseling*	*Immunizations*
Heart disease	**History**	**Diet and Exercise**	Tetanus-diphtheria (Td)
Lung cancer	Dietary intake	Fat (especially saturated fat),	booster[**]
Cerebrovascular disease	Physical activity	cholesterol, complex	*High-risk groups*
Breast cancer	Tobacco/alcohol/drug use	carbohydrates, fiber, sodium,	Hepatitis B vaccine (HR26)
Colorectal cancer	Sexual practices	calcium[¶]	Pneumococcal influenza
Obstructive lung disease		Caloric balance	vaccine (HR27)
	Physical Exam	Selection of exercise program	Influenza vaccine (HR28)[††]
	Height and weight		
	Blood pressure	**Substance Use**	**Remain Alert for:**
	Clinical breast exam[†]	Tobacco cessation	Depressive symptoms
	High-risk groups	Alcohol and other drugs:	Suicide risk factors (HR17)
	Complete skin exam (HRI)	Limiting alcohol consumption	Abnormal bereavement
	Complete oral cavity exam	Driving/other dangerous	Signs of physical abuse or
	(HR2)	activities while under the	neglect
	Palpation for thyroid nodules	influence	Malignant skin lesions
	(HR3)	Treatment for abuse	Peripheral arterial disease
	Auscultation for carotid bruits	*High-risk groups*	(HR18)
	(HR4)	Sharing/using unsterilized	Tooth decay, gingivitis, loose
		needles and syringes (HR19)	teeth

Table 3-7 (*Continued*)

Preventive services*			
Screening	*Counseling*		
Laboratory/Diagnostic Procedures Nonfasting total blood cholesterol Papanicolaou smear‡ Mammogram§ *High-risk groups* Fasting plasma glucose (HR5) VDRL (HR6) Urinalysis for bacteriuria (HR7) Chlamydial testing (HR8) Gonorrhea culture (HR9) Counseling and testing for HIV (HR10) Tuberculin skin test (PPD) HR11) Hearing (HR12) Electrocardiogram (HR13) Fecal occult blood/ sigmoidoscopy (HR14) Fecal occult blood/ colonoscopy (HR15) Bone mineral content (HR16)	**Sexual Practices** Sexually transmitted diseases: partner selection, condoms, anal intercourse Unintended pregnancy and contraceptive options **Injury Prevention** Safety belts Safety helmets Smoke detector Smoking near bedding or upholstery *High-risk groups* Back-conditioning exercises (HR20) Prevention of childhood injuries (HR21) Falls in the elderly (HR22)	**Dental Health** Regular tooth brushing, flossing, and dental visits **Other Primary Preventive Measures** *High-risk groups* Skin protection from ultraviolet light (HR23) Discussion of aspirin therapy (HR24) Discussion of estrogen replacement therapy (HR25)	

High-risk categories

HR1: Persons with a family or personal history of skin cancer, increased occupational or recreational exposure to sunlight, or clinical evidence of precursor lesions (e.g., dysplastic nevi, certain congenital nevi).

HR2: Persons with exposure to tobacco or excessive amounts of alcohol, or those with suspicious symptoms or lesions detected through self-examination.

HR3: Persons with a history of upper-body irradiation.

HR4: Persons with risk factors for cerebrovascular or cardiovascular disease (e.g., hypertension, smoking, coronary artery disease, atrial fibrillation, diabetes) or those with neurologic symptoms (e.g., transient ischemic attacks) or a history of cerebrovascular disease.

HR5: The markedly obese, persons with a family history of diabetes, or women with a history of gestational diabetes.

HR6: Prostitutes, persons who engage in sex with multiple partners in areas in which syphilis is prevalent, or contacts of persons with active syphilis.

HR7: Persons with diabetes.

HR8: Persons who attend clinics for sexually transmitted diseases, attend other high-risk health care facilities (e.g., adolescent and family planning clinics), or have other risk factors for chlamydial infection (e.g., multiple sexual partners or a sexual partner with multiple sexual contacts).

HR9: Prostitutes, persons with multiple sexual partners or a sexual partner with multiple contacts, sexual contacts of persons with culture-proven gonorrhea, or persons with a history of repeated episodes of gonorrhea.

HR10: Persons seeking treatment for sexually transmitted diseases; homosexual and bisexual men; past or present intravenous (IV) drug users; persons with a history of prostitution or multiple sexual partners; women whose past or present sexual partners were HIV infected, bisexual, or IV drug users; persons with long-term residence or birth in an area with high prevalence of HIV infection; or persons with a history of transfusion between 1978 and 1985.

HR11: Household members of persons with tuberculosis or others at risk for close contact with the disease (e.g., staff of tuberculosis clinics, shelters for the homeless, nursing homes, substance abuse treatment facilities, dialysis units, correctional institutions); recent immigrants or refugees from countries in which tuberculosis is common (e.g., Asia, Africa, Central and South America, Pacific Islands); migrant workers; residents of nursing homes, correctional institutions, or homeless shelters; or persons with certain underlying medical disorders (e.g., HIV infection).

HR12: Persons exposed regularly to excessive noise.

HR13: Men with two or more cardiac risk factors (high blood cholesterol, hypertension, cigarette smoking, diabetes mellitus, family history of coronary artery disease); men who would endanger public safety were they to experience sudden cardiac events (e.g., commercial airline pilots); or sedentary or high-risk males planning to begin a vigorous exercise program.

HR14: Persons aged 50 and older who have first-degree relatives with colorectal cancer; a personal history of endometrial, ovarian, or breast cancer; or a previous diagnosis of inflammatory bowel disease, adenomatous polyps, or colorectal cancer.

HR15: Persons with a family history of familial polyposis coli or cancer family syndrome.

HR16: Perimenopausal women at increased risk for osteoporosis (e.g., Caucasian race, bilateral oophorectomy before menopause, slender build) and for whom estrogen replacement therapy would otherwise not be recommended.

HR17: Recent divorce, separation, unemployment, depression, alcohol or other drug abuse, serious medical illnesses, living alone, or recent bereavement.

HR18: Persons over age 50, smokers, or persons with diabetes mellitus.

HR19: Intravenous drug users.

HR20: Persons at increased risk for low back injury because of past history, body configuration, or type of activities.

Table continues on following page

Table 3-7 (*Continued*)

High-risk groups (*continued*)

HR21: Persons with children in the home or automobile.

HR22: Persons with older adults in the home.

HR23: Persons with increased exposure to sunlight.

HR24: Men who have risk factors for myocardial infarction (e.g., high blood cholesterol, smoking, diabetes mellitus, family history of early-onset coronary artery disease) and who lack a history of gastrointestinal or other bleeding problems, and other risk factors for bleeding or cerebral hemorrhage.

HR25: Perimenopausal women at increased risk for osteoporosis (e.g., Caucasian, low bone mineral content, bilateral oophorectomy before menopause or early menopause, slender build) and who are without known contraindications (e.g., history of undiagnosed vaginal bleeding, active liver disease, thromboembolic disorders, hormone-dependent cancer).

HR26: Homosexually active men, intravenous drug users, recipients of some blood products, or persons in health-related jobs with frequent exposure to blood or blood products.

HR27: Persons with medical conditions that increase the risk of pneumococcal infection (e.g., chronic cardiac or pulmonary disease, sickle cell disease, nephrotic syndrome, Hodgkin's disease, asplenia, diabetes mellitus, alcoholism, cirrhosis, multiple myeloma, renal disease, or conditions associated with immunosuppression).

HR28: Residents of chronic care facilities and persons suffering from chronic cardiopulmonary disorders, metabolic diseases (including diabetes mellitus), hemoglobinopathies, immunosuppression, or renal dysfunction.

* This list of preventive services is not exhaustive. It reflects only those topics reviewed by the US Preventive Services Task Force. Clinicians may wish to add other preventive services after considering the patient's medical history and other individual circumstances.

† Annually for women.

‡ Every 1–3 yr for women.

§ Every 1–2 yr for women beginning at age 50.

¶ For women.

** Every 10 yr.

†† Annually.

Table 3-8 Leading Causes of Death for Ages 65 and Over and Preventive Services

Schedule of visits

Schedule every year. The recommended schedule applies only to the periodic visit itself. The frequency of the individual preventive services listed in this table is left to clinical discretion, except as indicated in footnotes.

	Preventive services*		
Leading causes of death	*Screening*	*Counseling*	*Immunizations*
Heart disease Cerebrovascular disease Obstructive lung disease Pneumonia/influenza Lung cancer Colorectal cancer	**History** Prior symptoms of transient ischemic attack Dietary intake Physical activity Tobacco/alcohol/drug use Functional status at home **Physical Exam** Height and weight Blood pressure Visual acuity Hearing and hearing aids Clinical breast exam[†] *High-risk groups* Auscultation for carotid bruits (HR1) Complete skin exam (HR2) Complete oral cavity exam (HR3) Palpation for thyroid nodules (HR4) **Laboratory/Diagnostic Procedures** Nonfasting total blood cholesterol Dipstick urinalysis Mammogram[‡] Thyroid function tests[§]	**Diet and Exercise** Fat (especially saturated fat), cholesterol, complex carbohydrates, fiber, sodium, calcium[§] Caloric balance Selection of exercise program **Substance Use** Tobacco cessation Alcohol and other drugs: Limiting alcohol consumption Driving/other dangerous activities while under the influence Treatment for abuse **Injury Prevention** Prevention of falls Safety belts Smoke detector Smoking near bedding or upholstery Hot-water-heater temperature Safety helmets *High-risk groups* Prevention of childhood injuries (HR12) **Dental Health** Regular dental visits, tooth brushing, flossing	Tetanus-diphtheria (Td) booster[**] Influenza vaccine[††] Pneumococcal vaccine *High-risk groups* Hepatitis B vaccine (HR16) **Remain Alert for:** Depressive symptoms Suicide risk factors (HR11) Abnormal bereavement Changes in cognitive function Medications that increase risk of falls Signs of physical abuse or neglect Malignant skin lesions Peripheral arterial disease Tooth decay, gingivitis, loose teeth

Table 3-8 (*Continued*)

	Preventive services*	
	Screening	*Counseling*
	High-risk groups Fasting plasma glucose (HR5) Tuberculin skin test (PPD) (HR6) Electrocardiogram (HR7) Papanicolaou smear[¶] (HR8) Fecal occult blood/ sigmoidoscopy (HR9) Fecal occult blood/ colonoscopy (HR10)	**Other Primary Preventive Measures** Glaucoma testing by eye specialist *High-risk groups* Discussion of estrogen replacement therapy (HR13) Discussion of aspirin therapy (HR14) Skin protection from ultraviolet light (HR15)

High-risk categories

HR1: Persons with risk factors for cerebrovascular or cardiovascular disease (e.g., hypertension, smoking, coronary artery disease (CAD), atrial fibrillation, diabetes) or those with neurologic symptoms (e.g., transient ischemic attacks) or a history of cerebrovascular disease.

HR2: Persons with a family or personal history of skin cancer or clinical evidence of precursor lesions (e.g., dysplastic nevi, certain congenital nevi), or those with increased occupational or recreational exposure to sunlight.

HR3: Persons with exposure to tobacco or excessive amounts of alcohol, or those with suspicious symptoms or lesions detected through self-examination.

HR4: Persons with a history of upper-body irradiation.

HR5: The markedly obese, persons with a family history of diabetes, or women with a history of gestational diabetes.

HR6: Household members of persons with tuberculosis or others at risk for close contact with the disease (e.g., staff of tuberculosis clinics, shelters for the homeless, nursing homes, substance abuse treatment facilities, dialysis units, correctional institutions); recent immigrants or refugees from countries in which tuberculosis is common (e.g., Asia, Africa, Central and South America, Pacific Islands); migrant workers, residents of nursing homes, correctional institutions, or homeless shelters; or persons with certain underlying medical disorders (e.g., HIV infection).

HR7: Men with two or more cardiac risk factors (high blood cholesterol, hypertension, cigarette smoking, diabetes mellitus, family history of CAD); men who would endanger public safety were they to experience sudden cardiac events (e.g., commercial airline pilots); or sedentary or high-risk males planning to begin a vigorous exercise program.

HR8: Women who have not had previous documented screening in which smears have been consistently negative.

HR9: Persons who have first-degree relatives with colorectal cancer; a personal history of endometrial, ovarian, or breast cancer; or a previous diagnosis of inflammatory bowel disease, adenomatous polyps, or colorectal cancer.

HR10: Persons with a family history of familial polyposis coli or cancer family syndrome.

HR11: Recent divorce, separation, unemployment, depression, alcohol or other drug abuse, serious medical illnesses, living alone, or recent bereavement.

HR12: Persons with children in the home or automobile.

HR13: Women at increased risk for osteoporosis (e.g., Caucasian, low bone mineral content, bilateral oophorectomy before menopause or early menopause, slender build) and who are without known contraindications (e.g., history of undiagnosed vaginal bleeding, active liver disease, thromboembolic disorders, hormone-dependent cancer).

HR14: Men who have risk factors for myocardial infarction (e.g., high blood cholesterol, smoking, diabetes mellitus, family history of early-onset CAD) and who lack a history of gastrointestinal or other bleeding problems, or other risk factors for bleeding or cerebral hemorrhage.

HR15: Persons with increased exposure to sunlight.

HR16: Homosexually active men, intravenous drug users, recipients of some blood products, or persons in health-related jobs with frequent exposure to blood or blood products.

* This list of preventive services is not exhaustive. It reflects only those topics reviewed by the US Preventive Services Task Force. Clinicians may wish to add other preventive services after considering the patient's medical history and other individual circumstances.

† Annually for women until age 75, unless pathology detected.

‡ Every 1–2 yr for women until age 75, unless pathology detected.

§ For women.

¶ Every 1–3 yr.

** Every 10 yr.

†† Annually.

Table 3-9 Preventive Services* for Pregnant Women

First prenatal visit		Follow-up visits (Schedule†: Wk 6–8, 8–10,‡ 14–16, 24–28, 32, 36, 38,‡ 39,§ 40,‡ 41†)	
Screening	*Counseling*	*Screening*	*Counseling*
History Dietary intake Tobacco/alcohol/drug use Risk factors for intrauterine growth retardation and low birthweight Prior genital herpetic lesions **Physical Exam** Blood pressure **Laboratory/Diagnostic Procedures** Hemoglobin and hematocrit ABO/Rh typing Rh(D) antibody test VDRL Hepatitis B surface antigen (HBsAg) Urinalysis for bacteriuria Gonorrhea culture *High-risk groups* Hemoglobin electrophoresis (HR1) Rubella antibodies (HR2) Chlamydial testing (HR3) Counseling and testing for HIV (HR4)	Nutrition Tobacco use Alcohol and other drug use Safety belts *High-risk groups* Discuss amniocentesis (HR5) Discuss risks of HIV infection (HR4) **Remain Alert for:** Signs of physical abuse	Blood pressure Urinalysis for bacteriuria **Screening Tests at Specific Gestational Ages** *14–16 Wk* Maternal serum alpha-fetoprotein (MSAFP)¶ Ultrasound cephalometry (HR8) *24–28 Wk* 50 g oral glucose tolerance test Rh(D) antibody (HR9) Gonorrhea culture (HR10) VDRL (HR11) Hepatitis B surface antigen (HBsAg) (HR12) Counseling and testing for HIV (HR13) *36 Wk* Ultrasound exam (HR14)	Nutrition Safety belts Discuss meaning of upcoming tests *High-risk groups* Tobacco use (HR6) Alcohol and other drug use (HR7) **Remain Alert for:** Signs of physical abuse

High-risk categories

HR1: Black women.

HR2: Women lacking evidence of immunity (proof of vaccination after the first birthday or laboratory evidence of immunity).

HR3: Women who attend clinics for sexually transmitted diseases, attend other high-risk health care facilities (e.g., adolescent and family planning clinics), or have other risk factors for chlamydial infection (e.g., multiple sexual partners or a sexual partner with multiple sexual contacts).

HR4: Women seeking treatment for sexually transmitted diseases; past or present intravenous (IV) drug users; women with a history of prostitution or multiple sexual partners; women whose past or present sexual partners were HIV infected, bisexual, or IV drug users; women with long-term residence or birth in an area with high prevalence of HIV infection in women; or women with a history of transfusion between 1978 and 1985.

HR5: Women aged 35 and older.

HR6: Women who continue to smoke during pregnancy.

HR7: Women with excessive alcohol consumption during pregnancy.

HR8: Women with uncertain menstrual histories or risk factors for intrauterine growth retardation (e.g., hypertension, renal disease, short maternal stature, low prepregnancy weight, failure to gain weight during pregnancy, smoking, alcohol and other drug abuse, and history of a previous fetal death or growth-retarded baby).

HR9: Unsensitized Rh-negative women.

HR10: Women with multiple sexual partners or a sexual partner with multiple contacts, or sexual contacts of persons with culture-proven gonorrhea.

HR11: Women who engage in sex with multiple partners in areas in which syphilis is prevalent, or contacts of persons with active syphilis.

HR12: Women who engage in high-risk behavior (e.g., IV drug use) or in whom exposure to hepatitis B during pregnancy is suspected.

HR13: Women at high risk (see HR4) who have a nonreactive HIV test at the first prenatal visit.

HR14: Women with risk factors for intrauterine growth retardation (see HR8).

* This list of preventive services is not exhaustive. It reflects only those topics reviewed by the US Preventive Services Task Force. Clinicians may wish to add other preventive services after considering the patient's medical history and other individual circumstances.

† The recommended schedule applies only to the periodic visit itself. The frequency of the individual preventive services listed in this table is left to clinical discretion (except for services indicated at specific gestational ages).

‡ Nulliparas only.

§ Multiparas only.

¶ Women with access to counseling and follow-up services, skilled high-resolution ultrasound and amniocentesis capabilities, and reliable, standardized laboratories.

cinoma is increased in women of lower socioeconomic status, women with herpes type II, prostitutes, and multiparous individuals. Uterine and ovarian masses should be evaluated carefully.

The rectal examination affords an opportunity to screen for prostate nodules and rectal masses, both of which are common carcinomas in persons over the age of 50. Irregularities should be followed with biopsies or appropriate diagnostic studies. The testes should be examined, particularly in young males, because the incidence of testicular cancer is markedly increased when there is an undescended testicle. Screening of the abdomen and chest has not been shown to be particularly effective in early detection, although suspected pathology should be evaluated further.

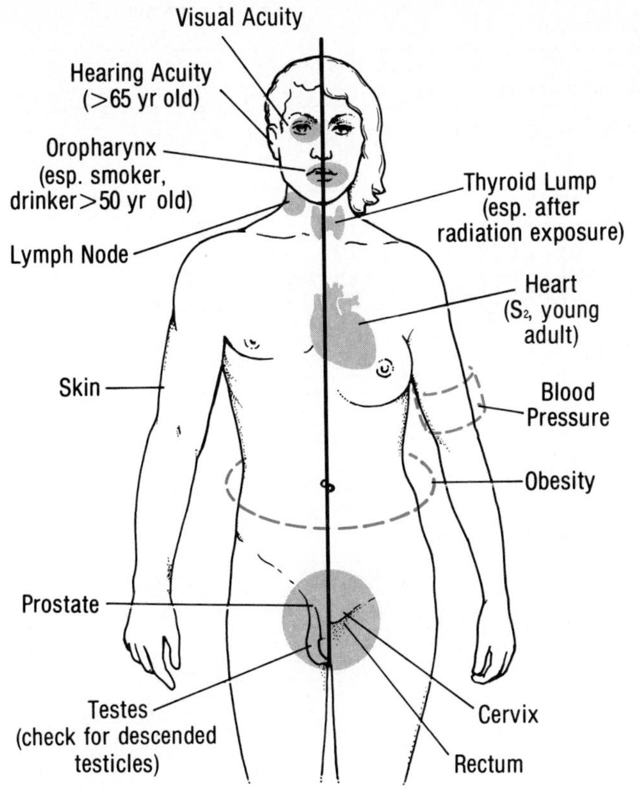

Figure 3-2 Physical examination as it relates to health maintenance and preventive care.

Screening Tests and Procedures

Laboratory tests and procedures that are to be included with screening must fulfill the criteria cited earlier. Mammography is a procedure well suited for screening because the disease it detects (breast cancer) has a high prevalence; it affects 7 percent of all women. Also, breast cancer has identifiable risk factors, and the 5-year survival is improved when the disease is detected in a localized stage. Although the cost of mammography is only approximately $50 to $100, one must also consider the cost of false reassurance for false-negative results and the cost of unnecessary biopsies and worry with a false-positive mammogram. Although some cases of breast cancer seem to be detected earliest by physical examination, others, particularly in women with pendulous breasts, are detected earliest by mammography. After correction for the lead-time bias and length bias, there appears to be a dramatic decrease in morbidity and mortality for women older than 50 years of age whose cancer is detected by screening mammography. Newer evidence suggests that this benefit may also extend to women as young as 40. The current American Cancer Society Guidelines suggest that women have a baseline mammogram between 35 and 40 years of age and every 1 to 2 years between 40 and 50 years of age. Yearly mammograms are recommended for women 50 years of age and older. More frequent screening may be recommended for high-risk women.

Screening for colorectal cancer has become part of the health maintenance approach because the incidence of colorectal cancer is high among adults more than 50 years old in this country, increasing age is a known risk factor, the disease has a long presymptomatic period, and early detection appears to be associated with improved outcome. Recommendations are to use impregnated guaiac slides to detect occult blood in the stool.

Table 3-10 Health Maintenance in the Asymptomatic Adult

Procedure	Age or other characteristic	Frequency
Immunizations		
Tetanus-diphtheria	First visit	Every 10 yr (after initial immunization)
Influenza	>65 yr old plus high risk	Every year
Pneumococcal	>65 yr old plus high risk	Once
Rubella	Before pregnancy	Once
Mumps	Not routine	—
Polio	Not routine	—
Physical Examination		
History and physical	First visit (18–22 yr old)	As occasion arises
Blood pressure	First visit	Every visit
Weight	First visit	Every visit
Oral examination	First visit	Every 2 yr >40 yr old*
Visual acuity	First visit	Every 2 yr >40 yr
Hearing acuity	>65 yr old	Every 1–2 yr
Patient Education for Self-Examination		
Breast self-examination	>18 yr old, female	
Testicular self-examination	18–40 yr old, male	
Skin examination	Fair-skinned, solar-exposed individuals	
Oral examination†	Smoker, drinker	
Specific for Women		
Breast examination	First adult visit (18–22 yr old)	Standard risk, <40 yr old: every 1–3 yr. Standard risk, ≥40 yr old: every year. High risk: at least annually.
Mammography	35–40 yr old	Baseline mammogram
	40–50 yr old	Every 1–2 yr
	Over 50 yr old	Yearly
	High risk	Every year
Pap smear/pelvic examination	First sexual encounter or first adult visit (18–22 yr old)	High risk: every year
Endometrial sampling	50 yr old, high risk	Needs further study
Colorectal Cancer Screening		
Stool for occult blood	≥40 yr old	Every year
Sigmoidoscopy	≥40 or 50 yr old	Every 3–5 yr
Rectal examination	≥40 yr old	Every year
Other Procedures		
PPD skin test	Health care worker	
	Lower socioeconomic status	
Serology	Multiple sexual partners	
Sickle cell trait	Blacks, at patient request	
Tay-Sachs serology	Ashkenazi Jews, at patient request	
Counseling		
Alcohol/drug use	Family planning	
Smoking	Sexual dysfunction	
Seat belts	Dietary	
Exercise	Disability	

* Frequency each visit as needed.
† For high risk (smoking/heavy ethyl alcohol).
‡ Depends upon relative risk and quality of physical examination.

A

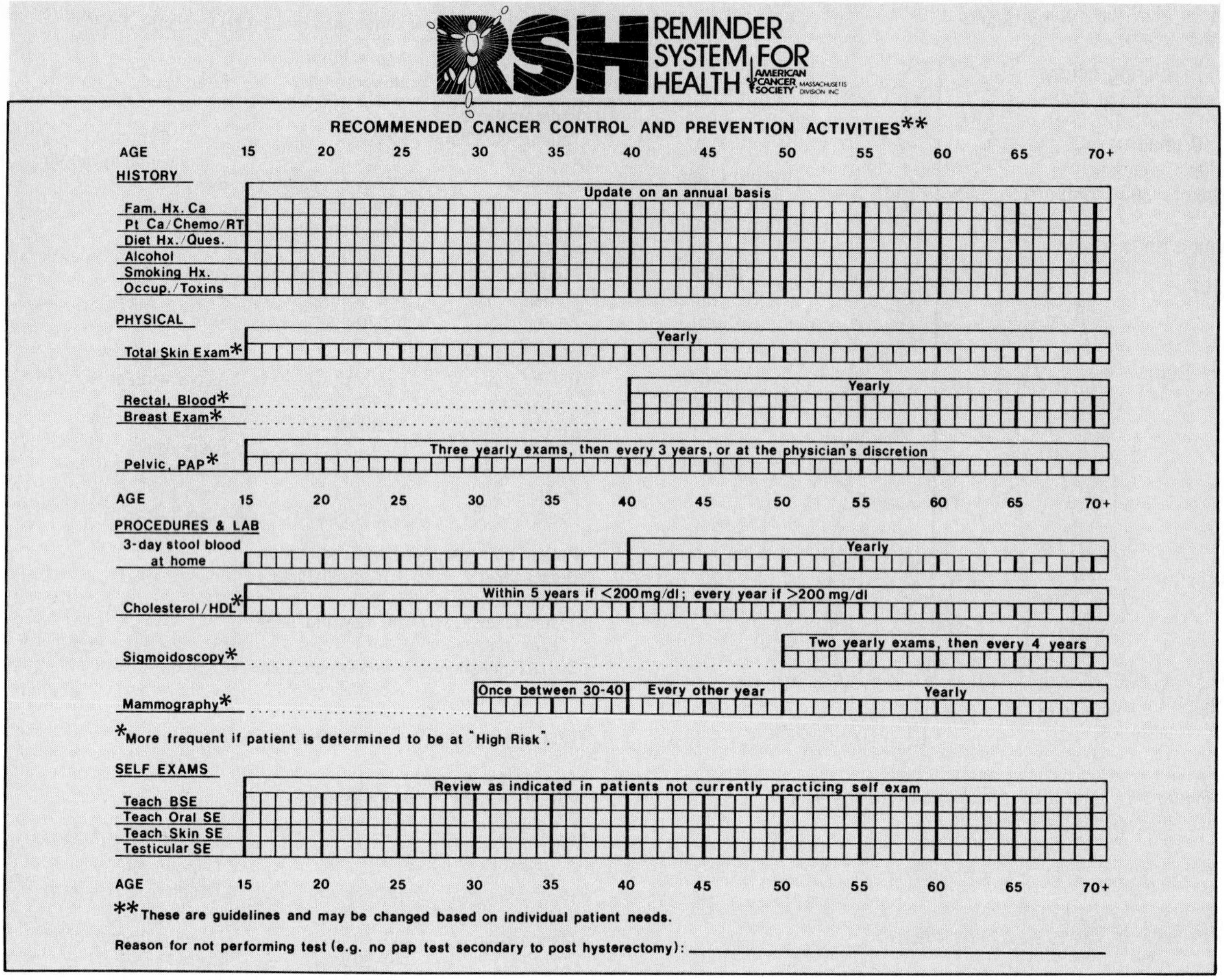

REMINDER SYSTEM FOR HEALTH — AMERICAN CANCER SOCIETY MASSACHUSETTS DIVISION INC

RECOMMENDED CANCER CONTROL AND PREVENTION ACTIVITIES**

AGE 15 20 25 30 35 40 45 50 55 60 65 70+

HISTORY — Update on an annual basis
- Fam. Hx. Ca
- Pt Ca/Chemo/RT
- Diet Hx./Ques.
- Alcohol
- Smoking Hx.
- Occup./Toxins

PHYSICAL
- Total Skin Exam* — Yearly
- Rectal, Blood* — Yearly (from 40)
- Breast Exam* — Yearly (from 40)
- Pelvic, PAP* — Three yearly exams, then every 3 years, or at the physician's discretion

AGE 15 20 25 30 35 40 45 50 55 60 65 70+

PROCEDURES & LAB
- 3-day stool blood at home — Yearly (from 40)
- Cholesterol/HDL* — Within 5 years if <200 mg/dl; every year if >200 mg/dl
- Sigmoidoscopy* — Two yearly exams, then every 4 years (from 50)
- Mammography* — Once between 30-40 | Every other year | Yearly

*More frequent if patient is determined to be at "High Risk".

SELF EXAMS — Review as indicated in patients not currently practicing self exam
- Teach BSE
- Teach Oral SE
- Teach Skin SE
- Testicular SE

AGE 15 20 25 30 35 40 45 50 55 60 65 70+

**These are guidelines and may be changed based on individual patient needs.

Reason for not performing test (e.g. no pap test secondary to post hysterectomy): ______

B

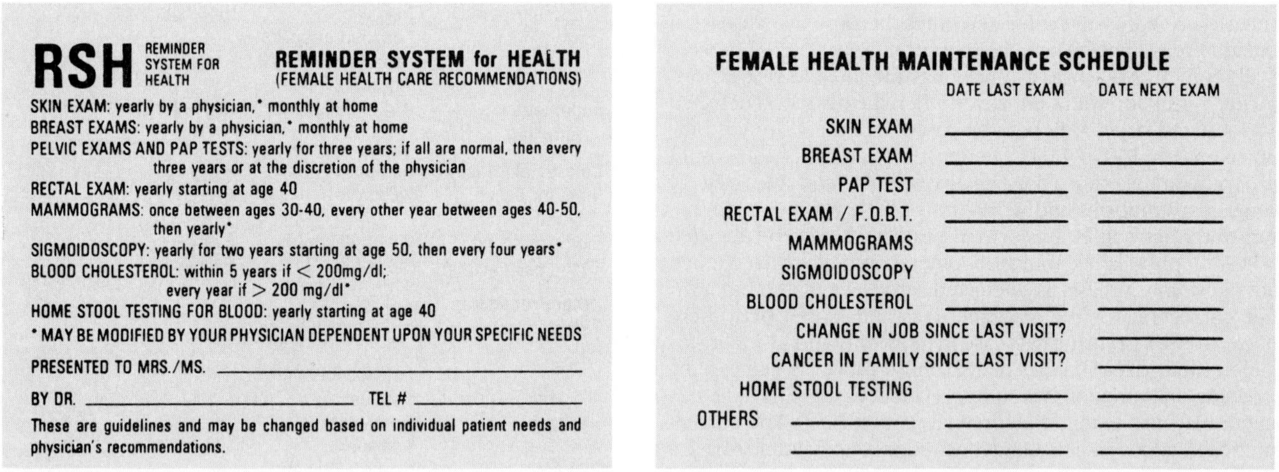

RSH REMINDER SYSTEM FOR HEALTH

REMINDER SYSTEM for HEALTH (FEMALE HEALTH CARE RECOMMENDATIONS)

SKIN EXAM: yearly by a physician,* monthly at home
BREAST EXAMS: yearly by a physician,* monthly at home
PELVIC EXAMS AND PAP TESTS: yearly for three years; if all are normal, then every three years or at the discretion of the physician
RECTAL EXAM: yearly starting at age 40
MAMMOGRAMS: once between ages 30-40, every other year between ages 40-50, then yearly*
SIGMOIDOSCOPY: yearly for two years starting at age 50, then every four years*
BLOOD CHOLESTEROL: within 5 years if < 200mg/dl; every year if > 200 mg/dl*
HOME STOOL TESTING FOR BLOOD: yearly starting at age 40
* MAY BE MODIFIED BY YOUR PHYSICIAN DEPENDENT UPON YOUR SPECIFIC NEEDS

PRESENTED TO MRS./MS. ______

BY DR. ______ TEL # ______

These are guidelines and may be changed based on individual patient needs and physician's recommendations.

FEMALE HEALTH MAINTENANCE SCHEDULE

	DATE LAST EXAM	DATE NEXT EXAM
SKIN EXAM		
BREAST EXAM		
PAP TEST		
RECTAL EXAM / F.O.B.T.		
MAMMOGRAMS		
SIGMOIDOSCOPY		
BLOOD CHOLESTEROL		
CHANGE IN JOB SINCE LAST VISIT?		
CANCER IN FAMILY SINCE LAST VISIT?		
HOME STOOL TESTING		
OTHERS		

Figure 3-3 (**A**) Office chart to remind physician and patient when screening is due. (**B**) Wallet-sized reminder for women.

The optimal schedule includes two specimens from separate sections of a stool specimen on three separate days. The use of the fecal slide for occult blood is associated with a 50 percent false-positive rate and a 30 percent false-negative rate. Of the truly positive stool samples that indicate occult blood, underlying diseases include diverticular disease, benign polyps, other benign diseases, and finally carcinoma in approximately 2 to 5 of 1,000 individuals screened initially. Follow-up of these positive stool samples will result in approximately 20 barium enemas for each cancer found. The low cost of the test and the high prevalence of the disease appear to make this a cost-effective screening technique. Although some epidemiologists are still uncomfortable with the available prospective data regarding the value of screening with sigmoidoscopy, it too has been included in many plans for health maintenance. Approximately 10 percent of colorectal cancers are palpable by digital rectal examination, and approximately 50 percent by the 25-cm rigid sigmoidoscope. Use of the sigmoidoscope for screening in adults older than 40 to 50 years of age yields approximately one case of invasive colorectal carcinoma per 667 initial exams. When we wait and evaluate patients only after symptoms of cancer have developed, 70 percent of the cancers have penetrated all layers of the bowel wall and two-thirds of the patients have regional metastatic disease. The combined 5-year survival for patients with colorectal carcinoma is 70 percent with disease localized to Duke's level A/B, but it drops to 40 percent for patients with disease categorized as Duke's level C/D. Because most patients with early and localized disease are asymptomatic, the stool test for occult blood and sigmoidoscopy have been evaluated as screening tools to allow early detection of colorectal cancer and thus decrease morbidity and mortality.

Counseling and immunizations are also important aspects of the health maintenance approach. Table 3-10 outlines a suggested approach to health maintenance.

One of the most challenging problems in health maintenance is the issue of remembering when screening is due. Screening is easily forgotten in the office encounter in which the patient has a complaint and screening is not on his or her agenda. New programs such as the Massachusetts Division of the American Cancer Society's Reminder System for Health seek to provide a reminder system for both the physician and the patient and thus create a memory alliance that ensures health maintenance activities. This system includes a wallet-sized card that is kept by the patient and an office chart to remind physician and patient when screening is due (Fig. 3-3).

References

American Cancer Society. Report on the cancer-related check up. Cancer 1980; 30:194.

Breslow L, Somer AR. The lifetime health monitoring program. N Engl J Med 1977; 296:60.

Canadian Task Force on the Periodic Health Examination: The periodic health examination. Can Med Assoc J 1979; 121:193.

Eddy DM. Screening for cancer: Theory, analysis, and design. Englewood Cliffs, NJ: Prentice-Hall, 1980.

Fletcher SW, Sptizer WO. Approach of the Canadian Task Force to the periodic health examination [editorial note]. Ann Intern Med 1980; 92:253.

Franc PS, Carlson SJ. A critical review of periodic health screening using specific screening criteria. J Fam Pract 1975; 2:29–36, 123–129, 189–194, 283–289.

Medical Practice Committee, American College of Physicians. Periodic health examination: A guide for designing individualized preventive health care in the asymptomatic patient. Ann Intern Med 1981; 95:729.

Mulley A. Health maintenance and the role of screening. In: Goroll A, et al., eds. Primary care medicine. Philadelphia: JB Lippincott, 1987:11.

Screening for disease. Lancet 1974; October 5–December 21 (18-part series).

U.S. Preventive Services Task Force. Guide to clinical preventive service: An assessment of the effectiveness of 169 interventions. Baltimore: Williams & Wilkins, 1989.

4 Genetic and Familial Aspects of Disease

R. Curtis Ellison, MD

Many diseases tend to cluster in families and are thus classified as *familial*. Although some of these diseases are inherited, genetic disorders, others may be due predominantly to a shared environment. In any case, obtaining a detailed family history on all patients, including those being seen for health maintenance, can provide information that will be of value in making a diagnosis, deciding on appropriate screening tests, and identifying individuals for special primary preventive efforts. This chapter focuses primarily on how to obtain an adequate family history and how to get the maximum benefit from it.

Obtaining a Family History

The time and effort devoted to obtaining a family history may vary from simply asking the patient whether "anything runs in the family" to spending a long time obtaining a complete family pedigree (Fig. 4-1). In general, a form such as that illustrated in Figure 4-2 may be used for grandparents and all first-degree relatives (parents, children, siblings), living or dead, of the patient being evaluated. Forms for each relative should be furnished to and completed by the patient prior to the office visit (see Fig. 2-1, pages 5 and 6). If one suspects genetic illness, it is desirable to obtain an evaluation of other second-degree relatives (uncles, aunts, nieces) and even third-degree relatives (first cousins), although this is often difficult. At the time of the visit, the physician should briefly review the forms, answer any questions the patient may have, and obtain additional details, when needed. Forms like the one illustrated in Figure 4-2 are useful for collecting the information; data may then be recorded in conventional pedigree form.

Completion of the forms prior to the office visit not only saves considerable time but also enables one to acquire more accurate information. Discussions with spouse, parents, or other relatives may be accomplished in anticipation of the visit and may yield information otherwise not known to the patient. The patient should be informed, in advance, of the steps that will be taken to ensure confidentiality of the information obtained.

Getting the Maximum Benefit from the Family History

In the evaluation of a patient, information from the family history, if obtained in sufficient detail, may be of value in the following ways:

1. *Assist in diagnosing an inherited disease.* Eliciting a family history of a specific inherited disease (e.g., Wilson's disease, Huntington's disease) may lead to an earlier diagnosis in the patient being evaluated. For example, one will be guided in the

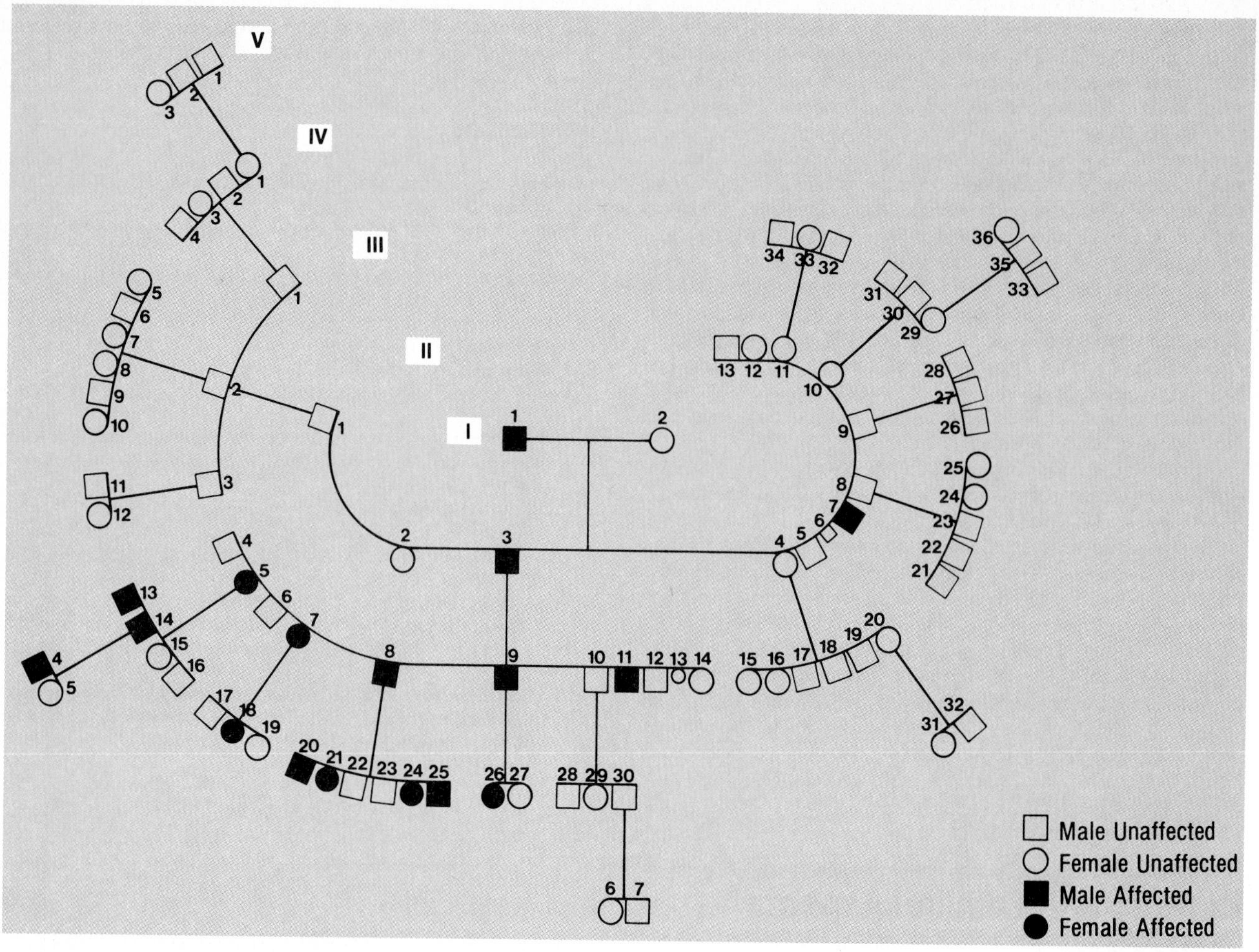

Figure 4-1 A sample pedigree showing autosomal dominant inheritance for myotonic dystrophy.

evaluation of a patient who exhibits muscle weakness if there is a family history of myotonic dystrophy. Similarly, one will be better able to assess abnormal movements in a patient who has a parent with Huntington's disease and to evaluate chest pain in a patient with a family history of Marfan's syndrome. Some common inherited diseases are discussed in the next section.

2. *Make the work-up of other "familial" diseases more efficient and cost-effective.* Given a number of potential diagnoses, one should initially focus the work-up on those conditions that have occurred in other members of the family. For example, when evaluating a breast mass in a woman, one may wish to proceed more rapidly to breast biopsy if there is a strong family history of cancer of the breast.

3. *Prompt appropriate screening procedures to detect early disease or risk factors for disease.* Significant weakness in the dorsiflexors of a child's foot that is producing difficulty in walking may cause suspicion of muscular dystrophy; the presence of a family history might prompt earlier muscle biopsy for diagnosis. A patient with long arms and lower limbs and a family history of Marfan's syndrome might undergo echocardiography to evaluate the aortic and mitral valves at an earlier stage. Although measuring cholesterol in all children is not generally considered to be cost-effective, such screening is warranted when there is a strong family history of heart disease.

4. *Identify individuals for special primary preventive efforts.* Given a family history of severe hypertension, for example, one may wish to make a particular effort to have a patient restrict salt intake and avoid excessive weight gain. By focusing specific preventive efforts on patients who know that they are at increased risk for a disease, one is more likely to elicit compliance with such measures and the cooperation of other family members, especially if the preventive efforts are presented as a family undertaking. Furthermore, because the individuals on whom the preventive efforts are focused are at higher risk of certain diseases, the potential benefits of such interventions are greater than when they are applied to the general public.

A guideline for use of information obtained from the family history is given in Table 4-1. Specified items from the family history are given in the first column. In subsequent columns, the table lists conditions for which the patient may be at increased risk, recommended screening procedures for such individuals, and some factors that have been proposed as possible means for the primary prevention of the disease. Some of the factors listed in the last column have strong scientific support as being effective in prevention of the disease; an example would be treating hypertension as a means of preventing stroke. Other factors, particularly those indicating dietary measures that may play a role in the prevention of certain cancers, are based primarily on animal research or epidemiologic data. Nevertheless, they are considered by some to be reasonable approaches, based on currently available information.

Indications for Consultation and Genetic Counseling

When there is a family history of a recognized genetic disorder, such as those listed in Table 4-2, a more intensive investigation

1. Patient's name ______
2. Patient's medical record no. ______
3. Name of relative ______
4. Address of relative ______
5. Relation of relative to patient ______
6. Blood relative? Yes ______ No ______
7. Year of birth ______ 8. Age (now or at time of death) ______
9. If dead, cause(s) of death ______

Complete Below for the Relative Listed in (3) Above

10. Has (did) this person ever had (have) any of the following problems?

Problem	No	Yes	Don't Know	Approximate Age When Diagnosis First Made	Comments
High blood pressure					
Medications for high blood pressure					
Diabetes					
Angina pectoris or other evidence of heart disease					
High blood cholesterol or blood fat (lipids)					
Heart attack (myocardial infarction)					
Coronary bypass surgery or angioplasty					
Stroke					
Bronchitis, emphysema, lung disease					
Peptic ulcer disease (stomach or duodenal ulcer)					
Psychiatric or mental disease					
Marked obesity (grossly overweight)					
Excessive alcohol intake					
Cigarette smoking (more than ½ pack per day for several years)					
Any congenital anomaly (specify under comments)					
Cancer, type unknown					
Cancer of breast					
Cancer of lung					
Cancer of colon (large bowel)					
Cancer of stomach or esophagus					
Cancer of uterus or cervix					
Malignant melanoma					
Any other skin cancers					
Other type of cancer (specify under comments)					
Other problem (specify under comments)					

Figure 4-2 Information to be obtained for all first-degree relatives, living or dead, of patients with genetic diseases. A separate form is used for each relative.

Table 4-1 Recommendations Based on Selected Items from Family History for Patient Being Evaluated

Taken from family history	Patient at increased risk for	Recommended screening procedures	Factors to emphasize for prevention
Coronary artery disease before age 55, hyperlipidemia	Premature coronary artery disease, hyperlipidemia	Serum lipids, blood pressure, smoking history, etc.	Diet low in saturated fat and cholesterol, high in fiber; weight loss, if obese; treat blood pressure if hypertensive; stop smoking; increase physical activity
Hypertension or stroke	Hypertension, stroke, premature coronary artery disease	Blood pressure, also serum lipids, smoking history, etc.	Reduce sodium in the diet (from birth); weight loss, if obese; also others listed above
Obesity	Obesity, diabetes, cardiovascular disease, cancer	Height, weight, waist-to-hip ratios, skin-fold thickness, blood glucose; assessment of other cardiovascular risk factors listed above	Weight control, if obese; primary prevention of obesity for infants and children in family; also others listed above
Diabetes	Diabetes	Height, weight, skin-fold thickness, glucose tolerance	Avoid obesity
Chronic lung disease	Lung disease	Smoking history, exposure to toxic inhalants	Stop smoking; avoid toxic inhalants
Peptic ulcer disease	Peptic ulcer disease	Careful gastrointestinal history	Stress management; stop smoking
Osteoporosis	Osteoporosis	Bone evaluation	Increase physical activity; high calcium intake; stop smoking
Alcoholism	Alcoholism, cirrhosis, cancer of liver, esophagus, and oropharynx	History of alcohol intake	Decrease alcohol intake if excessive; balanced diet
Mental illness, suicide	Mental illness	Social and psychiatric history	Stress-management techniques; develop support systems; counseling
Maternal exposure to diethylstilbestrol	Vaginal cancer	Pelvic exam at puberty and yearly thereafter	
Colonic polyps	Colonic polyps, cancer of colon	Sigmoidoscopy; radiographs	Avoid obesity; low-fat diet; high intake of fiber and cruciferous vegetables
Cancer			
Breast	Cancer of the breast, endometrial cancer	Repeated and careful breast examinations; teach self-examination; mammography; Pap smears	Avoid obesity; avoid high-fat diet
Lung	Cancer of the lung	Smoking history; cessation counseling	Stop smoking; high intake of vitamin A
Colon	Cancer of the colon	Periodic stool guaiac tests; sigmoidoscopy	Avoid obesity; low-fat diet; high intake of fiber and cruciferous vegetables
Esophagus, stomach	Gastrointestinal cancer	Careful gastrointestinal history	High intakes of vitamins A and C and cruciferous vegetables; limit intake of alcohol and nitrite-cured meats; stop smoking
Bladder	Bladder cancer	Genitourinary history; urinalysis	Stop smoking; avoid industrial toxins
Uterus	Cancer of the uterus	Periodic Pap smears	Avoid obesity; avoid estrogens
Prostate	Prostatic cancer	Prostatic examinations	—
Malignant melanoma	Malignant melanoma	Careful dermatologic examinations; early biopsy of suspicious lesions	Avoid excessive sun exposure; use sunblocks

Table 4-2 Prevalence of Selected Monogenic Disorders Among Liveborn Infants

Disorder	Estimated prevalence
Autosomal Dominant	
Familial hypercholesterolemia	1 in 500
Polycystic kidney disease	1 in 1,250
Huntington's disease	1 in 2,500
Hereditary spherocytosis	1 in 5,000
Marfan's syndrome	1 in 20,000
Autosomal Recessive	
Sickle cell anemia	1 in 625 (US blacks)
Cystic fibrosis	1 in 2,000 (whites)
Tay-Sachs disease	1 in 3,000 (US Jews)
Cystinuria	1 in 7,000
Phenylketonuria	1 in 12,000
Mucopolysaccharidoses (all types)	1 in 25,000
Glycogen storage disease (all types)	1 in 50,000
Galactosemia	1 in 57,000
Homocystinuria	1 in 200,000
X-Linked	
Duchenne muscular dystrophy	1 in 7,000
Hemophilia	1 in 10,000

From Wyngaarden JB. Human heredity. In: Wyngaarden JB, Smith LH Jr., eds. Cecil textbook of medicine. 18th ed. Philadelphia: WB Saunders, 1988:147; with permission.

may be warranted. The physician should consider early consultation with a specialist for appropriate genetic counseling and prenatal diagnostic approaches. Certain genetic diseases with autosomal inheritance appear in adulthood, and a search for affected individuals among family members is essential because the disorders may be either treatable or preventable. For example, siblings of patients with hemochromatosis should be evaluated by human leukocyte antigen (HLA) typing and liver biopsy to determine whether they have the disease, because early initiation of treatment may prevent liver, heart, and pancreatic complications. Family members of patients with either hereditary polyposis or Gardner's syndrome should undergo colonoscopy, since colectomy of affected individuals will prevent colonic cancer in these familial diseases. Several autosomal dominant syndromes lead to parathyroid dysfunction, including familial hyperparathyroidism and several types of multiple endocrine neoplasias. Early diagnosis and surgery of affected family members may prevent complications of hypercalcemia and hypertension, and even cancer. Screening of all family members of patients with familial hypercholesterolemia will lead to the early detection of cases; the initiation of dietary or drug therapy (or both) will diminish the risk of premature coronary artery disease in such individuals.

The investigation of the human genome is progressing at such a pace that the list of diseases that are caused, or at least influenced, by genes will undoubtedly increase dramatically during the next decade. Furthermore, it is expected that genetic engineering will make it possible to "correct" many of the genetically determined diseases that we see today. Collecting a detailed and complete family history on each patient will gain importance as such research makes possible the prevention of an increasing number of diseases.

References

McKusick VA. Mendelian inheritance in man. Baltimore: Johns Hopkins University Press, 1988.

Scriver CR, Beaudet AL, Sly WS, et al. The metabolic basis of inherited disease. New York: McGraw-Hill, 1989.

Vogel F, Motulsky AG. Human genetics: Problems and approaches. New York: Springer-Verlag, 1986.

Watson JD. The molecular biology of the gene, revised ed. Menlo Park, CA: Benjamin-Cummings, 1987.

5 Keeping Up to Date with the Medical Literature

Gertrude W. Manchester, MD

The absolute quantity of existing medical knowledge has increased dramatically during the twentieth century, and the ability of any given physician to read it, let alone learn it, has clearly been surpassed. This information overload is further compounded by continuing expansion of the medical database. Medical information doubles every 7 to 10 years, whereas the half-life of new information is estimated to be 3 to 5 years. As an example, the National Library of Medicine receives more than 20,000 serial publications each month and adds more than 250,000 new citations to the Index Medicus each year.

Clearly, the task of managing, analyzing, and organizing new medical information is an enormous one. Likewise, it is a particularly important task that, if mastered, allows a physician to continue to provide quality care throughout his or her career. Two important facts must be recognized. First, learning medicine is a life-long task. The process of studying and learning should not end with the completion of residency training. Second, keeping up to date requires a plan, expenditure of time, and commitment. It does not occur by chance alone.

In developing your own plan for keeping up to date and maintaining your level of competence, you should consider the steps discussed in the following sections.

Assess Your Personal Learning Style

Format. Do you learn better through active participation (as with home study courses, interactive computer software, workshops), or do you prefer passive learning (lectures, conferences)?

Time Frame. Can you concentrate and work efficiently during short blocks of time (perhaps ½ hour per day), or do you need to set aside larger blocks of time less frequently (perhaps 1 week, two or three times per year)?

Location. Are you able to concentrate on your learning program at the office or at home, or do you need to escape distractions by attending conferences or working at your hospital's medical library?

Be Selective in Your Choice of Information Sources

Selectivity is the key to success because you will have limited time to devote to your learning program. In addition to considering how, when, and where you learn best, consider the relevance, quality, accessibility, and cost of the information sources you will use. Availability of continuing medical education (CME) credits may also be a deciding factor if your state requires CME documentation for license renewal.

Original journal articles published in widely circulated general medical journals such as *The New England Journal of Medicine, Annals of Internal Medicine, Archives of Internal Medicine,* and *The Lancet* are among the best information sources. They are accessible, current, peer-reviewed, and compact. Be selective and critical in your choice of articles to read, however (see Chapter 7, "Critically Reviewing the Medical Literature"). Even for subspecialists, general medical journals are an important part of the learning program because articles of clinical importance are often published in the widely circulated general medical journals rather than the specialty journals.

Other information sources to consider include newsletters such as *The Medical Letter* (a biweekly newsletter providing updates on new medication), interactive computer CME programs (see Chapter 6, "Computer Applications in Internal Medicine"), and local, regional, and national conferences. Textbooks, home study courses, and annual reviews and reference summaries may also be considered but are often not as current as the other sources.

Develop Information-Retrieval Skills

Even the most conscientious physician who devotes time regularly to a well-tailored learning program will still encounter specific patient problems that require additional learning. The ability to retrieve specific information from the literature rapidly is just as important as history-taking and physical-examination skills.

Again, consider your information sources carefully. Sources should be evaluated for relevance (Is it current? Does it cover the areas where you are most likely to need help?), cost (either to obtain or to maintain), ease of use (How good is the indexing?), and accessibility. A medical library may be an excellent and comprehensive resource, but it is not useful for in-office problem solving if it is located on the other side of town!

Sources to consider include the following:

1. Your professional colleagues. This is often the most rapid means of getting information, but accessibility and credibility vary.
2. In-office textbook library. Texts are at least 2 years out of date when purchased, and cost is variable. They often are adequate for reviewing pathophysiology, differential diagnosis, and the like (see Huth, 1988, for suggested texts). The in-office textbook library may soon be replaced by a computer disk CD-ROM (see Chapter 6, "Computer Applications in Internal Medicine").

Table 5-1 Sample Three-Year Plan for a General Internist

Daily:	Take 30 minutes each day to review the patients you have seen and identify areas in which you need to learn more. Consult your textbook, library, or reprint file for general review of those areas. Do a literature search to locate more recent citations.
Weekly:	Attend one or two hospital conferences such as Medical Grand Rounds and Morbidity/Mortality Conference. Skim the journals that have arrived during the week. Select and read relevant original journal articles and reviews. Visit your local medical library to locate and read articles retrieved in your daily computer searches.
Yearly:	Attend two in-depth conferences covering your areas of weakness or perhaps new areas that you would like to learn about and master.
Every 3 Years:	Attend a comprehensive general medicine review course.

3. Personal reprint file. This may be a natural extension for those who read original journal articles and then file what they have read. The time expenditure to maintain the file may be prohibitive, however.
4. Computer literature search via personal computer (see Chapter 6, "Computer Applications in Internal Medicine"). Successful and efficient searching does require some training and/or practice, but through the computer, one has access to a wide range of the most current literature.

Periodically Assess Your Areas of Knowledge Deficit and Adjust Your Program Accordingly

This can be done in a rigorous fashion by working through the Medical Knowledge Self-Assessment Program (MKSAP) of the American College of Physicians (4200 Pine Street, Philadelphia, PA 19104). This comprehensive home study program covers general medicine as well as the subspecialty areas and is updated every 3 years. Perhaps a more relevant way to identify your weak areas is to review the questions and problems that arise in your practice. For instance, if you find yourself frequently consulting the *Physician's Desk Reference* to review indications, doses, and side effects of the newer antiarrhythmic drugs, you may wish to attend a conference on this topic.

Assign Time and Priority to Your Plan

Busy physicians recognize that their workload easily expands to fill the available time. The final key to a successful learning program is to set aside specific time blocks for this task and then prevent other obligations from interfering with your goal to keep up to date and maintain your competence (Table 5-1).

References

Garfield E. Which medical journals have the greatest impact? Ann Intern Med 1986; 105:313.

Govell DG, Uman GC, Manning PR. Information needs in office practice: Are they being met? Ann Intern Med 1985; 103:596.
Haynes RB, et al. Computer searching of the medical literature. An evaluation of Medline searching systems. Ann Intern Med 1985; 103:812.
Haynes RB, et al. How to keep up with the medical literature: I. Why try to keep up and how to get started. Ann Intern Med 1986; 105:149.
Haynes RB, et al. How to keep up with the medical literature: II. Deciding which journals to read regularly. Ann Intern Med 1986; 105:309.
Haynes RB, et al. How to keep up with the medical literature: III. Expanding the number of journals you read regularly. Ann Intern Med 1986; 105:474.
Haynes RB, et al. How to keep up with the medical literature: IV. Using the literature to solve clinical problems. Ann Intern Med 1986; 105:636.
Haynes RB, et al. How to keep up with the medical literature: V. Access by personal computer to the medical literature. Ann Intern Med 1986; 105:810.
Haynes RB, et al. How to keep up with the medical literature: VI. How to store and retrieve articles worth keeping. Ann Intern Med 1986; 105:978.
Horowitz GL, et al. Paper Chase—self-service bibliographic retrieval. JAMA 1983; 250:2494.
Huth EJ. A library for internists VI. Recommendations from the American College of Physicians. Ann Intern Med 1988; 108:497.
Marshall JG. Computers: How to choose the on-line medical database that's right for you. Can Med Assoc J 1986; 134:634.
Riegelman RK, Hirsch RP. Studying a study and testing a test. How to read the medical literature. Boston: Little, Brown, 1989.
Underhill LH, Bleich HL. Bringing the medical literature to physicians. West J Med 1986; 145:853.

Computer Applications in Internal Medicine

Gertrude W. Manchester, MD

6

The use of computers has dramatically affected many aspects of clinical medicine over the past 15 years. Automated cardiac dysrhythmia analysis and interpretation of standard 12-lead echocardiograms are commonly used. Noninvasive imaging techniques such as computed tomography, nuclear magnetic resonance imaging, and ultrasonography are all computer-based and have markedly expanded the physician's diagnostic repertoire. At the bedside, physiologic monitoring by means of computers has progressed from state-of-the-art to standard care in all intensive and cardiac care units. The ability to interface clinical laboratory equipment with computers has minimized errors and improved physician access to test results.

In each of these examples, data are obtained directly from the patient (or from the patient's body fluids) and then, via the computer, are presented to the physician in an easily interpretable form. Thus, the physician is not required to interact with (or even understand) the computer. Over the next 10 to 20 years, however, it is predicted that virtually every physician will be directly using a computer on a daily basis.

Computers are particularly well suited to storing, organizing, and to some extent analyzing data. Studies by Stross and Harlan (1979) and by Covell et al (1985) suggest that traditional information sources (textbooks, journals, conferences, consultation with colleagues) may be ineffective and inefficient in meeting the day-to-day information needs of clinicians. Thus, it is highly likely that physicians will come to depend on computers to assist with the information-overload problem and, ultimately, with diagnostic and management decisions in everyday practice.

Computers are likely to have significant impact on clinical practice in five basic areas, which are considered in the following sections.

Bibliographic Literature Search and Retrieval

The Index Medicus, which lists citations for a large portion of the published medical literature, was established by John Shaw Billings in 1879 and computerized in 1964. Each citation is classified and indexed by several topics within the MeSH system (*MeSH* stands for *me*dical *s*ub*h*eadings and includes more than 14,000 terms by which articles can be classified). Medline, established in 1971, enabled librarians in any remote library to gain access to the National Library of Medicine medical database via computer. The search program Elhill required intensive training and thus was used almost exclusively by librarians.

In 1980 a user-friendly search program called Paper Chase (Beth Israel Hospital, 330 Brookline Avenue, Boston, MA 02115) was developed and implemented at the Beth Israel Hospital in Boston (Horowitz, 1981). For the first time, physicians were able to conduct their own searches rather than using a medical librarian as an intermediary. Since that time, several commercial vendors have developed search software, with varying degrees of user friendliness, and subscribers are allowed to access Medline along with many other distinct databases, such as Cancerlit, Health Planning and Administration, or PsycINFO (psychological abstracts).

In each of these programs, the user utilizes a modem and communication software to connect to the database and then uses the vendor's software and MeSH to locate specific citations in the area of interest. In most cases, the citation (title of article, journal name, volume number, page number, and so on) and the abstract can be retrieved. With some vendors, such as BRS Colleague (1200 Route 7, Latham, NY 12110), and some common journals, the complete text of the article may be retrieved. This feature would be particularly useful for physicians who do not have access to a medical library.

CD-ROM (Compact Disc–Read Only Memory)

Compact discs have been in common use in the audio industry for some time. In addition to audible voice and music, the digital information on a disc can also be readily translated into text, diagrams, and graphs. Each 4.72-inch compact disc possesses enormous capacity; the American College of Physicians' recommended Library for Internists, comprising approximately 215,000 pages, would fit neatly on a single compact disc. As the cost of producing these discs comes down and as software is developed that allows for efficient retrieval of information from the disc, the physician's traditional (and usually limited) in-office textbook library will be replaced by a personal computer, a disc reader, and a single compact disc. As new texts are published, the on-disc library can be readily updated on a yearly basis.

At present, Medline is offered on CD-ROM by several companies. An annual fee entitles the subscriber to quarterly updates (i.e., every 3 months, the old disc is exchanged for a new one, which deletes the oldest citations and includes the most recent 3 months of citations). For a physician who requires frequent access to the most up-to-date information available in the journals, purchase of a CD-ROM Medline subscription may be more economical than use of Paper Chase or BRS Colleague (where the user pays a certain amount for each minute of on-line search time and for each citation displayed and printed).

Clinical Information Systems (Electronic Medical Records)

Many clinical information systems are currently in use within hospitals. The system at the Beth Israel Hospital in Boston is probably the most comprehensive and has been well described (Bleich, 1985). Although the standard paper chart is still used there, physicians and nurses in this hospital are able to utilize the computer terminals to retrieve data from the clinical laboratories, access reports from radiology and pathology, review demographic and outpatient-visit data, and look up prescriptions filled in the hospital's pharmacy. Data in the system are available throughout the hospital, are updated continually, and can be retrieved at the terminal much faster than via the telephone or the standard printed reports.

A similar comprehensive information system has been developed by Clement McDonald, M.D., in the outpatient clinic system of the Regenstrief Medical Institute and has been in use there since 1974. Clinical data, such as blood pressure, weight, and aspects of the physical examination, are recorded in the system along with laboratory results and prescriptions. Information is provided on paper in summary form at the time of a patient's encounter and can also be retrieved in a variety of formats at each physician's individual work station (McDonald et al, 1986).

A series of studies have been done utilizing the Regenstrief Medical Record (RMR) system to provide reminders to physicians. For instance, the summary sheet notifies the physician when a woman is due for a mammogram or that a potassium level should be checked if the patient is on diuretics. Physician compliance with certain accepted standards of care (e.g., the American Cancer Society's recommendations for screening mammograms) was markedly improved when the computer provided such reminders. McDonald (1976) hypothesized that, in the usual amount of time allotted for an outpatient encounter, most physicians could not adequately process all of the information available (review of problem list, medications, new symptoms, physical examination, results of recent laboratory tests, immunization and screening tests, and so on). The RMR reminder system clearly assisted physicians by retrieving clinical data and providing reminders on certain aspects of care.

Electronic record keeping for the private medical office is currently in development. Information-management systems advertised for the office setting have well-developed modules for billing, accounting, scheduling, and payroll, but most do not track clinical information per se—i.e., they do not record aspects of the physical examination, test results, and other like information. Given the usefulness of a computer-based reminder system in enhancing the quality and efficiency of medical care, it is likely that these office information systems will improve significantly in coming years.

Computer-Assisted Instruction and Continuing Medical Education

Computer-assisted instruction (CAI) has been used in medical education since the early 1960s, and the extent of use varies greatly. Some schools that lack resources and faculty commitment have virtually no CAI in the curriculum, whereas others, such as The Ohio State University College of Medicine (where 40 percent of each class learns the entire basic science curriculum by computer), utilize CAI heavily. The effectiveness of CAI and its acceptance by students as an alternative form of learning have been well established. The most widely used type of CAI consists of clinical simulation, in which the learner can be exposed to unusual clinical problems not likely to be encountered because of their rarity or severity and in which the learner can experiment with various diagnostic and management approaches in a no-risk setting.

As indicated in the previous sections, it is likely that physicians will have ready access via computer to both textbooks and recent literature. It is not likely that either of these modalities will replace traditional continuing medical education (CME), however. There will still be a need for physicians to review and update their medical knowledge and skills (perhaps as a requirement for relicensure or recertification), and there may be situations in which a physician wishes to master a new area of medicine. CME software developed for the personal computer may provide a more cost- and time-effective alternative to the traditional forms of CME, particularly for the individual who prefers a one-on-one, interactive form of learning. *Scientific American* publishes Discotest (415 Madison Avenue, New York, NY 10017), which consists of two case simulations each quarter. Each simulation is run once for credit and then may be repeated as often as desired, with or without feedback and critique. Another example of CME software for the practicing physician is *Cyberlog* (Cardinal Health Systems, Inc., 7562 Market Place Drive, Eden Prairie, MN 55344-3636), a quarterly software journal. Each issue covers one topic in detail through use of tutorials, animated graphics, case studies, and clinical tools for use in daily clinical practice. It seems likely that the number of CME software options will increase with time.

Artificial Intelligence and Expert Systems

Any discussion of the application of artificial intelligence to the field of medicine must be based on an understanding of the terms *data, information,* and *knowledge. Data* are noninterpretable items, such as a patient's weight or systolic blood pressure. *Information* is a collection of data elements organized in a manner that conveys meaning to the user. An example would be the automated medical record used at the Regenstrief Medical Institute. A simpler example might be a diabetic flow sheet that shows fasting blood sugar, glycosylated hemoglobin, and insulin dose against time. *Knowledge* is the formulation of the relationships, experience, rules, and so forth by which new information is created from existing data and information. An expert system, then, is a computer system that embodies the knowledge of a particular domain in conjunction with inference mechanisms that enable it to use this knowledge in problem-solving situations.

The most ambitious attempt to create a comprehensive internal medicine expert system has been the Internist-I project, conducted under the direction of Jack Myers, M.D., at the University of Pittsburgh (Miller, 1982) The goal of the project was to amass an extensive database that included symptoms, physical findings, and laboratory results for 750 specific diagnoses. Links among the data elements, in the form of causal, temporal, and probable interrelationships, were included in the database as well. When Internist-I was tested against clinicopathologic conferences (CPCs) from *The New England Journal of Medicine* in 1981, its performance was qualitatively similar to that of the clinicians at the Massachusetts General Hospital but inferior to that of the "experts," the case discussants.

A second project, called QMR (Quick Medical Reference), developed out of the experience with Internist-I (Miller, 1986). The goal of QMR was to develop a microcomputer-based system that could provide data, information, or knowledge rapidly and conveniently to the clinician. At its simplest level of operation, QMR can display a disease profile and links to other diagnoses or can provide a differential diagnosis for any given finding. At its most complex level, QMR can take all the known facts in a given case and then review diagnostic possibilities or critique diagnostic hypotheses. In essence, QMR and other similar expert systems are tools to extend a physician's capabilities rather than to replace the physician.

The computer applications discussed in these five sections all require active use by the physician. The following suggestions are made for physicians in training who would like to prepare themselves for a computer-assisted practice of medicine.

1. Become familiar with the general concepts of database management, spread sheets, and word processing. A relatively inexpensive personal computer and a single integrated software package such as Microsoft Works; Symphony, by Lotus; or PFS: First Choice, by Software Publishing, can be utilized for this purpose.

2. Read a publication about computers in medicine (such as *MD Computing*) on a regular basis. Exellent reviews and reports of new developments of interest to the individual practitioner are found in such publications.

3. Develop and refine your interpersonal skills. Computers are likely to take over the major task of organizing and retrieving medical information but will never be able to replace the human interactive aspect of clinical medicine.

4. Be cognizant of the process of decision making in medicine and take advantage of educational opportunities that will enhance your own decision-making abilities. Despite considerable progress in the development of expert systems, the physician is likely to retain full responsibility for making decisions. The physician of the future must successfully integrate information from all sources (including the patient, the literature, and the computer) to arrive at proper diagnostic and management decisions.

5. Begin now to utilize the computer-based literature search option to help answer clinical questions about the patients you care for. Like the studied use of the stethoscope, facility with computer searches will distinguish the clinician of the future. If you do not own a personal computer and modem, you may consult your medical librarian. Many medical libraries now have facilities for computerized literature searches, and this is an excellent way to experiment with different vendors before taking out your own subscription.

References

Anderson JG. Use and impact of computers in clinical medicine. New York: Springer-Verlag, 1986.

Bleich HL, et al. Clinical computing in a teaching hospital. N Engl J Med 1985; 312:756.

Blum BI, ed. Computers and medicine: Information systems for patient care. New York: Springer-Verlag, 1984.

Covell DG, Uman GC, Manning PR. Information needs in office practice: Are they being met? Ann Intern Med 1985; 103:596.

Horowitz GL, et al. Paper Chase: A computer program to search the medical literature. N Engl J Med 1981; 305:924.

Hunter TB. Keeping up with computers and their applications in medicine. Am J Res 1984; 143:678.

McDonald CJ. Protocol-based computer reminders, the quality of care and the non-perfectability of man. N Engl J Med 1976; 295:1351.

McDonald CJ, Tierney WM. The medical gopher—a microcomputer system to help find, organize, and decide about patient data. West J Med 1986; 145:823.

Miller RA, et al. Internist-I. Experimental computer-based diagnostic consultant for general internal medicine. N Engl J Med 1982; 307:468.

Miller RA, et al. The Internist-I/Quick Medical Reference Project—status report. West J Med 1986; 145:816.

Oberst BB, Reid RA, eds. Computer applications to private office practice. New York: Springer-Verlag, 1984.

Sox HC, et al. Medical decision making. Boston: Butterworths, 1988.

Stross JK, Harlan WR. The dissemination of new medical information. JAMA 1979; 241:2622.

7 Critically Reviewing the Medical Literature

Robert J. Goldberg, PhD

Physicians in training and practicing clinicians have been asked to acquire and continually update a diverse array of qualitative and quantitative skills in a multitude of areas. An integral part of the acquisition and development of these skills is reading the medical literature. Too often, however, peer-reviewed "expert" opinion is accepted uncritically and incorporated into the clinical decision-making process, with its attendant diagnostic and therapeutic implications in both healthy and diseased individuals. Given the burgeoning clinical literature and rapid turnover of novel diagnostic tests and promising therapeutic interventions, it is of fundamental importance, particularly for the busy clinician with limited reading time, to be able to understand and evaluate the medical literature. To this end, this chapter presents techniques that will enable you to assess the strengths and weaknesses of articles in the scientific literature and to judge their relevance for use in the clinical setting. Particular attention is devoted to the epidemiologic principles used in evaluating the validity of both screening and diagnostic tests as well as observational and experimental study designs, the collection of reliable and extrapolative information, and the analysis and interpretation of data. In addition, some tools for initiating and carrying out your own research are provided.

Before commencing, a word of caution: If one looks hard and long enough, some imperfections will be found in even the best of reported studies. This does not mean, however, that the reader should dismiss the overall study findings and their relevance. Human fallibilities and study logistics being what they are, the reader must be on guard when interpreting the printed word. Even with the realization that the "perfect" study may not exist, it is still possible to extract much useful and relevant data from studies appearing in the medical literature.

Basic Elements of an Article

Six major headings are typically present in a scientific article: the summary or abstract, introduction, materials and methods, results, discussion or conclusions, and references or bibliography. Too often, readers tend to concentrate on the abstract and discussion/conclusion sections and pay little attention to the methodology. This section describes the characteristics of the population of interest, the methods of information gathering, the study design format, and the analytic approaches employed in the study. The substance of the research report is contained within this section, and it is to this section that the trained critical reviewer allocates the majority of his or her reading time.

The major elements to consider in critically reviewing a scientific report are summarized in Table 7-1.

First, determine whether the objectives or hypotheses to be tested in a particular article are of interest and whether they are presented in a clear and succinct fashion. If the response is "no" to either of these items, proceed to other articles appearing in the journal.

If you are satisfied with the stated hypotheses and objectives, however, and decide to read on, approach the materials and methods section next. This section presents the details of the study population, including the sampling procedures used, the type of information collected and the method of collection, and the particulars of the study design. This is a critical juncture for the astute literature reviewer because a number of factors now need to be considered. Is the study population adequately described, and do the patients described reflect those seen in your own practice setting? Were the sampling procedures and sample size adequate to derive appropriate inferences? By what means were the data collected? Have these instruments been shown to have reliable predictability and validity, and were any independent validation checks performed? Were the data abstracters blinded to the hypotheses tested? If not, was the information obtained from the study and comparison groups collected in a similar manner? Finally, is this a descriptive or an observational investigation, or has a randomized controlled trial been undertaken? After pondering these questions, you must decide whether to read further, keeping in mind the relevance of the collected data to the management of your particular or potential practice population.

In examining the data analysis section, one that is often glossed over or neglected, you should decide whether the collected data are worthy of statistical manipulation and whether the methods of analysis were executed appropriately.

The results section is encountered next, and it is in this section that the reader must be particularly vigilant. Have the data been presented in a systematic and coherent fashion, and can the reader digest the facts presented? Have appropriate cut-off points been selected for the major independent and dependent factors to be examined, and have additional explanatory factors been satisfactorily taken into account? Are the tables presented in an objective and consistent fashion, or are there glaring errors of omission?

In the discussion section, determine whether the author's conclusions have been supported by the evidence presented or whether sweeping generalizations have been derived without appropriate supporting data. Are the conclusions placed in proper perspective, or should these conclusions be regarded as tentative, pending the results of further investigations?

After thoughtfully considering these and additional points of concern, you can then make a decision about the usefulness of the article and its potential relevance in the clinical work-up and management of patients with relatively similar conditions who are seen in your own practice.

Table 7-1 Outline for Critical Appraisal of Articles Appearing in the Medical Literature

1. Objectives or hypotheses to be tested
2. Study design features
   a. Description of the population of interest, including an appropriate comparison group
   b. Collection of data, including measurement instruments, reliability of collected information, and generalizability of ways in which information was obtained and validated
   c. Observational or experimental design approach
3. Data analysis
   a. Are methods used appropriate to the data collected, and have analyses been performed correctly?
4. Presentation of findings or results
   a. Are the data presented in a coherent, objective manner and in sufficient detail for the reader to derive independent conclusions?
5. Conclusions
   a. Are the conclusions supported by the data presented, and do they relate to the initial hypotheses posed?
   b. Should the reader accept the author's conclusions? If not, what additional information is needed?

Diagnostic or Screening Tests

Articles extolling the virtues of some newly developed diagnostic test appear regularly in the clinical literature. The tests typically use either clinical signs or symptoms or newly developed sophisticated technology to diagnose a relatively common or esoteric illness in less time and with more predictive accuracy than is possible with currently available diagnostic approaches. Before accepting these claims at face value, you should be familiar with the elements that constitute a systematic evaluation of a diagnostic test (Table 7-2).

Table 7-2 Elements to Consider in Evaluating the Clinical Utility of a Diagnostic Test

1. Was an independent and blinded comparison carried out with a "gold diagnostic standard"?
2. Did the patient sample studied include a diverse array of illness-severity states, or was it restricted to mild or severe cases?
3. Was the setting in which the new test was carried out sufficiently described, with observer bias minimized and reproducibility of the test examined?
4. Was "normality" defined on sensible clinical grounds?
5. Were the mechanics of carrying out the test described sufficiently to permit replication?
6. Was the utility of the test examined, and on what grounds does the new test propose to improve on previously employed diagnostic procedures (test accuracy, patient comfort, time involved, and associated costs)?

Table 7-3 Descriptive Characteristics of a Screening Test: "Gold Standard"

Proposed test results	Disease classification Diagnosed (+)	Diagnosed (−)	Totals
Screened positive	True positive (a)	False positive (b)	a+b
Screened negative	False negative (c)	True negative (d)	c+d
Totals	a+c	b+d	n

Sensitivity = a/a+c
Specificity = d/b+d

Positive predictive value = a/a+b
Negative predictive value = d/c+d

Prevalence of disease under study = a+c/n

When assessing the clinical usefulness of a new diagnostic test or constellation of symptoms, you should first compare its results with those of the definitive test, or "gold standard," as shown in Table 7-3. Basically, a number of both "ill" and "non-diseased" individuals (disease or health having been determined through the gold-standard test, e.g., coronary angiography, computed tomography, tissue biopsy) are also subjected to the new diagnostic test, results of which are then compared with those of the gold standard. The concepts of sensitivity, specificity, and predictive value emerge based on the comparison of these tests.

Sensitivity refers to the ability of the proposed test to identify correctly patients with disease that has been confirmed by the gold standard, whereas *specificity* refers to the ability of the new test to classify correctly those without disease. In the usual clinical situation, however, when a person is initially screened for disease or other health-related abnormality, the definitive diagnostic test or procedure has not yet been carried out. It is at this point that the negative or positive *predictive value* of the screening test becomes important: How conclusively has the test ruled in or ruled out the presence of disease? The practicing clinician is most typically concerned with the predictive value of a positive test, i.e., to what extent he or she will be successful in predicting the likelihood of disease on the basis of the results of the new diagnostic test. From the perspective of the patient's subsequent management and work-up, these results are important, because individuals with a positive test result typically need to receive further work-ups, with their attendant costs, risks, and compliance issues. Therefore, it is desirable to increase our predictive accuracy, and one way of doing this is to increase the prevalence of disease.

To accomplish this, other clinical signs and symptoms and laboratory test results are taken into account to identify those individuals who have an increased likelihood of disease; subsequently, our screening test is applied to these individuals. For example, if one developed a test to identify at an early stage those individuals with either acute or chronic coronary artery disease, one would use information that is currently known about the risk factors for coronary disease, its typical constellation of signs and symptoms, and the individuals in whom it is likely to occur. One could then apply the novel diagnostic test to these high-risk individuals (e.g., men older than 60 years of age with radiating chest pain and a positive history of two of the three major coronary risk factors) in order to increase the prevalence of suspect disease and decrease the likelihood of false-positive test results.

The second element of a useful screening or diagnostic test is its ability to discriminate between diseased and nondiseased individuals at various levels of disease severity. For example, a new diagnostic test that detects disease in its advanced stage, when cure is unlikely, may have limited usefulness, whereas a test that detects disease in an earlier or preclinical state may be of considerable clinical importance, particularly in assisting in the selection of appropriate therapeutic interventions.

The third element to assess is the setting in which the new test was applied. Does the setting described mirror your own clinical practice? You might also consider how reproducible the test results will be in less experienced hands.

The fourth element—the concept of "normality"—is extremely important but, at times, difficult to define. The definition of normality is instrumental in distinguishing a state of disease from that of nondisease; therefore, the parameters that constitute a normal value directly affect the sensitivity and specificity of the new procedure or clinical insight. How one chooses to define "normality" has a direct impact on both patient prognosis and management and test-related costs of either false-positive or false-negative findings. Typically, there is an inverse relationship between these two parameters and their attendant consequences.

Elements five and six (see Table 7-2) are relatively self-evident. They must be scrutinized before a decision is made to abandon clinical observations or diagnostic tests currently in use.

Observational Studies

In terms of the natural history of carrying out research in humans, observational studies (retrospective and prospective) are usually carried out first, followed by a randomized controlled trial, if the evidence obtained from previous studies suggests that such an extensive undertaking is necessary and may clarify the etiologic importance of a suspect risk factor or the costs and benefits of a selected therapeutic intervention. For most questions that arise in the context of clinical practice, however, observational studies may provide sufficient insights into observed clinical or etiologic associations.

Retrospective (Case-Control) Study

This study design, although probably unfairly maligned in the past, has had a recent resurgence in popularity, particularly given the significant costs and logistics involved in conducting long-term follow-up studies or randomized controlled clinical trials.

This design format is particularly appropriate when the disease or condition in question occurs rarely. It is relatively inexpensive to conduct, the number of study subjects needed is comparatively small, and it can be performed reasonably quickly. The retrospective study is ideally suited for the initial testing of hypotheses suggested by astute clinical observations. For example, this study design has been effectively utilized in evaluating the association between maternal exposure to diethylstilbestrol and the development of vaginal adenocarcinoma in their female offspring, between current use of oral contraceptives and the occurrence of acute myocardial infarction in young women, and between the use of certain tampons during the menstrual cycle and toxic-shock syndrome in young women. It has also been used to identify individuals at high risk for the development of acquired immunodeficiency syndrome (AIDS), such as homosexuals and intravenous drug abusers.

The basic design features of the case-control study are shown in Table 7-4. Essentially, the investigator first selects a number of patients with disease, preferably those with recently diagnosed, or incident, cases of illness, or some other health-related outcome and an appropriate comparison group of individuals without the condition under study. Each of the two study groups is then classified with regard to exposure to the putative factor under study. This information is usually obtained through

Table 7-4 General Design Features of a Retrospective (Case-Control) Study

	Study sample	
Determination of risk factor or exposure characteristic	*Cases (disease present)*	*Controls (disease absent)*
Exposed	a	b
Not exposed	c	d
Totals	a+c	b+d
Measures of association		
Proportions exposed	$\frac{a}{a+c}$	$\frac{b}{b+d}$
Odds ratio	$\frac{ad}{bc}$	

either personal interviews or review of medical records, with some validation attempted for questions asked of study respondents.

A 2 × 2 table is then constructed, consisting of the following four cells: diseased patients (cases) who were exposed to the factor of interest (a), ill patients who were not exposed (c), nondiseased or control subjects who were exposed (b), and control subjects who were not exposed (d). If exposure is associated with the disease or condition under investigation, there should be a greater proportion of diseased individuals exposed to the factor than controls.

We can also measure the strength of the association between exposure to the factor of interest and disease by calculating the odds ratio. This will provide an estimate of the odds of having the disease given a particular exposure as compared to the odds of disease without such exposure (odds ratio = ad/bc). An odds ratio close to 1 implies that there is no association between the factor of interest and the disease in question, and as the odds ratio increases, the exposure-related risk of having the disease likewise increases.

Let us further illustrate these design features through the use of a hypothetical example (Table 7-5) that will also be used in the other study designs in this chapter. In this example, we wish to study the association between the consumption of diets with varying intakes of salt and the occurrence of hypertension.

As seen in our example, we have selected 100 individuals with elevated blood pressure (cases), as defined on the basis of a specified number of blood-pressure readings, and a comparison group of 200 normotensive individuals (controls). Differences are then examined in both the case and control groups with regard to the exposure factor of interest, i.e., consumption of a diet high in salt. In this study hypertensives had a sixfold increased exposure to this diet as compared with normotensives. Confidence intervals could have been placed around this odds ratio to provide the reader with a degree of confidence in the observed results and upper and lower ranges of risk. This example illustrates numerous points to bear in mind when carrying out a study that utilizes this type of research design or when reviewing the use of this approach in a journal article.

Table 7-5 Example of a Retrospective Study Examining the Association Between Salt Intake and Risk of Hypertension

	Initially select	
Risk factor	*Hypertensives (disease present)*	*Normotensives (disease absent)*
Diet "high" in salt	80 (a)	80 (b)
Diet "low" in salt	20 (c)	120 (d)
Totals	100	200
Proportion exposed (%)	80	40
Odds ratio	$ad/bc = \frac{(80)(120)}{(80)(20)} = 6.0$	

Predefined selection criteria for both the case and control groups need to be specified a priori. For example, the study should state the cut-off point used to separate normotensives from hypertensives, the number of blood-pressure readings obtained, and whether the examination situations were standardized. It is also important to know whether these were newly diagnosed (incident) hypertensives or prevalent cases. The use of newly diagnosed cases minimizes the effect of other factors, such as recall bias, that may creep into the study and alter the etiologic importance of the risk factor under study in either a positive or negative direction.

The source of the case population strongly influences the extent to which the results of any study can be extrapolated. For example, hypertensives seen in a hospital setting may be quite different from those seen in the physician's office or in a neighborhood clinic, and patients selected from a tertiary-care hospital may differ in important respects from patients seen in a community hospital. The more representative the study population, the more likely that the results can be extrapolated to others in the population who have the disease or condition under study.

The ideal control group consists of individuals who are representative of all persons without the disease in the community, with respect to the exposure factor under study. To approximate this ideal, many case-control studies use two comparison groups: a group consisting of persons hospitalized with conditions other than the disease under study and a community or neighborhood control group consisting of persons who reside in the same neighborhood as those in the case group but who do not have the disease (e.g., hypertension) under study.

Use of hospitalized controls affords ease of access and allows both cases and controls to be interviewed in a similar setting. However, hospitalized controls may not be truly representative of the population at large without the disease under investigation. For this reason, it may be desirable to have a neighborhood control group as an additional proxy measure of the frequency of the exposure factor in the community at large. The selection of this comparison group usually necessitates some type of survey, be it door to door, mailed, or over the telephone; thus, it may entail considerable costs and potential response problems. A ratio of two controls for each case is usually considered adequate.

Aside from the problems with the selection of the control group, collection of reliable and accurate data from both cases and controls is a difficult task. In gathering data on the exposure factor (in this example, consumption of dietary intake of salt), it is important to have some method of validating exposure. For example, interviewers blinded to the major hypothesis under study, so that cases and controls would be asked the same predetermined questions, could administer dietary questionnaires to members of the respective study groups using standardized instruments as well as food models. Despite the use of these instruments to quantitate exposure, however, it may be difficult to characterize accurately the dietary intake of individuals in the comparison groups.

Data collected from other sources (e.g., medical encounters, school records) might also be used to validate some of the information collected, but one must decide if these data have been collected in a reliable and standardized fashion.

In addition to the principal exposure factor under study, other factors that may confound its association with the disease in question must be defined and taken into account. For in-

Table 7-6 General Design Features of a Prospective Study

Initial selection of	Follow-up over time to examine: *Disease development*	*No disease development*	Totals	Incidence rates of disease
Exposed population	a	b	a+b	a/a+b
Nonexposed population	c	d	c+d	c/c+d
Measure of association	Relative risk = $\frac{\text{Incidence of disease among exposed}}{\text{Incidence of disease among nonexposed}} = \frac{a/a+b}{c/c+d}$			

stance, in examining the relationship between diets high in sodium and development of hypertension, the influence of other factors related to the risk of high blood pressure, such as family history, body weight, and other dietary nutrients, must be taken into account. Matching on these factors in advance may help to minimize their impact, but these factors may also be handled in subsequent data analyses by means of appropriate stratification and multivariate analytic approaches.

The case-control study does have a number of potentially serious limitations. It is rarely possible to obtain a truly representative control group, and the information obtained about past events or exposures may be subject to differential recall bias. This type of study is usually the first approach used in investigating the possible association between a risk factor and disease. If the results of this study suggest some relationship, the investigator may then decide to proceed to a prospective study.

Prospective Study

The basic outline of a prospective study is illustrated in Table 7-6. In this cohort, or longitudinal, approach, the investigator typically selects a nonrandom sample of individuals exposed and not exposed to some factor of interest (primary prevention study) or of diseased individuals treated and not treated with some therapeutic agent (secondary prevention). These two groups are then followed over time to see whether those exposed to the factor of interest (or treated) are more likely to develop the selected study endpoints than those not so exposed (or not treated). The relative risk is then calculated to provide a measure of the degree of the strength of the association between exposure (or treatment) and development of the disease or other health-related endpoint.

This study design is particularly attractive to the clinical researcher because it enables one to determine the incidence rates or comparative risk of disease in exposed versus nonexposed or treated versus untreated or conventionally treated groups. Unfortunately, the major chronic diseases of public health and clinical concern typically have long latency periods, so that many years may pass before study results are obtained.

Frequently, as a means of condensing these years of follow-up, a nonconcurrent or historical prospective approach is utilized (Table 7-7). The features of the prospective design format are retained, but the study initiation point is moved back in time. This may be accomplished by selection of the study population from past medical records or other sources of data that can be reliably utilized. The subjects are then traced from that point to the present or some recent point in time.

As an example, let us explore the association between dietary intake of salt and development of hypertension from the perspective of the prospective study design. In a concurrent prospective study, one would select individuals without elevated blood pressure and classify them with regard to varying levels of sodium intake. These differentially exposed groups would then be followed over time to examine the incidence rates or risk of hypertension in individuals classified according to sodium intake. In the nonconcurrent prospective study, one would attempt to go back in the past to some reliable source of data, classify individuals at that time with respect to their sodium ingestion, and follow them up to the present in order to examine the incidence rates of hypertension in the various exposed groups. Although this study design clearly condenses the years of follow-up necessary, past records that describe an individual's sodium intake in a reliable and standardized manner are unlikely to be available.

Aside from this concern, there are other problems to consider in critically reviewing the results of a prospective study. One must carefully consider the sociodemographic and clinical makeup of the sample population, the system of referral to the health-care facility from which the population of interest may be assembled, and other relevant characteristics in order to judge their similarities or dissimilarities to the reader's own practice.

The major problem in the prospective study is the loss of individuals to follow-up. Clearly, losses must be kept at a minimum for two reasons: not only do they reduce the absolute number of subjects available for purposes of analysis, but the reasons why individuals are lost to follow-up (e.g., illness, death) may be related to the hypothesis under study and thus add a potential source of bias. These concerns should be addressed in any article reviewed.

The prospective study also has a number of disadvantages and limitations that should be considered in the results and conclusions of any written report utilizing this design approach. Because most diseases are relatively rare, a large study population, with its attendant costs and problems of logistics, is needed. Subjects may change their exposure status (e.g., from a low-salt to a high-salt diet) over the course of the study. Finally, there is a

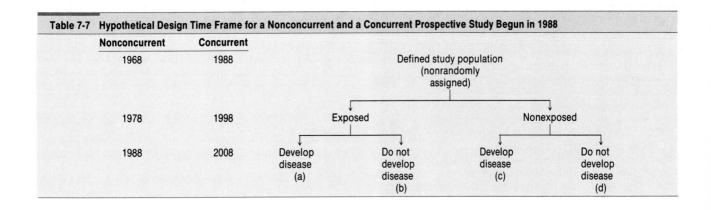

Table 7-7 Hypothetical Design Time Frame for a Nonconcurrent and a Concurrent Prospective Study Begun in 1988

Nonconcurrent	Concurrent				
1968	1988	Defined study population (nonrandomly assigned)			
1978	1998	Exposed		Nonexposed	
1988	2008	Develop disease (a)	Do not develop disease (b)	Develop disease (c)	Do not develop disease (d)

potential for surveillance bias. This may be introduced if the investigator has searched more diligently for the outcome event in the exposed than in the nonexposed cohort.

On the other hand, the prospective study has several distinct advantages over the retrospective study. It allows an estimation of the risk of disease in exposed and nonexposed individuals; it introduces less bias in the assessment of the risk factor of interest; it provides meaningful results when exposure is rare; it permits assessment of multiple health or disease outcomes (e.g., risk of stroke, renal failure); and it provides better data on the time relationship between exposure and the onset of disease.

Randomized Clinical Trials

These trials are usually undertaken only after sufficient evidence has been obtained from observational epidemiologic studies that have suggested a possible association between a specific risk or protective factor and the occurrence of disease. Randomized trials are also typically undertaken to evaluate the potential merits of a therapeutic intervention. The study design is essentially the same as that of the concurrent prospective study, the major difference being the random allocation of subjects to intervened and nonintervened groups.

Randomization is carried out to ensure the nonpredictability of assignment to study groups. This quality is desirable in a clinical trial because (1) investigators tend to have certain preconceived notions about patients and therapies and may unwittingly assign markedly different types of individuals to the study and control groups, and (2) randomization minimizes the effect of self-selection and attempts to balance both measurable and unmeasurable factors between intervened and nonintervened groups. The actual randomization process attempts to avoid investigator bias through treatment assignment by use of a table of random numbers or by other rigorous methods of allocation. In reviewing clinical trials reported in the literature, it is important to determine whether random assignment to intervened and nonintervened groups actually took place and whether differences between groups were examined after randomization, because differences may still exist in selected factors between the primary comparison groups, even after random assignment of treatment.

Clinical trials may employ different types of patient and investigator blindness to enhance the scientific quality of the trial, ranging from single blindness (e.g., patient) to triple blindness (e.g., patient, investigator, biostatistician), with either a placebo or conventional therapy employed in the comparison group.

Patient compliance with the prescribed therapeutic regimens is frequently a problem in clinical practice, and it may be even more so in the conduct of a clinical trial. If a significant proportion of subjects in the study do not comply with either the active therapy or the placebo regimen, the results of the study may be virtually useless. Therefore, some method of compliance assessment (e.g., blood or urine tests, pill counts) should be built into the study design. In reviewing the intervention employed, one must consider its utility and costs in one's own patient population as well as the impact of competing interventions that may blur the study findings.

In the analysis of a clinical trial, it is important to collect data on noncompliant subjects and those lost to follow-up. An "intent-to-treat" statistical analysis takes these factors into account in order to make the results of the trial reflect, as far as possible, the realities of clinical practice.

The disadvantages of the randomized controlled clinical trial are similar to those of the prospective trial, but the clinical trial poses some additional problems. The expenses can be great and the logistics involved in carrying out a multicenter trial can be complicated. Use of standardized protocols and adherence to these guidelines are of crucial importance in order to pool the findings from various participating centers.

Some of the major points to consider when reviewing the results of a randomized clinical trial are shown in Table 7-8.

Table 7-8 Elements to Consider When Reviewing the Results of a Randomized Controlled Trial

1. Is the study population described in adequate detail, and are inclusion and exclusion entry criteria carefully specified?
2. Is the treatment reproducible in actual clinical practice, and is enough information provided for its use in various patient subsets?
3. Is compliance bias potentially operative, and have adequate measures of compliance been developed?
4. Are competing interventions also being utilized, and are they evenly distributed between intervened and nonintervened subjects?
5. Has a formal randomization process been carried out, and are the study groups comparable at the time of trial initiation?
6. Have losses to follow-up been minimized and taken into account in the data analysis?
7. Has follow-up been long enough to detect a clinically or statistically important effect, and has surveillance bias been examined?

References

Bailar JC III, Mosteller F. Medical uses of statistics. Waltham, MA: NEJM Books, 1986.
Diamond GA, Forrester JS. Analysis of probability as an aid in the clinical diagnosis of coronary-artery disease. N Engl J Med 1979; 300:1350.
Feinstein AR. Clinical biostatistics. St. Louis: CV Mosby, 1977.
Gehlbach SR. Interpreting the medical literature: A clinician's guide. Lexington, MA: Collamore Press, 1982.
Goldberg R, Szklo M, Tonascia J, Kennedy H. Acute myocardial infarction. Prognosis complicated by ventricular fibrillation or cardiac arrest. JAMA 1979; 241:2024.
Hayden GF, Kramer MS, Horwitz RI. The case-control study. A practical review for the clinician. JAMA 1982; 247:326.
Haynes RB. Clinical epidemiology rounds. How to read clinical journals: II. To learn about a diagnostic test. Can Med Assoc J 1981; 124:703.
Haynes RB. Clinical epidemiology rounds. Clinical disagreement: II. How to avoid it and how to learn from one's mistakes. Can Med Assoc J 1980; 123:613.
Hulley SB, Rosenman RH, Bawol RD, Brand RJ. Epidemiology as a guide to clinical decisions: The association between triglyceride and coronary heart disease. N Engl J Med 1980; 302:1383.
Koran LM. The reliability of clinical methods, data and judgements. N Engl J Med 1975; 293:642–646, 695–701.
Multiple Risk Factor Intervention Trial Group. Risk factor changes and mortality results. JAMA 1982; 248:1465.
Ransohoff DF, Feinstein AR. Problems of spectrum and bias in evaluating the efficacy of diagnostic tests. N Engl J Med 1978; 299:926.
Riegelman RK, Hirsh RP. Studying a study and testing a test. Boston: Little, Brown, 1989.
Sackett DL. Bias in analytic research. J Chron Dis 1979; 32:51.
Sackett DL. Epidemiology rounds. Clinical disagreement: I. How often it occurs and why. Can Med Assoc J 1980; 123:499.
Sartwell PE. Retrospective studies: A review for the clinician. Ann Intern Med 1974; 81:381.
Spodick DH. The randomized controlled clinical trial. Scientific and ethical bases. Am J Med 1982; 73:420.
Trout KS. Clinical epidemiology rounds. How to read clinical journals: IV. To determine etiology or causation. Can Med Assoc J 1981; 124:985.
Tugwell PX. Clinical epidemiology rounds. How to read clinical journals: III. To learn the clinical course and prognosis of disease. Can Med Assoc J 1981; 124:869.

Interacting with Other Health Care Professionals

8

Nursing

Julie A. D'Andrea, RN, MA, MSN

Linda C. Greene, RN, BSN

Nurses make up the primary work force in every patient care area. Often they are the only professionals present on site and accountable for delivery of total patient care on a 24-hour-a-day, 7-day-a-week basis. Therefore, an understanding and appreciation of the professional nurse as an essential member of the health care team is vital to your growth and success as a medical student.

Definitions

Registered Nurse (RN). The RN is registered by the Board of Registration in Nursing after she or he has successfully passed a state board examination. There are three educational routes to qualify for examination by the board: BSN graduates have completed 4 years of college including nursing courses and have a Bachelor of Science degree in nursing; diploma graduates have completed a 3-year hospital-based program and hold a diploma in nursing; and an Associate Degree nurse has completed a 2-year program and has an Associate Degree in nursing. After successful completion of the board exam, all are considered RNs. The RN provides comprehensive, quality nursing care in accordance with licensure as well as the policies and procedures of the hospital or facility with which affiliated.

Licensed Practical Nurse (LPN). The LPN is a licensed technical nurse who functions under the direction and supervision of an RN to provide direct patient care.

Nursing Assistant (NA). The NA assists nursing personnel with routine care activities. He or she always works under the direction and supervision of an RN.

Nurse Manager. The nurse manager is responsible and accountable for the 24-hour-a-day, 7-day-a-week clinical management of a specific patient care unit. He or she promotes appropriate utilization of personnel, equipment, and supplies and works within the primary nursing model to ensure the practice of professional nursing and the delivery of quality patient care on the assigned unit.

Head Nurse. The head nurse is responsible for the delivery of nursing care to patients on a specific patient care unit for an 8- to 24-hour period. He or she coordinates activities within the nursing station and acts as the primary liaison between nursing staff and physicians.

Team Leader. The team leader is an RN or LPN who works under the direction and supervision of the head nurse. He or she coordinates the nursing care of a group of patients through specific patient assignments and the distribution of specific patient care tasks to different team members.

Primary Nurse. The primary nurse is a staff RN who assumes responsibility and accountability for assessing and coordinating the total nursing care needs of a patient in collaboration with other pertinent health team members, patient, and family, from the time of admission to the time of discharge.

Associate Nurse. The associate nurse is a staff RN who works with the primary nurse and assumes responsibility for supporting the plan of care established by the primary nurse for his or her primary care patient.

Assigned Nurse. The assigned nurse is an RN or LPN who cares for the patient and supports the established plan of care when the primary and associate nurses are unavailable.

Nursing Care Delivery Systems

Nursing care can be delivered in different ways, depending on the philosophy of the nursing department of the particular institution with which one is affiliated. Therefore, in order to achieve the communication necessary to realize the desired level of patient care, it is important to learn the particular method of nursing care delivery in each patient care area in which you practice. Two commonly practiced systems of nursing care delivery are *team nursing* and *primary care nursing.*

Team Nursing

In team nursing the traditional head nurse is in charge of a staff of RNs, LPNs, and NAs (Fig. 8-1). The head nurse helps to facilitate a system in which the nursing staff utilizes a team approach, with one or more nurses being given the title of team leader. The team leader is the nurse responsible for seeing that each member of the team has a patient care assignment and that specific patient care tasks, such as vital signs, medications, and treatments, are assigned to specific team members. In such a system a variety of personnel are responsible for different aspects of each patient's total care. Fragmentation of essential information can result, and it may become difficult for nursing staff to possess a true grasp of the patient's clinical presentation and overall needs. In addition, this type of nursing care delivery usually supports few professional RN staff members. Therefore, the health team member present at the bedside frequently may not be the most appropriate or the most informed member with whom to discuss a patient care concern. You must identify the key professional nursing personnel on each patient care unit, because they serve as the essential communication liaisons between you, the physician, and other staff members in the delivery of care to the patients on that unit. A major advantage of this system is that it tends to be less costly.

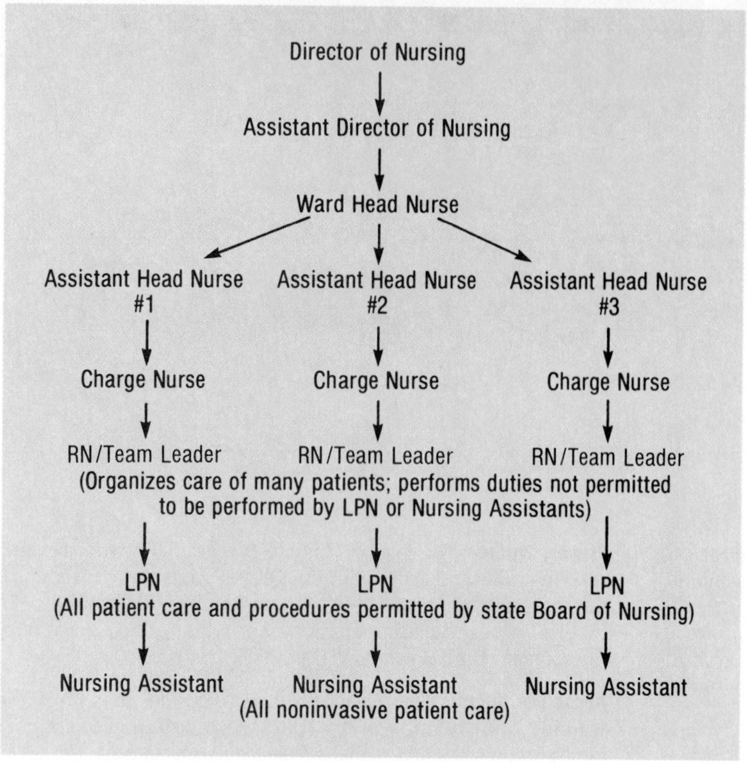

Figure 8-1 The team-nursing approach to patient care.

Primary Care Nursing

Primary care nursing is a more comprehensive style of patient care delivery than the team approach (Figs. 8-2 and 8-3). The nurse manager is responsible for the 24-hour staffing, organizing, planning, and budgeting of the patient care unit. The manager's staff RNs are the key people responsible for the delivery of quality patient care. This system necessitates a higher percentage of professional RN staffing. Each RN works in the capacity of primary/associate or assigned nurse. In the role of primary nurse, the staff RN faces the greatest challenge as well as the greatest opportunity for realizing his or her potential as a professional care provider. The primary nurse becomes identified as the staff member responsible for the total care of the patient from the time of admission to the time of discharge. He or she is responsible for being informed and keeping up to date with pertinent information and related patient care issues. The primary nurse is responsible for assessing patient care needs, collaborating with other members of the health team, and then documenting, implementing, evaluating, and updating a plan of care that clearly communicates to colleagues the nursing approach necessary to meet these individual needs at a particular time of hospitalization. Although another staff member may be requested to perform certain tasks, the primary nurse retains ultimate responsibility and accountability for that patient's care on a 24-hour basis. The primary nurse encourages the involvement of both patient and family and focuses on their emotional and educational needs as well as the physical care components. Because of his or her investment of much time, energy, and professional commitment, the primary nurse is indeed the key nursing resource for the physician to seek out on the patient care unit.

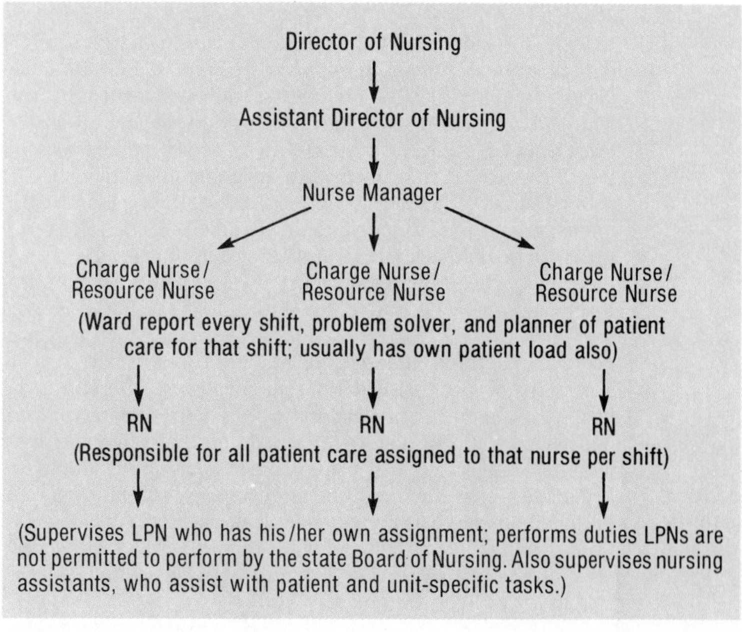

Figure 8-2 The primary-care approach to patient care.

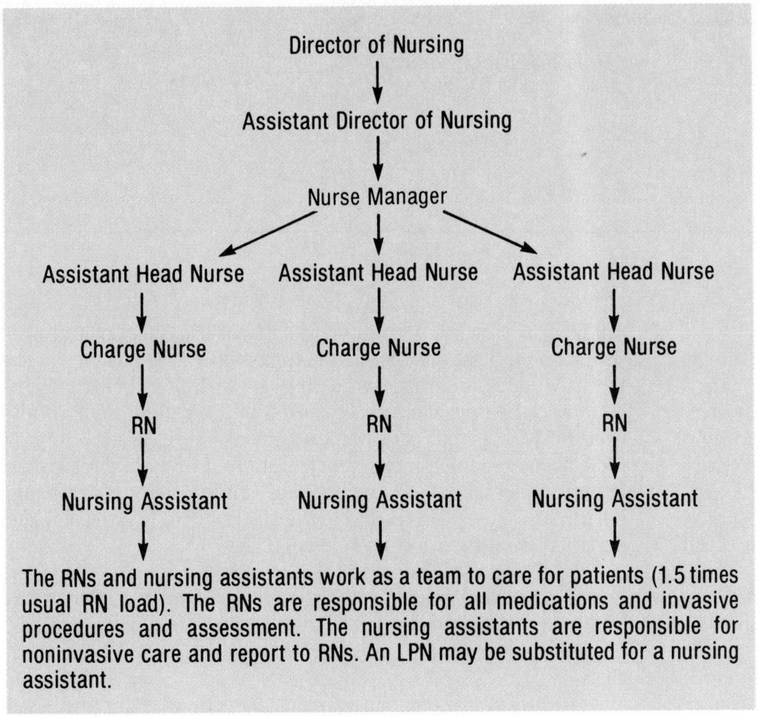
Director of Nursing
Assistant Director of Nursing
Nurse Manager
Assistant Head Nurse
Assistant Head Nurse
Assistant Head Nurse
Charge Nurse
Charge Nurse
Charge Nurse
RN
RN
RN
Nursing Assistant
Nursing Assistant
Nursing Assistant
The RNs and nursing assistants work as a team to care for patients (1.5 times usual RN load). The RNs are responsible for all medications and invasive procedures and assessment. The nursing assistants are responsible for noninvasive care and report to RNs. An LPN may be substituted for a nursing assistant.

Figure 8-3 The modified primary-care approach to patient care.

Summary

The primary objectives of the medical student who is working on any patient care unit are to learn and grow in the practice and art of medicine. It is important, then, that you recognize your own strengths and limitations and seek advice or direction from available resources as needed. Nurses can provide a tremendous resource for learning and will be eager to help, if you approach them with the professional courtesy they deserve. Through mutual respect, support, and collaboration, nursing and medical professionals can work together to deliver quality patient care in any patient care environment.

Clinical Dietetics

Sherri F. Murkland, RD, MEd, CNSD

Nutritional care of a hospitalized patient encompasses a broad area ranging from treatment of the severely malnourished patient to obesity management. For these reasons, the clinical dietitian is an essential member of the health care community.

Definition

The clinical dietitian is generally a registered dietitian (RD). This means that a bachelor of science degree in nutrition has been earned from an accredited college or university, an internship (or its equivalent) has been completed, and a national examination has been passed. Continuing-education credit is required to maintain registration. Many dietitians continue their education to the master's degree level and beyond. The academic background of the RD includes extensive study in general science as well as nutrition.

Responsibilities

The clinical dietetic staff (which includes both in-patient and outpatient dietitians) is responsible for all aspects of nutritional care of the hospitalized patient. This care includes nutrient calculation, specialized diet instruction, nutritional assessment and recommendations, and home support. The professional role of the dietitian is not limited to patient management, however. Public and professional education as well as research and publication are continuing responsibilities of the clinical dietitian.

Because the field of nutrition is such a large one, the move in recent years has been to make further use of the dietitian's expertise by encouraging specialization. Some of the more common nutrition specialties that can be found today in the hospital setting include oncology, cardiac rehabilitation, nutrition support (enteral and parenteral nutrition), pediatrics, diabetes, renal nutrition, and geriatrics.

The Pharmacist

Kenneth J. Tabor, PharmD

Definition

Stedman's dictionary defines a pharmacist as a druggist, pharmaceutist, an apothecary, or one who prepares and dispenses drugs and has knowledge of their properties. Today, the majority of graduating pharmacists have spent 5 years obtaining the education necessary to practice this profession. During those 5 years, the pharmacy student must take courses in social, preclinical, and biomedical sciences, including inorganic and organic chemistry, physics, biochemistry, medical chemistry, anatomy, physiology, pharmacology, pathophysiology, clinical pharmacy, biopharmaceutics, and pharmacy law. In many cases, the courses in pharmacology and medical chemistry are each 1 full year in duration. While in school, pharmacy students must complete an internship to be eligible for licensure. Their internship program is analogous to that of physicians, with practical, hands-on experience being obtained by working under the supervision of preceptors. After achieving the necessary academic requirements (i.e., graduation from a school of pharmacy with a bachelor of science in pharmacy) and internship hours, the student pharmacist may then take the Board of Registration in Pharmacy Examination to become a registered pharmacist (RPh). Once registered, he or she may enter the professional work force in one of several areas, which are discussed in the section, "Practice Areas."

Even though the majority of registered pharmacists graduate with a BS degree, some schools also offer the doctor of pharmacy (PharmD) degree, either as an entry-level degree in lieu of the BS degree or as an extension of the BS degree, with an emphasis on clinical training and research. Pharmacists who obtain the PharmD degree undergo additional training over 1 to 3 years, depending on the program. Course work during the first year often includes pathophysiology curricula at affiliated medical schools as well as advanced training in therapeutics, clinical pharmacology, clinical pharmacokinetics, physical assessment, drug-literature evaluation, drug information, and drug-research design. The second year is usually spent in the hospital in a clinical-residency setting, again similar to that which the physician-in-training experiences. Some of the activities during this period include rounding with medical teams as a drug therapy consultant, providing patient monitoring, acting as a drug-information resource, analyzing and interpreting drug concentrations using the principles of clinical pharmacokinetics and therapeutic drug monitoring, and conducting drug research.

Practice Areas

After formal education and licensure, pharmacists can enter a variety of practice areas. The most common and highly visible practitioner is the retail pharmacist, whose major function is to fill prescriptions brought by patients. Within this context, the pharmacist's duties may also include interpreting the prescription, with an emphasis on ensuring that a safe and effective dose is being prescribed; contacting the physician if clarification of a prescription is necessary; selecting a bioequivalent generic medication if the physician has indicated that substitution is possible; reviewing with the patient over-the-counter and prescription medications that he or she may be taking to screen for possible drug interactions; acting as a drug-information resource to the physician; and counseling the patient on administration, storage, and possible side effects of medications. Many pharmacists in this practice environment are very interested in becoming involved "clinically" and commonly answer drug-information questions posed to them. They also help to educate patients about their medication regimens.

A second career opportunity is that of hospital pharmacist. The functions and responsibilities of a hospital pharmacist can be diverse, but they may be divided into essentially three areas: (1) administrative, (2) traditional services, and (3) clinical services.

Administratively inclined pharmacists may be departmental directors, associate directors, assistant directors, and coordinators. These individuals are responsible for the overall direction of the pharmacy department, maintaining appropriate records and licenses, providing quality assurance, purchasing and pricing pharmaceuticals, monitoring purchase and distribution of controlled substances, and supervising departmental members. Because the pharmacy manager's administrative role is becoming increasingly complex, many of these individuals have obtained advanced training in business and health administration.

Some of the "traditional" pharmacy services that may be obtained within the hospital setting are described in this section. Delivery of the correct drug to the right patient at the proper time is the cornerstone of any therapeutic regimen. Unit dose dispensing facilitates this process. Preparation of intravenous medications and total parenteral nutrition solutions is also an important function of the hospital pharmacist. These pharmacists are an excellent source of information about intravenous medication compatibility and are also usually capable of advising the best way to provide a patient with nutritional support (calories, solution composition, and so forth). An efficient purchasing and pharmaceutical inventory control program is a major asset to the pharmacy department and hospital, particularly in this age of cost containment and prospective pricing. Pharmacists in this role are experts at keeping costs down and inventory turnover at an optimal rate. Another major responsibility of the institutional pharmacist is to screen for drug interactions and adverse drug reactions. Finally, hospital pharmacists contribute to the development and use of formulary systems to control costs and provide for improved drug therapy.

In general, the pharmacist with a BS degree is most often associated with "traditional" pharmacy services, whereas the pharmacist with a PharmD degree has been more likely to be involved in clinical services. However, the extent to which pharmacists with either educational background perform within each area depends largely on their level of enthusiasm about getting involved with patients and their department's willingness to support that interest.

"Clinical" involvement by the hospital pharmacist has expanded greatly over the last 10 to 20 years and is likely to continue to do so over the next decade. The "clinical" pharmacist will enjoy an ever-increasing role as an information source about drug therapy.

Clinical pharmacists are in an excellent position to help the physician with therapeutic-management decisions or drug-information questions. Within the hospital environment, they perform a variety of functions, including obtaining medication histories; providing consultation on therapeutic, pharmacokinetic, and drug- and poison-information topics; reviewing patients' medication regimens; and participating in medical rounds.

In addition, clinical pharmacists often have teaching responsibilities, and many hold academic appointments on the staffs of medical, pharmacy, and nursing schools. They teach, both formally (lectures, seminars, and continuing education) and informally (work rounds, answering drug-information questions), and many provide drug-therapy-oriented programs to the public. Various committees within a hospital also utilize their expertise. Pharmacy and Therapeutics, Quality Assurance, Drug Utilization Review, Resuscitation, and Investigational Review Boards frequently have clinical pharmacists as members.

Finally, some hospital and clinical pharmacists are involved in drug-research studies, and in some states clinical pharmacists are now being allowed to prescribe medications by protocol, under the supervision of a physician.

Hospital and clinical pharmacy are the two most common career paths taken by pharmacists. An alternative career path involves the pharmaceutical industry, in which pharmacists may function as salespersons, research monitors, formulations experts, or drug- and toxicology-information specialists.

In any case, no matter what type of position a pharmacist selects, he or she has a unique body of knowledge that should be utilized to its fullest. That individual has a strong desire to provide quality care to patients and can be a major asset to the physician.

References

American Association of Colleges of Pharmacy. Preparing students for the realities of contemporary pharmacy practice. Am J Hosp Pharm 1984; 41:269.

Biles JA. The doctor of pharmacy. JAMA 1983; 249:1157.

Brodie DC, Benson RA. The evolution of the clinical pharmacy concept. Drug Intell Clin Pharm 1976; 10:506.

Herfindel ET, Bernstein LR, Kishi DT. Effect of clinical pharmacy services on prescribing on the orthopedic unit. Am J Hosp Pharm 1983; 40:1945.

McKenney JM, Wyant SL, Atkins D, et al. Drug therapy assessments by pharmacists. Am J Hosp Pharm 1980; 37:824.

Smith WE. Clinical pharmacy in the 1980's. Am J Hosp Pharm 1983; 40:223.

Stimmel BL, McGhan WF. The pharmacist as a prescriber of drug therapy: The USC pilot project. Drug Intell Clin Pharm 1981; 15:665.

Occupational Therapy

Deborah M. Dufresne, MS OTR/L

Occupational therapy is the use of purposeful activity in order to maximize independence, prevent disability, and maintain health in individuals who are limited by physical injury or illness, psychosocial dysfunction, developmental or learning disabilities, poverty and cultural differences, or the aging process. The primary focus of occupational therapy is the development of adaptive skills and performance capacity. Occupational therapists are concerned with factors that serve as barriers or impediments to the individual's ability to function in his or her current role in life. *Occupation* refers to the use of purposeful activity, not necessarily gainful employment.

Definitions

Registered Occupational Therapist (OTR). An OTR is a graduate of an accredited college or university occupational therapy program who has obtained (1) a bachelor's degree in occupational therapy; (2) a certificate in occupational therapy, if a bachelor's degree in a related area is already held; or (3) an entry-level master's degree in occupational therapy. In addition to the academic work, 6 to 9 months of full-time supervised field work is required in a variety of settings. Upon completion of these requirements, it is necessary to pass a national certification examination for OTRs. Some states also require licensure.

Certified Occupational Therapy Assistant (COTA). The COTA is a graduate of an accredited occupational therapy assistant's program who has obtained either (1) an associate degree in occupational therapy or (2) a certificate from 1-year program in occupational therapy. In addition, 2 months of supervised field work is required. Upon completion of these requirements, it is necessary to pass the national certification examination for COTAs. Some states also require licensure. Certified occupational therapy assistants work under the supervision of registered therapists.

Occupational Therapy Aide (OTA). The OTA has a high-school diploma or the equivalent, with on-the-job training.

Responsibilities

In the treatment of the hospitalized patient, the goal of the occupational therapist is to increase or maintain the patient's physical, psychological, and functional abilities through an ongoing, carefully planned treatment program. An occupational therapy consultation is indicated whenever a concern arises about a patient's self-care capabilities, upper-extremity function, developmental status, perceptual cognitive status, psychosocial functioning, need for adaptive equipment, or need for upper- or lower-extremity splints. Occupational therapy evaluation and treatment generally concentrate on one or more of the following areas, depending on diagnosis and evaluation results.

Activities of daily living include issues such as bathing, dressing, feeding, personal-hygiene activities, bed mobility, transfers, functional mobility (including driving), homemaking skills, and community-living skills. Also included are provision of adaptive equipment and recommendations for environmental adaptations.

Assessment of the physical and functional status of the upper extremities entails evaluating the patient's range of motion and determining if this range is active, passive, or active assistive by means of goniometry. Also, the patient's strength and endurance may be measured by manual muscle testing and use of dynamometer (grasp meter) and pinch meter. The patient's light touch discrimination, sharp-dull discrimination, pain, temperature discrimination, proprioception, and kinesthesia are assessed to determine status. Coordination and dexterity are assessed by means of standardized fine-motor assessments.

The occupational therapist also evaluates the patient's need for upper- or lower-extremity plastic splints or adaptive-positioning devices and may be responsible for their fabrication. Evaluation of the patient's status and treatment activities are aimed at remediation or compensation in the areas of visual perception, eye-hand coordination, spatial relations, judgment, memory, and insight.

Prevocational assessment includes evaluation of the patient's physical, functional, and emotional strengths and weaknesses; exploration of his or her interests; and development of appropriate treatment activities based on the occupational therapist's evaluation of the patient. The occupational therapist assists the patient in the acquisition of basic prevocational skills.

Occupational therapy after the vocational evaluation includes work-simulation activities, work-hardening programs, and adaptation of the work environment as needed.

After the evaluation, occupational therapy treatment of the upper extremities includes range-of-motion exercises, which may be incorporated into a purposeful activity, and strength and endurance exercises to address general and specific muscle groups based on determinations made during the evaluation. The occupational therapist also instructs the patient in sensibility exercises, including monitoring of return, and protective methods, and provides a desensitization program. Coordination and dexterity exercises may include activities to facilitate fine-motor skills.

Structured, purposeful activities that are designed and used therapeutically in group and one-on-one situations provide patients with the opportunity to gain vocational, avocational, physical, emotional, and interpersonal skills that are necessary for the achievement of more independent functioning.

References

Hopkins H. Willard and Spackman's occupational therapy. 7th ed. Philadelphia: JB Lippincott, 1988.

Resolution Q. Definition of occupational therapy for licensure: Minutes of the 1981 AOTA Representative Assemby. Am J Occup Ther 1981; 35:798.

Physical Therapy

James A. Michaels, PT, MS

Kathleen F. Erickson, PT, MS

"Physical therapy is the promotion of optimum human health and function through the application of scientific principles to prevent, identify, correct, or alleviate acute or prolonged movement dysfunction of anatomic or physiologic origin" (Physical Therapy Association House of Delegates, 1983).

As a key member of the health care team, the physical therapist seeks to improve movement and function, relieve pain, and expand movement potential. The physical therapist attempts to maximize health through the use of various forms of exercise, education, special manual techniques, and modalities that employ the physiologic principles of heat, cold, and electricity.

Educational Requirements

The registered physical therapist (RPT) has an extensive educational background that combines academic study and clinical experience within an accredited university physical therapy program. It can be fulfilled at either a bachelor of science or basic master's degree level.

Also required for practice is the successful completion of a state licensure examination. Specific areas of study include gross anatomy, physiology, neuroanatomy, and kinesiology as well as course work in the principles and techniques of physical therapy practice. The physical therapy curricula have expanded to accommodate advances in medicine, science, and technology. Subsequently, in 1990, the entry-level educational requirement of all physical therapy educational programs will be the basic master's degree, and more emphasis will be placed on research and clinical experience. As in the medical profession, specific areas of clinical specialization have been established in physical therapy, including cardiopulmonology, clinical electrophysiology, neurology, orthopedics, pediatrics, geriatrics, and sports physical therapy. Many of these physical therapists have board certification as clinical specialists.

Physical therapists often work with supportive personnel: the physical therapy assistant and the physical therapy aide. The *physical therapy assistant* (PTA) is a licensed graduate of an associate's degree program in physical therapy that emphasizes knowledge of the basic sciences and many of the technical physical therapy skills. Under the supervision of a physical therapist, the assistant performs delegated physical therapy procedures. The *physical therapy aide* (PT aide) is trained on the job to assist physical therapists and physical therapy assistants in patient care and to carry out routine operational tasks.

Professional Affiliation

The American Physical Therapy Association (APTA) is a national professional organization representing physical therapists, physical therapy assistants, and students in the United States. Members comply with the APTA code of ethics and standards of conduct, which serve as the chief means of self-regulation of physical therapy practice. The APTA is the accrediting body for physical therapy educational programs.

Evaluation

Through a comprehensive evaluation process, the physical therapist assesses movement dysfunction, identifies problems, sets treatment goals, and establishes a specific treatment plan. During the evaluation process, the physical therapist performs special tests to measure the functional status of the musculoskeletal, neurologic, pulmonary, and cardiovascular systems as related to the patient's functional mobility and independence.

Specific areas of interest to the physical therapist include postural alignment, joint mobility, muscle strength and tone, integrity of sensation and perception, balance, coordination, endurance, the ability to alter postural positions, and the ability to ambulate. The need for assistive or adaptive devices such as ambulatory aids and orthotics is also evaluated. Through frequent consultation with physicians and other health care professionals, the physical therapist works to establish a comprehensive treatment plan to meet specific treatment goals.

Treatment goals may involve correction of movement dysfunction, promotion of the healing process, alleviation of pain, prevention of disability, and restoration of function. Treatment plans are implemented by employing varied therapeutic techniques such as individualized exercise programs, joint mobilization, gait training, biofeedback, retraining in activities of daily living, chest physical therapy, and therapeutic massage. Physical modalities such as ultrasound, traction, electrotherapy, and hydrotherapy are commonly used to help achieve treatment goals. Patient education is an integral part of the treatment process, and patients are encouraged to participate actively in their rehabilitation program.

Referral

Because physical therapists work with patients of all ages and levels of health and ability, the scope of their practice is broad. Physical therapists work with health care professionals in many disciplines, such as cardiology, dentistry, family practice, general surgery, neurology, neurosurgery, obstetrics, orthopedics, oncology, pediatrics, plastic surgery, pulmonology, podiatry, psychiatry, and sports medicine. Problems treated include spinal cord injury, cerebrovascular accidents, cardiopulmonary disease, soft-tissue injury, developmental delay, spinal dysfunction, and cancer. The early identification and referral to physical therapy for evaluation and treatment of patients with movement dysfunction or the potential of developing movement dysfunction, such as patients who require prolonged immobilization or bed rest, greatly enhance the rehabilitation prognosis.

The physical therapy profession is expanding to meet the challenge of today's health care system. In addition to the hospital, therapists practice in home health agencies, school systems, industry, nursing homes, academic and research institutions, sports and fitness facilities, and in their own private practices. The physician has been the traditional point of entry into the physical therapy system for patients who require services. Today, 21 states have enacted legislation that establishes direct access to physical therapy services; 16 additional states have legislation pending that would permit practice without referral by physician, dentist, or podiatrist (Henke, 1989).

References

American Physical Therapy Association House of Delegates. Philosophical statements on physical therapy, 1983.

Henke C. The brave new world of direct access. Rehab Manag 1989; February/March: 24.

Respiratory Therapy

Daniel E. Pritchard, BS, RRT

Respiratory therapy is an allied health specialty employed with medical direction in the treatment, management, control, diagnostic evaluation, and care of patients with deficiencies and abnormalities of the cardiopulmonary system. Its scope of services includes the therapeutic use of medical gases, administration apparatus, environmental control systems, humidification, aerosols, medications, ventilatory support, bronchopulmonary drainage, pulmonary rehabilitation, cardiopulmonary resuscitation, airway management, and pulmonary function testing.

Definitions

Registered Respiratory Therapist (RRT). The RRT is registered by the National Board for Respiratory Care. This individual has 2 to 4 years of formal instruction and training at the undergraduate level, provides all respiratory care modalities in accordance with physicians' orders, and works under the general supervision of the clinical respiratory therapy supervisor.

Certified Respiratory Therapy Technician (CRTT). The CRTT is certified by the National Board for Respiratory Care. This individual has 1 or 2 years of formal instruction and training and, depending upon his or her hospital's policies, provides most or all respiratory care modalities in accordance with physicians' orders and works under the general supervision of the clinical respiratory therapy supervisor.

Summary

The profession of respiratory therapy began in the 1940s and has gone through an impressive period of growth and development which has culminated in the present era of cost containment. Because there is considerable controversy regarding the efficacy of many respiratory therapy modalities, you are strongly urged to consult the pulmonary specialist, the professional literature, or a respiratory therapist when contemplating the use of one or more of the available modalities.

Social Service

Judith P. Stone, MSW, LICSW

Judith Freiman Olson, MSW, LICSW

Social work departments offer a variety of clinical services, including patient and family counseling and assistance in making use of community resources. Social workers, as nonmedical health professionals, bridge the gap between the hospital and the community.

Definitions

Social work departments include staff in some or all of the following classifications:

Social Worker with Master's Degree. An MSW social worker has completed a 2-year graduate program. Training includes courses in human behavior, research, social policy, and clinical treatment methods. Two supervised internships complete the program. Many hospital social workers have specialized in a health care concentration in graduate school. The MSW is the major professional degree.

Social Worker with Bachelor's Degree. These staff have a general understanding of community resources and interviewing skills. They work under the supervision of an MSW. These individuals may be graduates of an accredited BSW program or be college graduates with a liberal arts and science background.

Social Work Intern. This person is in an accredited BSW or MSW program and is fulfilling intensive practice requirements. Social work interns are supervised by MSWs.

Social Worker with Doctoral Degree. A DSW may be employed in a hospital setting where practice includes research and teaching.

Social Work Specialist. Social workers in health care may have training and experience that enable them to specialize in specific fields. Examples are oncology, renal, pediatric, and psychiatric social workers, as well as administrators, discharge planners, and rehabilitation and long-term care social workers.

Social Work Licensure. Most states have various levels of licensure in which education, experience, and examinations are the criteria for credentialing. There are usually bachelor's, master's, and senior clinical (experienced MSW) levels. Continuing education and supervision are required for licensure.

Responsibilities

Social work treatment begins with an assessment of the psychological and social situation of the patient and his or her family. The focus is on the impact of illness and the ability to cope. The elements of a psychosocial assessment should include information about the patient's living situation, family composition, financial and work status, and culture. The quality of relationships and support also is important. Does this person have social supports? Are there family problems that interfere with treatment or recovery? Are there significant persisting patterns of behavior (e.g., a history of chemical dependency or chronic psychiatric illness) that may affect compliance with the treatment plan? What are the the psychosocial problem areas that lend themselves to social work treatment?

Counseling generally comprises two aspects that may overlap. Supportive counseling is more common in in-patient medical settings with a limited length of stay. This type of counseling builds on the strengths of the individual as identified in the evaluation. Crisis intervention is a form of supportive counseling. Isolated patients may be particularly responsive to supportive treatment.

A more recent modality is psychoeducational support, which is basically a group method. This concept has tremendous potential and lends itself to a wide range of diagnostic or problem groups (e.g., living-with-cancer groups, support groups for families of Alzheimer's or chronic psychiatric patients, or parenting-skills groups). The goals are treatment as well as prevention. These groups are equally helpful for intact and seriously disturbed populations. It should be noted that this model is distinguished from self-help groups by its professional-leadership component.

Insight-oriented treatment is designed to heighten the individual's awareness of his or her behavior patterns, which may be dysfunctional. An example would be incest victims or victims of child abuse who may, as adults, seek abusive relationships or repeat pathologic behavior patterns and themselves become abusive. Although insight-oriented treatment is most commonly found in psychiatric settings, individuals in need of these services may present in medical settings.

Social work services consider the patient and family in relationship to the community and its resources. Ruth Cowin, an eminent social work educator, refers to community resources as the "pharmacopoeia of social work." As the bridge between the hospital and the community, social workers recognize the importance of environmental factors and the supports that assure optimal functioning. A comprehensive view of discharge planning includes such areas as services for children, financial resources (including public assistance and private charities), and traditional long-term and home-care resources.

Social work departments are also involved in consultative, educational, and planning functions in the health care setting. Consultation includes advocacy, understanding of dynamics of behavior and family systems, and service needs. Education involves training social work interns as well as assisting in the education of other health care professionals. Social workers frequently identify and understand gaps in service or dysfunctional systems or programs. This understanding can contribute to the planning of patient care delivery.

These indirect services are provided both informally and formally. The latter includes participation on committees concerning issues such as ethics, cancer management, quality assurance, utilization review, and patient care.

Social work contributions in research and grant writing may be related to programs or projects within the department.

These contributions may also be interdepartmental or in collaboration with community agencies.

The social work (or social service) department should be organized to respond efficiently to service needs throughout the hospital. Both in-patient and ambulatory areas of the hospital should have plans for putting patients in touch with social services. Comprehensive patient care should incorporate psychosocial dimensions of illness. This is best achieved by utilizing the skills of the professional social work department.

References

Bracht NF. Social work in health care: A guide to professional practice. New York: Haworth Press, 1978.

Carlton TO, et al. Clinical social work in health settings: A guide to professional practice with exemplars. Springer Series on Social Work, vol. 4. New York: Springer, 1984.

Miller RS, Rehr H, eds. Social work issues in health care. Englewood Cliffs, NJ: Prentice-Hall, 1983.

Optimal Utilization of the Laboratory 9

The Clinical Chemistry Laboratory

F. John Krolikowski, MD

Thomas E. Ukena, MD, PhD

The modern clinical chemistry laboratory has developed numerous and complex procedures to aid the clinician in various approaches to the patient, including diagnostic testing, monitoring of physiologic functions, prognostic signs, and emergency patient care. This section considers the approaches to the chemistry laboratory that will maximize the effectiveness and productivity of the clinician.

Laboratory Function

Keys to optimal utilization of the laboratory include a basic knowledge of the functioning of the laboratory and an understanding of how information can be retrieved expeditiously (Table 9-1). The duties and activities of a laboratory may be found in most hospital laboratory manuals. These handbooks are usually present at nursing stations, administrative areas, and laboratories within the hospital. The contents usually include a listing of all tests and their synonyms; interpretive data, including reference ranges; use of tests and their limitations; and specimen requirements, such as tubes to be used to obtain a specific sample, minimum volumes required, methodology employed, interfering substances, and methods of transporting specimens to the laboratory. Also included in a laboratory manual are criteria for specimen rejection and specimen storage, and the types of reports that are generated and when they are charted. Other general information includes laboratory location and hours of operation as well as what to do in off hours in order to have specimens analyzed. Many institutions list the costs of tests.

Table 9-1 Clinical Chemistry Functions

Electrolyte determinations	Lipid and liproprotein profiles
Enzyme, protein, and carbohydrate analyses	Urine evaluation
Drug and toxicology testing	Arterial blood gas quantitation
Body fluid measurements	Hormone and trace-metal evaluation
Analysis of cerebrospinal, amniotic, and seminal fluids	Immunochemical determinations
Gastric and bowel content testing	

It is important to highlight certain aspects of laboratory functions in order to better utilize services. The time elapsed between submission of a sample to the laboratory and the reporting of results (the turnaround time) is variable, depending on the type of test, the status of the test order, and whether the test is performed within the hospital or must be sent to a second "reference" laboratory. Every chemistry laboratory offers a limited menu of tests that can be performed with a very rapid turnaround time. These tests are generally referred to as STAT tests and are performed immediately when the specimen reaches the laboratory. The use of STAT tests is intended only for emergency situations. Performance of tests on a STAT basis consumes inordinate amounts of time and materials and interrupts the normal flow of work in the laboratory. Because of these factors, STAT tests are, in general, more expensive. Most chemistry laboratories also offer many tests on a "do today" or "as soon as possible" basis, which generally indicates that the test result will be available within a few hours after the sample reaches the laboratory. The majority of clinical chemistry testing is done on a "routine" basis, in which results are available within 24 to 48 hours. This "routine" system allows testing of large numbers of patient specimens in a single batch, which is the most efficient and economical approach.

Only the largest chemistry laboratories perform most test procedures; most laboratories send many specimens to a reference laboratory. Turnaround times are usually 2 to 3 days. These large facilities also have manuals that provide information similar to that described in the chemistry laboratory manual.

Cost Containment

Increasing pressures toward cost containment are directed to the clinical chemistry laboratory; as a result, the quantity and type of tests ordered will be increasingly monitored by the laboratory administration and regulatory agencies. In general, excessive use of STAT testing and repetitive daily testing is discouraged. When deciding to order a specific test, the clinician should have in mind the purpose of the test and the way in which the test result will affect patient management. Consideration of these two criteria could eliminate unnecessary cost to the patient and increase efficiency and productivity of the laboratory (see Chapter 11, "Cost Containment"). In the future, justification for tests ordered will be mandatory. Texts such as those by Fischbach (1988), Statland (1983), Tilkian (1983), Wallach (1983), and Widmann (1983) are useful guides. In many cases, however, appropriate documentation for their recommendations is absent.

Laboratory Interpretation

Interpretation of a test value usually involves comparing it to a predetermined value, often referred to as the "normal" or "reference" range. (The latter term is preferred.) The reference range is obtained by testing samples from persons judged to be free of disease. It is set, in general, as the average (mean) test result from this group, plus or minus two standard deviations (SD). Although this method provides a convenient guide for comparison with patient results, two SD represents 95 percent of the population. Therefore, 5 percent of the disease-free group will have test values that fall outside this range (1 out of 20, 1/20). Also, not all patients with test results within the reference range are necessarily free of disease; other variables, such as age, may have to be considered. An interesting example is alkaline phosphatase, a serum enzyme that is elevated in growing children, then declines in adulthood, and slowly rises again with aging. Table 9-2 lists causes of test variabilities.

Direct interaction between the clinician and the clinical chemistry laboratory often occurs in the setting of an unexpectedly normal or abnormal test result. In most cases, skepticism is a wise response to laboratory data that are inconsistent with the overall clinical picture. Could the test value be the effect of analytical error? In general, the validity of the test results is assured by an elaborate system of intra- and interlaboratory quality control that is based on statistical analysis of daily test samples. Additionally, most laboratories have a confirmatory procedure to recheck inconsistent results at no additional charge to the patient. If the clinician is attempting to assess whether a changed test result in an individual patient is biologically significant, a good "rule of thumb" is that the results are biologically different (95 percent chance) if the test differs by more than three SD from the baseline (comparison) value.

Despite numerous checks and balances, errors can occur, although they are rare (Table 9-3). Thus, it is of critical importance for the care of individual patients that, in cases of unexpected normal or abnormal results, the physician consult with the clinical pathologist before altering therapy. Consultation should also take place in nonquantitative situations that require interpretation. The laboratory will then take the responsibility for verifying the result and obtaining additional testing as necessary.

Table 9-2 Parameters Associated with Test Variability

Age, sex, race
Exercise
Drugs
Posture
Specimen collection, preparation, processing, and storage
Analytical variation

Table 9-3 Considerations in Specimen Testing

Physician orders test
Nurse records order
Ward secretary prepares requisition
Requisition transmitted to laboratory
Patient identification
Phlebotomy
Specimen preparation
Specimen analysis
Quality control data analyzed
Report preparation
Report transmitted to floor
Report charted
Physician interprets results

Laboratory Reports

Two basic types of reports are issued by a chemistry laboratory. The *ward report* (*interim report*) is issued several times a day. It is a status report of the various laboratory test requests and results of the completed analyses. Abnormal results are highlighted. The *summary* or *cumulative report* summarizes the laboratory data on a given patient in a manner convenient for review and includes the results of tests taken several days previously. The format of this report differs from laboratory to laboratory.

Additional reports may include a *discharge summary report*, which is similar to the cumulative summary report. This report is generated only after all tests that have been ordered are completed.

Many institutions also provide a *report by doctor*. This is a summary of tests on ambulatory and, at some institutions, in-house patients, and it is either "preliminary" or "complete" based on the requested analyses. Generally, these reports are issued daily.

Telephone inquiries are discouraged, not only because of potential misinterpretations of oral reports but also because anything that limits access to the chemistry laboratory prevents true emergency calls from being acknowledged.

The clinical chemistry director reviews laboratory data daily. One mechanism used by some clinical pathologists is called the *delta check*, a sensitive device that compares percentage change between similar tests. For example, if a potassium value from the previous day(s) had changed by 15 percent or more, a review process would be instituted.

Panic values are preset limits for tests that represent results incompatible with normal physiology and require immediate action. The laboratory verifies the results and immediately notifies the clinician.

All specimens must be labeled with the following information: (1) patient name, (2) patient hospital number, (3) date and time specimen was collected, and (4) signature of the phlebotomist. This will help prevent misidentification and provide information necessary for appropriate testing and interpretation. An example is a drug level obtained from a patient who has the same name as another patient on a different floor; without *all* the previously noted information, a serious error could occur. Unlabeled specimens as well as specimens not in proper containers are not processed, and the physician is so notified.

Cerebrospinal fluid is a unique specimen that requires prompt delivery and processing in order to maintain quality patient care. This specimen should be taken to the appropriate laboratory as soon as possible and handed to a supervising technologist.

Sometimes a situation arises involving the clinical staff and the chemistry laboratory for which there is no apparent solution. Such cases should be referred to the director of chemistry or his or her designee, who is on call at all times.

Clinical chemistry is a dynamic field with a future that portends a more highly automated environment. Ordering of tests and reporting of results by computer as well as robotics are shaping our future laboratories. New technologies utilizing DNA probes and other methods are becoming standard procedures in most laboratories. Clinicians must keep abreast of these changes in order to maximize their efficiency and productivity.

References

Fischbach FT. A manual of laboratory diagnostic tests. 3rd ed. Philadelphia: JB Lippincott, 1988.

Henry JB, ed. Todd-Sanford-Davidsohn clinical diagnosis and management by laboratory methods. 17th ed. Philadelphia: WB Saunders, 1984.

Statland BE. Clinical decision levels for lab tests. 2nd ed. Oradell, NJ: Medical Economics, 1988.

Tietz NW, ed. Textbook of clinical chemistry. Philadelphia: WB Saunders, 1986.

Tilkian SM, Conover MB, Tilkian AG. Clinical implications of laboratory tests. 4th ed. St. Louis: CV Mosby, 1987.

Wallach J. Interpretation of diagnostic tests: A handbook synopsis of laboratory medicine. 4th ed. Boston: Little, Brown, 1986.

Widmann FK. Clinical interpretation of laboratory tests. 9th ed. Philadelphia: FA Davis, 1983.

Handling of Laboratory Specimens

Richard I. Rothstein, MD

Brian J. Keroack, MD

Diagnosing a patient's problem(s) requires integration of the history, physical examination, and relevant laboratory data. The utility of the laboratory data is directly related to their reliability. Therefore, it is incumbent upon the health care team to limit sources of error that can make laboratory data less reliable and diagnosis more difficult. Sources of error include (1) incorrect preparation of the patient (i.e., special diet, drug ingestion history, informed consent), (2) improper collection techniques (i.e., position of the patient at collection, aseptic or anaerobic techniques), (3) improper handling of the laboratory specimens (i.e., methods of transport, storage), and (4) inappropriate laboratory processing of the sample (i.e., human or machine error). This chapter focuses on the proper handling of laboratory specimens.

Specimen collection involves procedures that are sometimes invasive and often unpleasant. Unnecessary repetition of such procedures (because of disorganization or improper labeling, handling, or transport) not only increases the risk of complication but also does not endear you to the patient! Therefore, before a patient is subjected to collection procedures, it is imperative to plan carefully all of the tests to be conducted on the specimens obtained. All tubes, containers, swabs, slides, and other equipment needed for proper collection should be obtained before the time of specimen collection. If required, special fixatives, culture media (i.e., viral, Thayer-Martin agar) or ice should be ready at hand.

Successful collection is only the first step. Proper processing of specimens requires labeling by the collector, with date, time of collection, and identifying data (patient name, physician, location, and hospital number). Furthermore, all specimens should be bagged as part of the universal blood and body fluid precautions recommended by the Centers for Disease Control. Although some specimens, such as admission venipuncture or a urine culture, can be sent to the lab via the routine channels, specimens obtained by "invasive methods" (i.e., lumbar puncture, paracentesis, thoracentesis, transtracheal aspirate) must be hand delivered. Such techniques should **never** have to be repeated because the specimen was lost en route. After prompt delivery to the laboratory, attention should be focused on correct storage of the specimens in the laboratory, such as the need for centrifugation, incubation, or refrigeration.

Blood Specimens

Whole blood consists of cellular elements and plasma. The straw-colored supernatant left when the cellular elements clot is *serum*. When whole blood is anticoagulated, then centrifuged, the supernatant is *plasma*. Certain testing procedures require whole blood (e.g., complete blood count) or plasma, while others use serum (electrolytes). Attention to these needs will determine whether the blood sample should be collected with or without anticoagulant. Most blood samples may be collected from either venipuncture or arterial puncture; however, a few tests require arterial blood (e.g., blood gases, serum ammonia). The most common tests performed on blood samples are listed in Table 9-4.

Specimens for a complete blood count (CBC) should be processed within 1 to 2 hours after collection; while stored, they require constant mixing. Blood samples for CBC should be drawn into a tube containing ethylenediaminetetraacetic acid (EDTA) (purple-top tube). This same anticoagulant is used for sample collections for the erythrocyte sedimentation rate (ESR), because other anticoagulants will affect the cell size and hence the ESR. Refrigeration of the sample for ESR determination, without allowing it to rewarm fully before testing, will increase the viscosity and falsely lower the value.

A critical and often overlooked facet in assessing whole blood is examination of the peripheral smear. The smear is a thin layer of whole blood on a slide that has been Wright's stained to highlight the cellular elements. It should be viewed under oil immersion for size, shape, and characteristics of all of

Table 9-4 Tests Commonly Performed on Blood Samples

Whole Blood
Blood cultures
Complete blood count
Differential blood count
Reticulocyte count
Platelet count
Erythrocyte sedimentation rate
Plasma
Prothrombin time
Partial thromboplastin time
Cold agglutinins
Serum
Electrolytes (sodium, potassium, chloride, bicarbonate)
Chemistry profiles
Renal function tests (blood urea nitrogen, creatinine)
Liver function tests (SGOT [AST], SGPT [ALT], alkaline phosphatase, gamma glutamyl transpeptidase, bilirubin)
Thyroid function tests (T_4, T_3 resin uptake, TSH)
Cardiac enzymes (LDH, CPK, SGOT [AST])
Visceral proteins (albumin, transferrin, total protein, protein electrophoresis)
Pancreatic tests (amylase, lipase)
Rheumatologic tests (RF, ANA, aldolase, CRP)
Metabolic tests (glucose, lactate, ammonia, cholesterol, calcium, phosphorus, magnesium, uric acid)
Vitamin and mineral levels (B_{12}, folate, iron, total iron-binding capacity, vitamin D)
Endocrine, oncologic, and infectious disease tests (hormone levels, alpha-fetoprotein)
Drug levels (antibiotics, cardiac medications, salicylate, overdose determinations)
Arterial Blood
Arterial blood gases
Ammonia
Carboxyhemoglobin

Abbreviations: ALT = alanine aminotransferase, ANA = antinuclear antibody, AST = aspartate aminotransferase, CPK = creatine phosphokinase, CRP = C-reactive protein, LDH = lactate dehydrogenase, RF = rheumatoid factor, SGOT = serum glutamic-oxaloacetic transaminase, SGPT = serum glutamic-pyruvic transaminase, TSH = thyroid-stimulating hormone.

the cell types. Proper diagnosis and management of hematologic abnormalities may hinge on information obtained when viewing the smear.

Coagulation Studies

Determinations of the prothrombin time (PT) and partial thromboplastin time (PTT) are done on blood collected into tubes containing 3.2 percent sodium citrate (blue-top tube). The collection tubes must be filled accurately with the correct volume, because overfilling or underfilling will alter the determinations of these clotting parameters. The specimen does not have to be stored or transported on ice, provided that the ambient temperature does not vary substantially from room temperature.

Determinations of fibrinogen or fibrin degradation products are done on samples collected in a tube containing thrombin to enhance clotting and trypsin inhibitor to prevent fibrin degradation in the specimen after collection ("special" blue-top tube).

Cryoglobulin protein studies should be performed on serum or plasma that is maintained at body temperature from the time of collection until the time of testing. Blood drawn into a prewarmed syringe should be placed into the appropriate tubes and transported directly to the lab while immersed in a warm bath. Cryoglobulin and cryofibrinogen studies are done at 40°C. A "bedside" test for cold agglutinins can be done by immersing a blue-top tube of blood into ice water for 15 to 30 minutes. Agglutination within that time is a positive test.

Chemistry Specimens

Blood chemistry analysis is done on serum (red-top tubes). One common problem in the handling of blood specimens for chemical determinations is hemolysis of red blood cells at the time of, or subsequent to, collection. Hemolysis causes elevations of the levels of serum potassium, phosphorus, and lactic dehydrogenase. Care must be taken when transferring blood from a syringe into the stoppered vacuum tubes, because forceful injection or handling or use of too small a needle can cause hemolysis. Prolonged storage of blood samples can also alter test results; for example, glycolytic bacteria or an elevated leukocyte count can falsely lower the level of glucose in blood samples held in storage for excessive periods. To combat this problem, some hospitals utilize a gray-top tube containing potassium oxalate and sodium fluoride, which arrest the metabolic processes that lead to a decrease in the measured glucose. In addition, delayed processing of samples from patients with severe thrombocytosis can falsely elevate serum potassium.

Aseptic techniques must be used while handling whole blood drawn for cultures. One set of blood cultures, aerobic and anaerobic, results from one venipuncture insertion at one site. To avoid bacteriostasis by faulty technique, allow the antiseptic (used to clean the rubber stoppers) to dry completely before inserting the needle into the media bottles. Some hospitals now use a "vacutainer" culture tube, which becomes one set of cultures when divided in the lab into the appropriate media. When separate bottles are used, needles should be changed between skin puncture and entry into the bottles to avoid possible contamination with skin organisms.

Arterial Blood Gases

Arterial blood for blood gas analysis is drawn into a syringe containing a small amount of heparin. After all the air bubbles are carefully expelled, the needle is removed and the syringe is capped and placed on ice. In general, glass syringes should be used, because oxygen has been shown to diffuse out of standard plastic syringes, even within 60 seconds after collection; however, special plastic syringes that resist oxygen diffusion are acceptable. Enough blood should be allowed to enter the syringe to eliminate the effect of heparin dilution in a small sample (reduction of P_{CO_2} and bicarbonate). Blood should enter the syringe spontaneously and actively and not be aspirated during the collection, which might artificially raise the oxygen content (P_{O_2}). Icing the sample arrests cellular metabolism and prevents spurious hypoxemia. Even when the sample is stored on ice, however, "leukocyte larceny" has been shown to be a cause of spurious hypoxemia in patients with extreme leukocytosis.

Urine Samples

Skillful interpretation of the urinalysis is a crucial step in the differential diagnosis of renal disease; however, urine samples are often neglected or analyzed casually. The result is a "rubber stamp" urinalysis report to the physician: occasional red blood cells, white blood cells, few hyaline casts (Levinsky, 1967). This leads the clinician to believe that urinalysis is of little value. On the contrary, urinalysis almost always reveals renal parenchymal disease when it is present.

Urine can be collected in many ways: spontaneous voiding, catheter specimen, or percutaneous bladder aspiration. Specimens for culture should be obtained aseptically or by "clean catch." Once collected, urine should be examined within an hour, preferably while the specimen is still warm. Gross inspection should include observation of color, amount, odor, and clarity. Specific gravity should be measured on a warm sample, as refrigeration spuriously elevates this value. The urine dipstick provides information about pH and the presence of protein, glucose, occult blood, ketones, bilirubin, and leukocytes. Some new dipsticks even give an estimate of specific gravity. If proteinuria is suspected but the dipstick results are negative, the sample can be exposed to 5 percent sulfosalicylic acid to precipitate protein (albumin). In multiple myeloma, light-chain proteins can be precipitated by the Bence-Jones method (boiling and acidification with acetic acid); however, urine electrophoresis is frequently required for definitive diagnosis.

For examination of cellular elements, the urine is swirled gently, placed in a 12-cc centrifuge tube, and spun at full speed for 5 minutes. Once the supernatant is carefully discarded, the small button of cellular elements at the bottom of the tube is resuspended by gently tapping the side of the tube with a finger. A Pasteur-type pipette can be used to transfer the material to a slide. A coverslip is then placed over the sample. Examination should begin under low-power/low-light microscopy and proceed to high dry (45×) microscopy to identify important elements (i.e., casts, cells, or crystals). Errors in this process can occur from inadequate sediment resuspension, contamination with foreign material, drying of the specimen on the slide, and refrigeration, which alters cellular elements and causes precipitation of $CaPO_4$ crystals, obscuring cellular elements.

Collection of urine over 24 hours requires the addition of a preservative, which varies depending on the substances being tested. The specific needs for each determination should be clarified with the investigating laboratory.

Sputum

The first examination of sputum was recorded in the fifth century BC. At that time, Hippocrates' gross observations of the sputum included color, taste, and smell. Today it is clear that gross inspection does correlate with microscopic observations. Thus, inspection of sputum for amount, color, odor, consistency, and presence of blood has a scientific basis (Henry, 1984).

Collection of sputum, as a rule, requires a cooperative patient. If sputum induction or transtracheal aspiration is required to collect sputum, nonbacteriostatic saline must be employed to preserve the flora. The specimen should be collected in a sterile, impermeable container with a tight-fitting lid or cover, and should be processed as soon as possible. Specimens awaiting microbiologic analysis should be refrigerated. A variety of examinations are performed on a sputum specimen, including routine culture and Gram stain, special stains and cultures (acid fast, fungal, viral), and Wright's stain and cytologic examination. Pulmonary secretions must be differentiated from saliva before these tests are performed. In 1974, Bartlett defined a "culture-worthy" sputum as one having fewer than 25 epithelial cells and more than 10 leukocytes per 100× power field. On cytologic examination, the presence of alveolar macrophages indicates an adequate sample.

Although Gram stain of sputum is frequently done by lab personnel, the physician should review the smear. Unfortunately, interpretation of Gram stains is fraught with difficulty. The best correlation between Gram stain and sputum culture exists with gram-positive organisms (62 percent in one study) (Rein et al., 1978). Gram-negative organisms are frequently overlooked because nonbacterial elements stain gram-negative. Under- or overdecolorization of the smear can also affect interpretation.

When malignancy is suspected, cytologic examination of sputum is indicated. Yield is best if a single early-morning, deep-cough sputum is obtained for three to five consecutive mornings. As noted previously, the presence of alveolar macrophages indicates a good specimen. Wright's staining of sputum can yield information about nonmalignant bronchopulmonary diseases (e.g., eosinophils in asthma).

Synovial Fluid

These fluids, which are obtained by sterile aspiration, should be processed with minimal delay. Repetition of this uncomfortable procedure can be obviated by pretest planning and proper handling. Although color, clarity, viscosity, and mucin clots should be recorded, Gram stain and crystal analysis are the two tests that help with immediate diagnosis of acute arthritis (Ward, 1988).

Clinicians often need to tailor tests on synovial fluid according to the amount aspirated (clearly, a large knee effusion will yield more fluid than a wrist effusion). Therefore, if a small volume is obtained, it is best to use a few drops for cell count and differential, a few drops for crystal analysis, and a few drops for bacteriologic examination. If a larger volume is aspirated, Ward (1988) suggests the following:

1. Instill 2 to 5 ml in a sterile heparinized test tube, and send it immediately for culture. If gonococcal infection is suspected, plate immediately in chocolate agar for carbon dioxide incubation.
2. Instill another 2 to 5 ml in a tube with sodium heparin for total and differential white blood cell counts and crystal examination.
3. Place 3 to 5 ml of fluid in a test tube with fluoride for estimation of its glucose content.
4. Use 2 to 5 ml in a tube without anticoagulant to evaluate the fluid for specific macroscopic and microscopic features.

Microscopic examination for crystals should be done on a freshly obtained specimen, because leukocyte digestion of crystals will decrease the yield over time. If the sample is not processed quickly, its glucose concentration will decrease as a result of white blood cell catabolism, especially with very pronounced elevations of leukocytes.

The complete cell count and Gram stain should be reviewed by the clinician obtaining the synovial fluid, in order to interpret the results in the clinical setting.

Cerebrospinal Fluid

Although relatively simple to perform, the collection of cerebrospinal fluid (CSF) by lumbar puncture involves invasive techniques and patient discomfort. Using sterile technique, the spinal needle is introduced. Once the opening pressure is measured, 6 to 8 ml of CSF is removed and inspected for color and clarity. The CSF is collected in four separate tubes. Generally, the first and fourth tubes are sent for cell count and differential. The second and third tubes are sent for biochemical analysis (glucose, protein, immunoglobulins), bacteriologic analysis (Gram stain, culture, viral culture or stains, and, if indicated, latex agglutination or counterimmunoelectrophoresis for bacterial or fungal antigens), serology (VDRL), and cytology.

Performing cell counts on fluid in the first and last tubes collected can help to clarify the problem of the "traumatic" spinal tap. A traumatic tap differs from hemorrhagic spinal fluid (i.e., subarachnoid bleeding) in two respects: (1) the number of red blood cells will be roughly the same in the first and last tubes collected in true cerebrospinal bleeding, whereas the number of red cells should be diminished significantly in the final tube collected after a traumatic tap; and (2) following centrifugation, the CSF will be xanthochromic when blood has been present in the fluid for at least 8 to 12 hours, whereas the supernatant will be clear after a traumatic spinal tap.

As with other body fluids, the clinician performing the collection should review the Gram stain as soon as it is prepared. In addition, the cell count, if not performed by the clinician, should be reviewed as soon as it is completed.

Cavitary Fluids

Like lumbar punctures, paracentesis and thoracentesis are invasive procedures that are often uncomfortable for the patient. Special care should be taken to avoid unnecessary repetition of these procedures. Once fluid is collected, it should be inspected for color, clarity, amount, and color. Fluid is sent in the appropriate tubes for total and differential cell counts, chemical analysis as indicated (sugar, protein, lactate dehydrogenase, amylase, lactate, pH, rheumatoid factor), cytology, Gram stain, acid-fast bacillus stain, and routine and special cultures. Concurrent serum samples will need to be obtained for selected chemistries in order to compare serum to fluid levels. Fluid for complete cell count should be put into an EDTA-containing tube (purple-top tube) for transport. Samples for pH determination are transported in heparinized glass syringes, stoppered and on ice. Chemistry and culture tubes have no additives and are treated in an aseptic fashion. Anaerobic samples are to be stoppered after all the air is removed from a syringe, and taken directly to the lab for processing.

It is common practice to add heparin, up to 3 units per milliliter of fluid, to the specimens for cytologic investigation, in order to prevent agglutination of the cellular elements. Some labs, however, prefer that the cells clump, which may facilitate the cellular analysis. Discuss this issue with the lab before initiating the collection.

Stool

Stool obtained by recent defecation or digital rectal examination is recorded for color, consistency, presence of gross blood or mucus, and presence of occult blood. Fecal occult blood test tapes and cards rely on a guaiac-peroxidase reaction that turns the paper blue in 30 to 60 seconds in the presence of blood-containing stool exposed to hydrogen peroxide developer. To maximize the reliability of this test, it is important that the developer and cards not be used after their expiration dates. The cards should be developed as soon as possible after collection, although the manufacturer (Hemoccult) states that they may be stored for up to 12 days before developing.

Freshly collected stool specimens should be transported to the lab with little delay for determinations of the presence of ova and parasites, fecal leukocytes, qualitative fat, or *Campylobacter* forms and for routine or special cultures. Special cultures (e.g., *Yersinia*) require notificaton of the lab personnel for proper processing, and this should be clearly indicated on microbiology requisition slips. *Clostridium difficile* titers are helpful when pseudomembranous colitis is suspected.

Enteric Fluids

Indications for gastric juice analysis include documenting recent or active hemorrhage, evaluating the degree or presence of acid, and performing toxic screen analysis after planned or accidental ingestions.

Gastric fluid is recorded for obvious blood, either fresh or the acid-bathed "coffee grounds," pH, bile, and guaiac testing. Following an overdose, gastric contents are sent to the lab for drug analysis in an additive-free container. Testing for pH can be done at the bedside with a commercially available paper tape and pH color scale.

Testing for occult blood, utilizing the guaiac cards used for fecal occult blood, may require the addition of 0.1 N sodium hydroxide to neutralize gastric acid, which if unbuffered might alter the peroxidase reaction.

Duodenal fluid, called succus entericus, is analyzed for parasitic or bacterial infection, depending on the clinical situation. Fluids obtained by intubated aspirate or on a "string" test can be quickly transported to the lab to be examined for *Giardia* organisms. Duodenal fluid can also be obtained, utilizing careful endoscopic technique, and processed for routine and anaerobic cultures in the work-up of malabsorption that is presumed to be due to bacterial overgrowth. Fluid is carried to the lab in a stoppered, sterile, air-free syringe.

Vaginal Secretions

A swab of vaginal contents can be placed on two slides. Both potassium hydroxide (KOH) and saline are added, and then the slides are coverslipped and examined under high-dry power. The KOH slide is viewed for the presence of fungal forms. The wet preparation is analyzed for the presence of trichomonads or clue cells (*Haemophilus vaginalis*). These findings, if present, will direct the therapy for abnormal vaginal discharge (see Chapter 162, "Vaginitis").

Vaginal secretions should be cultured when toxic shock syndrome or pelvic inflammatory disease (PID) is suspected. *Neisseria gonorrhoeae* and *Chlamydia*, the two most common pathogens in PID, are collected in a specific fashion. *Chlamydia* cultures are obtained using a cotton-tipped wire swab and are placed in a special medium. *N. gonorrhoeae* cultures are obtained with standard swabs and are quickly plated onto chocolate agar. The Papanicolaou smear of cervical and vaginal samples requires immediate fixing of the cellular material after placement on clean, dry slides, with subsequent transport to the cytology laboratory for interpretation.

Semen

Special techniques are required for semen analysis, which is often done as a part of fertility studies or to determine the effectiveness of vasectomies. A clean, sterile glass vial is used for collection of the sample. The specimen should be analyzed promptly, and it should be handled and stored at body temperature until examination.

Biopsy Specimens

Most specimens are sent to the histology laboratories after placement in formalin. Small samples are placed on Gelfoam, with attention paid to correct orientation of the material. This is important for skin and small biopsies, in which analysis of the specimen requires specific cutting of the sample.

Specimens may also be divided for placement in glutaraldehyde for future electron-microscopic processing, and in sterile containers for routine or special stain and culture. Some laboratories use Carnoy's fixative for liver biopsies instead of formalin; this should be determined before obtaining the specimen. Liver biopsies for quantitative iron determination (i.e., suspected hemochromatosis) need to be transported in an iron-free buffer and jar. Liver biopsy specimens for copper determinations (i.e., Wilson's disease) must be transported in copper-free solution and container. Discuss these special requirements with the laboratory before initiating the procedure.

Skin scrapings can be looked at with KOH for fungal elements or with saline for scabies. Samples from a skin vesicle can be dried on a slide and processed on the Wright's staining machine and then reviewed as a Tzanck smear for multinucleated giant cells or inclusions.

Miscellaneous Cultures

In order to avoid desiccation of the specimen, material obtained from throat, urethral, cervical, or nasal swab or from an abscess or wound must be transported to the microbiology lab without delay for Gram stain and routine and special cultures. In some clinical settings, a culture tube is used in which the swab is transported sealed and immersed in a sterile medium. In the lab, the specimen is then placed on specific media (Thayer-Martin, fungal, viral, routine bacterial). Material for culture may be inhibited by bacteriostatic saline if it is used during the collection process; therefore, nonbacteriostatic saline should be used for collection and transport.

References

Chodosh S. Examination of sputum cells. N Engl J Med 1970; 282:854.

Fox MJ, et al. Leukocyte larceny: A cause of spurious hypoxemia. Am J Med 1979; 67:742.

Hansen JE, Simmons DH. A systematic error in the determination of blood PCO_2. Am Rev Respir Dis 1977; 115:1061.

Harbell RA, Frestein GS. The effective scutboy. New York: Anco Publishing, 1981.

Henry JB, ed. Todd-Sanford-Davidsohn clinical diagnosis and management by laboratory methods. 17th ed. Philadelphia: WB Saunders, 1984.

Janis KM, Fletcher G. Oxygen tension measurements in small samples. Am Rev Respir Dis 1979; 106:914.

Levinsky NG. The interpretation of proteinuria and the urinary sediment. Disease-a-Month. March 1967.

Miale JB. Laboratory medicine: Hematology. 6th ed. St. Louis: CV Mosby, 1982.

Page LB, Culver PJ. Laboratory examinations in clinical diagnosis. Cambridge, MA: Harvard University Press, 1966.

Rein MF, et al. Accuracy of Gram's stain in identifying pneumococcus in sputum. JAMA 1978; 239:2671.

VanderSalm TJ, et al. Atlas of bedside procedures. 2nd ed. Boston: Little, Brown, 1988.

Wallach J. Interpretation of diagnostic tests. 4th ed. Boston: Little, Brown, 1986.

Ward JR. Achieving optimal diagnostic yield from arthrocentesis. Emerg Med Rep 1988; 9(22).

Anatomic Pathology: Biopsy and Cytology

Carolyn C. Compton, MD, PhD

Biopsy

For many disease processes, the biopsy is the "gold standard" of diagnosis. For some disorders, especially malignancies, the biopsy is an absolute prerequisite to specific therapy. The amount of information derived from the biopsy and the accuracy of the diagnosis depend on three major factors: (1) the skill of the pathologist, (2) the pathologist's knowledge of the clinical features of the case, and (3) the quality of the specimen he or she must interpret. The latter two ingredients depend greatly on the person taking and submitting the biopsy specimen.

Taking the Biopsy Specimen: Points to Remember

1. Be sure to get *enough* tissue. Adequacy of the specimen is essential; this may mean obtaining either a generous piece of a focal lesion or multiple small "random" samples of a diffuse process. Especially if the process is suspected to be inflammatory, samples should include areas that appear less clinically involved to evaluate the early features of the disease. Specimens taken from the interface between the visible lesion and the surrounding "normal" tissue are frequently most helpful to the pathologist, especially with skin lesions.

2. Be sure to get the *proper* tissue. If you are not certain you have succeeded in obtaining the desired tissue or an adequate sample, you may wish to call a pathologist to examine the specimen. Frozen section may be required for confirmation.

3. Place the tissue in proper fixative **as soon as possible**. Be **gentle** in handling the tissue and do **not** allow the tissue to dry out. Directions for submitting specific tissues appear in the section "Handling of Specimens," but if you are uncertain or if a delay in proper disposition arises, place the specimen on a piece of saline-moistened filter paper in a covered Petri dish and call the pathologist to help you.

Informing the Pathologist

Fill out the pathology request form fully and accurately, providing an adequate history and pertinent lab and radiographic findings. A histologic appearance may raise a differential diagnosis, just as a clinical presentation might. Knowledge of the clinical parameters of the patient's illness is required for accurate interpretation of the specimen. Be sure to indicate the clinical diagnosis on the request form. Failure to provide this information may delay the pathology report.

If the specimen represents a diagnostic emergency, let the pathologist know by either calling ahead of time or writing "Rush" on the request form, or both.

Handling of Specimens

In all cases, label the specimen containers clearly and accurately, exactly as the specimens are listed on the pathology request form. The label should include the patient's name, unit number, name of physician sending specimen, and clinical diagnosis. By including your phone number and paging unit (beeper) number, you can ensure more rapid feedback.

Specific Types of Biopsies

Bone Marrow Biopsy. Depending on the institution, routine bone marrow biopsies may be submitted in 10 percent formalin or in Zenker's solution (a fixative with mercuric chloride). Check with the pathologist for special instructions. Because they require time-consuming decalcification, bone marrow biopsies should be submitted as early in the day as possible for processing. Otherwise, the diagnosis may be delayed. Check with the pathologist about time constraints on processing.

Endomyocardial Biopsy. Place directly into EM fixative, which can be obtained from the pathology laboratory.

Endoscopic Gastrointestinal Biopsies. Submit in 10 percent formalin on filter paper. If possible, orient the specimen with the mucosal side up and the base of the resected sample down. This is most important for small-bowel biopsies. Biopsy samples from separate sites or lesions of interest should be submitted in separate containers.

Liver Biopsy. Submit in 10 percent formalin on filter paper.

Lung Biopsy. Lung biopsies may be endoscopic, transbronchial, or percutaneous. For information on bronchial brushings and washings, see the section on cytology. If immunologic lung disease is suspected, a frozen section may be required for immunofluorescent staining for immunoglobulins and complement; call the pathologist. Otherwise, submit in 10 percent formalin on filter paper.

Lymph Node Biopsy. Notify the pathologist, because these samples require special handling. The tissue should be examined fresh by the pathologist, and if infectious disease is suspected, portions should be selected under sterile conditions for cultures. A portion may be frozen for T- and B-lymphocyte marker studies if a hematologic malignancy is suspected. A portion may be fixed in glutaraldehyde for electron microscopy, particularly if metastatic disease is suspected. The remainder will be fixed in formalin for routine histology and special stains.

Pleural Biopsy. Submit in 10 percent formalin.

Renal Biopsy. Notify the pathologist; these specimens require special handling. The fresh biopsy will be partitioned for immunofluorescent studies, electron microscopy, and light microscopy. These studies require frozen tissue, glutaraldehyde, fixed tissue, and formalin-fixed tissue, respectively.

Skin Biopsy (Punch or Curettage). Submit in 10 percent formalin, unless bullous disease, lymphoma, autoimmune disease, or immune-complex disease is suspected. In these cases, immunohistochemical studies require fresh frozen tissue.

Tumor Biopsy. The parameters vary widely here. Especially if the tumor is metastatic from an unknown primary lesion, tissue must be set aside for electron microscopy, immunohistochemistry, and light microscopy. This means keeping the tissue moist (not wet) until the pathologist arrives to prepare the tissue. As described earlier, place the tissue on a piece of saline-moistened filter paper in a covered Petri dish until the pathologist comes. It is essential that the exact location and gross description of the tumor be communicated to the pathologist.

Synovial Biopsy. Place in 10 percent formalin.

Reports

The schedule of reading biopsies varies from institution to institution. In general, more time (about 12 to 24 hours) is required for reports to be issued in teaching institutions than in private facilities, because pathology house officers read the slides prior to official sign-out of cases with a staff pathologist. In any case, rush samples (diagnostic biopsies) are usually read the following day. Weekend delays may be a problem in institutions that do not provide technical staffing on weekends.

Immediate verbal communication of the diagnosis can be provided by the pathologist, if your name and a way of reaching you (phone extension or page code) are written on the pathology request form along with your request for such action. If you wish to review the slides with the pathologist, call ahead to the department and set an appointment. Inquiries at night or on weekends should be directed to the pathology house officer on call in teaching institutions or to the staff pathologist on call in private institutions.

Cytology

Cytologic examination can often substitute for biopsies in diagnosis. Material for cytology requires half the preparation time of biopsy material as well as far less biologic material. It also has the advantage of providing the ability to examine the cell content of body fluids. Table 9-5 lists the types of materials that can be examined by cytologic techniques.

Handling of Specimens

Adhere to the following guidelines when handling any type of specimen:

1. Do not add fixatives or heparin to any cytology specimen.
2. Send only fresh material.
3. Label specimen containers or prepared slides with the patient's name and medical record number.
4. Complete the cytology request form (Fig. 9-1) and provide clinical information.
5. Transport the specimen immediately to the cytology laboratory, if possible; otherwise, refrigerate it to preserve cell morphology.

Types of Cytologic Specimens

Breast Secretions. Spread on slide and fix immediately with 95 percent ethanol or Aquanet hair spray (available at most drug stores).

Table 9-5 Materials Examined by Cytologic Techniques

Fluids	**Scrapings of Surface Cells**
Spinal fluid	Cervical epithelium
Pleural effusion	Bronchial washings
Ascites	Gastrointestinal mucosa
Joint fluid	
Pericardial effusion	**Fine-Needle Aspirations**
Cyst fluid (any source)	Percutaneous lung biopsies
Bronchial and gastric washings	Thyroid biopsies
Cul de sac fluid	Breast biopsies
Urine	

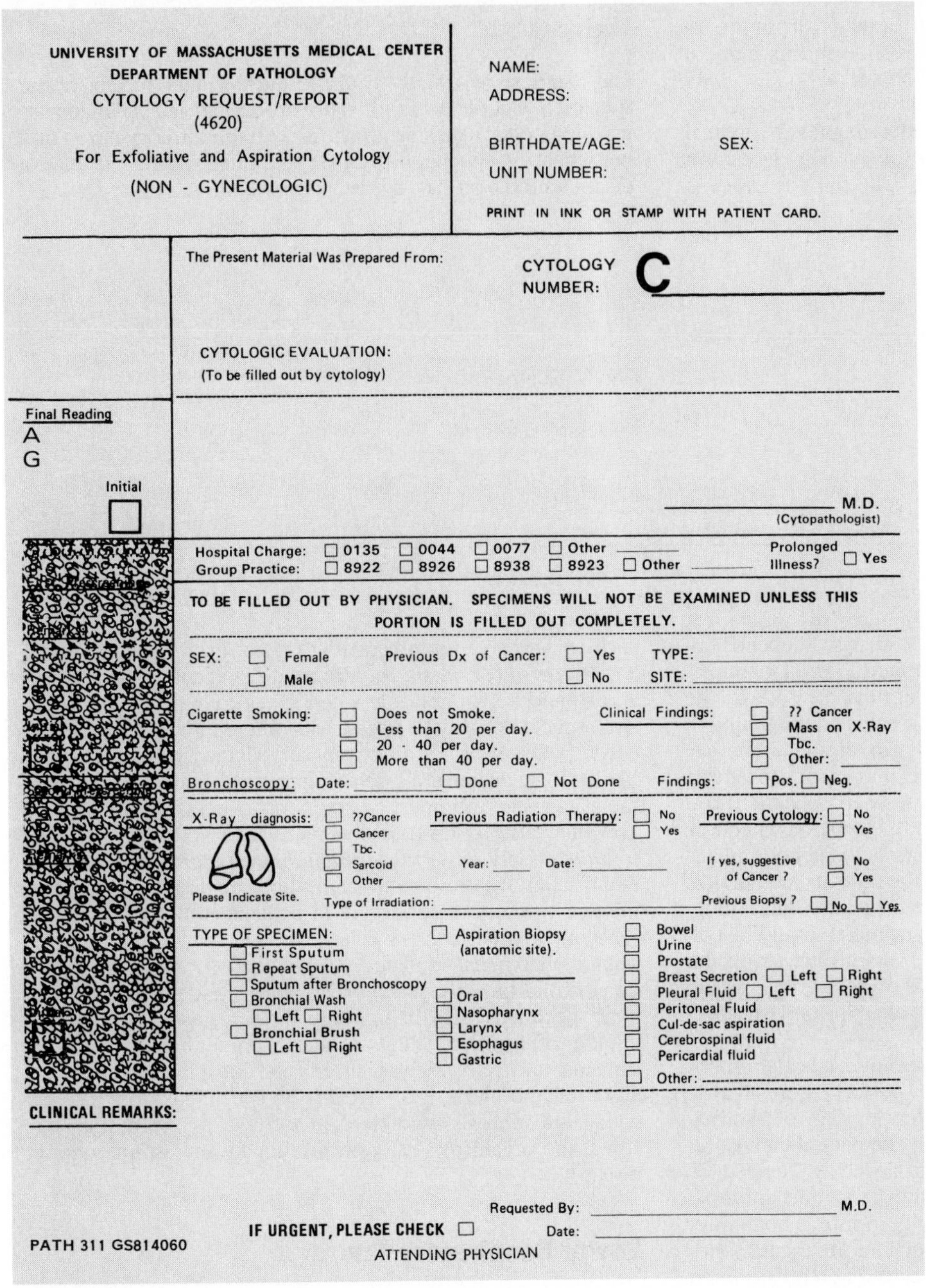
UNIVERSITY OF MASSACHUSETTS MEDICAL CENTER
DEPARTMENT OF PATHOLOGY
CYTOLOGY REQUEST/REPORT
(4620)
For Exfoliative and Aspiration Cytology
(NON - GYNECOLOGIC)

NAME:
ADDRESS:
BIRTHDATE/AGE: SEX:
UNIT NUMBER:
PRINT IN INK OR STAMP WITH PATIENT CARD.

The Present Material Was Prepared From:
CYTOLOGY NUMBER: C

CYTOLOGIC EVALUATION:
(To be filled out by cytology)

Final Reading
A
G
Initial

M.D.
(Cytopathologist)

Hospital Charge: ☐ 0135 ☐ 0044 ☐ 0077 ☐ Other
Group Practice: ☐ 8922 ☐ 8926 ☐ 8938 ☐ 8923 ☐ Other
Prolonged Illness? ☐ Yes

TO BE FILLED OUT BY PHYSICIAN. SPECIMENS WILL NOT BE EXAMINED UNLESS THIS PORTION IS FILLED OUT COMPLETELY.

SEX: ☐ Female ☐ Male
Previous Dx of Cancer: ☐ Yes ☐ No
TYPE:
SITE:

Cigarette Smoking: ☐ Does not Smoke. ☐ Less than 20 per day. ☐ 20 - 40 per day. ☐ More than 40 per day.
Clinical Findings: ☐ ?? Cancer ☐ Mass on X-Ray ☐ Tbc. ☐ Other:
Bronchoscopy: Date: ☐ Done ☐ Not Done Findings: ☐ Pos. ☐ Neg.

X-Ray diagnosis: ☐ ??Cancer ☐ Cancer ☐ Tbc. ☐ Sarcoid ☐ Other
Please Indicate Site.
Previous Radiation Therapy: ☐ No ☐ Yes
Year: Date:
Type of Irradiation:
Previous Cytology: ☐ No ☐ Yes
If yes, suggestive of Cancer ? ☐ No ☐ Yes
Previous Biopsy ? ☐ No ☐ Yes

TYPE OF SPECIMEN:
☐ First Sputum
☐ Repeat Sputum
☐ Sputum after Bronchoscopy
☐ Bronchial Wash ☐ Left ☐ Right
☐ Bronchial Brush ☐ Left ☐ Right
☐ Aspiration Biopsy (anatomic site).
☐ Oral
☐ Nasopharynx
☐ Larynx
☐ Esophagus
☐ Gastric
☐ Bowel
☐ Urine
☐ Prostate
☐ Breast Secretion ☐ Left ☐ Right
☐ Pleural Fluid ☐ Left ☐ Right
☐ Peritoneal Fluid
☐ Cul-de-sac aspiration
☐ Cerebrospinal fluid
☐ Pericardial fluid
☐ Other:

CLINICAL REMARKS:

Requested By: M.D.
IF URGENT, PLEASE CHECK ☐ Date:
ATTENDING PHYSICIAN
PATH 311 GS814060

Figure 9-1 Cytology request form.

Brush Samples. Spread cell film on slide and fix immediately in 95 percent ethanol or Aquanet hair spray. Send the brushes themselves to cytology in saline.

Fine-Needle Aspirates. For optimal results, it is recommended that a cytotechnologist be on hand to assist during this procedure. If no cytotechnologist is available, slides should be processed as follows:

1. Aspirate material from tissue, expel onto labeled glass slides (previously labeled), and spread with another slide as though it is a blood film.
2. Fix immediately with 95 percent ethanol or Aquanet hair spray. If a lymphoma or leukemia is suspected, one air-dried slide should be made.
3. After making whatever number of slides the amount of cell material permits, aspirate approximately 3 ml of saline through the needle into the syringe.
4. Remove the needle from the syringe and label the syringe with the patient's name and medical record number.
5. Bring the prepared slides and the syringe to the laboratory.

Fluids (Other Than Urine). Send 300 to 1,000 ml (typically an optimal specimen); otherwise, send whatever is available. Also, note that vacuum packs do *not* yield adequate specimens because degeneration occurs at room temperature.

Urine. Fresh specimens are optimal. Twenty-four-hour urine collections are *not* useful because of cell degeneration and bacterial growth.

Papanicolaou Smears. Samples should be taken from the vagina, cervix, and endocervix. Spread on slide and fix immediately in 95 percent ethanol or Aquanet hair spray.

Sputum. Three consecutive cough sputum samples are optimal. The fresh samples should be sent to the cytology laboratory immediately. Twenty-four-hour sputum collections are *not* useful because of degeneration of cells.

The Diagnosis

The diagnosis is usually available the day after receipt of the specimen. Cut-off times for daily processing of specimens are usually in effect. Be sure to check with the cytology lab to find out when the specimen must be submitted in order to have a diagnosis the next day, if this is important.

The Clinical Bacteriology Laboratory

Gary V. Doern, PhD

Nelson M. Gantz, MD

The value of essentially all bacteriologic analyses depends entirely on the quality of specimen submitted to the laboratory. The quality of an individual specimen, in turn, depends on the manner in which it is collected, in some cases on the timing of collection, on the volume of specimen obtained, and on the way it is transported to the laboratory. Specimens come in three general forms: tissue, fluid, and swabs. Swab specimens are usually the least appropriate and should be avoided whenever possible. Because the human host harbors an indigenous microflora that is present on the skin and on the mucous membranes of the oral cavity, upper respiratory tract, distal ileum and colon, anterior urethra, and genital tract, all specimens should be collected in such a way as to minimize contamination with the host's commensal flora. To that end, we present some specific recommendations regarding specimen collection and transport of individual specimens.

Upon receipt of a representative specimen, it is the responsibility of the microbiology laboratory to perform those analytic procedures which will maximize the clinical utility of information derived from specimen processing. The natural inclination to do "everything" in the laboratory is balanced by the need for cost-effectiveness and the irrefutable fact that too much information can often be clinically misleading (i.e., more is not always better). Summarized in the following sections are the bacteriologic procedures that should be applied to different specimen types. This discussion is restricted to bacteriologic analyses. Other microbiologic disciplines, such as virology, mycology, mycobacteriology, parasitology, microbial serology, and antibiotic testing, have not been addressed.

Upper Respiratory Tract

Pharyngeal swab specimens should be obtained by vigorously swabbing the posterior pharynx and both tonsils. Nasal swab specimens may be collected by inserting a single swab consecutively through both nostrils, at least to the level of the anterior nares, and rotating three to four times. Nasopharyngeal swab specimens are collected by inserting a small calcium alginate swab attached to a flexible wire through either of the nasal passages until the nasopharynx has been contacted. In all cases, the swab is placed into swab transport medium and sent to the laboratory within 2 hours of collection.

Pharyngeal swab specimens should be processed routinely only for beta-hemolytic streptococci (group A as well as non–group A strains). Other bacterial causes of acute pharyngitis, such as *Neisseria gonorrhoeae, Corynebacterium diphtheriae,* and *Bordetella pertussis*, require specialized culture techniques and should be sought only when specifically requested. Nasal swab specimens may be used to document carriage of *Staphylococcus aureus* or for infection surveillance in patients with hematologic malignancies. Nasopharyngeal swab specimens are the diagnostic specimen of choice in patients with pertussis. They may also be used to document carriage of *Haemophilus influenzae* and *Neisseria meningitidis* in epidemiologic surveys. Gram stains are of no value with upper respiratory tract specimens. The single exception is in patients suspected of having Vincent's angina (fusospirochetal disease), in which case Gram stain of pharyngeal exudates may be diagnostic. With the exception of children with cystic fibrosis, the age-old practice of using swab specimens from the upper respiratory tract to ascertain the etiology of respiratory illnesses such as pneumonia, otitis media, sinusitis, and retropharyngeal and peritonsillar abscesses has absolutely no merit. Pharyngeal swab specimens from patients with cystic fibrosis who have bronchitis or pneumonia may reveal the organism(s) responsible for lower respiratory tract disease.

Lower Respiratory Tract

The most convenient means of collecting lower respiratory tract specimens is by expectoration. Patients should be instructed to rinse their mouths vigorously with tap water and then to produce a deep-cough specimen. In patients who are intubated, suction specimens may be obtained through endotracheal, nasotracheal, or tracheostomy tubes. Lower respiratory tract secretions may also be obtained during bronchoscopy by suction, by instillation of washing fluids, or by bronchoalveolar lavage. In all cases, these specimens are likely to be contaminated to some degree with the microbial flora of the oral cavity, the oropharynx, or the pharynx. Transtracheal aspiration, open lung biopsy, protected bronchial brush biopsy, and percutaneous needle aspiration remain the only techniques capable of yielding uncontaminated specimens. All lower respiratory tract specimens should be transported to the laboratory in sterile, screw-capped containers within 1 hour after collection.

Gram stains should be performed routinely on all sputum specimens. They may be diagnostic, and they are useful in assessing the quality of the specimen. Gram stains that reveal numerous squamous epithelial cells and mixed microbial flora indicate a contaminated specimen. When seen on Gram stain, numerous polymorphonuclear neutrophils, a single or predominant organism, pulmonary macrophages, and columnar epithelial cells suggest a representative specimen. Culture is aimed at recovering lower respiratory tract pathogens.

Urinary Tract

The easiest approach to collecting urine specimens is by midstream clean void. In women, the vaginal orifice should first be cleaned with a disinfectant soap and then sterile water or saline. With the labia held securely apart, the first 25 to 50 ml of urine is passed, and then 20 to 30 ml of urine, the mid-stream specimen, is voided directly into the collection container. The end-stream specimen is then passed. In men, the glans of the penis is thoroughly washed with sterile water, and then the specimen is collected as described previously for women. The foreskin should be retracted manually in uncircumcised men. Alternatively, urine specimens may be obtained by catheterization (i.e., straight catheter or catheter aspiration via cystoscopy). In patients with an indwelling Foley catheter, specimens should be aspirated from the urine port site and not from the collecting bag. The magnitude of contamination of catheter specimens is less than that of clean-voided specimens; however, some contamination with the commensal microbial flora of the anterior urethra is likely to occur in all cases. The only means of collecting a completely uncontaminated urine specimen is by percutaneous suprapubic needle aspiration. Two techniques have been advocated for collecting urine specimens representative of infection of the upper urinary tract: sequential specimens collected through ureteral catheters and the bladder washout technique. Specific instructions for performing these procedures should be obtained from the clinical microbiology laboratory, infectious-disease consultants, or urology specialists.

Urine specimens should be collected during the first morning void or at least 4 hours after the most recent urination and transported to the laboratory in sterile, screw-capped containers within 2 to 4 hours after collection. Specimens held longer than 2 to 4 hours may be refrigerated for up to 48 hours. A variety of preservative urine transport media have been devised; their use is discouraged, however, as there is some evidence that they may diminish bacterial viability.

Urine Gram stains are of little value in establishing a diagnosis of urinary tract infection per se; however, when the diagnosis has already been made, such stains may help in determining the nature of the infection (i.e., gram-positive cocci versus gram-negative bacilli). Culture is performed quantitatively. A single organism, assuming it is a recognized urinary pathogen, present in quantities of 10^5 or more organisms per milliliter of clean voided specimen should always be considered clinically significant. The clinical significance of smaller quantities, such as 10^2 to 10^4 organisms per milliliter of clean voided specimen, must be viewed in light of other factors such as symptoms, presence or absence of pyuria, history of antecedent urinary tract infections, and predisposition. Significant bacteriuria with catheterized specimens may be defined as 10^3 or more organisms per milliliter. Any organism recovered from a urine specimen obtained by suprapubic needle aspiration should be considered significant. It should also be recognized that not all significant bacteriuria is monomicrobic; in rare cases, two and even three organisms may cause infection of the urinary tract simultaneously. Because of this, mixed cultures do not necessarily signify contamination. A repeat culture is often helpful in assessing the meaning of mixed cultures or those with low colony counts. Finally, it should be recognized that routine urine cultures are intended to document bacteriuria with the most common urinary pathogens. Rare causes of urinary tract infections such as anaerobes, *Chlamydia*, and genital *Mycoplasma* will not be recovered with routine urine culture procedures. When suspected, these organisms require special culture techniques.

Normally Sterile Body Fluids

Specimens such as cerebrospinal fluid, pleural fluid, peritoneal fluid, pericardial fluid, and synovial fluid should be collected by needle aspiration only after the overlying skin has been thoroughly disinfected. With cerebrospinal fluid, at least 5 ml of specimen should be submitted whenever possible. With other normally sterile body fluids, as much specimen as possible should be submitted. Specimens should be placed in a sterile screw-capped container and hand carried immediately to the laboratory. When sequential tubes of cerebrospinal fluid are collected, the third tube should be submitted to the microbiology laboratory.

Gram stains are performed routinely on all normally sterile body fluids. Culture techniques are designed to recover essentially all organisms. Culture results, however, may not be available in a clinically relevant time frame. As a result, a number of procedures have been devised to detect bacterial antigens directly in body-fluid specimens. These include counterimmunoelectrophoresis, latex agglutination, and coagglutination. These procedures, which yield results in 10 to 30 minutes, are useful in detecting *H. influenzae, Streptococcus pneumoniae, N. meningitidis,* and group B streptococci. They are extremely specific (i.e., a positive result is diagnostic) but relatively insensitive (i.e., a negative result means little).

Genital Tract

Endocervical and urethral specimens should be collected on flexible wire calcium alginate–tipped swabs and submitted to the laboratory in swab transport media within 2 hours after collection. In women, samples are obtained by rotating the swab three to four times within the endocervical canal or urethra. In men, the urethra is milked by manual stripping of the shaft of the penis, and the swab is inserted approximately 2 cm into the urethra, rotated three to four times, and withdrawn.

Specimens collected and transported in this manner should be processed only for *N. gonorrhoeae*. A Gram stain is performed routinely and examined for the presence of *intracellular* gram-negative diplococci. Approximately 95 percent of men with acute gonococcal urethritis have this finding. Gram stain is much less sensitive in women. Culture remains the definitive diagnostic test and takes 1 to 3 days. Other causes of acute urethritis and cervicitis, such as *Chlamydia* and genital *Mycoplasma*, necessitate special laboratory techniques and are sought only on request. The same is true for herpes simplex virus, another important cause of cervicitis.

Vaginal discharge specimens from patients with vaginitis should *not* be submitted to the microbiology laboratory for analysis. The etiologic diagnosis of vaginitis is best made by performing a few simple procedures in the clinic. The discharge is first examined for its gross appearance. A wet prep is then examined microscopically for *Trichomonas vaginalis*. A drop of 10 percent potassium hydroxide (KOH) is mixed with two to three drops of discharge on a glass slide, and its odor is characterized. A "fishy" amine odor is characteristic of *Gardnerella vaginalis* nonspecific vaginitis. The KOH prep is then examined microscopically for the presence of abundant yeast with pseudohyphae, which is indicative of yeast infection. Finally, a Gram stain of the discharge is performed. The presence of "clue" cells (i.e., squamous epithelial cells coated with gram-variable pleomorphic bacilli) and the complete absence of lactobacilli confirm the diagnosis of nonspecific vaginitis (bacterial vaginosis); gram-positive yeast with pseudohyphae confirms yeast vaginitis.

Stool Specimens

Feces are the optimal specimen. They should be collected into a screw-capped container and then transported to the laboratory within 1 hour after collection. When feces cannot be obtained, a rectal swab specimen, transported in swab transport medium within 2 hours after collection, suffices. Stool specimens are routinely processed for *Salmonella, Shigella*, and *Campylobacter*. A single negative stool specimen does not rule out *Salmonella* or *Shigella*. Three specimens, preferably obtained during the first morning bowel movement, should be collected on consecutive days. Gram stains of stool specimens are of little value. Other bacterial causes of gastroenteritis, such as *Yersinia enterocolitica*, enterotoxigenic and enterohemorrhagic *Escherichia coli, Vibrio cholerae, Vibrio parahaemolyticus, Clostridium difficile*, and the common agents of food poisoning, require special culture techniques and are therefore sought only on request.

Biopsy, Exudate, and Wound Specimens

Tissue specimens collected using strict aseptic technique are placed into sterile screw-capped containers and transported to the laboratory within 30 minutes after collection. Fluid specimens such as exudates, the fluid contents of abscesses, and cellulitic fluid aspirates are collected with a syringe using aseptic techniques, transferred into sterile screw-capped containers, and transported to the laboratory within 30 minutes after collection. Swab specimens, as discussed previously, should be avoided; however, when it is necessary to use them, they may be placed in swab transport media and submitted to the laboratory within 2 hours after collection.

Gram stains are performed routinely. Culture techniques are intended to recover all bacteria. Quantitative cultures of wound biopsy specimens have been advocated as a possible means of ascertaining the clinical significance of organisms that frequently contaminate or colonize certain wound sites. This approach to wound cultures, however, remains controversial; therefore, it should be applied only in selected circumstances by personnel fully acquainted with quantitative cultures and the limitations of the clinical information derived from them.

Blood Cultures

The optimal volume of blood that should be collected per adult blood culture is 20 ml. Because most bacteremias are not continuous, multiple blood cultures are indicated for all patients suspected of being bacteremic. Multiple blood cultures are also helpful in ascertaining the clinical significance of blood culture isolates thought to be contaminants. A total of three blood cultures will document nearly all bacteremias. The precise timing of collection depends on a number of clinical variables. If immediate antibiotic administration is necessary, three blood cultures should be collected from different sites consecutively. If a patient has chills or temperature elevations, specimens should be obtained during a chill or fever spike. When none of these conditions exist, three blood cultures should be collected at equally spaced intervals, over a 12- to 24-hour period.

Blood should be collected from peripheral venous sites using standard venipuncture techniques. Arterial blood offers no advantage over venous blood in the detection of bacteremia. The skin overlying the venipuncture site should be thoroughly cleansed with 70 percent ethanol and then scrubbed concentrically from the center laterally with an iodophore disinfectant such as 2 percent tincture of iodine. After the iodine has dried, the blood specimen is obtained. Blood may be collected into a syringe and then transferred directly into blood-culture bottles at the patient's bedside, or it may be collected into sterile yellow-topped vacutainer tubes and transported to the laboratory for inoculation of the blood-culture bottles. A conventional culture consists of two bottles, one aerobic and the other anaerobic, each containing 50 to 100 ml of culture medium. When bottles are to be inoculated at the patient's bedside, an equal aliquot (i.e., 10 ml) of blood from the initial 20-ml sample is distributed into each bottle. The rubber septa of either blood-culture bottles or yellow-topped tubes should be thoroughly scrubbed with 70 percent ethanol before entry. Blood for culture should not be collected through indwelling vascular cannulae or via femoral venipuncture because these specimens are more likely to be contaminated.

Blood cultures are maintained in the laboratory for at least 7 days before being discarded as negative. Blood-culture techniques are aimed at recovering those bacteria commonly associated with bacteremia. Because blood cultures are performed in broth, and because most conventional identification and susceptibility procedures can be performed only on organisms growing on solid medium, there is usually a 1-day delay in providing this information with positive blood cultures as compared with other specimen types. Gram stains of buffy coats prepared directly from patient blood have been advocated as a means for direct detection of bacteremia. Buffy-coat Gram stains, however, have not proved to be a reliable means of detecting bacteremia and therefore should not be performed routinely.

Anaerobic Cultures

Anaerobic cultures should be performed only on appropriately collected specimens that are transported in such a way as to avoid exposure to atmospheric oxygen and the resultant loss of viability of anaerobic bacteria. In addition, specimens must be collected in a manner that avoids contamination with the commensal human anaerobic flora. Acceptable specimens include transtracheal aspirates, suprapubic bladder taps, tissue specimens, fluid specimens collected by aspiration, and swab specimens of nonsuperficial sites in areas that are not contiguous with a mucous membrane normally colonized with anaerobes. Tissue specimens are submitted to the laboratory in toto in sterile screw-capped containers immediately after collection; the larger the specimen, the better. Fluid specimens should be submitted in the syringe in which they were collected, with a sterile rubber plug inserted firmly into the needle. Care must be taken to expel air bubbles trapped in the syringe prior to transport. Alternatively, fluid specimens may be transferred into sterile glass anaerobic vials for transport to the laboratory. Such vials are usually available in the laboratory. In either case, fluid specimens should also be transported immediately after collection. Swab specimens are always inferior; when necessary, however, the swab should be placed into an anaerobic swab transport device and submitted to the laboratory immediately. A variety of anaerobic swab transport devices have been developed and can usually be obtained from the microbiology laboratory.

Gram stains are performed routinely. Culture techniques are aimed at recovering strictly anaerobic organisms. Because of the fastidious nature of anaerobic bacteria, the results of cultures are frequently not available for 3 to 5 days and, in many cases, organisms present in the original specimens are not recovered in culture. In such cases, Gram stain becomes an invaluable tool. Assuming suitable aerobic culture techniques have been applied, an organism seen on Gram stain but not recovered from either aerobic or anaerobic cultures can usually be assumed to be an anaerobe.

Uncommon Organisms

Because of unusual growth characteristics, a number of bacteria not discussed previously will not be recovered using conventional aerobic or anaerobic culture techniques. Included in this group are *Francisella tularensis, Legionella* spp., *Brucella* spp., *Leptospira* spp., *Borrelia* spp., nutritional-deficient streptococci, and cell-wall defective variants. The laboratory should be notified when these organisms are suspected, so that appropriate culture techniques can be applied.

References

Bartlett RD. Making optimum use of the microbiology laboratory. JAMA 1982; 247:857.

Glecker RW, et al. Clinical value of paired sputum and transtracheal aspirates in the initial management of pneumonia. Chest 1985; 87:631.

Guerrant RL, et al. A cost effective and effective approach to the diagnosis and management of acute infectious diarrhea. NY Acad Sci 1987; 63:484.

Hayward RA, Shapiro MF, Oye RK. Laboratory testing on cerebrospinal fluid. Lancet 1987; 1:1.

Kass EH, Finland M. Asymptomatic infections of the urinary tract. Trans Assoc Am Phys 1956; 69:56.

Rothernberg RB, Simon R. Efficacy of selected diagnostic tests for sexually transmitted diseases. JAMA 1976; 235:49.

Stamm WE, et al. Diagnosis of coliform infection in acutely dysuric women. New Engl J Med 1982; 307:463.

Washington JA. Blood cultures: An overview. Eur J Clin Microbiol Infec Dis 1989; 8:803.

The Hematology Laboratory

Liberto Pechet, MD

In order to maximize the efficiency of obtaining laboratory information, a systematic decision-implementation process is necessary. The components of this process, as they apply to the hematology laboratory, are described here.

Ordering of Hematology Tests

In addition to the clinical considerations that lead one to order specific tests, a number of other elements must be kept in mind. One of the first considerations is how fast the results are needed. Is this an emergency (STAT) situation, in which event the results would be needed immediately, ahead of any other tests in the whole hospital? If the situation is not a dire emergency, are the results needed as soon as possible (ASAP)? Or is this a routine test, the results of which can wait for a few hours? The abuse of STAT test orders results in an excessive number of STAT tests being processed by the laboratory, so that the true *emergency* STAT tests do not receive the priority they deserve.

Consider also the cost of each test, so that whenever reasonable, the number of tests ordered can be reduced.

Avoid duplication of tests. If certain tests were ordered on the patient's admission, they should not be reordered the next day, unless the initial results or a change in the clinical situation necessitate retesting. Whenever a test is ordered on a daily basis, the order should be canceled when the need for daily results no longer exists. Complete blood counts (CBCs) should not be ordered if only red cell values are needed, at which time a hematocrit or hemoglobin reading can be obtained, usually at a lesser cost. Similarly, if only platelet counts are needed, there is no reason to order a CBC. For patients receiving oral anticoagulants, only prothrombin time (PT) should be ordered; for those receiving heparin alone, only partial thromboplastin time (PTT) should be ordered.

Finally, tests should not be ordered in the afternoon to be performed the same evening, unless they are really needed the same day and the ordering physician plans to examine them that evening. All laboratories are short staffed in the evening and at nights. It is preferable to order most routine tests for the morning workload. For similar reasons, ordering of laboratory tests on weekends and holidays should be minimized.

Who Fills in the Requisitions?

Once the physician has decided which tests are wanted and how soon the results are needed, an order is written in the patient's chart and the chart flagged so that the unit's clerk transfers the order on special laboratory requisitions, which vary with the test ordered. The requests should be written very clearly in order to avoid mistakes. For example, the clerks may order an alkaline phosphatase, a common test, when in fact the ordering physician wanted a leukocyte alkaline phosphatase, a hematology test, but did not write the order clearly. This will result in excess cost and delays. The clerks in nursing stations have a special form for every laboratory. Most hematology laboratories require requisition forms as follows: a special form for CBCs, another form for most coagulation tests, and a miscellaneous form for body fluids and a few special tests, such as hemoglobin electrophoresis, plasminogen, heparin levels, alpha-2 antiplasmin, and a few others. In most cases, the clerk will know which form to use.

Occasionally, when the clerk is not available, or if a physician collected the blood and is in a hurry to transfer it to the lab, he or she may have to fill in those forms. For STAT or ASAP tests, the physician requesting them will want to be informed of the results as soon as they become available. For this, his or her name and paging number should be clearly marked on the requisition form.

Who Collects the Blood?

In most hospitals, specially trained phlebotomists or laboratory technicians make rounds at predetermined hours and pick up all the requisition slips from the nurses' station, then collect the blood. In some institutions, nurses perform this function. Occasionally, particularly in emergency situations, such as when STAT or ASAP tests are required, the physician on the floor or a student (if properly trained) will collect the blood. It is conceivable that in most cases in which emergency tests are ordered, one may not want to wait for a phlebotomist's arrival, because this wastes precious time, if indeed the tests are to be done immediately.

What Test Tubes Are Used for Hematology?

Except for body fluids and a few special tests, vacutainers are used by the majority of hospitals. Each tube contains a specified anticoagulant, which can be recognized by the color of the stopper (Table 9-6). For instance, tubes containing ethylenediaminetetraacetic acid (EDTA) have a purple top; those containing citrate, a blue top; and those containing sodium heparin, a green top. Tubes with red tops contain no anticoagulant; hence, they are used for serum (serum is rarely used in the hematology laboratory). The vacuum in these test tubes predetermines the volume of blood to be aspirated. If the vacuum fails, because the test tubes are defective or too old, the tubes should not be used under any circumstance, because a lesser volume of blood means higher dilution and hence inaccurate results. It is also important that the blood be well mixed with the anticoagulant after filling of the vacutainer tube, in order to ensure its fluidity. The presence of clots, even very small ones, will vitiate the results, particularly in coagulation studies. On the other hand, mixing of the blood should not be too vigorous, because this may result in red cell hemolysis. All tubes with anticoagulant in them should be *inverted* five to six times to assure proper mixing.

Table 9-6 Types of Vacutainers Used for Hematology

Color of stopper	Anticoagulant	Tests
Purple	EDTA	CBC, hemoglobin and hematocrit, platelets, differential, sedimentation rate, body fluids
Blue	Sodium citrate	PT, PTT, thrombin time, clotting factor quantitation, coagulation inhibitors, plasminogen, heparin, antithrombin III, D-dimers
Green	Sodium heparin	Lymphocyte markers
Red	None	Type and cross match, Coombs, serology, body fluids
Special tubes containing thrombin	—	FSPs
Special tubes containing tissue culture medium	—	Cytogenetics

Abbreviations: CBC = complete blood count, FSPs = fibrinogen split products, PT = prothrombin time, PTT = partial thromboplastin time.

All CBCs, including platelet counts and differentials, or hemoglobins or hematocrits, as well as the Westergren sedimentation rates, use tubes with EDTA as the anticoagulant. Most coagulation studies, including PT, PTT, thrombin time, antithrombin III, euglobulin lysis time, D-dimers, fibrinogen, and clotting factors, use citrate as an anticoagulant. Two important exceptions are fibrinogen split products (FSP or FDP), for which special tubes containing thrombin are supplied by the laboratory, and platelet functional studies such as aggregation, release, and ristocetin cofactor. These have to be collected by a laboratory technician in citrated tubes without vacuum to ensure the functional integrity of platelets. Bleeding times are done by phlebotomists or laboratory personnel, using a standardized template. For body fluids such as spinal fluid or other small-volume sterile fluids, sterile tubes included in the respective kits should be used. For large-volume fluids, such as those obtained by thoracentesis or pericentesis, both red-top (no anticoagulant) and purple-top tubes should be used. In most cases, blood banking requires clotted blood; hence, red-top tubes are used.

Labeling of the Tubes Is of Utmost Importance

The phlebotomists who collect the specimens are well trained in precise labeling. If physicians or students obtain the blood, they must ensure that stickers with the patient's name and hospital number, the date, and the initials of the person collecting the blood are properly placed on every test tube obtained. This is particularly important if specimens are sent to the blood bank, because improper identification may have catastrophic results. It should also be noted that the laboratory will *never* accept a test tube that is improperly labeled or that has no label, even if the physician who drew the blood brings it to the laboratory.

Special studies such as cytogenetics, lymphocyte markers, or studies for gene rearrangement, which are analyzed in the cytogenetic or specialized hematopathology laboratories, should be collected in special tubes provided by these laboratories.

How Do the Test Tubes Reach the Laboratory?

When specimens are collected by a phlebotomist or laboratory technician, he or she will personally bring them to the laboratory. If, however, the tests were ordered ASAP or STAT and were obtained by a physician or student, the test tubes may be transported by a carrier or sent by a mechanical conveyance in pneumatic tubes or via a dumb waiter. They may then reach a triage station, where they are logged and separated for the various laboratories, and again distributed by carrier. In cases in which the STAT request represents an immediate emergency, it is highly desirable that the person who obtains the blood and labels the test tubes take them personally to the laboratory, rather than relying on people who may not be fully aware of the imminent emergency that these tests reflect.

How Does the Hematology Laboratory Function?

The director of the laboratory, who generally is a hematologist or a clinical pathologist, is the person responsible for all functions of the laboratory. The person immediately in charge under the laboratory director is a supervisor, and in some laboratories there is also an assistant supervisor. They supervise the daily work of a number of well-trained technicians, most of whom have obtained a special degree from a school of medical technology.

A hematology laboratory is usually divided into three components. The first component performs the routine CBCs, differentials, and platelet counts, which constitute the greatest volume of any hematology workload. In the majority of laboratories, the CBCs are performed on automated equipment that gives at least seven parameters: hemoglobin, hematocrit, red blood cell count, the three indices, and platelet count. Modern equipment also provides a preliminary three-cell differential, dividing the white cells into three categories: small (lymphocytes), medium (monocytes), and large (polys and bands) cells (recently, five-cell differentials have become available). Scaterograms (histograms) can be obtained on request; they describe the size distribution of red cells, white cells, and platelets. In some institutions, complete differential counts are done by special instruments, but because of the high cost of this equipment and certain imperfections, most hospitals do not possess automated differentials, which are done on each sample by light microscopy.

The second component of a hematology laboratory performs coagulation tests (most often PT and PTT), usually with semiautomated or automated equipment. In some institutions, the coagulation section of the laboratory also performs specialized tests, such as quantitation of individual clotting factors, fibrinogen, thrombin times, FSPs, fibrinolytic assays, inhibitor assays, and, in some instances, blood heparin levels. Most advanced laboratories will perform platelet aggregation and release, studies to evaluate von Willebrand factor, such as platelet agglutination with ristocetin, and immunologic studies for the quantitation of factors VIII and IX, protein C, and protein S antigens. Both factors VIII and IX antigens are helpful in determining the carriership state for hemophilia A and B.

The third component of some hematology laboratories performs "special" tests, such as hemoglobin electrophoresis with identification of abnormal hemoglobins, red cell enzymes, and white cell histochemistry, using special stains, and certain nonradioactive immunologic techniques, using a radial immunodiffusion method (haptoglobins and antithrombin III).

Reporting

In most hospitals the results of STAT and ASAP tests are reported to the floors as soon as they become available, and the ordering physician is paged or called. All other results are available on manual or computer printouts (wherever available) every few hours. In most teaching hospitals, cumulative sheets generated by computer are included daily in the patient's chart. Note that some complex, rarely performed tests, such as hemoglobin electrophoresis, may be batched and performed only on certain days.

Bone Marrow Aspirations and Biopsies

Bone marrow aspirations and biopsies are performed under sterile conditions, with trays containing special needles as well as the other materials necessary, such as Novocain, syringes, and needles. The location of these trays may vary depending on your hospital's practice. They are usually available on the floors or are brought up by a hematology technologist. In some hospitals the bone marrow aspirations and biopsies may be performed under supervision of a hematology/oncology fellow or an attending physician in hematology, oncology, or pediatric hematology/oncology, and with the help of a hematology laboratory technologist. In most cases, the bone marrows are stained within 1 or 2 hours after they reach the laboratory, but special stains (histochemistry) may take 1 to 2 days. Bone marrow biopsies are processed in the hematology department or in the pathology department and require 24 to 48 hours for completion.

10 Scheduling of Tests

Jonathan S. Appelbaum, MD

The approach to a particular diagnostic problem involves a carefully planned work-up using various diagnostic tests. This may include the use of the clinical laboratory, the radiology department, and various consultants, if necessary. The work-up should be planned efficiently, keeping in mind that the goal is to reach a diagnostic endpoint in the shortest possible time, with the least amount of discomfort to the patient, using the most cost-effective techniques. Other chapters provide information about the work-up of individual problems. This chapter provides some general guidelines to follow when planning the work-up.

Laboratory Studies

Certain laboratory tests should be performed when the patient is in a fasted state. Fasting blood sugars, triglycerides, and lipid profiles are the most common examples. Most other routine laboratory tests are not affected by meals.

At this point, it should be noted that some insurance companies are starting to deny payment for routine screening profiles unless they are clearly indicated by a diagnosis. It becomes cost-effective to order a "panel" of tests, if you would be ordering three or more of the separate tests contained in the panel.

Should any stool studies be desired, samples should be obtained prior to any radiographic studies of the gastrointestinal (GI) tract, because the barium used for these studies will interfere with stool cultures and determination of the presence of parasites.

Radiographic Studies

Barium will interfere with almost all other diagnostic modalities, both invasive and noninvasive, until it has been removed. After an upper GI series, this may take several days. Keep this in mind when planning a work-up. For example, if you are planning to evaluate an alcoholic patient with mid-thoracic back pain, guaiac-positive stools, mildly elevated amylase level, and microscopic hematuria, an abdominal ultrasound examination to evaluate the pancreas, an upper GI series to evaluate the gastrointestinal tract, and an intravenous pyelogram (IVP) to evaluate the urinary tract system might be considered. The most efficient sequence for ordering this series of tests would be to perform the ultrasound and IVP before the upper GI series. Barium will also interfere with the newer diagnostic modalities, such as computed tomography (CT) scanning, and will prevent adequate examination of a hollow viscus by fiberoptic technique. If endoscopy is planned, the barium study should be postponed. An upper GI series should be performed after a barium enema, because it is much easier to evacuate the barium from the lower GI tract than from the upper.

If a myelogram is to be done as part of a work-up, the spinal tap should be done at that time rather than subjecting the patient to two uncomfortable invasive procedures. In addition, the rent in the dura from the prior puncture may cause leakage of the contrast into the epidural space.

Most of the preceding studies need to be performed with the patient in a fasted state, and some require elaborate bowel preparation, including clear-liquid diets and cathartics. Each radiology department has its own guidelines for this preparation, which you should review before scheduling the tests. Other medical problems should be considered when evaluating your patient; for example, diabetics may need adjustment of oral hypoglycemic agents or insulin for these tests.

Most radiologists and gastroenterologists agree that abdominal ultrasound has supplanted oral cholecystography (OCG) as the diagnostic procedure of choice for evaluating cholelithiasis. This test requires little preparation, but it may be as much as two times as expensive as the OCG. The advantage of ultrasound is that it is simple and will provide results in those instances in which the OCG shows no function of the gallbladder. Unfortunately, bowel gas may interfere with this test. The procedures of choice to evaluate gallbladder function and obstruction are now iodinated hippuric acid (HIDA) and technetium-99-DISIDA scanning. These tests may be done even with elevated bilirubin levels. Magnetic resonance imaging (MRI) may prove to be superior to CT scanning for evaluation of tumors of the brain, herniated disks, and hepatic metastasis, to name a few. This test does not require contrast, and other contrast materials do not interfere with this test, but the patient cannot have any metal in the body or brain (such as a pacemaker or orthopedic screws).

Summary

In planning the diagnostic work-up of a patient, it is worth taking a moment to think about the tests to be ordered and how they might best be coordinated to alleviate any patient discomfort or to prevent unnecessary expense.

Cost Containment

Helen Beattie, MPH, EdD

David S. Hatem, MD

11

Over the last decade, medical knowledge and the environment in which medicine is practiced have changed dramatically. Routine breast biopsies and cardiac catheterizations are now 1-day ambulatory surgical procedures in many institutions. Such seemingly drastic alterations in the delivery of medical care aimed at minimizing cost will continue to increase because of growing concern by federal and state governments, the business sector, and the insurance industry. In the coming years some basic tenets of traditional medicine will be challenged, and a host of clinical and ethical dilemmas will be created in the process of seeking to balance patient care and cost considerations.

Adapting to these changes is a challenge that you will unquestionably face as you undergo medical training and ultimately enter practice. There are few role models to guide you through these issues, which can seem far removed from what you have learned thus far. However, your clinical and financial success will rest largely on your understanding of these complex issues and your willingness to address them. This chapter briefly reviews the current system, identifies where costs can be reduced without compromising care, and offers a strategy to help integrate cost awareness into the development of clinical skills.

The Problem

The cost of medical care in 1990 consumes over 11 percent of the gross national product and has increased at an annual rate far above that of general inflation. Numerous attempts are being made to curb this rapid escalation of costs, centering on the effort to convert medical finances from an unlimited budget system to one with a budget ceiling. This is most evident in the dramatic change in physician reimbursement, with a shift from retrospective reimbursement, in which the physician is paid for actual services rendered, to a prospective reimbursement system. This means that an insurance company or state or federal agency makes a decision concerning the average cost for any given disease or medical problem, which then becomes the flat rate reimbursed to the hospital or physician. The costs of additional testing or procedures or extended lengths of stay will no longer be paid by the private insurance companies or government-subsidized programs, regardless of need. It is clear that the primary incentive with prospective payment is to minimize the cost of care expended per patient. The financial ramifications of this shift in funding foreshadow a general period of crisis for hospitals and physicians, especially as the general population of the country ages and the proportion of elderly patients with significant medical problems increases.

The Current System: A Time of Transition

Health maintenance organizations (HMOs) have become established throughout the country. This form of medical care delivery aggressively seeks methods to reduce costs, primarily by minimizing hospitalization. Because of the cost of HMOs, these plans are competitive with many insurance companies. Therefore, increasing numbers of employers are choosing them as a major insurer of their employees. The HMOs designate a limited number of hospitals where the cost of care for their patients is covered and also limit reimbursement, primarily to physicians within their practice. This means that, increasingly, a hospital's census and potential patient population will depend upon the insurance decisions of business and industry. Industry therefore has become a major factor in shaping the delivery of health care in any given community. Insofar as arrangements between industry and health care delivery systems are mutually advantageous, this system will flourish, but the goals of the two may be incompatible. The limitation of spending on health care encouraged by an industry that is trying to cut costs may be at odds with the increasing expense of more advanced technologies being utilized today in medicine. Thus far, it is believed that quality of care will not be compromised by these changes, but conclusive studies have not been done to document this belief. Studies that have looked at the nature of health care delivery as HMOs and prospective payment systems have become established have yielded some interesting observations, as detailed later in this chapter. These trends will require close monitoring to ensure that if costs are to be cut, the system's goal becomes more efficient delivery of quality care, not just a decrease in the amount of care.

Another reality of the changing system is a trend for insurance copayment, which requires that the patient bear responsibility for a greater portion of the medical bills. Additionally, a general decrease in the range of coverage of existing plans is becoming evident, making the patient fully responsible for payment if he or she elects to utilize certain services.

Thus, it is evident that changes in reimbursement, HMOs, the steady growth of proprietary hospital corporations, the development of "emergency" medicine free-standing clinics, and a host of other factors are challenging the traditional system of medical care delivery. As a physician, you will predictably experience a great deal of pressure to minimize the cost of medical care, not only from the institutions in which you will practice but also from your patients, who are fast becoming cost-conscious as they face paying greater portions of their medical bills.

Cutting Costs: Target Areas

Where can costs be cut without compromising care? It has been shown that increasing hospital services does not guarantee improvement in quality of care or patient outcome. Numerous reports that carefully review routine tests (complete blood counts, biochemical profiles, blood and throat cultures) and their indications have proliferated. A critical look at these tests reveals that potential savings may be realized by decreasing the number of relatively inexpensive but frequently ordered tests, as well as limiting the use of expensive technologies.

Several studies also suggest that substantial savings can be realized by decreasing the ordering of diagnostic and therapeutic procedures. Ordering of procedures has escalated at a rate almost double that of other hospital services. Substantial documentation indicates that as many as 95 percent of tests ordered are never referred to in the clinical decision-making process, yet they constitute up to 25 percent of the total hospital bill. Excessive testing can lead not only to iatrogenic disease, but also to false-positive results that require further testing, which ultimately proves wasteful. So, the potential for substantial savings in cost and health by reducing diagnostic and therapeutic procedures is unquestionable. Equally important, the available literature indicates that using fewer procedures will not have an adverse impact on the quality of care. The challenge is to develop a better balance between ordering indicated tests and limiting useless procedures. This can be done only by having clear-cut reasons for ordering a test and knowing what information the test is capable of providing. A system that keeps this in mind promises to meet both the medical and financial needs of the patient in a more efficient manner.

In a similar vein, when a study of surgical rates was conducted, striking regional differences were found, with no clear reason for the extent of variation. The highest amount of variaion was noted for surgical procedures whose indications were debated (i.e., hysterectomies, tonsillectomies, and cataract surgery). For example, one study showed that in one town 25 percent of the women had undergone hysterectomies by age 75. In a town 30 miles away, the percentage climbed to 70 percent. These findings suggest that the potential exists to reduce health care costs by critically examining the relative value and indications for the performance of a surgical procedure. In a study looking at cesarean section, another procedure that has widely disparate performance rates in various settings, successful reduction of the rate of cesarean section was achieved without adverse consequences to mother or child. This was done by instituting a system of obtaining a second opinion, well-defined objective criteria for performance of cesarean section, and continued review of all cesarean sections and individual physicians' rates of performing them.

Appropriateness of the decision to admit a patient to a hospital also is being reviewed in an increasing number of instances. In a study conducted in England, in which patients with a suspected uncomplicated myocardial infarction were randomized to either home care or hospitalization, it was found that those at home had no significant difference in mortality. Some studies also indicate that length of stay for many patients can be shortened without compromising care. Vast amounts of money can be saved by decreasing the number of inappropriate admissions and days of hospitalization. Interestingly, however, studies looking at how HMOs save money, while agreeing with this in principle, have suggested that the reality is somewhat different. HMOs have saved money largely by decreasing the number of hospitalizations of their members as compared with those of enrollees in more conventional insurance programs. Generally, however, there have been no reductions in the length of hospital stays or the percentage of admissions deemed inappropriate, including the percentage of admissions for discretionary surgical procedures such as hysterectomy, cataract surgery, and hernia repairs. Money saved on in-patient care was not matched by an increase in outpatient expenditure or services. Finally, in a study of patients with hip fractures in which length of hospitalization was reduced and physical therapy services were decreased, a greater proportion of patients were discharged to nursing homes, and the proportion of patients remaining in the nursing homes 1 year after hip fracture rose significantly. There is also a greater percentage of deaths occurring in the nation's nursing homes, especially in areas where length of hospital stay has been reduced. This presumably reflects the transfer of terminally ill patients from acute care hospitals to nursing homes. The ability of the nation's nursing homes to handle these cases has yet to be determined. We must be careful to institute programs that reduce cost, not simply shift it to another agency or organization.

Another critical element in the changing health care system is the desire for the quality of health care to be maintained in the face of growing concerns about cost. *In no instance* should a decision to order an indicated diagnostic test, to perform necessary surgery, to prolong a hospital stay for continued care not available outside the hospital, or even to admit a patient who requires in-patient hospitalization, be tempered by cost factors. Conversely, the decision to order tests that may be interesting or helpful but not essential to decision making, to perform surgery of marginal benefit, or to allow days of hospitalization with limited value must be seriously questioned in terms of clinical benefit versus expense.

Admittedly, there are a number of disincentives for physicians to confront cost-containment issues, not the least of which is the reality of the malpractice epidemic. One study revealed that 8 percent of lab studies and 15 percent of radiographs were due to defensive medicine. Faced with uncertainty or ambiguity in clinical diagnosis or treatment, Pineault found marked increases in physician test-ordering patterns. A general lack of understanding or consensus on the sensitivity and specificity of tests, measures that must be considered in test interpretation, often aggravates clinical uncertainty. Another reality is that patients often demand more costly diagnostic procedures in search of definitive answers to their problems. These issues are real and must be factored into any attempt to bring cost containment to medical care.

The focus of medical care—that physicians have a primary responsibility to deliver the best patient care possible—must not change. It is reassuring that the literature suggests that the cost of medical care can, in certain situations, be decreased without a negative impact on the quality of care. Once again, the goal is to develop a plan of more efficient care, not simply less care. Unfortunately, the literature has not yet documented how best to integrate cost awareness into the development of clinical skills.

The Solution

How can cost awareness be integrated into medicine? Traditional teaching in medicine has focused on the correct practice of medicine without concern for cost. This means that as a physician in training, you may have few, if any, role models who will discuss cost. The challenge you face is to integrate the acquisition of clinical skills with an understanding of the financial impact of care in the absence of formal programs to assist you in this task.

Where do you start? The first step is no different from what you have already been doing in your first 2 years of medical school. You need to acquire a broad knowledge base through careful study of disease processes and their pathophysiology. Knowing the characteristic features of a disease allows you to form an educated opinion about its likelihood given a particular patient presentation. Study of diagnostic tests, including the information that they are able to provide as well as their sensitivity and specificity, will allow you to select diagnostic tests intelligently. Medicine has many tests that yield similar information, and given this, the issue of cost can then be factored in to help you decide which test or procedure, of two equivalent ones, should be performed.

Another factor that must be considered is physician education of patients and the increasingly cooperative relationship between physicians and their patients that must occur if cost containment is to be achieved. The reality of the current health care system is that there are spiraling costs but increasing numbers of people (roughly 35 million) who have no insurance or other coverage. Because of this and many other considerations, individuals are going to have to pay increasing proportions of their medical bills; thus, they too will have a vested interest in cost containment. Your role is to educate your patients and, where appropriate, to point out that additional testing, which is increasingly expensive as technology advances, will add nothing to what is already known about their disease. Just as good judgment dictates that necessary tests must be performed regardless of expense, unnecessary tests cannot be performed simply because patients insist that you do so. However, you must then discuss your reasoning with the patients and bring them to understand that fewer tests do not translate into inadequate care.

With this background, a number of practical steps can be taken. You should begin to familiarize yourself with the costs of tests, procedures, hospital room charges, and medications. This will help you form some criteria on which to judge clinical benefit versus expense. A review of the bills of the patients you treat is a good starting point.

Another piece of necessary information is a broad understanding of insurance coverage for the major health plans. Assessment of insurance status should become a basic component of a patient's history and physical. Knowledge of insurance coverage will allow you to estimate roughly the financial implications of a given course of action and will give you an opportunity to discuss this with the patient. If finances pose a major problem, or if complex questions arise that you cannot answer, you can then refer the individual to the social service department for further help. Social workers have an in-depth understanding of the intricacies of insurance coverage and are trained to deal with involved questions and concerns. The social service department is also a logical place for you to ask for help in understanding the similarities and differences of insurance plans (see Chapter 8, "Interacting with Other Health Care Professionals: Social Service").

Cost awareness is as complex as understanding the hundreds of different applications of prospective reimbursement or as simple as one basic question: Will this test, procedure, or hospitalization alter the patient's health outcome in any meaningful way? If you continually preface your clinical decisions with this question, you will set precedent in integrating cost awareness into medical care. You will serve as a role model to faculty, residents, and medical students. Finally, you will be capable of delivering the highest-quality medical care that minimizes both the physical and financial impact of disease and illness.

References

Cebul RD, Beck JB. Biochemical profiles: Applications in ambulatory screening and preadmission testing of adults. Ann Intern Med 1987; 106:403.

Dixon RH, Lazlo J. Utilization of clinical chemistry services by medical house staff. Arch Intern Med 1974; 1134:1064.

Enthoven A, Kronick R. A consumer-choice health plan for the 1990's: Universal health insurance in a system designed to promote quality and economy. N Engl J Med 1989; 320:29–37, 94–101.

Fineberg HV, Pearlman LA. Low-cost medical practices. Ann Rev Pub Health 1982; 3:225.

Garg ML, Gliebe W, Elkhatib M. Diagnostic testing as a cost factor in teaching hospitals. J Am Hosp Assoc 1978; 52:97.

Himmelstein DU, Woolhandler S. A national health program for the United States: A physician's proposal. N Engl J Med 1989; 320:102.

Luft HS. How do health-maintenance organizations achieve their "savings"? Rhetoric and evidence. N Engl J Med 1978; 298:1336.

Martin AR, et al. A trial of two strategies to modify the test ordering behavior of medical residents. N Engl J Med 1980; 303:1330.

Pineault R. The effect of medical training factors on physician utilization behavior. Med Care 1977; 15:51.

Russell LB, Manning CL. The effect of prospective payment on Medicare expenditures. N Engl J Med 1989; 320:439.

Sager MA, et al. Changes in the location of death after passage of Medicare's prospective payment system. N Engl J Med 1989; 320:433.

Schroeder SA, et al. Use of laboratory test and pharmaceuticals: Variation among physicians and effect of cost audit on subsequent use. JAMA 1973; 225:969.

Shapiro MF, Greenfield S. The complete blood count and leukocyte differential count: An approach to their rational application. Ann Intern Med 1987; 106:65.

Siu AL, Sonnenburg FA, Manning WG. Inappropriate use of hospitals in a randomized trial of health insurance plans. N Engl J Med 1986; 315:1259.

Stoline A, Weiner JP. The new medical marketplace: A physician's guide to the health care revolution. Baltimore: Johns Hopkins University Press, 1988.

Writing Orders for Hospitalized Patients

Arthur R. Russo, MD

12

Writing orders for the diagnosis and management of patients is one of the most important functions that a physician routinely performs. Physicians' orders indicate what the physician believes to be the major reason for a patient's hospitalization and indicate the seriousness of the problem. The orders outline the diagnostic evaluation and therapeutic interventions that may eventually lead to the patient's recovery or stabilization. Potential problems that may arise and indications for notification of the physician by the nursing staff of a change in the patient's clinical condition are also included in the orders. Order writing is a function that physicians carry out many times daily. Orders should be reviewed daily and updated as necessary. Because physicians' orders are so important, they must be legible and clearly conveyed so that there can be no misinterpretation of the intended plans.

Writing of orders must be undertaken in a logical and deliberate manner. There is no one format that must be followed; however, a commonly used approach to order writing is generally followed. You should develop an order-writing style that you are comfortable using, that is easy to interpret, and that is used consistently. In this chapter, an approach to writing orders, particularly hospital admission orders, is presented.

Throughout medical training, mnemonics are recommended so that important lists can be easily recalled. The mnemonic for admission orders is *A.D.C.Van Disal.* A sample set of admission orders is shown in Figure 12-1.

Admit. By convention, the first order written is that to admit the patient to the hospital. Included in this order is the name of the attending physician to whose service the patient is to be admitted (e.g., "Admit to Dr. John Smith").

Diagnosis. The next order that should be written is the admitting diagnosis or diagnoses (e.g., appendicitis). If a diagnosis cannot be given, i.e., it is not known, the chief complaint can be used (e.g., "Abdominal pain of unknown etiology" or "Chest pain, rule out myocardial infarction").

Condition. This is a clinical estimate made by the admitting physician, which should be updated as the patient's clinical condition changes. Some institutions have specific criteria for categorizing a patient's condition; others leave this judgment to the physician. Commonly used statements include the following: *good,* which implies that the patient is stable and that there are no anticipated complications; *fair,* which implies that the patient is ill and may have complications but has a good chance for recovery; *poor,* which implies that the patient is very ill, may have complications, and is not very stable, or that the patient is chronically or terminally ill and is not expected to do well; *serious,* which implies that the patient is very ill and not very stable, and that the clinical outcome is not predictable; *critical,* which usually implies that the patient is desperately ill, very unstable, and may not recover. In many institutions, patients in critical condition are placed on a "danger list," and this too can be written as an order (e.g., "Critical—place on danger list").

Vital Signs. Routine vital signs include temperature, pulse, respiratory rate, and blood pressure. The frequency with which these signs are obtained by the nurse is up to the physician and must be ordered. The clinical condition of the patient warrants the frequency; the vital signs of a critically ill patient may need to be obtained every 10 to 15 minutes, whereas those of very stable patients may need to be taken only every 8 hours (or once per shift). By convention, a lower-case "q" is placed before the number of hours between vital signs, and the number is followed by a lower-case "h"; e.g., q4h means "every 4 hours," and q15min means "every 15 minutes" (for further abbreviations, see Table 12-1 and Appendix III). It is important that these orders be reviewed daily, so that if lesser frequency is appropriate, it is written. This allows the nursing staff to focus on the patients who need more nursing care.

Activity. The amount of activity that a hospitalized patient may be allowed is also prescribed by the physician. The amount of activity is decided by the physician and is based on the patient's clinical status; it may range from strict bed rest to out of bed with assistance (abbreviation: OOB c̄ assist) to unimpeded activity (ad lib). Included in this order is whether the patient may have

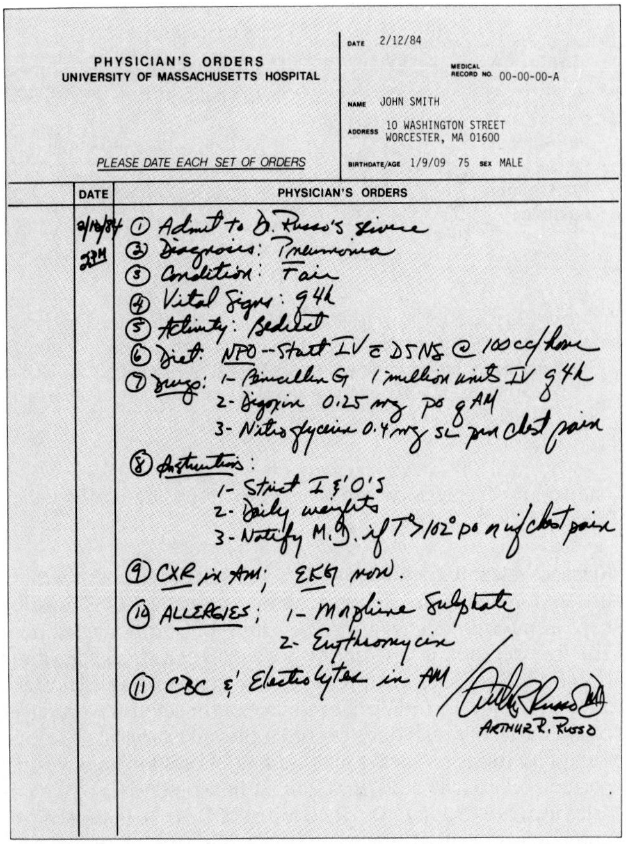
DATE 2/12/84

PHYSICIAN'S ORDERS
UNIVERSITY OF MASSACHUSETTS HOSPITAL

MEDICAL RECORD NO. 00-00-00-A

NAME JOHN SMITH

ADDRESS 10 WASHINGTON STREET
WORCESTER, MA 01600

PLEASE DATE EACH SET OF ORDERS

BIRTHDATE/AGE 1/9/09 75 SEX MALE

DATE	PHYSICIAN'S ORDERS
2/12/84 2PM	① Admit to Dr. Russo's Service
	② Diagnosis: Pneumonia
	③ Condition: Fair
	④ Vital Signs: q4h
	⑤ Activity: Bedrest
	⑥ Diet: NPO—Start IV c̄ D5NS @ 100cc/hour
	⑦ Drugs: 1- Penicillin G 1 million units IV q4h
	2- Digoxin 0.25 mg po qAM
	3- Nitroglycerin 0.4 mg SL prn chest pain
	⑧ Instructions:
	1- Strict I & O's
	2- Daily weights
	3- Notify M.D. if T > 102° po or if chest pain
	⑨ CXR in AM; EKG now.
	⑩ ALLERGIES; 1- Morphine Sulphate
	2- Erythromycin
	⑪ CBC & Electrolytes in AM — Arthur R. Russo MD, ARTHUR R. RUSSO

Figure 12-1 A sample set of admission orders.

Table 12-1 List of Abbreviations Commonly Used When Writing Orders and Prescriptions*

Diagnoses	Dx	Diagnosis
	ALL	Acute lymphocytic leukemia
	AML	Acute myelogenous leukemia
	CLL	Chronic lymphocytic leukemia
	CML	Chronic myelogenous leukemia
	COPD	Chronic obstructive pulmonary disease
	DVT	Deep venous thrombosis
	R/O MI	Rule out myocardial infarction
	TIA	Transient ischemic attack
Nutrition	NPO	Nothing by mouth
Drugs		
Dosages	gr	Grains
	mcg	Micrograms
	mg	Milligrams
	gm	Grams
	tabs	Tablets
	caps	Capsules
Time intervals†	qod	Every other day
	qd	Every day
	bid	Twice a day
	tid	Three times a day
	qid	Four times a day
Routes of administration	PO	By mouth
	SC	Subcutaneously
	IM	Intramuscularly
	IV	Intravenously
	PR	Per rectum
Instructions	I & O	Total daily intake and output
Intravenous solutions	D5W	5% dextrose and water
	D5NS	5% dextrose and normal saline
	NS	Normal saline
Special studies	CT scan	Computed tomography (specify body part)
	CXR	Chest x-ray film
	Echo	Echocardiogram
	EEG	Electroencephalogram
	EKG (ECG)	Electrocardiogram
	EMG	Electromyogram
	IPG	Impedance plethysmography
	IVP	Intravenous pyelogram
	KUB	Kidneys, ureters, bladder (abdominal x-ray film); also known as "flat plate" of the abdomen
	L/S scan	Liver/spleen scan (nuclear)
	RVG	Radionuclide ventriculogram (nuclear)
	V/Q scan	Ventilation and perfusion lung scan (nuclear)
Laboratories	CBC	Complete blood count
	'lytes	Electrolytes
	BS	Blood sugar
	BUN	Blood urea nitrogen
	Hgb	Hemoglobin
	Hct	Hematocrit
	U/A	Urinalysis
Phrases	$\bar{c}$	With
	$\bar{s}$	Without
	w/o	Without
	ac	Before meals
	pc	After meals
	hs	At bedtime
	$\bar{p}$	After
	prn	As needed

* Countless abbreviations are available. Most hospitals are required by the Joint Committee on Accreditation of Healthcare Organizations to have a list of approved abbreviations, but these should be used sparingly, with caution, and should be written clearly and carefully. When in doubt, write it out! This can save countless interruptions and prevent mistakes. See Appendix III for a more extensive list of abbreviations.

† It is important to know the exact time of each dose for your institution; i.e., qid does not necessarily mean every 6 hours, but q6h does.

bathroom privileges or is restricted to a bedside commode or bedpan.

Nutrition. Each patient admitted to a hospital must have written orders for nutritional support. Many patient variables must be kept in mind in determining the nature of nutritional support. The first decision is whether or not a patient may take anything by mouth. There are many reasons why a patient should not take anything orally, including altered state of consciousness and fear of aspiration of oral liquids or solids, planned surgical or laboratory procedures requiring withholding of oral feedings, or suspected abdominal pathology that may be worsened by eating or drinking (see Chapter 10, "Scheduling of Tests"). In these situations, an order must be written restricting intake to nothing by mouth (abbreviation: NPO). If this order is written, an alternative form of maintaining favorable hydration and nutritional status (intravenous therapy) should be considered. The patient's need for fluid, calories, and medications must be assessed and an appropriate order written.

For short-term intravenous therapy, peripheral intravenous therapy containing various solutions of electrolytes and fluid is probably adequate. If long-term intravenous therapy is anticipated, solutions containing electrolytes, fluids, vitamins, proteins, and lipids (hyperalimentation) should be considered. This may be delivered peripherally in moderate volumes and concentrations or in higher volumes and higher concentrations through catheters into large central veins (internal jugular or subclavian).

If a patient is a candidate for oral feedings, many dietary choices are available as dictated by the clinical situation. A patient may be restricted to clear liquids or advanced to a full liquid diet. A patient may be able to tolerate only a soft diet if he or she is recovering from a gastrointestinal problem, or may require a pureed diet if he or she has difficulty chewing or swallowing. Finally, a patient may be able to eat anything, and this is usually ordered as a "regular" or "house" diet.

Once a diet has been chosen, the physician must determine whether there should be any restrictions to this diet. If a patient is diabetic, appropriate restriction of calories and carbohydrates should be prescribed. If a patient has hypertension or congestive heart failure, a limit on the amount of sodium in the diet should be ordered. If a patient has renal disease, the maximum allowable amount of sodium, potassium, and protein contained in the patient's daily diet should be determined and then ordered. Patients with hepatic disease may require diets that are high in carbohydrates and low in protein. Other disease states may also require specific limitations of one or more components of the patient's diet.

Drugs. Every medication, including nonprescription drugs, that the patient will be taking while hospitalized must be ordered in writing. The medications are divided into two categories: those that the patient must take on a regular basis and those that may be required on an intermittent, as-needed (abbreviation: prn) basis. When writing for a medication, the drug name (generic or trade) is written first. This is followed by the dosage, the route of administration (orally, intramuscularly, intravenously, rectally, intranasally, insufflation, or aerosol inhalation), and the frequency with which it should be given (e.g., "hydrochlorothiazide 25 mg PO qd" [see Table 12-1]). If a drug is to be administered on an intermittent, as-needed basis, the order should be written as above and be followed by prn plus the indication for administration (e.g., "codeine 15 mg PO q6h prn headache"). Upper use limits may be included, if needed (e.g., "not to exceed 60 mg per 24 hours").

It is important that medication orders be reviewed frequently (preferably each day) during the patient's hospital stay and be updated as needed. Each institution has specific regulations regarding medication orders. Some require that these orders be written on a regular basis (e.g., once a week). Many institutions require that narcotic analgesic prescriptions be rewritten more frequently—sometimes as often as every 24 to 48 hours.

Instructions. This section of the admitting orders is directed at specific nursing duties (other than vital signs) that the physician believes must be carried out meticulously. The list of possible special instructions is endless, but some of the more common ones are listed in this section. The physician may order that the nurse frequently and accurately record the patient's intake of fluids and output of urine, the patient's weight on a daily basis, or the presence or absence of occult blood in a patient's stool.

Special instructions for nurses may include guidelines that specify when the nurse should notify the physician if specific changes occur in the patient's clinical status. Examples of orders for such notification may include one for notification if the patient develops chest pain, another if the patient's temperature rises above a certain level, another if the pulse rises above a certain maximum or falls below a predetermined minimum, or if the patient's systolic or diastolic blood pressure rises above a predetermined maximum or falls below a predetermined minimum (e.g., "Notify the physician if the temperature rises above 38.5°C rectally or if the pulse rate is greater than 100").

Special Studies. At this point in the admitting orders, special diagnostic studies could be ordered. Included here are orders for radiographic studies, such as chest radiographs; cardiovascular studies, such as electrocardiography, echocardiography, and impedance plethysmography; neurologic studies, such as electroencephalography and electromyography; and other studies.

Allergies. All medications or foods that the patient is allergic to should be listed in the admitting orders. Some physicians put this right after the order to admit and write it in *red ink*.

Laboratories. When a patient is admitted to a hospital, multiple diagnostic laboratory studies are often needed. Usual admitting laboratory studies include complete blood count with differential (this includes white blood cell count, red blood cell count, hemoglobin, hematocrit, and red cell indices), platelet count, prothrombin time, partial thromboplastin time, electrolytes (including sodium, potassium, chloride, and bicarbonate), a chemistry profile (including liver function tests, glucose, blood urea nitrogen, creatinine, cholesterol, and uric acid), serology for syphilis, and a urinalysis. Other studies may be indicated on admission. It is important to think about each test and whether or not it is needed. If you can't justify it, wouldn't change your management because of it, or if it has recently been done on an outpatient basis, don't order it. A few extra tests per patient can increase the cost of health care by millions of dollars, not to mention the additional patient discomfort it creates. Depending upon the institution, a variety of chemistry profiles are available, and you should be familiar with what is included in the profile of the institution in which you practice medicine. Some physicians write routine or "standing" orders for daily blood work; this is usually not optimal. Orders for blood work should be written daily or as needed to prevent unnecessary blood tests from being performed and to prevent anemia from excessive phlebotomy.

Discharge Orders

An important component of writing orders on hospitalized patients is the writing of discharge orders. When a patient is ready for discharge from the hospital, an order must be entered by the attending physician authorizing such a discharge. Multiple components of the discharge orders are listed in this section. In some settings, a physician may choose only to write the simple order to discharge the patient and then enter the remainder of the discharge order information into the last progress note of the chart. For the purpose of this textbook, the convention of writing complete discharge orders in the order section of the patient's medical record is used.

Discharge Order. An order authorizing the discharge must be entered. This order should include the location to which the patient will be discharged (e.g., "Discharge patient to home" or "Discharge patient to Quality Nursing Home").

Discharge Diagnosis. The discharge diagnosis for the patient's hospital admission is entered at this point. This may be the same as the admission diagnosis, although in many cases it may differ depending on the outcome of the hospital stay. An example of a discharge diagnosis would be "Pyelonephritis."

Condition on Discharge. The patient's condition at the time of discharge (e.g., "Good") is entered at this point. The rules listed previously for categorizing a patient's condition apply here as well.

Discharge Medications. A complete listing of all the medications for the patient, including dosages and time interval, is entered. This may include new medications that the patient should be taking at the time he or she is discharged. Also, at the time of writing this order, the physician should write out all necessary prescriptions and enter an order into the chart stating "Prescriptions Written." An example of a listing of discharge medications is as follows:

1. Isordil 20 mg q8h
2. Captopril 25 mg tid
3. Ampicillin 500 mg qid
4. Colace 100 mg bid

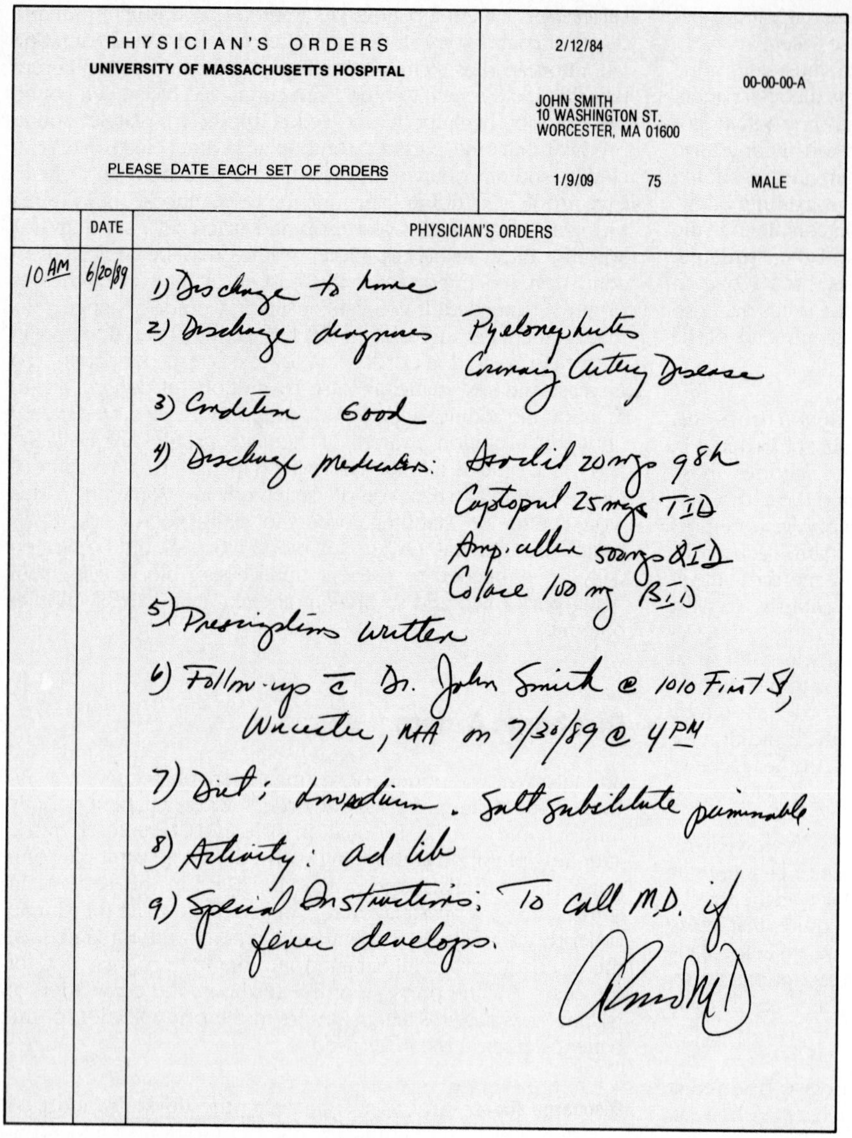

PHYSICIAN'S ORDERS
UNIVERSITY OF MASSACHUSETTS HOSPITAL
PLEASE DATE EACH SET OF ORDERS

2/12/84
00-00-00-A
JOHN SMITH
10 WASHINGTON ST.
WORCESTER, MA 01600
1/9/09 75 MALE

DATE		PHYSICIAN'S ORDERS
10 AM	6/20/89	1) Discharge to home
		2) Discharge diagnoses Pyelonephritis, Coronary Artery Disease
		3) Condition Good
		4) Discharge medications: Isordil 20 mgs q8h; Captopril 25 mgs TID; Ampicillin 500 mgs QID; Colace 100 mg BID
		5) Prescriptions written
		6) Follow-up c̄ Dr. John Smith @ 1010 First St, Worcester, MA on 7/30/89 @ 4PM
		7) Diet: low sodium. Salt substitute permissible
		8) Activity: ad lib
		9) Special Instructions: To call MD. if fever develops.
		[illegible] MD

Figure 12-2 A sample set of discharge orders.

Follow-up. At this point in the orders, specific instructions pertaining to medical follow-up for this patient should be entered (e.g., "Follow-up with Dr. John Smith at 1010 First Street, Worcester, MA, on July 30, 1989 at 4:00 PM").

Diet. The type of diet that the patient should be following at home is entered next (e.g., "Low sodium diet; salt substitute may be used").

Activities. An order should be entered describing the physical activities in which the patient may participate. This may be as simple as "ad lib," indicating that the patient may resume normal activities, or it may be more complicated, such as "May be out of bed to chair for 1 hour three times per day."

Special Instructions. Finally, any special instructions that the patient is to follow should be entered (e.g., "Patient is to notify attending physician if fever develops or if shortness of breath occurs"). A multitude of special instructions may be entered at this point, depending on the patient's diagnosis, condition, and prognosis. It is assumed that patient and physician have discussed these special instructions in detail prior to discharge. This pertains to all of the preceding categories as well. At the time the physician is discharging the patient from the hospital, time should be spent with the patient reviewing his or her diagnosis, condition, prognosis, discharge medications, activity, diet, and any special instructions that the physician may have for the patient. The fact that these specific discharge orders have been entered into the order section of the chart allows the patient's primary nurse to review all discharge orders with the patient. The nurse may be able to answer any questions the patient has just prior to discharge and help ensure that the patient will comply with those instructions. A sample set of discharge orders is included in Figure 12-2.

Writing a Prescription

Arthur R. Russo, MD

13

The writing of prescriptions is an extremely important function that a physician routinely performs for patients. A prescription results from the physician's assessment of the patient's clinical condition after a careful history and physical examination and review of indicated laboratory studies. It is the physician's order to initiate therapeutic intervention aimed at controlling or curing a disease state or ameliorating a symptom. Because this is such an important function, it should not be performed without careful thought about the disease state, the risks of therapy, and the risks of no therapy, an assessment of concomitant disease states, review of other medications that the patient is taking that may interact with the newly prescribed medication, a careful history of possible allergies to drugs, and consideration of the cost of the medication.

Nearly half of all medications used in the United States are available without a prescription. These are the over-the-counter (OTC) drugs, such as aspirin, that patients routinely use for minor, self-limited illnesses, usually without the advice of a physician. Physicians frequently recommend some of the OTC drugs to their patients and should therefore be familiar with their contents; however, a formal prescription for these drugs is not necessary.

Because the writing of a prescription for a medication that is not available without a physician's authorization is such an important task, it must be done carefully. The prescription must clearly state exactly what the physician wants the patient to receive. It must be legible, so that no misinterpretation on the part of the pharmacist is possible. Physicians whose handwriting is difficult to read should consider printing or typing prescriptions. The prescription should be written in indelible ink to prevent it from being altered. Furthermore, it is good practice for physicians to keep an exact copy of every prescription on file, although this is required by law only for Schedule II drugs (controlled substances).

The Prescription

In this section, the essential parts of a prescription are discussed and the mechanics of writing a prescription are detailed (Fig. 13-1).

Patient's Name. Use the patient's full legal name, including a middle initial. The full name may help to prevent errors in medication use between family members in the same household. Avoid nicknames. The name should be clearly written, printed, or typed.

Patient's Address. The patient's address should be completely listed and legible. This may help to avoid inadvertent errors with refills. It is a legal requirement on prescriptions for all Schedule II drugs.

Age. Although not required by law, the patient's age is an important addition to a prescription. It helps the pharmacist to recognize dosage errors, especially in the pediatric population, and may help jog the physician's memory about dose alterations for geriatric patients. Also, it serves to further identify the patient.

Sex. The patient's sex is not required, but it helps with patient identification.

Date. The date that a prescription is written should be on all prescriptions. It is a legal requirement for all Schedule II, III, and IV drugs. Also, it is important in patient care. If a prescription was written long before it is presented to the pharmacist, the pharmacist may require proof of identity of the patient (in the event that the prescription was lost, stolen, or inappropriately passed on to another person), or may request authorization from the physician to fill this dated prescription. The physician may then decide that the prescription is no longer valid because of the

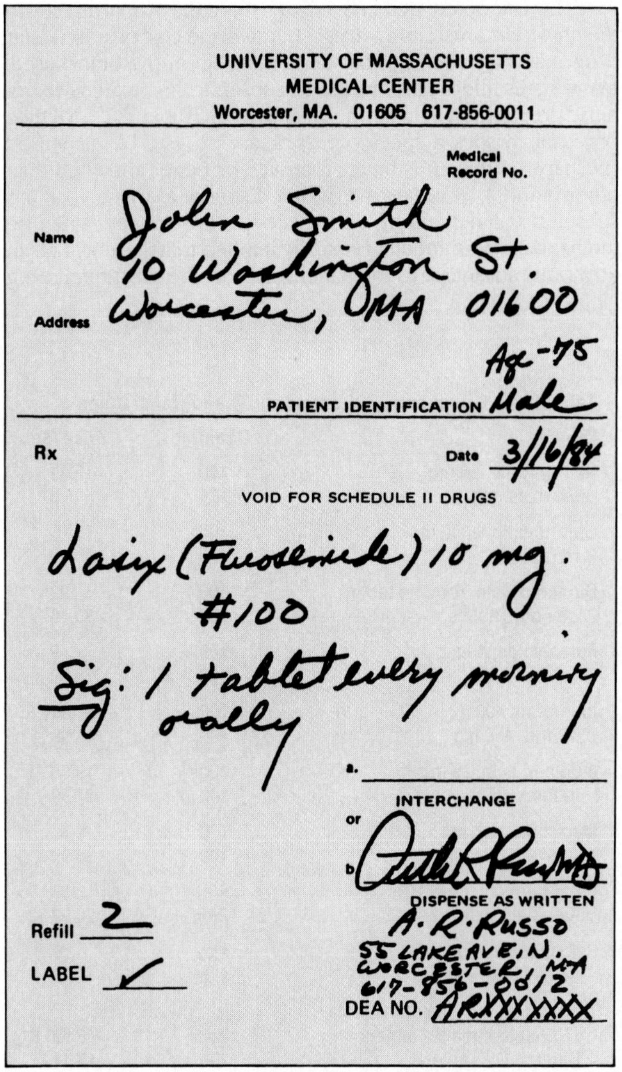
UNIVERSITY OF MASSACHUSETTS
MEDICAL CENTER
Worcester, MA. 01605 617-856-0011

Medical Record No.

Name John Smith
10 Washington St.
Address Worcester, MA 01600
Age-75
PATIENT IDENTIFICATION Male

Rx Date 3/16/84

VOID FOR SCHEDULE II DRUGS

Lasix (Furosemide) 10 mg.
#100
Sig: 1 tablet every morning orally

a. ______
INTERCHANGE
or
b. ______
DISPENSE AS WRITTEN
A. R. Russo
55 Lake Ave, N.
Worcester, MA
617-856-0012

Refill 2

LABEL ✓

DEA NO. ARXXXXXX

Figure 13-1 Preprinted prescription form.

time elapsed and may wish to re-examine the patient before authorizing the dispensing of the drug.

R_x. This is an abbreviation for *recipe* taken from the Latin for "take then." Classically, this is referred to as the superscription, and it signals the start of the body of the prescription (i.e., the part of the prescription dealing with the drug itself and the instructions to the patient). The term *recipe* was formerly more applicable in this situation. Prescriptions used to contain an elaborate recipe written by the physician for formulation of a drug. Now this is rarely done. Rather, most physicians now write prescriptions for drugs that are ready-made, i.e., compounded in standard dosages by the pharmaceutical companies. Therefore, in this chapter, reference is made only to prescriptions for standard drugs. Instructions for recipes for compounding medications are not included. (Appendix II presents the most frequently prescribed medications and their dosage forms.)

Drug Name. The drug name should be the first item written in this section. When prescribing a drug, the physician may choose to write either the trade or brand name (proprietary name) or the generic name (nonproprietary name). In recent years, there has been a major effort to control medical costs. Because the cost of medications is a major component of medical care costs, much controversy has centered on the merits of prescribing generically versus prescribing by trade name. Therefore, various states have adopted methods to bring this controversy directly to the physician prescribing drugs. Because the cost of a particular drug may vary considerably depending upon the brand used, many states allow pharmacists to substitute less expensive generic drugs when a prescription is written (Table 13-1). When a physician wishes a specific proprietary drug to be dispensed (perhaps because it is better tolerated or better absorbed than other brands), he or she may write "dispense as written" or "no substitution," depending upon state-specific statutes. When interchange is permitted, it is usually implied that there will be an economic advantage to the patient and that the substituted drug has equivalent properties in terms of efficacy. Some subsidized health care programs and most Veterans Administration pharmacies require that the pharmacist dispense the least expensive equivalent medication. Because there may be considerable state-to-state variation in prescribing regulations, physicians should become familiar with those in the states in which they practice. They also should be well aware of differences in bioavailability between the brands of drugs that they prescribe.

Table 13-1 Comparison of Generic and Brand-Name Drugs

Drug*	Quantity	Price ($)
Amitriptyline, 50 mg	100	12.49
Elavil, 50 mg	100	54.49
Chlorthalidone, 50 mg	100	9.95
Hygroton	100	40.89
Diphenoxylate-atropine tablets	100	8.99
Lomotil Tablets	100	35.49
Furosemide, 40 mg	100	7.49
Lasix, 40 mg	100	12.69
Ibuprofen, 400 mg	100	11.99
Motrin, 400 mg	100	14.99
Indomethacin, 25 mg	100	19.39
Indocin, 25 mg	100	37.99
Meclizine, 12.5 mg	100	4.81
Antivert, 12.5 mg	100	28.99
Potassium chloride, 10% elixir	Pint	3.29
Kay Ciel Elixir	Pint	20.99
Selenium shampoo	4 oz	4.29
Selsun Shampoo	4 oz	12.89
Trimethoprim-sulfamethoxazole double-strength tablets	20	8.99
Bactrim DS Tablets	20	17.11

*Note that the generic drug is cited first. The brand-name preparation is indented below.

Table 13-2 Dosage Equivalents

1 grain	=	0.065 gram
1 ounce	=	31.1 grams
1 kilogram	=	2.2 pounds
1 fluid ounce	=	29.57 milliliters
1 quart	=	946.4 milliliters

Dosage. In general, it is best to use the metric unit when prescribing medications (Table 13-2). Because the majority of physicians now choose to prescribe commercially available formulations rather than recipes for compounding individualized medications, the physician should be familiar with the dosages available for a particular drug. Many drugs are manufactured in multiple dosage sizes, and this information is available from multiple sources (e.g., *The United States Pharmacopeia* or *The Physicians' Desk Reference*). The combination of the drug name plus the dosage is referred to as the "inscription" part of the prescription.

Quantity to Be Dispensed. The amount of medication (e.g., number of pills, volume of liquid) to be dispensed by the pharmacist should be written next. This is referred to as the "subscription." This can be written out (e.g., # fifty), or Arabic numerals (e.g., # 50 or # 100 cc) can be used. When writing for a medication that has a potential for abuse (e.g., a narcotic), it is preferable to write out the amount to be dispensed. This helps to prevent the prescription from being altered, thereby limiting the amount dispensed to exactly what the physician desires.

When deciding how much medication to dispense, consider several factors. First, if this medication is for treatment of an acute, limited disorder (e.g., streptococcal pharyngitis), the amount dispensed should be exactly enough for one course of therapy. Second, if this medication is for a chronic disease or long-term therapy (e.g., treatment of hypertension), but this particular drug has not been used by this patient previously, a small amount of medication should be dispensed. If the patient were not to tolerate the medication, and therapy was discontinued or another medication substituted, the patient would not be left with a large supply of medication he or she could not use. In general, medications cannot be returned to the pharmacy. Third, if the medication has been well tolerated and the patient will require long-term therapy, it is often beneficial to prescribe larger quantities of medication, because there is often a financial benefit to the patient if a particular drug is purchased in bulk. Fourth, if the patient is suspected to be noncompliant in terms of seeking medical follow-up, it may be preferable to prescribe smaller quantities of medications in order to help ensure that the patient returns for periodic follow-up so that you can monitor therapy. Fifth, if the patient has an emotional or psychiatric problem and may attempt lethal ingestion (even if the possibility is remote), as in the case of a patient being started on medical therapy for depression, it is generally recommended that very small amounts of medication be dispensed. This helps prevent access to lethal amounts of medication and requires that the patient return frequently for careful monitoring of clinical status and efficacy of therapy.

Directions for Use. This section of the prescription may be the most important, because it is the physician's direct instructions to the patient for use of the medication. What the physician writes here, the pharmacist will place on the container. On the prescription, these directions are introduced by one of two words. The first is "sig," which stands for signature (*not* the physician's signature), and is taken from the Latin "signa." The other option is to write "Label:" and then follow with the directions. Many sources recommend the second choice, because the use of the English language is preferable and abbreviations can be avoided.

It is imperative that the actual directions for use be legibly written, clear, and very precise. In order to improve patient compliance, it is better to prescribe exact times for use (e.g., "8 AM, 1 PM, 6 PM, and 11 PM") rather than vague times (e.g., "four times a day" or "after meals" or "at bedtime"). Directions for use should never be written as "use as directed," because this implies that the physician has clearly and precisely given these instructions to the patient orally, that the patient understood the directions, and that the patient remembers them. Exceptions to this would be complex instructions (e.g., for chemotherapy) that are too extensive to type on the space available and can be given as separate written instructions.

Number of Refills. A physician may choose to permit a number of refills or may choose not to permit refills. These choices must be written on the prescription. Refills can be written either by number (e.g., 6 refills) or by time (e.g., refill for 6 months). For Schedule II drugs, no refills are permitted without another new prescription being written.

Physician's Signature. The physician must sign the prescription with his or her legal signature, including the appropriate suffix, e.g., MD, DO, DMD.

Physician's Name. The physician's name should be imprinted on the prescription. If a prescription does not have the name preprinted, the physician should print his or her name under the signature.

Drug Enforcement Administration Number. Federal law requires that any prescription for a Schedule II drug have the physician's Drug Enforcement Administration (DEA) registry number clearly printed on the prescription. A DEA number may be required in other circumstances as well, such as on prescriptions for patients on Medicare. (For a description of the classes of drugs needing a DEA number, see Appendix II and below.)

Physician's Address. The physician's professional address should be printed on the prescription. Prescriptions provided by hospitals usually have the hospital's name and address preprinted on them.

Physician's Telephone Number. So that the pharmacist may easily contact the physician in the event that a question arises, the physician's office telephone number should be included on preprinted prescription forms (see Fig. 13-1).

Scheduled Drugs

In an effort to combat drug abuse, the Controlled Substances Act of 1970 was passed. Drugs with a potential for abuse came under the jurisdiction of the Controlled Substances Act and were divided into five categories. The DEA, organized in 1973, eventually became responsible for overseeing, administering, and policing the Controlled Substances Act. The five categories are as follows:

Schedule I. These drugs have no accepted medical use and have a high potential for abuse (e.g., heroin and mescaline). Special licensing is required for use of such agents in research settings.

Schedule II. These drugs have a high potential for abuse as well as for psychic and physical dependence. They do, however, have accepted medical uses in the United States. Drugs in this category include some narcotics, stimulants, and depressants (e.g., morphine, amphetamines, and secobarbital).

Schedule III. These drugs have a potential for abuse, but it is less than that for drugs of Schedules I and II. Included in this category are drugs with small amounts of narcotics and certain other non-narcotic drugs (e.g., glutethimide).

Schedule IV. These drugs have a potential for abuse, but it is less than that for drugs of Schedule III. Multiple classes of drugs are in this category, including the benzodiazepines, dextropropoxyphene, and pentazocine.

Schedule V. These drugs have a potential for abuse, but it is less than that for drugs of Schedule IV. These drugs also contain small amounts of narcotics and are usually used as antidiarrheal and antitussive agents.

Drug Interactions

It has long been recognized that there are significant physical and chemical incompatibilities between various drugs. Those incompatibilities were very important to individual physicians when it was common practice for physicians to write prescriptions ordering the compounding of multiple drugs. Now, these properties are more important to pharmaceutical companies that compound unit-dosed drugs. In recent years, however, it has become well recognized that many drugs interact in many ways. This has become very clear with the advent of assays for in vivo drug levels that have shown that one drug may act to increase the blood level of a concomitantly administered drug, often causing the level of one or both drugs to reach toxic levels, even when administered in acceptable individual doses (e.g., digoxin and quinidine interactions). Physicians must be well aware of these potential interactions when prescribing multiple drugs for a patient or when prescribing a new drug for a patient who is already receiving other medications. It is implicit, therefore, that a physician must know all the drugs that a patient is taking. When administering drugs that are known to interact, the physician must carefully monitor for clinical signs of toxicity and obtain periodic blood levels, if indicated (see Chapter 14, "Adverse Drug Reactions," and Chapter 15 "Adverse Drug Interactions").

A rapidly growing volume of literature deals with drug interactions. Physicians must familiarize themselves with the available information. As a rule, it is worthwhile to review the product information when writing for a medicine that one is unfamiliar with or that one has not prescribed or reviewed for the last year. This keeps one up to date on newly recognized drug interactions or reactions.

Compliance

Good compliance by the patient is as important to a successful therapeutic intervention as the appropriate choice of a medical regimen. If a patient is noncompliant, therapy will probably fail, and the end result may be a disease state that is more refractory to treatment than the original problem.

The physician can do many things to help improve patient compliance. The physician must make an attempt to explain thoroughly to the patient the nature of his or her illness, its expected course, the benefits of therapy, and the result of noncompliance. The physician should review the prescription with the patient, explaining how and when to take the drug and what may be expected in terms of typical side effects. The doctor should, in some manner, make sure that the patient understands the instructions and then allow the patient to ask questions. One should legibly and precisely write the directions for use on the prescription. These directions should exactly repeat what the physician has already told the patient. You may wish to write out instructions on a separate sheet so that the patient has another source, besides the medication bottle, to refer to in case questions arise. This is particularly important when a patient is taking multiple medications. In these cases, the physician or nurse should write out a schedule for all the medications. Finally, the physician should choose medications that the patient can comply with easily. It is known that as the number of doses per day increases, compliance dramatically decreases.

Computerized Prescription Writing

Personal computers are becoming commonplace additions to medical offices. Billing functions as well as medical record keeping are being computerized, even in small offices. Software programs are now being developed to aid the physician in prescription-writing duties. This is likely to lead to better record keeping, as well as save time. Possibilities for "automatically" checking for drug interactions, assisting in dosage calculations, reviewing drug efficacy in certain disease states, and reviewing side-effect profiles are endless. The ability to generate detailed printed patient instructions is also possible. During the next several years, computerized prescription-writing programs are likely to become an important component of everyday medical practice.

References

Abramowicz M, ed. Adverse interactions of drugs. Med Lett 1981; 23(5):17.

Abramowicz M, ed. Drug interactions update. Med Lett 1984; 26:11.

Allen SI, et al. Prescription-writing with a PC. Comput Methods Programs Biomed 1986; 22(1):127.

American Pharmaceutical Association and American Society of Internal Medicine. Prescription writing and prescription labeling. J Pharm Assoc 1974; NS14(12):654.

Billings PR. Preventing tampering with prescriptions: The Marton method [letter]. Ann Intern Med 1988; 108:637.

Brown CS, et al. A computerized prescription writing program for doctors. Methods Inf Med 1985; 24(2):101.

Drug Enforcement Administration and the DEA/Practitioners Working Committee, A Joint Statement. Guidelines for prescribers of controlled substances. Ohio State Med J 1981; 77(5):312.

Gilman AG, et al, eds. Goodman and Gilman's the pharmacological basis of therapeutics. 7th ed. New York: Macmillan, 1988:1660.

Ingrim, NB, et al. Physician noncompliance with prescription-writing requirements. Am J Hosp Pharm 1983; 40:414.

Katzung BG, ed. Basic and clinical pharmacology. 4th ed. Los Altos, CA: Appleton & Lange, 1989:748.

Phillips D. Guidelines for prescribers of controlled drugs. J Arkansas Med Soc 1985; 81:463.

Salberg DJ, Frey DR. Prescription writing habits of physicians in postgraduate training. Am J Hosp Pharm 1982; 39:129.

Silverman HM, ed. The proper time for taking drugs. Pharm Facts 1971; 6(10):18.

Adverse Drug Reactions 14

Steven D. Reich, MD

Brian F. Johnson, MD

A drug is any chemical or natural product (or combination) that is used to modify physiologic systems or pathologic states for the benefit of the patient. Adverse drug reactions are a group of pathologic states induced by drug therapy. For most individual drugs, the incidence of serious adverse effects is low. However, because so many people take drugs for prolonged periods and because "polypharmacy" (multiple drug therapy) is so common, the chance that an individual patient will experience an adverse drug reaction is high. Because not all adverse drug reactions are recognized, and because those that are noted are not always reported, the number of adverse drug reactions can only be estimated. Also, incidence is not calculable, as the number of patients at risk for an adverse reaction to a particular drug (i.e., the number of people taking a drug) is rarely known. It is estimated, however, that 15 percent of hospitalized patients develop adverse reactions ranging from mild to fatal. About 85 percent of these reactions will occur during the first 2 weeks of hospitalization. One hospital calculated that about 5 percent of hospital costs resulted from adverse drug reactions. Another estimate is that about 6 million people a year suffer adverse drug reactions in the United States, and these reactions cost our society hundreds of millions, if not billions, of dollars annually in direct costs of additional treatment and in loss of productive work.

Because there is a finite risk of a drug reaction in any situation in which drugs are given, it is important to weigh risks versus benefits. The risk of a serious reaction is acceptable if the disease being treated is serious, but it is unacceptable if the disease is trivial. This means that before prescribing any drugs, the clinician must be familiar with its potential to cause toxicity. The clinician must also have a basic knowledge of the pharmacokinetic properties of the drug, factors that affect the susceptibility of a patient to a drug reaction, and the mechanisms of adverse reactions. Important factors that have an impact on the incidence and severity of adverse drug reactions include nonindividualized dosing, prolonged therapy, age, allergic history, and the pathophysiologic state of the patient as a result of the disease.

Adverse drug reactions may be difficult to recognize. The problem is that the human body has a limited number of ways it can react to damage. Degenerative changes and necrosis may occur in one or more anatomic sites, antibodies may form that lead to hypersensitivity reactions, or an adverse drug reaction

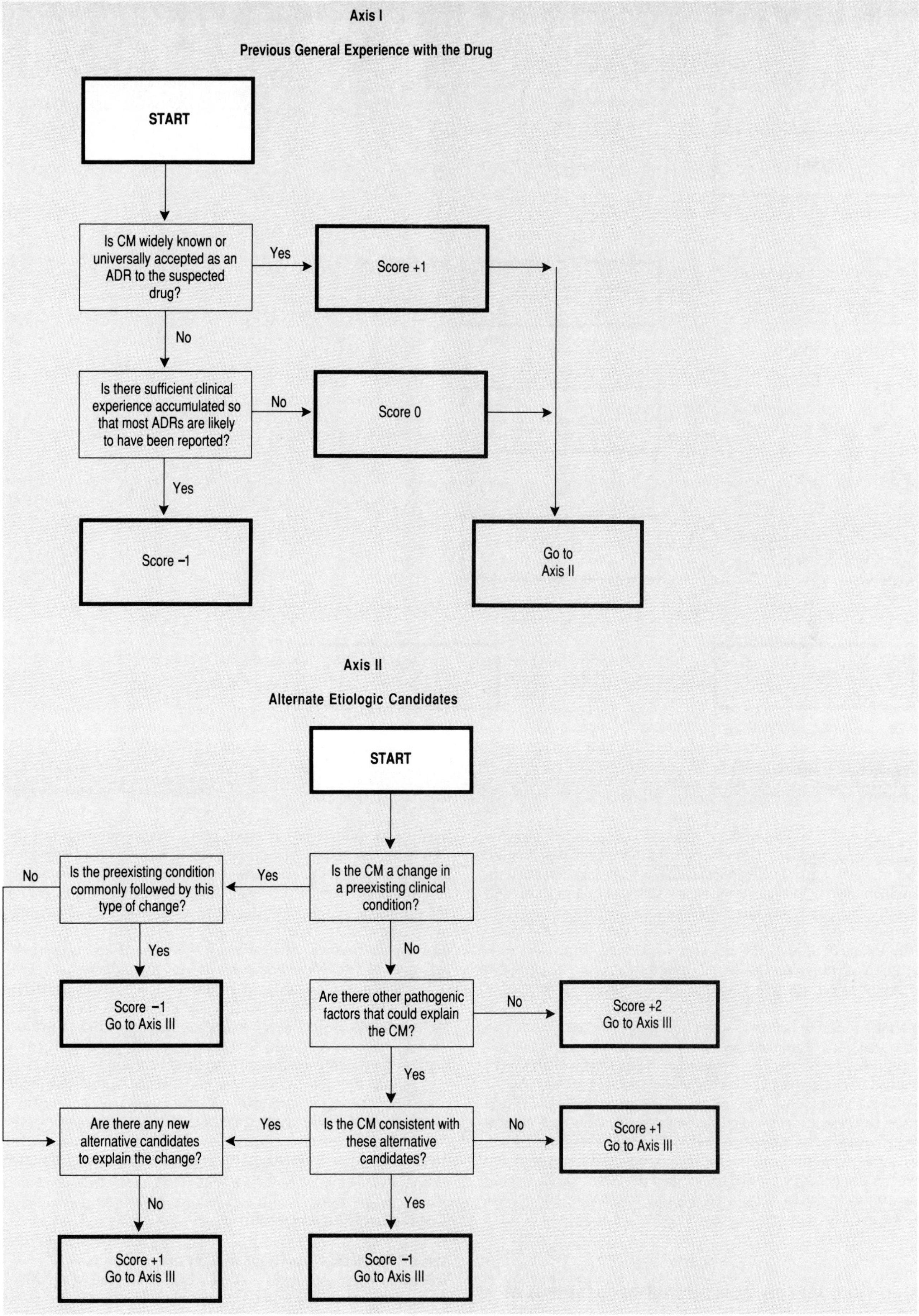

Figure 14-1 Algorithm for the evaluation of suspected drug reactions. ADR =adverse drug reaction, CM = clinical manifestation.

Figure continues on following page

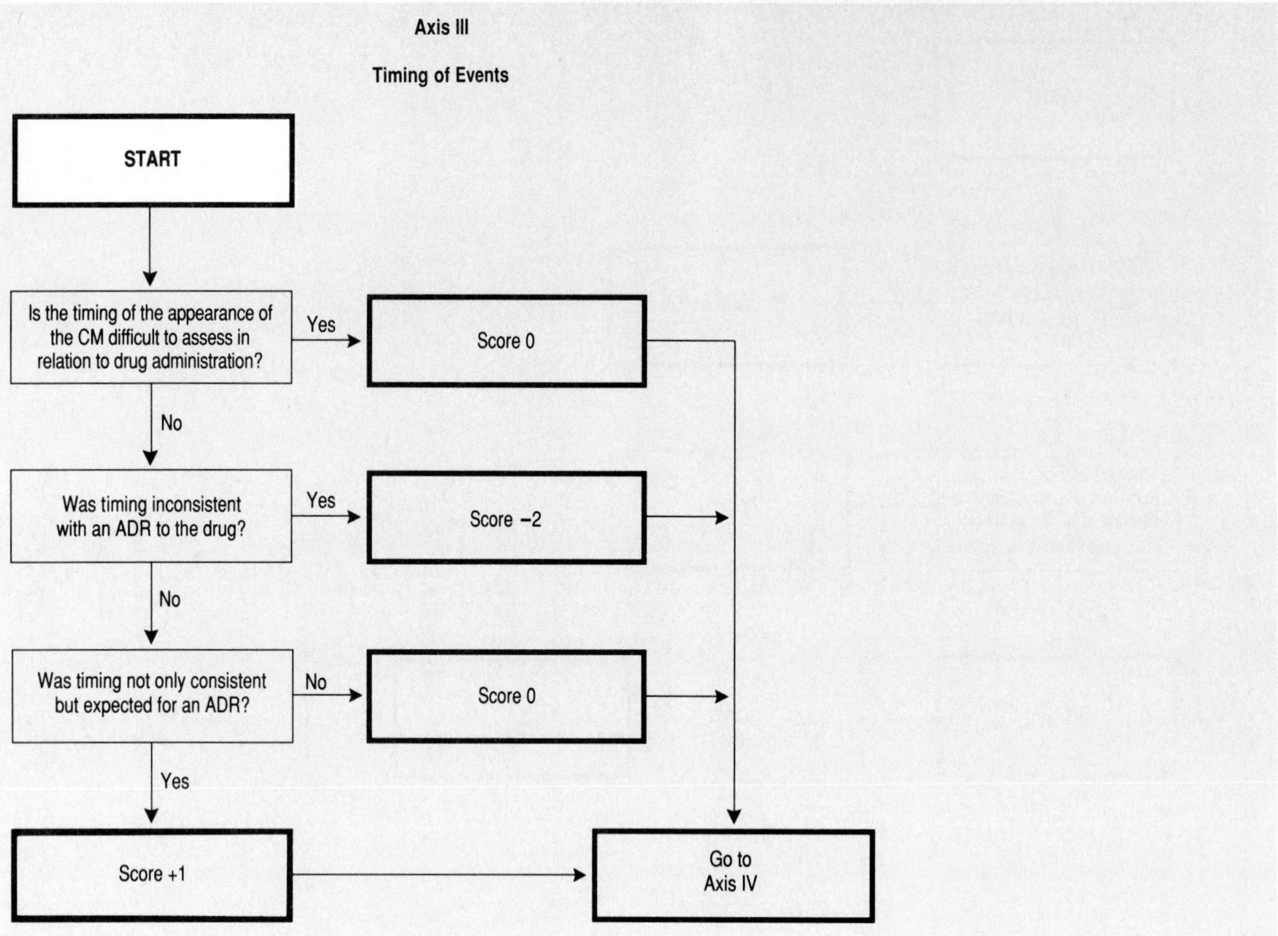

Figure 14-1 *Continued*

Figure continues on opposite page

can mimic well-known disease patterns. These disease patterns include congenital and developmental abnormalities, benign and malignant tumors, hyperplasias, hypoplasias, aplasias, inflammations including granuloma, vascular alterations, and functional changes without evident morphologic variations from normal. Hence, drug-induced illnesses often resemble non–drug-induced illness. No features of adverse drug reactions uniquely identify them as being caused by drugs. The problem of identifying an adverse drug reaction is reflected in the fact that a drug is rarely identified as the definite causative agent. In one analysis of 2,500 cases of suspected drug reaction, only 17.5 percent were considered definite, and another 30 percent were considered probable. This means that the majority of cases were evaluated as negative (5 percent), coincidental (14.5 percent), or possible (33 percent). Agreement among individuals evaluating cases of adverse drug reactions is poor. In studies of clinical pharmacologists who evaluated cases in which the clinical manifestations suggested an adverse drug reaction, these presumed experts disagreed one-third to one-half the time. The amount of disagreement can be decreased, although not totally eliminated, by the use of algorithms designed for the assessment of adverse drug reactions.

Algorithm for the Operational Assessment of Adverse Drug Reactions

Several algorithms for the evaluation of suspected drug reactions have been devised, and, to a greater or lesser extent, they have been validated as reproducible. When tested against the judgments of experts, they fare well. The focus of these algorithms varies, but they have many features in common; a simplified version of the algorithm by Kramer et al (1979) is shown in Figure 14-1. Although the use of complex algorithms may be best left to experts, the logic involved must be used by all those who evaluate adverse drug reactions if an accurate assessment of a suspected drug reaction is to be made.

The algorithm shown in Figure 14-1 comprises six major axes of decision strategy, with a scoring system incorporated into each axis. A final score is determined from the individual scores for each axis, and this final score is translated into a degree of certainty for the adverse drug reaction.

Before the algorithm is used, a reaction must have been observed. Some clinical manifestation must have alerted the patient or the health care providers that something is amiss. Failure to recognize a clinical manifestation as unusual for a patient with a particular disease complex will result in the failure to recognize an adverse drug reaction.

Contents of the Algorithm

Axis I: Prior Clinical Experience with the Drug

Some clinical manifestations of an adverse reaction to a particular drug are well known and are reported in standard pharmacology texts or textbooks of therapeutics; others are more obscure. Reasons for the obscurity include low incidence of the reaction, a drug that is seldom used, clinical manifestations that were first thought to be disease related and not drug related (as

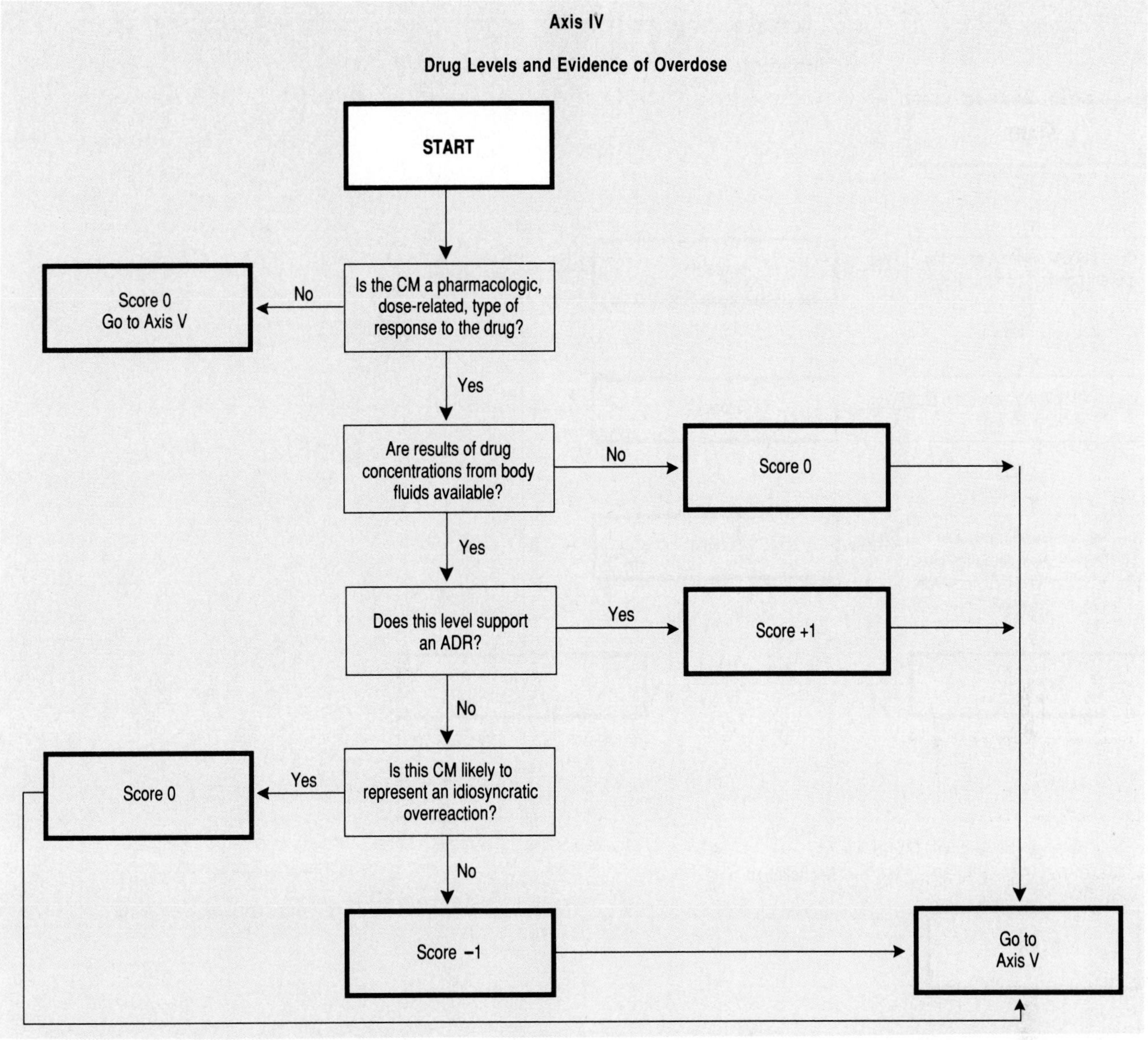

Figure 14-1 *Continued*

Figure continues on following page

in the case of Reye's syndrome and aspirin), or a drug so new that relatively few patients have been treated with it. With the use of computer searches of large databanks of indexed material on drug reaction, it is now easier to find single reports of suspected drug reactions. A case for a drug reaction is strengthened by previous reports of clinical manifestations similar to those of the suspected case, and it is weakened when the clinical manifestations have not been reported for a drug with which there is considerable clinical experience.

Axis II: Alternative Etiologies

Clinical manifestations may or may not be consistent with the natural history of a patient's disease complex. The purpose of this axis is to distinguish among the administered drug, underlying clinical conditions, and diagnostic or therapeutic interventions that might be responsible for causing the clinical manifestations. A new illness must also be considered.

Axis III: Chronologic Order of Events

Timing of events is critical to the assessment of a suspected adverse drug reaction. It is surprising how often a drug is considered the causative agent, although the drug was not given until after the start of the new clinical problem. By the same token, drugs have been accused of causing a reaction when in fact they were not given to or taken by the patient.

Axis IV: Drug Concentrations and Evidence of Overdose

The analysis of body fluids or tissues can be helpful. Adverse drug reactions that are known to be related to drug levels can be evaluated by measurement of drug concentrations. The classic example is the determination of serum digoxin concentrations in patients with cardiac arrhythmias. Because a diseased heart can produce arrhythmias resulting from either too much or too little digoxin, drug levels can help sort out problems of inadequate dosing from those of overdosing.

Axis V: Dechallenge

Dechallenge, or discontinuation of the drug in question, may lead to improvement in the clinical manifestations that led to the suggestion of a drug reaction. This is good, but not conclusive, evidence that the clinical manifestation was due to the drug. Spontaneous remissions of a disease state coincidental with

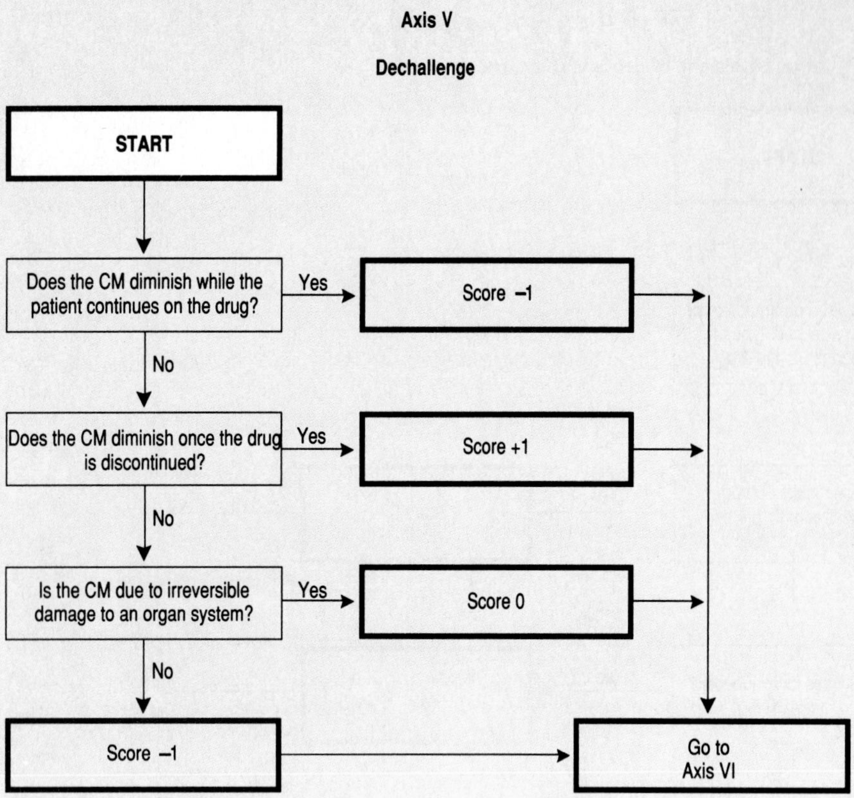

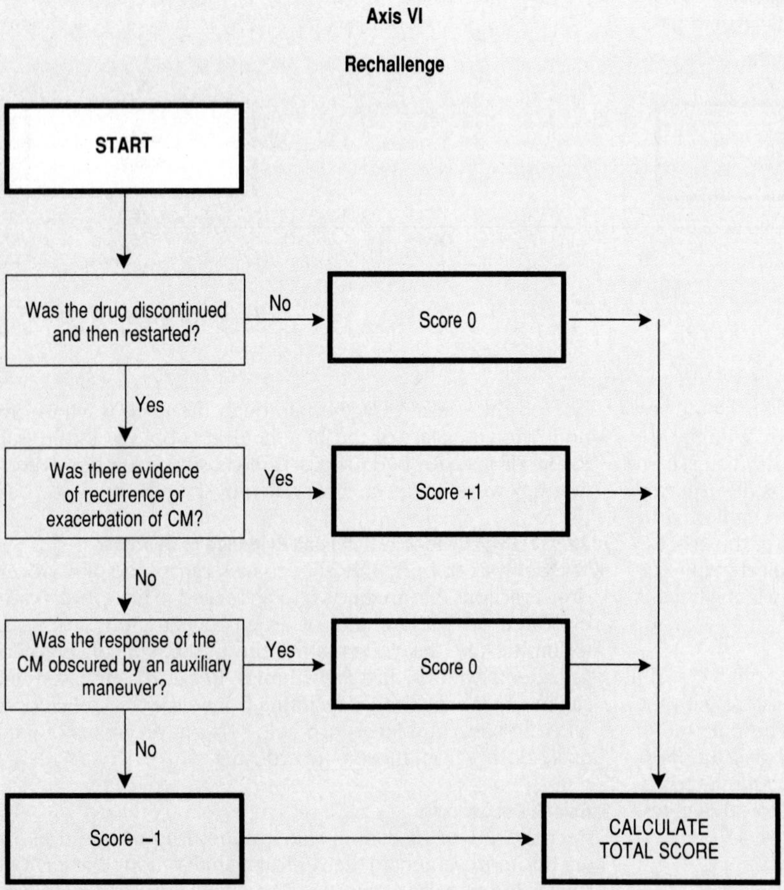

Figure 14-1 *Continued*

Table 14-1 Scoring System of the Algorithm for Assessment of Adverse Drug Reactions

Likelihood	Points
Definite	+6 or more
Probable	+4 or +5
Possible	0 to +3
Unlikely	Negative score

dechallenge can produce the same results. If the manifestations do not improve with dechallenge, this is evidence that the drug was not causative. Some clinical manifestations are irreversible, however. One might expect, for example, no improvement in liver cirrhosis with dechallenge.

Axis VI: Rechallenge

Recurrence of clinical manifestations after reinstituting the drug is good evidence for a drug-related event. Other reasons for the renewed clinical manifestations are still possible, but usually unlikely. Rechallenge is rarely done because it is usually not worth the trouble to rechallenge someone for minor reactions to a drug that has multiple alternatives. For severe or life-threatening reactions, rechallenge is rarely acceptable practice. Rechallenge is appropriate in those cases of mild to moderate suspected reactions in which the drug in question is clearly the optimal choice for the underlying disease.

Use of the Algorithm

Once thought processes are guided by the algorithm, a conclusion can be drawn regarding the likelihood of certain clinical manifestations being due to a drug. For the majority of cases in which a drug reaction is suspected, after careful analysis the drug will be determined to be possibly or probably the causative agent. The scoring system is shown in Table 14-1.

Although alcohol and "recreational" drugs like caffeine are not usually prescribed for the benefit of patients, the algorithm can be used to help ascertain whether these agents were responsible for clinical manifestations. However, the clinical manifestations due to drugs that are taken intentionally in overdose are not considered adverse drug reactions.

Conclusions

The use of drugs is increasing, as is the incidence of adverse drug reactions. It is important to be aware of such reactions because some patients may be harmed more by the effects of drugs than by the disease processes that the drugs were intended to treat. On the other hand, it is important not to withdraw optimal drug therapy because of incorrect attribution of a complex of signs, symptoms, or laboratory findings to a drug reaction. Although an operational approach to evaluating a case of a suspected adverse drug reaction can be helpful, the important point is to think logically and to have pertinent facts about the disease and the available drug. Once the clinician has decided that a drug has caused an adverse reaction, it is the responsibility of that physician to warn the patient about future use of the drug. It is also the responsibility of the clinician to report major suspected drug reactions. This can be done by notifying the hospital pharmacy or pharmacy and therapeutics committee, the drug manufacturer, or the U.S. Food and Drug Administration. Unusual clinical manifestations thought to be due to a drug reaction should be well documented and reported in the medical literature, so that the information can be used in the analysis of future suspected adverse drug reactions.

References

Hutchinson TA, et al. An algorithm for the operational assessment of adverse drug reactions II. Demonstration of reproducibility and validity. JAMA 1979; 242:633.

Irey NS. Diagnostic problems and methods in drug-induced disease. American Registry of Pathology. Armed Forces Institute of Pathology, 1966: part 1; 1967: part 2; 1968: part 3.

Karch FE, Lasagna L. Toward the operational identification of adverse drug reactions. Clin Pharmacol Ther 1977; 21:247.

Karch FE, et al. Commentary: Adverse drug reactions—A matter of opinion. Clin Pharmacol Ther 1976; 19:489.

Koch-Weser J, Sellers EM, Zacest RR. The ambiguity of adverse drug reactions. Eur J Clin Pharmacol 1977; 11:75.

Kramer MS, et al. An algorithm for the operational assessment of adverse drug reactions I. Background, description, and instructions for use. JAMA 1979; 242:623.

Leventhal JM, et al. An algorithm for the operational assessment of adverse drug reactions III. Results of tests among clinicians. JAMA 1979; 242:1991.

Levy M, et al. Hospital admissions due to adverse drug reactions: A comparative study from Jerusalem and Berlin. Eur J Clin Pharmacol 1980; 17:25.

Matthews SJ, Scheiweiss F, Cerosimo RJ, A clinical manual of adverse drug reactions. Norwalk, CT: Appleton-Century-Crofts, 1986.

Seidl LG, Thornton GF, Cluff LE. Epidemiological studies of adverse drug reactions. Am J Public Health 1965; 55:1170.

Venulet J. Methods of monitoring adverse reactions to drugs. In: Jucker, E. ed. Progress in drug research. Basel: Birkhauser Verlag, 1977:233.

Venulet J, Ciucci A, Berneker, GC. Standardized assessment of drug-adverse reaction associations—rationale and experience. Int J Clin Pharm Ther Toxicol 1980; 18:381.

Adverse Drug Interactions

Brian F. Johnson, MD

Steven D. Reich, MD

15

An adverse drug interaction occurs when the effect of one drug is increased, inhibited, or otherwise modified by another drug, resulting in a clinically unfavorable response. Clinical manifestations of an adverse effect vary and can consist of symptoms exclusively, new physical findings, abnormal laboratory or radiologic determinations, or some combination of these.

Mechanisms of Drug Interactions

Pharmacodynamic

A drug can interfere with the molecular, cellular, or physiologic basis of another drug's effect. Minor actions of a drug may become important by affecting the desired action of another drug at the same receptor site; e.g., streptomycin may potentiate the effect of some muscle relaxants. Other drugs may interact through entirely different sites of action; e.g., steroids inhibit the hypoglycemic effect of tolbutamide.

Pharmacokinetic

A drug can alter the absorption, transport processes, or elimination of another drug, and therefore modify its effects. Absorption of one drug may also be modified by the capacity of another to alter gastric emptying, bowel motility, or mesenteric blood flow, or drugs may form complexes in the intestine. The amount of free drug available to penetrate into target organs may be increased as a result of other drugs competing for the binding sites on plasma proteins. This effect is important only for drugs like warfarin, which is highly protein bound. The elimination of a drug may be greatly reduced if other drugs compete for transport systems in the renal tubules. By this mechanism, the uricosuric drug probenecid can increase the effects of penicillin, salicylates, or indomethacin. Metabolic elimination of drugs by hepatic enzymes may be inhibited by other drugs, as, for example, tolbutamide clearance is reduced by chloramphenicol or phenylbutazone. Many drugs can induce enzyme activity. By this process, several drugs, including hypnotics, anticonvulsants, phenylbutazone, rifampin, and spironolactone, may increase the rate of elimination of a wide variety of other agents.

Recognition of an Adverse Drug Interaction

Some drug interactions are clinically useful, as in the combined use of nitrites and beta-blockers in angina; however, the clinician should pay particular attention to those that can be harmful. The decision process about the probability that any clinical manifestation is due to a drug interaction is basically similar to that for recognizing adverse reactions to a single drug. This has been described in detail in Chapter 14, "Adverse Drug Reactions." The modified process is summarized in the sections that follow.

Previous General Experience. If the clinical manifestation is widely known and accepted as an interaction in the doses used, score +1. If not, score −1. If too little experience with the drug has been accumulated at present, score 0.

Alternate Etiologic Candidates. If the clinical manifestation is a worsening, recurrence, or complication of a preexisting condition, and if this change is commonly seen to occur naturally, score −1. If there are other possible pathogenetic factors, such as new disease or other interventions, score −1. If neither, score +2.

Timing of Events. If the clinical manifestation diminishes while the patient continues to take the drugs, score −1 (unless tolerance is common, or another treatment is given). If the clinical manifestation substantially diminishes with withdrawal of one or more drugs, and there is no obvious change in any other possible etiologic agent, score +1. If the effect of rechallenge is not measurable (e.g., death, episodic or irreversible clinical manifestation), score 0.

Rechallenge. If the clinical manifestation reappears or worsens with readministration of one or more drugs in similar dosage, score +1. If not, score −1. If there is no rechallenge, score 0.

Degree of Certainty for Adverse Drug Interactions. A final score is determined from the individual scores, and this final score is translated into a degree of certainty for the adverse drug interaction. A total score of 0 to +3 = possible; +4 to +5 = probable; and +6 to +7 = definite.

Examples of Important Adverse Drug Interactions

Central Nervous System Depressants. The depressant effects of a wide range of drugs may combine to produce coma with respiratory depression. Although narcotics and hypnotics are usually prescribed with appropriate care, the potential interaction between drugs like diazepam (Valium), propoxyphene (Darvon), alcohol, antihistamines, phenothiazines, and tricyclic antidepressants may be overlooked, with drastic consequences.

Anticoagulants. Dangerous bleeding may follow enhancement of the effects of warfarin by aspirin, clofibrate, chloral hydrate, or phenylbutazone. Any of the liver enzyme inducers (e.g., barbiturates, rifampin) may increase warfarin elimination. The resulting loss of control of prothrombin time will often be compensated by increased dosage. Bleeding can subsequently result if the interacting drug is discontinued without a reduction in the dose of warfarin.

Oral Hypoglycemics. The hypoglycemic effects of tolbutamide or chlorpropamide may be increased by phenylbutazone or reduced by steroids or thiazide diuretics.

Cytotoxics. The depressant effects upon bone marrow function and the other toxic effects of drugs like 6-mercaptopurine or azathioprine are increased by allopurinol, which inhibits their elimination.

Digoxin. The risk of cardiac toxicity is increased by hypokalemia induced by diuretics and by concurrent quinidine or verapamil therapy, which reduces digoxin elimination.

Monoamine Oxidase Inhibitors. Patients taking one of this group of drugs become highly responsive to tyramine-containing foods and to sympathomimetic drugs often used as nasal decongestants, appetite suppressors, and bronchodilators. Hypertensive crises and intracerebral bleeding may result. Hyperpyrexia with delirium may result if tricyclic antidepressant drugs, such as imipramine, are given to patients taking a monoamine oxidase inhibitor.

Liver Enzyme Inducers. Hypnotics, anticonvulsants, phenylbutazone, rifampin, and spironolactone are some of the inducing agents that may enhance elimination and therefore nullify the effects of steroids or oral contraceptives.

Spironolactone. When given in conjunction with oral potassium preparations, potassium-sparing diuretics can induce potentially dangerous hyperkalemia.

Guanethidine. The uptake of guanethidine into adrenergic nerve endings is blocked by tricyclic antidepressants (imipramine, amitriptyline, doxepin), with resulting loss of control of hypertension.

Conclusions

Because the average hospital patient in the United States is given about eight drugs in an admission period, there is ample opportunity for drug interactions to occur. The important adverse interactions involve commonly prescribed drugs that have a relatively low safety margin between effective and toxic dose.

However, the risks of adverse drug interactions should not be overstressed. It is often justified to use several drugs concomitantly, because patients commonly have multiple diseases, and some drug interactions are beneficial. Many drug interactions are minor when compared with other sources of variation in drug response. Genetic variations in pharmacokinetics, thyroid status, level of hepatic or renal function, age, and other factors can often affect drug action to a much greater extent. In many cases, the effects of drug interaction can be compensated by altering the dose of one of the drugs.

Recognition of an adverse drug interaction requires availability of good sources of information. Unfortunately, many supposed interactions are based on theoretical concept, in vitro studies, or unsubstantiated studies in healthy volunteers. The clinician should use only those sources of information that distinguish between theoretical and clinically relevant interactions. No one can be expected to remember all of the possible drug interactions, but appreciation of the few potentially life-threatening ones is essential. Appendix II reviews commonly prescribed medications and lists the common interactions. It is imperative that you review the *recent* literature for each new drug you prescribe and that you keep abreast of older drugs and their relationship to the newer ones by reviewing the *Medical Letter,* product inserts, *Physicians' Desk Reference, current* pharmacology texts, and medical morbidity and mortality reports as part of your regular reading.

References

Cadwallader DE. Biopharmaceutics and drug interactions. 3rd ed. New York: Raven Press, 1983.
Cluff LE, Petrie JC. Clinical effects of interaction between drugs. Amsterdam: Excerpta Medica, 1975.
Grahame-Smith DG. Drug interactions. London: Macmillan, 1977.
Griffin JP, D'Arcy PF, Speirs CJ. A manual of adverse drug interactions. 4th ed. London: Wright, 1988.
Hansten PD. Drug interactions. 6th ed. Philadelphia: Lea & Febiger, 1989.
Petrie JC, Cluff LE. Clinically important adverse drug interactions. New York: Elsevier North-Holland, 1985.

Overdoses and Poisons

Morris Ostroff, MD, MPH, MBA, FACEP

16

Poisonous plants and animals have been known to affect man for thousands of years. References to medicinal plants and herbs as well as poisons abound in the ancient writings of the Bible and of the Greeks and Romans. Numerous examples of intentional poisonings exist in ancient Greek and Roman literature and history. As the science of medicine developed during the 18th and 19th centuries, therapeutic drug overdoses began to be recognized. During the 20th century, numerous new therapeutic drugs were discovered and eventually introduced into clinical practice. The toxic effects of intentional and accidental overdoses as well as side effects and cumulative effects of drugs began to warrant greater attention. Suicide attempts with drugs, accidental overdoses, and substance abuse became epidemic during the 1970s and 1980s and will doubtless continue through the 1990s.

The intent of this chapter is to outline the general management of all patients with overdoses (Fig. 16-1). Some specific references are made to individual drugs or chemicals. Numerous recent reviews as well as monographs and books have appeared that specifically review individual chemical exposures.

Primary Medical Management

The primary goal in the initial management of any patient with suspected overdose or chemical exposure is to support the vital functions. As with all comatose patients presenting to emergency facilities, the ABCs (airway, breathing, and circulation) must be rapidly assessed and appropriately managed. Start intravenous fluids immediately, and save samples of blood, urine, and gastric

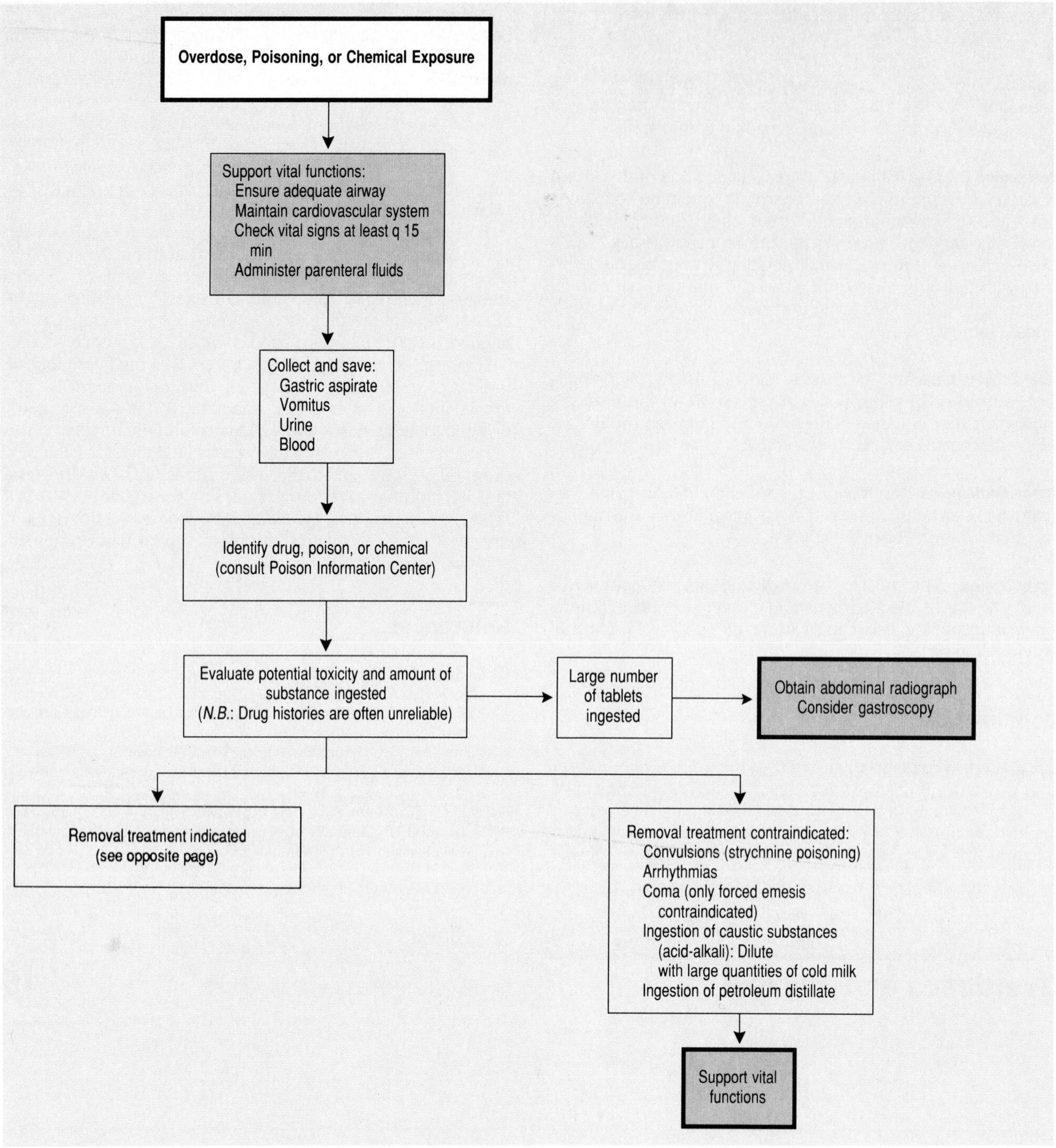

Figure 16-1 Algorithm for the treatment of a patient with an overdose, poisoning, or chemical exposure.

contents for toxicologic analysis. Infuse naloxone, thiamine, and 50 percent dextrose immediately in unconscious patients. Hypoxemia should be avoided, and blood gas determinations or peripheral oximetry performed in the comatose or agitated patient. Agitation may be the earliest sign of hypoxemia. The airway must be scrupulously maintained; in patients with decreased gag reflex, fluctuating mental status, progressive lethargy, somnolence, or coma, an endotracheal tube should be placed to protect the airway from aspiration. Blood pressure frequently needs to be monitored or maintained in these patients; fluids, rather than vasopressors, should be tried first. In elderly patients or those with compromised cardiovascular status, hemodynamic monitoring may be necessary. The use of specific vasopressors depends on the specific chemicals the patient has taken as an overdose. The use of norepinephrine bitartrate (Levophed) or metaraminol bitartrate (Aramine) may be preferred in patients who have taken an overdose of a psychotropic drug.

Agent Identification

Although trying to identify the specific drug or chemical to which the patient was exposed is important, one should not let the patient's vital functions deteriorate while spending excess time in this endeavor. Partially emptied bottles of medications, known drugs, or chemicals are often easy to identify. However, many patients brought to emergency departments are lethargic,

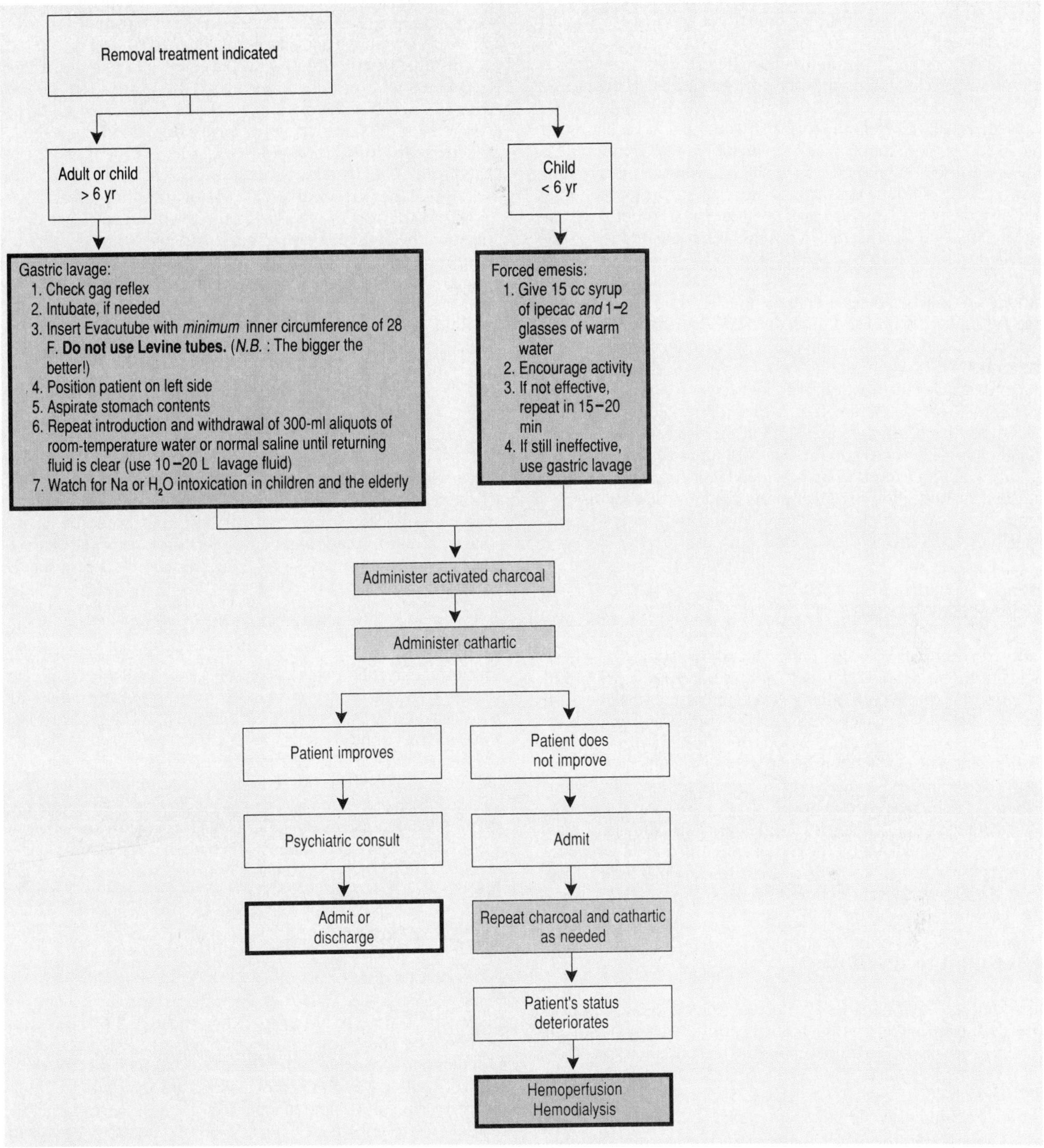

Figure 16-1 *Continued*

stuporous, comatose, or uncooperative and will not or cannot identify the drugs or chemicals to which they were exposed. Other patients may readily disclose what they have taken, but you may discover later, by toxicologic analysis, that their confession was false. Many patients take numerous drugs.

The physical examination may help in defining some drug categories. The pupils may be dilated and not reactive in patients who have been exposed to barbiturates, carbon monoxide, methanol and other alcohols, cocaine or belladonna derivatives, camphor, cyanide, and sympathomimetic or parasympatholytic agents. Miosis or pinpoint pupils are frequently seen in patients taking narcotic or morphine derivatives, as well as in patients who have some types of mushroom poisonings or who have taken cholinesterases, parasympathomimetics, chloral hydrate, ergot, nicotine, propoxyphene, or heroin. The respirations may be decreased after an overdose of narcotics or barbiturates. The skin may be flushed with alcohol, phenothiazines, or atropine. Red discoloration of the skin may occur with carbon monoxide poisoning. The patient may appear cyanotic because of methemoglobinemia due to phenacetin, lidocaine, para-aminosalicylic acid (PAS), antimalarial drugs, or the nitrates/nitrites. Large blisters or blebs of the skin are frequently caused by barbiturate poisoning, but they may also be seen with methadone, hydrocodone, meprobamate, imipramine, or glutethimide. Needle tracks in drug addicts may be found in the antecubital fossa, dorsum of the hands or feet, or other areas with easy vascular access. Alkali or acid burns may be seen in the mouth or on the face, and in these cases, esophagoscopy and gastroscopy should be performed.

Once the type of poison has been determined, a number of important specific issues about the drug or chemical should be elicited. The chemical nature of the substance should be reviewed, as well as its lethal potential. The actual dose exposure received by the patient may be difficult to determine, unless reliable witnesses were present when the overdose or exposure was received. Some drugs taken alone, even in large doses, may not be fatal; these same drugs, if combined with other drugs or alcohol, may be fatal in small amounts. The route of administration or exposure is important because some chemicals are rapidly absorbed through the skin or the gastrointestinal tract; others can only be absorbed intravenously. Some specific drugs may be rapidly eliminated from the body or metabolically converted into either less or more dangerous substances. Acetaminophen and methyl alcohol are examples of drugs that produce toxic substances when metabolized.

Choice of treatment will be greatly influenced by the excretion dynamics of each substance. Will the drug be excreted by the gut, lung, kidneys, or in the bile? Will there be enterohepatic circulation? Can excretion be hastened by the use of purgatives, diuresis, acidification or alkalinization of the urine, dialysis, ionic exchange, or blood exchange? Specific references should be sought for individual drugs or chemicals.

Laboratory Studies

Laboratory studies are also important in the evaluation of patients with overdoses, although most studies are not helpful early in the course of treatment. Toxic screens or specific drug levels may be sought, depending on the clinical situation. Baseline studies such as complete blood count, electrolytes, glucose, liver function tests, renal function tests, and urinalysis should be drawn early and be available for comparison throughout the patient's hospital course. Arterial blood gases should be followed if the patient's mental or pulmonary status deteriorates. Institute electrocardiographic monitoring in patients who may have ingested drugs with significant cardiovascular side effects (e.g., digoxin or tricyclic antidepressants).

Approach to the Patient

In addition to maintenance of the vital signs as described previously, the following actions should be instituted routinely in all patients with possible drug overdoses. The substance should be removed, be neutralized, or have its adverse effects reversed. In the case of skin exposures to dusts, powders, or liquids, the patient's clothing should be removed first, and the skin washed with copious amounts of plain water delivered by high-volume, low-pressure hoses or showers.

Removing the Substance

If the patient comes to the hospital within 60 minutes after the overdose, the substance may be removed by emesis with ipecac. The adult patient should be given 30 cc of syrup of ipecac, followed by six to eight glasses of water or juice. Do not use carbonated beverages. If emesis is not produced within 15 to 20 minutes, a second dose may be given. If this does not result in emesis, institute gastric lavage to prevent cardiac irritation resulting from the ipecac.

Syrup of ipecac may be contraindicated in several instances: (1) if substances are nontoxic in the existing dose range; (2) if the ingested substance is a caustic alkali or acid; (3) if a petroleum distillate was ingested (controversial); (4) if the patient is comatose, has a depressed gag reflex, or his or her mental status is deteriorating; and (5) if the ingested substance has a strong antiemetic property (e.g., phenothiazines).

Institute gastric lavage with a large-bore Evacutube or Ewal for patients who present more than 1 hour after ingestion or those whose time of exposure is unknown. In patients who are drowsy, stuporous, comatose, or have a depressed gag reflex or a decreasing level of consciousness, the airway must be protected with a cuffed endotracheal tube, and the patient placed on the left side, before one attempts to evacuate the stomach.

Gastric lavage may be performed with either water or saline, but the volumes being placed in the stomach and the quantity recovered must be carefully monitored. About 300 ml is placed in the stomach at one time and then removed, using low-pressure suction. This process is repeated until the returning fluid is clear. A minimum of 10 L of lavage fluid should be used; up to 20 L may be needed. In elderly patients or those with metabolic, renal, or cardiac diseases, pay special attention to fluid or salt overloading. The initial material removed from the stomach should be saved for analysis as necessary.

After lavage or administration of ipecac, instill activated charcoal in the stomach, using 50 to 100 g of charcoal mixed in a slurry with water or 50 percent sorbitol solution. Do not use activated charcoal in patients who have possible acetaminophen overdoses, because the charcoal will inactivate the acetylcysteine that is used to treat those overdoses. Activated charcoal may be used to inactivate syrup of ipecac that has not caused the patient to vomit.

Reversing Action

Specific agents that reverse drug action are available for a number of overdoses. Oxygen may be used in carbon monoxide overdoses; digitalis antibodies (Digibind), in digitalis preparations; and naloxone (Narcan), in narcotics overdoses. Atropine is used to counteract the cholinergic properties of mushrooms and organophosphate insecticides. Physostigmine has been used to reverse the anticholinergic properties of drugs such as the tricyclic antidepressants, but is itself fraught with danger. It should be used only in patients who have cardiac arrhythmias or seizures due to tricyclics that are not reversed by conventional therapy.

Hastening Excretion

Excretion of a drug or chemical in the gastrointestinal tract can be accelerated wth cathartics such as magnesium sulfate or magnesium citrate. Avoid castor oil, because of the risk of causing vomiting with aspiration and pneumonia. Forced diuresis with mannitol or furosemide (Lasix) helps only when the drugs ingested will have significantly increased excretion with increased urine flow. The dangers of forced diuresis include (1) electrolyte imbalance, (2) pulmonary edema, (3) water intoxication, and (4) cerebral edema.

Alkalinization of the urine with intravenous sodium bicarbonate assists in the removal of phenobarbital, salicylates, or butabarbital. Acidification of the urine using ascorbic acid speeds elimination of amphetamines or quinine.

Use of hemodialysis, ionic-exchange resins, or peritoneal dialysis is indicated in only 3 to 5 percent of patients taking overdoses. These procedures may assist in the removal of salicylates, phenylbutazones, phenobarbital, sulfonamides, sulfonylureas, and methanol.

Psychiatric Consultations

Psychiatric consultation should be sought for all patients taking intentional overdoses and for those whose accidental overdoses are suspicious. In hospitalized patients, psychiatric consultations should be sought before discharge, when the patient is able to participate with the psychiatrist in the evaluation.

References

Arena JM, Drew RH, eds. Poisoning: Toxicology, symptoms, and treatments. 5th ed. Springfield, IL: Charles C Thomas, 1986.

Barret SM. Poisoning. Prog Crit Care 1985; 2:316.

Bayer M, Rumack B. Poisoning and overdoses. Germantown, MD: Aspen Systems Corporation, 1982.

Bryson PD. Comprehensive review in toxicology. 2nd ed. Rockville, MD: Aspen Publishers, 1989.

Gosselin RE, Smith RP, Hodge HC. Clinical toxicology of commercial products. 5th ed. Baltimore: Williams & Wilkins, 1984.

Tobin MJ. Essentials of critical care medicine. New York: Churchill Livingstone, 1989.

Nuclear Medicine Studies 17

Dennis D. Patton, MD

Paul W. Doherty, MD

Nuclear medicine utilizes radioactive tracers for the diagnosis and treatment of diseases. Table 17-1 illustrates some of the tests, procedures, and therapies that are encompassed by nuclear medicine.

The major difference between the clinical use of nuclear medicine and other imaging modalities such as ultrasound and computed tomography (CT) is that nuclear medicine is based on *function* rather than morphology. For this reason, many nuclear medicine studies are quantitative and computer-assisted. Many can give differential right/left function.

Many nuclear medicine studies are available on an emergency basis, e.g., lung scans (for pulmonary embolism), biliary studies (for acute cholecystitis), testicular scans (for torsion), and others. Some procedures require special-order radiotracers and may not be routinely available.

Nuclear medicine studies are either imaging or nonimaging. Nuclear medicine images are made with position-sensitive radiation detectors called gamma cameras. Some gamma cameras can give tomographic images of the body similar to those obtained with CT and magnetic resonance imaging (MRI) (Fig. 17-1). Nonimaging studies in nuclear medicine include measurement of plasma volume, total red blood cell mass, blood volume, vitamin B_{12} absorption, red blood cell survival, thyroid iodine uptake, tests for malabsorption, and others.

The radiation dose from nuclear medicine studies is low, made possible by improved gamma cameras and by the use of the radioisotope technetium-99m (Tc-99m), which has a half-life of only 6 hours, decays almost entirely by gamma emission (beta or other particulate radiation delivers a high local radiation dose without contributing to the image), and has a gamma energy just high enough to get out of the body and low enough to be detected with nearly 100 percent efficiency. A patient undergo-

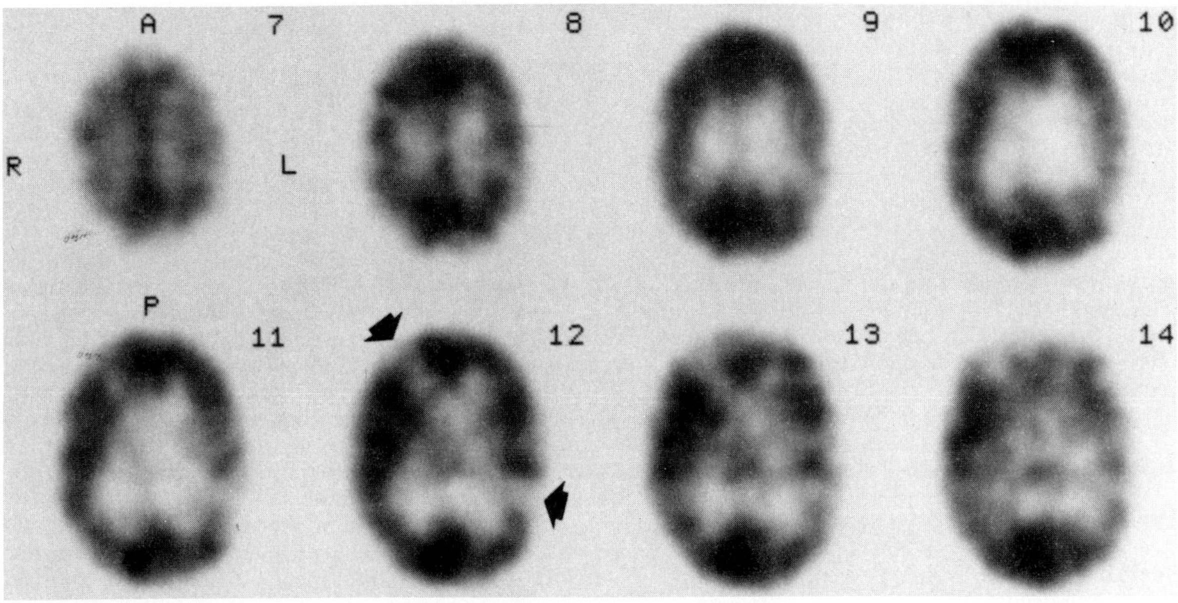

Figure 17-1 Some nuclear medicine cameras can make tomographic images similar to those from computed tomography (CT) or magnetic resonance imaging (MRI), although they are functional rather than morphologic images. This is a study of regional brain perfusion using Tc-99m HMPAO in a patient with multiple cortical strokes (*arrows*) following cocaine use.

Table 17-1 Nuclear Medicine Procedures

Cardiovascular
Cardiac ejection fraction: global/regional, right ventricular/left ventricular, first-pass/gated equilibrium ("MUGA"), rest/exercise, cardiac hemodynamics
Cardiac output
Cardiac wall motion
Dynamic vascular studies
Myocardial infarction/injury study (pyrophosphate)
Myocardial perfusion study (thallium-201), rest/exercise
Regurgitant fraction
Shunt quantitation: left-to-right, right-to-left
Vascular transit times
Vena cavagram: superior, inferior
Venogram

Endocrine and Metabolic (See *Therapy*)
Adrenal scan (baseline, dexamethasone)
Extracellular fluid space determination
MIBG scan (adrenergic tumors)
Parathyroid scan
Radiocopper turnover (Wilson's disease)
Thyroid cancer metastatic search
Thyroid scan
Thyroid uptake: standard, perchlorate washout, TSH stimulation, T_3 or T_4 suppression
Total body water determination

Gastrointestinal
Bile acid breath test
Biliary tree/gallbladder study (Tc-99m IDA or equivalent)
Esophageal motility study
Gallbladder emptying study
Gastric bile reflux
Gastric emptying time: solid, liquid
Gastroesophageal reflux/tracheal aspiration
Gastrointestinal bleeding: location of bleeding site
Gastrointestinal blood loss, quantitative
Gastrointestinal protein loss
LeVeen shunt patency study
Liver scan: standard/limited
Meckel's diverticulum study
Plasma albumin leak rate
Salivary gland study

Genitourinary
Effective renal plasma flow determination
Glomerular filtration rate determination
Renal scan and vascular study
Renogram
Residual bladder volume
Testicular scan
Ureteral reflux study (voiding cystoureterogram)

Hematology (See *Therapy*)
Bone marrow scan (In-111 chloride)
Bone marrow scan (Tc-99m sulfur colloid)
Blood volume
Ferrokinetics
Oral iron absorption
Plasma iron clearance
Plasma volume
Platelet deposition/survival
Red blood cell iron utilization
Red blood cell sequestration
Red blood cell survival
Red cell mass, total
Schilling test (parts 1 and 2)
Spleen scan (Tc-99m sulfur colloid)
Spleen scan (heat-damaged red blood cells)

Infectious Disease
Localization of infection (Ga-67 or In-111 white blood cells)

Musculoskeletal
Arthrogram
Bone scan: standard/limited/three-phase
Joint scan
Skin blood flow study

Neurology and Neurosurgery
Brain death study
Brain scan: standard/limited
Cerebral blood flow study (Xe-133 washout)
Cerebrospinal fluid shunt patency study
Cerebrospinal fluid study (cisternogram)
Dacryocystogram
Regional cerebral perfusion (HMPAO, IMP)

Oncology (See *Therapy;* see also specific organ scans)
Hepatic artery perfusion study
Lymph node scan (lymphoscintigram)
Lymphangioscintigraphy
Tumor scan (Ga-67)
Tumor scan (radiolabeled monoclonal antibodies)

Pulmonary
Deep vein thromboscintigram
Localization of bleeding site
Lung scan, perfusion
Lung scan, ventilation
Pulmonary alveolar permeability
Ventilation/perfusion ratio, global or regional ($\dot{V}/\dot{Q}$)

Therapy
I-131 (hyperthyroidism, toxic nodule, thyroid ablation, thyroid cancer)
P-32 soluble (polycythemia vera, thrombocytosis, intractable bone tumor pain)
P-32 colloid (intracavitary metastases, malignant effusions)

ing an average nuclear medicine study typically receives about the same radiation dose to the organ receiving the maximum dose as he would from one radiograph of that organ (with the exception of the lungs; a chest radiograph delivers a very low dose of radiation).

Diagnostic Nuclear Medicine

Nuclear Medicine in Cardiovascular Disease

Myocardial Perfusion. The myocardium actively takes up potassium, but nature has given us no radioactive isotopes of potassium that are suitable for nuclear medicine imaging. Biochemically close to potassium (K^+) is thallium (Tl^+), which is avidly taken up by the myocardium and other muscles. Thallium-201 (chloride) is injected at the end of the treadmill exercise, which dilates those coronary arteries that are capable of dilatation. In those patients who cannot or should not exercise, dipyridamole (Persantin) pharmacologically stresses the coronary circulation to produce maximal vasodilatation and can be used in lieu of exercise with equally good results. Images of the myocardium show which areas are being adequately perfused; both ischemic and infarcted areas show up as "cold" lesions. The size and distribution of these defects indicate the severity of the disease and the vessels involved.

Images are taken again at rest a few hours later. On the delayed images, there is filling in of the defects in reversible ischemia, and lack of filling in areas of frank infarction. Thallium studies have a sensitivity of 85 percent in detecting coronary artery disease, and a specificity of about 90 percent.

Thallium studies may be useful in patients with known or suspected myocardial ischemia or infarction when any of the following questions need to be answered: Where is the lesion?

Which arterial territory is involved? What is the extent of the ischemia or infarction? What is the extent of myocardium at risk? What is the clinical significance of lesions seen at coronary arteriography? (i.e., what is the perfusion in the involved myocardium?) In atypical angina, or resting electrocardiographic (EKG) abnormalities, is there really significant myocardial ischemia? Is there objective evidence of improved myocardial perfusion after coronary angioplasty or bypass surgery? In patients about to undergo major surgery, what is the risk of perioperative infarction?

Ventricular Function. Left ventricular function (ejection fraction, normal 55 to 80 percent) can be measured either by a first-pass study (tracer is rapidly injected as a bolus and its first pass through the left ventricle is analyzed; see Fig. 17-2) or by a gated equilibrium blood pool study in which some red blood cells are labeled, reinjected, and imaged after mixing is complete, using the EKG to trigger each set of frames showing the heart in motion. Right ventricular function (ejection fraction, normal 40 to 60 percent) can be measured only with the first-pass study, because in the equilibrium study there are too many overlapping structures. Both left and right ventricular cardiac output can be estimated from the first-pass study.

The gated blood pool study gives much more information than ejection fraction: it yields mean and maximum emptying and filling rates, emptying and filling times, and other quantitative data on ventricular function. Left ventricular volume can be estimated. The cine replay gives information on wall motion and chamber size; can reveal areas of hypokinesia, akinesia, and dyskinesia; and can localize aneurysms.

The major indications for gated blood pool scanning are to evaluate left ventricular function as an index of prognosis in patients after myocardial infarction, to differentiate between the different forms of cardiomyopathy, to evaluate the ventricular effects of valvular disease and potentially cardiotoxic drugs such as doxorubicin, and to assess the effectiveness of drugs in con-

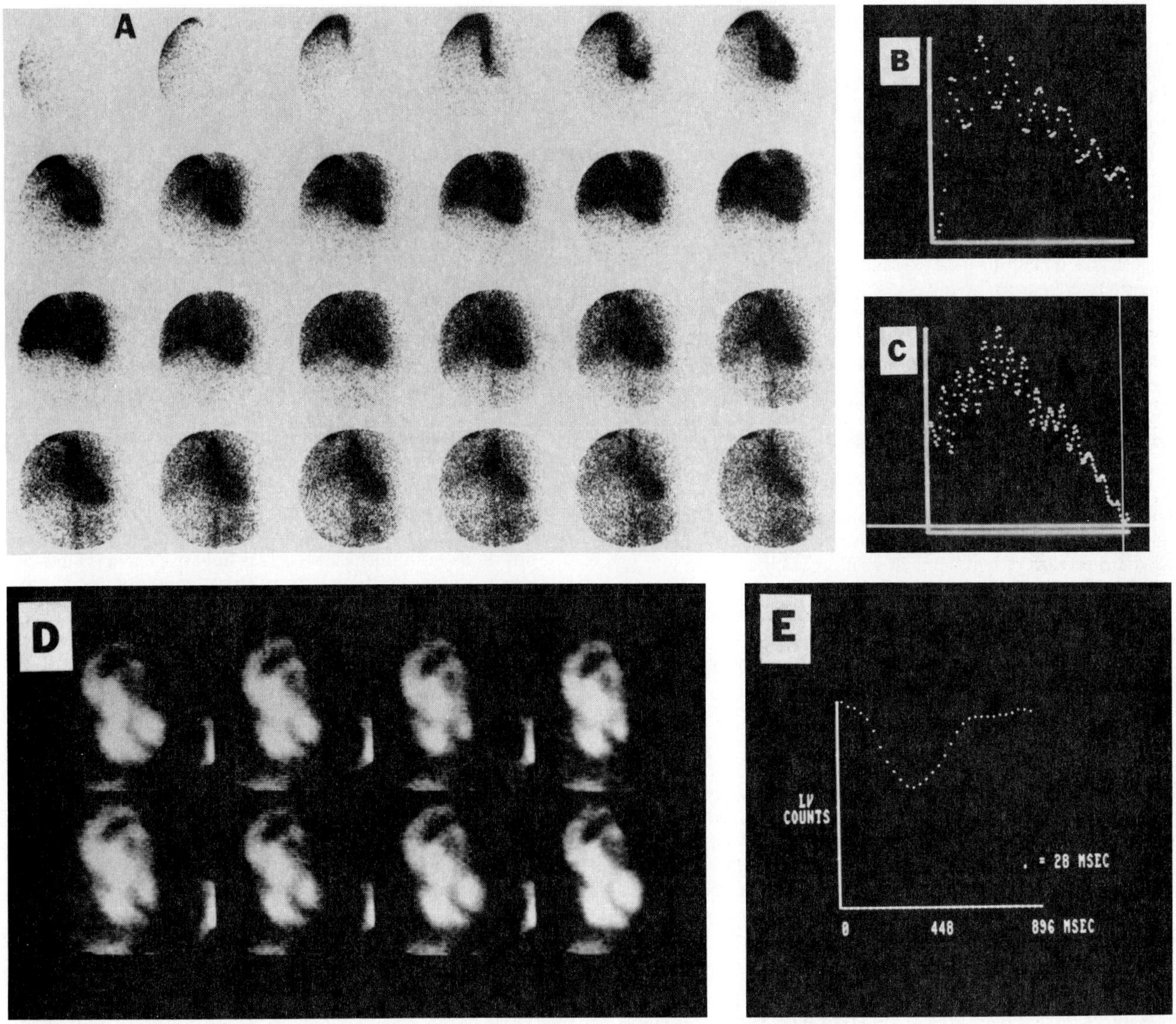

Figure 17-2 (**A**) First-pass study, right anterior oblique (RAO) projection, two frames per second. Note superior vena cava, right atrium, right ventricle, main pulmonary artery, right pulmonary artery (left not seen well in RAO projection), lungs, left ventricle, and abdominal aorta. (**B**) Time-activity curve of right ventricle (seven beats); beat-by-beat ejection fraction can be calculated. (**C**) Time-activity curve of left ventricle (15 beats). (**D**) Gated equilibrium blood pool study, left anterior oblique view; cardiac cycle is broken into eight frames. Normal motion in right and left ventricles. Note also aorta, left pulmonary artery, septum. (**E**) Time-activity curve of left ventricle starting with R wave. Normal emptying and filling. Note subtle atrial "kick" at end of cycle.

gestive cardiac failure and in the diagnosis of left ventricular wall motion abnormalities and aneurysms. The study gives objective evidence of cardiac function after revascularization procedures and cardiac transplants.

Infarct-Avid Agents. Two imaging agents are available that are actively taken up by infarcted myocardium: Tc-99m pyrophosphate and antimyosin. Pyrophosphate follows calcium into necrotic calcifying myocardial tissue. Tc-99m pyrophosphate (PyP) myocardial scans are positive from 12 hours to about 2 weeks after an acute infarction and can therefore help distinguish recent from remote myocardial infarction. Labeled antimyosin is a labeled antibody that binds to myosin. Normally the myosin of the myocardium is protected from direct contact with circulating antibodies, but in damaged myocardium this mechanism breaks down and the circulating antibody becomes bound. Images show the location and extent of myocardial damage.

Shunt Detection. Right-to-left shunts are detected by injecting labeled particles slightly larger than capillaries. Normally these would be trapped in the capillaries of the lung, but if there is an intracardiac or intrapulmonary right-to-left shunt, some of the particles will go through the shunt and appear in the systemic circulation (brain, kidneys, spleen). The ratio of extrapulmonary body counts to total body counts is the degree of the right-to-left shunt.

Left-to-right shunts are measured by an entirely different technique. Normally an injected bolus of radiotracer would pass rapidly through the lungs and on to the left side of the heart; the time-activity curve (TAC) of lung activity would show a single peak. If there is an intracardiac left-to-right shunt, some of the tracer will appear in the lungs a second time, forming a second (and sometimes even a third) peak in the lung TAC. Comparing the primary lung flow (Qp) and the systemic flow (Qs), which is calculated from the secondary shunt curve, gives the left-to-right shunt ratio (Qp/Qs). Normal values are 1.10 or less.

Lymphoscintigraphy and Lymphangioscintigraphy. A tracer is injected into the web spaces of the toes or fingers, or other appropriate places in the body, and finds its own way to the lymphatics; it is not necessary to cannulate a lymphatic vessel. The radiocolloid collects in lymph nodes along the way, outlining the direction of lymphatic flow. If ordinary albumin is used instead of colloid, the lymphatic trunks (but usually not the nodes) will be demonstrated. Radiocolloid injected directly into a tumor will likewise show the lymphatic drainage from the tumor, information that may be helpful in planning surgery and radiotherapy.

Bone Scans

Technique. Imaging of bone is done by using phosphate tagged with Tc-99m. The tracer is taken up by osteoblastic activity, and is also dependent on bone blood flow. (Note that about half of the tracer is excreted by the kidneys; always look for them on bone scans.) Increased osteoblastic activity is seen in primary and metastatic bone tumors, infection, trauma, degenerative disease, and almost any bone condition associated with the bone's attempt to heal itself.

Metastases. The most common indication for bone scanning is a search for metastases, in which there is almost always some increase in osteoblastic activity (Fig. 17-3). The sensitivity of bone scanning in detecting osseous metastases is about 98 percent for most of the common tumors (breast, prostate, lung) but is lower for melanoma, and multiple myeloma may be missed.

Even though bone scanning is sensitive, it usually cannot classify a lesion once it is found. Suspected metastases to bone are investigated by means of a whole-body bone scan; if it is negative, the chance that the patient has osseous metastases is very small. If the scan shows a lesion or lesions, radiographs usually enable one to determine what it is (e.g., trauma). If the radiograph is negative, the probability that the bone scan lesion represents metastasis is *increased,* because the bone scan may show metastases 3 to 6 months before they appear on radiographs. The whole-body radiographic "bone survey" is rarely done now, because the bone scan is more sensitive and can image the entire body.

Benign Bone Disease. Fractures are usually positive within 24 hours. The first test for suspected fracture is the radiograph, but if it is negative and fracture is strongly suspected, a bone scan may be helpful. Radiograph-negative stress fractures and periosteal reactions seen in athletes are usually well shown by bone scans. The scan is usually not useful in determining the age of a fracture.

Spondylolysis and spondylolisthesis are conditions in which bone scanning may be helpful in patient management. If the scan is negative, the spondylolysis is not likely to be the cause of the pain; if the scan is positive, it is.

Bone scans are extremely sensitive in detecting subacute and chronic osteomyelitis. Osteomyelitis in the very early stages may be missed. Septic and inflammatory arthritis are also usually well seen on bone scans (Fig. 17-4). Infection in a prosthetic joint can often be distinguished from loosening by a dual study (bone scan plus gallium or labeled white blood cell study). Avascular necrosis of the femoral head usually can be detected with tomographic imaging, as can degenerative or inflammatory diseases of the temporomandibular joint.

Bone scans can play a role in soft-tissue disorders. They can detect myositis ossificans and heterotopic bone and determine whether it is active.

Pulmonary Studies

Pulmonary Embolism. Nuclear medicine tests are used for two lung functions: perfusion and ventilation. These tests are most often requested to rule out pulmonary embolism. Perfusion lung scans show the distribution of blood flow from the pulmonary arteries. The lungs are imaged in several projections, and any area of nonperfusion such as lung distal to a pulmonary embolism shows up as a defect. This test is not specific for pulmonary embolism, however, and many other pulmonary conditions (e.g., pneumonia, effusion, tumor, emphysema) can cause defects. Most of these conditions show up as abnormalities on either the chest radiograph or the ventilation lung scan. The scan can be abnormal in ways that strongly suggest pulmonary embolism ("high probability") or strongly lead away from it ("low probability"). Although no pattern is pathognomonic for pulmonary embolism, a normal perfusion lung scan essentially rules out pulmonary embolism.

Ventilation lung scans show which parts of the lung are being adequately ventilated. Usually lung distal to a pulmonary embolism has no more than a moderate ventilation loss, whereas emphysema, asthma, and so forth usually show marked abnormalities.

The ventilation-perfusion lung scan should be requested early in the work-up of a patient suspected of having pulmonary embolism. The scans must be interpreted with a current chest radiograph (Fig. 17-5). A negative study rules out pulmonary embolism, and there are no clinical or laboratory tests sufficiently accurate to rule it in or out with certainty. A positive test does not establish the diagnosis, but it does justify further work-up such as pulmonary angiography.

Keep in mind that if venous disease is suspected in the lower extremities or pelvis, the perfusion lung scan can be done in conjunction with a radionuclide venogram.

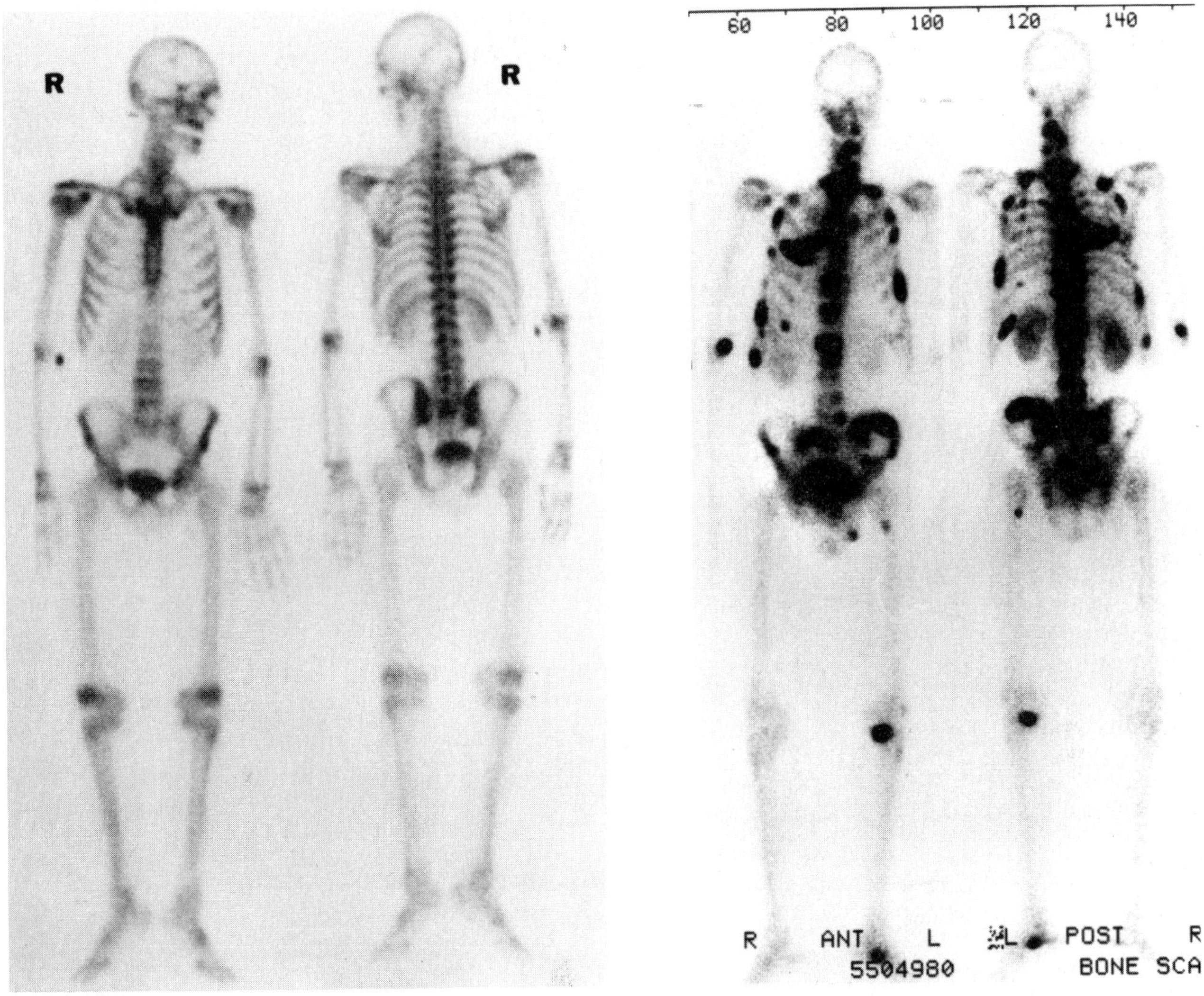

A B

Figure 17-3 (**A**) Normal whole-body bone scan, anterior and posterior views. Note activity in kidneys and bladder, and tracer injection site at right elbow. (**B**) Anterior and posterior whole-body bone scan of patient with widespread bone metastases from lung cancer. Lesions in left knee and ankle are unusual; metastases usually have an axial skeletal distribution, as shown here.

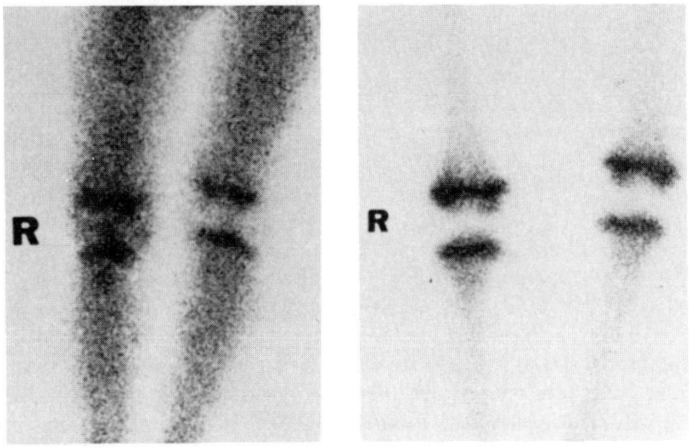

A B

Figure 17-4 Septic arthritis or osteomyelitis? Bone scan in a 3-year-old child who had had a painful right knee for 1 day. (**A**) Blood-pool image taken shortly after tracer injection shows a hypervascular right knee joint (next to *R* marker). (**B**) Delayed images show only minimal bone involvement (i.e., osteomyelitis is unlikely). Joint aspiration confirmed septic arthritis.

Other Pulmonary Questions. Ventilation-perfusion lung scans are also useful in the quantitative measurement of regional ventilation and perfusion, to predict which patients will be suitable for either a lobectomy or pneumonectomy. The relative contribution of each lung to total ventilation and perfusion and the ventilation/perfusion ratio can be determined globally and regionally. This determination can be useful in assessing treatment options in patients with emphysema (including congenital lobar emphysema) or congenital vascular anomalies.

An area of increasing interest is the use of gallium (Ga-67) scanning in patients with inflammatory lung disease (alveolitis, sarcoid, *Pneumocystis carinii* pneumonia, idiopathic pulmonary fibrosis). A quantitative index of the extent of Ga-67 uptake has been shown to be useful in predicting the response of the patient to steroid therapy, and it can also be used as a guide to when to stop treatment. For a discussion of Ga-67 in inflammatory disease, see the section on detecting and localizing infections.

Endocrine Studies

Thyroid Function Studies and Thyroid Scans. Thyroid scanning is useful in evaluating palpable nodules, in screening patients

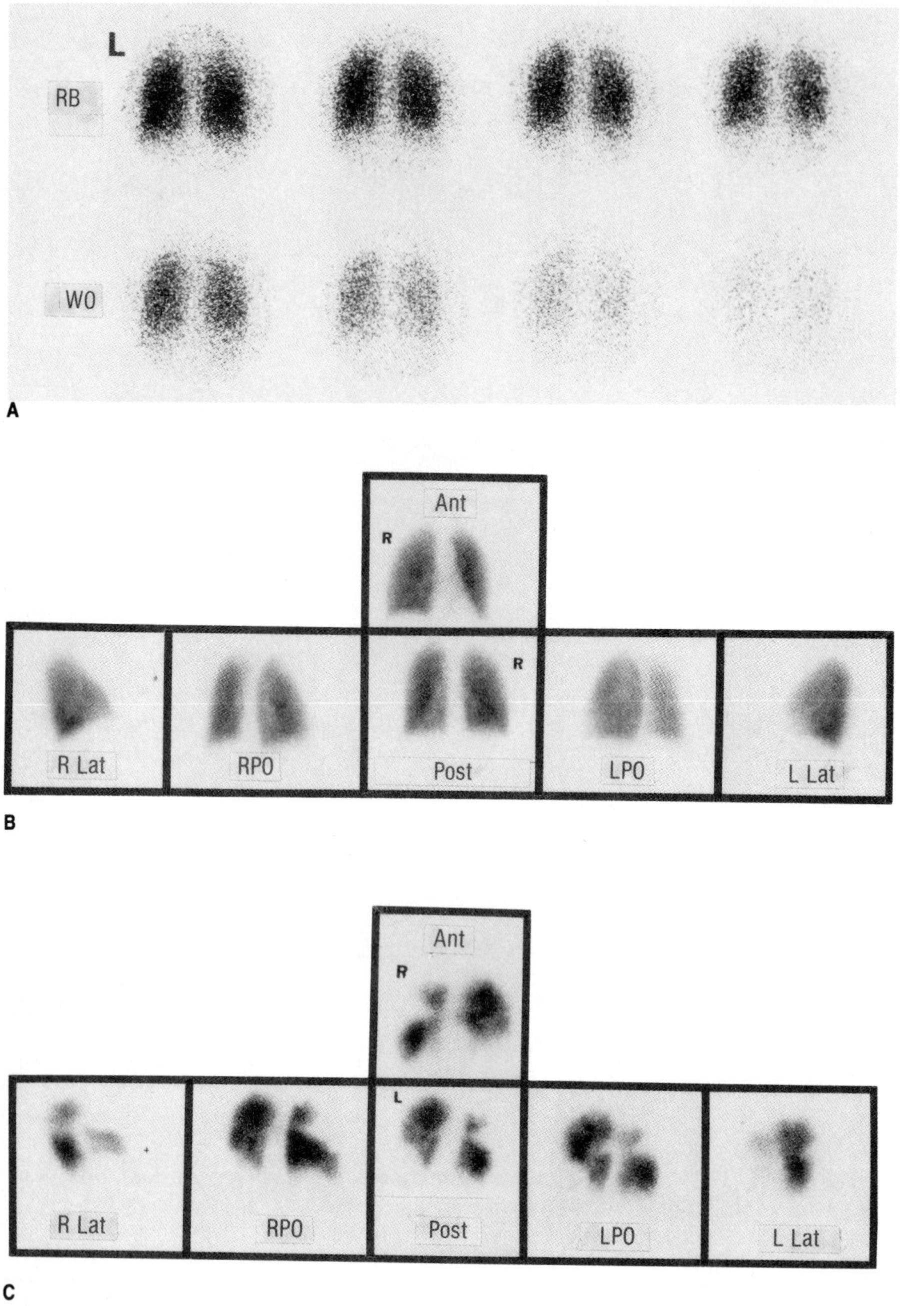

Figure 17-5 (**A**) Normal ventilation study (posterior view). Patient is sitting erect. RB = rebreathing, WO = washout. (**B**) Normal perfusion study. Ant = anterior, R/L Lat = right/left lateral, RPO/LPO = right/left posterior oblique, Post = posterior. Patient was injected while supine and imaged while sitting erect. (**C**) Perfusion study of patient with multiple pulmonary emboli. Note wedge-shaped, pleural-based segments of absent perfusion. Ventilation study and chest radiograph were normal.

who have been exposed to radiation and who are at risk for developing thyroid nodules that may be malignant, and in patients with a family history of medullary carcinoma (Fig. 17-6). If a nodule is nonfunctioning ("cold") on radioiodine (or pertechnetate) scan, it should be aspirated or biopsied. Other indications for thyroid scanning include demonstrating sites of ectopic thyroid such as lingual or retrosternal.

Hyperthyroidism has several forms: Graves' disease, toxic nodular goiter (Plummer's disease), subacute thyroiditis (Hashimoto's disease), and others. The first two cause the thyroid to take up more iodine than normal and can often be treated with radioactive iodine (I-131). The chance of successful I-131 treatment of Graves' disease and Plummer's disease is close to 100 percent, and the treatment is essentially free from side effects other than possible hypothyroidism (see the section on I-131 treatment of thyroid disease).

Parathyroid Imaging. Parathyroid adenomas can often be visualized and located by a dual-isotope technique. Parathyroid glands normally take up thallium, the tracer used in myocardial perfusion studies. Because the thyroid also takes it up, a second tracer is given (Tc-99m pertechnetate) that is also taken up by the thyroid, but not by the parathyroid. The thyroid-only image is subtracted from the thyroid-parathyroid image, so that only the parathyroid activity remains. Adenomas larger than 1 cm and adenomas outside the thyroid gland are usually well visualized with this technique, but false-negative results do occur.

Adrenal Imaging. Two radiotracers are available for adrenal imaging: I-131 iodonorcholesterol (NP-59), for imaging the adrenal cortex, and I-123 meta-iodo-benzylguanidine (mIBG), for imaging the adrenal medulla. With NP-59, we can quantitate the adrenal uptake of tracer and can differentiate among uni-

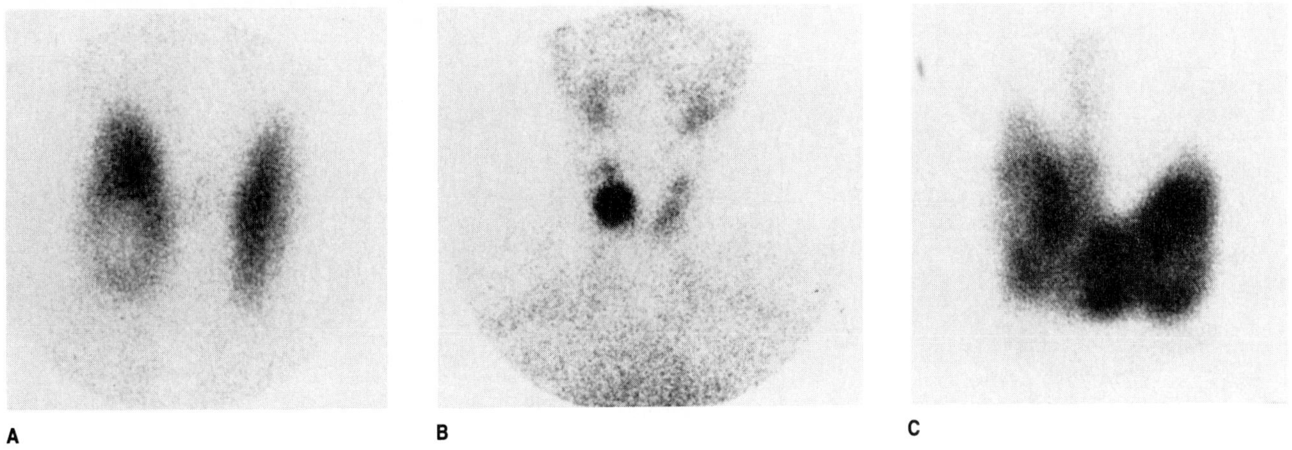

Figure 17-6 Thyroid scans (Tc-99m pertechnetate) in patients with palpable thyroid nodules. (**A**) Solitary nonfunctioning adenoma. Scan shows it to be solitary; only biopsy can distinguish it from carcinoma. (**B**) Toxic nodule suppressing remainder of gland (Plummer's disease). (**C**) Multinodular goiter showing both hyperfunctioning and hypofunctioning foci.

lateral hyperplasia, bilateral hyperplasia, and hyperfunctioning adenoma. Scans can show the location of functioning adrenal cortex.

The new tracer mIBG competes with norepinephrine for binding on catecholamine receptors. It is actively taken up by pheochromocytoma, paraganglioma, and neuroblastoma. In patients suspected of having pheochromocytoma, a whole-body mIBG scan may show the locations of all tumor sites, although tumors less than 1 to 2 cm in diameter will be poorly detected.

Gastrointestinal Studies

Biliary Studies. To visualize the flow of bile through the biliary tree, we use an organic tracer that is excreted into bile. The tracer (e.g., HIDA, DISIDA) is imaged as it is taken up by the hepatocytes and then progresses through the hepatic biliary radicles, common hepatic duct, cystic duct, gallbladder, common bile duct, and small intestine (Fig. 17-7). This entire process takes about 1 hour in normal individuals. Delayed flow, or obstruction, can be localized in most cases. If the gallbladder is not visualized within the first hour, delayed images are important, because a thick, noncompliant gallbladder involved with chronic cholecystitis might show activity only on delayed images. With modern tracers, this study performs well even in patients with hyperbilirubinemia.

The most common use of a biliary study is in diagnosing or ruling out acute cholecystitis, which in most cases (95 to 98 percent) means obstruction of the cystic duct from stone or edema. In this condition, the tracer is taken up by the hepatocytes and excreted into the biliary tree but never enters the gallbladder (Fig. 17-7*B*). The differential diagnosis of gallbladder nonvisualization is (1) cystic duct obstruction, (2) nonfunctioning or sludge-filled gallbladder, (3) acalculous cholecystitis, (4) prior cholecystectomy, and (5) gallbladder agenesis or ectopy (rare). To rule out a nonfunctioning or sludge-filled gallbladder, cholecystokinin is given before the study, to contract the gallbladder and expel its contents so it can fill again during the study. In the patient who has not eaten for 24 hours or is receiving parenteral alimentation, the gallbladder is usually nonfunctioning. Acalculous cholecystitis is a rare form of acute cholecystitis (1 percent) and cannot be positively diagnosed by any known test. A prior cholecystectomy is usually ruled out by history, but a look at the patient's right upper quadrant is *always* a good idea.

The most common clinical setting for the biliary study is the acutely ill patient with right upper quadrant pain and other signs or symptoms suggesting acute cholecystitis. The primary question is usually whether immediate operation is necessary. If the patient has acute cholecystitis, i.e., cystic duct obstruction, immediate operation is usually indicated, as there is a significant risk of perforation and bile leak leading to bile peritonitis. If the patient has chronic cholecystitis, operation can usually be deferred until antibiotic therapy and supportive measures have reduced the surgical risks.

What study should be done first in a patient thought to have acute cholecystitis? The answer depends on the specific question: ultrasonography to detect stones and morphologic changes suggesting inflammation, or biliary scintigraphy to detect cystic (as well as intrahepatic, hepatic, or common) duct obstruction and biliary function. Because 6 to 10 percent of the adult population in the United States has gallstones, an ultrasound study showing stones must be cautiously interpreted in the light of clinical data, unless a stone is seen actually obstructing one of the ducts. Biliary scintigraphy specifically shows whether the cystic duct is patent, but it requires more time (1 hour, and often longer) and is costlier than ultrasound. In the detection of acute cholecystitis, biliary scintigraphy has an overall accuracy of 98 percent.

The biliary study can be modified by cholecystokinin, as described previously, and in other ways. Gallbladder filling can be enhanced by morphine, which constricts the sphincter of Oddi. Careful imaging can reveal bile leaks not detectable by other methods. It is useful in the evaluation of patients with atypical gallbladder symptoms in whom a diagnosis of biliary dyskinesia, cystic duct syndrome, or sphincter of Oddi obstruction is suspected. In these patients, after the gallbladder is filled with tracer, cholecystokinin is injected; gallbladder emptying is measured and passage of the tracer through the biliary tree is assessed. The gallbladder "ejection fraction" can be determined.

Gastrointestinal Bleeding. A frequent clinical problem is localizing the source of lower gastrointestinal bleeding. The blood is labeled with autologous red blood cells, and the patient is imaged for about 1 hour. In many cases, the site of bleeding can be found from the images alone. Cine images obtained with a computer are helpful in verifying the site. This study is safer and more sensitive than angiography, and a positive study can help the angiographer or the surgeon plan the approach. A negative study indicates that the patient is not bleeding significantly at that time and that angiography would probably not be helpful. This study is of limited value in small-intestinal bleeding and of little value in upper gastrointestinal bleeding.

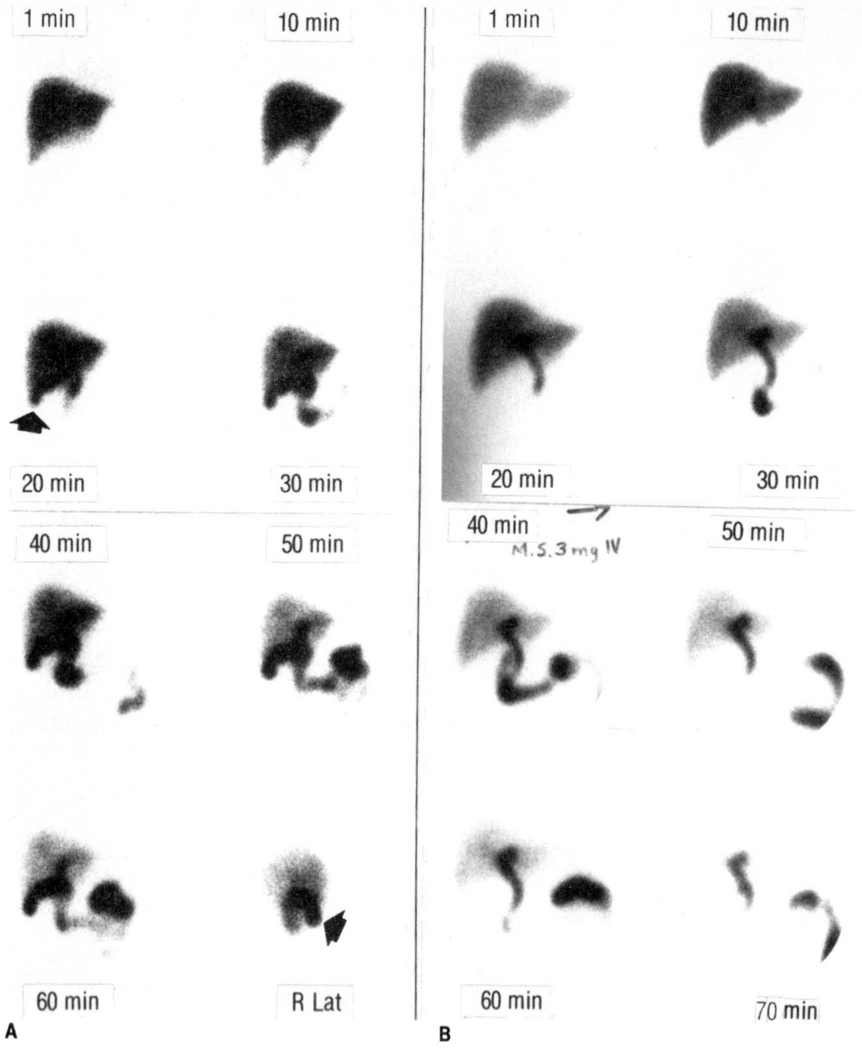

Figure 17-7 (**A**) Normal biliary study. Note rapid clearance of tracer into liver and rapid appearance of biliary tract, including gallbladder (*arrow* on 20-minute image). Tracer proceeds through common bile duct into duodenum and jejunum. Following the 60-minute image, a right lateral (R Lat) view confirms gallbladder position (*arrow*). (**B**) A 45-year-old woman with pain in right upper quadrant and fever. Although there is rapid clearance and transit through the biliary tree, the gallbladder is never visualized. At surgery, the cystic duct was blocked by stone.

Liver-Spleen Scan. A radiocolloid is injected and is taken up by the Kupffer (reticuloendothelial) cells in the liver and spleen (and bone marrow in reticuloendothelial insufficiency). Images show the size, shape, position, and degree and uniformity of uptake in the liver and spleen. It is an effective and inexpensive way to screen patients with hepatomegaly or abnormal findings of liver function tests. Liver-spleen scanning is useful in documenting hepatic hemangiomas, distinguishing hepatic adenomas from focal nodular hyperplasia, and in detecting liver or spleen laceration when other imaging studies are inconclusive. In trauma, it can be used to show which areas of the liver or spleen are no longer vascularized.

Spleen Scans. Heat-damaged red blood cells can be used to image the spleen preferentially; this test is useful in evaluating regional splenic vascularity in trauma or torsion and in assessing the spleen for laceration or fracture. It is sensitive in detecting accessory spleen(s), in identifying splenic tissue in trauma and congenital malformations (e.g., polysplenia), and in following splenectomy to identify splenic remnants.

Gastric Emptying Studies. The rate of gastric emptying of solids or liquids can be measured with ingested tracers. For solid-emptying studies (a more sensitive indicator of abnormality than liquid), the patient is given cooked egg or meat containing a tightly bound radiocolloid, and activity in the stomach is measured over the next 1 or 2 hours. The indication is usually to assess some form of obstruction, whether mechanical (duodenal ulcer, gastric cancer, hypertrophic pyloric stenosis) or functional, associated with abnormal gastric motility (vagotomy, diabetic gastroparesis, progressive systemic sclerosis). In diabetics, the study can be used to assess the response to metoclopropamide.

Gastroesophageal Studies. Esophageal motility can be studied as the patient swallows tracer. Gastroesophageal reflux can be demonstrated in this way. This test is useful in disabled adults with recurrent pneumonia or other problems suggesting reflux, and/or aspiration.

Meckel's Diverticulum. Approximately 20 to 30 percent of Meckel's diverticula contain gastric mucosa. This figure rises to 60 percent in symptomatic and 95 percent in bleeding diverticula. Because the pertechnetate ion (TcO_4^-) is actively secreted by mucoid cells of gastric mucosa, it is useful in detecting Meckel's diverticula. The patient should be placed on cimetidine for at least 24 hours (preferably 48 hours) prior to imaging, to prevent pertechnetate from leaving the stomach during the study and obscuring the abdomen. Constant gastric suction may be necessary in some patients.

The Genitourinary System

Renal Flow and Function. Renal functions can be measured using radiotracers, e.g., renal blood or plasma flow, glomerular filtration rate (GFR), proximal tubular cell function, distal tubular cell function, urinary concentration, and urinary transit. Renal vascularity can be assessed by imaging the kidneys following a rapidly injected bolus of radiotracer. The function measured here is transit time (aorta→kidneys→inferior vena cava) and not flow (Fig. 17-8). Renal artery stenosis, abdominal aortic aneurysm, renal edema, parenchymal disease, urinary tract obstruction, and renal vein thrombosis all cause abnormalities of transit, some showing a characteristic pattern.

Proximal tubular cell function is measured using I-123 or I-131 ortho-iodohippurate sodium (OIH, Hippuran). Effective renal plasma flow can be calculated from this study.

The term *renogram* refers to the OIH study. The renogram is indicated in the evaluation of patients with suspected renal failure, urinary tract obstruction, or vascular abnormalities. It is sensitive in the detection of unilateral renal artery stenosis as a cause of hypertension, especially when renal blood flow is challenged with captopril. A decline in renal blood flow after captopril indicates that the hypertension is probably due to renal artery stenosis. A negative result indicates the opposite, and suggests that renal arteriography will probably not be helpful.

In urinary tract obstruction, it is often necessary to distinguish mechanical obstruction (e.g., stone, stenosis) from functional obstruction (e.g., dilatation). A renogram is done, and when the renal pelvis is filled with tracer, an injection of furosemide is given. The diuretic "pushes" fluid through the kidney into the renal pelvis. If the obstruction is mechanical, the tracer activity in the pelvis will remain the same, whereas if it is functional, the extra pressure will drive the tracer down the urinary tract and the pelvic activity will drop.

The renogram is useful in measuring the contribution of each kidney to total renal function, e.g., when considering nephrectomy. It is a standard technique for evaluating renal function in transplants and in distinguishing rejection from acute tubular necrosis. It is useful in evaluating differential renal function prior to the use of nephrotoxic agents such as cyclosporin A.

Two radiotracers are handled more slowly by the kidney and can be used for morphologic imaging in patients in whom radiography with iodinated contrast agents is contraindicated: Tc-99m glucoheptonate can be used to visualize the renal parenchyma and collecting system, whereas Tc-99m DMSA (dimer-

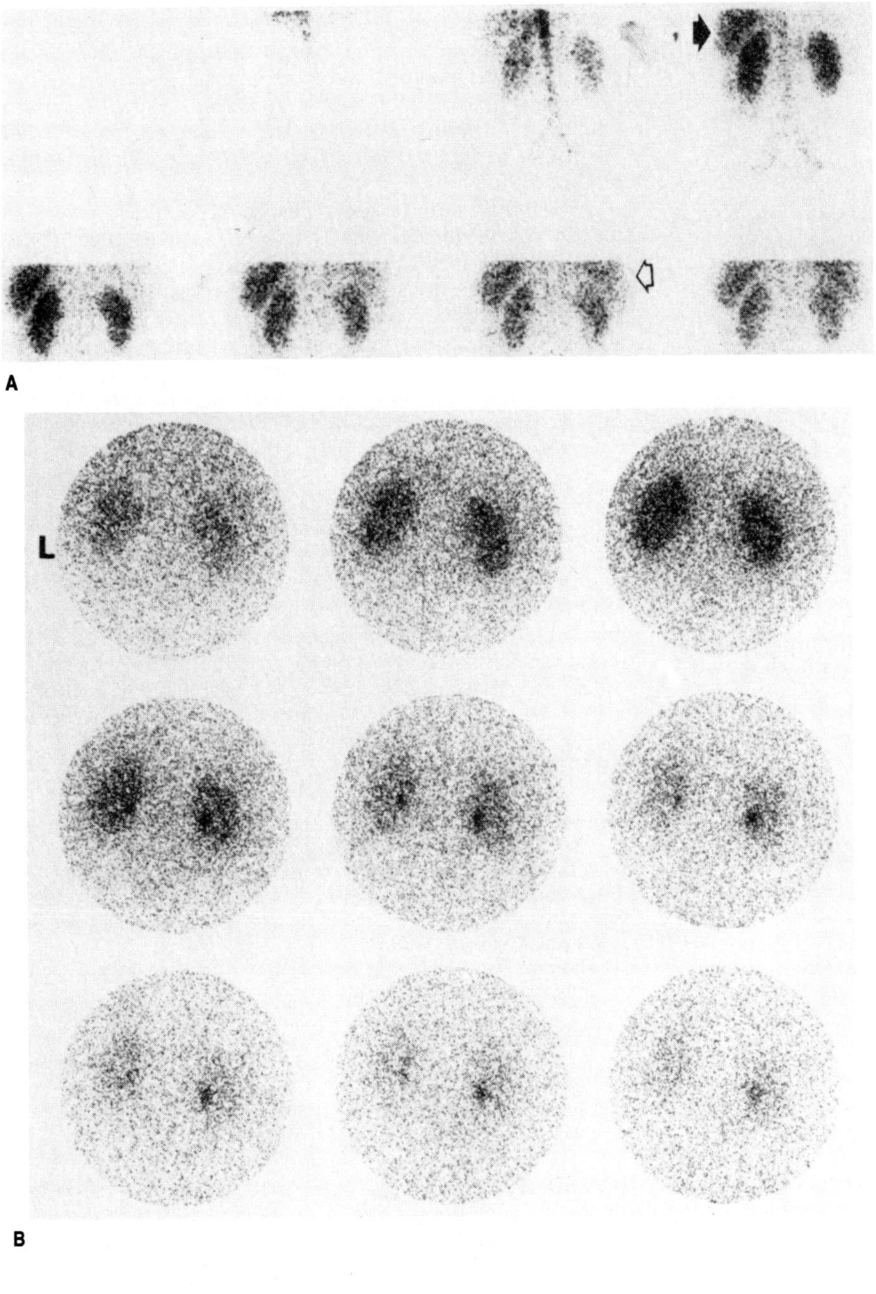

A

B

Figure 17-8 (**A**) Normal renal "flow" study; first passage of tracer after injection. Note abdominal aorta and bifurcation, prompt visualization of both kidneys, spleen (*solid arrow*), and liver (*open arrow*), whose delayed appearance results from its portal blood supply. (**B**) Normal OIH renogram; prompt appearance and excretion of tracer into bladder (not shown). Modern tracers soon to be available will give images of much greater clarity. L = left.

captosuccinate) is handled so slowly that only the renal cortex is imaged. These agents are useful in distinguishing functioning renal tissue (e.g., column of Berthin) from nonfunctioning masses needing further evaluation.

Ureteral Reflux. In patients with recurrent urinary tract infection or other indications of possible ureteral reflux, the (radiographic) voiding cystourethrogram (VCUG) is a standard test. An alternative test is the radionuclide voiding cystogram (RNVCG), in which the bladder is filled with radiotracer, either indirectly (via renogram) or directly (via catheter). The patient is positioned in front of the gamma camera and instructed to void whenever he or she wishes. With the computer running, and in privacy and quiet, it makes little difference when voiding occurs; the camera will detect *any* activity that appears in either ureter, and the reflux can be quantitated.

Testicular Torsion. In acute testicular pain, with or without trauma, it is often necessary to distinguish torsion, usually a surgical emergency, from epididymitis or other medical condition. A bolus of Tc-99m (any form) is rapidly injected, and the vascularity of the scrotal contents is assessed. Acute torsion presents as a hypovascular testis, whereas most of the inflammatory conditions show increased vascularity. Missed (late) torsion has an intermediate pattern. If this test is being considered, it must be requested as soon as possible.

Detecting and Localizing Infections

The patient with fever of undetermined origin (FUO) presents a challenge: the disease (infection) is presumed to exist, and the question is its location. Two nuclear medicine tests are available: the Ga-67 scan and the indium (In-111) white blood cell scan. Gallium is generally more sensitive for chronic infections.

In-111 labeled white blood cells are prepared from the patient's own white blood cells after centrifugation and separation; they are usually predominantly granulocytes and behave like them after labeling and reinjection. The mechanism of Ga-67 has not been elucidated. Either tracer will accumulate in inflammatory tissue, although In-111 white blood cells are more specific for infections. Because Ga-67 is normally excreted through the large intestine, In-111 white blood cells are more suited to imaging the abdomen.

Ga-67 and In-111 white blood cell studies are used in localizing suspected abscess and other foci of infection and in osteomyelitis, septic arthritis, infected vascular grafts, sarcoidosis, idiopathic pulmonary fibrosis, *Pneumocystis carinii* pneumonia, and septic emboli. In-111 white blood cells have been reported to be useful in diagnosing acute appendicitis and in assessing the activity of Crohn's disease and ulcerative colitis.

Central Nervous System Studies

Cerebral Perfusion. The tracers currently used for imaging regional cerebral perfusion are Tc-99m HMPAO (hexamethylpropylene amine oxime) and I-123 IMP (iodoamphetamine), both of which distribute rapidly after injection according to regional blood flow (see Fig. 17-1). They can be used to assess regional cerebral perfusion in strokes and to help distinguish Alzheimer's disease from multi-infarct dementia. Epileptogenic foci can often be shown; this is especially useful when surgical resection is being considered.

Cerebrospinal Fluid Studies. Communicating hydrocephalus can usually be demonstrated clearly by injecting a tracer (e.g., In-111 DTPA) into the cerebrospinal fluid (CSF) in the lumbar subarachnoid space and imaging its subsequent appearance in the head. Normally, the flow of CSF down the aqueduct of Sylvius is strong enough to block transit of tracer up into the lateral ventricles, but in communicating hydrocephalus the flow is arrested or even reversed, allowing "penetration" to occur. Whether the ventricles then empty spontaneously may be of great significance in neurosurgical management.

It is also possible to tell whether a CSF shunt is *working* (actually transporting CSF) or merely *patent* (open throughout) by injecting tracer percutaneously into the reservoir and imaging the subsequent flow. By knowing the volume of the reservoir and the rate of tracer disappearance from it, one can calculate the CSF shunt flow in milliliters per minute.

Making the Best Use of a Nuclear Medicine Service

First, define the clinical problem and determine what you know, what questions you want to answer, and what information you need. You should be reasonably familiar with all the diagnostic tests available that pertain to your questions. Keep your threshold for ordering expensive tests high, but have a low threshold for consulting with imaging specialists, especially if more than one test will be required. The *order* in which tests are done can be critical; an angiogram with an iodinated contrast agent can interfere with a thyroid radioiodine uptake test for weeks to months. A barium enema can interfere with a labeled white blood cell study.

Diagnostic tests perform different services. Do you need the test to *detect* an abnormality, to *classify* it, to *localize* it, or to *quantitate* it? You must know how to interpret test performance in terms of sensitivity, specificity, predictive value, accuracy, and rate of inconclusive results. You should have some idea of the kind of information the test gives, and the likelihood that the test will yield the information you need. To maximize this, it is essential to give the imaging physician enough clinical data to steer his or her interpretation along the right line. Interpretation is best done with clinical information and other relevant test results available. Go interpret the study with the imaging specialist; you will both benefit from this collaboration, and so will your patient.

Be prepared to say what you plan to do next if the test is positive, negative, or inconclusive. You should be familiar with the costs and risks of doing a test, as well as the costs and risks of not doing it. The power of diagnostic tests is rising, and so are the complexity and costs. As physicians ordering tests, we will be called upon to know how to use the available services wisely.

References

Alazraki NP, Mishkin FS, eds. Fundamentals of nuclear medicine. New York: Society of Nuclear Medicine, 1988.

Beierwaltes WH. The treatment of hyperthyroidism with iodine-131. Semin Nucl Med 1978; 8:95.

Gottschalk A, et al, eds. Diagnostic nuclear medicine. Baltimore: Williams & Wilkins, 1988.

Harbert J, da Rocha AFG, eds. Textbook of nuclear medicine. Philadelphia: Lea & Febiger, 1984.

Matin P. Clinical nuclear medicine imaging. New York: Medical Examination Publishing Co., 1986.

Mettler FA, Guiberteau MJ. Essentials of nuclear medicine imaging. New York: Grune & Stratton, 1983.

Walker JM, Margouleff D. A clinical manual of nuclear medicine. Norwalk, CT: Appleton-Century-Crofts, 1984.

Radiology and Magnetic Resonance Imaging

Carl J. D'Orsi, MD

18

The discovery of x-rays in 1895 by Dr. Wilhelm Conrad Roentgen heralded a new and exciting era in medicine. It was now possible to examine the skeletal system and other internal structures directly without surgical intervention. From this rather modest foundation the discipline has expanded rapidly, with the use of computerized methods and therapeutic techniques such as angioplasty and drainage procedures, which can be performed in the modern diagnostic radiology department.

The X-Ray Requisition

The formal link between the radiologist and the clinician is the x-ray requisition. In essence, this is a request for a consultation and should be regarded as such. Basic information, including the patient's age, primary diagnostic possibilities, and any known allergies, should be clearly stated. Most important is a list of questions to be answered by the study. The request must be filled out by the physician requesting the examination and should not be delegated to the nursing staff or ward clerk.

Basic Examinations

Five types of examinations are almost always ordered by the clinician without prior consultation with a radiologist. They constitute the framework that may lead to more sophisticated examinations and often serve as screening procedures.

The Chest Examination: Posteroanterior and Lateral Views (Fig. 18-1)

This study is by far the most common examination done in any radiology department and possibly one of the most difficult to interpret. The routine views are an upright posteroanterior, or PA (describing the path of the x-ray beam) (Fig. 18-2) and a left (describing the side against the film) lateral view. In certain circumstances, oblique PA views are also obtained to clarify a confusing density on the standard examination.

Remember that the heart, mediastinum, portions of the abdomen and neck, the bony thorax, and the lung parenchyma are all portrayed on the routine chest examination. Thus, when the films from this study are analyzed, all of the systems mentioned must be scrutinized. A valuable technique for the neophyte reader is to study the areas most likely to be omitted and work toward the lung parenchyma. This method ensures that the wealth of anatomy presented on the chest examination will be appreciated.

The chest examination should be used whenever there are any signs or symptoms related to the chest or thorax. It should also be the first radiographic examination in any investigation of symptoms related to the lung or thorax.

The Skeletal Examination

Examination of the skeletal system is usually straightforward from a clinical point of view. The majority of these films are

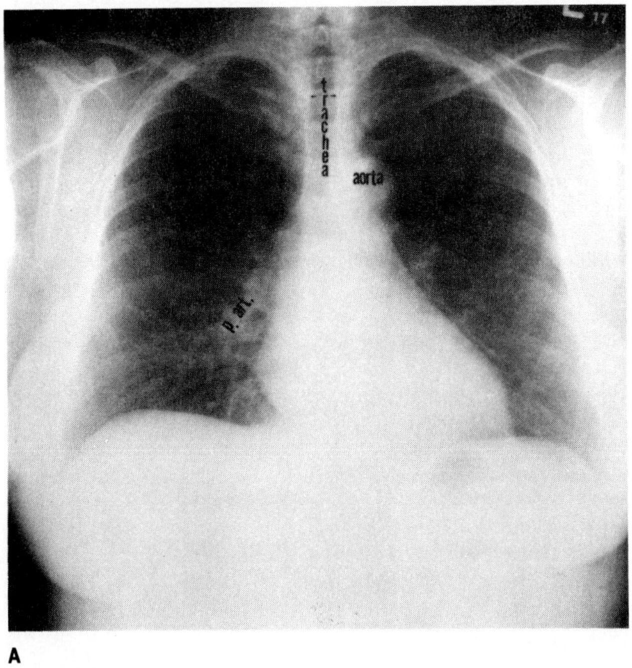

A

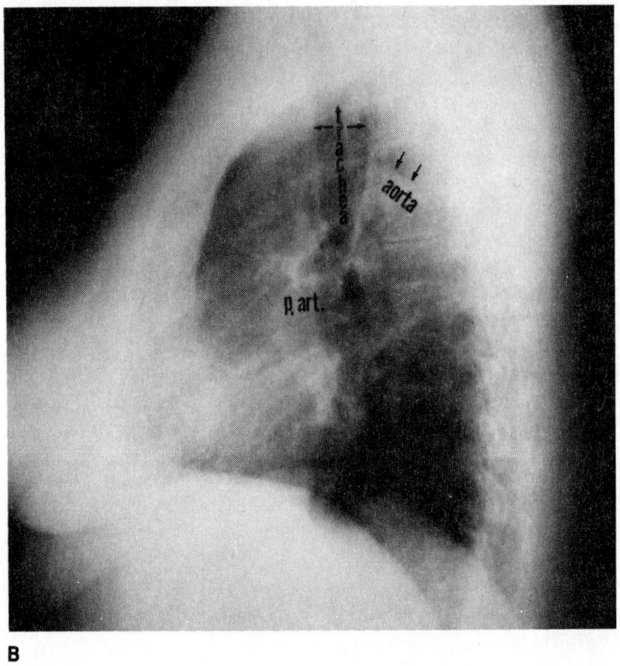

B

Figure 18-1 (**A**) Posteroanterior (PA) view of the chest. The pulmonary artery (P. art.), aorta, and trachea are indicated. (**B**) Lateral view of the chest. By convention, this film is usually taken with the patient's left side adjacent to the x-ray film cassette.

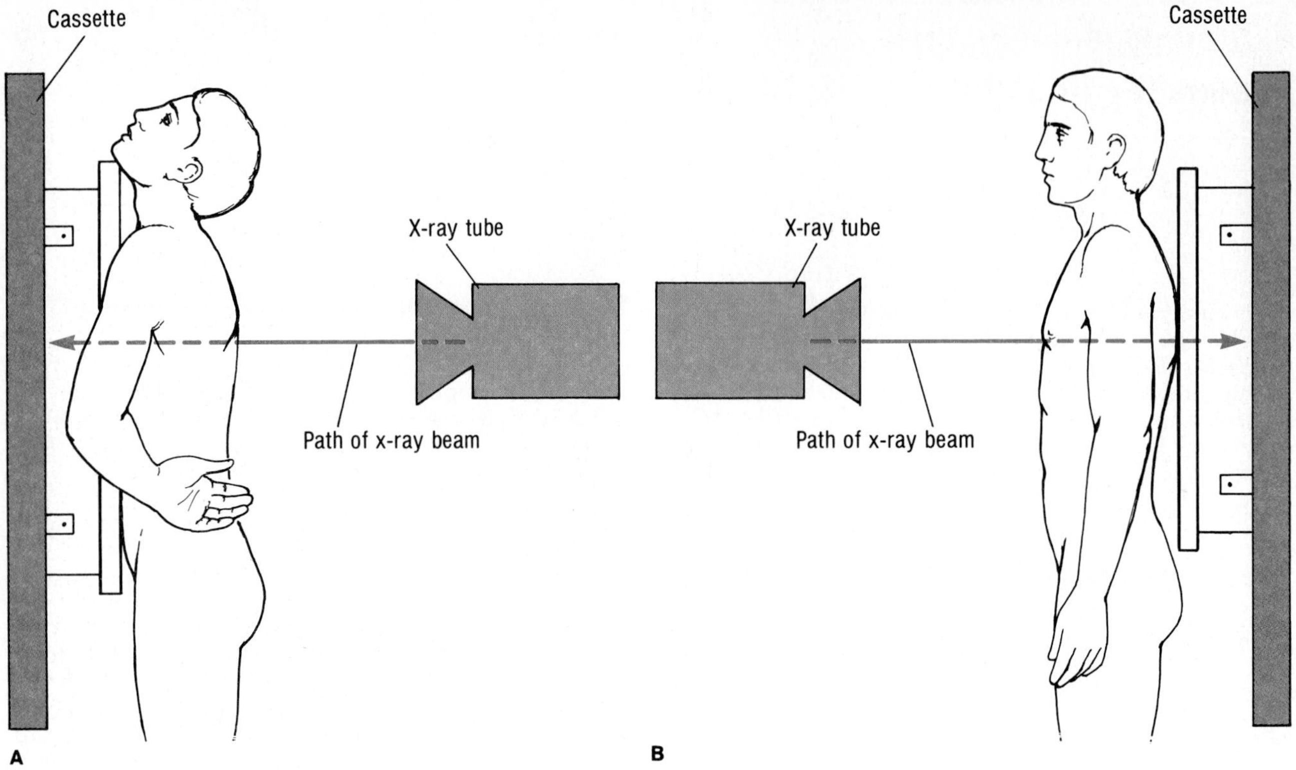

Figure 18-2 (**A**) Schematic diagram of conventional PA view of the chest. (**B**) Schematic diagram of AP view of the chest, which may be done to better visualize certain areas of the lungs, particularly the apical regions.

requested to rule out fractures in cases of trauma. The physician should be familiar with the standard radiographic views of the axial skeleton and vertebral bodies. Most studies include at least anteroposterior (AP) and lateral views of the bony structure in question. A list of the radiographic procedures performed and the standard views for each can be obtained from any radiology department.

Special mention should be made of cervical spine radiography for acute trauma, because the potential for tragic complications is great. The most crucial films for the severely injured patient with acute cervical spine trauma are the cross-table lateral and 45-degree oblique views, which are done with the patient in the supine position. Patients who have sustained major head and neck trauma, are unconscious or paralyzed, or have multiple regions involved with significant trauma should have these initial views. The less severely injured patient should have the previously mentioned studies; if they prove normal, an AP 20-degree angled cephalad view, an "open-mouth" view for C1–C2, and a posterior 35-degree angled caudad AP view should be added. If these views demonstrate a definite abnormality, flexion and extension views are contraindicated.

Gastrointestinal Contrast Studies

Radiographic studies of the gastrointestinal (GI) tract include the barium swallow, upper GI series, small bowel series, small bowel enema, and barium enema. For the most part, these examinations should serve as initial screening tests for patients with symptoms and physical findings referable to the esophagus, stomach, small intestine, or colon (Fig. 18-3).

The successful completion of these examinations relies heavily on proper preparation of the patient. No specific preparation is needed for the barium swallow alone. If an upper GI series is to follow, however, the patient should not take anything by mouth after midnight prior to the examination. If a small bowel series is to be done, any drugs that affect bowel motility should also be discontinued 12 to 24 hours before the examination, if possible. Colonic preparation must be meticulously followed, or residual fecal material can mimic pathologic processes. The patient should have a liquid diet 1 day prior to the barium enema. Drinking at least six glasses of fluid should be encouraged. A barium enema preparation kit is then used. The patient ingests the Phosphosoda 30 minutes before the evening meal. The Bisacodyl tablets are taken before retiring for the night, and the Bisacodyl suppository is used approximately 1 hour before the patient leaves for the examination.

The contrast agent used in all routine GI examinations is barium mixed with appropriate amounts of water for each particular study. Most modern radiology departments use a "double-contrast" technique for GI imaging. Air, introduced either rectally for the colon or via gas-producing tablets for the stomach, along with the barium allows for a very detailed examination of the mucosal lining of the GI tract.

The order of the examinations should be dictated by the clinical findings. The examination most likely to answer the primary clinical question should be done first. Computed tomography (CT) scans to visualize bony structures of the abdomen and pelvis and nuclear medicine exams should be ordered prior to any GI study.

The Intravenous Pyelogram

Intravenous pyelography (IVP) is an examination done to visualize the kidneys, ureters, and bladder (Fig. 18-4). Very often, it is the initial study for genitourinary symptoms. Once again, this examination functions as an initial screening procedure for the genitourinary tract.

The contrast agent used is a large molecule to which or-

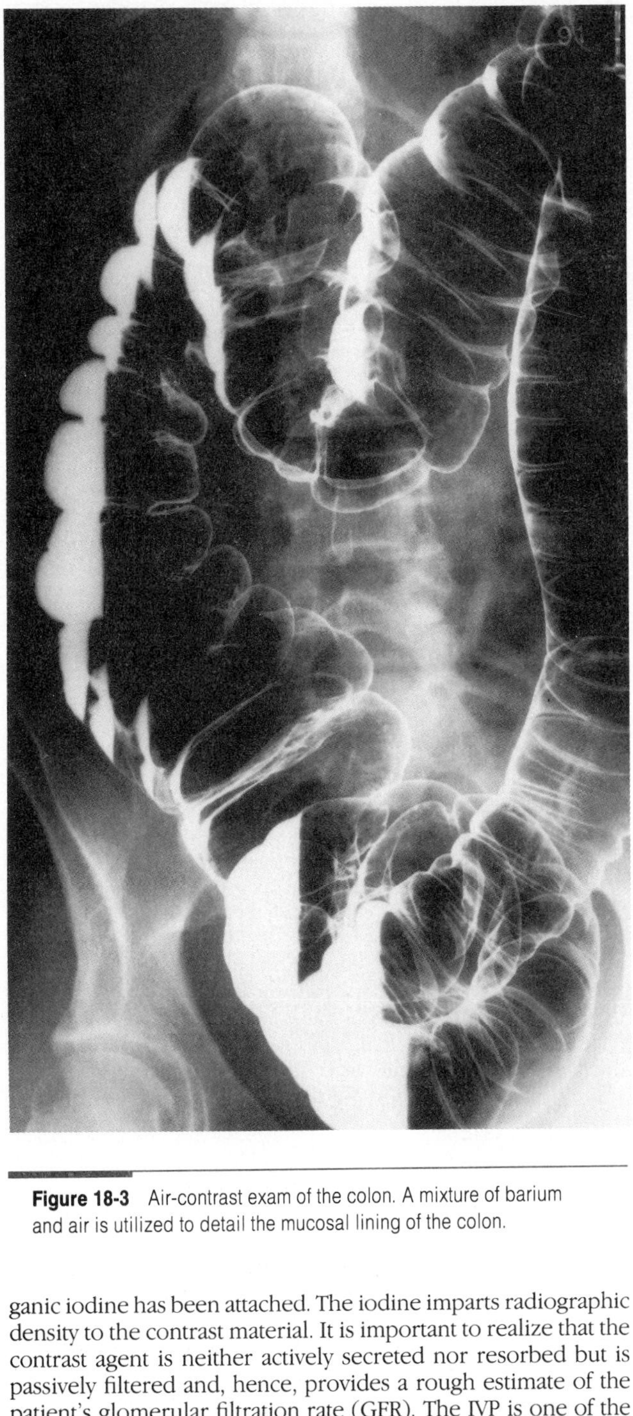

Figure 18-3 Air-contrast exam of the colon. A mixture of barium and air is utilized to detail the mucosal lining of the colon.

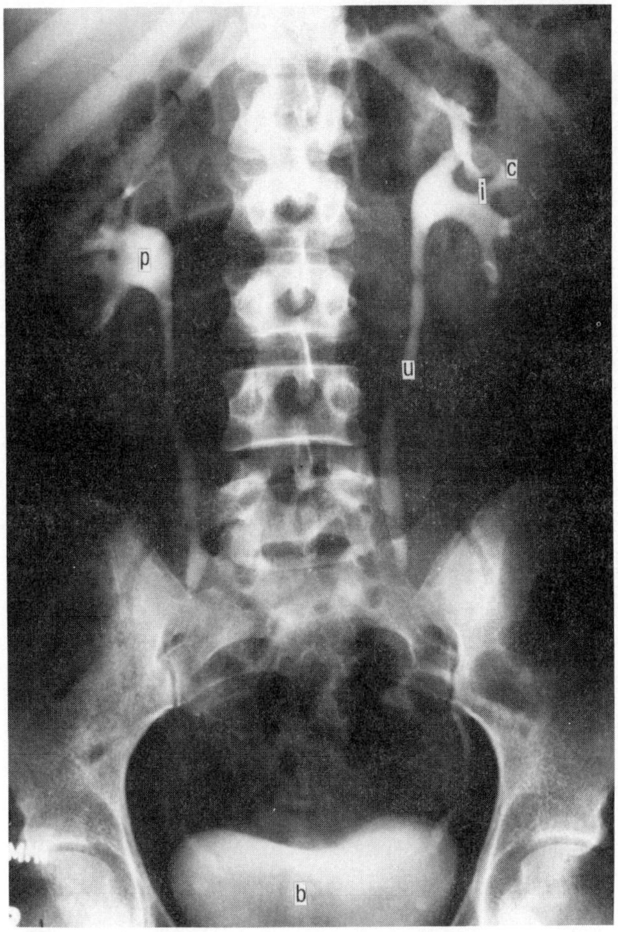

Figure 18-4 Single abdominal film from an IVP. Note the visualization of the calyx (c), infundibulum (i), pelvis (p), ureter (u), and bladder (b) by the injected contrast material.

ganic iodine has been attached. The iodine imparts radiographic density to the contrast material. It is important to realize that the contrast agent is neither actively secreted nor resorbed but is passively filtered and, hence, provides a rough estimate of the patient's glomerular filtration rate (GFR). The IVP is one of the few examinations that is timed. In this manner, the contrast can be visualized in various compartments of the kidney as a function of time. Thus, in the initial films before contrast reaches the renal collecting system, the contrast can be seen to be evenly distributed in the collecting tubules. This imparts a homogeneous and increased density to the kidney and usually occurs 1 minute after the injection.

Unfortunately, this injected contrast material is not innocuous. Three types of reactions may occur. The first is minor, consisting of occasional hives, sneezing, and nausea. The second is more severe and usually requires treatment. The symptoms consist of difficulty in breathing (probably secondary to laryngospasm) and massive production of hives. The third and, fortunately, least common is an anaphylactic type of reaction leading to immediate cardiovascular collapse. Thus, when any contrast agent is administered, a "crash cart" (resuscitation capabilities) containing drugs and equipment necessary to treat cardiovascular collapse should be immediately available. Despite this precaution, the death rate from administration of these contrast materials is about 1 in 50,000. A new class of contrast agents that are nonionic and have a lower osmolality than the more traditional ionic agents have a markedly diminished incidence of reactions. They will probably replace the ionic media, even though they are three to four times as costly. From a clinician's standpoint, it is essential that a history of prior contrast reaction be investigated and the type of reaction documented. Reactions in the same patient tend to be similar, so a previously minor reaction will tend to recur rather than escalate to the type of major reaction described previously. Obviously, this information should be clearly noted on any requisition for studies in which contrast agents are to be used. Indeed, if a severe reaction has occurred in a patient, the clinician and the radiologist should carefully consider options available to avoid future contrast delivery, if at all possible. Another caveat for the clinician is to ensure that the patient's blood urea nitrogen (BUN) and creatinine levels are normal prior to studies that use contrast material. There is both clinical and experimental evidence to show that renal function can be affected deleteriously after the use of contrast material. These values should also be included on the patient's requisition.

Special note should be made of patients with multiple myeloma and diabetes mellitus, especially those in renal failure. It is known that contrast agents precipitate the abnormal Tamm-Horsfall proteins in renal tubules in patients with multiple my-

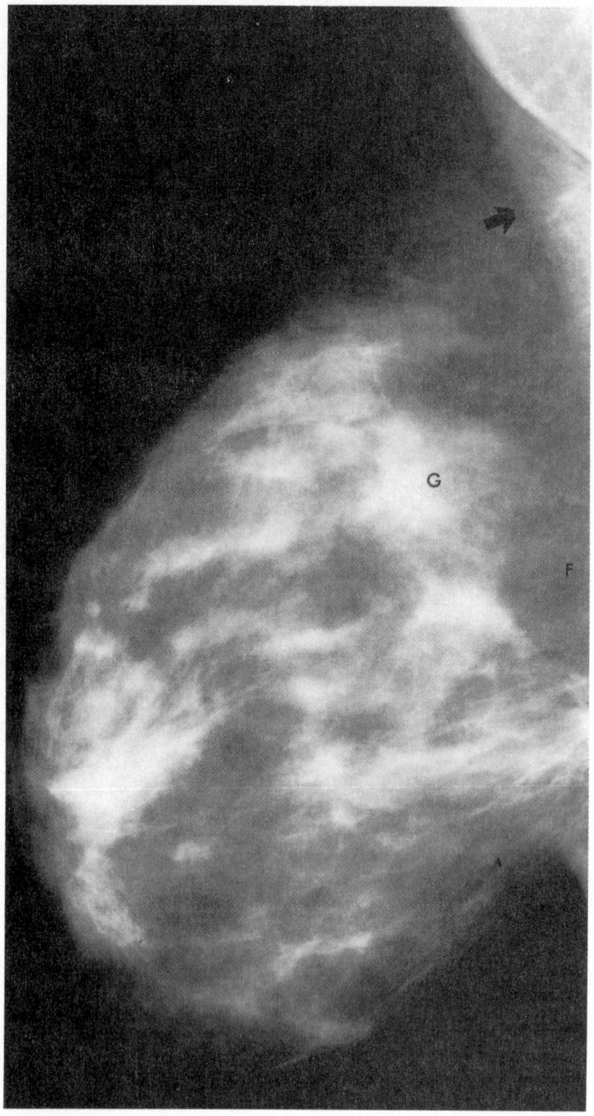

Figure 18-5 Lateral view of the breast done with film technique. The lighter areas seen represent glandular tissue (G); the gray regions represent fatty tissue (F). The pectoralis muscle (*arrow*) is clearly seen highlighted against the adjacent fat within the breast.

eloma and that similar events tend to occur more frequently than generally expected in diabetic patients, especially those with a degree of cardiac failure. As a matter of fact, these diagnoses have been considered contraindications to contrast administration. Recent work, however, has shown that it is the relative fluid restriction as much as the contrast administration that causes tubular protein precipitation. Thus, if there is no alternative to the administration of contrast to these patients, they should be well hydrated both before and after the examination.

Patient preparation for the IVP is relatively simple and includes no food after midnight and no breakfast on the morning of the examination. Clear fluids may be taken up until 2 hours before the exam. If patients with intravenous lines are to be examined and the intravenous administration cannot be discontinued, realize that renal enhancement will be diminished secondary to a dilution effect. There is no need for enemas or cathartic bowel preparation.

Mammography

This is the radiographic examination of the breast using either a film or a xeroradiographic technique (Fig. 18-5). It is beyond the scope of this chapter to list the pros and cons of each technique; however, most exams are done with a film-screen system.

It has been well established that mammograms can detect carcinoma earlier than the clinical examination. In fact, in recent studies, 50 percent of patients with breast carcinoma were diagnosed solely by mammography. It was equally clearly demonstrated that the benefit accrued from screening for breast cancer with mammography far outweighs the potential risk for development of breast cancer by the radiation from this technique.

The following guidelines are recommended by the American Cancer Society. Any patient with symptoms referable to the breast or with high-risk status should undergo mammography. Obviously, this must be tempered by the patient's age, and consultation with a radiologist will produce satisfactory compromise. All women, regardless of symptoms, should have a baseline study done between the ages of 35 and 40. All women between the ages of 40 and 50 should have an exam yearly or every other year, depending on presence of risk factors. All women over age 50 should have yearly mammograms.

Special Radiographic Procedures

In general, these studies should be ordered only after consultation with a radiologist. Thus, they are rarely used for screening. Space limitations preclude a discussion of every procedure, but the ones in common usage are reviewed.

Tomography

Tomography is a technique for visualizing more clearly a particular plane within the body. It can be used in almost any anatomic area of interest. As can be seen in Figure 18-6, the x-ray tube and film-holding device are attached to each other and pivot about a fulcrum. This fulcrum can be raised or lowered as desired. The patient is placed on the x-ray table between the x-ray tube and the attached film cassette. When the x-ray tube and film cassette move about the pivot or fulcrum, anatomic detail is blurred,

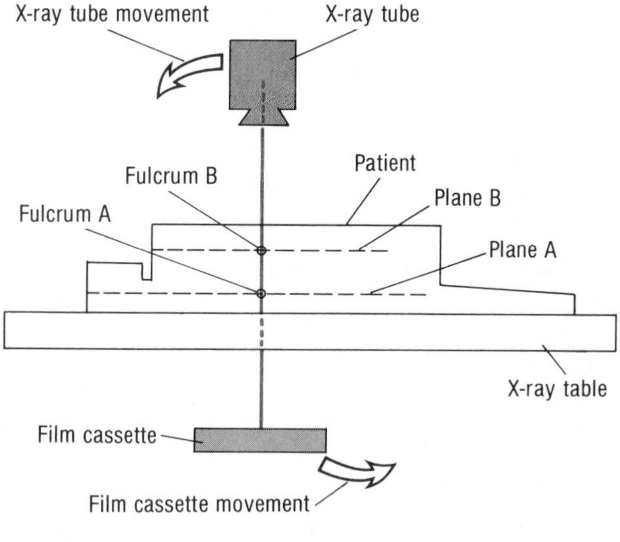

Figure 18-6 Schematic diagram of the physical principles involved in tomography (see text for discussion).

except for anatomy contained within a plane that includes the fulcrum. Thus, if the fulcrum is placed at the level of the kidneys, these organs will be clearly seen, whereas planes above and below will be blurred. By altering the fulcrum it is possible to select any plane in the body and highlight it by blurring "extraneous" anatomy above and below the desired plane.

Tomography is typically used for examining the chest and kidneys. No special patient preparation is necessary, and again, this technique should be considered when a particular area needs further delineation.

Angiography

Angiography is a method of studying the aorta, the inferior and superior vena cava, and their major branches using iodinated contrast material (the same as used for IVPs). A percutaneous arterial or venous puncture, usually in the femoral artery or vein, is done with an 18-gauge needle after appropriate local anesthesia is given. A guidewire resembling piano wire is introduced through the needle into the femoral vessel and then into the major vessel. The needle is then removed, and a hollow tube with multiple holes at its distal end is threaded over the guidewire into the aorta or inferior vena cava. The guidewire is then removed, leaving a hollow tube in the vessel to deliver contrast material so that the great vessels and their branches may be visualized. By using appropriately curved catheters and fluoroscopy, the angiographer can insert the catheter into virtually any branch of the aorta or inferior and superior vena cava (Fig. 18-7).

These tests are employed basically for determining the extent of disease, less often for diagnosis, and most recently for therapy. Through analysis of vascular displacement and deformity, the extent of known disease can be established. In the era before ultrasound and CT, angiography often was the major modality for confirming a diagnosis suspected clinically or suggested by a prior radiographic examination. Today, however, angiography is often used to map peripheral vascular disease

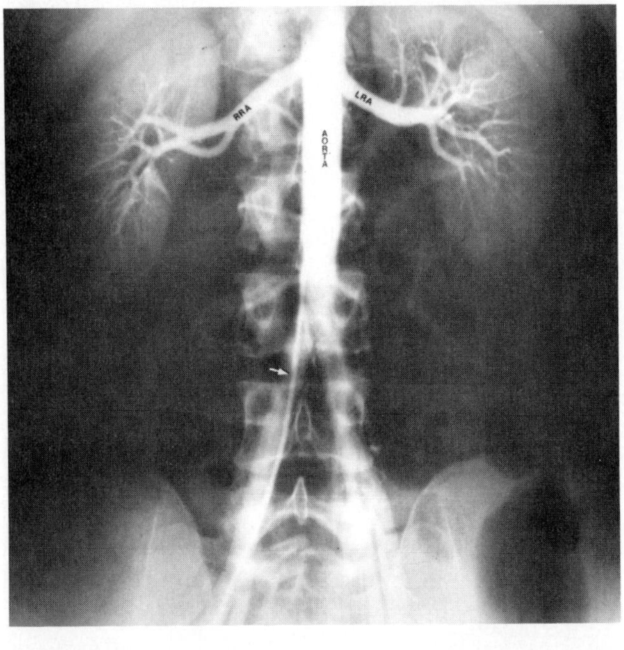

Figure 18-7 Abdominal aortogram. The aorta as well as the right (RRA) and left (LRA) renal arteries and their branches are clearly depicted. The hollow catheter (*arrow*) used to deliver the contrast into the aorta is seen ascending from the right femoral artery into the right common iliac artery to the aorta.

and to supply a vascular "road map" for the surgeon. Its more recent and exciting application involves using angiographic technique to widen areas of vascular stenosis percutaneously, a practice called percutaneous transluminal angioplasty (PTA). By the addition of an inflatable balloon incorporated into its tip, the catheter may be guided into an area of narrowing and inflated for variable periods of time, producing long-lasting patency in the area formerly strictured. This technique has now extended beyond the vascular system, having been tried in ureteral and biliary duct strictures as well.

Another form of therapy using angiographic technique is in the control of vascular bleeding secondary to a multitude of causes. Placing a catheter in the bleeding vessel, followed by the injection of microparticles of various materials, can cause a thrombus to form in that vessel and bleeding to cease. The matching of the type of injected material to the specific case can lead to thrombosis of varying duration.

Patient preparation for these examinations should be clearly understood. Only clear liquids should be given to the patient after midnight prior to the exam. A recent prothrombin time (PT), partial thromboplastin time (PTT), platelet count, BUN, and creatinine should be in the chart. A hypocoagulable state (i.e., PT greater than 10 above control, PTT greater than 1.5 times control, and low platelets), severe congestive failure, and renal failure all constitute relative contraindications to the procedure. More than any other study, this procedure requires close consultation between the angiographer and the clinician, with the purpose of the study clearly outlined on the requisition.

After the angiographic examination is completed, vital signs should be checked every 15 minutes for the first hour and then every hour for the next 4 hours. The puncture site should be examined frequently, especially in the first hour after the study. Note should be made of any frank hemorrhage or swelling in the area. The pulse at the puncture site and distal to it should be evaluated at the time of vital-sign checks. The patient should be on complete bed rest for the remainder of the day and night after the examination, and if the femoral artery was punctured, the groin on that side should remain extended for 6 hours. If an axillary artery was punctured, the axilla on that side should remain adducted for 6 hours.

Ultrasonography

A relatively new procedure in diagnostic radiology, ultrasonography has dramatically altered diagnosis in several areas. Ultrasonography depends on high-frequency sound (ultrasound) to produce echoes and uses these echoes to depict anatomy within the body. As such, it does not use ionizing radiation, and, to date, no definite deleterious effects attributable to ultrasound have been detected.

In general, ultrasonography is not a screening procedure, and consultation with the radiologist on individual cases is encouraged. However, there are instances when ultrasonography serves as the initial diagnostic radiologic screening procedure: in obstetrics and pelvic pathology (Fig. 18-8), and in gallbladder and biliary duct disease.

One should realize the limitations of ultrasound examinations and the importance of proper patient preparation. Because of the high frequency of these sound waves (on the order of 2 to 3 million cycles per second, with the highest audible sound about 20,000 cycles per second), they will not penetrate air, bone, or calcium-containing structures. If barium is present in the GI tract, it should be eliminated before the study. If large amounts of gas are present in the GI tract, the examination may have to be repeated after a trial of simethicone. Patients receiving a pelvic ultrasound examination should usually have a full bladder prior to this study.

Patients scheduled for ultrasonically guided aspirations or

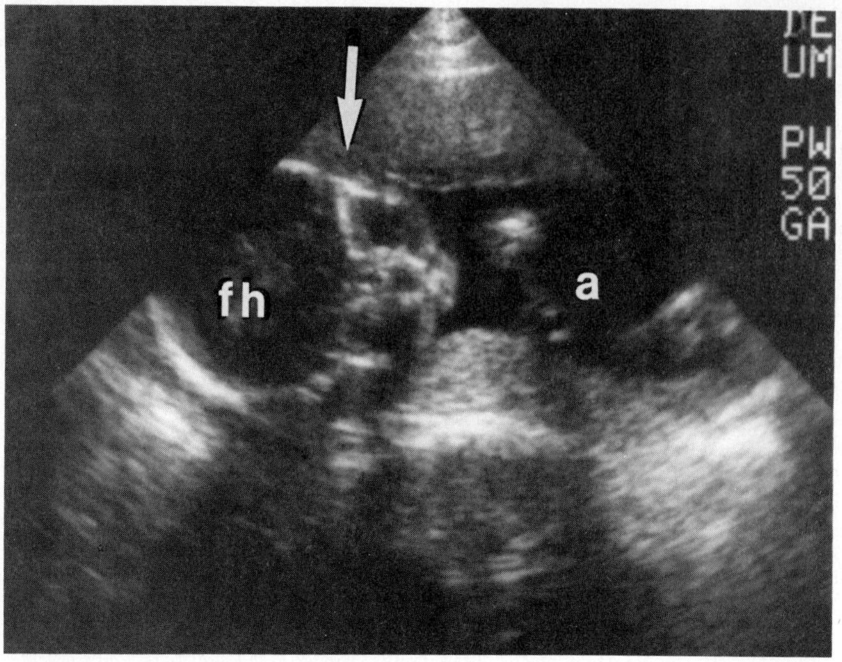

Figure 18-8 Sonogram of a gravid uterus. The fetal head (fh) can be seen surrounded by amniotic fluid (a). The placenta (*arrow*) is visualized adjacent to the fetal head.

biopsies must sign a consent form and have a bleeding work-up completed (PT, PTT, hemoglobin, hematocrit, and platelets). Once again, consultation with the radiologist is imperative in planning a biopsy.

Computed Tomography

Few diagnostic techniques in recent times have excited as much interest and affected diagnosis as dramatically as CT. Indeed, this technology led to a Nobel Prize for its creator, Dr. Geoffrey Hounsfield. Basically, an x-ray source and x-ray detectors rotate about the area of interest, producing thousands of bits of x-ray density information per slice or rotation, called *pixels*. Density information is present in each pixel (fat, bone, soft tissue, or air), and its exact location in that slice is known by the computer. From this information, a two-dimensional plane is reconstructed, portraying all of the anatomy within the area under investigation (Fig. 18-9). Because of the geometry of the scanner at present, only direct transverse sections may be done. However, reconstructions from the transverse plane to any other plane may be done, although these planes do not have the detail of the original, directly obtained transverse scan.

Again, CT focuses on answering specific questions rather than serving as a general screening procedure. There are regions, however, where CT may serve as the initial study in searching for disease. These regions include the head, the mediastinum and hilar areas of the lung, the liver parenchyma, and the pancreas.

Because the examination requires the patient to be relatively motionless, pediatric patients present a unique problem and usually must be sedated for both the cranial and body CT examinations. Thus, when pediatric patients are to have a CT scan, parents should be told that mild anesthesia will be used. It is also important to note the pediatric patient's weight on the request, so that the proper amount of anesthetic can be given.

In abdominal CT examinations, a very dilute mixture (2 percent) of barium and fruit juice is given to opacify the bowel. Loops of bowel can be very confusing when seen in cross section and may be mistaken for masses or adenopathy. Note that the dilution is vastly different from the barium used in GI studies (80 percent). If the abdomen and pelvis are to be visualized, the mixture is started the night before the exam to ensure that the colon is opacified. Otherwise, the drink is given on the day of the exam. Most patients receive intravenous contrast administration, so all the precautions outlined in the IVP section regarding these agents apply here as well. Women who require a pelvic scan should have a tampon inserted before arriving in the CT section.

As with ultrasound-guided biopsies, biopsies done with CT should have a completed bleeding work-up.

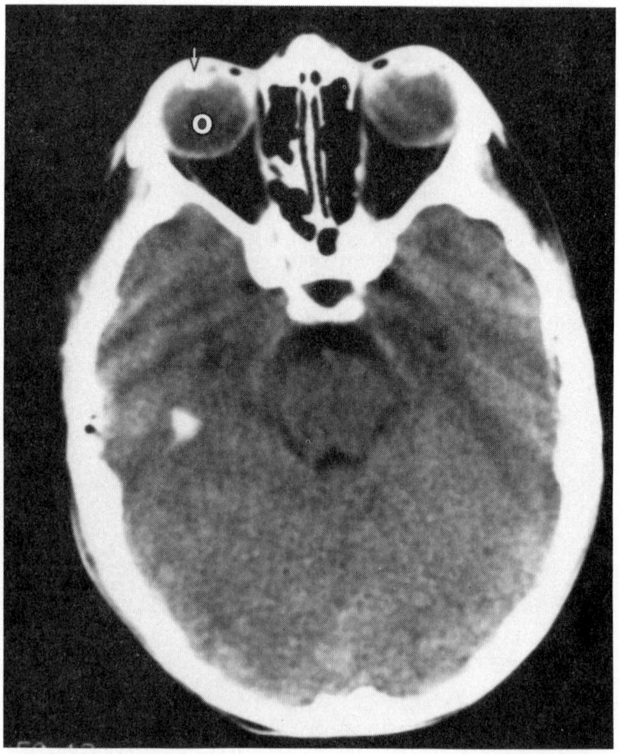

Figure 18-9 Axial scan of the brain. A scan oriented in the axial plane through the level of the orbits (o). The biconcave white area (*arrow*) represents the lens.

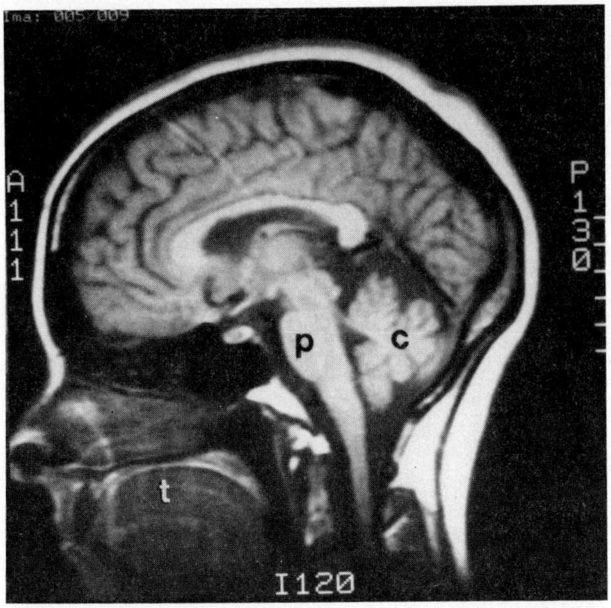

Figure 18-10 Midline sagittal section of the skull. High-contrast depiction of the brain and facial structures in the sagittal plane. Note pons (p), cerebellum (c), and tongue (t).

Magnetic Resonance Imaging

Magnetic resonance imaging (MRI) could represent the most significant advance in medicine since the discovery of x-rays. The principles of MRI have been understood for some time, beginning in 1924, when Wolfgang Pauli first observed the magnetic properties of certain nuclei. With this technology, it is possible to observe and quantify magnetic characteristics of certain atomic nuclei when they are in various energy states. Only atomic nuclei with an odd number of protons or neutrons have magnetic properties. When we see images generated by MR, we are looking at hydrogen nuclei because of their abundance in the body and the presence of a magnetic field.

When a body is placed within an external magnetic field, magnetic nuclei tend to align with and rotate about the axis of the external magnetic field. If at this time an appropriate radiofrequency (RF) signal is introduced into the body, hydrogen nuclei will absorb this energy and alter their position and direction, or "resonate," with the RF signal. When this signal is stopped, the nuclei will "relax" toward their equilibrium state and release energy, which can be detected as a signal. The relaxation depends on the chemical structure or lattice surrounding the excited nuclei (T1 relaxation) and on the effect one excited nucleus has on other surrounding excited nuclei (T2 relaxation). The emitted signal can be detected by an antenna and, by complex maneuvers, can be processed by a computer into an image (Fig. 18-10). Because, as stated previously, the signals emitted depend heavily on the local molecular environment, they provide an excellent depiction of body anatomy. The modality has several advantages over currently used imaging modalities. Superior soft-tissue contrast is present and is under direct control of the user by varying several technical factors. It is also possible to scan directly in any image plane, unlike CT, which requires reconstruction from a transverse plane. Thus, anatomy is now clearly appreciated in direct axial, sagittal, or coronal sections. The inherent properties of nuclei in cortical bone prevent a signal produced from this portion of bone. However, fatty marrow will produce a signal. Thus, there is high artifact-free contrast between cortical bone, on the one hand, and marrow and soft tissue, on the other. Because of the flowing nature of blood in vessels, no signal is detected from this blood, which acts as a natural "contrast agent" for vessels. The potential for great specificity exists because we are analyzing signals that depend on the molecular environment of the excited

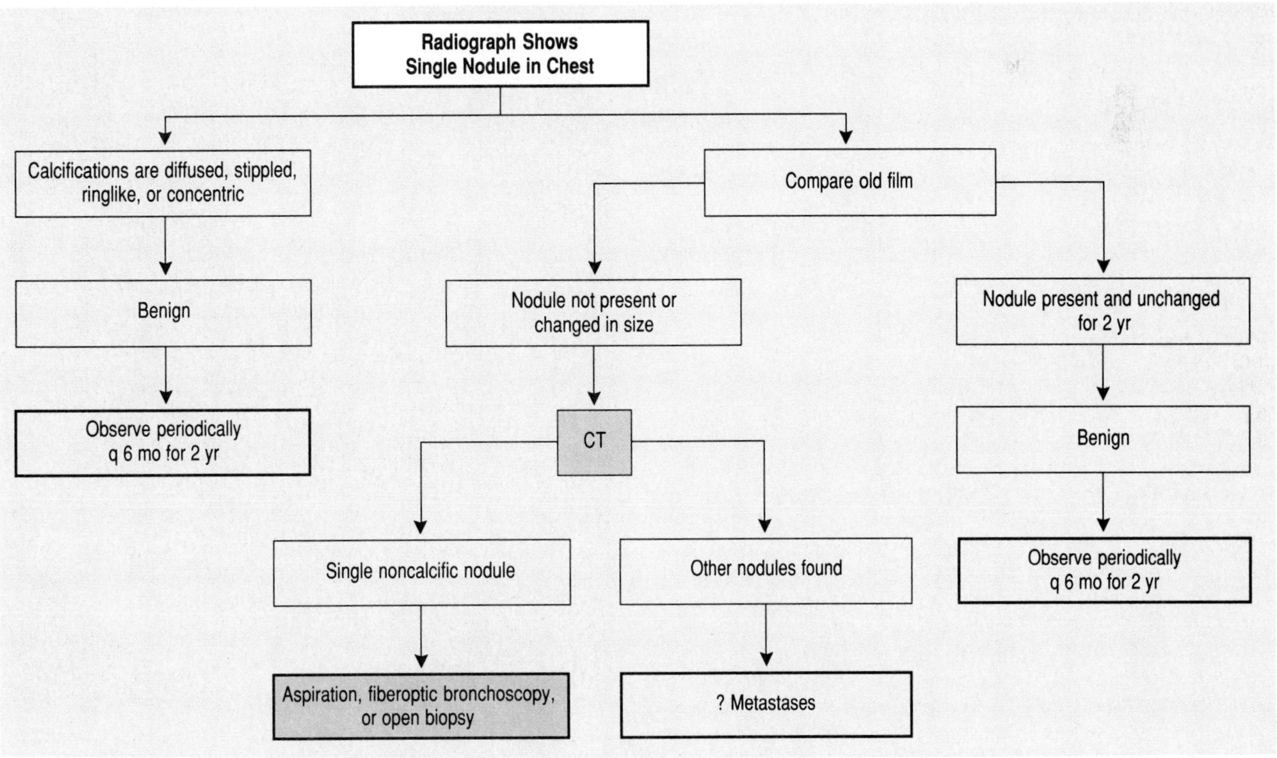

Figure 18-11 Algorithm for the diagnostic evaluation of a solitary pulmonary nodule. CT = computed tomography.

nuclei. To date, no adverse affects have been reported in association with MRI. We are merely at the threshold of potential for this exciting new modality. The ability to visualize altered chemical states, heretofore only analyzed in the basic science laboratory, has not yet been tapped by the clinician.

The scope of the chapter precludes a detailed study of diagnostic radiographic work-ups. However, a guide for the evaluation of a solitary pulmonary nodule is presented (Fig. 18-11).

References

Balter S. An introduction to the physics of magnetic resonance imaging. Radiographics 1987; 7:371.

Black WC, Armstrong P, Daniel TM. Cost effectiveness of chest CT in T1N0M0 lung cancer. Radiology 1988; 167:373.

Brooks FP. Radiologic exploration of the gastrointestinal tract: An interdisciplinary enterprise. Radiographics 1986; 6:160.

Chezmos JL, et al. Liver and abdominal screening in patients with cancer: CT versus MR imaging. Radiology 1988; 168:43.

Feig SA. Decreased breast cancer mortality through mammographic screening: Results of clinical trials. Radiology 1988; 167:659.

Goldkrand JW, Benjamin DS, Contro DM. Role of ultrasound in obstetric management. J Clin Ultrasound 1986; 14:589.

Pavlicek W. MR instrumentation and image formation. Radiographics 1987; 7:809.

Raptopoulos V, et al. Clinicians' appraisal of sonography. Radiology 1987; 105:237.

Ritchie WW, et al. Evaluation of azotemic patients: Diagnostic yield of initial ultrasound examination. Radiology 1988; 167:245.

Tabar L, Dean PB. Control of breast cancer through mammography screening: What is the evidence? Radiol Clin North Am 1987; 25:993.

Tobin RS, et al. Comparative study of computed tomography and ERCP in pancreatico-biliary disease. CT 1987; 11:261.

van Sonnenberg E, Casola G. Interventional radiology, 1988. Invest Radiol 1988; 23:75.

II Internal Medicine: A Signs and Symptoms Approach

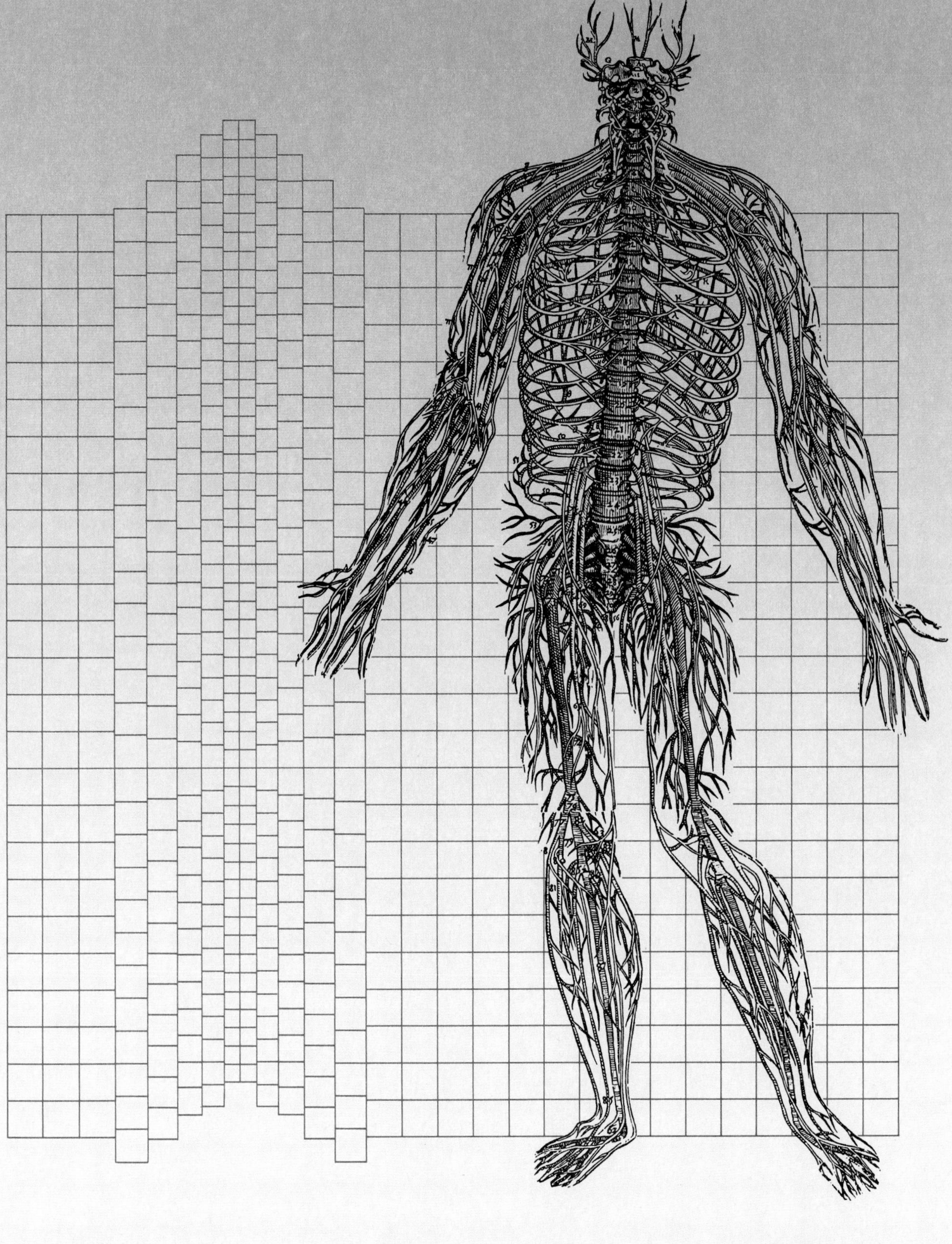

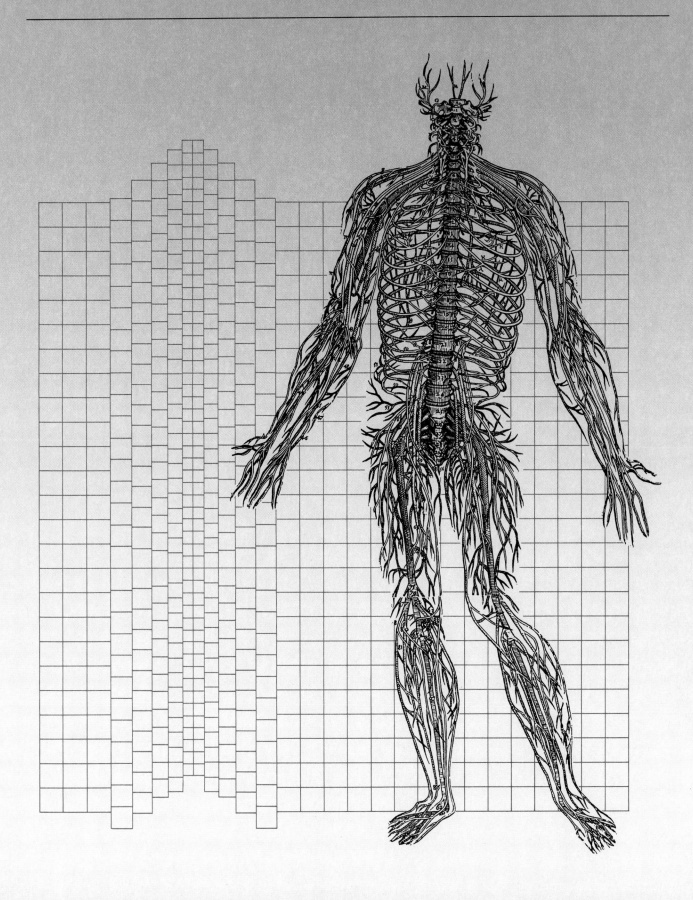

Cardiovascular

Elevated Serum Cholesterol and Other Lipid Disorders

Harry L. Greene, MD

Dennis Davidson, MD

19

Coronary heart disease is the leading cause of premature death and disability in the United States and throughout much of the rest of the world. A major reduction in the incidence of this disease can be achieved by altering its associated risk factors. Elsewhere in this text, we address decreasing the risk due to cigarette smoking (Chap. 147), controlling obesity (Chap. 45), and detecting and treating hypertension (Chap. 23). In this chapter, we discuss the identification of disorders of lipid and lipoprotein metabolism. The major focus is on serum cholesterol and its components because of their critical contributions to heart disease.

Definitions

Cholesterol is a relatively insoluble lipid that is a sterol and is needed for the formation of cell membranes, steroid hormones, nerve sheaths, and bile acids. It is carried in the plasma as a spherical particle composed of lipid and protein, and its components can be categorized by their density.

High-Density Lipoprotein

As the most dense of the three major classes of lipoproteins, high-density lipoprotein (HDL) comprises roughly 25 percent of the total serum cholesterol. HDL is produced by both the liver and the intestine, and its property of reverse cholesterol transport may account for its protective effect with respect to heart disease. The Framingham study showed an inverse relationship of HDL to fatal cardiac events and nonfatal heart attacks. Conditions that are associated with a low HDL level include primary hypoalphalipoproteinemia (a genetic factor), cigarette smoking, obesity, sedentary lifestyle, hypertriglyceridemia, and use of anabolic steroids, progestational agents, and some beta-blocking agents.

Low-Density Lipoprotein

Low-density lipoproteins (LDLs) constitute about 70 percent of the total serum cholesterol and are believed to be the most atherogenic of the cholesterol subgroups. The Framingham heart study showed a positive relationship between LDL and cardiac events that becomes linear at levels above 160 mg/dl. LDL is made from products of very low density lipoprotein metabolism (see following section) and can be increased from overproduction or from a defect in removal through altered number or affinity of receptors for LDL removal. It is believed that these LDL particles interact with platelets, damaged arterial endothelium, and smooth muscle cells beneath the damaged endothelium to set up a cascade of events leading to atherosclerosis. Macrophages move into the region of damage and ingest the LDL, forming "foam cells." This collection of cells, along with platelets, cholesterol, fibrin, and smooth muscle cells, can narrow or totally occlude the vessel.

Very Low Density Lipoprotein

The very low density lipoprotein (VLDL) fraction carries 15 percent of the total cholesterol and the majority of the triglycerides from the liver. The VLDLs are made in the liver and metabolized in adipose tissue or muscle by lipoprotein lipase. The triglycerides are released and intermediate-density lipoprotein remains to be returned to the liver to produce more LDL.

Intermediate-Density Lipoprotein

The lipoprotein fraction remaining after VLDL interacts with lipoprotein lipase is known as intermediate-density lipoprotein (IDL).

Lipoprotein Metabolism

The two major pathways in lipoprotein synthesis and transport are the exogenous and the endogenous systems. The *exogenous pathway* is involved in the handling of dietary lipids. Ingested lipid passes through the stomach and is acted upon in the duodenum by pancreatic lipase. These lipids are then taken into the cells in the intestinal wall, where they become chylomicrons. The chylomicrons are transported from the intestinal cells via lacteals that coalesce to form the larger lymphatic system, which joins at the thoracic duct, and ultimately empty into the peripheral venous system. From there the chylomicrons proceed through the circulation to the arterial system to systemic capillaries, where chylomicrons come in proximity to muscles or adipose tissues. Endothelial cells in muscle and adipose tissue capillaries contain lipoprotein lipase, which hydrolyzes the triglycerides to produce fatty acids for energy conversion (muscle) or for storage (adipose tissue). For the lipoprotein lipase to be effective, a cofactor, apolipoprotein CII, which comes from HDL, must be present. Those components that are not utilized for energy or storage return to the liver, where these chylomicron remnants are removed from the circulation and utilized in the production of bile acids or coupled with triglycerides to form VLDL.

The *endogenous pathway* begins in the liver with the production of VLDLs, which enter the circulation and are metabolized by muscle and adipose tissue lipoprotein lipase in the presence of apolipoprotein CII from HDL. IDL, the remnant left from this process, can be used for the production of LDL in the liver. The LDL pathway in the liver, shown in Figure 19-1, is dependent upon the liver's need for cholesterol production. This process, which requires LDL, can be regulated by increasing or decreasing the LDL receptor in the liver cells. The LDL that is not taken up by the liver passes through a nonreceptor pathway and is ingested by macrophages. Normal cells can produce LDL receptors when they need to make cholesterol for steroid hormone or bile acid production, or when cell or neuronal mem-

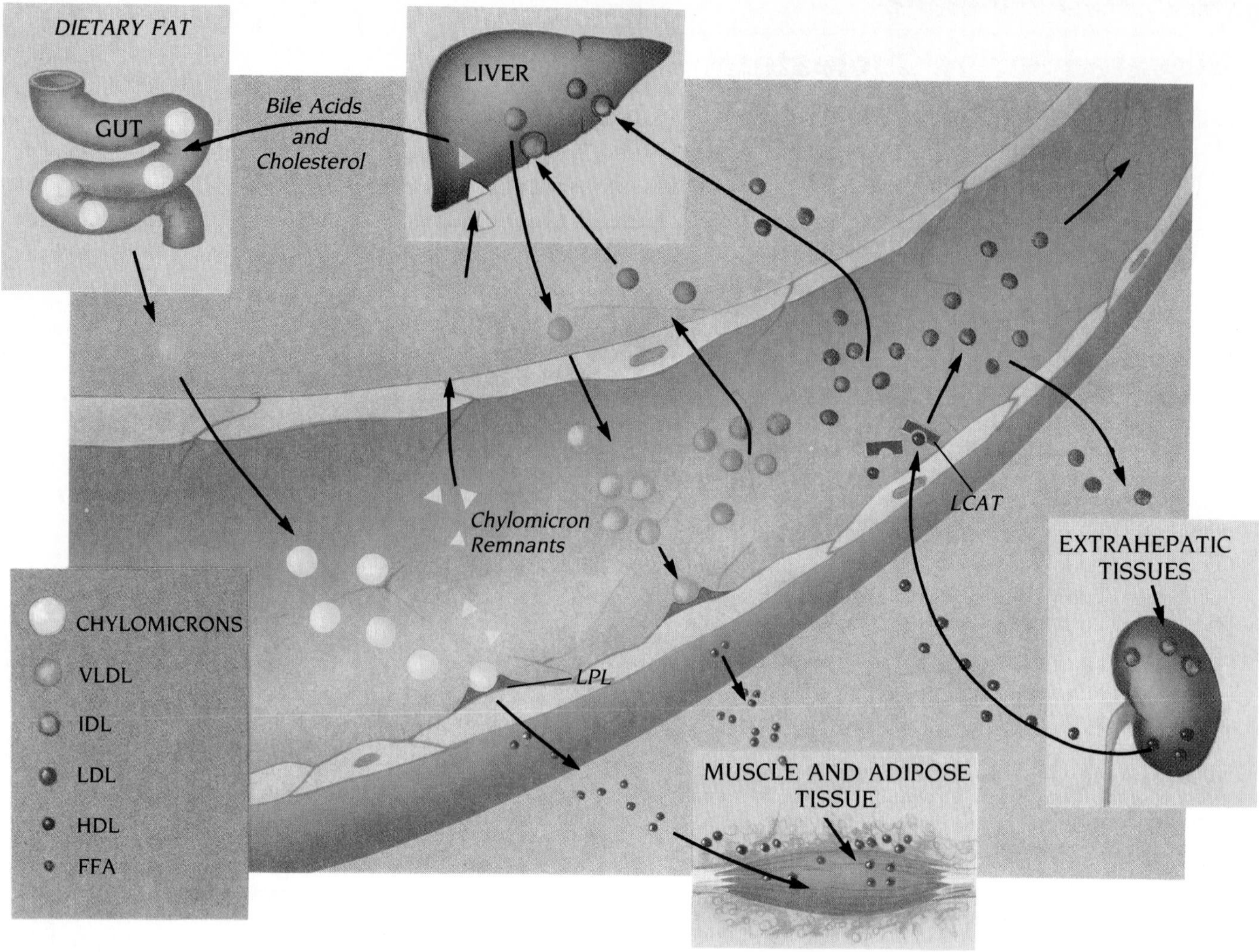

Figure 19-1 Schematic overview of lipoprotein metabolism. FFA = free fatty acids, HDL = high-density lipoproteins, IDL = intermediate-density lipoproteins, LCAT = lecithin : cholesterol acyltransferase, LDL = low-density lipoproteins, LPL = lipoprotein lipase, VLDL = very low density lipoproteins. (From Kalant H, Roschlau WHE. Principles of medical pharmacology. 5th ed. Toronto: BC Decker, 1989; with permission.)

branes are needed. This receptor protein binds apolipoprotein B (a component of LDL) to facilitate uptake by the cell.

HDL acts as a cholesterol scavenger. It reaches the circulation from both liver and intestine and removes cholesterol first by absorption onto its surface. HDL then facilitates enzymatic conversion to cholesterol esters, which move to the core of the HDL particle and return it to the liver. This property of removing cholesterol from peripheral tissues is thought to give HDL its cardioprotective properties.

Rationale for Lowering Serum Cholesterol

The association between elevated levels of serum cholesterol and coronary heart disease has been shown in numerous epidemiologic studies and clinical trials. High levels of blood cholesterol have been demonstrated to be an independent risk factor like smoking and high blood pressure. Investigations in Oslo, Norway, showed that modifying the diet and smoking habits of men with elevated levels of cholesterol could decrease their risk of heart attacks and sudden death by 47 percent. The Lipid Research Council's Coronary Primary Prevention Trial demonstrated a 2 percent reduction in coronary artery disease risk for every 1 percent reduction in cholesterol. Further enthusiasm for lowering cholesterol came from the Cholesterol Lowering Atherosclerosis Study. In this study, serum cholesterol was lowered using colestipol and nicotinic acid. The treatment group experienced a 26 percent reduction in total plasma cholesterol, with a 46 percent reduction in LDL cholesterol and a 37 percent increase in HDL. Coronary angiograms done before and after the intervention showed a significantly greater regression and a slower progression of lesions in subjects receiving the cholesterol-lowering drugs when compared with the usual care group.

In 1984, an expert panel was convened by the National Heart, Lung and Blood Institute to evaluate the data regarding cholesterol and heart disease and to consider making national recommendations, similar to those developed by a consensus panel for the National High Blood Pressure Education Program. The National Cholesterol Education Program (NCEP) issued their recommendations in 1987 with a focus on adults. The NCEP estimated that up to 25 percent of the population in the United States may fall into the borderline or high cholesterol groups defined below. This would encompass 40 million people!

Guidelines for Serum Cholesterol

The NCEP classification used to identify and treat elevated blood cholesterol is based on the total cholesterol and the LDL cholesterol for individuals over 20 years of age. A desirable total cholesterol level is one that is less than 200 mg/dl. Those individuals having levels in this range are given advice and educational material on the current dietary recommendation and are encouraged to have their cholesterol levels rechecked in 5 years (Fig. 19-2). They also should be questioned to determine the presence of any other risk factors for coronary heart disease such as family history of coronary heart disease (myocardial infarction or sudden death before age 55 in a parent or sibling), cigarette smoking (more than 10 cigarettes per day), hypertension, an HDL cholesterol level below 35 mg/dl, male gender, diabetes mellitus, history of cerebrovascular or occlusive peripheral vascular disease, and obesity (more than 130 percent of ideal total body weight).

Although there is an association between total cholesterol and risk of coronary heart disease, the LDL lipoprotein subfraction carries the greatest proportion of this risk. Given the total cholesterol, the HDL cholesterol, and the triglycerides, the LDL cholesterol can be calculated as follows:

LDL cholesterol =

$$\text{Total cholesterol} - \text{HDL cholesterol} - \frac{\text{Triglycerides}}{5}$$

The initial classification and management of patients based on total cholesterol and LDL cholesterol are shown in Figures 19-2 and 19-3.

Those patients with blood cholesterol levels from 200 to 239 mg/dl are termed *borderline-high*. If these individuals have no coronary heart disease and have fewer than two other risk factors, they are instructed on a diet to lower their cholesterol (Fig. 19-4) and are given an annual follow-up examination and a repeat cholesterol determination at that time. If the borderline-high patient has two or more risk factors or has definite coronary heart disease, a lipoprotein profile is done to determine the LDL cholesterol, HDL cholesterol, and triglyceride levels. In a similar manner, those with a blood cholesterol level of 240 mg/dl or greater are classified as having *high blood cholesterol* levels and should have a lipoprotein profile done regardless of other risk factors.

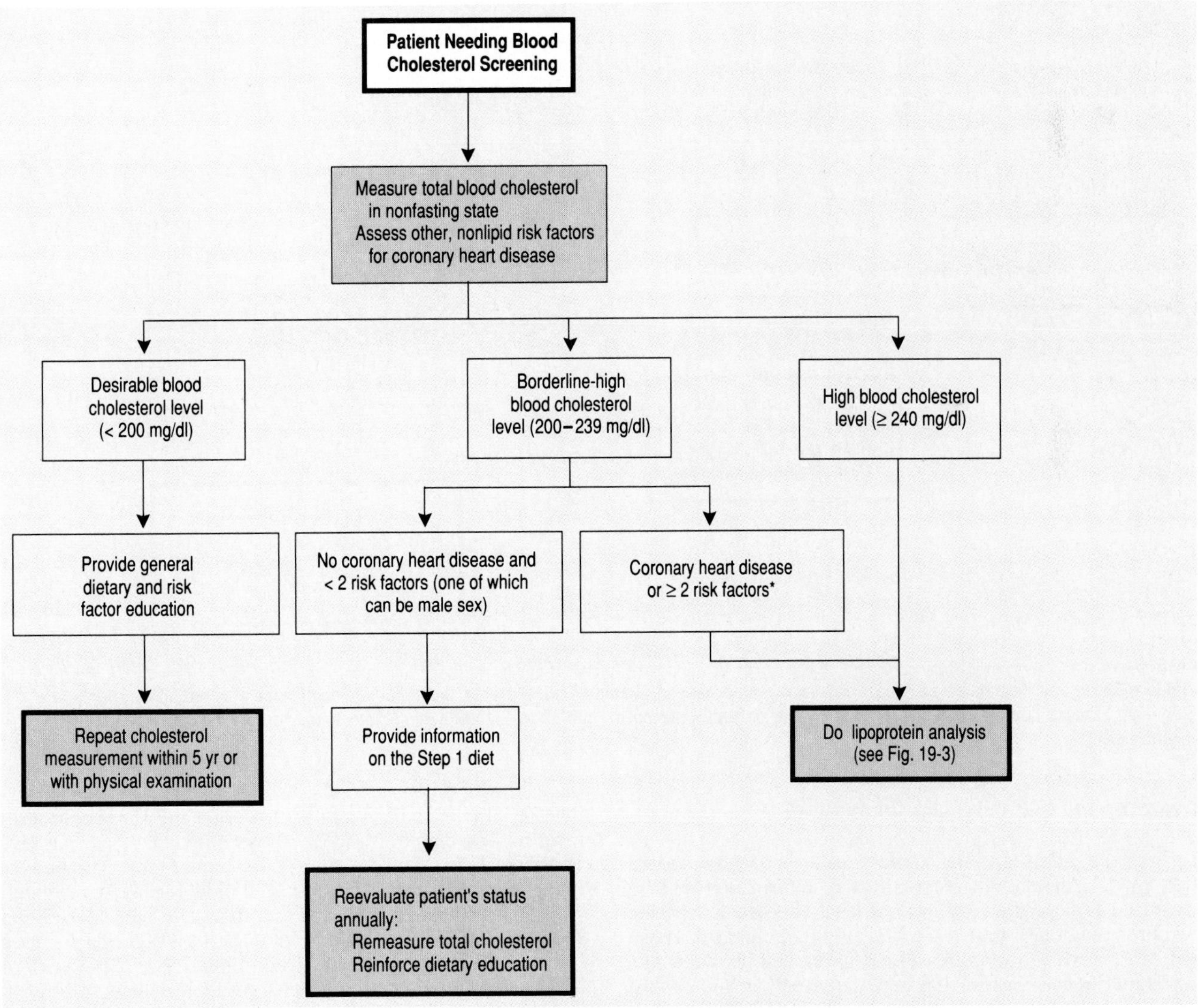

Figure 19-2 Initial classification based on total cholesterol. Assignment of a patient to the borderline-high category must be confirmed by repeat measurement; use average value. (*Modified from* Goodman DS, et al. The expert panel. Report of the National Cholesterol Education Program Expert Panel on Detection, Evaluation, and Treatment of High Blood Cholesterol in Adults. Arch Intern Med 1988; 142:36; with permission.)

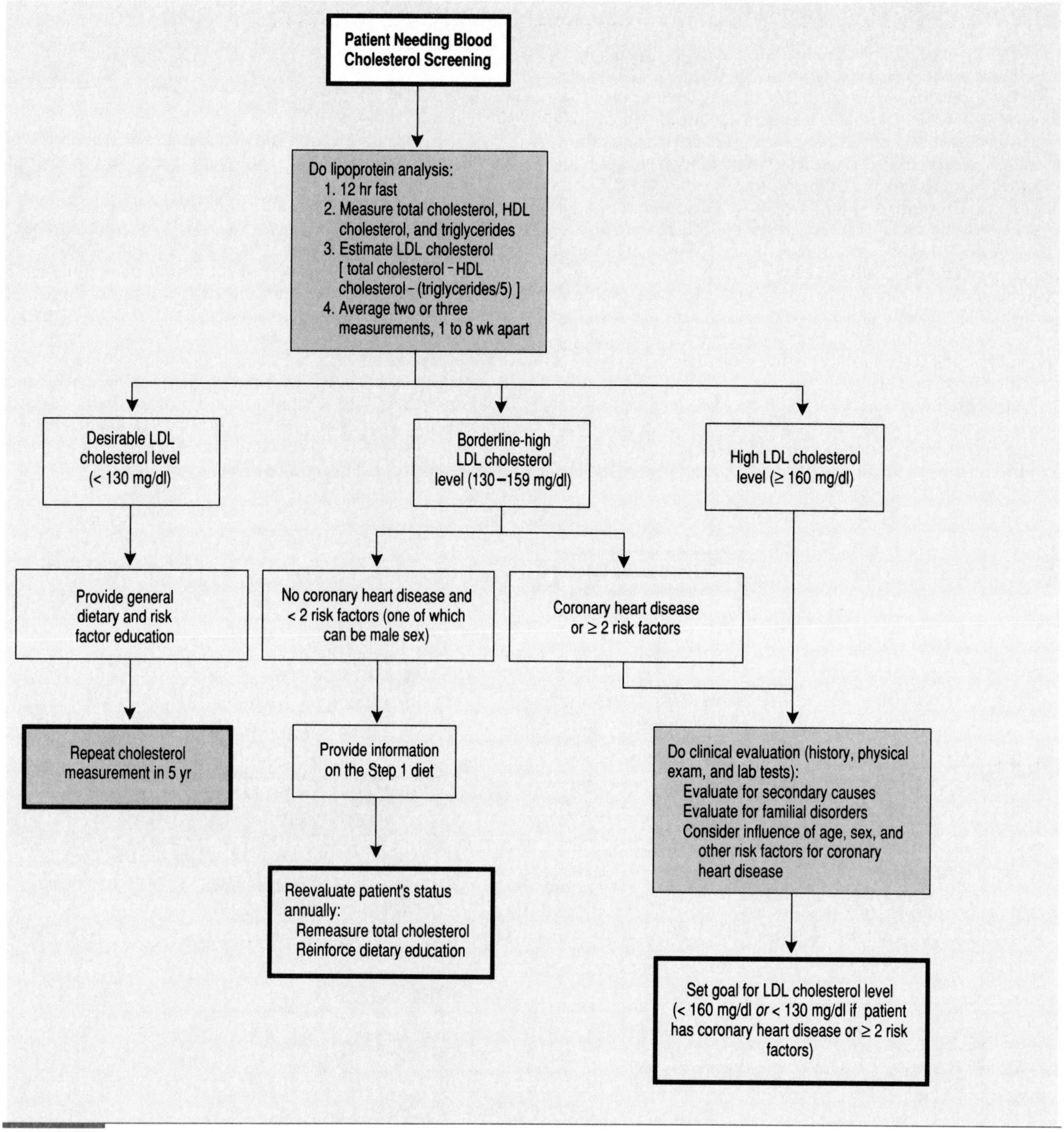

Figure 19-3 Classification based on LDL cholesterol. (*Modified from* Goodman DS, et al. The expert panel. Report of the National Cholesterol Education Program Expert Panel on Detection, Evaluation, and Treatment of High Blood Cholesterol in Adults. Arch Intern Med 1988; 142:36; with permission.)

Classification Using the LDL Cholesterol

Patients with a desirable LDL cholesterol level (defined as less than 130 mg/dl) should receive dietary information and be instructed to have their cholesterol level checked in 5 years. Borderline-high LDL values are from 130 to 150 mg/dl. Those with no coronary heart disease and fewer than two risk factors should receive instruction in a diet low in fat and cholesterol (Table 19-1). They should be seen by their physician and have their lipid levels rechecked annually. Those individuals with borderline-high LDL levels who have clinical coronary heart disease or more than two risk factors should receive a more rigorous program consisting of dietary treatment (see the Step 1 diet) with a goal of lowering the LDL cholesterol level to less than 160 mg/dl. Those individuals with an LDL cholesterol level of 160 mg/dl or higher are classified as being in a high-risk group. They should receive a thorough clinical examination focusing on the heart and peripheral vascular system and should be evaluated for secondary causes of an elevated cholesterol level (Table 19-2). The goal of treatment is an LDL cholesterol level of less than 160 mg/dl for those in the borderline-high LDL group. A more strenuous goal of an LDL cholesterol level of less than 130 mg/dl is indicated for borderline-high patients with coronary heart disease or more than two risk factors and patients in the high-risk LDL group.

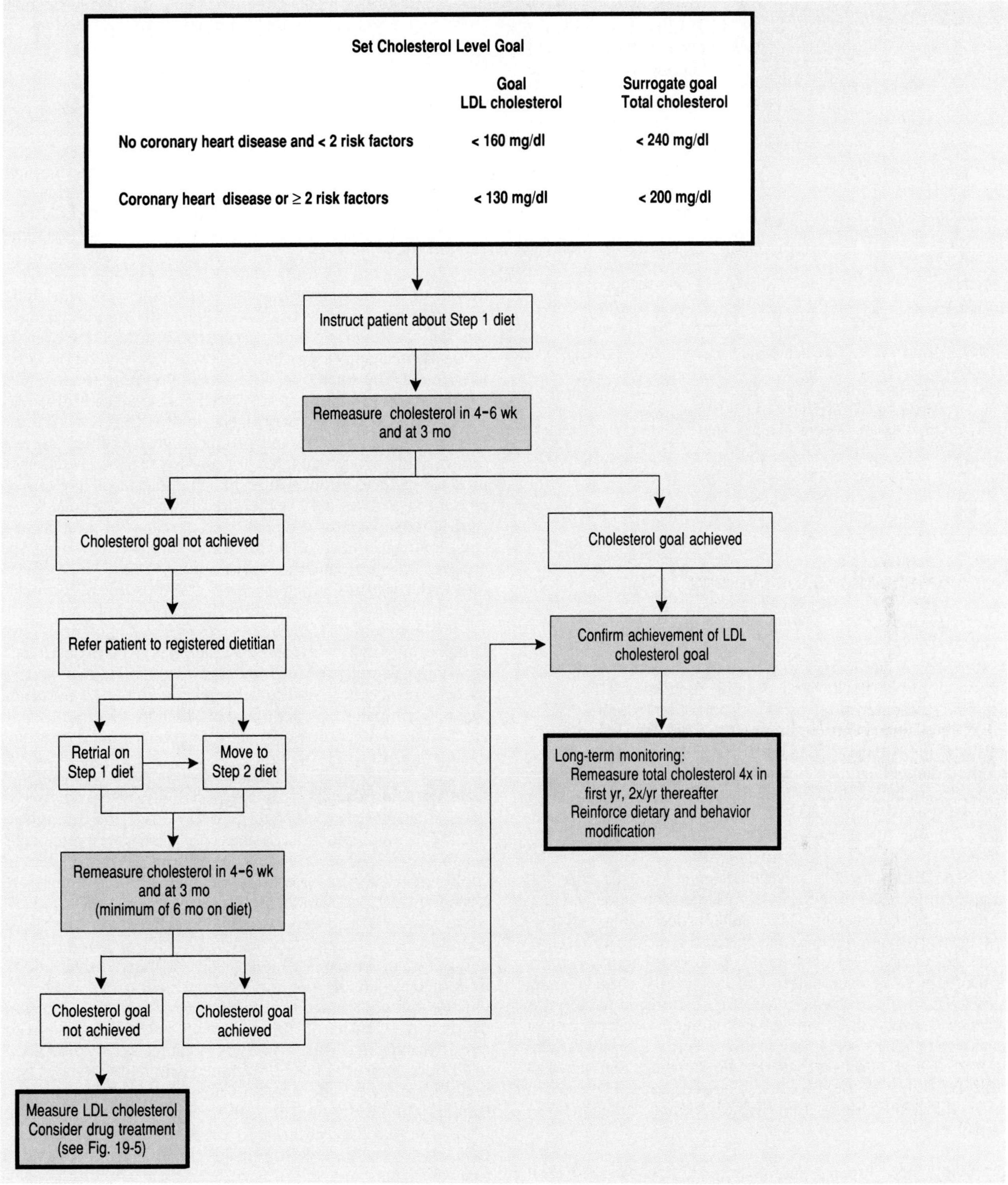

Figure 19-4 Dietary treatment of elevated serum cholesterol. (*Modified from* Goodman DS, et al. The expert panel. Report of the National Cholesterol Education Program Expert Panel on Detection, Evaluation, and Treatment of High Blood Cholesterol in Adults. Arch Intern Med 1988; 142:36; with permission.)

Table 19-1 Dietary Therapy of High Serum Cholesterol

Nutrient	Recommended intake: Step 1 diet	Step 2 diet
Total fat	Less than 30% of total calories	
Saturated fatty acids	Less than 10% of total calories	Less than 7% of total calories
Polyunsaturated fatty acids	Up to 10% of total calories	
Monounsaturated fatty acids	10 to 15% of total calories	
Carbohydrates	50 to 60% of total calories	
Protein	10 to 20% of total calories	
Cholesterol	Less than 300 mg/day	Less than 200 mg/day
Total calories	To achieve and maintain desirable weight	

From Goodman DS, et al. The expert panel. Report of the National Cholesterol Education Program Expert Panel on Detection, Evaluation, and Treatment of High Blood Cholesterol in Adults. Arch Intern Med 1988; 142:36; with permission.

Recommendations for Therapy

Diet Therapy

A fat-modified diet has been advocated for all Americans as an important public health goal. Support for this goal has come from the National Institutes of Health and other federal agencies, as well as voluntary agencies such as the American Heart Association and the American Cancer Society. The adoption of this prudent diet will significantly lower the incidence of coronary heart disease in the entire population. With national acceptance of these goals, perhaps fast-food stores, the airlines, and restaurants will offer more prudent meal choices.

The Step 1 Diet. The Step 1 diet is designed to be palatable and to reduce the intake of cholesterol, saturated fatty acids, and total fat as well as total calories. This is done by decreasing consumption of food containing butter fat, decreasing red meat consumption, and replacing it with skinned chicken and fish. Consumption of egg yolks is curtailed, and individuals who eat organ meats (i.e., liver, pancreas, brain) are encouraged to stop this practice. Grocery label reading is encouraged so that the patient can avoid products containing saturated fatty acids such as palm oil, coconut oil, or others that are altered through partial hydrogenation. Table 19-2 shows specific foods to emphasize and others that should be avoided. This chart can be copied for the patient.

The Step 2 Diet. Patients should have their cholesterol level checked 4 to 6 weeks after starting the Step 1 diet and again after 3 months, at which time cooking and dietary practices can be reviewed. If the target goals are not met after 3 months, a Step 2 diet should be prescribed and implemented with the collaboration of a registered dietitian. The Step 2 diet involves reducing intake of saturated fatty acids to below 7 percent of calories and lowering cholesterol intake to less than 200 mg per day. Studies done on metabolic wards have shown that a decrease in total cholesterol of 30 to 40 mg/dl (10 to 15 percent) may be achieved on the Step 1 diet, although free-living persons usually make lesser reductions. The Step 2 diet may provide a further reduction in total cholesterol of 15 mg/dl, most of the change being in the LDL fraction. Patients are encouraged to maintain or move toward an ideal body weight by adding exercise to the diet.

Medications

The addition of medication to dietary therapy should be considered when target goals have not been met by diet alone after an appropriate interval. However, dietary therapy must be continued when drugs are added. Figure 19-5 shows an algorithm for approaching the drug treatment of elevated cholesterol.

There are four classes of drugs to choose from: cholesterol binding resins, nicotinic acid, HMG CoA reductase inhibitors, and fibric acid derivatives.

Resins. The cholesterol binding resins colestipol and cholestyramine are the drugs of choice. These two are interchangeable, but cost differences may prompt selection of one over the other. These agents lower LDL cholesterol by binding bile acids in the gastrointestinal tract. They are contraindicated for those with levels of serum triglycerides greater than 500 mg/dl. Cholestyramine was the primary agent in the Coronary Primary Prevention Trial (CPPT) and produced an overall 20 percent reduction in myocardial infarction and coronary-related deaths. In those able to reduce their blood cholesterol level by 25 percent, there was a 49 percent reduction in heart attack and cardiac-related deaths. As mentioned previously, colestipol was combined with nicotinic acid in the Cholesterol Lowering Atherosclerosis Study, and the study population achieved a 26 percent reduction in total cholesterol, a 43 percent reduction in LDL, and a 37 percent increase in HDL cholesterol.

Cholestyramine is given in doses of 12 to 24 g per day two or three times daily with meals. Colestipol is given in doses of 15 to 30 g per day with meals. The drugs are supplied in 4- and 5-g packets, respectively, and in bulk containers with a measured scoop. Constipation, bloating, and binding of other medications are commonly encountered, but they can be lessened by adding dietary fiber or stool softener.

Nicotinic Acid (Niacin). This agent has also been shown to lower mortality over a long-term follow-up period through reduction in total and LDL cholesterol. This experience makes niacin a preferred second agent in the drug therapy of elevated cholesterol. It acts by lowering adipose tissue lipoprotein lipase, lowering VLDL production, and lowering plasma VLDL and LDL while raising HDL. It may also inhibit cholesterol synthesis. An additive effect is seen when it is given with one of the resins mentioned previously. Although niacin is inexpensive, side effects such as flushing, tingling, gastric irritation, hyperuricemia, glucose intolerance, and liver toxicity may necessitate discontinuation in many patients. The flushing and tingling can be ameliorated by taking niacin after meals or by taking 650 mg of aspirin 1 to 2 hours before the niacin. Sustained-action preparations generally have fewer side effects. Niacin should not be used in patients with liver dysfunction, diabetes, or peptic ulcer disease. It is administered by starting with low doses (50 mg three times a day) and gradually increasing the dose by 150 mg per day every 1 to 2 weeks until a dose of 1.5 to 2 g per day is reached. Niacin may reduce total cholesterol by 15 to 20 percent and LDL by about 20 percent, and it has the salutary effect of raising HDL 10 to 20 percent.

HMG-CoA Reductase Inhibitors. 3-Hydroxy-3-methylglutaryl coenzyme A reductase (HMG-CoA reductase) is a key enzyme for cholesterol synthesis in the liver. Lovastatin suppresses the activity of this enzyme, thus depriving the liver of cholesterol production. The hepatocyte responds by increasing the number of LDL receptors, which in turn increases the rate of removal of LDL from the plasma. Lovastatin is available in tablet form and can be prescribed in doses ranging from 10 to 80 mg per day, starting at

Table 19-2 Recommended Diet Modifications to Lower Serum Cholesterol: The Step 1 Diet

	Choose	Decrease
Fish, chicken, turkey, and lean meats	Fish, poultry without skin, lean cuts of beef, lamb, pork or veal, shellfish	Fatty cuts of beef, lamb, pork, spare ribs, organ meats, regular cold cuts, sausage, hot dogs, bacon, sardines, roe
Skim and low-fat milk, cheese, yogurt, and dairy substitutes	Skim or 1% fat milk (liquid, powdered, evaporated), buttermilk	Whole (4% fat) milk (regular, evaporated, condensed), cream, half and half, 2% milk, imitation milk products, most nondairy creamers, whipped toppings
	Nonfat (0% fat) or low-fat yogurt	Whole-milk yogurt
	Low-fat cottage cheese (1% or 2% fat)	Whole-milk cottage cheese (4% fat)
	Low-fat cheeses, farmer or pot cheeses (all of these should be labeled no more than 2–6 g fat/oz)	All natural cheeses (e.g., blue, Roquefort, Camembert, cheddar, Swiss)
		Low-fat or "light" cream cheese, low-fat or "light" sour cream
		Cream cheeses, sour cream
	Sherbet, sorbet	Ice cream
Eggs	Egg whites (2 whites = 1 whole egg in recipes), cholesterol-free egg substitutes	Egg yolks
Fruits and vegetables	Fresh, frozen, canned, or dried fruits and vegetables	Vegetables prepared in butter, cream or other sauces
Breads and cereals	Homemade baked goods using unsaturated oils sparingly, angel food cake, low-fat crackers, low-fat cookies	Commercial baked goods: pies, cakes, doughnuts, croissants, pastries, muffins, biscuits, high-fat crackers, high-fat cookies
	Rice, pasta	Egg noodles
	Whole-grain breads and cereals (oatmeal, whole wheat, rye, bran, multigrain, etc.)	Breads in which eggs are a major ingredient
Fats and oils	Baking cocoa	Chocolate
	Unsaturated vegetable oils: corn, olive, rapeseed (canola oil), safflower, sesame, soybean, sunflower	Butter, coconut oil, palm oil, palm kernel oil, lard, bacon fat
	Margarine or shortening made from one of the unsaturated oils listed above	
	Diet margarine	
	Mayonnaise, salad dressings made with unsaturated oils listed above	Dressings made with egg yolk
	Low-fat dressings	
	Seeds and nuts	Coconut

From Goodman DS, et al. The expert panel. Report of the National Cholesterol Education Program Expert Panel on Detection, Evaluation, and Treatment of High Blood Cholesterol in Adults. Arch Intern Med 1988; 142:36; with permission.

20 mg each evening. In those patients receiving 40 mg twice a day, total cholesterol may be lowered by 20 to 30 percent, LDL by 20 to 40 percent, and triglycerides by 20 to 30 percent, whereas HDL may be increased by 10 percent. Lovastatin is extremely well tolerated, but it is relatively expensive and there have been no long-term trials to evaluate its toxicity or efficacy. It is contraindicated in liver disease, in pregnancy, and during lactation. Adverse effects include liver toxicity, myositis, and (rarely) rhabdomyolysis. It should not be given with cyclosporine.

Fibric Acid Derivatives. Gemfibrozil is approved for use in treatment of hypertriglyceridemia. In the Helsinki Heart Study, doses of 60 mg twice a day produced a decrease in total and LDL cholesterol and triglyceride levels and increased HDL levels, while reducing coronary heart disease events by 34 percent. Adverse effects include gastrointestinal distress, rash, muscle pain, blurred vision, anemia, leukopenia, and an increased risk of gallstone formation. Gemfibrozil can inhibit insulin or oral hypoglycemic agents and potentiate oral anticoagulants.

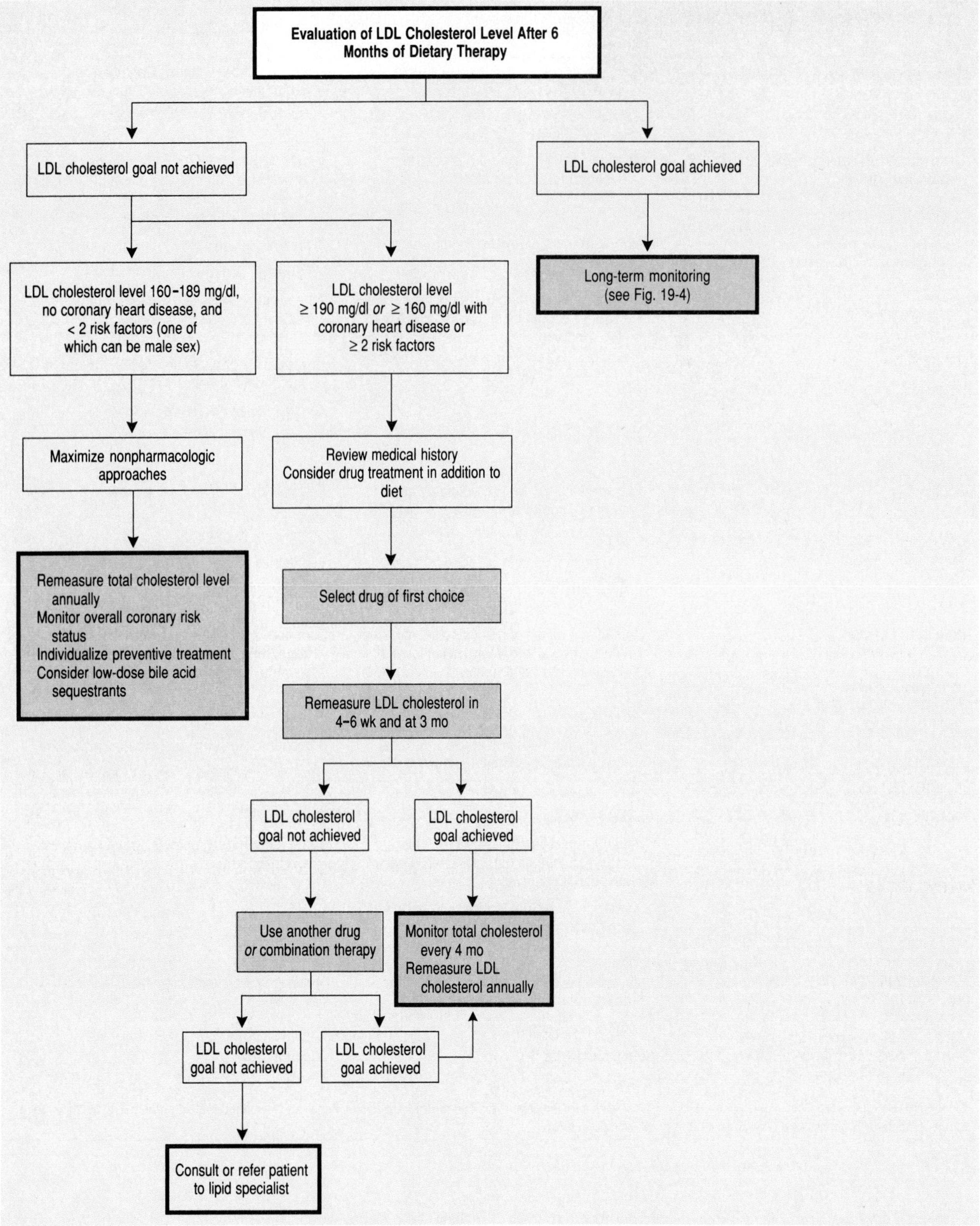

Figure 19-5 Drug therapy of elevated serum cholesterol. (*Modified from* Goodman DS, et al. The expert panel. Report of the National Cholesterol Education Program Expert Panel on Detection, Evaluation, and Treatment of High Blood Cholesterol in Adults. Arch Intern Med 1988; 142:36; with permission.)

Table 19-3 Characteristics of the Primary Hyperlipoproteinemias

Type	Names	Clinical presentation	Risk of coronary heart disease	Plasma cholesterol level	Plasma triglyceride level	Genetic form	Secondary causes	Treatment
I	Exogenous hypertriglyceridemia Familial hyperglyceridemia Familial chylomicronemia Fat-induced hyperlipidemia Hyperchylomicronemia	Pancreatitis Eruptive xanthomas Hepatosplenomegaly Lipemia retinalis	Risk not increased	Normal or slightly increased	Very greatly increased	Autosomal recessive; rare	Systemic lupus erythematosus; dysgammaglobulinemia; insulinopenic diabetes mellitus	Dietary: low intake of fat; no alcohol
II	Familial hypercholesterolemia Familial hyperbetalipoproteinemia Familial hypercholesterolemic xanthomatosis	Accelerated atherosclerosis Xanthelasma Tendon and tuberous xanthomas Juvenile corneal arcus	Very strong risk, especially for coronary atherosclerosis	Greatly increased	a. Normal b. Slightly increased	Autosomal dominant; common	Excess dietary cholesterol; hypothyroidism; nephrosis; multiple myeloma; porphyria; obstructive liver disease	Dietary: low-cholesterol, low-fat diet Drugs: cholestyramine, colestipol, niacin, probucol Possible surgery
III	Broad beta disease Familial dysbetalipoproteinemia Floating betalipoproteinemia	Accelerated atherosclerosis of coronary and peripheral vessels Planar xanthomas Tuboeruptive and tendon xanthomas	Very strong risk for atherosclerosis, especially in peripheral and coronary arteries	Greatly increased	Greatly increased	Mode of inheritance unclear; uncommon but not rare	Dysgammaglobulinemia; hypothyroidism	Dietary: reduction to ideal weight; maintenance of low-cholesterol, balanced diet Drugs: niacin, clofibrate
IV	Endogenous hypertriglyceridemia Familial hyperprebetalipoproteinemia Carbohydrate-induced	Possible accelerated atherosclerosis Glucose intolerance Hyperuricemia	Possible risk, especially for coronary atherosclerosis	Normal or slightly increased	Greatly increased	Common, often sporadic when familial; genetically heterogeneous	Excess alcohol consumption; oral contraceptives; diabetes mellitus; glycogen storage disease; pregnancy; nephrotic syndrome; stress	Dietary: weight reduction; low-carbohydrate diet; no alcohol Drugs: niacin, gemfibrozil
V	Mixed hypertriglyceridemia Combined exogenous and endogenous hypertriglyceridemia Mixed hyperlipidemia	Pancreatitis Eruptive xanthomas Hepatosplenomegaly Sensory neuropathy Lipemia retinalis Hyperuricemia Glucose intolerance	Risk of atherosclerosis not clearly increased	Normal or slightly increased	Very greatly increased	Uncommon but not rare; genetically heterogeneous	Alcoholism; insulin-dependent diabetes mellitus; nephrosis; dysgammaglobulinemia	Dietary: weight reduction; no alcohol Drugs: niacin, gemfibrozil

Modified from Fredrickson DS, Levy RI. Familial hyperlipoproteinemia. In: Stanbury JB, Wyngaarden JB, Fredrickson DS, eds. The metabolic basis of inherited disease. 5th ed. New York: McGraw-Hill, 1982.

References

Blankenhorn DH, et al. Beneficial effects of combined colestipol-niacin therapy on coronary atherosclerosis and coronary venous bypass grafts. JAMA 1987; 257:3233.

Denke MA, Grundy SM. Hypercholesterolemia in elderly persons: Resolving the treatment dilemma. Ann Intern Med 1990; 112:780.

Frick MH, et al. Helsinki Heart Study: Primary prevention trial with gemfibrozil in middle-aged men with dyslipidemia. N Engl J Med 1987; 317:1237.

Goodman DS, et al. The expert panel. Report of the National Cholesterol Education Program Expert Panel on Detection, Evaluation, and Treatment of High Blood Cholesterol in Adults. Arch Intern Med 1988; 142:69.

Gordon DJ, Rifkind BM. High-density lipoprotein: The clinical implications of recent studies. N Engl J Med 1989; 321:1311.

Jacobs DR, Mebane IL, Bangdiwala SI. High density lipoprotein cholesterol as a predictor of cardiovascular disease mortality in men and women: The follow-up study of the Lipid Research Clinics prevalence study. Am J Epidemiol 1990; 131:32.

Abnormalities of Heart Rate and Rhythm

John C. Love, MD

James M. Rippe, MD

20

Palpation of the radial arterial pulse is an essential part of the physical examination. Within 30 to 60 seconds, the physician is able to assess the heart rate and rhythm and make observations that reflect the hemodynamic status of the cardiovascular system. Discussion in this chapter is limited to abnormalities in the heart rate and rhythm.

Definitions

The pulse has two variables: rate and regularity. The normal heart rate is determined by the frequency of depolarization of the sinus node and, by convention, is considered to have a normal range between 60 and 100 beats per minute (bpm). It is well known, however, that some normal individuals have heart rates above and below this "normal range," particularly during extremes of activity, such as exercise and sleep. The pulse is generally regular, but there is a modest phasic variation in the rate with the respiratory cycle, especially in younger healthy people. This physiologic "sinus arrhythmia" is characterized by a gradual decrease in rate during inspiration and an increase during expiration.

Abnormalities of rate are tachycardia (when the heart rate exceeds 100 bpm) and bradycardia (when the heart rate is less

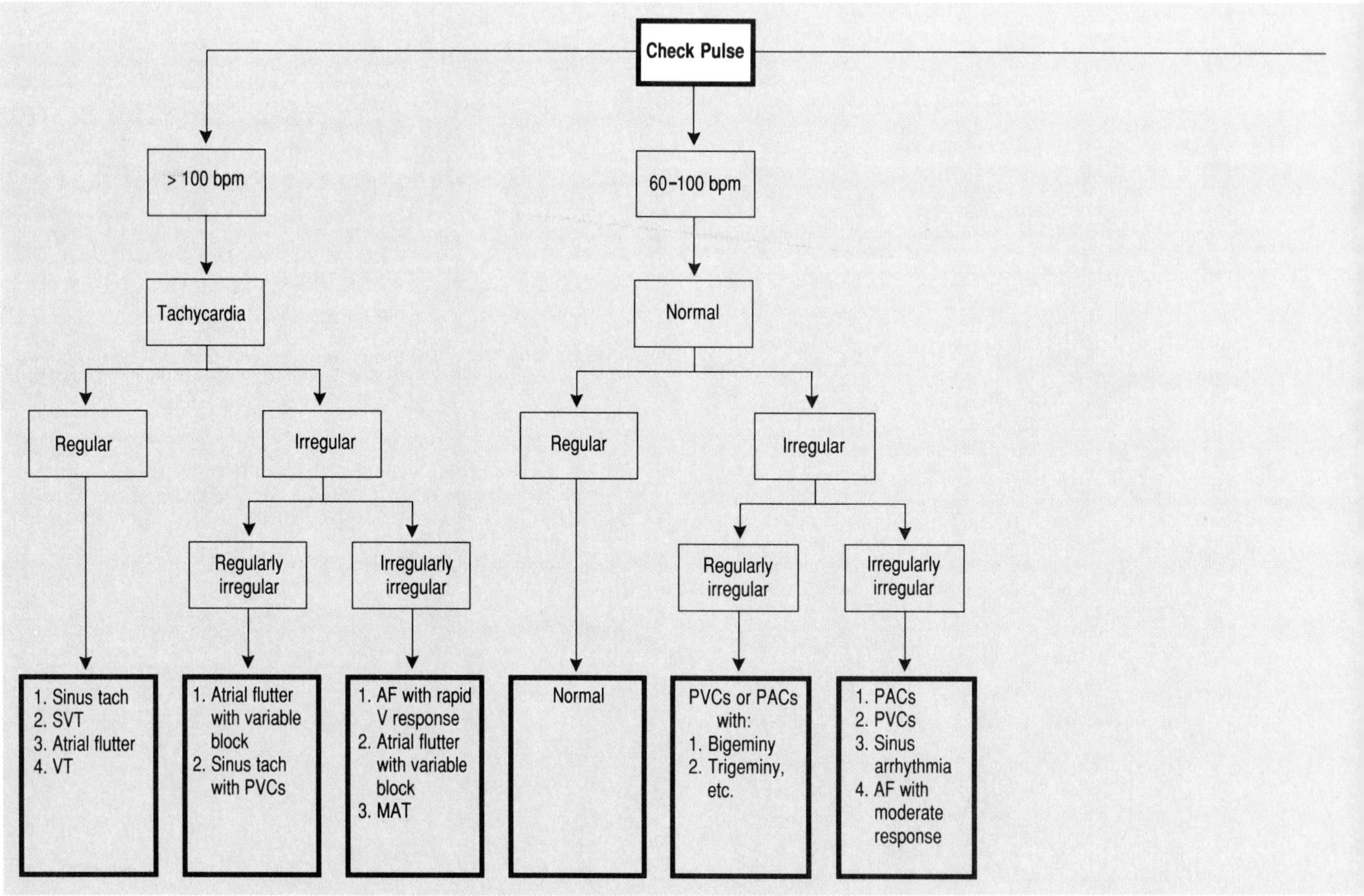

Figure 20-1 Differential diagnosis of an abnormal pulse as derived from rate and regularity. AF = atrial fibrillation, MAT = multifocal atrial tachycardia, PAC = premature atrial contraction, PVC = premature ventricular contraction, Sinus tach = sinus tachycardia, SVT = supraventricular tachycardias, V = ventricular, VT = ventricular tachycardia.

than 60 bpm). At any given rate, the pulse can be regular or irregular, and an irregular pulse can be further characterized as irregularly irregular or regularly irregular. An irregularly irregular pulse is one in which there is a changing and unpredictable variation between beats. A regularly irregular pulse, on the other hand, has a recognizable and predictable pattern.

Etiology

The algorithm in Figure 20-1 develops a differential diagnosis for the etiology of an abnormal pulse on the basis of the two variables: rate and regularity. Although an electrocardiogram (EKG) is needed to make a precise diagnosis, physical examination can provide major clues to the causes of most abnormalities of heart rate or rhythm.

Tachycardia

Regular Tachycardia

Sinus Tachycardia. Sinus tachycardia is the most common form of tachycardia with a regular rhythm. There is no intrinsic abnormality of sinus node function, but the sinus node is responding to any of a variety of extranodal cardioaccelerating influences. For this reason, the identification of sinus tachycardia should lead to a search for an underlying cause. Table 20-1 shows a partial list of etiologies of sinus tachycardia.

Supraventricular and Atrial Tachycardias. In supraventricular and atrial tachycardias (SVT), the atrial rate is no longer controlled by the sinus node, but is instead determined by an abnormal atrial pacemaker or reentry circuit. These may be related to a congenital abnormality in the cardiac conduction system (e.g., Wolff-Parkinson-White syndrome or dual atrioventricular [AV] nodal pathways) and can be associated with underlying cardiac structural defects. SVT may be exacerbated or caused by acute systemic illness, thyrotoxicosis, and drug toxicity (e.g., digitalis, theophylline).

Atrial Flutter. In atrial flutter, the atrium is contracting at a rate of 250 to 350 bpm and appears to be fluttering if observed in situ. It is associated with saw-tooth–like "flutter waves" on the EKG. The ventricular rate is determined by the rate at which these flutter waves can be conducted through the AV node. Usually,

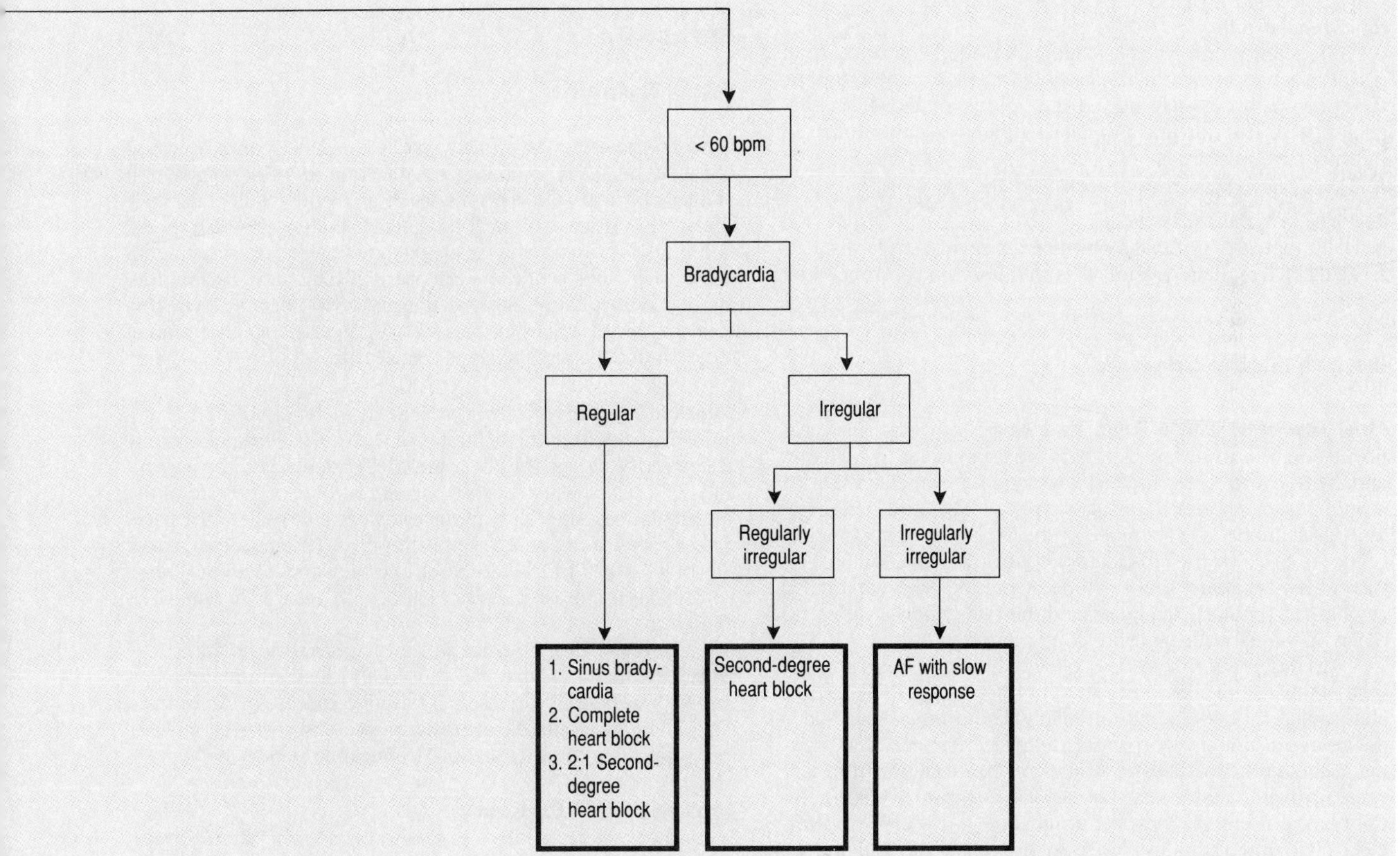

Figure 20-1 *Continued*

Table 20-1 Etiologies of Sinus Tachycardia

Excitement	Hypoglycemia
Stress	Thyrotoxicosis
Anxiety	Hypoxia
Exertion	Pheochromocytoma (catecholamines)
Fever or infection	Pregnancy
Decreased intravascular volume (bleeding, dehydration)	Congestive heart failure
	Drugs (caffeine, sympathomimetics, anticholinergics)

the atrial flutter rate is an even multiple of the ventricular rate (i.e., 1:1, 2:1, 4:1 conduction). If the ratio of atrial rate to ventricular rate is constant, the pulse will be regular. If the ratio changes erratically, the pulse will be irregularly irregular; if the ratio changes by a repetitive pattern, the pulse will be regularly irregular.

Atrial flutter may be caused by intrinsic disease in the atrial muscle or by extracardiac abnormalities similar to those discussed in relation to atrial fibrillation.

Ventricular Tachycardia. Ventricular tachycardia (VT) is an inherently unstable rhythm. It often degenerates into ventricular fibrillation and sudden cardiac death. Occasionally, however, VT is sustained and is detected by symptoms of hypotension and a rapid regular pulse.

VT is almost always associated with underlying myocardial disease such as myocardial infarction, ventricular aneurysm, or cardiomyopathy. It may be a complication of the congenital prolonged Q-T syndrome and can also, paradoxically, be caused by antiarrhythmic drugs.

Regularly Irregular Tachycardia

Atrial flutter with a variable AV block is a form of tachycardia with a regularly irregular rhythm. It is discussed in the preceding section.

Irregularly Irregular Tachycardia

Atrial Fibrillation with a Rapid Ventricular Response. In atrial fibrillation, the atrial muscle fibers are contracting in a chaotic and hemodynamically ineffective sequence, which gives the atrium the appearance of "a bag of worms." The ventricular rate, as in atrial flutter, is determined by the frequency of penetration of the AV node by the "fibrillatory waves." Because the fibrillatory waves bombard the AV node at random, the ventricular rhythm is irregularly irregular, and the rate depends upon the ability of the AV node to conduct frequent impulses.

Atrial fibrillation can be caused by intrinsic electrical disease of the atrium (i.e., "lone atrial fibrillation"), by any cardiac abnormality that involves the atrial muscle or causes dilatation of the atria (e.g., mitral regurgitation, mitral stenosis, cardiomyopathy, ischemic heart disease, congestive heart failure from any cause, or hypertensive heart disease), by pericardial disease, by pulmonary disease, or by systemic illness (e.g., hyperthyroidism, electrolyte abnormalities, fever, or drugs such as caffeine or alcohol).

Atrial Flutter with Variable Atrioventricular Block. This form of irregularly irregular tachycardia is discussed in the preceding section.

Normal Rate, Irregular Rhythm

Irregularly Irregular Rhythm

Extrasystoles. Premature atrial contractions (PACs) and premature ventricular contractions (PVCs) may be palpated as either a premature pulse ("extra beat") or a sudden pause ("skipped beat").

The etiologies of PACs are similar to the causes of atrial fibrillation and atrial flutter. PVCs are related to the etiologies discussed in relation to VT. It should be stressed, however, that both PACs and PVCs often occur in normal individuals and that they do not necessarily imply underlying heart disease or a poor prognosis.

When extrasystoles occur at a regular interval, the rhythm can be regularly irregular. When every second beat is an extrasystole, it is defined as "bigeminy," when every third beat is an extrasystole, "trigeminy," and so on.

Sinus Arrhythmia. As mentioned previously, there is a normal variation in sinus rhythm with the respiratory cycle. However, when the sinus node becomes erratic and has no relationship to other physiologic patterns, it signals intrinsic sinus node disease.

Atrial Fibrillation with Moderate Ventricular Response. This entity is discussed in an earlier section.

Regularly Irregularly Pulse. This entity is described in the section on extrasystoles.

Bradycardia

Regular Bradycardia

Sinus Bradycardia. As in tachycardia, the most common cause of a slow heart rate is an abnormal frequency of depolarization of the sinus node. Sinus bradycardia can be the result of intrinsic sinus node disease as well as the consequence of extranodal influences. Intrinsic sinus node disease may occur in such entities as sick sinus syndrome, myocardial infarction, and infiltrative cardiomyopathy. Athletic training, hypothermia, hypothyroidism, and drugs (e.g., beta-blockers, verapamil) are among the extranodal causes of sinus bradycardia.

Complete Heart Block. In complete heart block, the atrial impulse is blocked at the AV node or in the His-Purkinje system. The ventricular rate thus becomes dependent upon the appearance of a pacemaker "below" the site of block. The rate of the ventricular "escape" rhythm depends upon the site of the pacemaker focus. Junctional tissue is the most common pacemaker site in AV nodal block and has a rate between 40 and 60 bpm. Ventricular tissue, on the other hand, will "escape" at rates of 20 to 40 bpm.

Complete heart block can be congenital or acquired. Acquired heart block may be caused by degenerative changes (Lev's or Lenegre's disease), infiltrative diseases (sarcoidosis, amyloidosis, rheumatoid arthritis, myocardial abscess) or ischemic changes in the AV node or His-Purkinje system.

Regularly Irregular Bradycardia

Second-degree heart block is said to be present when conduction from the atria to the ventricles is only intermittently blocked. The regularity of the pulse is determined by the pattern of nonconducted atrial beats. For instance, if every other atrial beat is blocked, the resultant bradycardia will be regular. On the other hand, when every third impulse is blocked (3:2 block), there will be a regularly irregular pattern to the pulse.

Irregularly Irregular Bradycardia

Atrial fibrillation with slow ventricular response is discussed in a preceding section.

Diagnostic Approach

When palpation of the radial pulse reveals an abnormality of rate or regularity, the history, physical examination, and laboratory tests are directed to answering three questions: (1) What symptoms or physiologic consequences result from the abnormal rhythm? (2) What is the nature of the arrhythmias? and (3) What are the underlying causes of the arrhythmia?

Many patients are totally asymptomatic and may be unaware of their rhythm disturbance. The most common symptom is palpitation. It is important to note the frequency, duration, and mode of onset and termination of palpitations. The relationship of the palpitations to stress, sleep, exertion, and other symptoms is noteworthy. The character of the palpitations may help to identify the rate, regularity, and etiology of the rhythm. Arrhythmias can also be experienced as chest pain, shortness of breath, and, in some cases, loss of consciousness (syncope).

In addition to palpating the pulse, other clues on physical examination will help identify the rhythm. The neck veins may show flutter waves during atrial flutter or cannon "A" waves during the AV dissociation, which results from heart block and VT. The heart sounds may provide a clue to the nature of the arrhythmias. A variable S_1 intensity is common in atrial fibrillation. The heart examination will also identify possible underlying causes of the arrhythmia such as valvular heart disease, hypertrophic obstructive cardiomyopathy (formerly known as idiopathic hypertrophic subaortic stenosis), cardiac enlargement, pericarditis, and congestive heart failure.

Extracardiac etiologies and consequences of arrhythmias can also be identified from the general review of symptoms and physical examination. Signs and symptoms of thyrotoxicosis, anemia, lung disease, and infection, among others, have bearing on the arrhythmia. Evidence of congestive heart failure, systemic embolism, or neurologic symptoms may signify complications of the abnormal rhythm elicited by a history.

After the initial history and physical examination, the diagnosis of a particular arrhythmia can be confirmed by EKG. Occasionally, a prolonged EKG strip or 24-hour continuous EKG recording will be required to capture the abnormality of rate or rhythm that is suspected from the history. The remainder of the laboratory evaluation is guided by the EKG diagnosis. This might include blood electrolytes, a complete blood count, thyroid function tests, and a chest radiograph. In many cases, the workup may be limited to an EKG and a thorough history and physical examination. In severely symptomatic or life-threatening arrhythmias, a more extensive evaluation may be indicated. Echocardiography, radionuclear studies, and even invasive clinical electrophysiologic studies may be required in certain patients.

The choice of therapy depends not only upon adequate identification of the abnormal rhythm, but also upon its hemodynamic consequences. Some patients may require no treatment for their arrhythmia, but the finding of an abnormal pulse may lead to the discovery and treatment of a significant underlying illness.

References

Mandel WJ. Cardiac arrhythmias: Their mechanisms, diagnosis, and management. 2nd ed. Philadelphia: JB Lippincott, 1986.

Marriott HJL, Myerburg RJ. Recognition of cardiac arrhythmias and conduction disturbances. In: Hurst JW, et al, eds. The heart. 7th ed. New York: McGraw-Hill, 1990:489.

Massie E. Palpitations and tachycardia. In: Blacklow RS, et al, eds. MacBryde's signs and symptoms. 6th ed. Philadelphia: JB Lippincott, 1983.

Rippe JM. Arrhythmias. In: Alpert JS, Rippe JM, eds. Manual of cardiovascular diagnosis and therapy. 3rd ed. Boston: Little, Brown, 1988:44.

Zipes DP. Specific arrhythmias: Diagnosis and treatment. In: Braunwald E, ed. Heart disease. 3rd ed. Philadelphia: WB Saunders, 1988:658.

Chest Pain

Linda A. Pape, MD

21

Definitions

Chest pain usually refers to pain in the anterior thorax. *Angina pectoris* (or simply angina) is a common type of midthoracic retrosternal chest discomfort caused by myocardial ischemia. Although angina is commonly defined as chest pain, most patients who have angina actually deny pain and instead describe chest sensations of pressure, tightness, heaviness, or squeezing. These latter terms or the term *chest discomfort*, rather than chest pain, would therefore be considered better synonyms for angina.

Typical angina pectoris is retrosternal; may radiate to the jaw, shoulders, or ulnar aspect of the left arm; is provoked by exertion or emotion; and is relieved within minutes by rest or nitroglycerin. Episodes are usually less than 10 minutes in duration.

Atypical angina is not provoked by exertion or emotion, although the character of the chest symptom and its location suggest angina.

Stable angina occurs and is relieved by rest or nitroglycerin in a predictable pattern that has not changed significantly in a given patient over months or years.

Unstable angina refers to a marked increase in the frequency or severity, or both, of the patient's angina episodes and requires hospitalization. New-onset angina is also considered unstable angina. A gradual change over months is not considered unstable angina.

Pleuritic pain is usually sharp or stabbing in character and is characteristically aggravated by breathing and coughing. It may be caused by inflammation or trauma involving any of the thoracic structures affected by respiratory motion: ribs, cartilage, muscles, nerves, pleurae, sternum, or pericardium.

Table 21-1 lists the various etiologies of chest pain.

Table 21-1 Etiologies of Chest Pain

Cardiovascular	**Pulmonary**
Coronary artery disease (atherosclerotic, vasospastic)	Pleuritis (with or without pneumonia)
Hypertrophic obstructive cardiomyopathy (IHSS)	Pneumothorax
Aortic stenosis, regurgitation	**Neuromuscular**
Pericarditis	Neuritis
Aortic dissection	Skeletal muscle inflammation or spasm
Pulmonary embolism or infarction	Costochondritis
Pulmonary hypertension	**Other**
Gastrointestinal	Herpes zoster
Esophageal spasm	Broken rib
Gastric reflux	Mediastinal tumor
Gastritis	Coxsackievirus infection
Peptic ulcer disease	Hyperventilation syndrome
Pancreatitis	Unexplained
Cholecystitis	

Diagnostic Approach

The Patient with Acute Severe Chest Pain

Any patient who presents with the complaint of chest pain should be rapidly assessed for the presence of a serious condition and for the need for urgent medical treatment. For the patient who is in obvious severe distress, the diagnostic approach may begin with taking the patient's vital signs (measuring blood pressure, heart rate, respiratory rate, and body temperature) at the same time as the history is being elicited. In a patient with acute severe chest pain, acute myocardial infarction or ischemia is usually the first diagnostic consideration. The major differential diagnoses are aortic dissection, acute pericarditis, acute pulmonary embolism, acute pneumothorax, ruptured esophagus, and mediastinal emphysema (Table 21-2).

Certain classic features, when present in the history, physical, electrocardiogram (EKG), and chest radiograph, are very helpful in guiding one toward the correct diagnosis (Table 21-3). The diagnosis of acute myocardial infarction is suggested by a prior history of typical angina or infarction and oppressive retrosternal pressure or pain, accompanied by diaphoresis. The diagnosis of acute pericarditis is entertained when the pain is retrosternal and pleuritic, and there are associated symptoms of a viral illness. When the pain appears suddenly and is of maximum intensity at the onset, the diagnosis of aortic dissection should be considered carefully, particularly in a patient with a history of hypertension. Esophageal rupture is suggested by a tearing pain noted after forceful or protracted vomiting. The patient's age and sex help to establish the likelihood of a certain diagnosis. In the 50-year-old man presenting with severe chest pain, for example, the diagnosis of first exclusion is usually acute myocardial infarction. In an 18-year-old person of either sex, pericarditis or pneumothorax would be more likely.

If the history is classic, the diagnosis will often be secure prior to the physical exam. In cases of severe pain when the history and symptoms are either atypical or nonspecific, physical examination may pick up certain findings that, if present, are strongly suggestive of the proper diagnosis (see Table 21-3). Much of the time, however, the physical findings in the patient with chest pain are nonspecific, and great reliance must be placed on the history and laboratory tests.

The two most useful laboratory tests for evaluating a patient with acute severe chest pain are the EKG and the chest radiograph. The EKG finding, during pain, of ST-segment elevation or depression that disappears after the pain subsides is firm evidence for myocardial ischemia. The absence of ST-segment changes on EKG during an episode of severe pain does not exclude myocardial ischemia. Diffuse ST-segment elevations (involving nearly all EKG leads) may be seen in acute pericarditis. The changes in coronary artery spasm or acute myocardial infarction are usually ST-segment elevations of a more focal nature, i.e., involving only the anterior leads or only the inferior leads. An EKG taken when a patient is free of pain or has only mild symptoms is often normal and does not exclude the presence of severe obstructive coronary artery disease.

The chest radiograph is extremely useful in confirming the presence of pneumothorax or pneumomediastinum. In acute pericarditis or acute myocardial infarction, the chest radiograph is often normal or in the case of acute myocardial infarction may reveal evidence of pulmonary venous congestion. A normal chest radiograph with a normal mediastinum virtually excludes the diagnosis of aortic dissection. A widened mediastinum, on the other hand, is consistent with the diagnosis of aortic dissection but is not specific. The definitive diagnosis can only be made by angiography, computed tomography, echocardiography, or magnetic resonance imaging.

The Patient with Intermittent, Subacute, or Chronic Chest Pain

The evaluation of chest pain in the patient who is not acutely or gravely ill focuses almost entirely upon the history. Taking the history begins with determining some of the basic attributes of the pain (pleuritic or nonpleuritic, deep or superficial). Excluding large groups of diagnoses greatly simplifies the evaluation (Table 21-4).

Most of the neuromuscular or skeletal pains are easily recognized by their superficial quality. They often are somewhat pleuritic in nature. Physical examination should focus on finding localized tenderness over muscles, ribs, or cartilage to confirm the diagnosis. Herpes zoster may present as severe pleuritic pain, and one may need to search carefully to find the characteristic dermatome distribution of vesicles.

Pleuritic pain of a less superficial character may arise from any of the structures affected by respiratory movement: ribs, cartilages, muscles, nerves, pleurae, and pericardium. Involvement of the pleurae is suggested by sharp, shooting, or so-called *lancinating* pain and suggests pleuritis with or without accompanying pneumonia, pleurodynia, or pulmonary infarction. The pain of pericarditis may also be pleuritic, but its central, deep, oppressive quality tends to suggest acute myocardial infarction more than pleurisy. Radiation to the trapezius ridge is believed to be specific for pericardial pain and may help differentiate it from myocardial ischemia.

Deep or visceral retrosternal pain may be due to mediastinal or lung tumor, but most commonly it is of cardiac or gastrointestinal origin. Gastrointestinal pains are usually identified by their relation to eating and their association with upper abdominal pain, a characteristic not usually shared by cardiac pain. Relief with antacids suggests gastritis, esophagitis, or peptic ulcer disease. The pain of esophageal spasm may easily be con-

Table 21-2 Differential Diagnosis of Severe Chest Pain

Acute myocardial infarction	Acute pericarditis
Acute myocardial ischemia	Pneumothorax
Aortic dissection	Ruptured esophagus
Acute pulmonary embolism	Mediastinal emphysema

Table 21-3 Observations and Physical Findings in Patients with Severe Chest Pain

Finding	Suggested diagnosis	Also consider
Pericardial friction rub	Acute pericarditis	Acute myocardial infarction with associated pericarditis, aortic dissection extending into pericardial sac
Absent major arterial pulse, cardiovascular accident	Aortic dissection	Acute myocardial infarction with left ventricular thromboembolism
Marfan's syndrome	Aortic aneurysm rupture	Aortic dissection
Aortic insufficiency murmur	Aortic dissection	Infective endocarditis
Unilateral absent breath sounds, tracheal deviation	Pneumothorax	
Increased central venous pressure with systemic hypotension	Acute massive pulmonary embolism, acute right ventricular infarction	Aortic dissection with cardiac tamponade
Tachypnea with clear lungs	Acute pulmonary embolism	Cardiac tamponade secondary to acute pericarditis

fused with angina because of its location and its prompt relief by nitroglycerin.

The single most helpful clue to the diagnosis of angina pectoris is its precipitation by exertion and relief by rest or nitroglycerin. Typically angina lasts less than 10 minutes. If a classic history is obtained in a middle-aged man, the diagnostic accuracy of the history alone is 90 to 95 percent.

Another important diagnosis is variant angina. This pain is due to coronary artery spasm and is typical of myocardial ischemia, but it occurs at rest. Although usually associated with fixed coronary stenosis, spasm may be found in patients with otherwise normal coronary arteries. Diagnostic clues to the presence of coronary spasm are its frequent occurrence in the early morning hours and its prompt relief with nitroglycerin.

The physical examination in the patient with pleuritic pain would seem to confirm the presence of pleural or pericardial friction rubs. There may be associated findings of splinting, decreased diaphragmatic excursion, pulmonary consolidation, or rales. The examination of the patient with peptic ulcer disease, esophageal spasm, or reflux is likely to be unremarkable, as is the examination of the patient with angina pectoris. In a minority of patients with typical angina, the cause is not coronary artery atherosclerosis but rather valvular aortic stenosis, or hypertrophic obstructive cardiomyopathy (HOCM, formerly known as IHSS). In this latter group of patients, the physical examination may provide the first clue that the symptoms are not due to coronary artery atherosclerosis. Therefore, in all patients with angina, careful search for and evaluation of murmurs are essential.

Table 21-4 Causes of Chest Pain

Character of pain	Etiology	Differential diagnosis
Pleuritic	Pleural, pericardial	Pulmonary embolism or infarction Pneumonitis Pleurodynia Pericarditis
Superficial	Musculoskeletal	Intercostal muscle spasm Slipped rib Costochondritis Herpes zoster
Deep, visceral	Cardiovascular	Angina pectoris Acute myocardial infarction Acute pericarditis Pulmonary hypertension Aortic dissection Aortic aneurysm Massive pulmonary embolism
	Other	Herpes zoster
Gastrointestinal	Esophageal spasm	Gastric reflux Peptic ulcer disease, gastritis Pancreatitis Gallbladder disease
Other		Mediastinal tumor Unknown

The laboratory examinations necessary to evaluate chest pain may range from the simple chest radiograph and EKG to esophageal manometry, gastroscopy, or cardiac catheterization. Whereas in acute severe chest pain an EKG and chest radiograph are nearly always necessary, only one or neither may be needed in the more chronic and subacute types of chest pain. If the pain is obviously superficial, neither chest radiograph nor EKG is usually needed. In pleuritic pain, a chest radiograph may suffice to exclude underlying pneumonitis, infarction, or effusion.

For deep visceral pain, both EKG and chest radiograph are usually required, with numerous exceptions. For example, if a 26-year-old patient has nonexertional deep retrosternal or epigastric pain that is clearly related to eating and is relieved with antacids, and gives a past history of identical symptoms diagnosed and treated successfully as peptic ulcer disease, one could argue that an EKG is unnecessary. If, however, the patient were a 50-year-old hypertensive man with a history of heavy cigarette smoking and therefore at increased risk of coronary artery disease, an EKG would be indicated. Although the history may suggest a gastrointestinal origin of deep retrosternal pain, an EKG should be done in most middle-aged patients as part of the initial assessment.

Further testing for suspected peptic ulcer disease, esophageal spasm, or reflux usually begins with a barium swallow and an upper gastrointestinal series. If ischemic heart disease is suspected, an exercise treadmill test may be of great value. If pulmonary embolism or infarction is suspected, an arterial blood gas determination and a ventilation-perfusion scan should be ordered.

The approach to the diagnosis of chest pain is generally an attempt to find a reasonable explanation for a patient's symptoms and to exclude conditions requiring further testing or treatment. Remaining are the "other" chest pains for which causes may never be found. These include atypical aches that last all day; sharp, seconds-long shooting pains experienced in the inframammary region; and other atypical chest pains occurring in normal healthy individuals. Because nearly any chest pain may raise the concern of heart disease in a patient, it is especially important that the diagnostic approach to atypical chest pain be rapid and direct. The patient may be reassured as soon as possible that he or she does not have heart disease.

References

Braunwald E. Chest discomfort and palpitations. In: Harrison's principles of internal medicine. 11th ed. New York: McGraw-Hill, 1987:17.

DeGowin RL, DeGowin RL. Bedside diagnostic examination. In: The thorax and lungs. 5th ed. New York: Macmillan, 1987.

Edema

Katherine L. Kahn, MD

Harry L. Greene, MD

22

Definition

Edema is an excessive collection of fluid in the interstitial space, which may be generalized, involving the body's entire interstitium, or localized, affecting a particular body part. Edema is not a disease; it is a sign reflecting abnormal fluid shifts within the body. Edema results when increased hydrostatic pressure, decreased oncotic pressure, or disrupted capillary permeability allows fluid to shift from the intravascular to the extravascular space. Any mechanism that causes excess salt and water retention may contribute to formation of edema by increasing the fluid present in the interstitium.

Synonyms for edema include swelling; anasarca (dropsy), which is generalized body edema; ascites, which is edema localized to the peritoneal cavity; and hydrothorax (pleural fluid or effusion), which is edema fluid localized to the pleural space.

Etiology

The diagnostic approach to edema depends upon identifying the cause of the abnormal fluid shift. Increased capillary hydrostatic pressure results in edema formation as the high pressure of the intravascular space causes an excessive movement of fluid from the intravascular space to the low pressure of the interstitium.

Generalized edema commonly results from increased capillary hydrostatic pressure in congestive heart failure, renal failure with excess sodium and water retention, expansion of intravascular volume by large volumes of fluid at a rate faster than kidneys can excrete, sodium-retaining conditions (e.g., menstruation, pregnancy), use of sodium-retaining drugs (e.g., estrogens, corticosteroids), or pericardial disease (less common).

Localized edema is often due to increased capillary hydrostatic pressure in chronic venous insufficiency, in which incompetent venous valves prevent venous return and lead to venous stasis in the lower extremity with subsequent increased venous pressure and deep vein thrombophlebitis (DVT). Less commonly, localized edema results from increased capillary hydrostatic pressure in external compression of venous drainage by a mass effect (e.g., lymph node compressing iliac veins in lymphoma), external compression of lymphatic drainage (e.g., lymph node compressing lymphatic drainage in breast cancer), chronic lymphangitis, because the fluid return from the interstitium to the intravascular space is impaired by disrupted lymphatics, or after lymph node resection.

Decreased oncotic pressure results in edema formation by allowing transudation of fluid from the intravascular space to the interstitium. Normally, fluids remain intravascularly because of the oncotic pressure associated with serum proteins. When serum proteins, particularly albumin, are reduced, there is insufficient oncotic pressure within the intravascular space to hold the fluid there.

Common conditions that result in edema formation from a decrease in oncotic pressure include malnutrition with hypoalbuminemia (i.e., albumin generally less than 2.5 mg/dl), protein loss via the kidney (i.e., proteinuria of more than 3 g per day suggests nephrotic syndrome), liver dysfunction resulting in diminished production of albumin, *severe* catabolism, and protein loss via the gastrointestinal tract (i.e., protein-losing enteropathy [less common]).

Disruption of capillary endothelium results in increased vessel permeability and leakage of protein and fluid from the intravascular space to the extravascular space. *Generalized edema* results from disrupted capillary endothelium in immunologic injury with hypersensitivity and idiopathic edema. *Localized edema* commonly results from disrupted capillary endothelium after local injury to the capillary wall in infection, chemical injury, thermal injury (burns), mechanical injury (trauma), or decreased vascular tone (following central nervous system insult).

Certain miscellaneous conditions result in edema formation by a combination of mechanisms or unknown mechanisms such as *refeeding edema*, which occurs in the severely malnourished person after nutritional supplementation begins, and *idiopathic cyclic edema*, a condition affecting mainly women that is usually characterized by periodic edema, abdominal distention, diurnal weight changes, and a temporal relation to the menstrual cycle. The mechanisms for both refeeding and idiopathic cyclic edema remain unclear, but they may be related to a combination of salt retention and capillary permeability.

Myxedema causes swelling as a result of the abnormal accumulation of hyaluronic acid in the dermis of the hypothyroid patient.

Diagnostic Approach

To approach a patient with edema, study the data provided by the history, physical examination, and laboratory findings for clues about causes of the edema (Fig. 22-1). If the edema is localized, search for reasons for increased hydrostatic pressure,

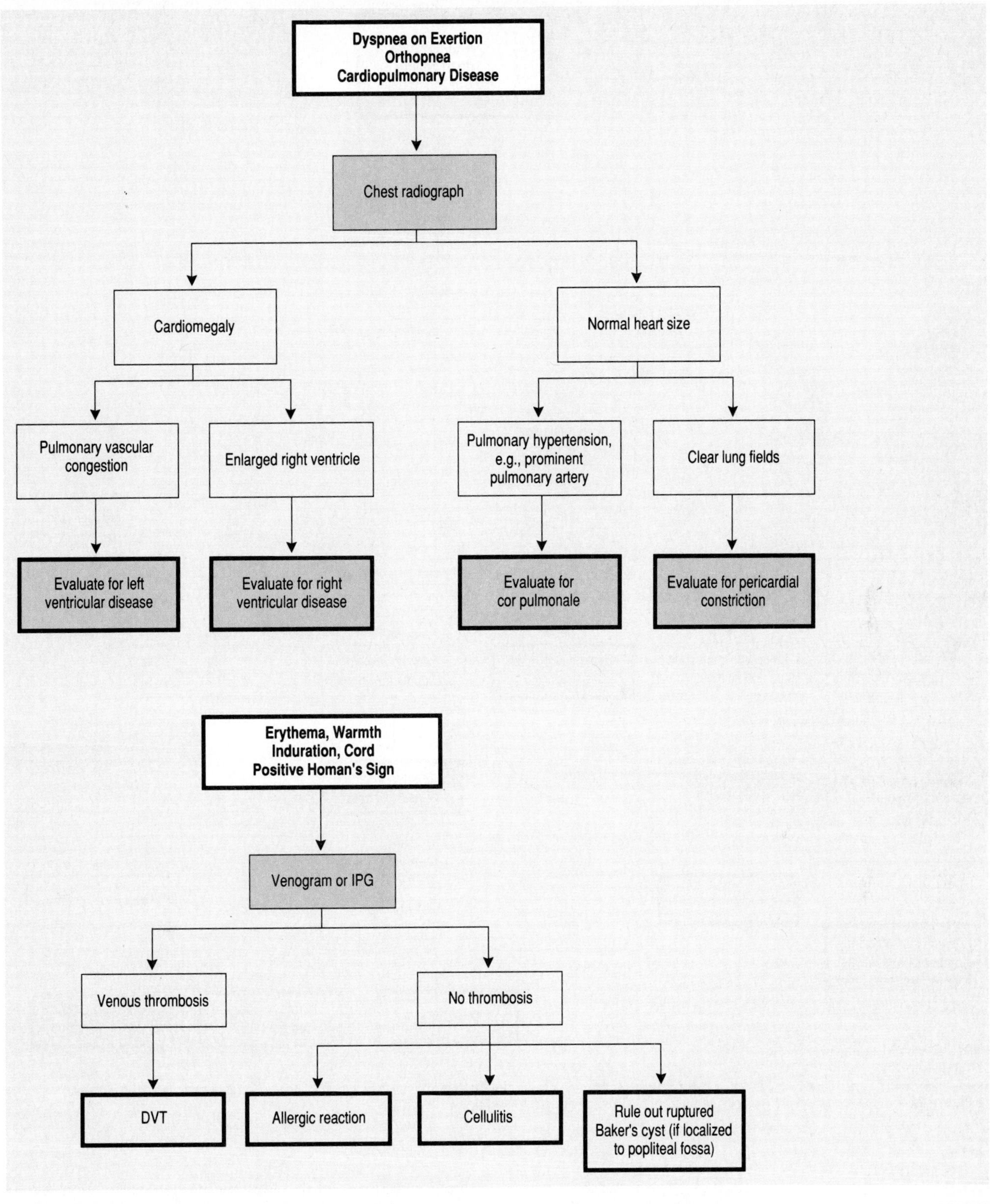

Figure 22-1 Algorithms for diagnostic approaches to the patient with edema. In all cases of edema the physician should consider deep vein thrombophlebitis (DVT), especially with unilateral edema, and should consider sodium retention as a contributing factor. IPG = impedance plethysmography.

Figure continues on following page

decreased oncotic pressure, or abnormal capillary permeability in the edematous region. If the edema is generalized, look for the mechanism of edema formation that would allow fluid shifts throughout the body. Edema formation of bilateral lower extremities is common and generally reflects generalized body edema, which is most obvious in the dependent lower extremities because of gravity. However, lower extremity edema occasionally represents truly localized edema resulting from pelvic disease that is causing obstruction to venous or lymphatic flow.

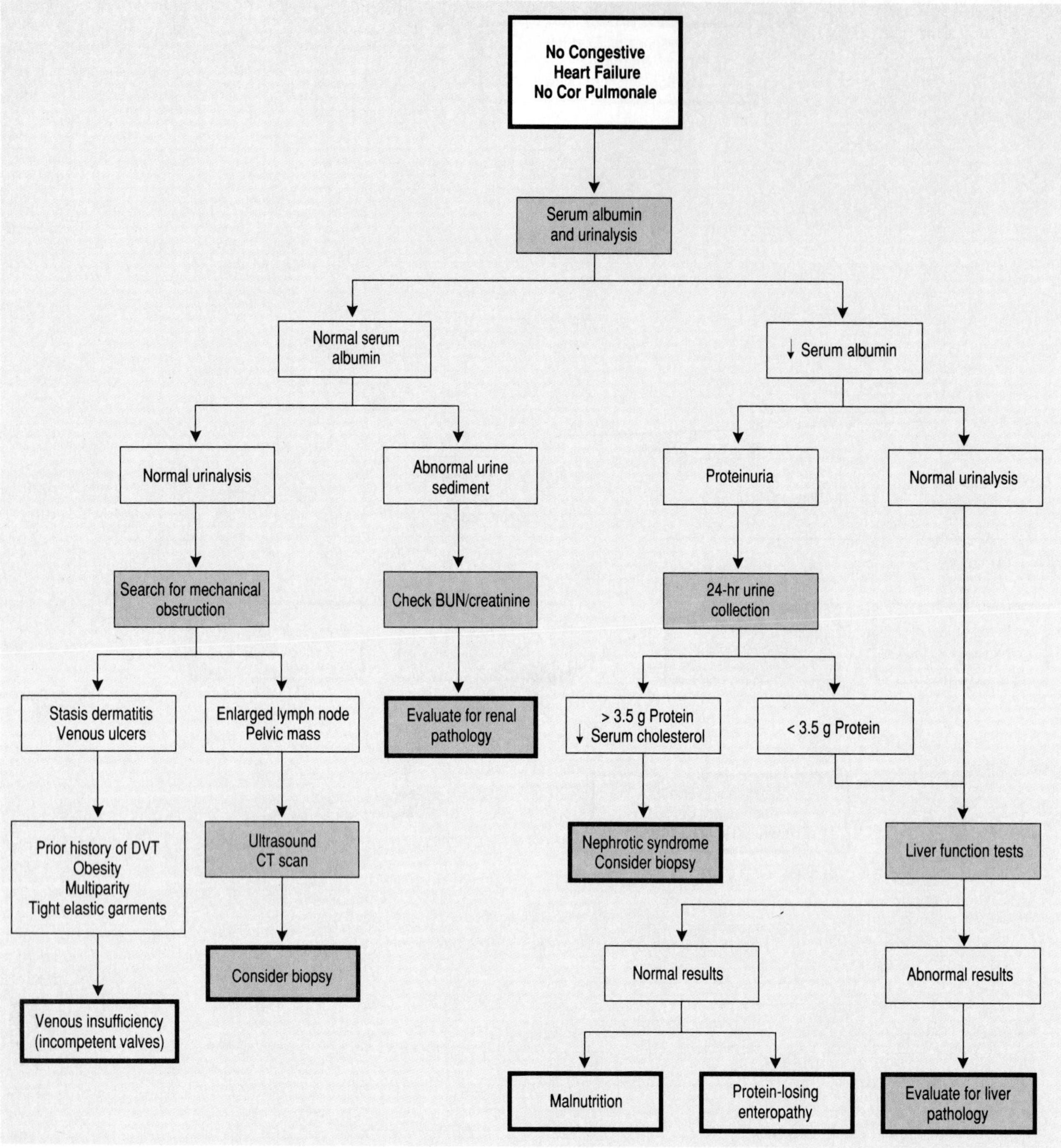

Figure 22-1 *Continued* BUN = blood urea nitrogen, CT = computed tomography

History

Interviewing the patient should characterize the edema and provide clues as to the underlying pathology that might be causing the edema.

Characterizing the Edema

Edema can be characterized by the extent of edema formation, the rapidity of edema onset, and the symptoms associated with the swelling. Edema formation can be quantitated by noting the extent of weight gain. Because the interstitial volume may increase by liters before edema is noted clinically, questioning should investigate subtle clues about edema formation. A tight ring, a new snug-fitting shoe, facial puffiness, or increased abdominal girth may provide an early clue to the presence of edema. Edema formation may be characterized by its tempo. The acute onset of swelling suggests a discrete new cause for the abnormal fluid shifts, whereas chronic edema is generally caused by long-standing pathology. For example, a history of acute onset of leg swelling suggests a possible diagnosis of DVT, whereas chronic edema is more characteristic of venous insufficiency. Cyclic episodes of edema in otherwise healthy women who admit to ingesting salt in their diet suggest idiopathic cyclic edema. Pain suggests that inflammation is accompanying the fluid shift and raises the diagnosis of DVT, trauma, or inflammation from other sources (e.g., infection).

Clues to the Etiology of Edema

When a patient presents with edema, review the complete history in search of information that may explain the presence of increased hydrostatic pressure, decreased oncotic pressure, or capillary fragility. Historical data generally offer sufficient information to clarify the cause of the edema.

A history of cardiac symptoms such as dyspnea, paroxysmal nocturnal dyspnea, and orthopnea suggests congestive heart failure as a cause of the edema. In the edematous patient with a history of smoking, cough, sputum production, or pulmonary disease, cor pulmonale must be considered, since in this setting it causes edema formation by increasing capillary hydrostatic pressure.

Data about dietary intake can offer clues to the cause of the edema. A rough quantification of salt intake is helpful because edema formation may be exacerbated with a large sodium intake. A lack of protein intake suggests protein malnutrition as a cause of edema, but this is unusual without overt cachexia. Information about the patient's alcohol intake offers an opportunity to anticipate liver dysfunction resulting in ascites formation through diminished protein intake, diminished protein synthesis, or portal hypertension. A history of diarrhea suggests protein-losing enteropathy, which is associated with a number of systemic diseases.

A personal or family history of renal disease, a change in urinary frequency, or the development of hematuria points to renal disease with abnormal salt retention as a possible cause for the edema. A recent history of strep throat or other infection also suggests renal disease as a mechanism for edema, because glomerulonephritis associated with strep throat infections may result in edema formation secondary to abnormal salt and water retention.

A history of ingestion of drugs that cause salt retention should be sought. Birth control pills, steroids, and estrogens are commonly used salt-retaining drugs. Certain nonsteroidal anti-inflammatory drugs may also cause edema through salt retention. Pregnancy and the premenstrual period are associated with salt retention because they are high estrogen states.

A history of blood clot, trauma, or infection suggests local venous or lymphatic obstruction or capillary disruption. A history of surgery or trauma to involved lymph nodes suggests a compromised lymphatic drainage, which may be the cause of an edematous limb.

A history consistent with neoplasm must be sought in the patient with edema of unknown cause, because common complications of malignant diseases may have edema as a primary symptom. Malignant tissue obstructing venous or lymphatic drainage is occasionally a presenting sign of cancer. Pericardial disease and superior vena cava syndrome are complications of carcinoma that can lead to complaints of generalized swelling. The chronic malnutrition of the cancer patient also may result in edema. The nephrotic syndrome is a condition that may be associated with cancer, and historical clues should be sought for a possible site of carcinoma in the edematous patient.

Physical Examination

The physician's examination of the patient with edema should focus on characterizing the distribution of the edema and obtaining data about underlying disease that causes the edema.

Characterizing the Edema

The distribution of the edema is assessed by physical examination and may be labeled as generalized or localized. The most severe form of generalized edema, anasarca, involves swelling throughout the body. Search for periorbital edema, presacral edema, edema of the labia or scrotum, pedal edema, and the presence of internal fluid collections, such as pleural effusions or ascites. When edema is generalized, a systemic process is the most likely cause. Edema from congestive heart failure, cor pulmonale, liver disease, kidney disease, and venous insufficiency is generally most prominent in the legs and most noticeable in the evening, if the patient has been upright during the day. Presacral edema is noted in patients with anasarca and in patients who remain recumbent (gravity localizes the interstitial fluid to the most dependent position). Edema resulting from decreased albumin is generalized but often most prominent in the periorbital area.

The presence of localized edema should prompt a search for a cause of localized increased hydrostatic pressure or capillary permeability. Edema of a limb suggests venous or lymphatic obstruction. Asymmetric edema raises the possibility that edema is forming in a limb that is positioned so that it is most affected by gravity. Unilateral edema occasionally occurs as a result of vasomotor instability associated with a nervous system lesion.

Local tenderness and heat suggest inflammation, which is often associated with DVT, allergic reaction, infection, burns, or trauma. Skin thickening, brawny discoloration from hemosiderin deposition, and the presence of ulcers above the ankle implicate chronic venous insufficiency.

Isolated facial edema is rare but occurs with trichinosis after pork ingestion, allergic reactions, myxedema, and superior vena cava syndrome.

Clues to the Etiology of Edema

A thorough physical examination must be performed in the patient with edema. Look for evidence of an underlying disease or condition that would result in edema formation.

Dyspnea, pulmonary rales, and an S_3 gallop with cardiomegaly suggest congestive heart failure. Abnormal lung sounds with an accentuated pulmonary component of the second heart sound suggest cor pulmonale. Both of these conditions increase capillary hydrostatic pressure with resultant edema formation in the lower extremity, with or without ascites. The presence of Kussmaul's sign (distention of neck veins with inspiration [less common]) and pulsus paradoxus (greater than 10 mm decrease in systolic blood pressure with inspiration) raises the possibility that pericardial disease may be restricting venous blood return to the heart. Estimation of an elevated systemic venous pressure by neck vein assessment supports the diagnosis of congestive heart failure, intravascular volume overload, or pericardial disease. The presence of collapsed neck veins suggests that the edema is not associated with an elevated systemic venous pressure. Collapsed neck veins in the presence of generalized edema of the lower extremities suggest liver disease or venous/lymphatic obstruction of the lower extremities. A pelvic or prostate examination is indicated to rule out a mass lesion producing obstruction of the venous or lymphatic channels. Cachexia suggests hypoalbuminemia, malnutrition, or neoplasm.

References

Braunwald E. Edema. In: Braunwald E, et al, eds. Harrison's principles of internal medicine. 11th ed. New York: McGraw-Hill, 1988:149.

MacGregor G, deWardener HE. Idiopathic edema. In: Schrier R, et al, eds. Diseases of the kidney. Boston: Little, Brown, 1988:2743.

Rose BD. Pathophysiology of renal disease. New York: McGraw-Hill, 1987.

Seiften JL, et al. Control of extracellular fluid volume and pathophysiology of edema formation. In: Brenner BM, Rector FC Jr, eds. The kidney. 3rd ed. Philadelphia: WB Saunders, 1986:360.

Hypertension

Harvey J. Kowaloff, MD

23

Definition

Arterial blood pressure normally varies with age. For most adults, aged 17 to 40, blood pressure in excess of 140 mm Hg systolic or 90 mm Hg diastolic is considered elevated. At ages 41 to 60, the pressure should be less than 150/90. Over age 60, pressure should be below 160/90.

It is common for individuals to experience a transient and moderate elevation of blood pressure when under stress, such as when visiting a physician or a hospital emergency room, or when in pain and hospitalized for acute illness. Elevated blood pressure found in this setting may be spurious; therefore, when patients are found to have mildly elevated blood pressure, in the range of 140 to 150 mm Hg systolic or 90 to 95 mm Hg diastolic, it is customary to document elevated blood pressure on three separate occasions before making a diagnosis of hypertension.

Although both systolic and diastolic pressures are elevated concomitantly in most patients with hypertension, there are many individuals in whom only the systolic pressure is found to be elevated. This is particularly true of the elderly. It is important to identify these people as hypertensive, so that appropriate diagnostic and therapeutic efforts can be undertaken.

Likewise, there are many young individuals whose blood pressure is found to be elevated at one time and within normal limits on another occasion. These individuals are said to have labile hypertension. Many of them will develop fixed hypertension in the future and therefore merit regular follow-up care, with appropriate diagnostic and therapeutic intervention if and when the blood pressure is found to remain elevated.

Etiology

The etiology remains unknown in approximately 95 percent of patients with arterial hypertension who are seen in a community setting. These individuals are considered to have essential (or idiopathic) hypertension. Clinically, they are viewed as a homogeneous group, although it is highly likely that several different pathophysiologic mechanisms operate in these patients, with a common result being the maintenance of chronically elevated blood pressure. Precisely which mechanisms are operational and why remains unknown, although one attractive possible mechanism is the kidneys' difficulty in handling sodium. In approximately 5 percent of hypertensive patients, on the other hand, the hypertension can be shown to be the result of a specific lesion, either metabolic or structural. These patients are said to have secondary hypertension. The hypertension in these cases is a secondary phenomenon related directly to physiologic alteration induced by the primary lesion. In these patients, the etiology of hypertension can be readily demonstrated using currently available biomedical technology. The causes of secondary hypertension are listed in Table 23-1.

Table 23-1 Secondary Causes of Hypertension

Endocrine	**Drug-Induced**
Hyperaldosteronism	Oral contraceptives
Cushing's syndrome	Steroids
Pheochromocytoma	Amphetamines
Adrenogenital syndrome	**Coarctation**
Licorice ingestion (only in imported licorice)	
Renal	
Renal parenchymal disease	
Renal artery stenosis	
Renal obstruction (acute)	

Diagnostic Approach

Although patients may complain of symptoms caused by their hypertension, chronic hypertension per se is asymptomatic. Headache, epistaxis, and dizziness are not symptoms of mild or moderate hypertension. Generally, individuals are discovered to be hypertensive during a routine physical examination, while being treated for an unrelated problem, through a blood-pressure screening program, or unfortunately, when they come to medical attention because of symptoms related to a complication of long-standing hypertension. They may have eyeground changes related to elevated blood pressure (Fig. 23-1). Hypertension is a major factor in the pathogenesis of coronary artery disease leading to myocardial infarction, angina pectoris, and congestive heart failure; cerebrovascular disease causing stroke and transient ischemic attack; and chronic renal failure. These are referred to as end-organ effects of hypertension. More rarely, patients who have secondary hypertension seek medical care because of symptoms related to the lesion underlying the hypertension. (These are discussed in a subsequent section.)

The history and physical examination provide invaluable information in planning a diagnostic and therapeutic approach to the hypertensive patient. When taking a history from a hypertensive patient, keep the following goals in mind: (1) specific questions should be asked to help rule in or out the various secondary causes of hypertension; (2) information should be obtained to help assess the degree of end-organ damage incurred by the hypertension; and (3) because hypertension is a major risk factor in the pathogenesis of arteriosclerotic vascular disease, the presence and severity of coexisting risk factors should be determined during the interview.

Figure 23-2 shows an algorithmic approach to the diagnosis of hypertension.

Historical Features Associated with Secondary Hypertension

Because the majority of hypertensive patients have essential hypertension, the history is useful in gathering data that may help to identify that minority of patients with secondary hypertension. The age and circumstances of onset of hypertension should be determined. Hypertension starting in the very young or elderly is not typical of essential hypertension. Additionally, the sudden onset of hypertension is not a common feature of

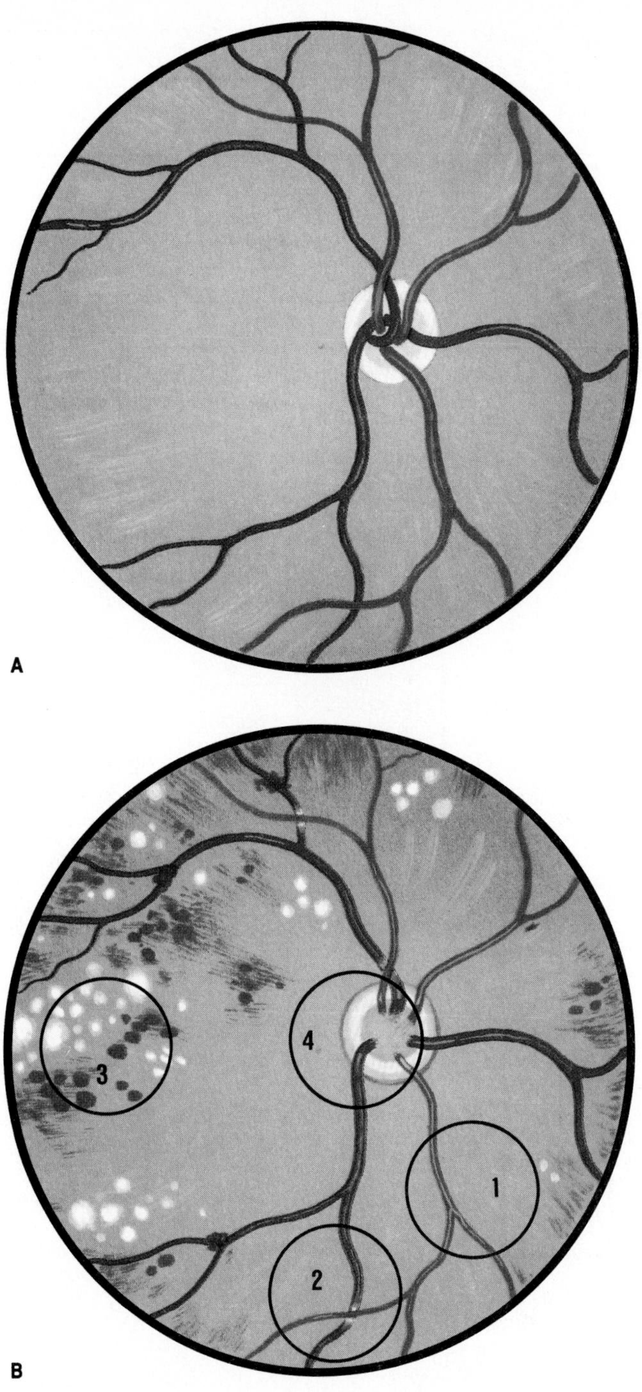

Figure 23-1 Eye-ground changes related to elevated blood pressure. (**A**) The normal retina. (**B**) Four stages of hypertensive retinopathy. See text for description of stages.

essential hypertension. The presence of a family history of hypertension is an important factor that supports the likelihood that a patient has essential hypertension.

Endocrine causes of secondary hypertension may be suggested by the presence of the following features. Hyperaldosteronism is often associated with muscle cramps, weakness, and polyuria due to the hypokalemia that accompanies hypertension in this syndrome. Patients with pheochromocytoma experience paroxysmal secretion of very high levels of catecholamines. Patients with pheochromocytoma may display wide swings in blood pressure when measured on several different occasions, often associated with palpitations, sweating, weight loss, or headaches. Cushing's syndrome, although more often suggested by characteristic physical findings, may be suspected in hypertensive patients who have had recent onset of diabetes, menstrual irregularities, proximal muscle weakness, easy bruising, or personality changes. These are all effects attributable to the elevated cortisol levels diagnostic of this syndrome.

The possibility that *renal disease* is responsible for hypertension is suggested by a history of prior abnormal urine sediment analysis, hematuria, or edema.

Renal artery stenosis, although not associated with any characteristic historical features, may be suggested by the following: (1) the development of hypertension in a young woman, which may indicate fibromuscular hyperplasia of the renal artery; (2) the sudden onset or the recent worsening of hypertension; and (3) in patients already taking medication for hypertension, the inability to control blood pressure on a standard multidrug regimen.

Finally, a history of medication and diet should be included. Specifically, women should be asked about use of oral contraceptives and estrogen preparations, because these agents are known to cause hypertension in some patients. Chronic use of amphetamine-type drugs and of over-the-counter nasal decongestants containing sympathomimetic agents can also cause hypertension. The dietary history should focus on sodium intake, alcohol, and obesity. These factors seem to aggravate hypertension in almost all cases.

Signs Associated with Secondary Hypertension

In observing the general appearance of the patient, note stigmata that suggest Cushing's syndrome, including truncal obesity, dorsal fat pad ("buffalo hump"), moon facies, plethora, acne, hirsutism, and violaceous abdominal striae. Measure the blood pressure in both arms while the patient is sitting and supine. Unequal pressures in the arms may suggest the presence of a coarctation of the proximal aorta. Palpate the pulse at both the radial and femoral locations. In patients with coarctation, there is a murmur during systole that may be heard best in the posterior midline between the scapulae; this murmur may extend into diastole if the obstruction is severe. In addition, there is a delay in the appearance of the femoral pulse relative to the radial, referred to as *radial-femoral lag.* Finally, auscultate the back at the level of L2 for a renal artery bruit, which may be heard in patients with renal artery stenosis.

Assessment of End-Organ Damage

The examination of the head and neck includes a thorough assessment of the retinal vessels. The retina is the only site in the body where the appearance of small vessels can be visualized, and damage seen here may reflect parallel changes in the renal and cerebral vessels. There are four grades of hypertensive retinopathy (see Fig. 23-1B): 1—arteriolar narrowing; 2—arteriovenous nicking; 3—hemorrhages, exudates; and 4—papilledema.

The cardiac examination is important because long-standing hypertension can cause left ventricular hypertrophy and congestive heart failure. Observe and palpate the apical impulse. In left ventricular hypertrophy, the impulse is forceful and sustained in quality. It may be displaced lateral to the midclavicular line, if there is left ventricular dilatation. On auscultation, pay attention to the presence or absence of an S_4, which may appear as a result of left ventricular hypertrophy with decreasing compliance of the hypertrophied myocardium. Likewise, the S_3 should be sought, because this may be the first sign of impending congestive heart failure.

When examining the lungs, note basilar rales, which may be heard in the presence of congestive heart failure.

The abdominal examination is not often helpful in the

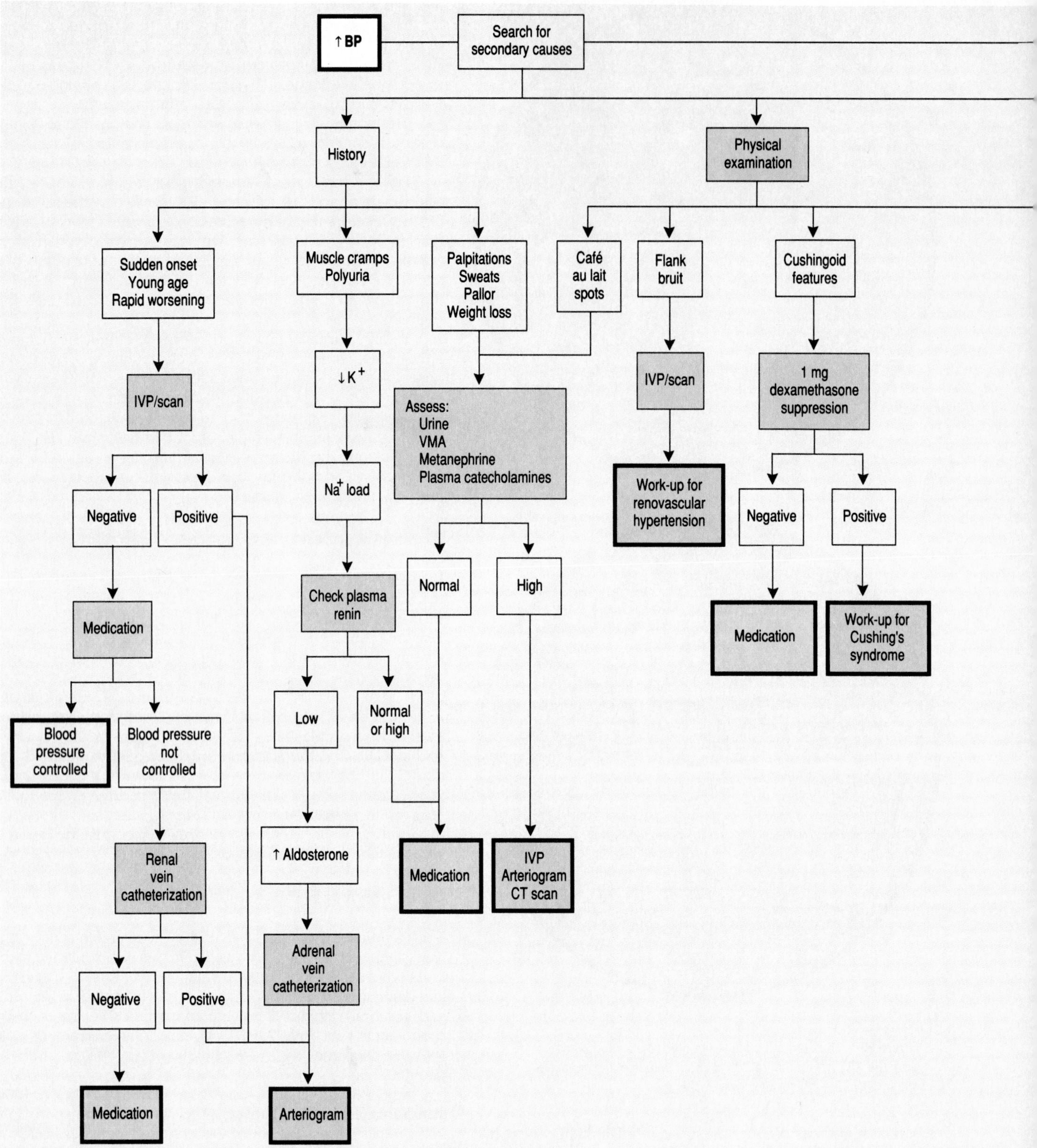

Figure 23-2 Algorithm for the evaluation of hypertension. CT = computed tomography, CXR = chest radiograph, IVP = intravenous pyelogram, VMA = vanillylmandelic acid.

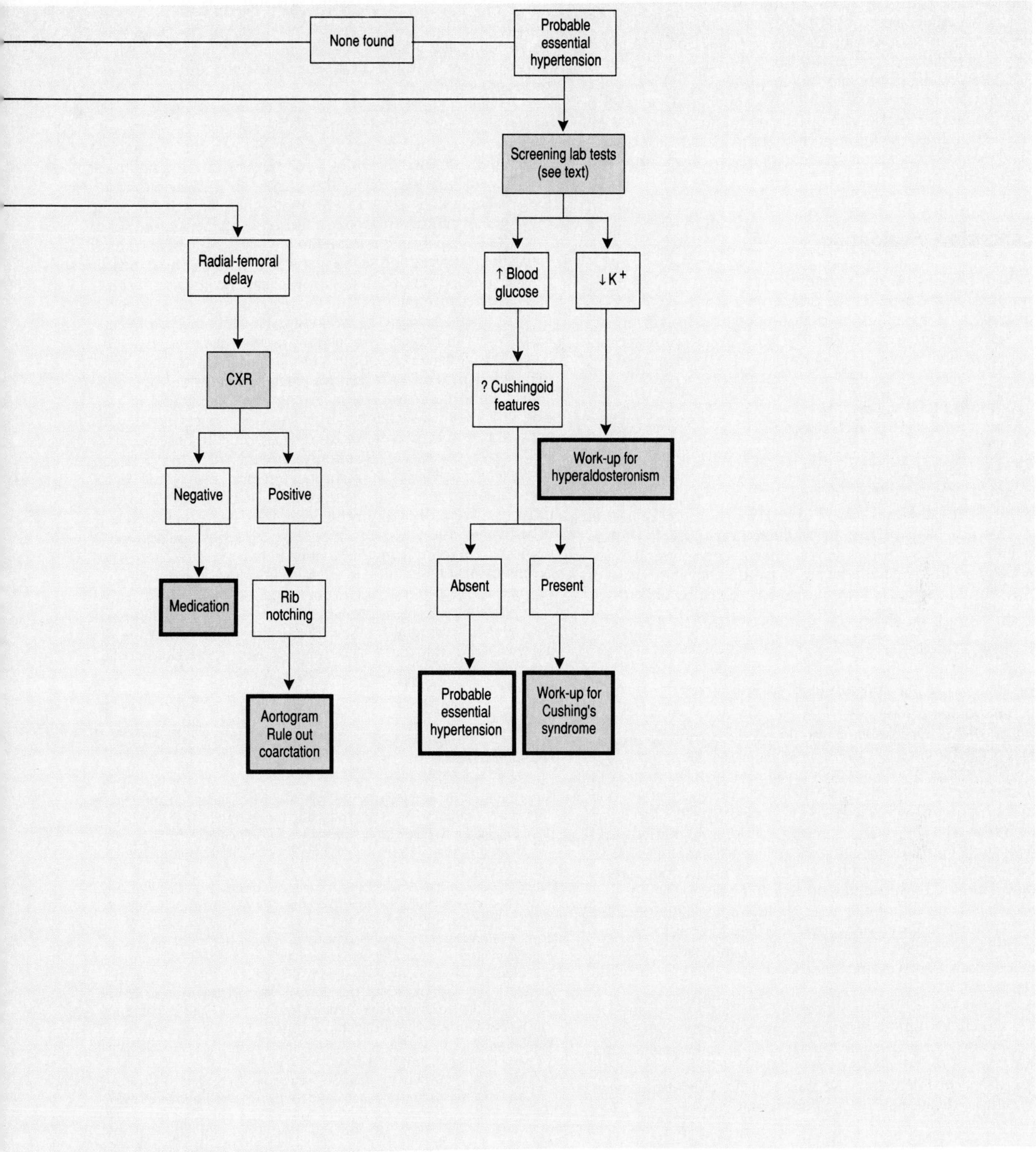

Figure 23-2 *Continued*

hypertensive patient. Palpate the epigastrium for aortic pulsation. Widening of this pulsation beyond 3 cm may indicate the presence of an abdominal aortic aneurysm. Abdominal masses may suggest polycystic renal disease.

Examine the extremities for the presence of edema, which is seen with congestive heart failure. Ascertain the adequacy of the peripheral circulation by palpating the femoral, popliteal, and pedal pulses. Finally, inspect the skin for xanthelasma about the eyes and xanthoma on the tendons, which suggest hypercholesterolemia.

Laboratory Evaluation

As with the history and physical examination, the laboratory evaluation of the hypertensive patient aims to screen for secondary causes of hypertension, evaluate end-organ function, and ascertain coexisting risk factors. The following lab studies constitute a sufficient database for all patients with hypertension:

1. Blood urea nitrogen
2. Fasting blood sugar
3. Serum cholesterol and potassium
4. Urinalysis
5. Electrocardiogram
6. Chest radiograph (optional)

These studies allow assessment of renal function, determination of left ventricular hypertrophy, and detection of occult diabetes mellitus or hypercholesterolemia. When history, physical examination, or clinical circumstances suggest a secondary cause of hypertension, additional specific studies should be obtained as indicated.

Evaluation for Secondary Hypertension

When hypertension and hypokalemia are found to coexist, evaluation should be undertaken to exclude primary hyperaldosteronism. (*Note:* Hypokalemia should be documented with the patient off diuretics.)

The work-up of these patients includes the measurement of plasma renin activity (PRA) with the patient on a normal diet and off antihypertensive medications for 3 weeks. The PRA should be measured with the patient supine for at least 30 minutes, and then after stimulation by either 40 to 80 mg of oral furosemide, followed by 4 hours upright, or 40 mg of intravenous furosemide, followed by 30 minutes upright. In addition, plasma aldosterone is measured simultaneously. The finding of low PRA and high plasma aldosterone suggests hyperaldosteronism as a cause for the hypertension. Diagnosis is confirmed by adrenal catheterization and computed tomography (CT) scanning of the abdomen.

Patients with features suggesting Cushing's syndrome are best screened with the overnight dexamethasone suppression test. Plasma cortisol is measured at 8 AM following a 1-mg oral dose of dexamethasone at midnight. Values greater than 5 μg/dl are considered positive and should be followed by more definitive evaluation of adrenal function.

Pheochromocytoma is screened by measuring urinary vanillylmandelic acid (VMA) and/or metanephrines on a 24-hour collection. If available, plasma catecholamines can be measured directly and may represent a better screening test for this disorder.

Finally, if renal artery stenosis is suspected, a rapid-sequence (timed) intravenous pyelogram may be obtained. This test is positive in approximately 80 percent of cases of renal artery stenosis. A positive test consists of three findings: (1) delayed opacification of the kidney on the stenotic side, (2) smaller kidney by 1 to 1.5 cm on the affected side, and (3) hyperconcentration of contrast material on the affected side.

The sensitivity of this test is limited in cases of both bilateral renal artery disease and segmental artery stenosis. The standard nuclear isotope renogram has been plagued with false-positive and false-negative rates that are too high (as high as 48 percent) to recommend its use as a screening test for renovascular hypertension. Sophisticated computer programs, however, may enhance the characteristics of this test as a tool for noninvasively identifying patients with renovascular hypertension. There is considerable controversy concerning the role of PRA in the diagnosis of renovascular hypertension because it is elevated in approximately 15 percent of cases of essential hypertension as well as in renovascular hypertension. When suspicion of renovascular hypertension is high, renal arteriography with a renal vein catheterization and measurement of renin levels in the renal vein are indicated for the definitive diagnosis of renovascular hypertension. This test is positive for renovascular hypertension if (1) renin from the stenotic kidney is 1.5 to 2 times or greater the level measured in the normal kidney, and (2) there is suppression of renin on the normal side.

Coarctation of the aorta, when suspected, can be diagnosed on the chest radiograph when there is prominent notching of the ribs. This is due to the presence of hypertrophied intercostal artery collaterals beyond the stenotic area.

References

Ferguson RK. Cost and yield of the hypertensive evaluation: Experience of a community-based referral clinic. Ann Intern Med 1975; 82:761.

Haber E, Slater E. High blood pressure. In: Rubenstein E, et al, eds. Scientific American medicine. New York: Scientific American, 1986: 1-VI and 1-33.

Hall WD, Wollam GL, Tuttle EP Jr. Diagnostic evaluation of the patient with hypertension. In: Hurst JW, et al, eds. The heart. 7th ed. New York: McGraw-Hill, 1990:1150.

Hypertension Detection and Follow-up Program—Cooperative Group. Reduction in mortality of persons with high blood pressure, including mild hypertension. JAMA 1979; 242.

Laragh JH. Symposium on hypertension. Vasoconstriction-volume analysis for understanding and treating hypertension: The use of renin and aldosterone profiles. Am J Med 1973; 55:261.

Weinberger MH, et al. Primary aldosteronism in diagnosis, localization and treatment. Ann Intern Med 1979; 90:386.

Working Group on Renovascular Hypertension. Detection, evaluation, and treatment of renovascular hypertension. Arch Intern Med 1987; 147:820.

Hypotension

Joseph R. Benotti, MD

24

Definition

Hypotension is a reduction in the arterial blood pressure. It assumes clinical importance when there is associated evidence of organ hypoperfusion or compensatory cardiovascular reflexes (diaphoresis, pallor, tachycardia). In the absence of clinical manifestations, hypotension is present when the systolic arterial blood pressure is consistently below 90 mm Hg in an otherwise asymptomatic patient.

Hypotension, rather than a specific disease entity, is a physical finding. It results from a variety of pathophysiologic processes. As with all symptoms and signs in medicine, hypotension demands determination of its cause as a prerequisite to successful management.

Shock is a clinical syndrome characterized by inadequate tissue perfusion, which is the inevitable consequence of declining blood pressure in conjunction with activation of compensatory cardiocirculatory reflexes. Although hypotension and shock are interrelated, a low blood pressure may be present in the absence of tissue hypoperfusion (shock); conversely, shock can be present despite reasonable preservation of the arterial pressure.

Pathophysiology

The arterial blood pressure is determined by the cardiac output (CO) and systemic vascular resistance (SVR). Mean arterial pressure (MAP) is the product of these two variables:

$$MAP = CO \times SVR$$

Systemic vascular resistance is predominantly influenced by arteriolar smooth muscle tone under adrenergic control, and cardiac output is determined by the product of stroke volume (SV) and heart rate (HR):

$$CO = HR \times SV$$

Arterial pressure is determined by stroke volume, heart rate, and systemic vascular resistance according to the following equation:

$$MAP = SV \times HR \times SVR$$

Reduced Cardiac Filling. Any impairment of stroke volume because of reduced venous return and cardiac filling elicits hypotension. Volume depletion resulting from hemorrhage or loss of plasma volume into the interstitium (e.g., thermal injury, anaphylaxis, or pancreatitis) commonly results in hypotension. Failure of autonomic tone may cause hypotension, in part related to inadequate vascular tone and venous return.

Obstruction to Central Blood Flow. Diseases that impede the flow of blood into and out of the heart and great vessels compromise stroke volume, eventuating in hypotension. Examples include cardiac tamponade, pulmonary embolism, left atrial myxoma, mitral stenosis, aortic stenosis, hypertrophic obstructive cardiomyopathy (HOCM, formerly known as IHSS), and aortic dissection.

Cardiac Dysfunction. Arrhythmias that result in excessively fast or slow heart rates or inappropriate timing of atrial systole reduce cardiac output and result in hypotension. Ventricular dysfunction from myocardial infarction may compromise stroke volume to the point of hypotension. Acute destruction of a cardiac valve due to infective endocarditis or trauma may result in aortic insufficiency, mitral regurgitation, or tricuspid regurgitation. The ensuing precipitous fall in stroke volume and cardiac output may result in hypotension.

Clinical Evaluation

The hypotensive patient may present with symptoms due to organ hypoperfusion or the underlying disease. Hypotension of sufficient magnitude causes symptoms resulting from cerebral hypoperfusion. These include dizziness and light-headedness progressing to obtundation and coma. Cerebral ischemia is often precipitated by the decline in venous return and cardiac output accompanying upright posture (orthostatic hypotension). The patient with hypotension consequent to intravascular volume depletion or arrhythmia is most symptomatic when upright (walking or standing). Symptoms are characteristically improved by recumbency, with the legs at or above the level of the heart.

The presence or absence of symptoms and signs consequent to the underlying disease process should always be determined in the hypotensive patient. A history of open or closed trauma points to possible blood loss resulting from hemorrhage (external or internal) as a cause of hypotension. Extensive burns implicate loss of colloid. History of exposure to a known or potential foreign substance capable of behaving as an antigen or hapten raises the likelihood of anaphylaxis (e.g., ingestion of a new medication, venomous insect bite). Therapy with diuretics or other antihypertensive drugs suggests volume depletion (diuretic induced) and excessive arterial or venular dilation (vasodilator induced). Less likely, a central defect in the sympathetic nervous system may be the cause.

Chest pain of an ischemic nature suggests myocardial dysfunction or infarction, aortic stenosis, HOCM, or pulmonary embolism as a possible explanation for hypotension. Sharper chest pain of a more positional nature (alleviated by sitting up and leaning forward and aggravated by lying flat) associated with shoulder pain points to pericarditis with effusion and tamponade as a possible explanation. Sharp upper abdominal discomfort of similar quality and radiation is characteristic of pancreatitis. Excruciating, searing chest pain or lower back pain in association with hypotension should alert the clinician to the possibility of thoracic aortic dissection or abdominal aortic aneurysm with retroperitoneal leakage and impending rupture into the peritoneal activity.

Dyspnea in conjunction with hypotension implicates pulmonary embolism or, less likely, severely impaired left ventricular function. The latter may be a result of cardiomyopathy, myocardial infarction, or acute bacterial endocarditis with valvular insufficiency. History of a febrile illness, infection elsewhere, intravenous drug abuse, or previous dental manipulation points to possible infective endocarditis.

Palpitation (awareness of an excessively fast, slow, irregular, or forceful heart beat) may suggest tachyarrhythmia (supraventricular or ventricular), bradyarrhythmia, or heart block as a cause of hypotension.

The passage of excessively black, foul-smelling stools with the appearance and consistency of tar (melena), frequent maroon stools, or a history of hematemesis, previous ulcer disease, or alcoholism suggests gastrointestinal bleeding.

Hypotension due to excessive urinary salt and water loss, as occurs with diabetes insipidus or poorly controlled diabetes mellitus, is heralded by polydipsia and polyuria. Generalized fatigue, weight loss, salt craving, postural hypotension, and skin hyperpigmentation point to adrenal cortical insufficiency.

Drug-induced hypotension must be suspected in any patient being treated with diuretics or other antihypertensive drugs. Patients treated with phenothiazine tranquilizers may experience postural hypotension as a side effect or as a result of purposeful overdose. Hypotension in conjunction with coma in a known drug abuser raises the possibility of heroin, barbiturate, glutethimide, or other sedative-hypnotic or tranquilizer drug overdose, almost always associated with excessive alcohol ingestion. Hypotension and coma occurring in a patient known to be previously depressed, or after an emotionally traumatic experience (e.g., argument with a loved one, sudden loss of a loved one), likewise implicate drug overdose as a suicidal gesture or true intent.

Low blood pressure may be seen as a manifestation of high spinal cord trauma. With damage to the cord in the neck or upper thorax, outflow of sympathetic nerve impulses along the thoracolumbar chain is impaired. The loss of sympathetically mediated arteriolar and venular tone results in inadequacy of peripheral vascular resistance, venous return, and cardiac output. Arterial pressure, the product of cardiac output and peripheral vascular resistance, likewise declines. Antihypertensive medications, particularly alpha-adrenergic receptor blockers (tolazoline, phentolamine), vasodilators (hydralazine, minoxidil), and, less likely, centrally acting sympatholytic agents (alphamethyldopa, clonidine), have similar effects.

The most common cause of drug-induced hypotension is excessive treatment with diuretic agents. Initially, the hypotensive effect of diuretics results from salt and water depletion, hypovolemia, and reduction in cardiac preload (venous return). Long-term diuretic therapy, probably by depleting arteriolar smooth muscle cells of salt and water, effects relaxation of vascular tone, reduces peripheral vascular resistance, and perpetuates the hypotensive effect. Organic nitrate preparations (nitroglycerin, isosorbide dinitrate) used in the treatment of angina and congestive heart failure exert their therapeutic effects primarily by reducing venular and arteriolar tone. Nitrate preparations not infrequently evoke hypotension and syncope. This is particularly common when these drugs are administered for the first time to hospitalized patients who may be volume depleted because of the natriuretic effect of bed rest. Vasodilator agents, including hydralazine, minoxidil, and the calcium-channel blocking drugs, particularly nifedipine, effect a reduction in arteriolar smooth muscle tone and peripheral vascular resistance. Hypotension, as a side effect, is really an extension of this therapeutic effect. Opiate narcotics, including morphine, pentazocine, and meperidine, cause a centrally mediated reduction in sympathetic venular and arteriolar tone, predisposing to hypotension. This is particularly frequent in volume-depleted patients. The fluid deficit may be consequent to blood, crystalloid, or colloid loss (e.g., the postoperative state, a restricted salt intake, or extensive thermal injury).

Hypotension resulting from medication(s) or volume depletion most commonly manifests as light-headedness, near syncope, or frank collapse soon after the patient stands up after lying or sitting for any length of time. Any postural stress activates sympathetic cardiovascular reflexes to preserve blood pressure by augmenting venular and arteriolar tone, heart rate, and myocardial contractility. A drug-induced hypotensive diathesis usually results first in a posturally related rise in pulse (rise of more than 10 beats per minute), then in posturally related hypotension (greater than 10 mm Hg decline in systolic pressure), and finally in a sustained reduction in arterial pressure. Likewise, sufficient volume depletion first manifests itself as postural hypotension. If the volume of blood in the venous (venular) reservoir is inadequate, the compensatory augmentation in venular tone with the upright posture is inadequate to maintain cardiac stroke volume, and hypotension ensues despite compensatory tachycardia.

Hospitalization and bed rest frequently lead to postural hypotension. Bed rest characteristically promotes natriuresis with contraction of the extracellular fluid and plasma volume compartments. Similarly, frequent phlebotomies for diagnostic purposes may further deplete the blood (plasma) volume. Patients are frequently treated with medications for hypertension and heart failure (diuretics and vasodilators). Elderly patients with diminished skeletal muscle mass often have insufficient augmentation of venous return (by the leg muscles and thoracoabdominal "pumping mechanism") when assuming the erect posture. Likewise, they are frequently treated with tranquilizing medications, a side effect of which is to reduce sympathetic outflow by effecting alpha-adrenergic receptor blockade. This impairs cardiovascular reflexes designed to preserve blood pressure in response to orthostatic stress. Elderly patients are frequently afflicted with overt or occult degenerative disease of the central nervous system. Although more obviously manifested as dementia, these may also impair the cardiovascular reflexes that are vital in the defense and preservation of the blood pressure against postural stress. These multiple factors associated with hospitalization and bed rest predispose patients, particularly the elderly, to postural hypotension and syncope.

Physical Examination

The physical examination is critical in identifying hypotension, assessing its severity (whether associated with organ hypoperfusion or shock), and determining its cause. The history is rarely obtainable immediately from the patient. The hypotensive patient with cerebral hypoperfusion is frequently agitated, uncooperative, lethargic, obtunded, or frankly comatose, depending upon the magnitude and severity of the hypotensive cerebral insult, the underlying illness, and the previous adequacy of the cerebral circulation.

Figures 24-1 to 24-3 are algorithms for the evaluation and treatment of hypotension.

Assessment of Vital Signs

Careful assessment of the vital signs is mandatory for the evaluation of hypotension. The pneumatic cuff of the sphygmomanometer must be deflated slowly to ensure that the blood pressure reading is not artifactually depressed. Similarly, if the patient is obese or very muscular, such that the arm is very thick, use of a standard-sized blood pressure cuff may cause artifactual overestimation of the blood pressure. In this case, accurate estimation of blood pressure requires use of a leg cuff. If the Korotkoff sounds are inaudible over the brachial area, the systolic blood pressure may be accurately measured by palpation of the radial pulse as the cuff is deflated. Alternately, the audible equivalent of the radial or brachial pulse may be detected with the aid of a Doppler stethoscope. If the radial and brachial pulses

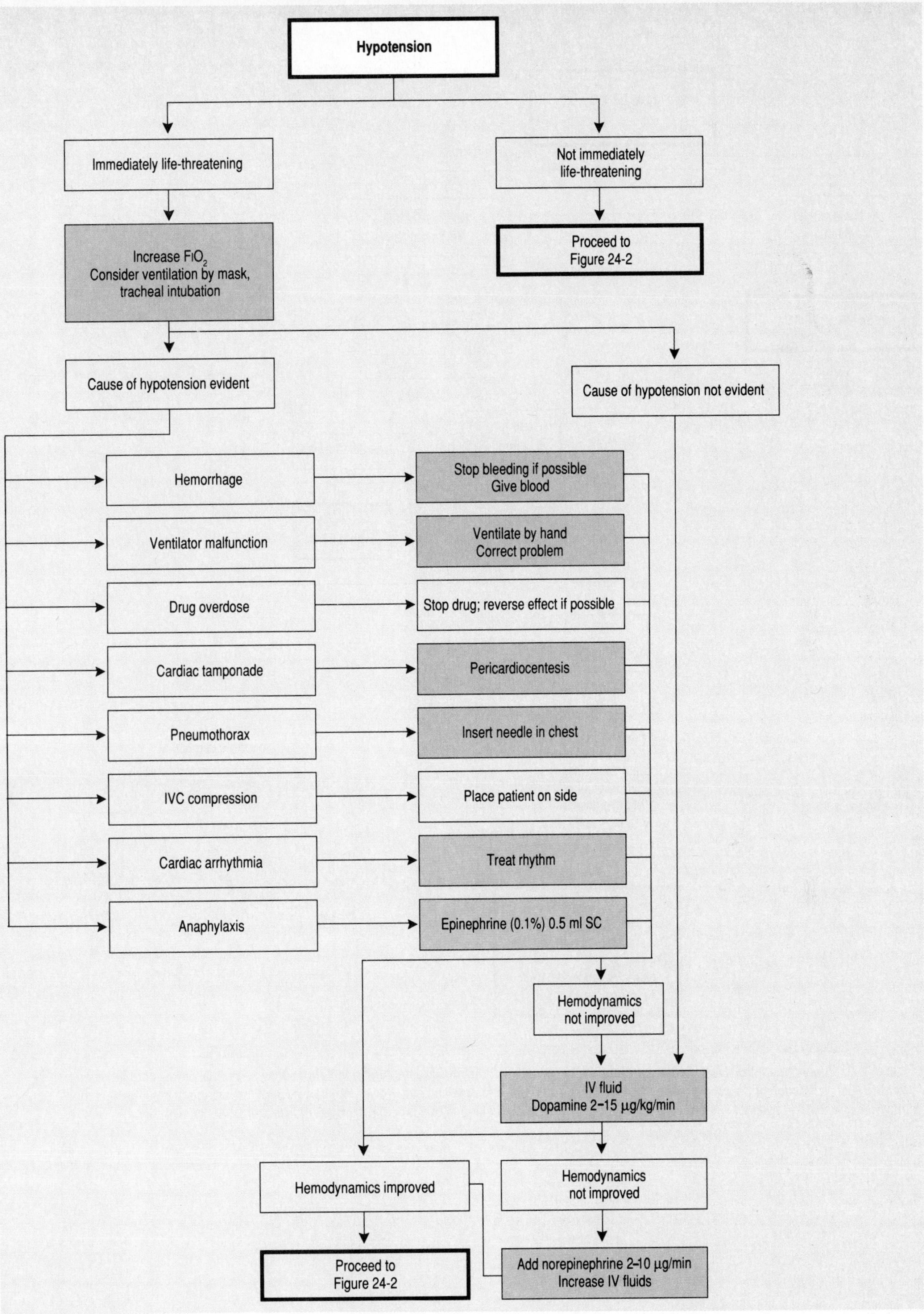

Figure 24-1 Algorithm for the evaluation of life-threatening hypotension. FIO_2 = fraction of inspired oxygen, IV = intravenous, IVC = inferior vena cava, SC = subcutaneous. (*From* Don H, ed. Decision making in critical care. Toronto: BC Decker, 1985:29; with permission.)

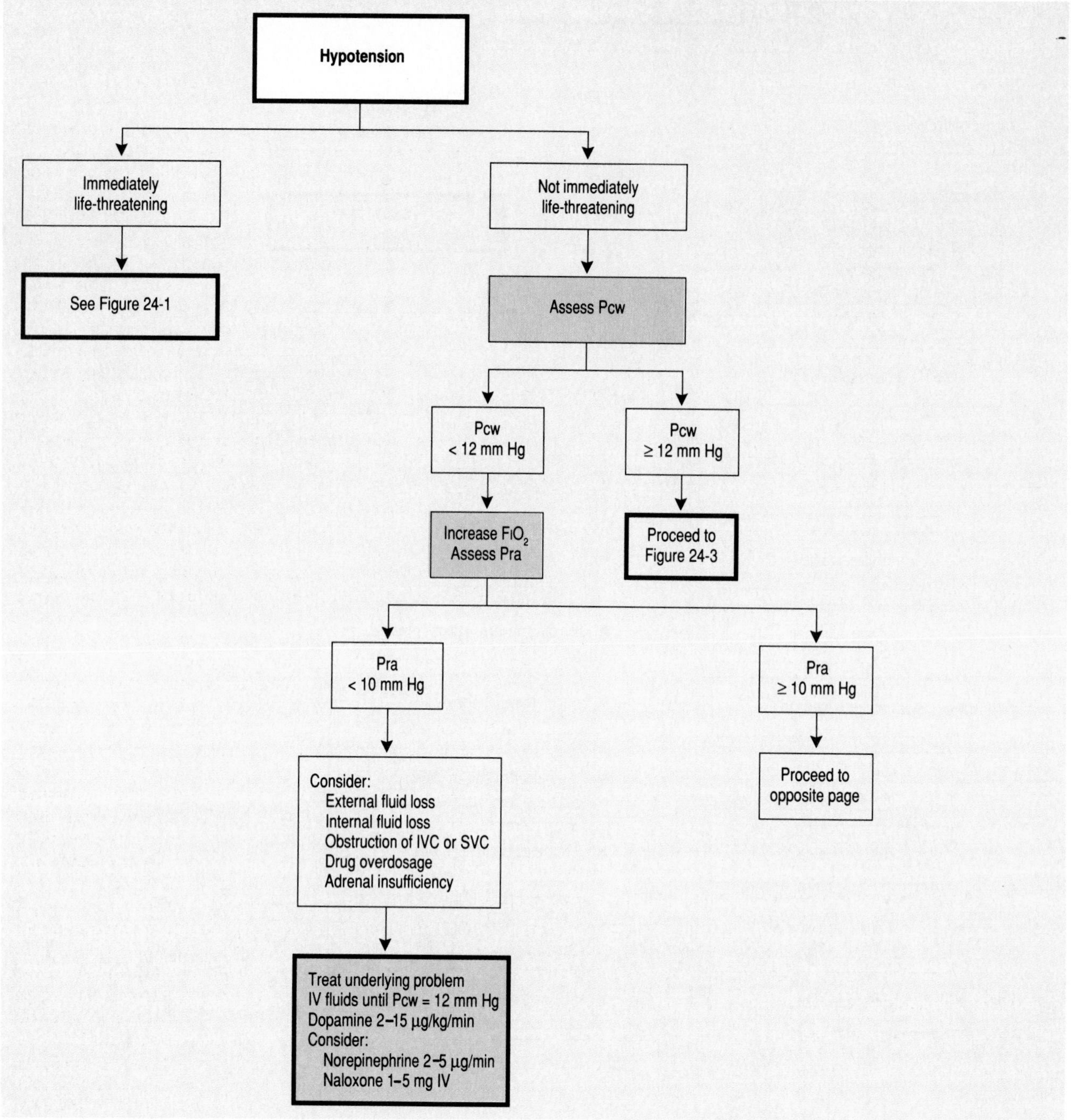

Figure 24-2 Algorithm for the evaluation of hypotension that is not immediately life-threatening in the patient with normal or low capillary wedge pressure. F_IO_2 = fraction of inspired oxygen, IV = intravenous, IVC = inferior vena cava, Pcw = pulmonary capillary wedge pressure, Pra = right atrial pressure, SVC = superior vena cava. (From Don H, ed. Decision making in critical care. Toronto: BC Decker, 1985:31; with permission.)

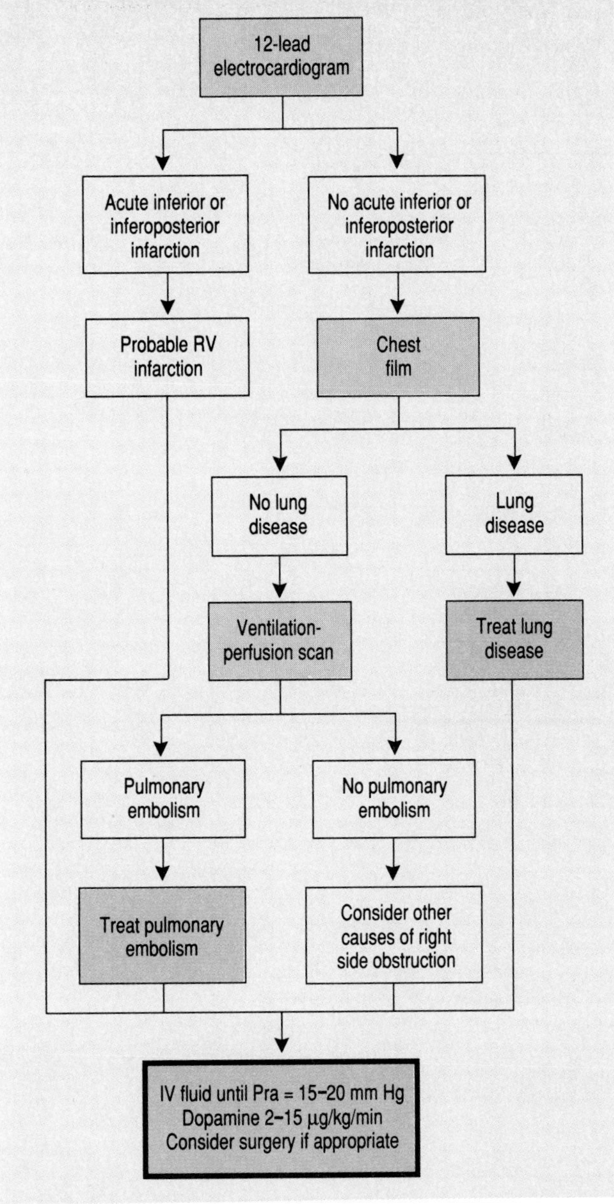

Figure 24-2 *Continued*

Table 24-1 Causes of Shock

Type of shock	Cause
Cardiogenic or vascular obstructive	Arrhythmias
	Obstructive outflow (valvular and perivalvular) lesions
	Atrial myxoma
	Acute myocardial infarction
	Severe congestive heart failure
	Cardiac tamponade
	Massive pulmonary embolism
Hypovolemic	Hemorrhage
	Vomiting
	Diarrhea
	Dehydration
	Diabetes (mellitus or insipidus)
	Addison's disease
	Burns
	Peritonitis, pancreatitis
Septic	Gram-negative or other overwhelming infections
Miscellaneous	Anaphylactic
	Neurogenic
	Drug overdose
	Hepatic or renal failure
	Myxedema

are not evident, a palpable carotid or femoral pulse guarantees a systolic blood pressure in excess of 60 mm Hg.

Shock, i.e., clinical evidence of inadequate blood flow to one or more organ systems, is often present in conjunction with hypotension (arterial pressures less than 90 mm Hg systolic) (Table 24-1). With extreme vasoconstriction that results in increased peripheral vascular resistance, however, the arterial systolic pressure is not infrequently maintained at or above 90 mm Hg, despite organ hypoperfusion. However, the arterial pulse pressure (systolic less diastolic pressure) is invariably narrowed (less than 25 mm Hg). Occasionally, patients with hypotension have clear mentation; warm, dry, normally suffused skin; and no evidence of organ hypoperfusion. The classic example is hypotension seen immediately after surgical sympathectomy or in association with the chemical sympathectomy resulting from rostral migration of spinal anesthesia, particularly in the volume-depleted patient. Hypotension in association with these findings invariably represents failure of the sympathetic nervous system.

With hypotension or shock, the pulse is usually rapid (more than 80 beats per minute) as the sympathetic nervous system effects acceleration of the heart rate to preserve cardiac output and blood pressure in the setting of a declining stroke volume. If the pulse is less than 80 beats per minute, adrenergic compensation for hypotension is inadequate or the cardiac impulse generation-conduction system is diseased. This may be due to pharmacologic blockade of the cardiac beta$_1$-adrenergic receptors consequent to treatment with propranolol, metoprolol, nadolol, atenolol, or another beta$_1$-adrenergic-blocking drug. "Inappropriate sinus bradycardia" may also result from injury or pharmacologic interruption of the adrenergic nervous system (e.g., cervical or high thoracic spinal cord trauma, spinal anesthesia). Intrinsic disease of the cardiac conduction system, particularly involving the sinoatrial node (sick sinus syndrome), consequent to ischemic, infiltrative, or primary disease of the myocardium may also be responsible for inappropriate sinus bradycardia. Extreme pyrexia associated with typhoid fever may be associated with an inappropriately slow heart rate. A rapid and irregularly irregular pulse implicates atrial fibrillation with hypotension consequent to extreme shortening of the diastolic filling period (rapid ventricular response) or as a result of loss of coordinated atrial systole with its booster pump function. Hypotension resulting from paroxysmal atrial fibrillation occurs only with an extremely rapid ventricular rate (more than 150 beats per minute) unless there is associated heart disease. A regular rate and rhythm in excess of 130 beats per minute is likely the cause of hypotension if it is ventricular tachycardia. Here the decline in stroke output is due to the rapid heart rate with inadequate diastolic filling, loss of effective atrial contraction, or asynchronous ventricular depolarization. There may also be ventricular dysfunction consequent to active ischemia, or underlying myopathic or structural heart disease. A rapid heart rate of 150 beats per minute suggests atrial flutter. A regularly irregular heart rate consequent to atrial or ventricular extrasystoles implicates underlying heart disease. However, the arrhythmias per se are not usually responsible for severe hypotension unless extremely severe underlying cardiac dysfunction is present.

Important clues to the cause of hypotension and shock may be gleaned from the temperature and respiratory rate. It is imperative that a rectal temperature be obtained, because hyperventilation with mouth breathing or insufficient mucocutaneous perfusion may invalidate measurements of oral temperature. The patient with shock may have a mild to moderate temperature elevation in the absence of infection (a temperature below 39.5°C implicates sepsis as the cause of hypotension). If the septic patient is in the process of generating a fever, peripheral

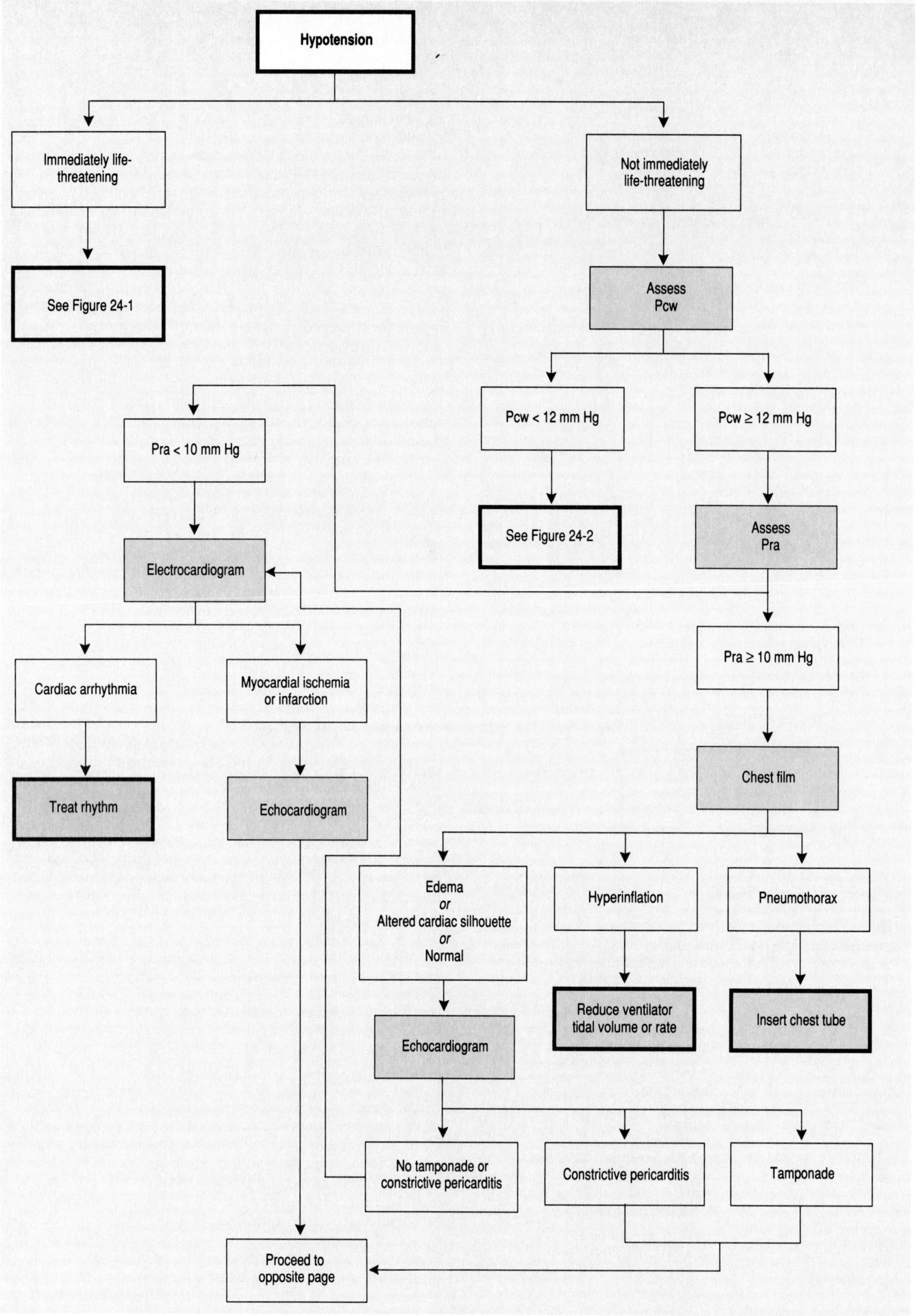

Figure 24-3 Algorithm for the evaluation of hypotension that is not immediately life-threatening in the patient with elevated capillary wedge pressure. Pcw = pulmonary capillary wedge pressure, Pra = right atrial pressure. (From Don H, ed. Decision making in critical care. Toronto: BC Decker, 1985:33; with permission.)

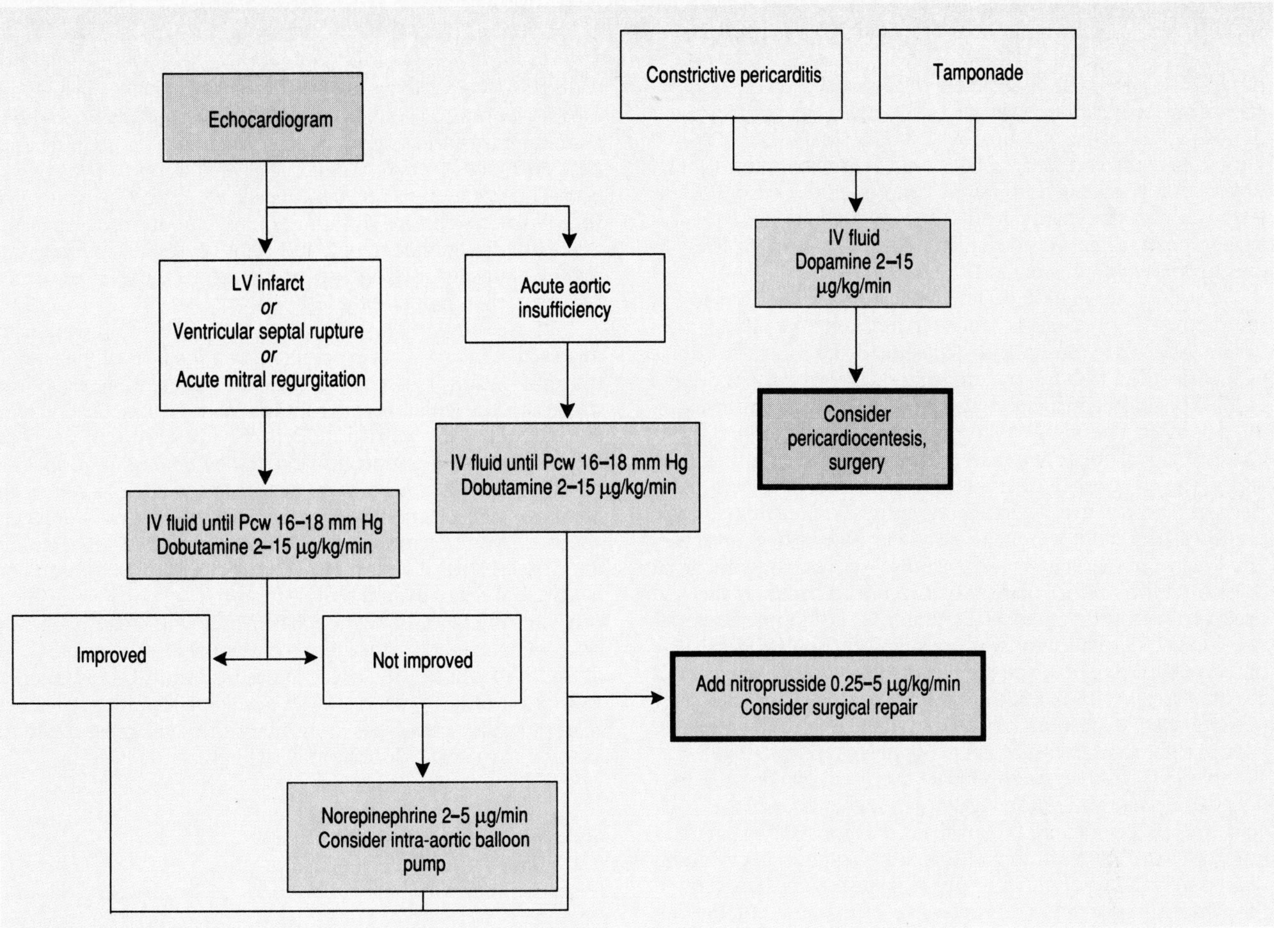

Figure 24-3 *Continued*

pallor and cool acrocyanotic extremities are prominent because of intense arterial vasoconstriction. The blood pressure is normal or moderately depressed, the pulse is thready because the pulse pressure is narrowed, the temperature is normal or moderately elevated, and shivering is usually present. The septic patient in the phase of defervescence is characterized by moist, hot, flushed skin and hypotension consequent to generalized vasodilation. In this case, hypotension is consequent to translocation of circulating blood volume into the cutaneous venous plexus and, later on, results from loss of salt and water (reduced preload) and reduced arteriolar tone (reduced systemic vascular resistance). Hypotension in association with rapid defervescence is particularly common when salicylates are used for control of pyrexia in the patient who is febrile for a sustained period. This is commonly seen with fever resulting from lymphoma or Hodgkin's disease.

The accurate quantification of hypothermia requires a special rectal thermometer graduated below 94°F. Hypotension may be a manifestation of hypothermia, which in turn may be due to cold exposure, myxedema, hypoglycemia, barbiturate or narcotic overdose, or overwhelming infection, particularly in elderly patients.

A rapid respiratory rate with deep breathing defines Kussmaul's respiratory pattern; this usually indicates respiratory compensation for an underlying metabolic acidosis. In conjunction with hypotension and shock, this results from respiratory stimulation consequent to lactic or diabetic ketoacidosis. A similar respiratory pattern of tachypnea and hyperpnea is responsible for the respiratory alkalosis associated with sepsis or hepatic failure (hyperammonemia). However, the latter condition is not predictably associated with hypotension unless something has occurred in the patient with underlying liver disease that could eventuate in hypotension and worsening hepatic encephalopathy. This includes sepsis, excessive paracentesis, diuretic therapy, or gastrointestinal bleeding.

Cutaneous Examination

During the cutaneous examination, attention should be directed at determining the adequacy of cutaneous perfusion. Evidence for impaired skin blood flow includes decreased skin temperature, pallor, and acrocyanosis. Acrocyanosis, present when the concentration of reduced hemoglobin in the cutaneous venous plexus exceeds 5 mg/dl, results from increased tissue extraction of oxygen from arterial blood to maintain regional oxygen delivery in the face of reduced arterial flow. It may be absent if there is significant anemia. Diaphoresis, mediated by cholinergic sympathetic discharge, occurs in association with the massive sympathetic outflow characteristic of the shock syndrome. Warm, dry, and normally colored or flushed extremities in the hypotensive patient are characteristically seen in association with a vasovagal episode. Similar findings are characteristic of hypotension resulting from precipitous failure of sympathetic autonomic tone, which occurs with spinal cord trauma and chemical or surgical sympathectomy.

Undue emphasis is often placed on assessing salt and water balance by estimating tissue turgor and moisture content of mucous membranes. This estimate of salt and water balance is neither sensitive nor specific. Most elderly patients have lax skin consequent to subcutaneous connective tissue atrophy in the absence of salt and water depletion. Conversely, obese patients may have seemingly normal skin turgor despite substantial salt and water (volume) depletion because of the excessive adiposity of their subcutaneous tissue. Patients who breathe through the mouth frequently have desiccated mucous membranes in the absence of volume depletion.

Palpation of Carotid Pulses

Palpation of the carotid pulses, like the arterial pulse pressure, provides a rough estimate of the stroke volume. In almost all forms of hypotension associated with reduced cardiac output and increased peripheral vascular resistance, the carotid pulse is diminished in volume ("thready"). A delay in the rate of rise of the carotid pulse pressure suggests left ventricular outflow tract obstruction consequent to aortic stenosis. In the setting of this lesion, any hemodynamic insult (myocardial infarction, hemorrhage, sepsis, or supraventricular arrhythmia) is more likely to eventuate in hypotension and shock.

Careful examination of the jugular veins with estimation of the right atrial pressure is crucial in assessing the adequacy of the intravascular volume and right ventricular function. This is best performed with the patient lying supine with the head in a relaxed position and angulated slightly toward or away from the the observer. The jugular venous meniscus is identified by its characteristic double impulse (representing the right atrial A and V waves) normally seen just above the medial aspect of the clavicle. The A wave, representing atrial systole, immediately precedes or occurs simultaneously with the carotid upstroke. The V wave of the jugular venous pulse, representing the atrial pressure during ventricular systole, occurs immediately after the peak of the carotid pulse. This timing is best appreciated by simultaneous palpation of the opposite carotid pulse. Estimation of the vertical height of the jugular meniscus above the level of the right atrium (5 cm vertically below the sternal angle) usually permits accurate estimation of the right atrial pressure. The normal right atrial pressure is 4 to 8 mm Hg (approximately 5 to 10 cm H_2O). Failure to appreciate the jugular meniscus in a nonobese patient in whom adequate examination of the neck veins can be performed means that the right atrial pressure is less than 5 cm saline (4 mm Hg) and that intravascular volume depletion is an important factor in the genesis of the hypotensive state. More important, in the absence of extreme volume depletion, a normal or low right atrial pressure reliably excludes massive pulmonary embolism or cardiac tamponade as the cause of hypotension. A jugular venous pressure exceeding 10 cm H_2O (8 mm Hg) likewise excludes volume depletion. It implicates cardiac tamponade, myocardial infarction involving the right ventricle, or cor pulmonale consequent to massive pulmonary embolism. With cardiac tamponade, the jugular venous pressure is elevated and there is no abrupt descent in the V wave (y component). If a substantial accumulation of pericardial fluid underlies tamponade, the left border of cardiac dullness is laterally displayed to percussion; however, the apical (left ventricular) and the left parasternal (right ventricular) impulses are usually very diminished, if at all palpable, and the heart sounds are soft. There is usually pulsus paradoxus (an inspiratory decline in peak systolic arterial pressure exceeding 10 mm Hg when the systolic pressure exceeds 100 mm Hg). Right ventricular infarction is characterized by impaired right ventricular function. Here the neck veins are distended and the heart sounds, particularly the pulmonic component of the second heart sound, are somewhat reduced in intensity. The right ventricular impulse is usually not obvious.

Massive pulmonary embolism, in addition to causing elevation in the jugular venous pressure, characteristically causes severe and otherwise unexplained dyspnea; i.e., there is no obvious pneumonia, atelectasis, or pleural effusion to explain the patient's extreme air hunger. Because of the moderate pulmonary hypertension consequent to massive pulmonary embolism, the pulmonic component of the second heart sound is somewhat increased in intensity. Similarly, because of the increased resistance to right ventricular ejection, its ejection time is prolonged. Underfilling of the left ventricle simultaneously shortens its ejection time. The net effect is that the second heart sound may be widely but physiologically split in massive pulmonary embolism; i.e., with inspiration, the aortic and pulmonic components of the second heart sound separate widely but do not fully move together to become a single sound during expiration. There may be a left parasternal lift, reflecting acute right ventricular distention. With pulmonary embolism, acute distention of the pulmonary trunk and right ventricular outflow tract may eventuate in a systolic ejection murmur at the base (particularly over the second left intercostal space).

In the patient who becomes hypotensive following acute myocardial infarction, the presence of a loud, harsh pansystolic murmur midway between the apex and lower left sternal border suggests ventricular septal rupture. Acute mitral insufficiency consequent to myocardial infarction with rupture of the papillary muscle may present similarly. In acute mitral regurgitation, however, the murmur is at or nearer to the apex, is softer, and often is more ejection in timing. Hypotension with unilateral absence of one or more arterial pulses implicates dissection of the thoracic aorta. In this instance, true central hypotension does not usually result from the dissection per se; rather, it is due to aortic insufficiency or hemopericardium with tamponade. Spurious hypotension consequent to regional arterial insufficiency of the limb where pressure is measured must be excluded by measuring blood pressure in all four limbs in the patient with suspected dissection. Any asymmetry in blood pressure so detected makes aortic dissection very likely.

Abdominal Examination

In the hypotensive patient, rebound tenderness on abdominal examination implicates peritonitis with crystalloid loss and, possibly, septic shock. Ecchymoses emanating from the flanks to the umbilicus anteriorly, Grey Turner's sign, may result from retroperitoneal rupture of an abdominal aortic aneurysm, from bowel infarction, or from hemorrhagic pancreatitis. Abdominal distention with preservation of the bowel sounds and minor direct tenderness may reflect retroperitoneal hemorrhage. This may be due to leakage from abdominal aortic aneurysm with impending rupture, or it may result from spontaneous venous hemorrhage consequent to anticoagulant therapy. A tender anterior abdominal mass or tender abdominal "distention" that does not disappear with active flexion of the abdominal muscle wall by elevation of the legs off of the bed suggests hematoma of the rectus sheath or anterior abdominal wall, another possible complication of anticoagulant therapy.

A careful history and physical examination usually identify the cause of hypotension. Careful estimation of the central venous pressure and adequacy of the intravascular volume serves as a guide to resuscitative and definitive therapy.

References

Ferguson DW, Abboud FM. The pathophysiology, recognition, and management of shock. In: Hurst JW, et al, eds. The heart. 7th ed. New York: McGraw-Hill, 1990:442.

Lipsitz LA. Orthostatic hypotension in the elderly. N Engl J Med 1989; 321:952.

McCall D, O'Rourke RA. Hypotension and cardiogenic shock. In: Stein J, et al, eds. Internal medicine. 3rd ed. Boston: Little, Brown, 1990:459.

Weil MH, Von Planta M. Clinical shock states. In: Braunwald E, ed. Heart disease. 3rd ed. Philadelphia: WB Saunders, 1988:568.

Systolic Heart Murmurs

25

Diana DeCosimo, MD

James E. Dalen, MD, MPH

Definition

Heart murmurs are a series of audible vibrations at a frequency of 50 to 1,000 cycles per second that occur during systole, during diastole, or continuously throughout the heart cycle. The work of Stein (1981) has shown that systolic murmurs are due to turbulent blood flow, which is an irregular eddying motion characterized by random fluctuations in pressure and velocity of blood flow. The factors that increase turbulence include increased velocity of blood flow, increased stroke volume, decreased blood viscosity, and structural abnormalities within the heart.

Systolic murmurs are classified into ejection murmurs, which begin after the first heart sound (S_1) and end before the second heart sound (S_2), and holosystolic (or pansystolic) murmurs, which begin with S_1 and persist throughout systole to S_2. Ejection murmurs may be of maximal intensity in early, mid-, or late systole. These murmurs are usually due to turbulence engendered by obstruction to ventricular outflow, dilatation or increased velocity of flow into the great arteries, or structural abnormalities of the aortic or pulmonic valve. Holosystolic murmurs occur when blood flows from a high-pressure chamber or artery into an artery or chamber that has a lower pressure throughout systole.

The most common murmurs are functional (or innocent) ejection murmurs that are due to turbulence caused by the projection of the free margins of the normal aortic valve into the stream of flow into the aorta. Functional murmurs become audible or louder when blood flow is increased as a result of anemia, fever, pregnancy, or hyperthyroidism.

Etiology

Evaluation of a systolic murmur is among the most challenging tasks for the physician. Systolic murmurs are highly prevalent, being present in nearly 50 percent of all children and many adults.

Systolic murmurs are often functional; i.e., they may occur in patients without organic heart disease. The prognosis of patients with functional heart murmurs is normal. They do not require therapy, further diagnostic studies, or special follow-up.

On the other hand, the presence of a systolic murmur, even in an asymptomatic patient, may be the first clue that the patient requires cardiac surgery (e.g., secundum atrial septal defect) or that life-long antibiotic prophylaxis for dental work or surgical procedures is indicated to prevent endocarditis in the patient whose systolic murmur is due to valvular heart disease (aortic stenosis, pulmonic stenosis, mitral insufficiency, or tricuspid insufficiency).

It is therefore clear that systolic murmurs, even when they occur in an asymptomatic patient, require definitive diagnosis. A false-positive diagnosis of organic heart disease can lead to iatrogenic cardiac neurosis. A false-negative diagnosis in patients with organic heart disease can lead to cardiac complications that might have been prevented.

A definitive diagnosis of the cause of a systolic murmur can usually be established by attention to the patient's history, general physical examination, and cardiovascular examination, including but not limited to careful evaluation of the murmur itself. The principal causes of a systolic murmur in an asymptomatic or minimally symptomatic adult are shown in Table 25-1.

Diagnostic Approach

History

The first question to ask is whether the patient has been told of a heart murmur in the past and, if so, at what age. A history of a heart murmur at birth or shortly after is highly suggestive of congenital aortic or pulmonic valve stenosis. A murmur first heard in childhood or adolescence suggests atrial septal defect.

The presence of symptoms of heart disease should be sought. A history of syncope suggests aortic stenosis or hypertrophic obstructive cardiomyopathy (HOCM; also called IHSS). Patients with congenital heart disease often deny dyspnea or decreased exercise tolerance. However, they may have unconsciously altered their lifestyle to compensate for their cardiac defect and may therefore be unaware of their limitation. It is important to determine whether their exercise tolerance was truly normal by asking if they participated in competitive athletics and if they were able to keep up with their peers when they were adolescents. Patients with congenital heart disease often recall that they could not keep up with their peers in high school, although they may deny dyspnea and easy fatigability per se.

A history of acute rheumatic fever or Sydenham's chorea in the past increases the probability that the systolic murmur is due to rheumatic heart disease that is causing mitral or aortic stenosis or mitral or tricuspid insufficiency.

Physical Examination

Blood pressure should be taken in both arms. If it is elevated in either arm, blood pressure in the lower extremities should be measured. Hypertension in either upper extremity with a lower systolic pressure in the legs makes it very likely that the patient has coarctation of the aorta. The systolic murmur may be due to the coarctation itself or to a bicuspid aortic valve, which is present in more than 50 percent of patients with coarctation.

Careful examination of the carotid pulses may yield important clues to the cause of the systolic murmur. A slow carotid upstroke and decreased pulse volume are highly consistent with aortic stenosis. A rapid carotid upstroke suggests HOCM.

The signs of left and right ventricular failure should be sought, but these are unlikely in an asymptomatic patient.

If the nail beds reveal cyanosis with or without clubbing, the systolic murmur may be due to a ventricular or atrial septal defect with pulmonary hypertension. Such patients would be expected to be symptomatic.

If examination of the upper extremities demonstrates skeletal abnormalities such as syndactyly, polydactyly, or a missing

Table 25-1 Differential Diagnosis of Systolic Murmurs

Location	Lesion	Timing and intensity	Other auscultatory findings	Other physical findings	Other
Right upper sternal border (second RICS)	Valvular aortic stenosis	Ejection grade 2–6; diamond-shaped	+/− Systolic ejection click; +/− AI murmur; S_2 may be absent	Carotid upstroke is small, delayed; +/− thrill; forceful apical impulse	Murmur radiates to carotids
	Aortic sclerosis	Ejection grade 1–3; peaks early systole		Carotid pulses normal or brisk	Common in elderly
Left upper sternal border (second to fourth LICS)	Functional murmur	Ejection grade 1–2; peaks in early systole	Intensity varies with respiration and position		
	Atrial septal defect	Ejection grade 1–3	Fixed split of S_2	Right parasternal heave; skeletal abnormalities in upper extremities	
	Pulmonic stenosis	Ejection grade 2–6; diamond-shaped	Systolic ejection click with inspiration; wide split at S_2	+/− thrill; right parasternal heave	
Lower left sternal border and apex	Ventricular septal defect	Holosystoloic (or ejection) grade 3–6; harsh	Wide split of S_2	+/− thrill; forceful diffuse apical impulse	
	Hypertrophic obstructive cardiomyopathy	Ejection may be holosystolic at apex	Murmur increases with Valsalva maneuver or standing; S_4 gallop	Rapid, double carotid upstroke; forceful apical impulse	
	Mitral regurgitation: valvular	Holosystolic grade 2–6; radiates to axilla	S_3 gallop; +/− diastolic murmur at apex	+/− thrill; hyperdynamic apical impulse	
	Mitral regurgitation: papillary muscle dysfunction	Ejection peaks in early systole or diastole	S_3 gallop		
	Mitral valve prolapse	Ejection peaks in late systole	Midsystolic click(s); murmur may become louder and longer with Valsalva maneuver or standing		
	Tricuspid regurgitation	Holosystolic grade 1–4	Murmur increases with inspiration	Pulsatile neck veins	Usually associated with mitral valve disease or pulmonary hypertension

Abbreviations: AI = aortic insufficiency, LICS = left intercostal space, RICS = right intercostal space.

radial head, the systolic murmur is almost certainly due to familial atrial septal defect (Holt-Oram syndrome).

Cardiac Examination

Palpation of the apical impulse may help in the differential diagnosis. A diffuse, heaving apical impulse suggests left ventricular volume overload and points to mitral insufficiency or ventricular septal defect. A sustained apical impulse of increased intensity suggests aortic stenosis or HOCM. A parasternal (right ventricular) heave is consistent with right ventricular volume overload due to tricuspid insufficiency or atrial septal defect.

The precordium should be palpated carefully for thrills. A thrill at the second right intercostal space is almost diagnostic of hemodynamically significant aortic stenosis, whereas a thrill in the second left intercostal space is usually due to pulmonic stenosis. A systolic thrill at the lower left sternal border indicates ventricular septal defect, whereas a thrill near the apex is associated with mitral regurgitation or HOCM.

The presence of a systolic click aids in the differential diagnosis. An early systolic ejection click is frequently heard in patients with mild aortic or pulmonic stenosis. An early systolic click that disappears during inspiration is nearly diagnostic of mild pulmonic stenosis. A mid-systolic click that becomes louder and earlier while the patient is standing is essentially diagnostic of mitral valve prolapse, which may also cause a late-systolic murmur due to mitral insufficiency.

The splitting of S_2 should be evaluated carefully. If the splitting is fixed, i.e., does not widen with inspiration, a diagnosis of atrial septal defect is virtually certain. Wide splitting of S_2 that increases with inspiration suggests ventricular septal defect or pulmonic stenosis.

Auscultation

By auscultation, one determines the location, timing, radiation, intensity, and quality of the systolic murmur. The location (Fig. 25-1) and timing of the murmur (Fig. 25-2) are particularly

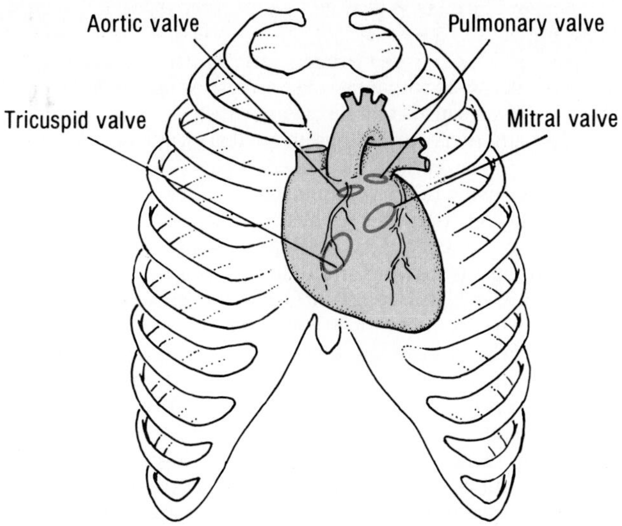

Figure 25-1 Precordial location of the cardiac valves and their associated murmurs.

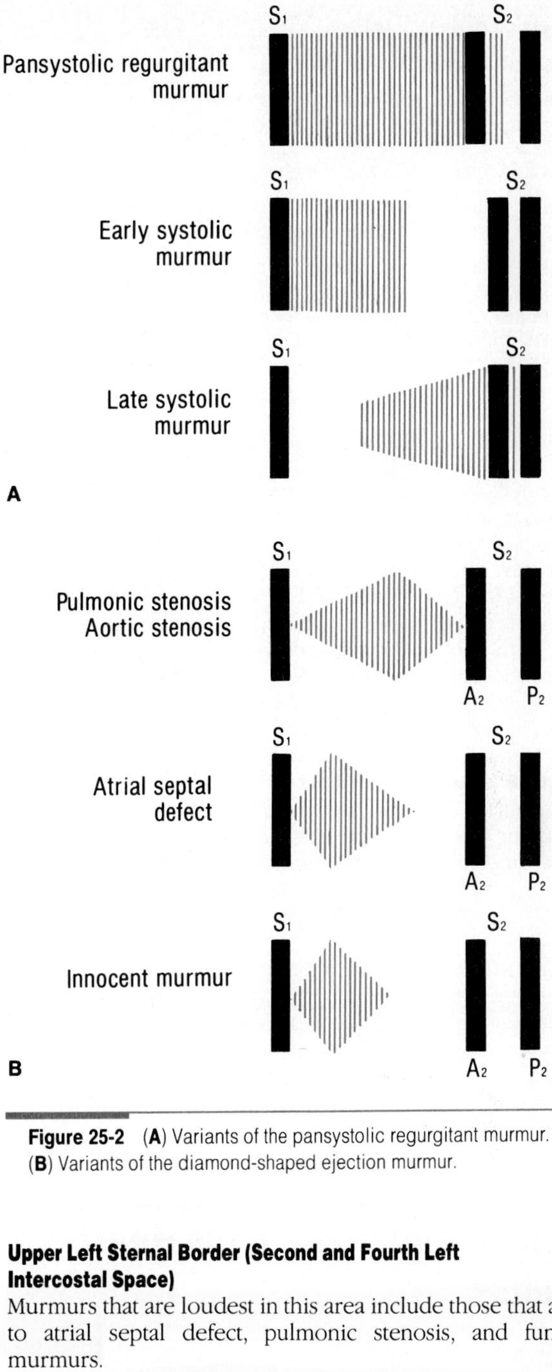

Figure 25-2 (**A**) Variants of the pansystolic regurgitant murmur. (**B**) Variants of the diamond-shaped ejection murmur.

important. These characteristics, coupled with the history, variation with physiologic maneuvers (Table 25-2), and other physical findings, usually allow the clinician to determine the origin of the murmur.

The location of the systolic murmur when it is of maximal intensity presents important clues to its etiology, as shown in Table 25-1. The grading of murmurs by intensity is described in Table 25-3.

Right Upper Sternal Border

Valvular aortic stenosis, aortic sclerosis, and bicuspid aortic valve without stenosis are the most common causes of murmurs in this location. These murmurs are of the ejection type.

The murmur of aortic sclerosis is due to turbulence caused by dilatation of the ascending aorta and is seen most frequently in the elderly. The murmur usually peaks in early systole and is usually grade 1 to 3 in intensity. The carotid upstroke is normal or brisk, and there are no systolic clicks or associated diastolic murmur. This murmur is a benign finding in the elderly.

The characteristics of the murmur of valvular aortic stenosis depend upon the severity of obstruction. If the stenosis is hemodynamically significant, the murmur peaks in mid- or late systole and radiates into the carotids. The carotid upstroke is delayed, and the pulse volume is decreased. With mild aortic stenosis, the murmur peaks in early systole, is softer (grade 1 to 3), and is less likely to radiate to the carotids, which have a normal upstroke and volume. An early systolic click is often heard in patients with mild aortic stenosis. An early, short, decrescendo diastolic murmur at the aortic area or along the left sternal border may accompany mild or significant aortic stenosis.

Upper Left Sternal Border (Second and Fourth Left Intercostal Space)

Murmurs that are loudest in this area include those that are due to atrial septal defect, pulmonic stenosis, and functional murmurs.

The most frequent murmurs in this area are functional. They are usually soft (grade 1 to 2) ejection murmurs that peak in early systole. The intensity of these murmurs often changes during respiration or with body position.

Table 25-2 Variation in Murmurs with Physical Maneuvers

	Aortic stenosis	Subaortic stenosis	Mitral regurgitation	Pulmonic stenosis	VSD
Inspiration	—	—	—	↑ or —	—
Valsalva release	↑	↓	↑ or —	↑	?
Post-extrasystolic beat	↑	↑	↓ or —	↑	?
Hand grip	↓	↓	↑	↑ or —	?

Key: No change, —; increase, ↑ ; decrease, ↓ .
Abbreviation: VSD = ventricular septal defect.

Table 25-3 Grading of Murmurs

Grade 1	The softest murmur that can be heard
Grade 2	A soft murmur heard by most observers
Grade 3	A murmur that is loud but without a thrill
Grade 4	A loud murmur associated with a thrill
Grade 5	A loud murmur with a thrill that can be heard from the edge of the stethoscope chestpiece
Grade 6	A murmur heard without the use of a stethoscope

Modified from Shah PM. Approach to the patient with heart murmurs. In: Kelley WN. Internal medicine. Philadelphia: JB Lippincott, 1989.

The murmur of atrial septal defect is ejection and is grade 1 to 3 in intensity. The key to its recognition is the associated fixed splitting of S_2. It is usually accompanied by a parasternal (right ventricular) heave due to right ventricular volume overload.

The auscultatory findings of pulmonic stenosis depend upon its severity. In mild pulmonic stenosis, the ejection murmur peaks in early systole and is accompanied by an early systolic click that disappears with inspiration. The ejection murmur of significant pulmonic stenosis is louder (grade 4 to 6), peaks in late systole, may obscure S_2, and may be accompanied by a thrill. An ejection click is not heard in severe pulmonic stenosis.

Lower Left Sternal Border and Apex

The murmur of ventricular septal defect is usually holosystolic, but it may be ejection in type. It is loud (grade 3 to 6), harsh, and often accompanied by a thrill at the lower left sternal border. The murmur of ventricular septal defect is often well heard over the lower sternum or to the right of the lower sternum. The second sound is widely split.

Hypertrophic obstructive cardiomyopathy usually causes an ejection murmur, but when it causes mitral insufficiency, the murmur may be holosystolic and loudest at the apex. The carotids have a rapid upstroke and may have a double impulse, and the apical impulse is usually forceful. An S_4 gallop is usually present and may be palpable. A very important clue to the presence of HOCM is that the murmur becomes louder when the patient stands or performs a Valsalva maneuver. All other murmurs decrease with these maneuvers, except the murmur of mitral valve prolapse, which may become louder and longer.

The auscultatory findings in patients with mitral insufficiency vary because of its diverse etiologies. Mitral insufficiency due to rheumatic heart disease usually causes a harsh blowing holosystolic murmur that is heard loudest at the apex with radiation to the axilla. An S_3 gallop is usually present, and the apical impulse is heaving and diffuse owing to left ventricular volume overload. An apical thrill may be present. A diastolic murmur may also be present at the apex.

When mitral insufficiency is due to an abnormality of the papillary muscles or chordae tendineae, the murmur is usually ejection in quality, peaking in early or mid-systole. An S_3 gallop is frequent.

Mitral insufficiency due to mitral valve prolapse produces distinct auscultatory findings. The systolic murmur is ejection in type and occurs in mid- to late systole. It is usually preceded by one or more clicks in mid-systole. When the patient stands or performs a Valsalva maneuver, the clicks may become louder and occur earlier, and the murmur is longer.

Tricuspid insufficiency causes a holosystolic murmur that is grade 1 to 4 in intensity. This murmur is recognized by its increase in intensity during inspiration. Severe tricuspid regurgitation causes visible systolic pulsations in the neck veins and a pulsatile liver.

References

Leatham A. Systolic murmurs. Circulation 1958; 17:601.

Levine SA, Harvey WP. Clinical auscultation of the heart. 2nd ed. Philadelphia: WB Saunders, 1959.

Perloff JK. Clinical recognition of congenital heart disease. 3rd ed. Philadelphia: WB Saunders, 1987.

Shaver JA, Salerni R. Auscultation of the heart. In: Hurst JW, et al, eds. The heart. 7th ed. New York: McGraw-Hill, 1990:175.

Stein PD. A physical and physiological basis for the interpretation of cardiac auscultation. Mt. Kisco, NY: Futura Publishing Company, 1981.

26 Diastolic and Continuous Heart Murmurs

Joseph S. Alpert, MD

Diastolic Murmurs

Diastolic heart murmurs occur during the time period between the second heart sound (S_2) and the first heart sound (S_1), i.e., during cardiac diastole. Diastolic heart murmurs are always organic; that is, they result from acquired or congenital anatomic derangements within the cardiovascular system. Innocent or benign diastolic murmurs do not exist.

Intensity or loudness of diastolic murmur is classified in the manner described previously for systolic murmurs (see Chapter 25, "Systolic Heart Murmurs"). Most diastolic murmurs fall within the range of grade 1 to grade 4. Grade 5 and 6 diastolic murmurs are very unusual.

Pathophysiology

Diastolic murmurs, like systolic murmurs, are caused by turbulent blood flow within the heart or great vessels. They can be classified into three groups: (1) early diastolic murmurs, (2) mid-diastolic murmurs, and (3) late diastolic or presystolic murmurs (Table 26-1).

Etiology

Diastolic murmurs are usually the result of semilunar valvular incompetence (aortic or pulmonic valvular regurgitation) or atrioventricular valvular stenosis (mitral or tricuspid valvular stenosis). Occasionally, they are due to markedly increased flow

Table 26-1 Classification of Diastolic Murmurs

Early Diastolic Murmurs
Aortic regurgitation
Pulmonary regurgitation secondary to pulmonary hypertension (Graham Steell's murmur)

Mid-Diastolic Murmurs
Mitral stenosis
Tricuspid stenosis
Increased flow across the mitral valve: mitral regurgitation, ventricular septal defect, patent ductus arteriosus
Increased flow across the tricuspid valve: tricuspid regurgitation, atrial septal defect
Pulmonic regurgitation (usually congenital) in the presence of normal pulmonary arterial pressure

Late Diastolic (Presystolic) Murmurs
Mitral stenosis (sinus rhythm)
Tricuspid stenosis (sinus rhythm)
Austin Flint murmur: resembles the murmur of mitral stenosis; it is the result of closure of normal mitral leaflets by a large aortic regurgitant jet (see text)
Left or right atrial myxoma

across the mitral or tricuspid valve. Semilunar valvular regurgitation usually produces a high-pitched, blowing murmur, whereas atrioventricular valvular stenosis causes a low-pitched, rumbling murmur.

Differential Diagnosis and Evaluation

Early Diastolic Murmurs

The most common diastolic murmur heard in developed countries is that of aortic valvular regurgitation (Fig. 26-1; also see Table 26-1). This murmur begins immediately following the aortic component of S_2. The murmur is decreasing, or decrescendo, in loudness or intensity. It is rather high-pitched and blowing in quality. On occasion, the murmur has a musical quality, particularly when aortic regurgitation is the result of cusp perforation or eversion. The murmur of aortic regurgitation usually lasts for the first one-third to one-half of diastole (depending on the chronicity and severity of valvular regurgitation, the state of left ventricular function, and the heart rate; the more acute the onset of aortic regurgitation, the shorter the murmur lasts into diastole). Individuals with very severe but acute aortic regurgitation often have murmurs that are heard only during the earliest part of diastole.

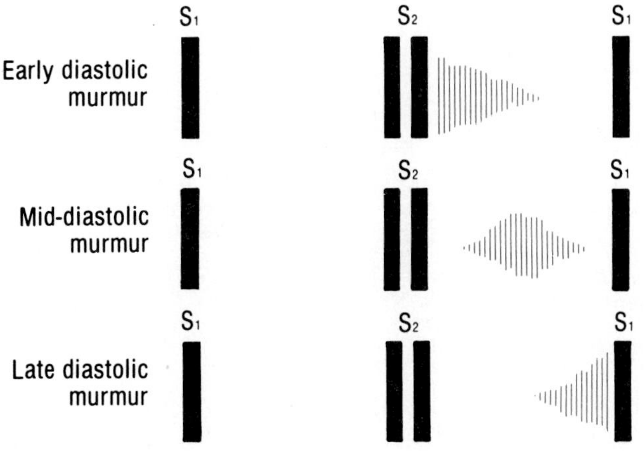

Figure 26-1 Diastolic murmurs.

Rapid heart rates shorten diastole, so that relatively short murmurs of aortic regurgitation occupy a greater percentage of the diastolic period. Patients with long-standing, mild to moderate aortic regurgitation have left ventricular diastolic pressures that are low. Aortic diastolic pressure is therefore higher than left ventricular diastolic pressure throughout diastole, producing a murmur that lasts for most of the diastolic period. Finally, patients with left ventricular dysfunction have high left ventricular diastolic pressures. The diastolic pressure gradient between the aorta and the left ventricle is present only during the initial phase of diastole. Hence, the aortic regurgitation murmur lasts for only a brief period at the onset of diastole.

The murmur of aortic regurgitation is frequently difficult to hear because it is soft and high-pitched. The murmur is best heard if one listens with the diaphragm of the stethoscope firmly applied to the mid-portion of the left sternal border, with the patient sitting forward and holding his or her breath in deep expiration. A clue to the etiology of aortic regurgitation can be obtained by noting whether the murmur is loudest at the right or left sternal border at the mid-sternal level.

Murmurs that are loudest along the right sternal border suggest the presence of disease entities that lead to aortic root dilatation, e.g., Marfan's syndrome. Rheumatic valvular disease produces an aortic regurgitant murmur that is loudest along the left sternal edge.

Soft murmurs of aortic regurgitation increase in intensity with firm, sustained hand grip or squatting, both of which increase aortic diastolic pressure and hence the aortic to left ventricular diastolic pressure gradient and the quantity of regurgitant blood flow (Table 26-2).

Pulmonic regurgitation produces a murmur that is often similar to that of aortic regurgitation. Pulmonic regurgitation may be secondary to severe pulmonary hypertension (Graham Steell's murmur), or it may be the result of a congenital abnormality of the pulmonic valve. Only Graham Steell's murmur resembles the murmur of aortic regurgitation (see Table 26-2). Congenital pulmonic regurgitation produces a mid-diastolic murmur; this entity is discussed in the next section.

Graham Steell's murmur is the result of marked pulmonary hypertension. Therefore, the pulmonic component of S_2 that accompanies this murmur is invariably loud. Graham Steell's murmur is high-pitched, decrescendo or decreasing in intensity, and often lasts through at least the first half of diastole or longer. It is often difficult or impossible to distinguish Graham Steell's murmur from that of aortic regurgitation (see Table 26-1).

Differentiation of aortic from pulmonic regurgitation often depends on associated clinical findings and the results of noninvasive cardiac examinations. Thus, the patient with left ventricular or aortic root dilatation and normal right-heart chamber size probably has aortic regurgitation as the cause of the early diastolic blowing murmur. By contrast, right ventricular hypertrophy and dilatation accompany pulmonary hypertension and secondary pulmonic regurgitation.

Mid-Diastolic Murmurs

Mid-diastolic murmurs result from obstruction of the mitral or tricuspid valves, increased blood flow across the mitral or tricuspid valves, or pulmonic regurgitation secondary to an abnormal valve and in the presence of normal pulmonary arterial pressure (see Table 26-1 and Fig. 26-1). Mitral and tricuspid valvular obstruction are often the result of rheumatic heart disease. These murmurs are low-pitched and rumbling in quality. They are best heard with the bell of the stethoscope applied lightly (not firmly) to the skin. The mid-diastolic rumble of mitral stenosis is best heard at the cardiac apex, whereas that of tricuspid stenosis is most clearly audible along the left sternal edge (half to two-thirds of the way down the sternum towards the xiphoid). The rumble of tricuspid stenosis increases in loudness during inspiration and decreases in intensity during expiration

Table 26-2 Characteristics of Diastolic Murmurs

Lesion	Location of murmur	Timing and intensity	Other auscultatory findings	Other physical findings	Other
Early Diastolic Murmurs					
Aortic regurgitation	Mid left sternal border	Begins right after S_2; decrescendo; increases in intensity with hand grip or squatting	High-pitched and blowing; occasionally musical	Left ventricular heave; bounding pulses	Search for clue to etiology, e.g., Marfan's syndrome
Pulmonic regurgitation with pulmonary hypertension (Graham Steell's murmur)	Mid left sternal border	Begins right after S_2; decrescendo	P_2 is loud; murmur is high-pitched	Right ventricular heave; normal peripheral pulses	Difficult to distinguish from murmur of aortic regurgitation
Mid-Diastolic Murmurs					
Mitral stenosis	Cardiac apex	Often soft; begins after opening snap	Low-pitched and rumbling; associated opening snaps; loud S_1	—	Exercise can increase intensity of murmur
Tricuspid stenosis	Half to two-thirds of the way down the left sternal border	Soft; begins after opening snap; increases in intensity during inspiration	Low-pitched and rumbling	—	Almost always associated with mitral stenosis
Increased mitral valve flow: mitral regurgitation, VSD, PDA	Cardiac apex	Short and in mid-diastole	Medium in pitch; often associated with S_3	Murmurs of VSD or PDA or mitral regurgitation	—
Increased tricuspid valve flow: tricuspid regurgitation, ASD	Lower edge of left sternal border	Short and in mid-diastole	Medium in pitch; often associated S_3	Murmurs of ASD or tricuspid regurgitation	—
Pulmonic regurgitation with normal pulmonary arterial pressure	Mid left sternal border	Crescendo-decrescendo and mid-diastolic	Low to medium in pitch; normal or soft P_2	—	—
Late Diastolic Murmurs					
Mitral and tricuspid stenosis (see above)	—	—	—	—	—
Austin Flint murmur (aortic regurgitation)	Cardiac apex	Crescendo and rumbling; occurs just before S_1	Murmur of aortic regurgitation	—	—
Myxoma	Cardiac apex	Crescendo and rumbling; occurs just before S_1	Murmur changes in character and intensity as patient changes position	—	Can be associated with systemic symptoms, e.g., fever, myalgias

Abbreviations: ASD = atrial septal defect, PDA = patent ductus arteriosus, P_2 = pulmonic second sound, S_1 = first heart sound, S_2 = second heart sound, S_3 = third heart sound, VSD = ventricular septal defect.

as a result of increased right-heart venous return during inspiration (see Table 26-2).

Mid-diastolic murmurs also occur when there is a marked increase in flow across the mitral or tricuspid valves. Markedly increased mitral valve flow can occur in patients with mitral regurgitation, ventricular septal defect, or patent ductus arteriosus; markedly increased tricuspid valve flow may be present in patients with tricuspid regurgitation or atrial septal defect (see Table 26-1). Mid-diastolic flow murmurs are medium in pitch (as opposed to the low-pitched murmurs of mitral and tricuspid stenosis) and are often preceded by a third heart sound (rapid filling sound). The Austin Flint (see the following section on late diastolic murmur) murmur is occasionally located in mid-diastole, although it usually occurs in late diastole.

The mid-diastolic murmur of pulmonic regurgitation in the presence of normal pulmonary arterial pressure (usually congenital in origin) is quite different from the murmur of pulmonic regurgitation in the presence of pulmonary hypertension (Graham Steell's murmur). Congenital pulmonic regurgitant murmurs are low to medium in pitch, whereas Graham Steell's murmurs are high-pitched (see Table 26-2). Congenital pulmonic regurgitation produces a mid-diastolic murmur; the murmur that is caused by pulmonary hypertension occurs in early diastole. Congenital pulmonic regurgitation produces a low-pitched murmur because the diastolic pressure gradient between the pulmonary artery and the right ventricle is small, resulting in a low rate of regurgitant flow and a low-pitched murmur. The opposite is true for Graham Steell's murmur. Finally, the murmur of congenital pulmonic regurgitation is crescendo-decrescendo (rising and falling) in intensity (loudness), whereas Graham Steell's murmur is decrescendo (see Table 26-2).

Late Diastolic (Presystolic) Murmurs

Late diastolic murmurs (see Table 26-1 and Fig. 26-1) occur in late diastole when atrioventricular valvular flow is increased by atrial systole (in patients who are in sinus rhythm). Mitral and tricuspid stenosis produce typical crescendo (increasing loudness) presystolic murmurs in patients who are in sinus rhythm. Rarely, patients with mitral stenosis in atrial fibrillation with short cycle lengths also demonstrate the presystolic crescendo murmur. The presystolic murmur of tricuspid stenosis increases in intensity with inspiration, when venous return to the heart increases.

The Austin Flint murmur is almost always presystolic in location and occurs in patients with severe aortic regurgitation (see Tables 26-1 and 26-2). In these patients, the aortic regurgitant jet partially closes the mitral valve during diastole at a time when forward flow across the mitral valve is occurring. The Austin Flint murmur is therefore the result of continuing antegrade flow across a partially closed but otherwise normal mitral valve. The Austin Flint murmur is a rumbling, presystolic murmur that is best heard at the cardiac apex, with the bell of the stethoscope lightly applied to the skin.

Left or right atrial myxomas can obstruct the atrioventricular valves, giving rise to late diastolic (rarely mid-diastolic) murmurs. These murmurs can change markedly in character and intensity as the patient's position is altered, thereby changing the position of the tumor in the orifice of the atrioventricular valve (see Table 26-2).

Diagnostic Approach

In evaluating a diastolic murmur, pay careful attention to the patient's history and noncardiac physical examination. Important clues concerning etiology, severity, and associated abnormalities are overlooked if traditional history taking and physical examination are ignored. For example, does the patient with an aortic regurgitant murmur exhibit other features of Marfan's or Ehlers-Danlos syndrome? Is the patient truly asymptomatic? Is there a history of rejection from military service because of the murmur? Are there associated systemic manifestations of endocarditis or atrial myxoma? Does the patient have a history of acute rheumatic fever? As is the case with systolic murmurs (see Chapter 25, "Systolic Heart Murmurs"), a full understanding of the pathophysiology of a particular murmur can be obtained only after a careful history and physical examination.

Laboratory investigations are often of considerable use in defining the etiology and severity of a diastolic murmur. Electrocardiographic or roentgenographic evidence of cardiac-chamber enlargement is most helpful. For example, electrocardiographic or radiologic left atrial enlargement points to mitral stenosis as the cause of a rumbling, mid-diastolic murmur. Plethoric lung fields in the chest radiograph imply that a mid-diastolic murmur is the result of increased flow across the mitral or tricuspid valve secondary to a large left-to-right shunt. A widened mediastinal shadow in the chest radiograph points toward dissection of the aorta as the cause of an aortic regurgitant murmur. Finally, specialized noninvasive cardiac examinations (echocardiography, pulse tracings, radionuclear ventriculography) can, in selected patients, define the exact site of origin and the severity of the cardiac abnormality that is producing the diastolic murmur. For example, an echocardiographic study can demonstrate quite clearly the stenotic mitral valve that is generating a rumbling, mid-diastolic murmur. Bear in mind, however, that noninvasive testing can be expensive and redundant if ordered before a careful history and physical examination have been obtained.

Continuous Murmurs

Continuous murmurs begin in systole and persist without interruption through S_2 and into diastole (Fig. 26-2). These murmurs often end in mid-diastole; hence, they are not "continuous" in the strictest sense of the word. Continuous murmurs may be the result of benign disturbances in physiologic flow patterns in arteries or veins, or they may be due to abnormal connections between the aorta and the right heart or an artery and a vein.

The most common form of a continuous murmur is the benign venous hum. This murmur is frequently heard in children and is the result of rapid venous blood flow in the great veins of the neck and mediastinum. The hum is often a rough, noisy, high-pitched murmur that is truly continuous; i.e., there is no pause or fading of the hum at mid- or end diastole. The murmur is loudest in the supraclavicular region. The diagnosis is confirmed by abolishing the murmur with digital compression of the right internal jugular vein during auscultation. Continuous murmurs secondary to high blood flow in engorged breast arteries may be heard in an apparently healthy, normal, pregnant woman during routine precordial auscultation. These murmurs, known as mammary souffles, can be easily obliterated by pressing the stethoscope firmly into the breast tissue, thereby briefly compressing the breast arteries that are producing the murmur. They should not be considered pathologic.

Continuous murmurs may also result from severely nar-

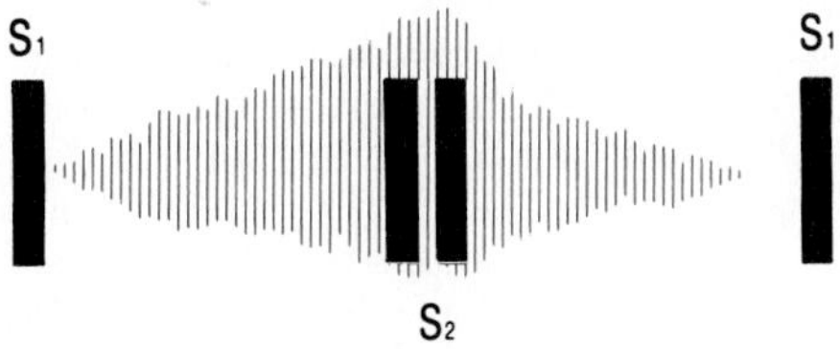

Figure 26-2 Continuous murmur.

rowed systemic or pulmonary arteries. Thus, both coarctation of the aorta and congenital pulmonary arterial branch stenosis can give rise to continuous murmurs heard over the posterior thorax. Similarly, a critically narrowed peripheral artery, e.g., the iliac or femoral artery, can also be the cause of a continuous murmur heard in the region of the arterial stenosis.

The most common cardiac etiology for a continuous murmur is a patent ductus arteriosus. This entity produces a whirring, rough (commonly called "machinery-like") murmur that begins softly during early systole and increases in intensity, reaching its loudest point around the time of S_2. Thereafter, the intensity of the murmur diminishes, ending in mid-to-late diastole. The murmur is often quite localized and can best be heard along the upper left sternal border (second and third intercostal spaces).

Arteriovenous fistulae also produce continuous murmurs that can easily be heard if the stethoscope is placed over the abnormal vascular connection. A common cause for such a murmur is the forearm arteriovenous fistula that is constructed in patients with chronic renal failure for use in hemodialysis. Transient digital pressure on the fistula stops blood flow and obliterates the continuous murmur.

References

Braunwald E. Heart disease: A textbook of cardiovascular medicine. 3rd ed. Philadelphia: WB Saunders, 1988:29.

Constant J. Bedside cardiology. 3rd ed. Boston: Little, Brown, 1985.

Leatham A. Auscultation of the heart and phonocardiography. 2nd ed. New York: Churchill Livingstone, 1975.

Perloff JK. Physical examination of the heart and circulation. Philadelphia: WB Saunders, 1982:171–237.

Shaver JA, Salerni R. Auscultation of the heart. In: Hurst JW, et al, eds. The heart. 7th ed. New York: McGraw-Hill, 1990:175.

27 Syncope

Howard Kirshenbaum, MD

Definition

Syncope is a reversible loss of consciousness of rapid onset due to transient cerebral hypoperfusion. Syncope, commonly known as either "fainting" or "passing out," is distinguished from other types of loss of consciousness by its relative unpredictability, lack of obvious direct relationship to external causes (e.g., heat trauma, drug intoxication), lack of associated symptoms (e.g., seizure activity), and rapid reversibility (i.e., seconds to minutes). Because of the dramatic aspect of "passing out," syncope is generally a frightening symptom, even when clearly of a benign origin.

Etiology

Although there are multiple causes of syncope, many of which have nearly identical presentations, the history alone often provides the correct diagnosis. *Vasovagal syncope,* the common faint, is responsible for the vast majority of syncopal episodes. Vasovagal syncope appears to be due to reflex-mediated dilatation of peripheral arterial beds unaccompanied by a compensatory increase in either heart rate or venous return. The net result is a fall in blood pressure, with transient cerebral hypoperfusion. Vasovagal syncope typically occurs within a clearly apparent environmental backdrop, e.g., in a very hot room, during severe pain, or at the sight of blood.

There are several other benign forms of syncope. *Postmicturition syncope,* found occasionally in otherwise healthy men, occurs at night, immediately after or during voiding. This symptom generally does not recur. *Post-tussive syncope* is found typically in men with chronic pulmonary disease. Dizziness may commonly occur after a paroxysm of coughing in susceptible individuals. Loss of consciousness is much less common, but can be recurrent in certain patients. The mechanism has not been well defined in either postmicturition or post-tussive syncope, but it probably is predominantly a function of reflexes controlling venous blood return to the heart. In post-tussive syncope, increased intracranial pressure may also be a causative factor.

Manual pressure applied to either carotid sinus will normally result in an increase in vagal tone, with a resultant modest slowing of the heart rate and, less commonly, modest drop in blood pressure. *Carotid sinus hypersensitivity* in certain individuals can transform this asymptomatic reaction into syncope or marked dizziness.

Iatrogenic causes of syncope need to be included in the list of generally benign etiologies. Antihypertensive medications (e.g., alpha-methyldopa, prazosin, hydralazine) can cause syncope by an exaggeration of their intended pharmacologic effect, even in proper therapeutic dosages. Rapid changes in posture (supine to standing) will exaggerate the hypotensive effect of these drugs. Less commonly, diuretic drugs, especially the potent loop diuretics, can cause postural syncope due to dehydration. Indeed, hypovolemia of any sort, whether drug induced or secondary to illness (gastrointestinal tract blood or fluid loss, hemorrhage) is a common cause of a notable fall in blood pressure when the patient stands, or even sits, up (see Chapter 24, "Hypotension"). Although syncope can occur, lightheadedness without loss of consciousness is much more common.

Cardiac causes of syncope are common and become progressively more likely as the age of the patient increases. Cardiac etiologies of syncope are never benign; they generally require prompt diagnostic and, if available, therapeutic interventions. Most are distinguished from the previous listing of causes of syncope by the potentially life-threatening nature of cardiac syncope.

Complete heart block, the most common cardiac cause of syncope, is due to transient or irreversible interruption of atrioventricular conduction. Ventricular or junctional escape rhythms (20 to 40 beats per minute) can provide adequate cerebral perfusion, but slower rates or asystole can cause sudden death. Although occasionally congenital, complete heart block is generally related to degeneration of the conduction system (Lenegre's disease) in older individuals or massive myocardial infarction. There are many other far less common causes of complete heart block.

Many arrhythmias can cause syncope. Their causes can be numerous and lie outside the scope of this book; ischemia, valvular disease, cardiomyopathy, congenital heart disease, and drug intoxication (with either legitimate or illicit drugs) can all cause cardiac syncope due to arrhythmia. Infrequently, severe arrhythmias will occur in a person without demonstrable organic heart disease.

Ventricular tachycardia and ventricular fibrillation are the arrhythmias typically associated with syncope and sudden death. Ventricular tachycardia, at heart rates of 100 to over 200, can be asymptomatic or cause syncope owing to poor cerebral perfusion. This rhythm generally reverts to normal spontaneously, but

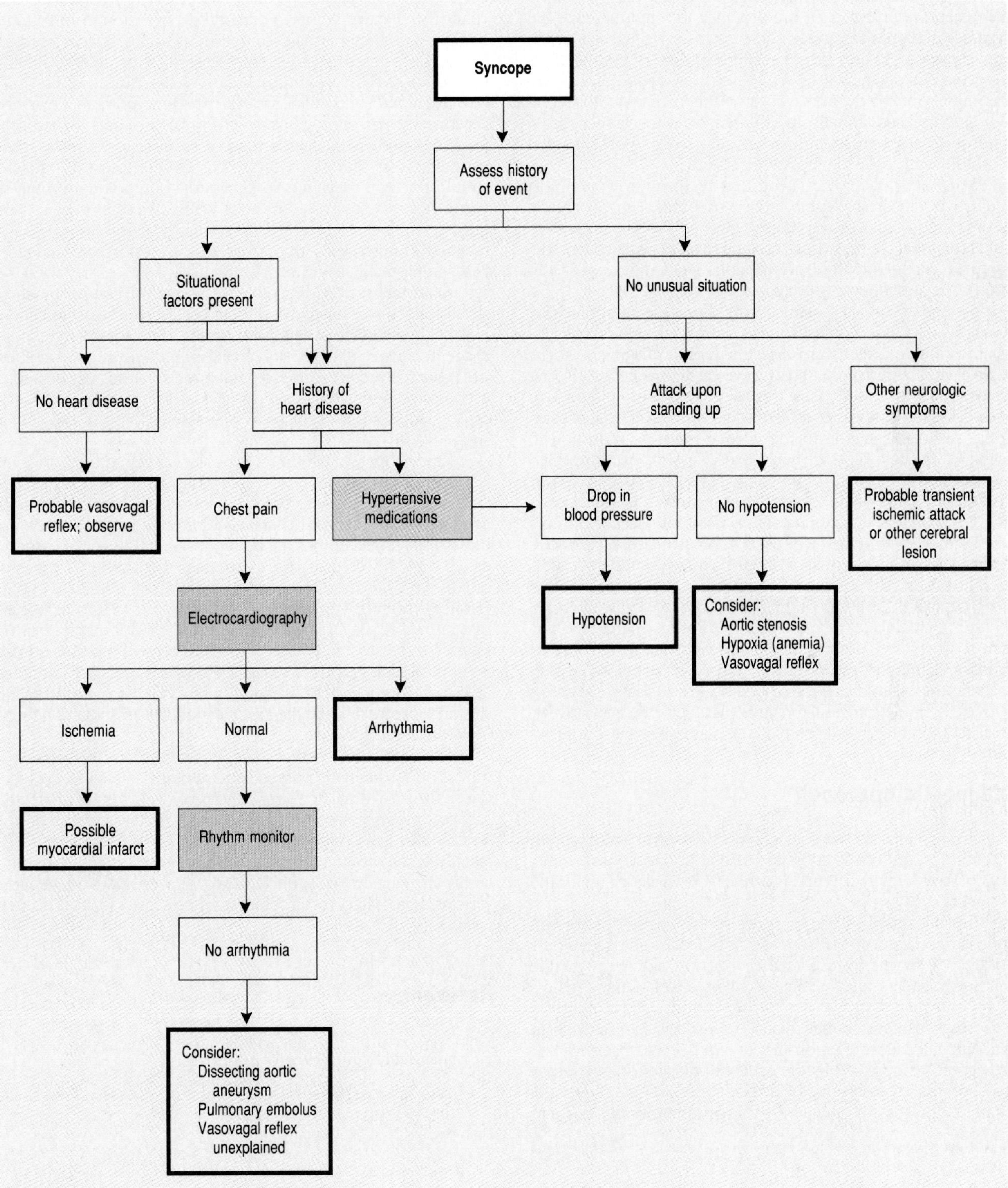

Figure 27-1 Algorithm for the diagnostic evaluation of syncope. (*From* Weisberg LA, Strub RL, Garcia CA. Decision making in adult neurology. Toronto: BC Decker, 1987:243; with permission.)

many patients degenerate to ventricular fibrillation and sudden death. Ventricular fibrillation, i.e., chaotic ventricular activity, is virtually always fatal unless it is terminated by cardiopulmonary resuscitation and electrical defibrillation. Very rarely, ventricular fibrillation reverts spontaneously to an organized cardiac rhythm (e.g., quinidine-induced syncope).

Tachyarrhythmias of atrial origin (atrial fibrillation and flutter) generally do not cause syncope because impulse conduction through the atrioventricular node assumes reasonable stability of ventricular contraction and acceptable cardiac output and cerebral perfusion. In the presence of a muscle tract that bypasses the atrioventricular node, however, ventricular activation at rates of 300 or more beats per minute is possible. Syncope may then occur. The Wolff-Parkinson-White and Lown-Ganong-Levine syndromes can cause this problem. Most commonly diagnosed initially in children or young adults, these syndromes may be asymptomatic or may result in considerable morbidity and, occasionally, sudden death.

Many pharmacologic agents can result in syncope. Most antiarrhythmic drugs (e.g., digoxin, quinidine, procainamide, disopyramide) can cause syncope if given to excess or to susceptible individuals. Other drugs include thyroid replacement, decongestants, theophylline preparations (including excess caffeine), and antihypertensive agents.

Several forms of organic heart disease commonly have syncope as a major manifestation. A careful history and physical examination frequently provide the correct diagnosis. Aortic stenosis and hypertrophic obstructive cardiomyopathy (HOCM, formerly known as IHSS) are the two most common lesions. In both diseases, syncope typically occurs immediately after exertion, presumably owing to the normal transient reduction in filling of the left ventricle after exercise. The hypertrophied myocardium's ability to pump sufficient blood past a fixed or dynamic obstruction is thereby compromised. In both aortic stenosis and HOCM, sudden death is common.

Pulmonic stenosis as well as other congenital lesions associated with pulmonic stenosis will cause syncope; sudden death is rare, however. Malfunction of a prosthetic cardiac valve due to clot or transient jamming of the poppet also can cause syncope. If not immediately fatal, this situation is always a surgical emergency. Much less commonly, left or right atrial myxoma or primary pulmonary hypertension causes syncope. Acute pulmonary embolism, frequent in bed-ridden patients, can cause syncope in rare instances if the embolus is sufficiently massive to obstruct blood flow transiently in the main pulmonary artery.

Diagnostic Approach

In a given patient, the etiology of syncope may be rapidly apparent, may require observation and careful testing for determination, or may remain obscure. Figure 27-1 is an algorithm for the evaluation of syncope.

Initially, the physician must determine whether or not syncope did in fact occur. The presence of head trauma generally points to a concussion rather than syncope, although syncope can precipitate a motor-vehicle accident. A well-defined neurologic abnormality, such as a hemiparesis or dysarthria, indicates a stroke, transient ischemic attack, or postictal state rather than syncope. Elicitation from observers of a history of seizure-like activity or incontinence by the patient implicates seizure rather than syncope as the cause of loss of consciousness. Repeated, multiple episodes of alleged loss of consciousness in a patient behaving bizarrely should raise the possibility that the symptom is hysterical. Light-headedness or loss of consciousness occurring repeatedly 1 to 2 hours after meals can point to reactive hypoglycemia, an early symptom of diabetes mellitus.

If syncope seems likely, and the cardiac monitor has not demonstrated a significant arrhythmia, a careful history and physical examination will provide the correct diagnosis in the majority of patients. Heart rate and blood pressure should be measured, with the patient both supine and standing. A substantial increase in pulse and drop in blood pressure with the change in posture points to postural hypotension from volume depletion; an appropriate cause should then be determined (drug, gastrointestinal bleeding, congenital or acquired autonomic insufficiency). Abnormalities of the carotid artery pulsations (diminished pulse, systolic bruit) can point to a primary cerebrovascular etiology (transient ischemic attack or stroke), but may simply be an aggravating factor of hypoperfusion from another cause. Therefore, the search for the cause of syncope should not stop when a carotid bruit is found. The murmur of aortic stenosis is always ominous when syncope is suspected. Further evaluation must be done promptly. Rarely, the click and murmur of mitral valve prolapse (Barlow's syndrome) may suggest symptomatic ventricular tachycardia.

Other physical findings are less likely to be helpful, but they should always be checked diligently. The rectal examination may be the first clue to a life-threatening gastrointestinal hemorrhage. Extensive diabetic skin changes in the lower extremities can point to syncope caused by diabetic autonomic denervation. A complete neurologic examination is critical in syncope, because evidence for a stroke may be present despite the lack of a suggestive history.

Laboratory evaluation of syncope, except in an obvious example of vasovagal syncope, should always include an electrocardiogram. A complete blood count, electrolytes, and blood drug levels (e.g., digoxin) are also often appropriate. Beyond these tests, however, lies the path of potential financial extravagance. On the cardiac side (generally the class of diagnosis pursued if evaluation has been negative so far) lie the 24-hour (Holter) monitor (up to $300), exercise test ($200), echocardiography ($200), or even cardiac catheterization and electrophysiology study ($2,000 to $4,000+). Neurologically, cranial computed tomography ($300 to $500), electroencephalography ($35 to $50), and cerebral angiography ($1,000) also are expensive and rarely yield the diagnosis if clinical suspicion of neurologic disease is low.

Although all the preceding tests may at times be necessary, they should usually be pursued after an initial syncopal episode only if the physician has a strong index of suspicion for a primary cardiac or neurologic event. If the history, physical examination, and simple tests have not suggested serious pathology, it is usually best to await a second episode of syncope before undertaking an extensive work-up. Most syncopal episodes are benign, vasovagal in origin (even without typical history), and do not recur.

References

Manolis AS, et al. Syncope: Current diagnostic evaluation and management. Ann Intern Med 1990; 112:850.

Weissler AM, et al. Syncope: Pathophysiology, recognition, and treatment. In: Hurst JW, et al, eds. The heart. 7th ed. New York: McGraw-Hill, 1990:581.

Dyspnea

Lewis Dexter, MD

28

Definition

Dyspnea is shortness of breath, and it can be defined as an abnormally uncomfortable awareness of breathing. It is not painful, but it has varying degrees of unpleasantness. It is a symptom elicited by taking the patient's history. Dyspnea is not a physical sign, although tachypnea and labored breathing may at times be observed without the patient complaining of shortness of breath. This chapter describes many types of abnormal breathing patterns of which the patient may or may not be aware.

Mechanism

Dyspnea is purely subjective. Its precise mechanism has eluded extensive investigation. Introspective individuals require less of a stimulus for dyspnea to appear than do extroverts. A number of different mechanisms undoubtedly operate to produce this symptom—receptors in lungs, upper airways, respiratory muscles, and respiratory center, with impulses originating in the vegetative nervous system and modulated by lower central and peripheral vagal pathways. The patient's own awareness of breathlessness originates in the cerebral cortex.

Types of Dyspnea

Exertional Dyspnea and Dyspnea at Rest

Patients describe dyspnea in a variety of ways ("I'm short of breath," "I cannot catch my breath," "I have difficulty getting air in," "I'm smothering," "My chest feels tight," "I feel pressure in my chest," "I feel as though my chest would burst"). Having determined that the patient is describing dyspnea, assessing the circumstances of its occurrence provides information about its significance as well as the severity of the underlying cause.

Dyspnea during exertion is the earliest symptom of left ventricular and pulmonary failure. At first, it occurs with moderately severe exertion, such as jogging, running for a bus, or walking up a steep hill. As the heart failure progresses, dyspnea occurs with less and less exertion. It may progress to the point of being produced by walking slowly on a level surface, necessitating frequent stops. Finally, the patient may become dyspneic at rest, in bed.

A careful history of the preceding progression of dyspnea reflects the progression of deterioration of cardiac or pulmonary function over time and gives an indication of future prognosis. Therapy or cessation of causative factors can interrupt the downward course, however, and dyspnea may be alleviated by further progression of heart failure, i.e., by right ventricular failure. Dyspnea may be made abruptly worse by such complications as a severe infection (e.g., pneumonia), arrhythmias (e.g., atrial fibrillation), or acute myocardial infarction.

Acute Pulmonary Edema

Attacks of acute pulmonary edema are due to the sudden intensification of pulmonary congestion, which is usually a result of failure of the left side of the heart. There is a rapid transudation of fluid out of the pulmonary capillaries into the alveoli.

Acute pulmonary edema may occur in individuals with heretofore normal hearts as a result of acute myocardial infarction, but usually it occurs in individuals with already compromised hearts. Common precipitating factors are sudden increases of blood pressure in hypertensive persons, sudden increases of pulse rate (e.g., arrhythmias), unusual exertion, rapid intravenous infusions of fluid, and a number of causes of sudden failure of valve function, such as rupture of chordae tendineae of the mitral valve.

During the attack of acute pulmonary edema, patients either sit bolt upright or stand. They are anxious, agitated, pale, and drenched with sweat. The skin may be cold, damp, and cyanotic. The respiratory rate is 30 or 40 per minute. All accessory muscles of respiration are used. There may be cough, wheezing, and rattling sounds in the trachea. Sputum may be profuse, pink, frothy, or blood streaked. The lungs contain bubbling rales, rhonchi, and wheezes. These symptoms may subside in 15 minutes or after several hours if left untreated, but they subside much faster when treated.

Orthopnea

Orthopnea is a form of dyspnea in which the patient must assume a sitting position to avoid respiratory distress. He or she sleeps propped up on pillows. When orthopnea is severe, the patient may sit on the side of the bed, with legs hanging down and hands clutching the side of the mattress to aid the accessory muscles of respiration. He or she may move to a chair for the night.

Orthopnea is a manifestation of advanced heart or pulmonary failure. The sitting position relieves dyspnea by lowering the diaphragm and by creating, in a sense, an internal phlebotomy (redistribution of blood to the lower extremities).

Paroxysmal Nocturnal Dyspnea

Paroxysmal nocturnal dyspnea usually occurs an hour or two after the patient has gone to bed and fallen asleep. The patient awakens with shortness of breath and anxiety. The breathing is often asthmatic (cardiac asthma). To obtain relief, the patient sits up in bed or on the side of the bed, with feet hanging down. He or she may open the window "to get more air." In mild cases, relief is obtained in a few minutes. In more severe attacks, respiratory distress may persist for an hour or two. With the return of breathing to normal, the patient usually has an undisturbed sleep for the rest of the night. In the most severe cases, the patient feels he or she is dying and is desperately trying to catch his or her breath. Breathing is asthmatic, bubbling, and gurgling. Sounds from fluid in the lung are clearly audible, and sputum may be pink and frothy or blood streaked. Occasionally, the attack is fatal.

The cause of the acute attack is that the patient is already on the borderline of pulmonary edema. In going to sleep in the recumbent position, there is a shift of fluid from the lower extremities to the upper, including the lung. The result is an increase of pulmonary capillary pressure and pulmonary edema. Being asleep, the patient does not notice the appearance of dyspnea until it is of moderate severity. He or she awakens in pulmonary edema and its syndrome of paroxysmal nocturnal dyspnea.

Cardiac Asthma

Cardiac asthma is asthmatic breathing in patients with heart disease. It is not allergic in origin. It is caused by congestion of the bronchial mucosa from heart failure. It frequently occurs during attacks of paroxysmal nocturnal dyspnea and, at other times, during attacks of pulmonary edema. It is often seen in patients with severe mitral stenosis, in whom it is likely to be mistaken for bronchial asthma because of the difficulty of hearing the mitral diastolic murmur in a noisy "asthmatic" chest.

Cheyne-Stokes Respiration

This periodic breathing waxes and wanes in depth and is marked by periods of apnea and hyperventilation. In the typical case, respirations are at first imperceptible, but then a gradual and rhythmic increase of respiratory excursions to normal, followed by deeper and deeper respirations, is observed. They then slowly subside until apnea recurs. Apneic periods may last for a few seconds to a minute or more. This crescendo-diminuendo cycle of breathing occupies up to 2 or 3 minutes. During the apneic period, the patient may become drowsy, cyanotic, and twitchy. In the hyperpneic phase, he or she may become agitated and frightened.

Cheyne-Stokes respiration is seen in patients with severe left ventricular failure; in patients with central nervous system disease, such as brain-stem disease; in patients receiving narcotics; and in normal individuals at high altitude, before they have adapted to the change in altitude.

Trepopnea and Platypnea

Trepopnea is dyspnea occurring in one lateral decubitus position, but not in the other. Platypnea is dyspnea occurring in the upright but not in the recumbent position. These breathing patterns are both too rare and too poorly understood to warrant further discussion.

Other

Other types of abnormal breathing patterns are seen in brain-stem disease. Central neurogenic hyperpnea consists of very rapid, deep respirations. In apneustic breathing, there is a pause of 2 to 3 seconds after a full inspiration. Biot's respiration consists of irregular periods of apnea that alternate with four or five respirations of identical depth. Ataxic breathing is chaotic with respect to both rate and depth.

Causes of Dyspnea

The most common causes of dyspnea are heart failure and pulmonary failure. There are a few other miscellaneous causes.

Heart

Cardiac dyspnea is due to the accumulation of fluid in the lungs. In left ventricular failure, myocardial contraction becomes impaired. By the Frank-Starling mechanism, the left ventricular diastolic pressure becomes elevated, with equal rises of pressure in the left atrium, pulmonary veins, and pulmonary capillaries. When the hydrostatic pressure in the pulmonary capillaries exceeds oncotic pressure of plasma (25 to 30 mm Hg), transudation of fluid from capillaries to alveoli takes place. Pulmonary congestion stimulates respiration by way of the Hering-Breuer reflex mediated by the vagus nerve. Cardiac dyspnea has a panting quality. Respirations are rapid and shallow.

Lung

Compromise of lung function leads to dyspnea. There is, however, a large respiratory reserve. Pneumonectomy, for example, does not produce dyspnea at rest or during heavy exercise in otherwise normal patients. A host of diseases afflict the lung, but there are too many to be discussed here. This section outlines salient points regarding dyspnea of pulmonary origin.

Obstructive Disease of Airways

Large airway obstruction produces a type of dyspnea (stridor) that is distressing. Acute obstruction is due to aspiration of food or foreign body, angioneurotic edema of the glottis, or infection of the epiglottis (epiglottitis). In the first case, relief is often obtained by the Heimlich maneuver; in angioneurotic edema, by the injection of epinephrine; in the last, with appropriate antibiotics. Chronic obstruction is due mainly to tumors and to fibrotic stricture of the trachea following tracheostomy or endotracheal intubation.

Obstruction of intrathoracic airways produces another type of dyspnea—asthmatic wheezing. In an acute asthmatic attack, the patient sits upright, using all accessory muscles of respiration, and complains of being unable to get air in, although the real problem is to get air out. In severe attacks, the patient is cyanotic and fearful, feeling that he or she is going to smother.

Chronic bronchitis and bronchiectasis are inflammatory disorders that wax and wane, and are accompanied by cough, expectoration of purulent sputum, and, depending on their severity, a wheezing dyspnea on exertion and, in advanced cases, at rest.

Emphysema

Emphysema is a slowly progressive disorder in which many years of exertional shortness of breath progress to dyspnea at rest and finally to orthopnea.

Diffuse Parenchymal Lung Disease

There are innumerable parenchymal lung diseases, varying from pneumonia to sarcoid to tumors to a wide variety of pneumoconioses. Each has its own distinctive clinical behavior. Suffice it to say that all are capable of producing dyspnea, depending on the extent to which the lungs have become involved.

Disease of Chest Wall and Respiratory Muscles

Kyphoscoliosis is the principal example of chest deformity producing dyspnea. Weakness and paralysis of respiratory muscles can lead to respiratory failure. One previously common example was poliomyelitis. Various myopathies and neuropathies can produce respiratory failure when respiratory muscles are sufficiently impaired.

Pulmonary Vascular Occlusive Disease

Principal causes are mitral stenosis, pulmonary embolism, intracardiac left-to-right shunts, and an idiopathic type. In all of these, dyspnea on exertion is the first complaint. As the vascular obstruction increases, dyspnea worsens. Terminally, it is agonizing. Lung volumes and arterial P_{O_2} are usually normal. P_{CO_2} is low as a result of hyperventilation.

Miscellaneous Causes of Dyspnea

Anxiety may give rise to frequent sighing respirations, and it may also produce episodes of bizarre hyperventilation, with very rapid irregular breathing, during which the patient appears to be hysterical and may show symptoms and signs of tetany during the acute attack, e.g., tingling around the mouth, spasm of muscles in hands, and a positive Chvostek's sign.

The hyperventilation of acidemia (e.g., diabetic acidosis), characterized by deep breathing, does not usually lead to a complaint of dyspnea by the patient, although there are exceptions.

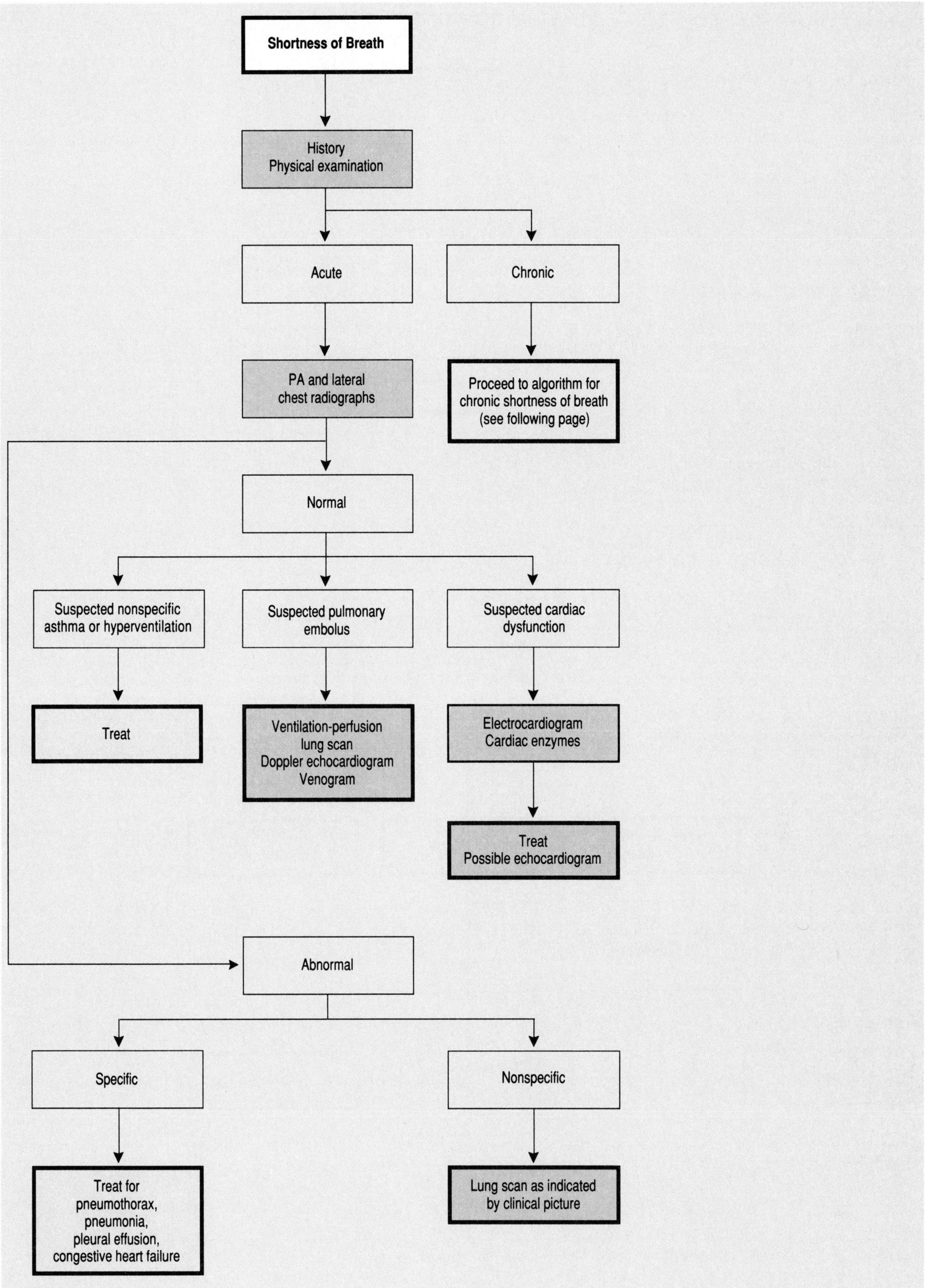

Figure 28-1 Algorithm for the evaluation of the patient with shortness of breath. (*From* Scott WW, Scott PP. Consultation in diagnostic imaging. Toronto: BC Decker, 1985:41; with permission.)

Figure continues on following page

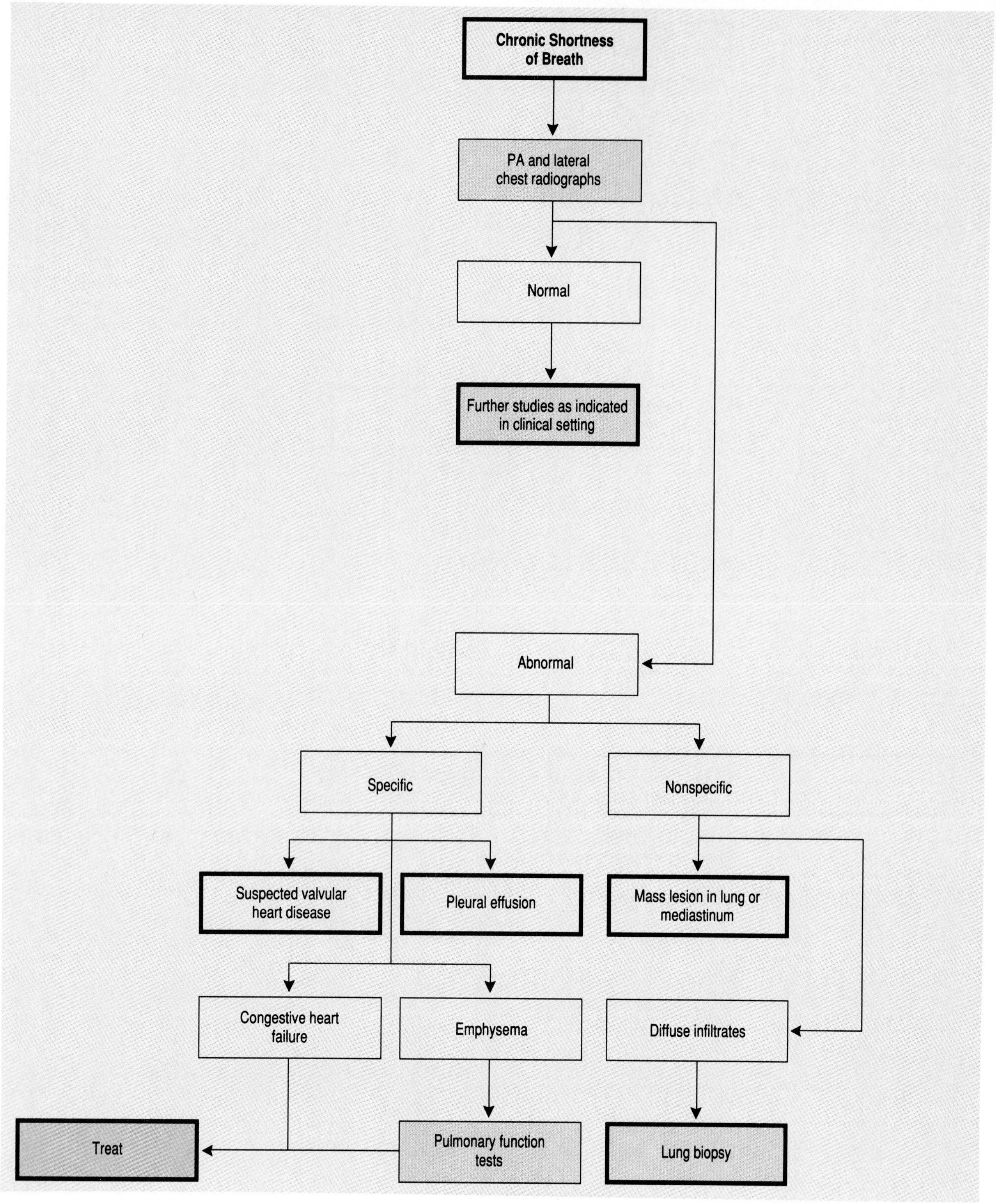

Figure 28-1 *Continued*

Severe anemia from blood loss (hematocrit in the 20s) produces exertional dyspnea.

Pregnancy

Hyperventilation during pregnancy elevates the arterial Po_2—a mechanism for maximally oxygenating the fetus. Low serum protein concentration and a tendency to retain fluid lead to edema, even pulmonary edema in mothers with perfectly normal hearts. All of this, plus the weight of the uterine contents, leads to exertional dyspnea, especially in the later months. One might think that lung volumes become reduced as pregnancy advances, but quite the contrary, they increase.

Physical Conditioning

A change from regular physical activity to a sedentary occupation results in poor muscular conditioning in a few months. The individual may complain of shortness of breath during an exertion that previously produced no dyspnea. This is seen not infrequently in students going from college to medical school and even more so in individuals going from medical school to internship.

Diagnostic Approach to a Dyspneic Patient

Because most dyspneic patients have heart or lung disease, the chief problem is to decide which of the two is responsible (Fig. 28-1). Usually history (including smoking history, environmental and occupational exposures, and cardiac risk factors), physical examination, and a radiograph of the chest are all that is needed. At times, however, the problem may be difficult. If, in such cases, the clinical problem is not too pressing, a therapeutic trial to correct heart failure may be instituted (salt restriction, digitalis, diuretics). If the patient was in heart failure, one would anticipate a weight loss of more than 4 or 5 pounds and simultaneous improvement in breathing. Such a regimen would not improve dyspnea of pulmonary origin.

Pulmonary function tests do not do a good job of differentiating cardiac from pulmonary etiologies. In cardiac failure, there is a reduction of vital capacity, total lung capacity, diffusion capacity, and compliance. Pulmonary function tests are, of course, of great value in patients with pulmonary disease.

Cardiac function tests for the determination of the cause of dyspnea might include electrocardiography, for arrhythmias and ischemia; Holter monitoring, for arrhythmias; echocardiography, if valvular disease is suspected; and cardiac catheterization, if corrective cardiac surgery is being considered.

References

Braunwald E. Clinical manifestations of heart failure. In: Braunwald E, ed. Heart disease. A textbook of cardiovascular medicine. 3rd ed. Philadelphia: WB Saunders, 1988:471.

Fishman AP. A first approach to the patient with respiratory signs and symptoms. In: Fishman AP, ed. Pulmonary diseases and disorders. New York: McGraw-Hill, 1980:3.

Gold W. Dyspnea. In: Blacklow RS, ed. MacBryde's signs and symptoms. 6th ed. Philadelphia: JB Lippincott, 1983:335.

Hurst JW, et al. The history: Symptoms and past events related to cardiovascular disease. In: Hurst JW, et al, eds. The heart. 7th ed. New York: McGraw-Hill, 1990:122.

Rees PJ, Clark TJH. Paroxysmal nocturnal dyspnea and periodic respirations. Lancet 1979; 1315.

Schlant RC, Sonnenblick EH. Pathophysiology of heart failure. In: Hurst JW, et al, eds. The heart. 7th ed. New York: McGraw-Hill, 1990:387.

Fever

Richard H. Glew, MD

Definition

For centuries, fever has been recognized as a sign of disease. Physiologically, fever represents a disturbance in normal thermoregulation in which there is an upward shift of the body's temperature setpoint as the body actively seeks to elevate its temperature.

Pathophysiology

Fever results when phagocytic leukocytes, in response to pyrogenic substances such as infectious agents, immunologic mediators, or toxic agents, release a protein known as endogenous pyrogen, which then interacts with specialized receptors in the thermoregulatory center of the anterior hypothalamus, ultimately resulting in shivering and vasoconstriction, thereby raising the body's temperature (Fig. 29-1). An individual's normal or baseline temperature varies with time of day (lowest on arising in the morning), activity (exercise), physiologic events (ovulation), and habits (smoking). Elderly patients tend to have lower baseline temperatures and often produce less impressive fever response to pyrogenic stimuli than younger patients—hence the clinical aphorism, "the older, the colder."

Lacking a facile criterion for normal human temperature, it is difficult to state a simple definition of fever. Moreover, the several methods of recording body temperature vary in their accuracy and reliability. When properly obtained with a standard glass mercury thermometer (good lip and tongue seal and left in place for several minutes) or when an electronic thermometer is employed, oral temperature recordings should produce values approximately equal to simultaneous rectal temperature readings. On the other hand, it is this author's experience that axillary temperatures are too unreliable to be recommended for common use. In most clinical settings, rectal temperatures are preferred because of optimal accuracy and reliability.

Carefully obtained oral or rectal temperature should be assumed to indicate fever when a reading of 38°C (100.4°F) is obtained. Furthermore, concern should be raised in the patient, particularly the elderly, in whom serial recordings over several days demonstrate a loss of normal diurnal periodicity, such that the morning nadir (usually to 37°C or 98.6°F or lower) is absent. For clinicians who are not fluent in metric-English conversions, it is helpful to memorize a few convenient equivalents (Fig. 29-2). Remember that patients with chronic renal failure or congestive heart failure, as well as patients at both extremes of age, may fail to mount a fever during illnesses usually associated with a febrile response. Moreover, numerous drugs can act as antipyretics, including salicylates, acetaminophen, nonsteroidal anti-inflammatory agents, corticosteroids, and quinine.

Etiology

Although infections generally are considered to be the most common causes of febrile reactions, fever frequently occurs in many noninfectious illnesses, including collagen vascular diseases (e.g., systemic lupus erythematosus, rheumatoid arthritis, Reiter's syndrome, vasculitides), hypersensitivity reactions (e.g., to medications, blood products), neoplastic diseases (especially lymphomas, primary and secondary tumors of the liver, and renal cell carcinoma), hemorrhage (especially retroperitoneal, subarachnoid, and intra-articular bleeding), microcrystalline arthritis (e.g., gout, pseudogout), and thromboembolic disease (e.g., thrombophlebitis, pulmonary embolism). Nevertheless, given the virulence but treatability of many microbial diseases, the examining physician is wise to assume that fever in the critically ill patient is due to infection until extensive diagnostic efforts have failed to document an infectious etiology.

Unfortunately, in most diseases capable of producing fever, the characteristics of the fever curve are of little or no help in suggesting the etiology of the fever. Even the four human malarias, known for their classic tertian or quartan periodicity, usually produce hectic, persistent fevers early in the course of infection in travelers from nonendemic areas such as North America. Moreover, although frank rigors are suggestive of bacterial infection, chills may also be seen in patients with nonbacterial diseases, including viral illnesses, protozoal infections (such as malaria), drug reactions, and inflammatory diseases.

Diagnostic Approach

The first priority in the evaluation of a patient with fever is to determine the degree of urgency suggested by the clinical presentation. A febrile patient who presents with a brief history of a rapidly evolving illness and who appears toxic and acutely ill warrants an urgent diagnostic evaluation, leading to prompt therapeutic intervention, in order to prevent a morbid or even fatal outcome from an acute, fulminant disease. In contrast, the chronically ill patient who describes a prolonged, lingering illness, with either unremitting fever or recurrent episodes of fever (commonly termed fever of unknown origin) is unlikely to exhibit a precipitous clinical deterioration or present a quick and easy solution as to etiology of the fever. Accordingly, in the patient with subacute-to-chronic presentation, the diagnostic approach should be more prolonged and meditative, with therapy delayed until a diagnosis is certain, in order to avoid further obscuration of the clinical picture by administration of antimicrobial agents. Despite these differences, similar areas of investigation are included in the history and physical examination of the acutely or chronically febrile patient.

History

Host Factors. Determine whether the febrile patient is predisposed to infections that are likely to be fulminant or fatal, and therefore must be detected and treated urgently: (1) gram-negative bacteremia in the patient with severe alcoholism, malignancy, or neutropenia; (2) *Staphylococcus aureus* bacteremia or endocarditis in the parenteral drug abuser, the hospitalized patient with indwelling plastic intravenous cannulas, or the patient on hemodialysis; and (3) fulminant bacteremia (usually

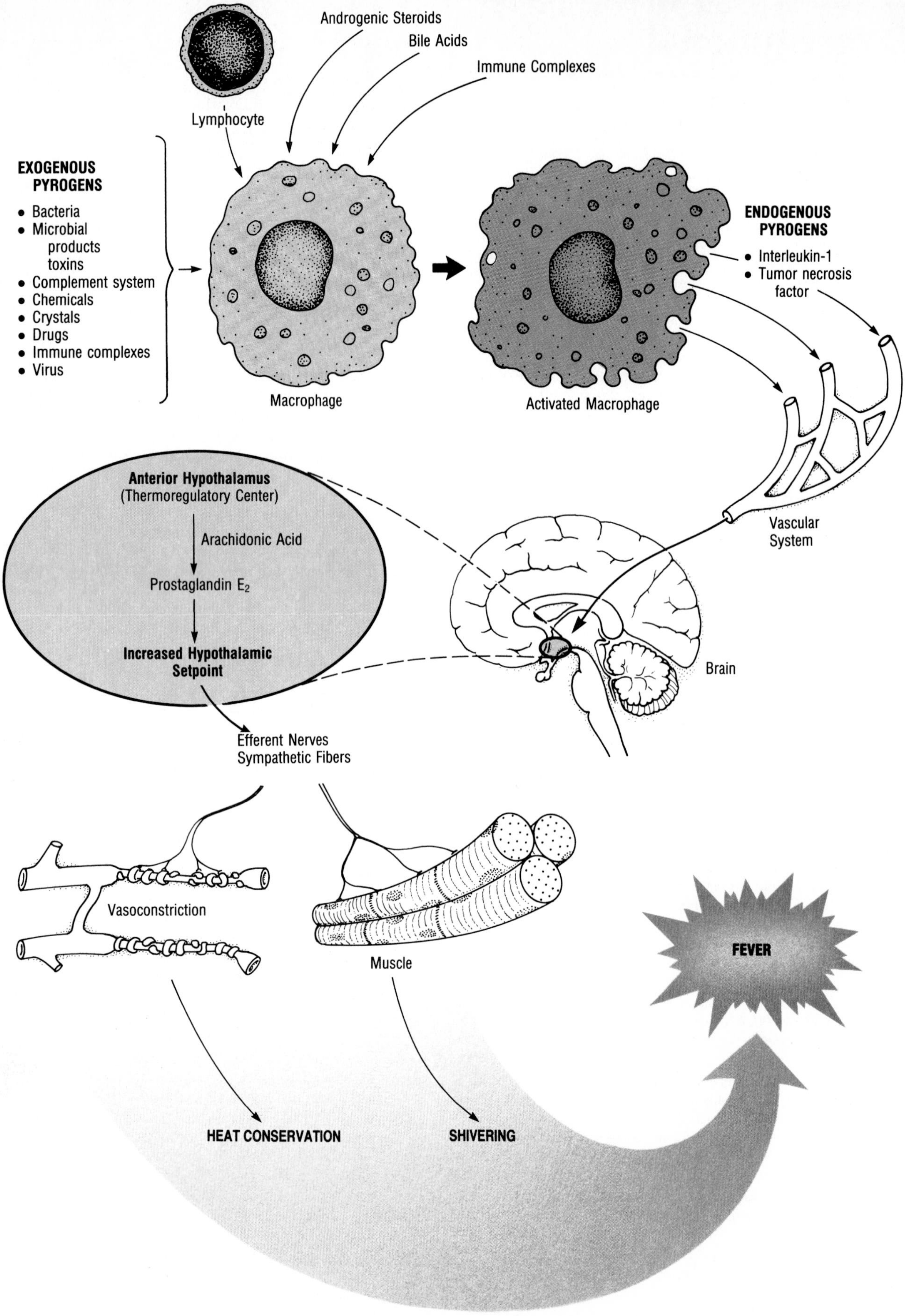

Figure 29-1 The pathogenesis of fever. (After Dinarello CA, Cannon JG, Wolff SM. New concepts on the pathogenesis of fever. Rev Infect Dis 1988; 10:168; with permission.)

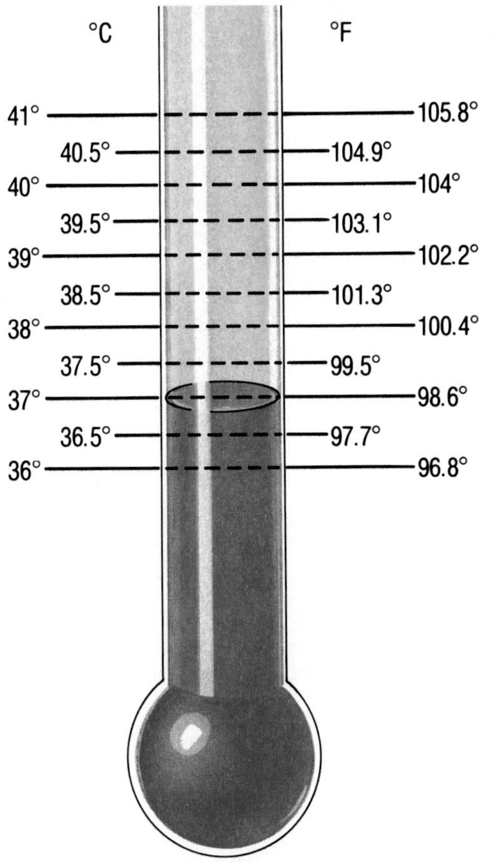

Figure 29-2 Celsius-Fahrenheit temperature conversions.

due to *Streptococcus pneumoniae, Haemophilus influenzae,* or *Neisseria meningitidis*) in the patient splenectomized surgically or spontaneously (due to a hemoglobinopathy, such as sickle cell disease). Serious infections commonly occur in other conditions, including (1) bacterial peritonitis in cirrhotic patients and in patients on chronic peritoneal dialysis; (2) pneumococcal peritonitis in children with nephrotic syndrome; (3) bacterial meningitis (usually due to *Streptococcus pneumoniae*) in patients with cerebrospinal fluid rhinorrhea or otorrhea; (4) pyelonephritis in patients with deranged urinary tract anatomy or dynamics, including neurogenic bladder, prostatic obstruction, indwelling Foley catheter, or nephrolithiasis.

Over the past decade, patients immunosuppressed as a result of infection with human immunodeficiency virus (those with acquired immunodeficiency syndrome or AIDS-related complex) have raised additional concerns in this area. These patients are susceptible to a variety of infections that can present subacutely or fulminantly owing to etiologic agents that span all of microbiology, including viruses, bacteria (common and uncommon), fungi, and protozoa (Table 29-1).

Mortality Factors. Is the patient's ability to tolerate various infections impaired by chronic medical conditions such as coronary artery disease, congestive heart failure, or chronic obstructive pulmonary disease? Does the patient have a medical illness known to be deleteriously affected by infection, including sickle cell disease, diabetes mellitus, or adrenal insufficiency? Positive answers to such questions should impart a sense of urgency to the evaluation of the patient.

Epidemiology (Table 29-2). Inquire about recent or past exposure to diseases via (1) travel to exotic lands as well as within

Table 29-1 Causes of Fever in Patients Immunosuppressed Owing to HIV-1 Infection

Neoplasia
Non-Hodgkin's lymphoma
Kaposi's sarcoma with liver involvement

Infections
Viral
- Cytomegalovirus—disseminated, enteritis, encephalitis
- Herpes simplex virus—extensive mucocutaneous lesions
- Varicella zoster virus—disseminated

Bacterial
- Pyogenic bacteria (*Haemophilus influenzae, Streptococcus pneumoniae*)—pneumonia, sinusitis, bacteremia
- *Salmonella* species—recurrent bacteremia
- *Listeria monocytogenes*—bacteremia, meningitis
- *Mycobacterium avium-intracellulare*—disseminated
- *Mycobacterium tuberculosis*—disseminated

Fungal
- Mucosal infection—*Candida* species, *Aspergillus* species
- Dissemination—*Cryptococcus neoformans, Histoplasma capsulatum, Coccidioides immitis*

Protozoal
- *Pneumocystis carinii*—pneumonia
- *Toxoplasma gondii*—encephalitis, disseminated
- *Cryptosporidium* species—enteritis

Table 29-2 Epidemiologic Clues in the Febrile Patient

Travel in the United States
Southwest: Coccidioidomycosis
Midwest (Ohio, Mississippi River Valleys): Histoplasmosis
Atlantic Coast states: Rocky Mountain spotted fever
Northeast Coast and islands: Babesiosis; Lyme disease (also Minnesota, Wisconsin, California)
Northern mountainous regions: Giardiasis

Foreign travel

Malaria	Amebiasis
Typhoid	Giardiasis
Brucellosis	Dengue
Hepatitis (A or B)	Leishmaniasis
Relapsing fever (borreliosis)	

Vocation/Habits/Diet
Dogs: Leptospirosis
Cats: Toxoplasmosis
Hiking: Rocky Mountain spotted fever, giardiasis
Hunting: Tularemia, Lyme disease
Abattoir (slaughterhouse) work: Brucellosis
Undercooked or raw meat: Toxoplasmosis, trichinosis, brucellosis
Raw milk: Toxoplasmosis
Raw eggs: Salmonellosis
Male homosexual: Hepatitis B, amebiasis, acquired immunodeficiency syndrome
Parenteral drug user: Hepatitis B, infective endocarditis, osteomyelitis/pyarthrosis, acquired immunodeficiency syndrome
Menstruation/tampon use: Toxic shock syndrome

Fellow Travelers (Family, Community Outbreaks)
Mycoplasma pneumoniae infection
Influenza
Enteroviral illnesses
Group A streptococcal illnesses (pharyngitis, scarlet fever, cellulitis)

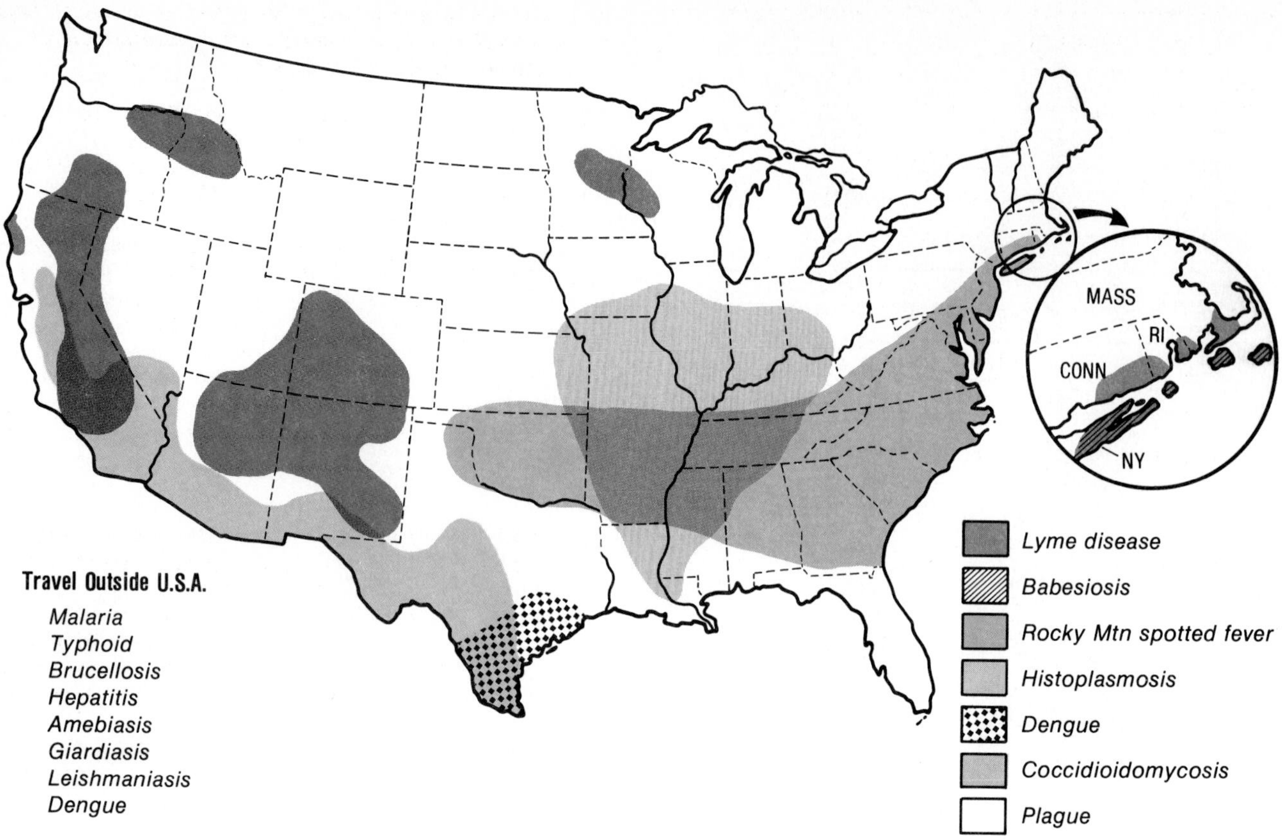

Figure 29-3 Infectious causes of fever in the United States.

temperate regions (Fig. 29-3), (2) occupations, (3) avocations, (4) unusual dietary habits, (5) exposure to animals, and (6) illnesses in family members and the local community.

Localization of Symptoms (Table 29-3). The site of infection or inflammation in a patient may be highlighted by focal complaints and may be referable to localized pain, organ dysfunction, or organ irritability. These leads should be pursued early in the evaluation of the febrile patient. Unfortunately, many febrile, systemic illnesses, including generalized viral illnesses and severe bacterial infections (endocarditis and protozoan infections), are marked by apparently spuriously localizing complaints, such as low back pain, arthralgias, headache, and abdominal pain.

Temporal Sequence. A careful history of the temporal evolution of symptoms and signs may provide useful clues. For example, the patient who presents with pain due to gonococcal pyarthrosis commonly relates a history of several days of antecedent migratory polyarthralgias and is noted to have acrally distributed, papulopustular skin eruptions, with or without a history of symptoms of prior or ongoing genital gonorrhea.

Physical Examination

The physical examination of the febrile patient begins with the skin and mucous membranes, including conjunctivae, oropharynx, and the anogenital region. Primary infection of the skin (e.g., cellulitis) may be detected. There may be integumentary evidence of disseminated infection (Fig. 29-4): (1) the petechial rash of meningococcemia or Rocky Mountain spotted fever, (2) embolic lesions of endocarditis, and (3) palpable purpura or necrotic papules of systemic vasculitis. Alternatively, exanthemas may reflect disease due to toxins (such as occur with scarlet fever and toxic shock syndrome) or immunologic mechanisms (drug reactions, collagen vascular diseases, vasculitis). Although the childhood exanthematous diseases produce rather classic eruptions in children, these can be simulated in adults by infections due to viruses (infectious mononucleosis) and spirochetes (secondary syphilis), or manifested in unusual or muted fashion in patients with prior immunization (atypical measles).

Direct particular attention to areas highlighted in the history. Careful examination should always be conducted of the chest, heart, and abdomen. Examination of the musculoskeletal system includes a search for local tenderness, warmth, swelling, or erythema, as well as manipulation of all accessible joints for presence of effusions or restriction of motion. A diligent search must be carried out for localized or generalized lymphadenopathy. Moreover, in the acutely ill, febrile patient, examination of the tympanic membranes, teeth, genitalia, rectum, and pelvis, as well as a neurologic assessment, should not be deferred, because one may stumble upon unsuspected causes of fever, including periapical dental abscess, sinusitis, otitis media, epididymitis or prostatic abscess, or pelvic inflammatory disease.

Laboratory Studies

General Approach. No laboratory test is routine in the evaluation of a febrile patient. In addition, the rate and extent of laboratory utilization should be determined by several factors, including (1) severity and acuteness of the patient's condition, (2) presence of debilitating or compromising underlying diseases, (3) occurrence of symptoms that require specific investigation (dysuria or flank pain, dictating urinalysis and urine cul-

Table 29-3 Localizing Symptoms

Symptoms	Possible diseases
Headache, stiff neck	Meningitis, brain abscess, encephalitis, central nervous system vasculitis, sinusitis, mycoplasma pneumonia, rickettsial infections
Sore throat	Parapharyngeal or retropharyngeal abscess, streptococcal pharyngitis, infectious mononucleosis, epiglottitis
Cough, tachypnea, chest pain	Pneumonia, pulmonary embolism, tuberculosis, lung abscess, esophageal rupture
Right upper quadrant pain	Hepatitis, cholecystitis, liver abscess, subdiaphragmatic abscess, right lower lobe pneumonia
Lower abdominal pain	Diverticulitis, appendicitis, pelvic inflammatory disease
Back pain	Pyogenic vertebral osteomyelitis, Potts' disease, epidural abscess, pyelonephritis, retroperitoneal abscess, endocarditis
Dysuria/frequency	Cystitis, pyelonephritis, urethritis, prostatitis
Constipation	Pyelonephritis
Diarrhea	Bacterial or amebic dysentery, pericolonic abscess, mesenteric ischemia, pseudomembranous (antibiotic-associated) colitis, inflammatory bowel disease, diverticulitis, gonococcal proctitis
Localized bone or joint pain, joint swelling, immobility	Osteomyelitis, pyarthrosis, inflammatory arthritis, Reiter's syndrome

ture; cough, sputum production, or pleurisy, suggesting the need for a chest radiograph), (4) physical findings that establish a virtually certain diagnosis with little need for laboratory assistance (classic measles in an unvaccinated child, typical herpangina in a child, or typical dermatomal shingles due to herpes zoster), and (5) the likelihood that presumptive antibiotic therapy will be instituted before the diagnosis is confirmed. Because antibiotics may inhibit the growth of bacteria from subsequent blood cultures, at least two blood cultures should be obtained before instituting antibiotic therapy in certain outpatients (e.g., patients with organic valvular heart disease who are about to be given oral antibiotics for a febrile illness and who may be harboring bacterial endocarditis) and in virtually all hospitalized patients acutely ill enough to warrant parenteral antibiotic therapy.

A low threshold should be maintained for sampling abnormal collections of fluid (pleural and joint effusions and ascites) for examination and culture. More difficult is the question of whether or not to perform a lumbar puncture. Although headache may occur in many febrile illnesses without direct central nervous system involvement, cerebrospinal fluid should be sampled immediately in (1) patients with fever and severe headache, fever and altered mental status, or fever and stiff neck; (2) the febrile ill patient whose sensorium is difficult to interpret, such as infants and the demented; and (3) the patient with altered mental status and cutaneous manifestations compatible with disseminated bacterial infection.

Special Considerations in the Acutely Ill In-patient. The appearance of fever in a hospitalized patient not recently evaluated for fever merits at least a modest initial battery of laboratory tests, including white blood cell count with differential count, urinalysis, and chest radiograph. Two blood cultures, obtained from separate venipunctures, plus a mid-stream clean-catch or catheterized urine specimen should be sent for culture. As discussed earlier, the need for paracentesis and lumbar puncture is dictated by appropriate clinical indications. Patients with an endotracheal tube as well as any patient with cough or dyspnea should be sampled for a deep sputum specimen for Gram stain and culture. Abdominal findings may suggest the need for liver chemistries, amylase, and abdominal imaging, such as radiographs, ultrasonography, or computed tomography (CT) scanning.

Fever of Unknown Origin. Fever of unknown origin (FUO) generally is defined as an illness of at least 3 weeks' duration, with fever (temperature greater than 101°F, or 38.3°C, on several occasions), and no established diagnosis after 1 week of investigation. Application of these criteria will eliminate from study most self-limited pyrexic illnesses of viral or indeterminate etiology and will allow many pyrogenic diseases to declare themselves.

Evaluation of the patient with an FUO requires a structured, meticulous approach. Although the classic, lengthy list of differential diagnoses should be kept in mind, it is prudent to begin with a more limited, stratified list of possible etiologies that are ranked according to certain principles.

First, keep in mind that the primary categories of disease responsible for most cases of FUO are (1) infections, including generalized infections such as the various forms of tuberculosis, endocarditis, and the infectious mononucleosis syndrome (Epstein-Barr virus, cytomegalovirus, toxoplasmosis), as well as localized pyrogenic infection, such as abscesses; (2) neoplasia, especially the lymphomas, carcinoma of the liver, colon, or kidney, or tumors associated with obstruction or perforation; and (3) inflammatory diseases, including medication reaction, collagen vascular diseases such as systemic lupus erythematosus and rheumatoid arthritis, and the various vasculitides, such as giant cell arteritis and Wegener's granulomatosis.

Second, Sutton's law ("go where the money is") dictates that one first pursue diagnoses suggested by the epidemiologic history, past medical history, evolution of the present illness, or by the presence of abnormalities detected by the physical examination or routine laboratory studies.

Third, consider risk-benefit factors. It is judicious to pursue most aggressively those diagnoses that are (1) most immediately fatal or morbidly destructive if appropriate treatment is delayed or if confounding nonantibiotic therapy (e.g., corticosteroids) is to be begun; (2) most easily and efficaciously treated once diagnosed; and (3) diagnosable by the least dangerous or unpleasant tests. For example, in an elderly woman with underlying rheumatic valvular heart disease who presents with several weeks of unexplained fever and weight loss, the diagnosis of infective endocarditis should take precedence over lymphoma, because the former diagnosis may be confirmed simply by blood cultures, whereas entertaining the latter can generate large expenses and iatrogenic morbidity in laboratory testing, including biopsies or even exploratory laparotomy. Fortunately, the abdominal CT scan has largely replaced laparotomy in searching for occult abscess or tumor in the patient with an enigmatic FUO.

Finally, remember that the least expensive and most pleasant diagnostic test available is the careful, thorough, compassionate history and physical examination conducted anew.

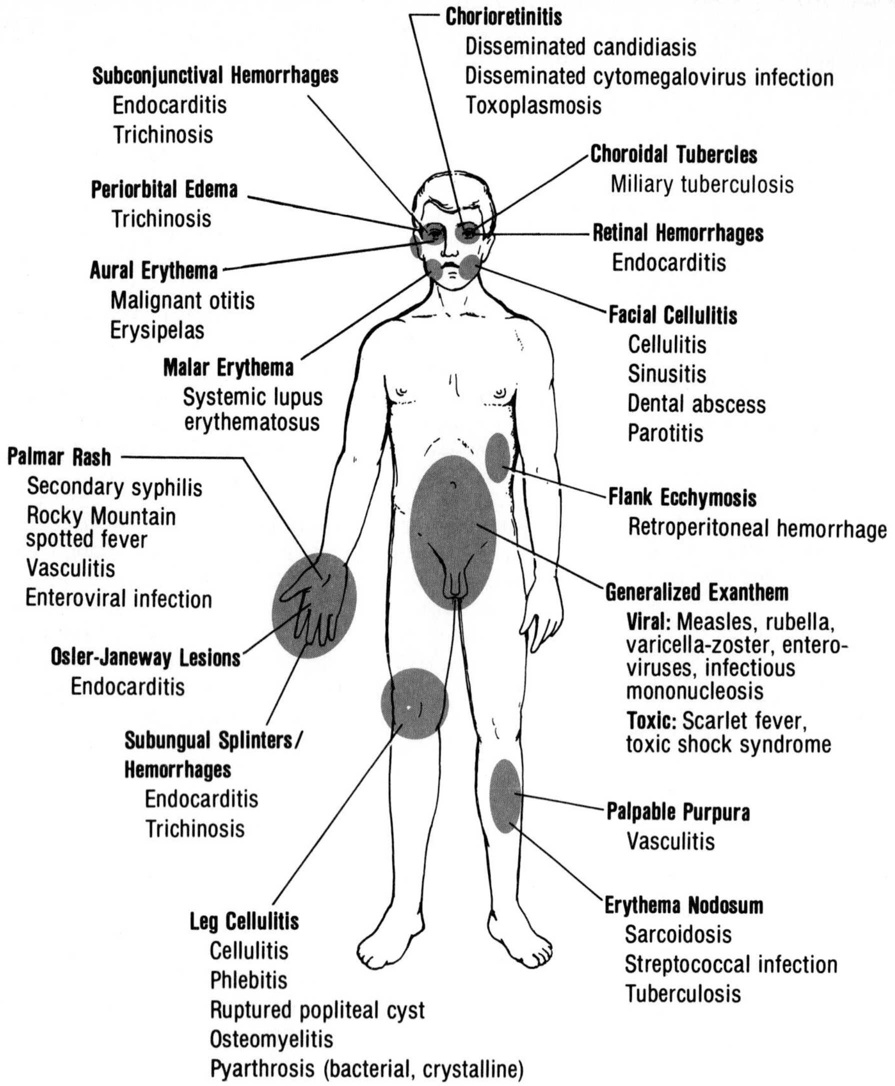

Figure 29-4 Integumentary evidence of disseminated infections.

References

Bernheim HA, Block LH, Atkins E. Fever: Pathogenesis, pathophysiology and purpose. Ann Intern Med 1979; 91:261.

Dinarello CA, Cannon JG, Wolff SM. New concepts on the pathogenesis of fever. Rev Infect Dis 1988; 10:168.

Fauci AS, Haynes BF, Katz P. The spectrum of vasculitis: Clinical, pathologic, immunologic, and therapeutic considerations. Ann Intern Med 1978; 89:660.

Gleckman RA, Esposito AL. Fever of unknown origin in the elderly: Diagnosis and treatment. Geriatrics 1986; 41:45.

Glew RH. The acute infectious disease syndrome. In: Conn HF, Conn RB Jr, eds. Current Diagnosis 6. Philadelphia: WB Saunders, 1980:6.

Jacoby GA, Swartz MN. Fever of undetermined origin. N Engl J Med 1973; 289:1407.

Larson EB, Featherstone HJ, Petersdorf RG. Fever of undetermined origin: Diagnosis and follow-up of 105 cases, 1970–1980. Medicine 1982; 61:269.

McGowan JE Jr, et al. Fever in hospitalized patients with special reference to the medical service. Am J Med 1987; 82:580.

Petersdorf RG, Beeson PB. Fever of unexplained origin. N Engl J Med 1961; 40:1.

Seligmann M, et al. Immunology of human immunodeficiency virus infection and the acquired immunodeficiency syndrome: An update. Ann Intern Med 1987; 107:234.

Steere AC. Lyme disease. N Engl J Med 1989; 321:586.

Weinstein MP, et al. The clinical significance of positive blood cultures: A comprehensive analysis of 500 episodes of bacteremia and fungemia in adults. I. Laboratory and epidemiologic observations. Rev Infect Dis 1983; 5:35.

Weinstein MP, et al. The clinical significance of positive blood cultures: A comprehensive analysis of 500 episodes of bacteremia and fungemia in adults. II. Clinical observations, with special reference to factors influencing prognosis. Rev Infect Dis 1983; 5:54.

Fatigue

Francis J. Gilroy, MD

30

Definition

Fatigue is a commonly stated or implied complaint that brings the patient to a physician's attention. Often the patient does not use the word *fatigue* but uses a synonym such as "all-in," "exhausted," "all used up," "run down," or "just plain weak." Fatigue can be a normal and physiologic consequence of physical and mental exertion (Table 30-1). When physiologic, it is usually relieved by an appropriate period of physical or mental rest. Because it is sometimes difficult to distinguish physiologic or appropriate fatigue from pathologic fatigue, it is often helpful to quantify in detail the patient's stresses and activities as well as the recuperative attempts.

Etiology

Although fatigue may be a symptom of most illnesses, several studies have shown that the major cause of chronic fatigue as an isolated symptom is psychologic. If the patient has both psychologic and physiologic reasons for fatigue, attention to both of these mechanisms will allow a more productive diagnostic approach and therapeutic outcome.

Diagnostic Approach

The history is often the most helpful tool in diagnosing the etiology of fatigue. The first priority is to confirm that the symptom in question is truly fatigue, and not weakness, paresis, paralysis, or another problem that would require a separate and distinct diagnostic approach. Documentation of the amount of exertion and rest that the patient describes should be compared with what he or she thinks was done previously and what could be done if he or she were feeling better. The extent to which the fatigue has altered the patient's life and that of his or her family may offer clues to why the symptom has become prominent.

Although some patients "overuse" the term *fatigue,* others avoid the term, even when it is a significant symptom. This most often occurs when patients with several symptoms assume that the fatigue is an expected corollary of their symptoms. An unfortunate example of this is the fatigued geriatric patient with depression or anemia who does not seek medical evaluation because of a belief that the fatigue is a result of aging. Such an approach delays or avoids the appropriate diagnostic work-up.

Although fatigue as a manifestation of psychologic problems is often an isolated symptom, patients with fatigue of psychologic origin often have associated symptoms. These may include nervousness, irritability, insomnia, muscle tension, headaches, difficulty in concentrating, sexual disorders and maladjustments, loss of appetite, curtailment of social involvements, or decrease in job performance. With further questioning, the patient may complain of boredom, lack of interest in the environment, a monotonous or routine lifestyle, or a sense of being "trapped" in an unpleasant life situation. Insomnia, in spite of fatigue, and awakening feeling more tired than before retiring are frequent complaints. Fatigue may relate to specific events, such as a grief reaction to the death of a spouse or other relative, or to a medical illness or surgical procedure. Financial insecurity or sudden translocations of social contacts can produce anxiety, depression, and dissatisfaction with life situations, which may manifest themselves as fatigue. Each patient undergoes a series of disappointments and frustrations in life. The physician must know enough about the patient's lifestyle to be able to evaluate the extent to which the fatigue is an emotional problem (see Chapter 140, "Anxiety," and Chapter 142, "Depression").

The many organic diseases that produce fatigue can usually be identified by history and physical examination (Table 30-2).

Heart disease associated with a decrease in cardiac output, inadequate tissue perfusion, and oxygenation results in generalized fatigue and lowered tolerance of exertion. Valvular heart disease, coronary artery disease, or cardiomyopathy may cause the patient to seek medical attention because of fatigue. Many patients with moderate or advanced degrees of chronic pulmonary insufficiency complain of fatigue or weakness in addition to dyspnea. Usually such patients have significant hypoxia, carbon dioxide retention, and abnormal pulmonary function tests. Fatigue is especially common in patients with pulmonary disease associated with polycythemia or cor pulmonale.

Patients with azotemia and uremia often complain of fatigue, especially when the blood urea nitrogen (BUN) is greater than 50 mg/dl. Unfortunately, the fatigue is sometimes not relieved by hemodialysis or peritoneal dialysis. Fatigue may be associated with anemia, necessitating additional investigations for a source of blood loss or other cause of anemia. Fatigue is more commonly a presenting sign of anemia when the anemia is chronic in onset. A more acute drop in hemoglobin may be associated with fatigue, but commonly has other symptoms.

Although most acute infectious diseases are accompanied by fatigue, other symptoms of the process are generally more prominent. The following infectious diseases commonly have fatigue as a prominent symptom, sometimes persisting for protracted periods: infectious mononucleosis, cytomegalovirus disease, acquired immunodeficiency syndrome (AIDS), hepatitis, and influenza. Significant fatigue may also occur in the prodromal stage of tuberculosis or rheumatic fever, but as the disease

Table 30-1 Diagnostic Grouping of 300 Patients Complaining of Lethargy

Diagnostic group	Number of cases
No organic cause found	187 (62.3%)
Infection or postinfection	38 (12.7%)
Circulatory disorders	28 (9.3%)
Iatrogenic	15 (5%)
Endocrine disorders	15 (5%)
Anemia	11 (3.7%)
Uremia	3 (1%)
Others	3 (1%)

From Jarrett WA. Lethargy in general practice. Practitioner 1981; 225:731; with permission.

becomes more overt, fever and more obvious symptoms and signs usually develop.

Endocrine disease is a common cause of fatigue of organic origin. Although hypothyroidism is commonly associated with fatigue, hyperthyroidism also may present with fatigue, particularly in the elderly. Other manifestations are usually present, but in the elderly they may be inconspicuous and require astute questioning, careful physical examination, and a high index of suspicion. Appropriate laboratory procedures may be needed to confirm the clinical suspicion. Adrenal insufficiency may present initially with fatigue, which may be present for long periods before weight loss, hypotension, skin pigmentation, and more classic symptoms and signs appear. Although diabetes mellitus commonly presents with a triad of polydipsia, polyphagia, and polyuria, onset is sometimes insidious, with fatigue as the initial symptom. Non–insulin-dependent diabetes in older patients may present with fatigue as a major complaint, with neither the traditional triad nor significant weight loss. Testing of blood and urine samples for hyperglycemia and glycosuria may be necessary to arrive at the proper diagnosis. Hypercalcemia, although less common, may also be accompanied by fatigue. Symptoms and physical findings may be minimal and subtle or easily overlooked, i.e., muscle weakness, anorexia, nausea, or constipation. As the patient worsens, confusion, stupor, or coma demands more searching investigation and treatment. Hypopituitarism may also produce fatigue, usually resulting from secondary deficits of thyroid and adrenal hormones.

Patients with primary muscular diseases may present with the complaint of fatigue, which, on close questioning, is more accurately found to be weakness or even varying degrees of paralysis. Myasthenia gravis is characterized by weakness with repetitive motions and usually is confirmed by an edrophonium test, with or without electromyographic testing. Polymyositis is characterized by weakness of proximal muscle groups, an elevated sedimentation rate, and elevated levels of creatine phosphokinase and aldolase. Various muscular dystrophies produce muscular weakness that may cause the patient to complain of fatigue. Patients with neurologic disorders such as amyotrophic lateral sclerosis, multiple sclerosis, and periodic paralyses may present with the initial complaint of fatigue, whereas paresis or paralysis is the actual problem.

Nutritional deficiencies can be responsible for complaints of fatigue, but they are usually associated with other findings. Alcoholism, food faddism, and ill-advised diets can result in varying degrees of malnutrition that result in easy fatigability. The role of vitamin deficiency in production of fatigue is not entirely clear at present, but it is being re-examined.

Unexplained fatigue can be seen in the presence of occult

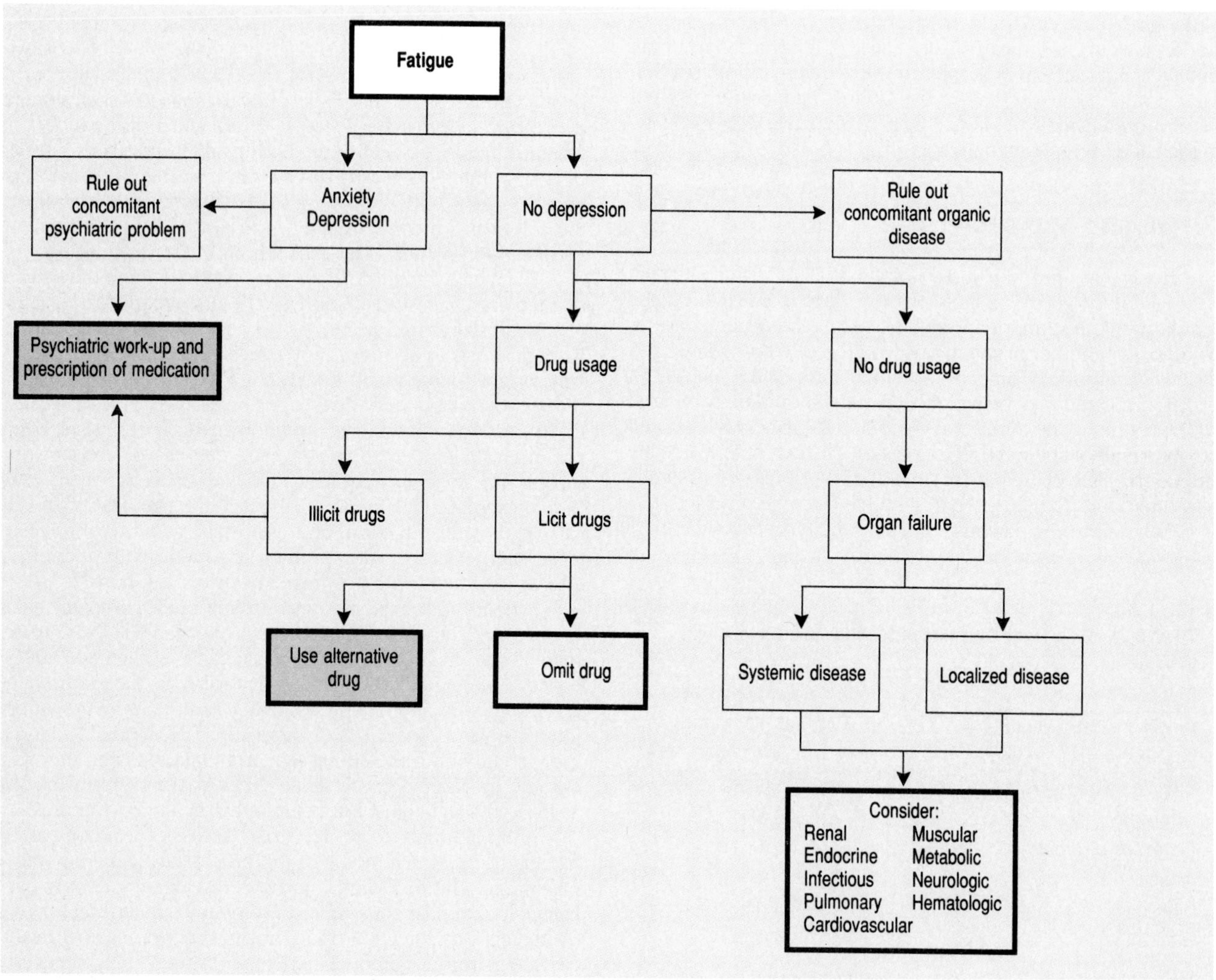

Figure 30-1 Algorithm for the diagnostic approach to fatigue.

Table 30-2 Diseases That May Be Associated with Fatigue

Malignancy	Chronic psychiatric disease and medications
Autoimmune disease	Endogenous depression
Localized infection	Hysterical personality disorder
Occult infection	Anxiety
Chronic or subacute bacterial disease	Neurosis
Endocarditis	Schizophrenia
Lyme disease	Tranquilizers
Tuberculosis	Lithium
Fungal disease	Antidepressive medications
Histoplasmosis	Chronic inflammatory disease
Blastomycosis	Sarcoidosis
Coccidioidomycosis	Wegener's granulomatosis
Parasitic disease	Chronic hepatitis
Toxoplasmosis	Neuromuscular disease
Amebiasis	Multiple sclerosis
Giardiasis	Myasthenia gravis
Helminthic infestation	Endocrine disease
Human immunodeficiency virus (HIV) infection	Hypothyroidism
Drug dependency and abuse	Addison's disease
Alcohol	Cushing's syndrome
Controlled prescription drugs	Diabetes mellitus
Illicit drugs	Other known or defined chronic disease
Side effects of chronic medication	Pulmonary
Other toxic agents	Cardiac
Chemical solvents	Gastrointestinal
Pesticides	Hepatic
Heavy metals	Renal
	Hematologic disease

From Holmes GP, et al. Chronic fatigue syndrome: A working case definition. Ann Intern Med 1988; 108:387; with permission.

malignant tumors. Usually weight loss, anorexia, malnutrition, or anemia is present, but at times, the initial complaint is fatigue without other overt findings. Fatigue may be associated with the production of an ectopic hormone by a malignant tumor.

In searching for an explanation for the sole complaint of fatigue without other evidence of disease, it is important to question the patient carefully regarding use of licit or illicit drugs. Antihistamines, tranquilizers, sedatives, many antihypertensives, opiates, and hallucinogens are widely used and commonly produce fatigue. Beta-blocking drugs are also commonly associated with fatigue.

Figure 30-1 presents an algorithm of the diagnostic approach to fatigue.

Summary

In summary, fatigue is a symptom capable of being produced by a wide variety of illnesses. Identification of the etiology of the fatigue requires careful history taking and physical examination. Quantification of changes in activity level over time may offer the most important diagnostic clue. The need for laboratory studies is generally dictated by the signs and symptoms that accompany the complaint of fatigue.

References

Adams RD. Anxiety, depression, asthenia, and personality disorders. In: Petersdorf RG, et al, eds. Harrison's principles of internal medicine. 10th ed. New York: McGraw-Hill, 1983:68.

Goroll AH, May LA, Mulley AG. Evaluation of chronic fatigue. In: Goroll AH, May LA, Mulley AG, eds. Primary care medicine: Office evaluation and management of the adult patient. 2nd ed. Philadelphia: JB Lippincott, 1987:25.

Holmes GP, et al. Chronic fatigue syndrome: A working case definition. Ann Intern Med 1988; 108:387.

Jarrett WA. Lethargy in general practice. Practitioner 1981; 225:731.

Manu P, Lane TJ, Matthews DA. The frequency of the chronic fatigue syndrome in patients with symptoms of persistent fatigue. Ann Intern Med 1988; 109:554.

Minden SL, Reich P. Nervousness and fatigue. In: Blacklow RS, ed. MacBryde's signs and symptoms. 6th ed. Philadelphia: JB Lippincott, 1983:615.

Weight Loss

George H. Eypper, MD

31

Unexplained significant involuntary weight loss is frequently a clue that a patient has serious disease. The importance of this symptom is supported by the observation that approximately one-fourth of such patients die within a year of their initial evaluation.

Definition

A useful working definition for involuntary weight loss is the loss of 5 percent of usual body weight over the previous 6 months, documented by medical records. If medical documentation is unavailable, patients may be considered to have significant weight loss if two of the following three criteria are met: (1) change in clothing (including belt) size, (2) verification of weight loss by a friend or relative, (3) ability to give a numerical estimate of weight loss. It is useful as well as cost efficient to document the patient's story carefully because weight loss cannot be verified in up to one-half of patients presenting with this symptom.

Approximately one-third of patients with weight loss identify this symptom as their chief complaint. The remainder may present with other symptoms such as pain, weakness, pulmonary complaints, a change in bowel habits, neuropsychiatric problems, fevers, sweats, chills, nausea, vomiting, dysphagia, early satiety, or other complaints, but a clue to the seriousness of their illness is loss of weight.

Etiology and Pathogenesis

Although weight loss is a symptom of a great many diseases, those that present with weight loss as an initial symptom representing a diagnostic problem form a much smaller subset. These diseases are listed by pathophysiologic mechanism in Table 31-1. A number of diseases cause weight loss by more than one mechanism and therefore appear more than once in the table. Several causes of involuntary weight loss warrant further discussion.

Cancer

In addition to mechanical obstruction of the gastrointestinal tract by tumor, malignancy also can cause weight loss by poorly understood mechanisms such as those producing anorexia. For example, it has been postulated that some cancers elaborate humoral factors that act on the hypothalamus to decrease appetite. Also, alterations in taste, including an aversion to meat, are often encountered. Lastly, some patients with occult malignancy become depressed, and this can contribute to the anorexia. Decreased intake alone, however, does not always account for the degree of weight loss. It is thought that decreased efficiency of glucose utilization resulting from insulin resistance, increased Cori cycle activity, and increased gluconeogenesis account in part for this discrepancy.

Drugs

Many medications lead to impaired nutrient intake for a variety of reasons. Some of the more common are outlined here. Digoxin in toxic doses may produce anorexia, nausea, and finally vomiting by direct stimulation of the chemoreceptor trigger zone on the floor of the fourth ventricle in the medulla. Nonsteroidal anti-inflammatory drugs, theophylline, quinidine, and procainamide, even with nontoxic blood levels, may produce nausea. Angiotensin-converting enzyme inhibitors may alter taste and smell. Tricyclic antidepressants, diuretics, and clonidine may cause dry mouth, making swallowing difficult. Weight loss resulting from amphetamine use is due almost entirely to inhibition of the feeding center of the hypothalamus. Alcohol may inadequately replace normal food intake. Numerous other medications may serve to decrease intake in individual patients.

Cardiac Cachexia

Advanced congestive heart failure is associated with an increased metabolic rate secondary to increased work of breathing and increased levels of circulating catecholamines. Reduced cardiac output leads to tissue hypoxia, which in turn forces an increased percentage of energy production to occur via the less efficient anaerobic pathways. Increased venous pres-

Table 31-1 Pathophysiologic Classification of Weight Loss

Decreased Intake	
Anorexia	Cancer, depression, anorexia nervosa, alcoholism, cardiac cachexia, chronic obstructive pulmonary disease, drugs (theophylline, digoxin, amphetamines, angiotensin-converting enzyme inhibitors), pyloric obstruction (peptic ulcer, gastric cancer), uremia, Addison's disease, AIDS-related syndromes
Nausea	Drugs (theophylline, digoxin, nonsteroidal anti-inflammatory drugs, quinidine, procainamide), pyloric obstruction (peptic ulcer, gastric cancer), diabetic gastroparesis, uremia, Addison's disease
Dysphagia	Pharyngeal motor disorder (due to stroke, Parkinson's disease, myasthenia gravis), esophageal obstruction (carcinoma, peptic stricture, web), esophageal motor disorder (achalasia, scleroderma), drugs causing dry mouth (tricyclic antidepressants, diuretics, clonidine)
Discomfort worsened by food	Poor dentition, ill-fitting dentures, odynophagia due to peptic esophagitis, chronic pancreatitis, intestinal angina, esophageal or gastric cancer, aspiration of food, minor degrees of chronic diarrhea or fecal incontinence
Social/adjustment reaction	See text
Loss of Nutrients	
Vomiting	See under Nausea; also bulimia
Maldigestion	Pancreatic insufficiency
Malabsorption	Many causes, including Crohn's disease
Increased motility	Laxative abuse, hyperthyroidism, dumping syndrome
Loss in urine	Uncontrolled diabetes mellitus
Other	Gastrointestinal losses of blood and protein, as seen in inflammatory bowel disease
Increased Energy Expenditure	
Hypermetabolism	Hyperthyroidism, chronic inflammatory disease (rheumatoid arthritis, ulcerative colitis, Crohn's disease), chronic infection (tuberculosis, abscess), chronic obstructive pulmonary disease, cardiac cachexia, amphetamine abuse, pheochromocytoma
Decreased metabolic efficiency	Cancer, diabetes mellitus

sure produces congestion in the mesenteric vascular bed. Anorexia and low-grade malabsorption ensue. The net result is weight loss, ultimately including myocardial atrophy and worsening of the heart failure. Keep in mind that weight loss secondary to therapeutic diuresis should not be attributed erroneously to cardiac cachexia.

Chronic Obstructive Pulmonary Disease

Severe airway obstruction causes increased work of breathing. Sympathomimetics and bronchodilators contribute to increased adrenergic tone. The result is hypermetabolism, but this may be compensated for by increased food intake. Acute exacerbations of chronic obstructive pulmonary disease produce anorexia, despite the increased metabolic rate, causing rapid weight loss during illness. This weight is often not completely regained before the next exacerbation.

Hyperthyroidism

In hyperthyroidism there are multiple mechanisms of weight loss whose relative contributions are unclear. Elevated amounts of thyroid hormone have been shown to increase membrane sodium-potassium ATPase activity as well as membrane uptake of multiple metabolic substrates. Although both protein synthesis and catabolism occur more rapidly, catabolism predominates. Fat degradation and oxidation are increased. Mitochondria appear to be stimulated directly to consume more oxygen and to form more ATP. The net result of these processes is greater energy utilization and loss of weight. In addition, low-grade fat malabsorption, probably due to faster gastrointestinal motility, contributes to the weight loss.

Diabetes Mellitus

In uncontrolled diabetes mellitus, relative or absolute insulin deficiency, together with glucagon excess, results in increased catabolism of fat and protein and loss of weight. This is compounded by loss of calories in the form of glucose in the urine. Weight loss is aggravated by dehydration resulting from the osmotic diuresis produced by the glycosuria.

Inflammatory Bowel Disease

Widespread inflammation in ulcerative colitis and Crohn's disease produces hypermetabolism. Food may worsen symptoms in both diseases, causing fear of eating. Loss of blood and inflammatory exudate in the stool contribute to the negative caloric balance. In addition, Crohn's disease may produce carbohydrate malabsorption resulting from disaccharidase deficiency caused by inflammation. Lymphatic obstruction leads to fat malabsorption. Ileal disease causes impaired resorption of bile acids, leading to a decrease in the body's bile salt pool. This impairs micelle formation and worsens the fat malabsorption.

Psychosocial Causes

Depression is the psychologic problem most frequently cited as a cause of involuntary weight loss. In addition, dementia may cause weight loss because of concomitant depression, decreased sense of smell, various degrees of aspiration, and patients' decreased ability to feed themselves. However, adjustment reactions may be even more important, especially in the outpatient population. These may be impossible to diagnose unless an adequate functional and social history is taken. Examples may include insufficient income to buy adequate food, inability of a widower to prepare meals, lack of transportation to the store, and difficulty walking once at the store. Patients with only mild degrees of chronic diarrhea or fecal incontinence may purposefully limit their intake in order to minimize their symptoms. These problems become obvious only after the right questions have been asked.

Multifactorial Causes

Frequently, a given patient may have a combination of physical or psychosocial problems that, taken together, cause weight loss. The relative frequencies of various diagnoses causing weight loss are outlined in Table 31-2. It is worth pointing out that although cancer was a common diagnosis, only two truly occult malignancies were noted among the 439 patients studied.

Diagnostic Evaluation

A diagnostic strategy for evaluating patients with involuntary weight loss has been elucidated (Fig. 31-1). The three studies cited in the reference section all agree that patients with serious physical disease can almost always be identified quickly and easily. The key to rapid and cost-effective diagnosis is a careful history and physical exam, including a thorough review of sys-

Table 31-2 Frequencies of Involuntary Weight Loss in Different Populations

Cause	Marton and Sox VA hospital Male in-patients Mean age = 59 yr *n* = 91 Prospective study	Weinstein Medical center Outpatients M:F = 1:1.3 Mean age = 54.6 yr *n* = 117 Prospective study	Rabinowitz Israeli in-patients M ≅ F Mean age = 64 yr *n* = 154 Retrospective study	Wiley Medical center Outpatients M:F = 1:2 Mean age = 77 yr *n* = 67 Retrospective study
Physical total	65*	30	66	66
Cancer	19	7	36	
Gastrointestinal	14	9	17	—
Endocrine	4	4	4	—
Drugs/alcohol	10	4	0	—
Other	22	5	9	
Nonphysical total	35	70	34	22
Psychiatric	9	61	10	—
Unknown	26	9	23	19

* All frequencies are percents. Figures may total more than 100% because some patients had more than one diagnosis.

Constitutional

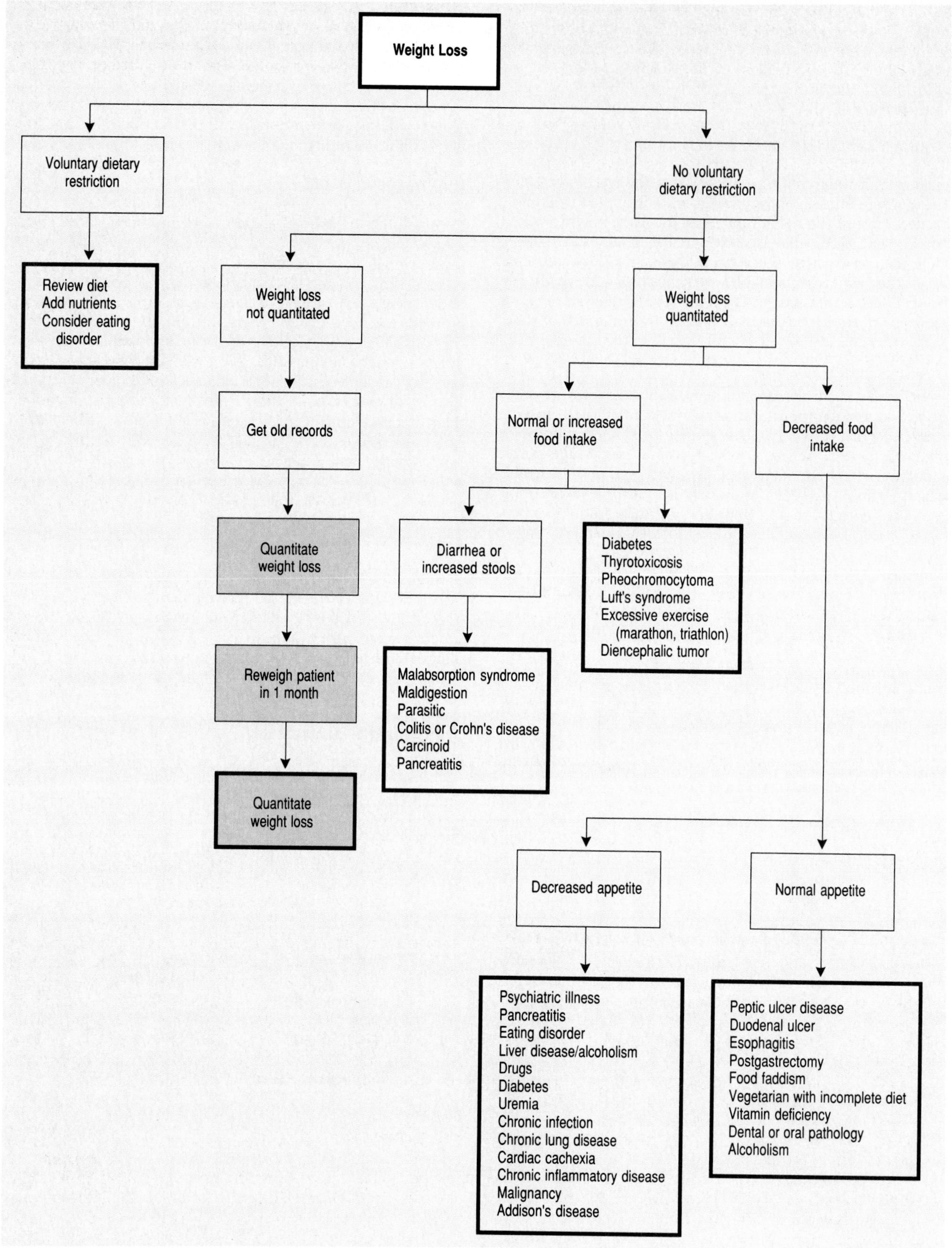

Figure 31-1 Algorithm for determining cause of weight loss.

tems, a careful drug history, a functional assessment, and an active search for psychosocial causes. The history and physical should be supplemented by a complete blood count, urinalysis, SMA-12, chest radiograph, and three stool specimens for occult blood.

If there is a physical cause for involuntary weight loss, clues are almost always present on the initial evaluation, which will focus further work-up and direct the ordering of subsequent studies leading to the correct diagnosis. If no clues are found, a reasonable next step is to review the chest radiograph again with a trusted radiologist, because incorrectly read chest radiographs delayed diagnoses in two of the three studies mentioned. If the work-up for physical causes remains negative at this point, there is a high likelihood that a nonphysical cause is present. Psychiatric disorders and decreased functional ability should be treated, and the patient should be followed over time. There is no evidence that further testing is warranted unless indicated by the finding of specific abnormalities among the tests already mentioned. In particular, nondirected ordering of contrast radiographs of the bowel and abdominal imaging studies in order to look for occult malignancies do not improve diagnostic outcome and do not save lives.

In conclusion, the diagnostic evaluation for physical causes of involuntary weight loss is straightforward. If it proves negative, the examiner should follow the patient with attention directed toward treatment of psychiatric, social, and functional causes. These nonphysical causes appear to be especially important among the ambulatory population. Occult malignancy is not a frequent cause of isolated involuntary weight loss in the ambulatory care population. Therefore, routine use of a nonfocused, nondirected approach to search for malignancy is not justified.

References

Braunwald E. Harrison's principles of internal medicine. 11th ed. New York: McGraw-Hill, 1987:175 (weight loss), 427 (cancer), 909 (cardiac cachexia), 911 (digoxin toxicity), 1769 (Addison's disease).

Marton KI, Sox HC, Krupp JR. Involuntary weight loss: Diagnostic and prognostic significance. Ann Intern Med 1981; 95:568.

Rabinovitz M, et al. Unintentional weight loss. Arch Intern Med 1986; 146:186.

Sleisenger MH, Fordtran JS, eds. Gastrointestinal disease. 4th ed. Philadelphia: WB Saunders, 1989:185 (anorexia), 200 (dysphagia), 488 (hyperthyroidism), 495 (diabetic gastroparesis), 708 (dumping syndrome), 932 (pyloric obstruction), 1340 (Crohn's disease), 1446 (ulcerative colitis), 1847 (chronic pancreatitis), 1908 (intestinal angina), 1236 (AIDS-related syndromes).

Wiley MK, Zahn PE. Evaluation of weight loss in the elderly [abstract]. Clin Res 1987; 35:93A.

Wilson JD, Foster DW, eds. Williams textbook of endocrinology. 7th ed. Philadelphia: WB Saunders, 1985:738 (thyroid), 854 (Addison's disease), 934 (pheochromocytoma).

32 Chronic Pain

W. Thomas Edwards, PhD, MD

Definition

Pain, one of the most ancient of animal experiences, is defined by the IASP Subcommittee on Taxonomy as "an unpleasant sensory and emotional experience associated with actual or potential tissue damage, or described in terms of such damage." Note that this definition implies that pain is a highly integrated phenomenon, so that the *experience* of pain is separated from the stimulus that leads to that experience. Acute pain occurs with a clear temporal relationship to an injury. Chronic pain persists beyond the time surrounding the original injury and persists into a time when it produces no beneficial effects. Most of our knowledge about the neurophysiology of pain is based on experiments with induced (acute) pain in animals. In life, the conditions that produce such pain often can be terminated quickly by escape or avoidance, which is not true in chronic pain states. Chronicity in any syndrome implies a certain time has elapsed since its onset. It is not possible to define a discrete time when a pain state becomes truly chronic, but generally one should look for elements of a chronic pain behavior in any patient whose pain has persisted for more than 6 months, particularly if evidence of the associated illness or injury has disappeared.

Acute pain serves many useful purposes, most of which have to do with the encouraging of inactivity that leads to healing of an injury. Quietude of the patient encourages redirecting of metabolic reserves toward the reparative process at cellular and tissue levels. Splinting of an injured part prevents further injury. These activities in patients with chronic pain states, whether or not there is ongoing nociception, lead to psychological and social dysfunction. Also, limitation of physical capacity can work to make the perception (pain) worse and further exacerbate the dysfunction, as in Figure 32-1. This results in an increasing downward spiral in physical and psychosocial functioning that can be likened to a marble rolling around the inside of a funnel. One of the most important distinctions to be made in the diagnosis of any pain state is that between acute and chronic pain. Table 32-1 lists some of the mechanisms whereby chronic pain syndromes may be initiated and maintained.

Pathophysiology

A *noxious stimulus* is any stimulus whose intensity is potentially or actually inimical to the integrity of tissue. *Nociception* is the process of detection and signaling of noxious stimulation. *Pain* (alternate definition) is the conscious perception of nociception. *Suffering* is a negative affective response generated at higher nervous centers by pain and such other situations as stress, anxiety, fear, depression, or loss of loved ones. *Pain-related behavior* is the reaction of the organism to the conscious perception of pain.

Chronic pain syndromes may include all of the above, but

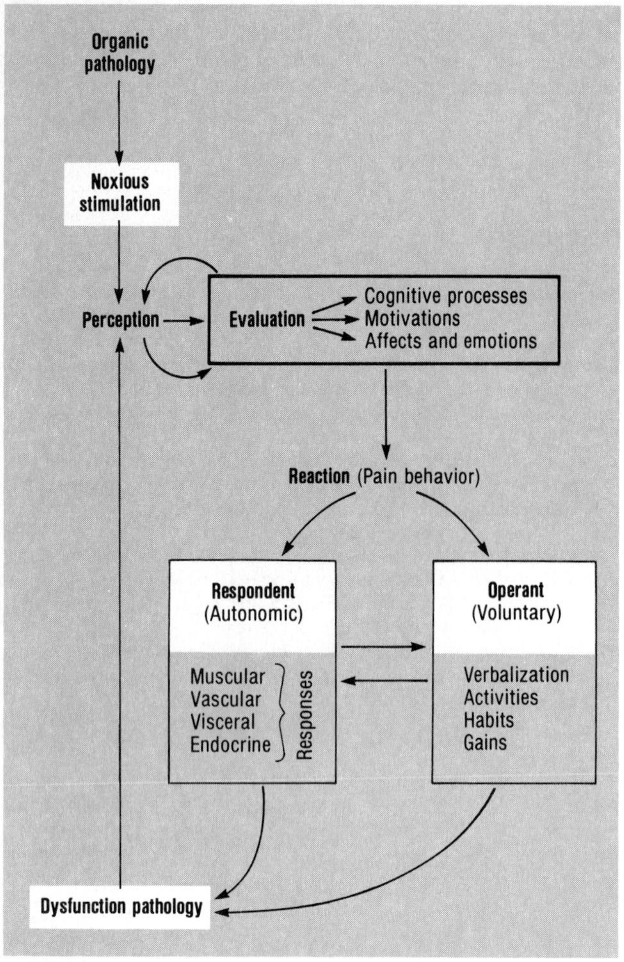

Figure 32-1 The pathway for the interaction of noxious stimulation and dysfunction pathology. Note that the reaction of the organism by operant conditioning mechanisms is the important route to dysfunction in chronic pain states, whereas the respondent reactions dominate acute pain states.

Table 32-1 Development of Chronic Pain Syndromes

Persistent Nociception
Chronic persistent stimulation of nociceptor (noxious stimulus persists)
Chronic muscle spasms (as in musculoskeletal back pain)
Persistent reflex muscle spasm (guarding)
Chronic sensitization of nociceptors by products of cellular breakdown (e.g., prostaglandins) or catecholamines
Derangements in Nociception
Decreased peripheral inhibition: Destruction of large, rapidly conducting sensory afferent fibers decreases their inhibitory influence on transmission from the dorsal horn of the spinal cord (peripheral neuropathies and phantom pain)
Decreased *ascending* central inhibition: Loss of sensory input to reticular formation leads to decreased central biasing (cordotomy and rhizotomy)
Decreased *descending* central inhibition (some midbrain and most thalamic infarcts)
Psychological Mechanisms
Emotional stress causes visceral dysfunction, vasoconstriction, and skeletal muscle tension, resulting in chronic pain, e.g., tension headache, spasm of muscles of back, chest, and shoulder girdle
Operant Mechanisms
Chronic pain follows minor injury or disease; reinforcement by favorable consequences leads to a pattern of pain behavior
Psychogenic and Psychiatric Pain Mechanisms (Rare)
A psychogenic process from early life associated with anxiety, fear of harm, and loss of love
Chronic pain may be caused by depression, hysteria, or other psychiatric disorders

sometimes the noxious stimulus and nociception have disappeared. When persistence of a noxious stimulus is suspected, look for some or all of the following hallmarks of acute pain:

1. Localized or segmental involuntary responses such as splinting, guarding, muscle spasms, or increased local vasomotor activity
2. Localized tissue reaction (inflammatory response)
3. Generalized increase in systemic sympathetic activity (sweating, hyperventilation, tachycardia, nausea)

Recently, information has begun to accumulate on the neurophysiology of chronic pain, which indicates that it is an even more complex problem than had been thought. Persistent stimulation of nociceptors and nociceptive afferents may be combined with an increase in localized sympathetic efferent activity, resulting in ongoing peripheral nociception. Loss of descending central pain-modulating mechanisms (as through cord transection, thalamic infarcts, and so forth) and psychological factors can also be central mechanisms for the development of chronic pain.

History is the clue to diagnosis because chronic pain always develops in the setting of antecedent injury or illness. The character of the pain (e.g., stinging, burning, aching), duration, onset, course, exacerbating and relieving factors, successful or unsuccessful past therapies, and so on will all suggest a diagnosis, and this will indicate further work-up and therapy, if they are indicated.

A complete pain history includes the usual patient description plus the following information specific to the pain problem.

At Onset. What were the date (approximate), the character intensity, location, radiating pattern, and precipitating event?

Prior Interventions. Ask about medications that have been tried, surgery, other therapies (acupuncture, chiropractic, physical or occupational therapy, and so on), and the effects of those interventions. Be certain to ask about psychological and behavioral management techniques that might have been tried, and whether or not a visit to a "pain clinic" has ever been suggested.

Course of Intensity Since Onset. Has the pain become better, worse, or has there been no change?

At Present. What are the character intensity, location, radiating pattern, exacerbating and relieving factors? Does the pain have a daily pattern of fluctuation in intensity, and what is that range on a scale of 0 to 10 (0 = no pain, 10 = the worst pain imaginable)? Inquire about the pattern of daily activities, including time spent in pain-relieving activities, the reactions of family and friends when the patient is "in pain," sleep pattern, current medications and patterns of use, interference with specific activities, feelings about the pain syndrome, outlook, and expectations for the future.

Additional components of the usual medical history, including other past medical and surgical problems, family and social histories, and review of systems, must also be included.

Some Common Conditions in Which Pain Is the Dominant Feature

Not all disease states are characterized by pain. Pain is a frequent concomitant of some diseases, however. A brief description of some chronically painful conditions and their principal features follows.

The Painful Peripheral Neuropathies (Degenerative)

The complaint is usually of burning or aching bilaterally in hands and feet, usually worse at rest than with activity. Many patients describe abnormal sensations (dysesthesias) in the area in which they experience pain. Chronic tingling or a sense of numbness may also be described. The history may include the associated diseases (diabetes mellitus, hypothyroidism, Paget's disease, syphilis) or a history of environmental exposure to neurotoxins such as lead or benzene. The physical examination usually includes decreased pinprick and light-touch sensation in a stocking-and-glove distribution, and very little else.

The Entrapment Neuropathies

The complaint is usually of pain at rest that is often severely aggravated by activity. Pain usually is unilateral and confined to a specific peripheral neurologic distribution, as in median nerve entrapment at the wrist (carpal tunnel syndrome). The history may include significant trauma (e.g., a fracture) or surgery in a compartment. Thoracotomies are sometimes associated with intercostal nerve entrapments, and herniorrhaphies are sometimes complicated by ilioinguinal nerve entrapments. The onset of an entrapment neuropathy may be insidious, however. The physical examination usually includes exquisitely sensitive trigger areas where slight pressure causes characteristic radiation of the pain in the distribution of the entrapped nerve.

The Radiculopathies (Nerve Root Compressions)

The complaint is of pain originating in the back and radiating in a dermatomal distribution. The history is not necessarily specific for onset. The pain may be insidious, as after a laminectomy or spinal fusion, or it may be sudden, as in acute disc ruptures or vertebral body collapse. Patients are usually unable to sustain one posture for long and usually say the pain gets worse as the day progresses. The physical examination usually discloses considerable associated paraspinus muscle spasm and exacerbation of pain during Valsalva maneuvers or any maneuver that puts traction on the affected root. For example, straight-leg raising, particularly if it is combined with dorsiflexion of the foot, markedly distorts a tethered or compressed lumbar root.

Much low back pain radiating into the leg is not radiculopathy, however (Table 32-2). Mechanical or musculoskeletal low back pain is much more common.

Table 32-2 Classification of Back Pain

Musculoskeletal	Hallmark is muscle spasm with diffuse tenderness of affected muscle
	Pain is largely confined to the back, but trigger points may be present that cause pain to radiate to buttocks or thighs
	Pain that radiates posteriorly to the knee only on extension of the back may point to a facet joint problem
Neurogenic	Usually radicular in character
	May arise from extruded or protruding discs, postsurgical perineural adhesions, arachnoiditis, or bony overgrowth in lateral neural foramina
Visceral	Often arises from pathology along the posterior peritoneum or in the retroperitoneal space such as abdominal aortic aneurysm, chronic pancreatitis, ureteral calculus, retroperitoneal fibrosis, lymphoma, etc.
Psychogenic	Complaints markedly outweigh historical and physical findings
	Look for secondary gain (financial, social, emotional) or factors such as medication use that reinforce pain-related behavior

Sympathetically Maintained Pain

Reflex sympathetic dystrophy, Sudeck's atrophy, shoulder-hand syndrome, and causalgia are all synonyms for sympathetically maintained pain. The syndrome is frequently misdiagnosed as malingering or neurosis because the complaint is so diffuse. Burning, tingling, aching, and throbbing of an entire extremity are common descriptions of the pain. This will not be in the distribution of any one nerve or root. The history is always one of an injury that produces traction or pressure on a peripheral nerve. The onset is often insidious and may follow the original injury by days or weeks. The pain is always worsened by any activity that increases local or systemic activity in the sympathetic nervous system. Fear, anger, fright, and extremely cold or hot environments all exacerbate the pain. These periods are often accompanied by color changes, such as blanching or reddening in the affected limb. The physical examination may show nothing, or there may be diffuse swelling, hair loss, and shiny skin. These changes are more evident when the syndrome is severe. Look for hypersensitivity of the skin in the affected area. Light touch (even of clothing) may be unbearably painful. Sweating and mottled skin color are often present. Strength and all active ranges of motion are impaired.

The Neuralgias

These may be paroxysmal (have a tic component) or nonparoxysmal. The complaint is of severe deep aching in the distribution of a nerve, commonly one division of cranial nerve V or cranial nerve IX. The history includes an insidious beginning, but there is early development of a trigger zone in the distribution of the affected nerve, the slightest stimulation of which always elicits the pain. In the paroxysmal neuralgias, stimulation of the trigger point usually brings on a lancinating pain that patients describe as "like a knife being stuck into the area." In contrast, postherpetic neuralgia is a nonparoxysmal pain described as itching or burning, and it follows a herpes zoster infection. Postherpetic neuralgias are most common in intercostal distribution and in the distribution of the ophthalmic division (division 1) of the trigeminal nerve (cranial nerve V). Chronic deep aching pain of insidious onset that is not clearly neurologically distributed in the head or neck is usually described as atypical facial pain. It is never paroxysmal in character. The physical examination of patients with neuralgias is usually unrevealing. There are often tender scars in the area affected by a postherpetic neuralgia. Muscle contraction under an area affected by a tic is often evident during the paroxysm. Examine for trigger zones very carefully; patients are not at all grateful for the eliciting of a tic.

Regardless of the mechanism by which the chronic pain state develops, there is no adaptation. The pain always becomes worse. Physical and emotional depletion, alteration of lifestyle, emotional changes, and economic and social debilitation become more pronounced the longer the pain state persists. Early recognition of clinical situations that herald the onset of a chronic pain state may help to abort the problem early in its course. The chronic pain states that respond to specific therapy respond more thoroughly the earlier the therapy is initiated.

Malignant Pain

Not all malignant conditions are characterized by the development of pain. When pain is a dominant feature of malignant disease, it often occurs fairly late in the course. It is best not to think of cancer pain as chronic pain, although there certainly are important behavioral components to any cancer pain syndrome. The term *acute recurring pain* best describes this particular clinical entity because the acute pain aspects, particularly ongoing nociception, are so prominent.

Cancer patients can have pain arising from many sources (Table 32-3). The pain of malignancy is often due to direct tumor involvement, so that early in the course of the disease, measures designed to relieve tumor bulk often alleviate the problem. It is pain that occurs after the first course of therapy, be it radiation, chemotherapy, or surgery, that presents the diagnostic dilemma. A good example of this diagnostic dilemma is the patient who presents with a complaint of arm pain 12 months after irradiation of the chest wall for carcinoma of the breast. Radiation fibrosis of the brachial plexus must be distinguished from recurrent tumor. A careful history that delineates the time course of onset of symptoms will usually give a better clue to the diagnosis than will any procedure.

The hallmark of direct tumor invasion is pain *before* the onset of any other signs of neuropathy, such as sensory or motor changes, whereas post-therapeutic neuropathies will likely present first as dysesthesias and in a more diffuse pattern. In the aforementioned example, one should look for sensory changes predominating in the C5 or C6 dermatome, with motor weakness in the deltoid and biceps progressing to a diffusely painful swollen and useless arm, if radiation fibrosis is suspected. Direct tumor invasion of the brachial plexus will also lead ultimately to a diffusely painful swollen and useless arm, but the progression of symptoms will usually be from painful dysesthesias in C8 and T1 distribution through distal sensory and motor changes to the more proximal findings. The presence of Horner's syndrome is strongly suggestive of direct tumor invasion, particularly if it appears early in the pain syndrome.

Leptomeningeal metastases usually present as pain that worsens when the patient lies down. Early on there may also be a radicular component, so that it is difficult to tell by history and physical exam whether this represents bony collapse with radicular compression or cord compression from metastatic disease. A conventional work-up by radiography and bone and computed tomography (CT) or magnetic resonance imaging (MRI) scans will usually sort things out properly. Because treatment is so different (radiation therapy or surgery for metastatic disease, analgesics and steroids or nerve blocks for root compression), it is important to make this distinction as early as possible.

The therapy-related causes of cancer pain are sometimes easier to diagnose than to manage. The neuropathies can usually be diagnosed by a combination of electromyelographic and nerve conduction studies with sympathetic and somatic nerve blocking procedures. If a major sympathetic component exists, as is often the case in postmastectomy pain, for example, repeated nerve block therapy may be indicated. Once the etiology of the pain has been sorted out, a logical approach to therapy based on the underlying pain mechanism can be designed.

Table 32-3 Mechanisms of Cancer Pain

Direct (caused by tumor pressure and invasion)
Localized neural compression and ischemia in a peripheral nerve
Invasion of a major neural plexus with traction, as in brachial, lumbar, or sacral plexopathy
Invasion of leptomeninges (root compression) or spinal cord (deafferentation)
Bony involvement—compression fractures or root compression
Indirect (related to treatment side effects or complications)
Radiation
Postradiation neuropathies (peripheral)
Radiation fibrosis of a major neural plexus
Radiation-induced myopathy with deafferentation
Surgical
Post-thoracotomy pain
Postmastectomy pain
Phantom limb pain
Chemotherapy
Peripheral neuropathies secondary to vinca alkaloids
Herpes zoster (acute) and postherpetic neuralgia
Pseudorheumatic pain secondary to steroid withdrawal

The Role of the Pain Consultant

Chronic pain can be a complex problem because it involves derangements of anatomy or physiology as well as emotional (suffering) and psychosocial (depression, anxiety, family dynamics, work disability) complications; therefore, it is often wise to invoke the help of a pain consultant in the diagnosis and development of a treatment plan for a chronic pain state. Often such a consultant will be allied with a team of chronic pain specialists that consists of a physician, nurse, psychologist, physical therapist, rehabilitation specialist, and others who can help to develop a comprehensive multidisciplinary evaluation and treatment plan for the patient. Sometimes the plan can be quite simple, but sometimes it is necessary to involve the patient in longer-term management through a comprehensive pain treatment center (often called a pain clinic), where the expertise of all these specialists can be brought to bear on the various aspects of the problem all at once. It is very unusual for a single approach—be it medical, as with drugs or nerve blocks, physical, as with exercise programs, or psychological, as with psychotherapy—to succeed in returning a patient with chronic pain to a full and rewarding lifestyle. Pain management specialists concentrate on the use of multilevel approaches to chronic pain problems for both diagnosis and treatment.

Example of a Chronic Pain History

Mr. P is a 42-year-old married white man who was in good health until 4 years ago, when he injured his back at work while lifting from the floor a box weighing approximately 75 pounds. He noted the sudden onset of stabbing pain across his mid-lumbar spine that radiated into his left buttock. Over the course of several weeks of bed rest, he failed to improve; in fact, the pain began to radiate into his left lower leg and occasionally would shoot into the fifth toe. This was particularly true when he would bend forward, sneeze, cough, or move his bowels.

He underwent myelography and CT scanning after 2 months, and ultimately had a laminectomy and disk excision at the L5-S1 level. This resulted in immediate relief of the leg pain, but over the next several months, the pain began to return in his leg and gradually became worse.

He describes that pain as different from the earlier leg pain. It is now more burning in character, involving the entire lower leg and always present in the fourth and fifth toes. A "numb" feeling is present all the time, but pain and a "buzzing" sensation are also present.

He has been treated with multiple narcotic medications and nonsteroidal anti-inflammatories. Narcotics make him nauseated, and nonsteroidal anti-inflammatory drugs upset his stomach. He has tried acupuncture. He has also had a course of physical therapy, most of which consisted of hot packs, ultrasound treatments, and stretching exercises, none of which helped his leg pain.

Mr. P is very discouraged and says he cannot do even simple household chores. Bending, sitting in a straight chair, standing, and riding in a car all make the pain worse. Lying down on his side, taking hot baths, and reading help him to feel somewhat better. Pain is better in the morning, worse toward evening. He spends much of the day in a lounge chair watching TV. He gets about 3 hours of interrupted sleep at night, after lying awake in bed for about an hour or so. Pain interferes with his life because he is unable to sustain an erection, and this is stressing his relationship with his wife. He rarely goes out to any social functions. He hopes to get some relief from his leg pain, to learn to cope with the remaining pain, and to return to some type of work.

References

Aronoff GM. The role of the pain center in the treatment for intractable suffering and disability resulting from chronic pain. In: Aronoff GM, ed. Evaluation and treatment of chronic pain. Baltimore: Urban and Schwarzenberg, 1985:503.

Bond MR. Pain: Its nature, analysis and treatment. 2nd ed. New York: Churchill Livingstone, 1984.

Cousins MJ. Introduction to acute and chronic pain: Implications for neural blockade. In: Cousins MJ, Bridenbaugh PO, eds. Neural blockade in clinical anesthesia and management of pain. 2nd ed. Philadelphia: JB Lippincott, 1988:739.

Fields HL. Pain. New York: McGraw-Hill, 1987.

IASP Subcommittee on Taxonomy. Pain terms: A list with definitions and usage. Pain 1979; 6:249.

Loeser J. Conceptual framework for pain management. J Burn Care Rehab 1987; 8:309.

Wall PD, Melzack R, eds. Textbook of pain. 2nd ed. New York: Churchill Livingstone, 1989.

Dermatology

Skin Lesions: Definition of Terms

Rita S. Berman, MD, MPH

33

Macule

A macule (Fig. 33-1) is a circumscribed flat lesion that may be any size or shape and that has a different color from the surrounding skin. Macular lesions may be due to abnormalities of the epidermis or the dermis. They may be the results of pigmentary alterations: hyperpigmentation (e.g., café au lait spots, seen in neurofibromatosis), hypopigmentation (e.g., ash leaf spots, seen in tuberous sclerosis), or depigmentation (e.g., vitiligo). Vascular abnormalities (e.g., port-wine stains, seen in Sturge-Weber syndrome), capillary dilatation (e.g., erythema, seen in some drug exanthemas), and extravasated red blood cells, seen as purpura (e.g., thrombocytopenic purpura), can also give rise to macular lesions. Petechiae are flat, pinpoint purpuric lesions, whereas ecchymoses are larger purpuric lesions. Pressing on a lesion with a glass slide, known as diascopy, can differentiate among erythema, vascular anomalies, and purpura because the red color of purpura remains, whereas in the other cases, it disappears.

Papule

A papule (Fig. 33-2) is a small (<1.0 cm) solid raised lesion. It may result from metabolic deposits in the dermis, seen in amyloidosis; from localized cellular infiltrates in the dermis, seen in xanthomas, or from an increase in the number of cells of the epidermis or dermis, seen in warts. It may have different shapes (e.g., pointed lesions, seen in acne; flat-topped lesions, seen in lichen planus; or rounded lesions with a central umbilication, seen in molluscum contagiosum). Different colors may give a clue to diagnosis. For example, copper-colored lesions may be seen in secondary syphilis; yellow lesions, in xanthomas; and violaceous lesions, in lichen planus. Papules may be smooth-topped, as in senile angiomas; scaly, as in psoriasis; or crusted, as in old lesions of chicken pox. Closely spaced projections on the surface of a papule (or plaque) are known as vegetation and can be seen in seborrheic keratosis. Although the term *maculopapular* is widely used, it is imprecise and should be avoided. The term *macular and papular eruption* is more accurate.

Plaque

A plaque (Fig. 33-3) is a lesion that is raised only slightly above the skin surface and has a surface area that is much greater than its height. Confluent papules may merge to form a plaque, as is sometimes seen in drug eruptions. Erythematous plaques with

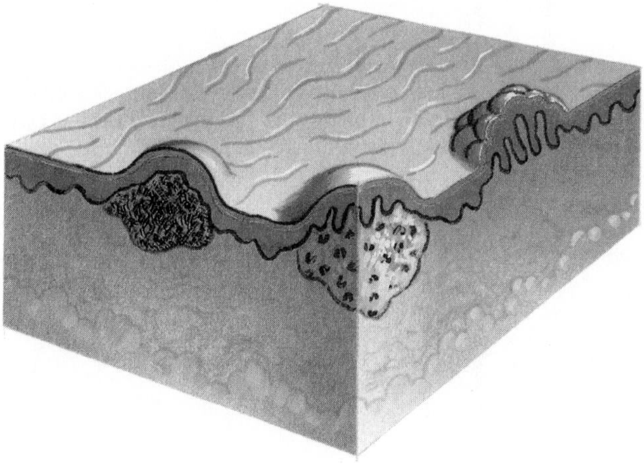

Figure 33-2 Papules.

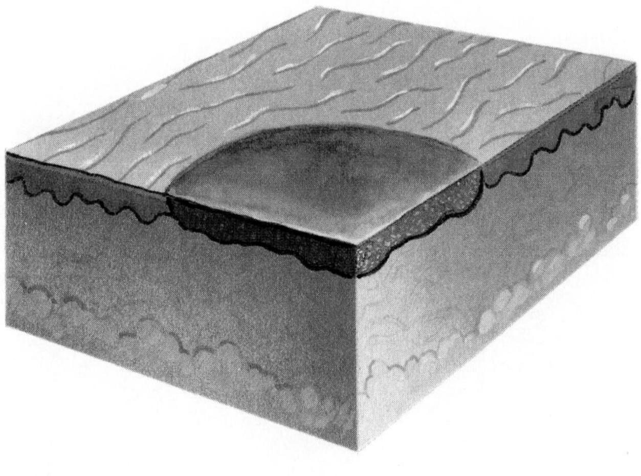

Figure 33-1 A macule.

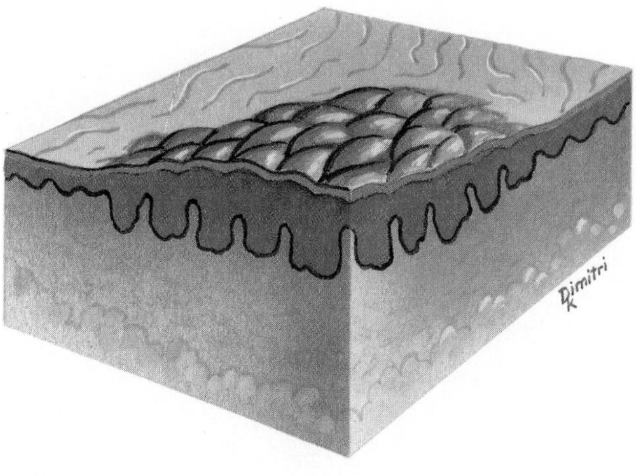

Figure 33-3 A plaque.

silvery scale are characteristic of psoriasis. Chronic rubbing, as seen in atopic dermatitis, can create thickened plaques with accentuated skin markings known as lichenification. This is produced by proliferation of the epidermis and changes in dermal collagen. When diascopy of a papule or plaque leaves a yellow-brown or "apple-jelly" color, this indicates a lymphomatous infiltration of the skin or a disease of granulomas (e.g., sarcoid, granuloma annulare, necrobiosis lipoidica diabeticorum, or tuberculosis of the skin, known as lupus vulgaris).

Wheal

A wheal (Fig. 33-4) or hive is a transient, raised, flat-topped, or rounded elevation of the skin caused by edema of the upper dermis. The color may vary from deep red to pink to white, and the size may be only a few millimeters to many centimeters. Its borders may be sharp or ill-defined, and they may move outward in a period of minutes to hours. Most lesions last less than 24 hours. If lesions last longer than 24 hours, a biopsy should be performed to rule out an urticarial vasculitis (inflammation of the blood vessels).

Wheals may result from an allergic response to many agents or from insect bites.

Angioedema is a deep and extensive urticarial reaction, occurring often on the lip or around the eyes. It is caused by massive edema into areas with loose connective tissue.

Nodule

A nodule (Fig. 33-5) is a solid, palpable, rounded or ellipsoidal lesion that may be located in the epidermis, dermis, or subcutis. Nodules may be benign or malignant. The word *tumor* is used to indicate a large nodule, which may be either benign or malignant. A nodule is differentiated from a papule because it is much firmer and not because of its diameter. Dermal or subcuticular nodules may indicate systemic disease, and may result from inflammations (as seen in erythema nodosum), infections (as seen in deep mycoses), neoplasms (as seen in malignant melanoma), or metabolic deposits (as seen in tophi of gout). Because nodules may indicate a systemic disease, biopsy and culture of undiagnosed lesions should be performed.

Cyst

A cyst (Fig. 33-6) is a sac that contains a liquid or a semisolid substance, including fluid, cells, and cell products. Epidermal (keratinous) cysts are common cysts that are lined with squamous epithelium and produce keratinous material. They are often found on the head and upper trunk.

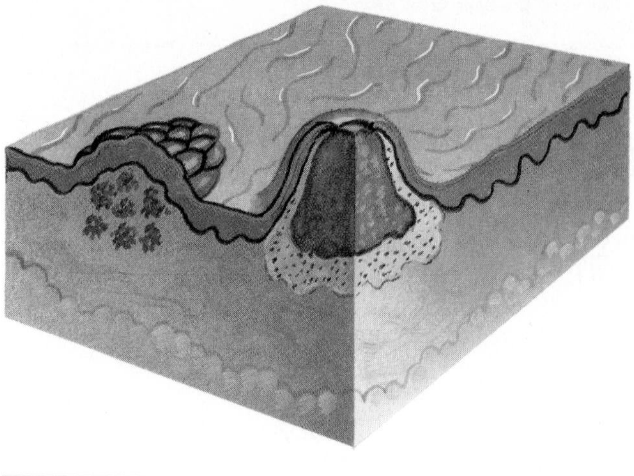

Figure 33-5 Nodules.

Vesicle and Bulla

A vesicle (Fig. 33-7) is a circumscribed raised lesion that contains fluid and is less than 0.5 cm in diameter. When the lesion is greater than 0.5 cm, it is called a bulla (Fig. 33-8). The term *blister* is a general word that refers to both vesicle and bulla. Cleavage at various levels of the skin causes accumulations of serum, blood, lymph, or extracellular fluid that can be visible through the thin walls of the lesion. Cleavage may be through the epidermis or through the dermal-epidermal junction. Subcorneal vesicles or bullae can occur just under the stratum corneum (an example of this is impetigo). Intraepidermal blisters may result from intercellular edema (spongiosis), as seen in allergic contact dermatitis; loss of cellular bridges or desmosomes (acantholysis), as seen above the basal layer in pemphigus vulgaris; and ballooning degeneration of epidermal cells, as seen in herpes simplex or zoster. Subepidermal vesicles and bullae result from dissolution of the basement membrane at the dermal-epidermal interface, such as that seen in bullous pemphigoid.

When part or all of the epidermis is lost as a result of a blister or other cause, a moist, slightly depressed area is left, known as an erosion (Fig. 33-9). Because they are so superficial,

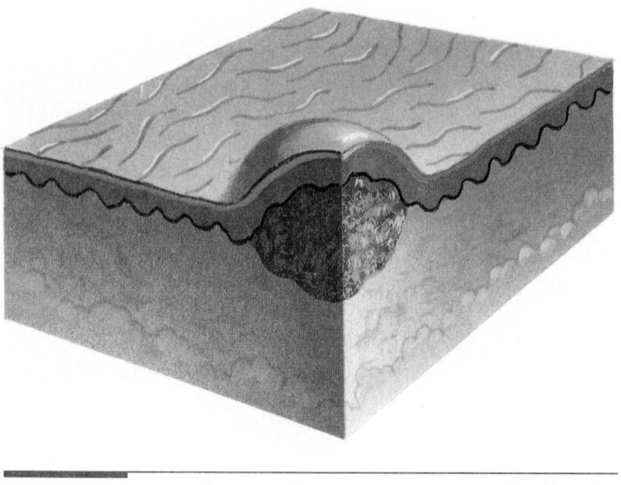

Figure 33-4 A wheal.

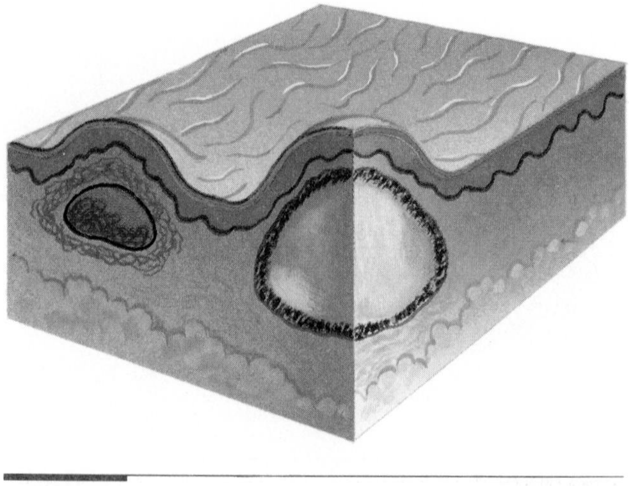

Figure 33-6 Cysts.

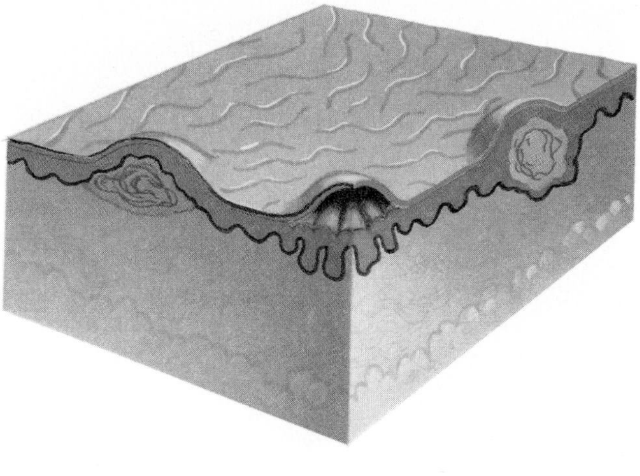

Figure 33-7 Vesicles.

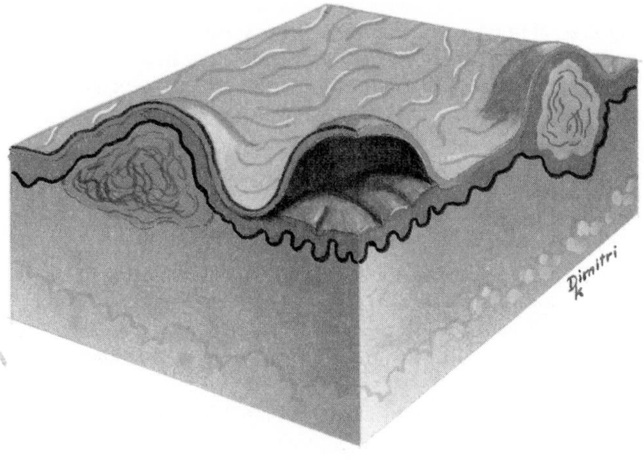

Figure 33-8 Bullae.

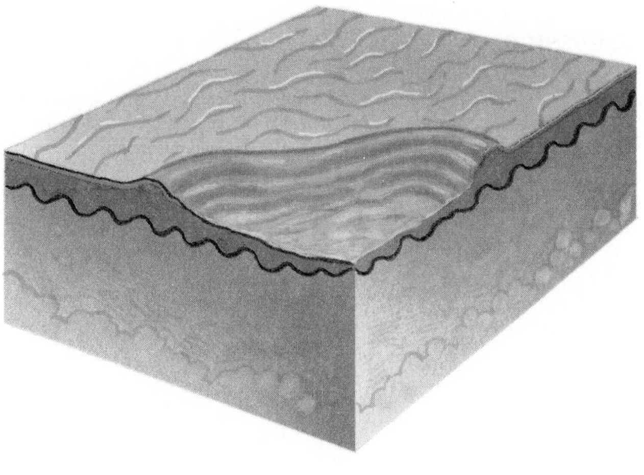

Figure 33-9 An erosion.

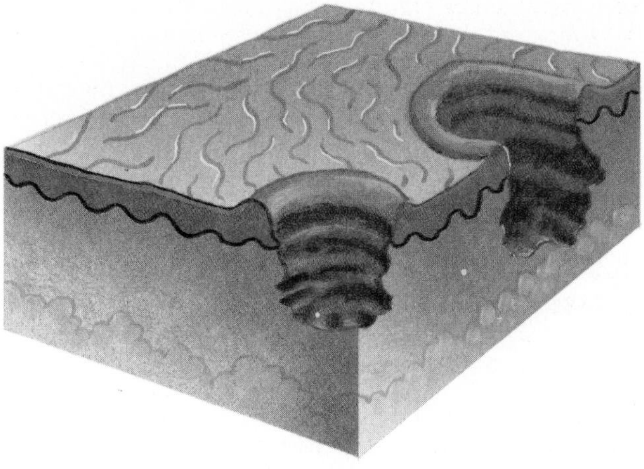

Figure 33-10 Ulcers.

erosions do not scar. Loss of tissue to the upper dermis or deeper is known as an ulcer (Fig. 33-10), and these lesions can scar.

Pustule

A pustule (Fig. 33-11) is a raised lesion of variable size and shape that contains polymorphonuclear leukocytes and cellular debris. Depending on the nature of the exudate, the color may vary from white, to yellow, to green. Some pustules may be sterile, such as those of pustular psoriasis, whereas others may result from bacterial infections. The blisters seen in some viral diseases, such as varicella, or in some dermatophytoses may become secondarily pustular. A Gram stain and culture of the pustule are necessary. Sometimes one should use a potassium hydroxide preparation to look for fungi or a Tzanck preparation to look for multinucleated keratinocytes, which are seen only in herpes simplex or varicella zoster.

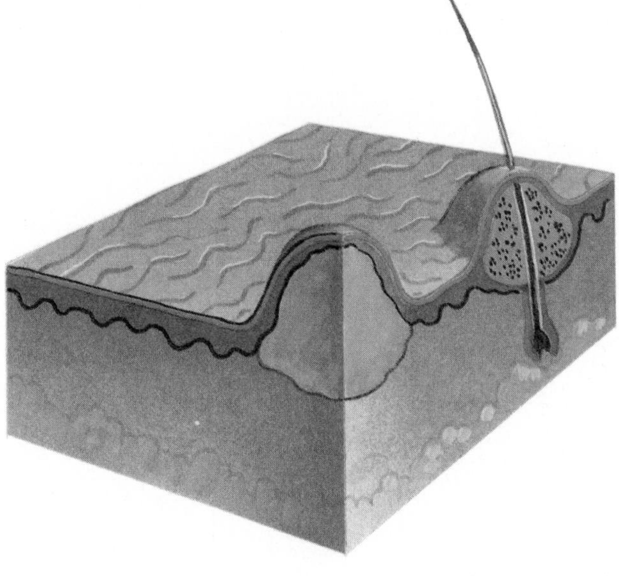

Figure 33-11 Pustules.

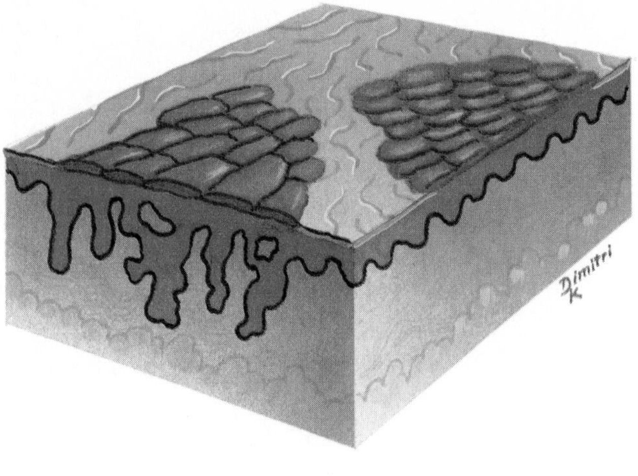

Figure 33-12 Desquamation (scaling).

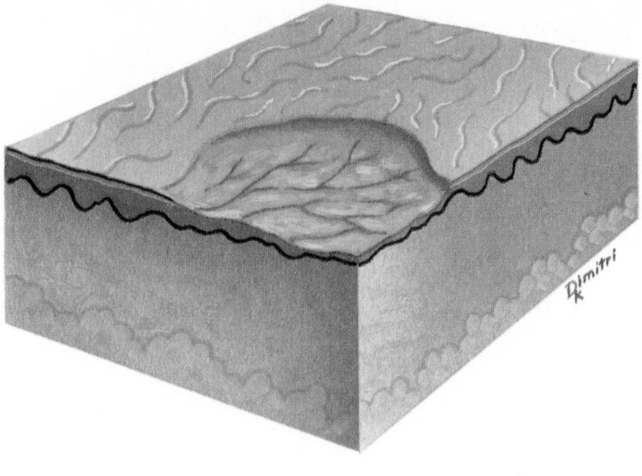

Figure 33-14 Atrophy.

Desquamation

Desquamation (Fig. 33-12) or scaling is the result of loss of the outermost layer of skin when there is abnormal keratinization and exfoliation of cornified epithelial cells. This outermost layer, the stratum corneum, does not ordinarily contain nuclei, but under abnormal circumstances, such as in psoriasis, the nuclei are retained, and this is known as parakeratosis. Parakeratotic cells accumulate and contribute to the formation of scales.

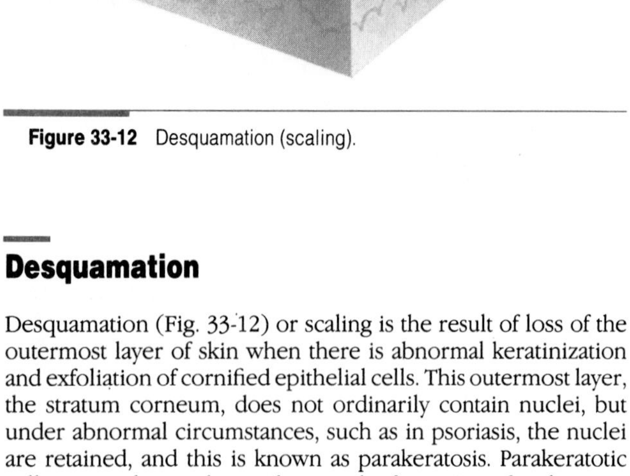

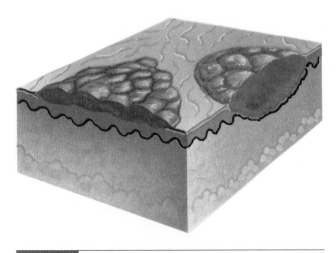

Figure 33-13 Crusts.

Crust

A crust (Fig. 33-13) is the result of dried serum, blood, or pus on the skin. When crusts originate from serum, they are yellow; when from pus, green or yellow-green; and when from blood, brown or dark red. Crusts may be thin and friable or adherent and thick. Honey-colored crusts may be seen in impetigo.

Atrophy

Epidermal atrophy (Fig. 33-14) refers to a thin epidermis and is due to a decrease in the number of epidermal cells. It may follow inflammation or trauma. Sometimes the normal skin lines are retained, as in senile skin; sometimes they are not, as seen in some types of inflammation (e.g., some lesions of discoid lupus erythematosus).

Dermal atrophy (Fig. 33-14) results from a decrease in the connective tissue of the dermis, and it usually is seen as a depression in the skin. Dermal atrophy may occur with or without epidermal atrophy. In the first case, loss of skin markings with increased translucence may occur, in addition to localized depression; this is seen in striae. When dermal atrophy occurs without epidermal atrophy, the surface of the skin may appear normal over a depressed area, as seen in the atrophic variety of lichen planus. Loss of the panniculus, as in progressive lipodystrophy, may also result in depression of the skin.

Reference

Fitzpatrick TB, Bernhard JD. The structure of skin lesions and fundamentals of diagnosis. In: Fitzpatrick TB, et al, eds. Dermatology in general medicine. 3rd ed. New York: McGraw-Hill, 1987:20.

Generalized or Widespread Eruptions

John R. Person, MD

34

A widespread or generalized rash or itching may accompany systemic disease or it may represent a cutaneous disease alone. A generalized, bilateral, and symmetric eruption is usually either of systemic etiology or an affliction of the entire skin.

The diagnosis of skin disease generally rests on three criteria: (1) the nature of the rash, (2) its distribution, and (3) the clinical setting in which it arises. The last criterion is rarely discussed in textbooks, but it is obvious that the patient's age, sex, occupation, allergic history, concurrent diseases, and other factors can be prejudicial in making a likely diagnosis from among several possibilities. Occasionally, distribution is paramount in diagnosis. Seborrheic dermatitis, for example, is usually diagnosed by its paranasal and scalp-margin localization. The most important criterion in the diagnosis of skin disease, however, is the local character of the eruption. Traditional dermatologic teaching stresses differentiating primary lesions (macules, papules, plaques, vesicles, bullae; see Chapter 33, "Skin Lesions: Definition of Terms") from secondary ones (excoriations, lichenification, crusting). Although helpful in fostering visual discipline, this approach often fails to help in diagnosis. The diagnosis of an eczematous eruption or neurodermatitis, for example, is often based purely on secondary lesions; sometimes the "primary lesion" is itch! Papulosquamous disorders are virtually impossible to diagnose when papular. The lesions must enlarge to guttate plaques before their scaly quality becomes evident. The diagnosis of some skin diseases depends not on the character of the eruption itself, but on the shape of the individual lesions. The annular plaques of tinea corporis and the oval plaques of pityriasis rosea are examples. A simplified approach to dermatologic diagnosis is to categorize the general reaction pattern of the eruption as eczematous, papulosquamous, vesiculobullous, pustular, purpuric, or dermal.

The accessibility of the skin also facilitates tissue diagnosis. Punch biopsy should be part of the procedural repertoire of all physicians. The differential diagnosis of a generalized rash and pruritus is shown in Table 34-1.

Eczematous Eruptions

Eczematous eruptions are the clinical equivalent of what is seen as spongiosis (intercellular edema) histologically. Erythema, scaling, and sometimes small vesicles are present. Eczema often appears slightly moist and itches. Eczemas are often multifactorial in etiology, but scratching, dry skin, and secondary infection play a role in most cases. Noneczematous conditions can become eczematous (e.g., psoriasis) if scratched sufficiently.

Atopic dermatitis is usually flexural in distribution and associated with other stigmata or family history of atopy. It is usually most severe in childhood (Atlas Figure 27).* In infancy, it is often predominantly facial. "Soft" signs of atopy include keratoses pilaris (follicular papules most prominent on the elbows and knees), Dennie's lines (double fold beneath eyes), allergic "shiners" (darkness around the eyes), dry skin, intolerance of wool, and pityriasis alba (faint white scaly patches on the cheeks and arms).

Nummular eczema is a descriptive term for an eczematous eruption that appears in coin-sized patches (Atlas Figure 28).

A diagnosis of *contact dermatitis* is usually made by distribution and history. If a dermatitis is generalized and affects the borders of axillae, waist, and upper thighs, a clothing-related allergy should be suspected. Rhus dermatitis (poison ivy, oak, or sumac) is by far the most frequent etiology (Atlas Figure 29). It is usually vesicular, linear, asymmetric, and in the distribution of plant contact (e.g., hands, ankles) and of "touching" one's self.

Papulosquamous Disorders

The papulosquamous disorders range in lesional size from individual papules to total-body confluence (exfoliative erythroderma). The scaly quality is difficult to appreciate in lesions smaller than 5 to 10 mm.

In *psoriasis* (Atlas Figure 9), thick silver-ivory scaly patches occur on an erythematous base and show a predilection for the elbows, knees, and scalp. Itching sometimes occurs. (Guttate psoriasis is a distinct clinical presentation usually in children or young adults. The lesions begin as papules, but are usually drop-sized ["gutta"] by the time the patient seeks medical attention. It is often triggered by streptococcal pharyngitis.) The lesions are usually round. Pitted nails and a family history of psoriasis may help in the diagnosis.

In *pityriasis rosea,* the scaly patches are usually 5 to 30 mm in diameter and occur predominantly on the neck and trunk.

Table 34-1 Differential Diagnosis of Generalized Rash and Pruritus

Eczematous Eruptions	**Purpura**
Atopic dermatitis	Purpura simplex
Nummular eczema	Thrombocytopenic purpura
Contact dermatitis	"Senile" purpura
Papulosquamous Disorders	Vasculitis
Psoriasis	Leukocytoclastic or hypersensitivity vasculitis
Pityriasis rosea	Small artery vasculitis
Lichen planus	
Lupus erythematosus	**Dermal Reaction Patterns**
Tinea versicolor	Urticaria and angioedema
Tinea corporis	Morbilliform ("measle-like") eruptions
Secondary syphilis	Cutaneous granulomas
Generalized Bullous Diseases	Hard vascular nodules
Erythema multiforme	
Toxic epidermal necrolysis	**Generalized Excoriations**
Staphylococcal "scalded skin" syndrome	Scabies
Viral exanthemas	Folliculitis
	Dermatitis herpetiformis
Pustular Eruptions	Manifestation of systemic disease
Acne	Neurotic excoriations and neurodermatitis
Folliculitis	
Candidiasis	**Generalized Itching Without Rash**
	Symptomatic dermatographia
	Dry skin

* Many of the conditions discussed in Chapters 34 to 36 are illustrated in the Atlas of Dermatology, which appears on pages 178 to 193.

The most important clues tò the diagnosis are the oval shape of some lesions and their long-axis orientation parallel to skin lines. A larger, often annular herald patch often precedes the generalized eruption by days or weeks (Atlas Figure 30). The disease usually occurs in healthy adolescents or young adults. Secondary syphilis must be ruled out if palmoplantar lesions are present.

In *seborrheic dermatitis* (Atlas Figure 26), erythema and scaling are ill-defined and preferentially affect the paranasal, brow, and scalp margins. The cutaneous yeast *Pityrosporum* is involved in its pathogenesis, and it is probably the most common cutaneous manifestation of the acquired immunodeficiency syndrome. Differentiation from psoriasis is not always possible.

Lichen planus usually appears as lilac-colored, flat-topped itchy papules with a predilection for the volar wrists and shins. The papules often are topped with faint white netlike lines called Wickham's striae (Atlas Figure 7). A biopsy is often necessary to make the diagnosis. A white, lacy eruption on the buccal mucosa is the most common oral presentation. A similar or identical eruption, but one that spares mucosal surfaces, can be seen as a drug reaction.

Lupus erythematosus is often papulosquamous, but generally also shows follicular plugging, atrophy, and telangectasia. Scarring may also occur. Many lesions also appear faintly eczematous. A photodistribution is characteristic. Any persistent photoeruption should be biopsied.

Tinea versicolor may best be called a "maculosquamous" eruption, because the lesions are only minimally elevated. The lesions are scaly and irregularly sized. They can be lighter (if the patient is tan or has a dark complexion) or darker (if the patient is white or untanned) than the surrounding skin (hence, "versicolor"). The neck and shoulders are the sites of predilection (Atlas Figure 31). The condition often flares with heat and often becomes more noticeable with sunbathing. Itching is uncommon.

Tinea corporis is usually annular and asymmetric (Atlas Figure 32). A potassium hydroxide (KOH) test should be performed in all annular rashes. This is done by placing scrapings from an infected area on a glass slide and adding a drop of 10 to 20 percent potassium hydroxide. A coverslip is placed on top and the slide is gently heated, then blotted dry. The fungi, if present, appear as refractile aqua-colored "wormlike" hyphae.

Secondary *syphilis* should be suspected whenever a papulosquamous eruption affects the palms and soles.

Generalized Bullous Diseases

Generalized bullous diseases are an important part of dermatology, but with the exception of varicella, they are rare. Despite their dramatic presentation, a biopsy is necessary to secure the diagnosis of most vesiculobullous eruptions. If an autoimmune bullous disease (pemphigus, pemphigoid, dermatitis herpetiformis) is suspected, direct (tissue) and indirect (serum) immunofluorescence should also be performed (see also the section on generalized excoriations).

As the name *erythema multiforme* implies, the disease has varied clinical presentations. The number of possible causes is legion. It is a hypersensitivity phenomenon. Drug hypersensitivity and antecedent herpes simplex virus infection are the most common causes.

Typical erythema multiforme shows urticaria-like but persistent and nonpruritic plaques, vesicles, or small bullae in a generalized but sparse distribution, and classically, "target lesions" on the palms and soles (Atlas Figure 33). Mucosal involvement is usually mild. By far the most frequent etiology is herpes simplex. The work-up should be individualized, but in the absence of a preceding herpes infection, it should include biopsy and throat culture.

Stevens-Johnson syndrome is a severe form of erythema multiforme with fulminant mucosal involvement. A drug etiology is most common. Because ocular involvement occurs, ophthalmologic consultation should be obtained. Bladder involvement may necessitate catheterization.

Toxic epidermal necrolysis (Lyell, "drug-induced" or "adult" type) is similar to Stevens-Johnson syndrome, but the bullae involve such large areas of the cutaneous surface that the patient almost molts, shedding large areas of epidermis, often including the nails (Atlas Figure 34). The risks of fluid and electrolyte imbalance, secondary infection, and septicemia are similar to those of burn patients.

Erythema multiforme, Stevens-Johnson syndrome, and toxic epidermal necrolysis are points on a spectrum of mucocutaneous disease.

Staphylococcal "scalded skin" syndrome (formerly called toxic epidermal necrolysis of the Ritter, or childhood, type) is caused by an exotoxin produced by some phage types (especially 71) of *Staphylococcus aureus*. The bullae are subcorneal and hence fragile and often unnoticed. Fluid and electrolyte problems are rarely associated. Usually the presentation is severe peeling, most severe on the palms, soles, and lips, with vivid redness underneath (Atlas Figure 35). The differentiation between scalded skin syndrome and toxic epidermal necrolysis is a dermatologic emergency. Frozen section of a biopsy is the most accurate technique.

The exfoliation in *toxic shock syndrome* is similar, but it is caused by an immunologically distinct toxin that also causes systemic illness.

Viral exanthemas, most notably varicella, are sometimes vesicular. This diagnosis is easily recognized by the presence of the accompanying systemic illness.

Pustular Eruptions

Pustular eruptions are generally an easy differential diagnosis. Biopsy is rarely necessary.

Acne consists of comedones and cysts in addition to pustules (Atlas Figure 36). The face, neck, chest, and back are the areas of predilection (see Chapter 33, "Skin Lesions: Definition of Terms"). The diagnosis is usually obvious, but an isolated lesion in a patient without a history of acne merits a culture. *Rosacea* is usually limited to the face and lacks comedones (Atlas Figure 37). It usually begins in mid-adult life.

Folliculitis is an infection usually caused by *Staphylococcus aureus,* but occasionally by other organisms, including tinea. The pustules are obviously follicular and most commonly on the lower arms and legs (Atlas Figure 22). Overlaps between furunculosis and impetigo are common. Shaving "nicks" may provide portals of entry, and hence the beard area of men and the legs of women are common sites. *Pseudomonas* folliculitis may occur in epidemics from hot tub or spa contamination. Gram-negative folliculitis is an occasional complication of long-term antibiotic therapy for acne.

Candidiasis is generally an intertriginous dermatitis with satellite pustulosis. Heat and moisture are predisposing factors. Candidiasis is often part of diaper dermatitis and intertrigo (Atlas Figure 23). Similar eruptions often occur on the backs and buttocks of bedfast patients.

Purpura

Purpura is an easy diagnosis in white skin because of the dramatic color. True purpura is purple and does not blanch (Atlas Figure 3).

Purpura simplex (Schamberg's pigmented purpura plus many other eponyms) is not purple but brick or rust-colored. It is a petechial eruption most common on the legs. It usually is an idiopathic capillaritis, but it can be a secondary phenomenon from stasis, trauma, and so forth. The diagnosis is usually made clinically. It has no systemic significance and requires no further evaluation.

As an oversimplified rule, *thrombocytopenic purpura* is usually petechial, whereas purpura secondary to clotting dysfunction (including disseminated intravascular coagulation) is usually ecchymotic; i.e., there are much larger areas of hemorrhage. A biopsy should be avoided.

"Senile" purpura is almost invariably on the forearms and is caused by trauma in skin that has undergone connective tissue atrophy due to aging and solar damage. *Steroid purpura* is caused by steroid-induced atrophy, but it is histologically identical.

In *vasculitis* the purpuric lesions are usually larger than petechiae, but smaller than coin-sized. Lesions are usually palpable ("palpable purpura") and sometimes bullous or ulcerative. The lesions are usually fairly round. Dependent areas are sites of predilection: usually the legs, but also the buttocks in bedfast patients. Diagnosis is confirmed by biopsy, preferably also by direct immunofluorescence.

Leukocytoclastic or *hypersensitivity vasculitis* is the most common type and is an immune complex disease (Atlas Figure 4). Leukocytoclasis is the rupture of neutrophil nuclei into "nuclear dust." *Cryoglobulinemic purpura* and *Henoch-Schönlein purpura* are subtypes caused by cryoglobulin and IgA-containing immune complexes, respectively.

Arthritis, nephritis, or gastrointestinal hemorrhage is the most common systemic manifestation. If a drug is not the obvious etiology, the work-up should include a complete blood count with platelets, urinalysis, creatinine, rheumatoid factor, antinuclear antibodies, cryoglobulins, CH50, sedimentation rate, stool guaiac, and immunoelectrophoresis in addition to skin biopsy.

Small artery vasculitis, such as Wegener's granulomatosis and periarteritis nodosa, usually results in more obvious nodules and ulcerations in addition to purpura. Scarring usually occurs. There is almost always systemic involvement.

Dermal Reaction Patterns

In assessing a generalized rash, it is important to inspect the integrity of the epidermis. If it is intact (although perhaps distended by underlying inflammation), the site of pathology is probably in the dermal vasculature. This generally means that the problem is systemic. (For information on vasculitis and erythema multiforme, see preceding sections.)

Urticaria (hives) and *angioedema* (hivelike tissue swelling) are easily diagnosed. Circumlesional pallor and dermatographia (whealing after the skin is vigorously stroked) are helpful confirmatory signs (Atlas Figure 10). They are caused by a variety of physical, infectious, dietary, or inhalant allergens. A dietary cause is most common. If the etiology is obscure and the urticaria is chronic, further investigation may be indicated. Testing should be selective and oriented toward "clues" provided by history and physical examination. If individual lesions persist for more than 12 hours, if they resolve with hyperpigmentation, if they are accompanied by systemic symptoms such as arthralgias, if the patient fails to respond to an antihistamine, or if the patient's sedimentation rate is elevated, a biopsy should be performed to rule out an urticarial leukocytoclastic vasculitis.

Morbilliform ("measles-like") eruptions are most commonly manifestations of drug allergy (Atlas Figure 39). The eruption begins within 1 to 2 days if the patient had already been sensitized to the offending agent. It begins in 1 to 2 weeks if primary sensitization has developed to a drug that the patient has continued to take (with ampicillin and amoxicillin, it often begins *after* the drug has been discontinued!). The lesions persist for 1 to 2 weeks after withdrawal of the offending agent. Similar eruptions are seen as viral and rickettsial exanthems, but the patient is systemically ill.

Multiple, persistent firm papules with a faint translucent quality and a tan color ("apple jelly") may represent *cutaneous granulomas* and merit a biopsy. The pattern recognition, however, is quite subtle. Cutaneous granulomas often also assume an annular pattern.

Hard dermal vascular nodules may represent *metastases* and should be biopsied if the clinician is suspicious. The skin should be examined carefully for suspicious lesions before an extensive malignancy work-up is begun.

Generalized Excoriations

Generalized excoriations are a frequent clinical problem. The search for primary lesions may be confusing when such lesions are rare. For example, if pustules are found on the back, they may not be primary lesions, but simply concomitant acne.

In *scabies,* the primary lesion is usually a papulovesicle (Atlas Figure 40). Often, the patient has excoriated all primary lesions. The excoriations are characteristically tiny, about 1 mm. Microscopic identification of the mite from a scraping of an unexcoriated papule is often possible. Linear burrows and interdigital location are seen in "textbook" cases. The beltline is probably the most common site. Sparing of the head and increased itching at night are significant clues, as is a history of acquaintances or family members who itch. If clinical suspicion is high, response to therapy is a reasonable diagnostic approach, but every attempt to confirm the diagnosis by microscopic examination of a scraping should be made first.

All patients with excoriations should be cultured to rule out folliculitis, even in the absence of pustular lesions.

Dermatitis herpetiformis classically presents as extremely itchy, grouped papulovesicles that share a predilection for the elbows, knees, and sacrum. Often, however, it presents as excoriations. Diagnosis is established by biopsy and immunofluorescence.

Systemic diseases such as anemia, cholestasis, renal failure, hyperthyroidism, hypothyroidism, and drug allergy can all cause pruritus with resultant excoriations. Most of these are easily ruled out by simple laboratory testing. A malignancy work-up is obviously more involved and should be done only if clinical suspicion justifies it.

Neurotic excoriations and *neurodermatitis* are common problems. Significant psychopathology is usually absent: these patients are usually just "pickers." The patient often admits to picking and denies primary lesions. If the patient lacks insight, however, neurodermatitis may be a diagnosis of exclusion.

Generalized Itching Without Rash

Generalized itching without rash can be caused by any of the systemic diseases mentioned under generalized excoriations, but two simple and common problems, symptomatic dermatographia and dry skin, ought to be ruled out.

Symptomatic dermatographia differs from asymptomatic dermatographia because the patient itches. Simply stroking the skin produces a wheal and establishes the diagnosis. It does not merit an evaluation as thorough as that for urticaria.

Any itchy patient with *dry skin* should be intensively treated with lubrication before a more esoteric cause is sought (Atlas Figure 41).

References

Bernhard JD. Itching as a manifestation of non-cutaneous disease. Hosp Pract 1987; 22:81.

Fitzpatrick TB, Bernhard JD. The structure of skin lesions and fundamentals of diagnosis. In: Fitzpatrick TB, et al, eds. Dermatology in general medicine. 3rd ed. New York: McGraw-Hill, 1987:20.

Pigmented Lesions

Gregory Bishop, MD

35

Definition

Pigmented lesions of the skin vary in color from tan to brown to black. The lesions may be macular, papular, or nodular with well- or ill-defined borders. The color may arise from the presence of increased melanin, increased number of melanocytes, and nevus cells. Hemoglobin, carotene, and a number of other pigments contribute to skin color and some pigmented lesions, but this chapter deals mainly with lesions that arise from nevus cells or melanocytes.

Etiology

The pigment as seen on the surface of the skin is a reflection of the depth of the melanin in the skin; i.e., superficial melanin in the epidermis gives a tan hue, as opposed to melanin deep in the dermis, which gives dark brown or black hues. Bluish colors represent the deepest levels of melanin deposit. Most pigmented lesions seen by the clinician will be among those listed in Table 35-1.

A *nevocellular nevus* is composed of collections of nevus cells (melanocytes) in the epidermis and dermis. If present at birth, it is called congenital; if it arises after birth, it is called acquired. This is an important distinction because, of the two types, the congenital nevus is more likely to evolve into malignant melanoma. When nevus cells and melanin are present deep in the dermis, the lesion may appear blue and is then called blue nevus.

A *melanoma* is a malignant tumor of melanocytes. It may arise from epidermal melanocytes or nevus cells. Melanomas may metastasize and are among the most malignant of all cancers.

In 1978, Clark et al described two families with a large number of melanomas. They were associated with numerous large irregular nevi that were believed to be precursors to melanoma because they had clinical and histopathologic features different from nevocellular nevi and suggestive, but not diagnostic, characteristics of melanoma. The term *dysplastic nevus* has been applied to this lesion. The dysplastic nevus syndrome may occur in a familial autosomal dominant pattern or sporadically in the population.

Freckles are created by increased amounts of melanin in the epidermis without increased numbers of melanocytes. On the other hand, a lentigo is due to increased numbers of melanocytes as well as melanin in the epidermis.

A *seborrheic keratosis* is a focal well-defined area of overgrowth of the epidermis that frequently contains melanin pigment.

Basal cell carcinoma is a malignant tumor of pluripotential epidermal basal cells that rarely metastasizes but shows aggressive local growth. It occasionally contains melanin and thus may be pigmented.

A *café au lait spot* is a coffee-colored macule with well-defined sharp borders. It is larger than a freckle and contains increased melanin and melanocytes in the epidermis.

Dermatofibromas are common, benign, fibrous tissue tumors of the dermis associated with increased thickness and pigmentation of the epidermis.

Finally, *urticaria pigmentosa* is a rare mast cell disorder in which tan macules that urticate when stroked are present.

Table 35-1 Differential Diagnosis of Pigmented Lesions

Nevocellular nevus*	Lentigo*
Congenital	Seborrheic keratosis*
Acquired	Pigmented basal cell carcinoma
Blue	Café au lait spot
Dysplastic nevus	Mongolian spot
Melanoma	Dermatofibroma
Freckles*	Urticaria pigmentosa

* Denotes more common conditions.

Diagnosis

The most important features of differential diagnosis relate to the physical characteristics of the lesions themselves. Freckles are usually multiple tan-to-brown macules with well-defined borders and are confined to sun-exposed areas. By contrast, nevi are scattered all over the body and may be flat, slightly elevated, papillomatous, dome-shaped, or pedunculated. With the exception of congenital nevi, which can be quite large, they are usually less than 1 cm in diameter. The pigmentation may be slightly darker in the center, but in general the color is fairly uniform. The outward contour is also regular, denoting an orderly growth pattern. In contrast, melanomas, being composed of malignant cells, display disorderly, haphazard growth patterns that manifest clinically as irregular pigmentation (Atlas Figure 42). Coal-black colors, which suggest deep penetration of the cells, lie next to tan or brown areas, which denote lesser penetration. There may even be red or white areas that reflect inflammation and regression as the individual's immune response tries and perhaps partially succeeds in eradicating the malignant cells. Sometimes melanomas are not pigmented and are then called amelanotic melanomas. Melanoma cells not only show irregular downward growth but also irregular growth outward across the skin surface. Clinically, this is expressed by an irregular outer margin, with projections of pigmentation creating indentations or notching of the border. Melanomas are frequently more than 1 cm in diameter.

The dysplastic nevus shows some features of both a benign nevus and a melanoma (Atlas Figure 43). The size generally ranges between 0.5 and 1.0 cm in diameter. It is located primarily on the trunk and arms. The color shows subtle variations of brown and pink and occasionally focal areas of black. The contour is slightly irregular and often poorly defined, diffusing into the normal surrounding skin. It is usually flat but may have a central papule. Although a dysplastic nevus can be suspected clinically, the definitive diagnosis rests on its pathology as characterized by cellular dysplasia, irregular nesting of nevus cells, and fibrous tissue reaction. It is suspected that the dysplastic nevus is more likely to evolve into melanoma than the common benign nevus.

Seborrheic keratoses may have a tremendously varied appearance. They usually have a soft surface that is crumbly and has the appearance of being stuck or plastered on the surface of the skin (Atlas Figure 44). Frequently, there are multiple lesions. The color varies from flesh color to jet black. They are more common in the elderly. A special type of seborrheic keratosis called dermatosis papulosa nigra, common on the faces of blacks, presents as shiny black papules.

For the most part, basal cell carcinomas have a pearly translucent nodular appearance (Atlas Figure 45). Often they ulcerate and bleed easily. When pigmentation is present, they are difficult to differentiate from melanomas (Atlas Figure 46). One helpful, but not conclusive, fact is that pigmented basal cell carcinomas usually occur in individuals with brown eyes and melanomas are more common in people with blue eyes.

Café au lait spots are distinctive, appearing as tan macules with well-defined borders. They are larger than freckles and lentigos. The presence of more than five with a size greater than 1.5 cm in diameter is very suggestive of neurofibromatosis. The café au lait spots of Albright's syndrome are generally larger and have a more jagged border than the smooth contour seen in those of neurofibromatosis.

The Mongolian spot typically is seen as bluish discoloration in the lumbosacral area. It is present at birth and represents a delay in disappearance of melanocytes from the lower dermis. Characteristically, it disappears in the third or fourth month after birth.

Dermatofibromas are firm nodules that may feel like "buttons" in the skin. They are usually less than 1 cm in size and have increased pigmentation in the overlying skin. With lateral pressure, they often "dimple," and this can help differentiate them from melanomas.

Urticaria pigmentosa may give rise to solitary or multiple uniformly tan lesions that are flat or slightly elevated above the skin surface (Atlas Figure 10). Because they contain large amounts of mast cells, scratching the surface of the skin will elicit an urticarial wheal in the brown pigmentation but not in the surrounding normal skin. This is known as Darier's sign.

Although the physical appearance is a fairly reliable method of distinguishing among pigmented lesions, certain historical information may be of importance. For example, freckles, nevi, café au lait spots, Mongolian spots, and urticaria pigmentosa usually arise early in life, whereas seborrheic keratosis is uncommon before midlife. Changing lesions are viewed with more suspicion for melanoma. A history of trauma may explain the bizarre appearance of a nevus or a seborrheic keratosis.

Diagnostic Procedures

Although in most cases the physical appearance and history reveal the nature of the pigmented lesion with confidence, even a pigment specialist cannot always distinguish between a melanoma and a nevus, seborrheic keratosis, dermatofibroma, and pigmented basal cell carcinomas. At times, even nonpigmented lesions such as venous lakes and thrombosed capillary aneurysms of the skin may mimic melanoma. If there is any question, a skin biopsy must be done to rule out a melanoma.

References

Fitzpatrick TB, et al, eds. Dermatology in general medicine. 3rd ed. New York: McGraw-Hill, 1987.

Maize JG, Ackerman AB. Pigmented lesions of the skin. Philadelphia: Lea & Febiger, 1987.

Moschella SL, Hurley HJ. Dermatology. 2nd ed. Philadelphia: WB Saunders, 1985.

Skin Ulcers

Steven A. Franks, MD

36

Definitions

An ulcer is a circumscribed loss of tissue in which the epidermis and at least the upper (papillary) dermis have been destroyed or removed. Ulcers may be superficial or may occur as massive defects involving the whole thickness of the skin and the tissues underlying it. Technically, an erosion is a lesion from which the epidermis alone has been removed, leaving a moist, denuded surface behind.

Diagnostic Approach

Ulcers are a reaction pattern, as are the papulosquamous diseases or the bullous processes. The patient's history and the clinical appearance, distribution, and configuration of their lesions are the keys to diagnosis.

The history may reveal an episode of preceding trauma, prior evidence of inflammation (redness, heat, swelling), or tumor. Careful questioning is important. Is this an acute process or has the area failed to heal over weeks to months? Is the area painful or not? Has the patient had similar ulcers before?

The primary configuration and number of lesions are important. Is it a single lesion with round, sharply defined borders? Are there multiple lesions with borders forming acute angles? Is there evidence of serous, purulent, or hemorrhagic exudate with crusting? Is there surrounding inflammation or heaped-up margins suggesting tumor? Where are the lesions located? Are there several ulcers on the leg, recurrent ulcers in the mouth or on the genitalia, or a single slowly enlarging ulcer on the forehead? Is it a persistent ulcer of the sacrum?

There are many ways to begin evaluating the nature of an ulcerating process; probably the best is the distribution of the lesions over the body. For example, many ulcerating processes are confined, more or less, to the lower extremities. Here, common types of lesions include ulcerations secondary to arterial insufficiency, stasis ulcers, ulcers associated with a vasculitis, pyoderma gangrenosum, ulcers in necrobiosis lipoidica diabeticorum, and neurotrophic ulcers. Painful lesions, a history of claudication and pain on walking, and pain on warming suggest *arterial ulceration.* Supporting physical findings include absent or decreased pulses, yellowing and thickening of all 10 toenails, and poor venous filling. With more advanced disease, a purplish blotchy discoloration of the skin may occur as well as loss of sensation. The ulcers themselves appear "punched-out." There may be undermining of the surrounding skin and islands of normal skin within the ulcer. Diabetes, hypertension, and arteriosclerosis are the most frequently associated underlying disorders.

Stasis ulceration occurs more frequently in women and is usually post-thrombotic, with venous insufficiency alone being a much less common cause. These ulcerations are much less painful and occur most frequently above or posterior to the medial malleoli. Surrounding hyperpigmentation, petechiae, edema, and induration are usually present.

Necrobiosis lipoidica diabeticorum is found in 0.1 to 0.3 percent of all diabetics. This condition usually occurs over the anterior aspects of the legs, beginning as asymptomatic dull red papules and plaques. As these lesions enlarge, central atrophy and induration develop. Often ulceration occurs in this central area.

The ulcer(s) of *pyoderma gangrenosum* are usually irregular in outline and often reach several centimeters in diameter. The initial papule or pustule is rarely seen. With enlargement, the suggestive bluish-red overhanging edge develops (Atlas Figure 19). The crater is red and edematous, with a necrotic base. Look for underlying ulcerative colitis, regional enteritis (granulomatous colitis), rheumatoid arthritis, and lymphoreticular malignancy.

Although most common on the legs, pyoderma gangrenosum and necrobiosis lipoidica may occur essentially anywhere on the body. This is also true of ulcers resulting from an allergic vasculitis. However, typical palpable purpura (vasculitic lesions) initially occurs on the dependent areas. Thus, lesions are first seen on the lower extremities in ambulatory patients and on the back in bed-ridden patients. These lesions may range from asymptomatic to extremely painful. There may be nonspecific "constitutional symptoms," such as fever, malaise, and myalgia. In addition, evidence of systemic involvement, especially renal, joint, and gastrointestinal, should be sought.

Forms of *necrotizing vasculitis* include allergic or "leukocytoclastic" vasculitis; Henoch-Schönlein purpura; serum sickness–like reaction; hypocomplementemia, or urticarial, vasculitis; and vasculitis associated with malignancy.

When a variety of *neurologic* disorders (e.g., those occurring secondary to diabetes, degenerative disorders, tabes dorsalis) result in a loss of pain sensation, local trauma is unrecognized and may continue until an ulcer has formed. Again, although this may occur on the face or hands, the foot is the most common site. Initially, prolonged pressure over the metatarsal heads or heel results in significant callus formation. This is followed by fissuring, possibly infection, and ulcer formation. Friction against shoes may accomplish the same thing. Although the ulcers are usually painless, deep or referred pain may be present. Underlying fascial, bone, and joint involvement are possible complications.

The mouth is another area where the differential diagnosis of ulcerated lesions is frequently encountered. The two most common entities are aphthous stomatitis and herpes simplex infection. Of unknown etiology, aphthae appear as discrete, shallow 1- to 10-mm ulcers with grayish-yellow bases and are accompanied by tenderness. They are seen most frequently on the tongue, labial and buccal mucosa, and mucobuccal fold. Healing occurs in 7 to 10 days, and irregular recurrences are common.

The stomatitis associated with the initial *Herpesvirus hominis* infection of the mucous membranes can occur in children and is usually accompanied by fever, headache, malaise, and regional adenopathy. The primary 2- to 5-mm vesicles on the lips, gingiva, and oral mucosa rapidly break to leave erosions and surrounding edema and erythema as well as local significant tenderness. They resolve within 2 weeks. Subsequent self-limited and irregular recurrences appear as closely grouped, short-lived vesicles with progression to ulceration and healing within 7 to 10 days. Factors provoking recurrences include fever, sunlight (lips), menstruation, ingestants, and emotional stress. Often, though, no inciting factor is identified. There may be premonitory itching or burning.

Other *viral diseases* can produce transient vesiculation and erosions of the oral mucosa. These include chicken pox (varicella) (Atlas Figure 15), herpes zoster (Atlas Figure 16), and coxsackievirus infection (hand, foot, and mouth disease and herpangina). Skin lesions, distribution, and epidemiologic considerations make the diagnosis in these infections.

When oral erosions persist or become unusually deep or necrotic, the blistering diseases should be considered. Erythema multiforme (Stevens-Johnson syndrome), toxic epidermal necrolysis, bullous pemphigoid (Atlas Figure 17), and pemphigus (Atlas Figure 18) are usually associated with typical skin lesions. However, oral lesions may be present alone. When in doubt, a biopsy of the skin or mucous membrane lesions for routine histologic examination as well as for direct immunofluorescence can be very helpful in confusing cases. Trauma, usually in the form of cheek biting, produces shallow erosions with ragged overhanging white margins horizontally along the buccal mucosa.

The genitalia is another area where ulceration is a commonly seen reaction pattern. As with the oral mucosa, trauma and viral infection (herpesvirus, coxsackievirus) are often considered in the differential diagnosis. In addition, one must keep in mind other sexually transmitted infections. The archetypal lesion here is the chancre of primary syphilis (Atlas Figure 20). This is the asymptomatic single ulcer with an indurated border and a relatively clean, nonpurulent surface. Unfortunately, extragenital lesions and multiple genital ulcers can be seen. Darkfield demonstration of *Treponema pallidum* makes the diagnosis. A positive nontreponemal test developing within 4 to 6 weeks is confirmatory.

The ulcers of chancroid, caused by *Haemophilus ducreyi*, typically are painful, shallow, ragged, and multiple, capable of increasing in number by autoinoculation. Thus, "kissing" ulcers on opposing skin surfaces are often seen. The base of the ulcer is soft. Gram stain of an early ulcer may show the small gram-negative rods, but Gram stain and cultures are most often negative. Clinical appearance and response to antibiotics are usually the basis for diagnosis. The possibility of coexisting chancroid and syphilitic chancre should always be considered.

The distribution of ulcers on other parts of the body can also be a clue to diagnosis. For example, the single ulcer in a papule with raised, translucent margins on sun-exposed skin suggests the presence of a basal cell or squamous cell carcinoma. Ulcers in sun-exposed areas may be seen with lupus erythematosus or following the vesicles of polymorphous light eruption. Ulcers may also develop in malignant melanoma.

Self-inflicted ulcerations have acutely angular margins and present as polymorphous lesions with haphazard distribution on reachable surfaces (Atlas Figure 21). The center of the back is usually spared. Hemorrhagic crusting may be seen beneath the patient's fingernails.

Pressure and friction are key etiologic factors in decubitus ulcers, where the sacrum, hips, heels, and elbows are common sites. The fragile skin associated with porphyria cutanea tarda often separates after minor trauma to form ulcers on the dorsum of the hands.

Finally, there are processes that may have a variety of distributions. Ulcers may result from direct injury or chemical or thermal burns. Infectious agents may produce single or multiple ulcerations. These include bacteria, usually *Staphylococcus aureus*, mycobacteria (atypical, *Mycobacterium tuberculosis*), fungi, and viruses (herpes simplex, herpes zoster). The gumma of tertiary syphilis can ulcerate. The blistering diseases can produce a variety of ulcerations following rupture of vesicles and bullae. In such cases, overhanging "collarette" scaling can be seen around the periphery of the lesion at the base of the prior blister. Pemphigus vulgaris, bullous pemphigoid, toxic epidermal necrolysis, erythema multiforme, dermatitis herpetiformis, and epidermolysis bullosa are diseases in the differential diagnosis of blistering conditions.

References

Bernhard JD, Mark EJ. Case records of the Massachusetts General Hospital. Case 17-1986. An 18-year-old man with cutaneous ulcers and bilateral pulmonary infiltrates. N Engl J Med. 1986; 314:1170.

Callen P. Cutaneous aspects of internal disease. Chicago: Year Book Medical Publishers, 1981:161.

Demis DJ, et al, eds. Clinical dermatology. 15th rev. ed. Philadelphia: JB Lippincott, 1988.

Fitzpatrick TB, et al, eds. Dermatology in general medicine. 3rd ed. New York: McGraw-Hill, 1987.

Moschella SL, Hurley J, eds. Dermatology. 2nd ed. Philadelphia: WB Saunders, 1985.

Pillsbury DM, Heaton CL. A manual of dermatology. 2nd ed. Philadelphia: WB Saunders, 1980.

Rook A, et al, eds. Textbook of dermatology. 4th ed. Oxford: Blackwell Scientific Publications, 1986.

Atlas of Dermatology

Mark J. Scharf, M.D.

The following 50 cases were chosen to give an introductory overview of some of the more common and important diseases in dermatology and to complement the accompanying chapters in this textbook.

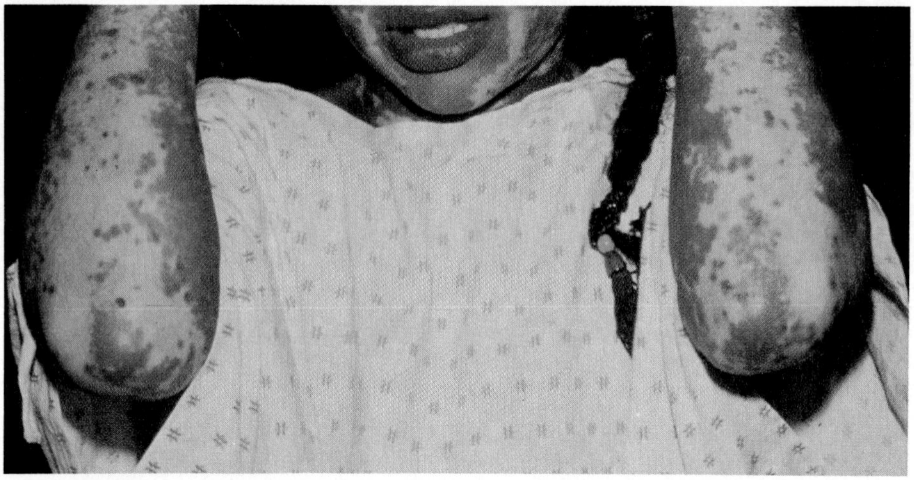

Figure 1. Sharply demarcated, irregularly bordered depigmented macules are characteristic of vitiligo.

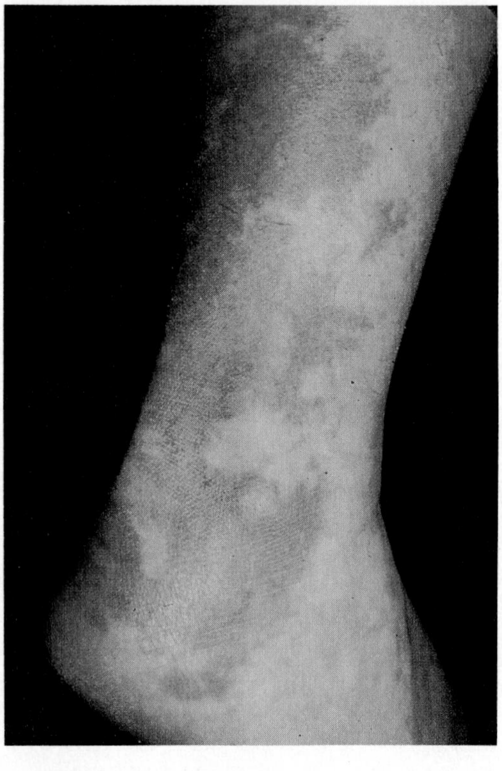

Figure 2. A reddish-purple blanchable port-wine stain macule on the lower extremity.

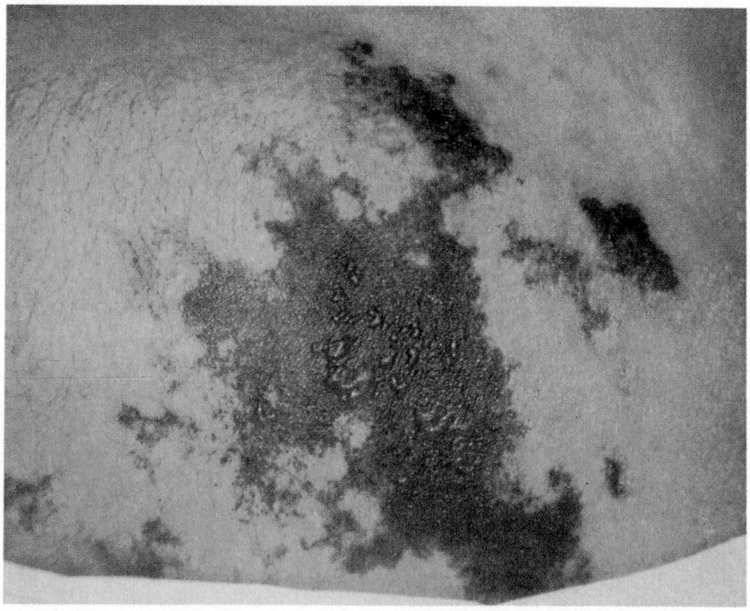

Figure 3. Large areas of nonblanchable purpura in a patient with overwhelming sepsis and disseminated intravascular coagulation. Hemorrhagic bullae in the center of the largest macule are a sign of epidermal necrosis and possible impending ulceration.

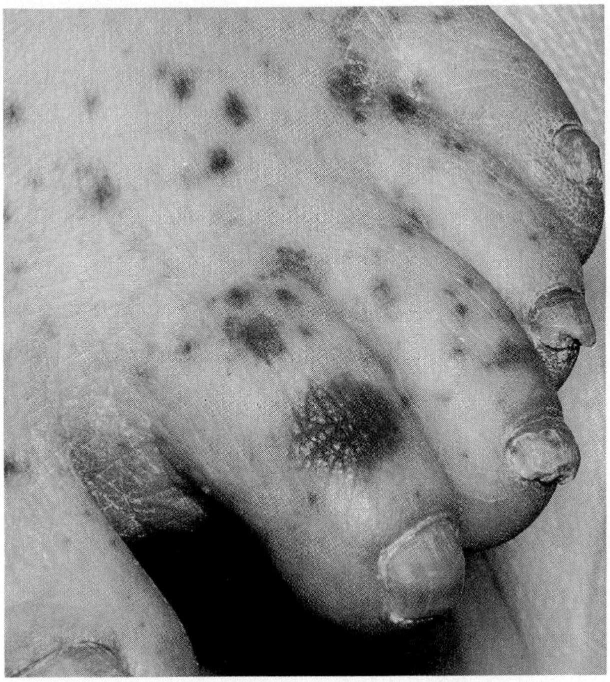

Figure 4. Nonblanchable petechial macules and palpable purpura in a patient with leukocytoclastic vasculitis due to immune complex deposition from her underlying subacute bacterial endocarditis.

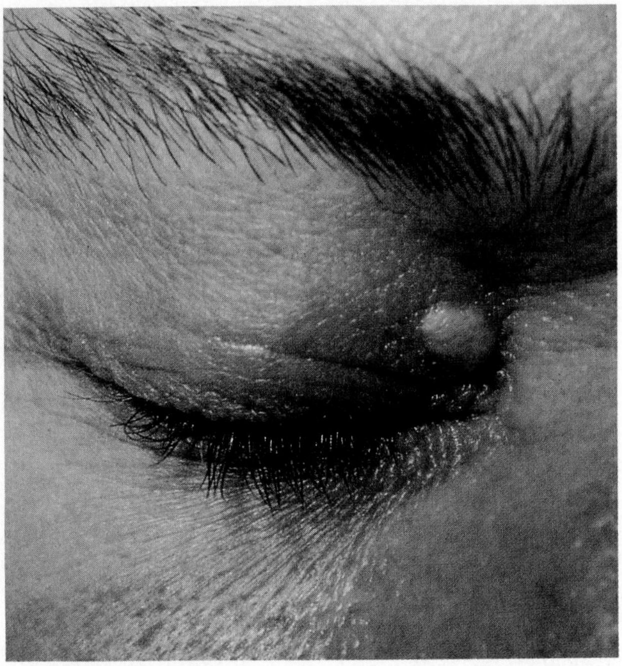

Figure 5. Waxy, dull yellow papules on the upper eyelids are a type of xanthoma known as xanthelasma. They are due to an excess accumulation of lipid deposits in the dermis.

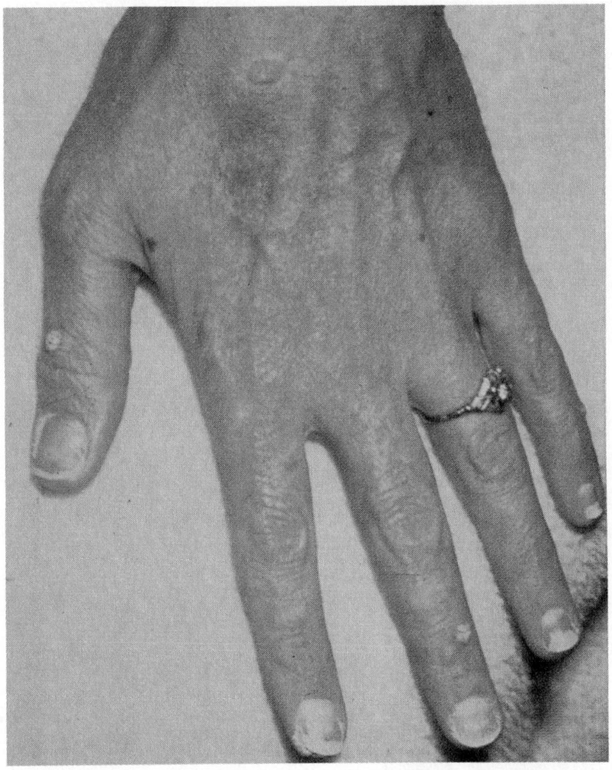

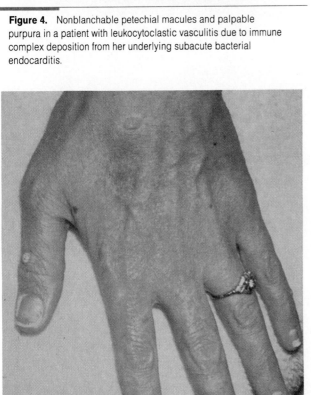

Figure 6. Multiple verrucous papules on the dorsum of the hand and fingers in a patient with common warts, or verruca vulgaris.

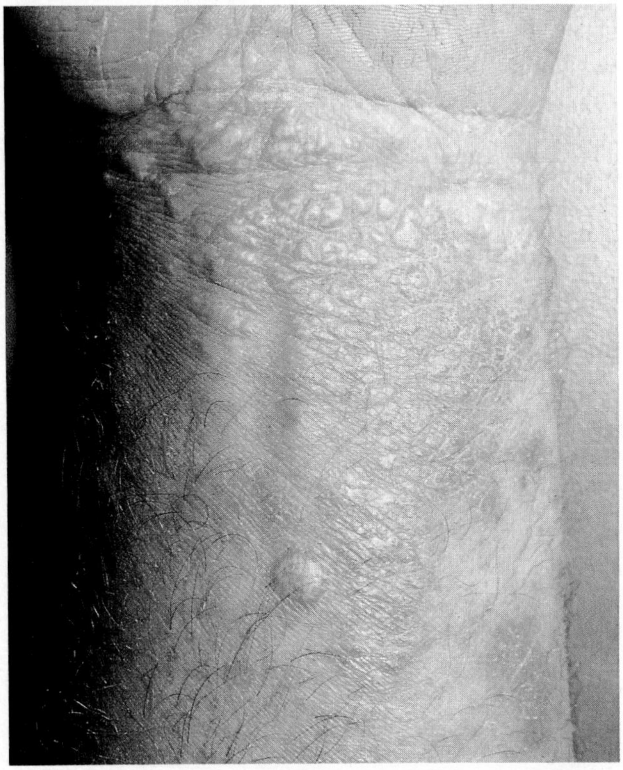

Figure 7. Flat-topped polygonal papules of lichen planus may coalesce to form larger lichenified plaques with accentuation of the skin markings. Some of the larger papules are topped with a lacy whitish pattern known as Wickham's striae, which is diagnostic for lichen planus.

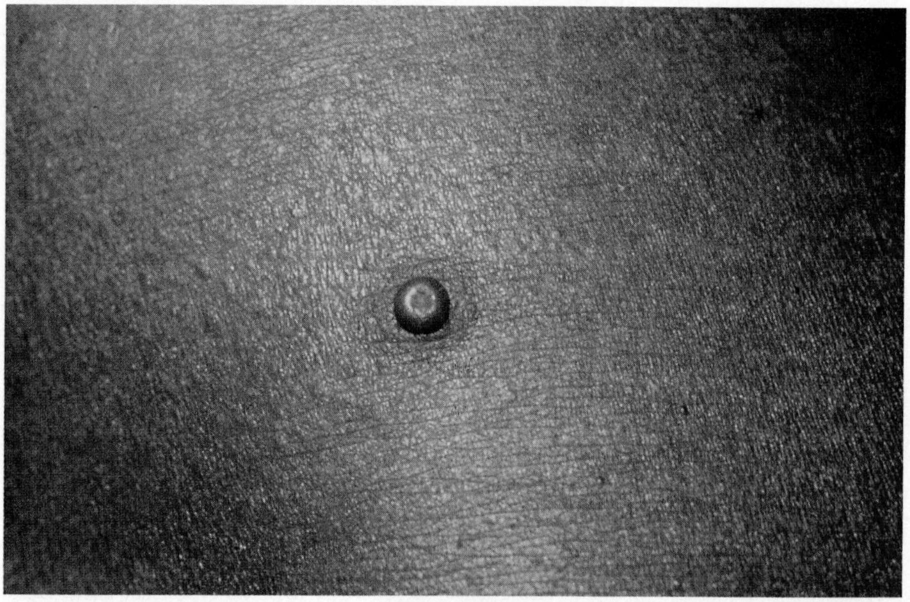

Figure 8. A single rounded umbilicated papule of molluscum contagiosum.

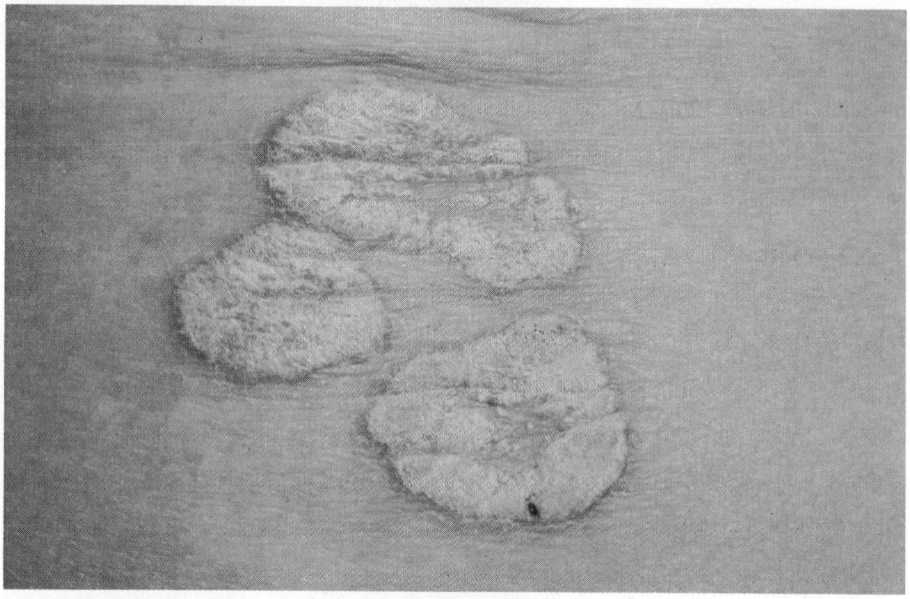

Figure 9. A group of well-demarcated erythematous plaques with silvery scale in a patient with psoriasis. Note the small area of crusted blood at the edge of the lowest plaque where the scales have been pulled away. This sign, called Auspitz's sign, is characteristic of psoriasis.

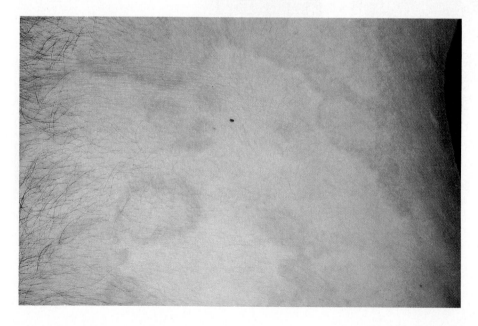

Figure 10. Large confluent polycyclic wheals with erythematous raised borders and central pallor in a patient with urticaria.

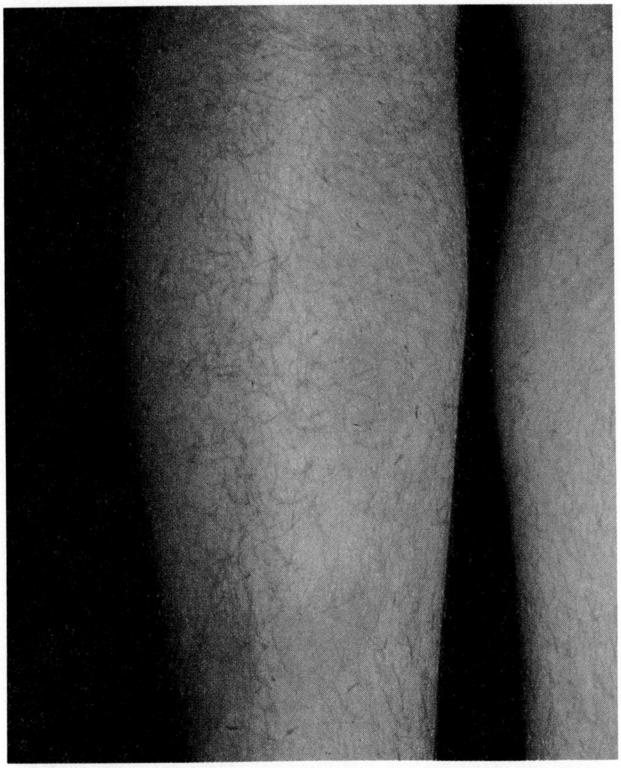

Figure 11. Painful, warm erythematous subcutaneous plaques or nodules of erythema nodosum are best appreciated by palpation.

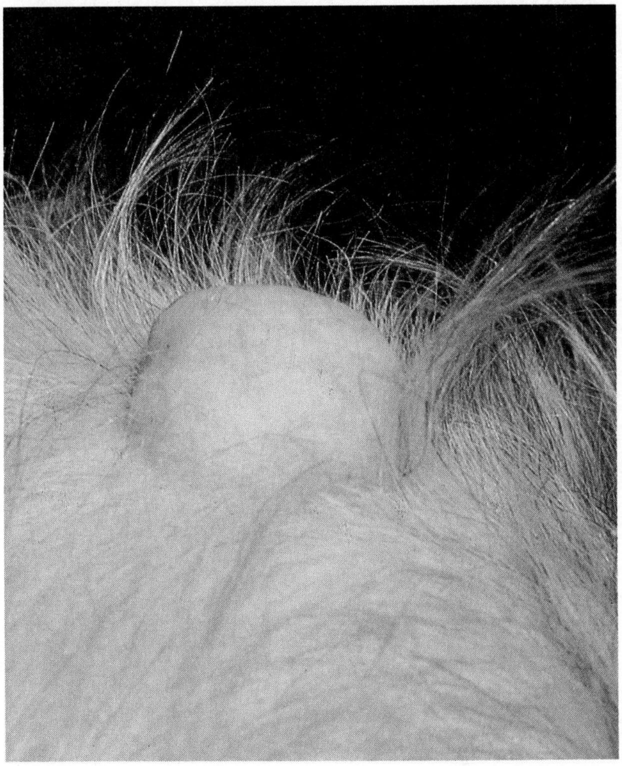

Figure 12. A large mobile epidermal cyst on the scalp.

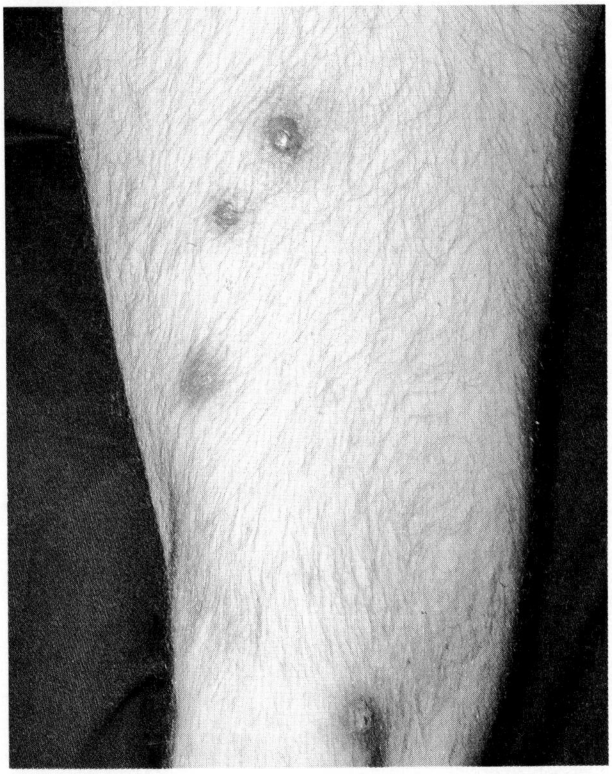

Figure 13. A localized group of bullae, some no longer intact, with underlying crusts are typical of bullous impetigo.

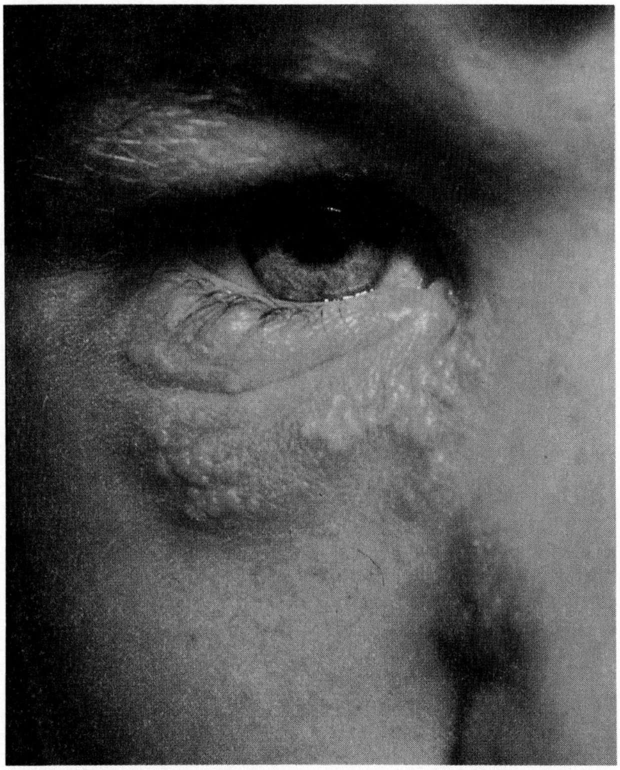

Figure 14. Grouped cloudy vesicles on an erythematous base are classic findings of herpes simplex infections. The diagnosis is confirmed by a positive Tzanck test or viral culture.

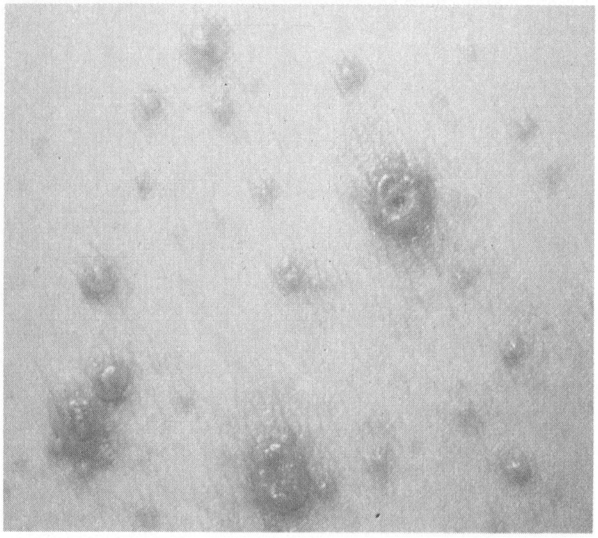

Figure 15. Chicken pox is characterized by a diffuse eruption of erythematous papules and vesicles. Note the central umbilication in the larger vesicles, which are beginning to form crusts.

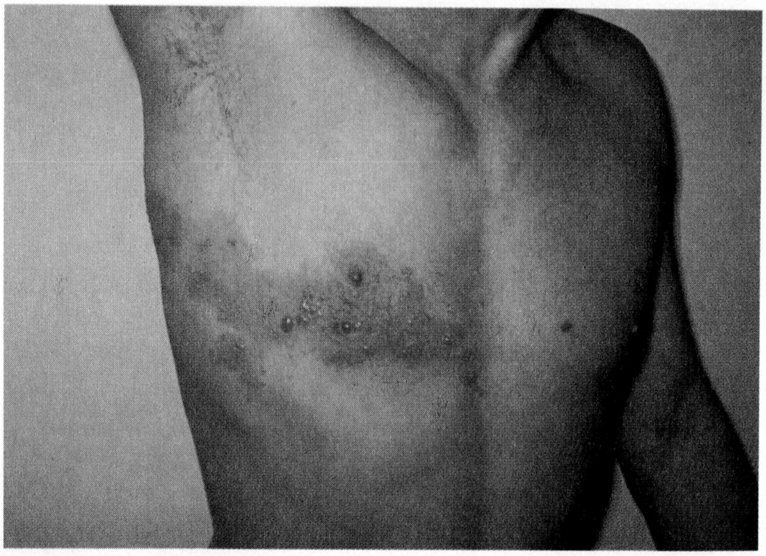

Figure 16. Painful erythematous plaques with vesicles and bullae present in a dermatomal distribution in herpes zoster.

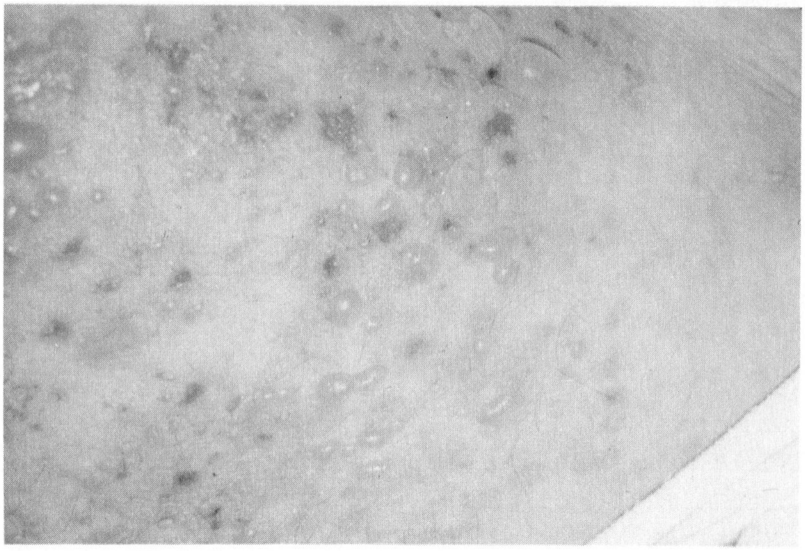

Figure 17. Diffuse tense pruritic bullae in a patient with bullous pemphigoid are often broken or excoriated, leaving shallow erosions.

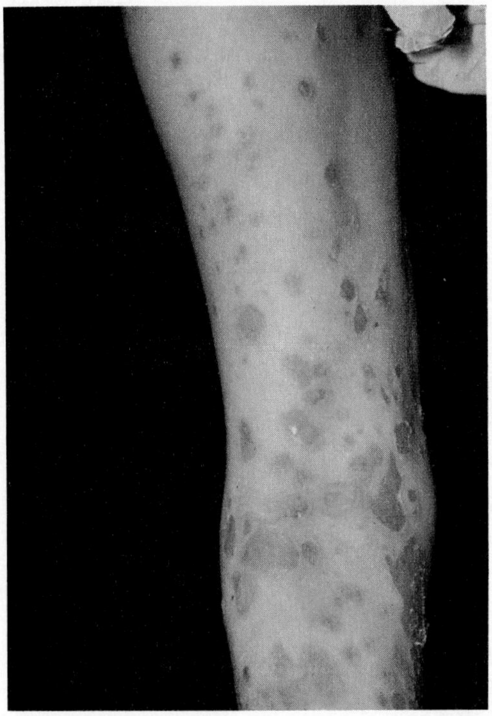

Figure 18. In some forms of pemphigus it may be difficult to find intact bullae. The majority of blisters in this patient have been broken, leaving large healing erosions.

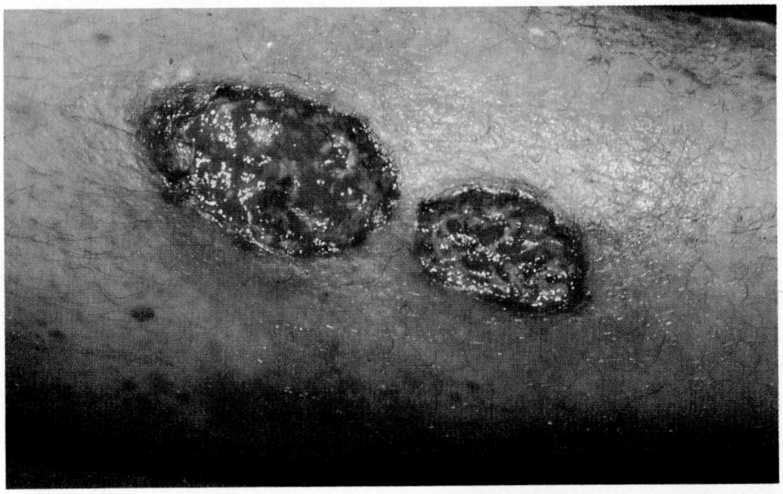

Figure 19. Ulcers in pyoderma gangrenosum have irregular borders with bluish-red overhanging edges.

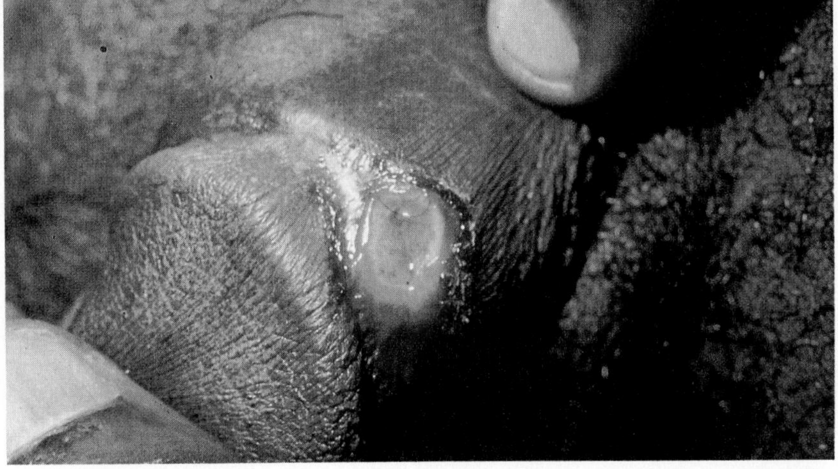

Figure 20. An indurated painless ulcer or chancre of primary syphilis.

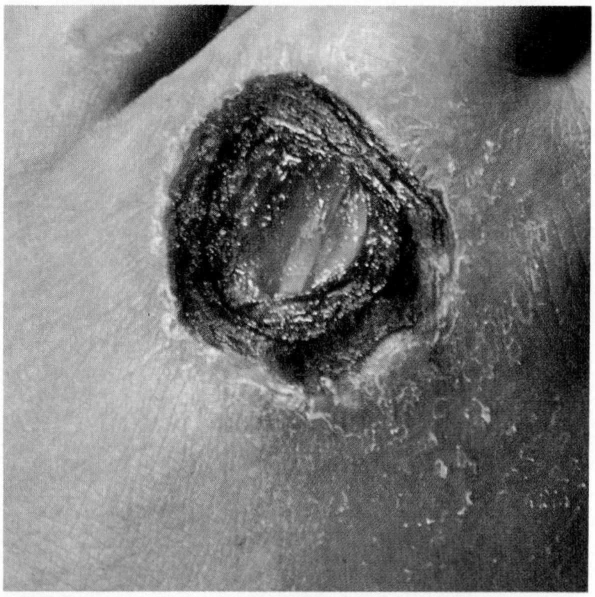

Figure 21. A factitial or self-inflicted ulcer often has sharp angular margins.

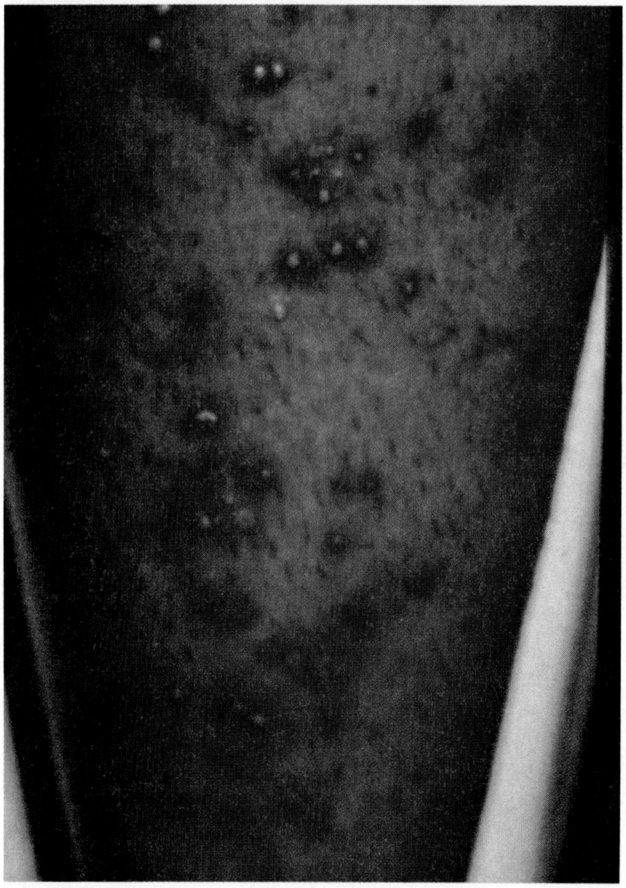

Figure 22. Follicular-centered pustules on an erythematous base should prompt the diagnosis of folliculitis.

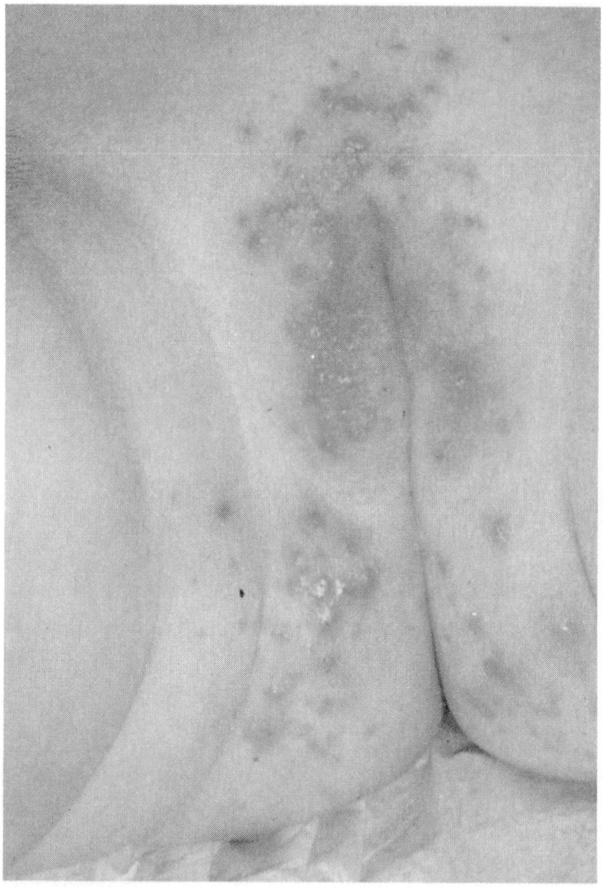

Figure 23. A case of *Candida* "diaper dermatitis" demonstrates characteristic satellite lesions of erythematous papules and pustules spreading out from the main body of the rash.

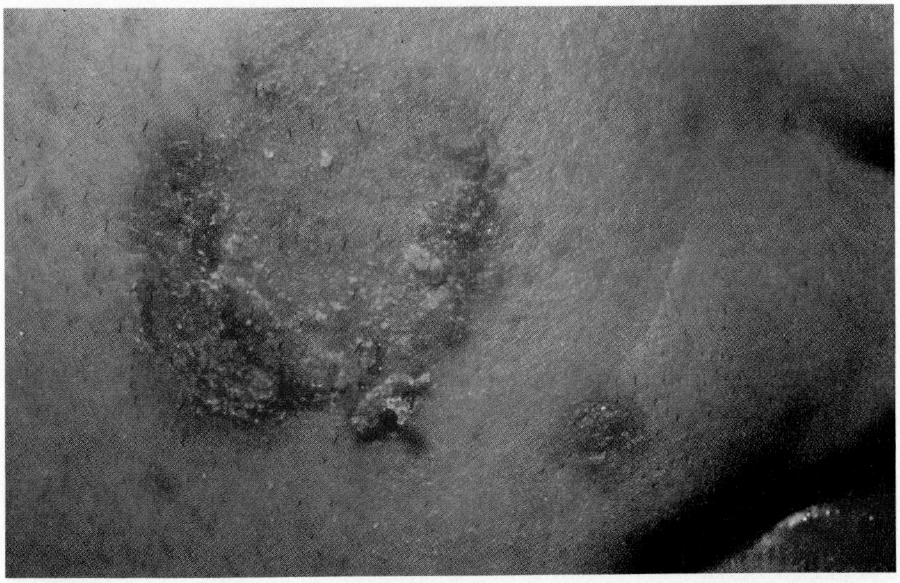

Figure 24. Honey-colored crusted papules and plaques are typical of impetigo.

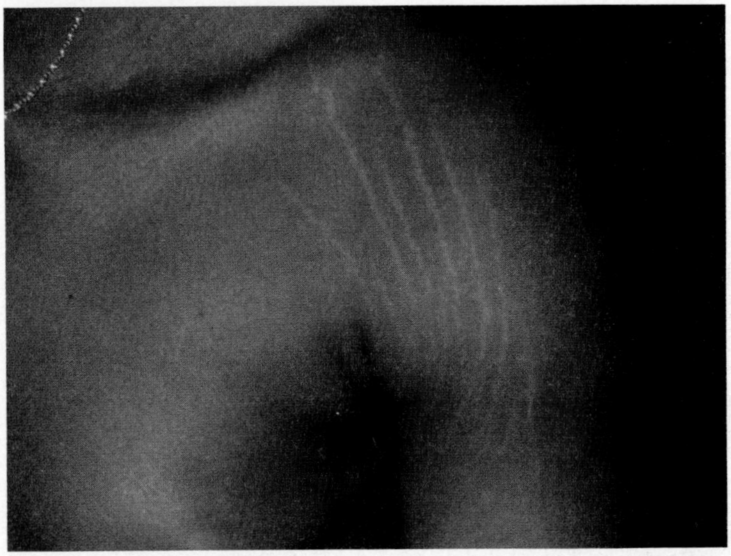

Figure 25. Striae are examples of epidermal and dermal atrophy.

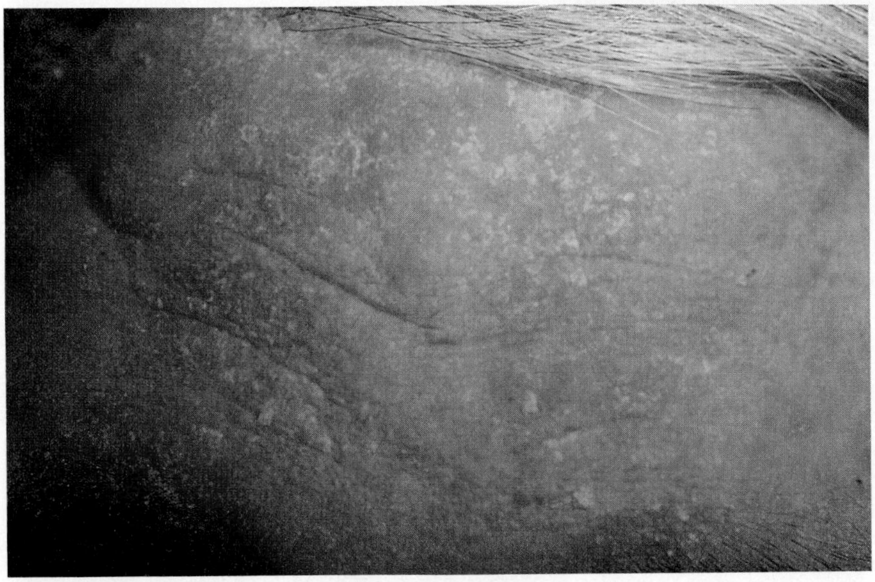

Figure 26. This patient has seborrheic dermatitis. The erythema and desquamative scale are typical.

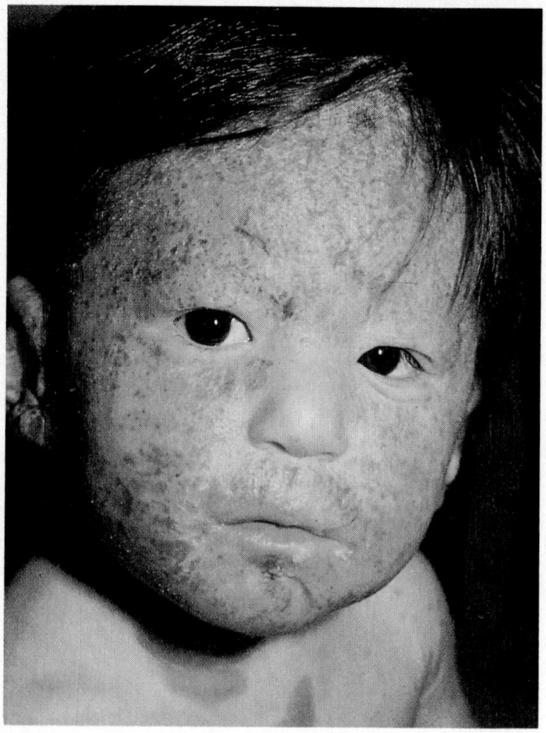

Figure 27. Patients with severe atopic dermatitis may develop diffuse erythema and edema with secondary excoriations, fissuring, and crusting.

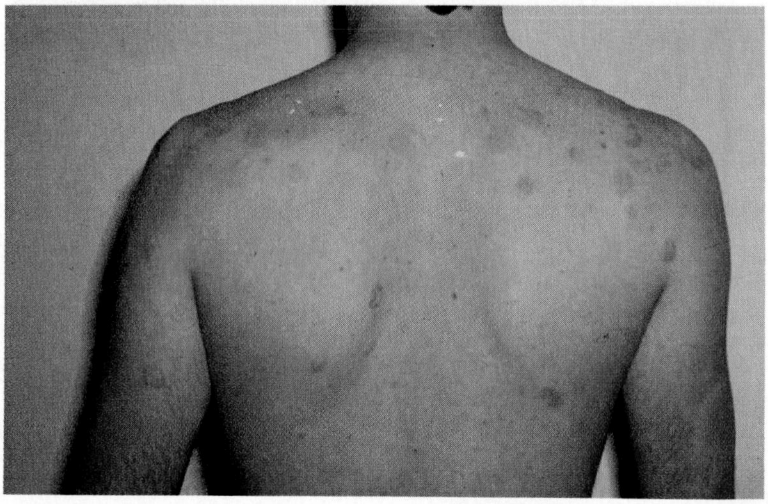

Figure 28. Round, coin-sized plaques of nummular eczema.

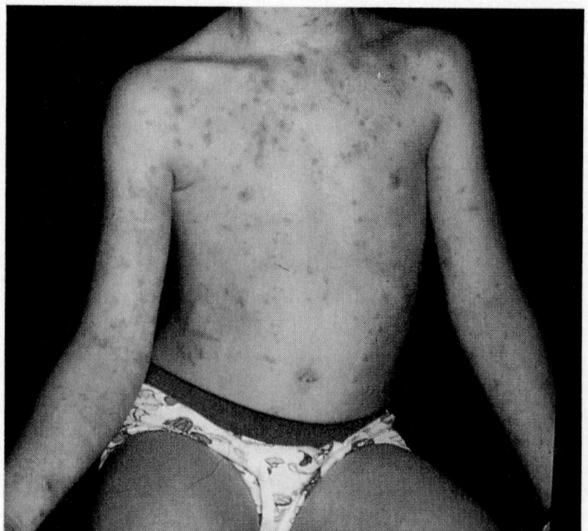

Figure 29. This young boy had an extensive exposure to poison ivy. Note especially the linear papulovesicular streaks, which are very helpful in making the diagnosis.

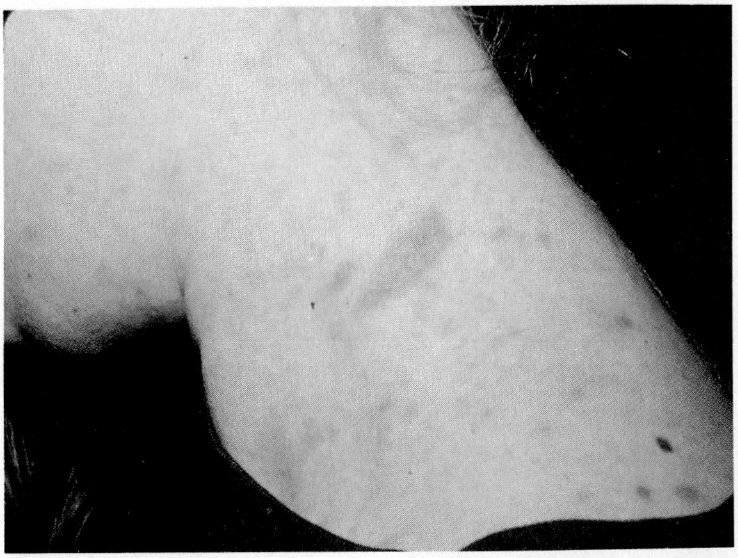

Figure 30. The large, oval, scaly plaque on this patient's neck is a herald patch of pityriasis rosea.

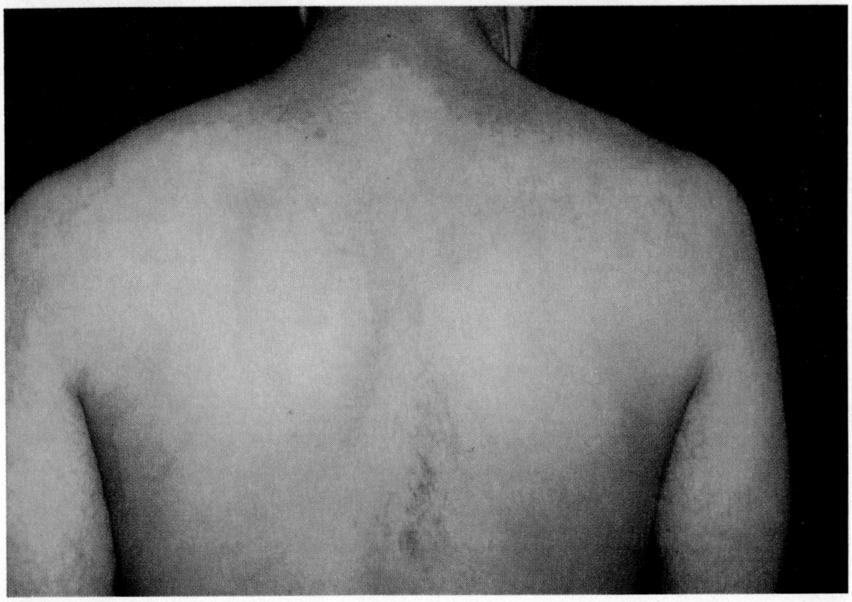

Figure 31. Large confluent patches of hypopigmentation with minimal erythema at the borders were diagnosed as tinea versicolor by a positive KOH exam.

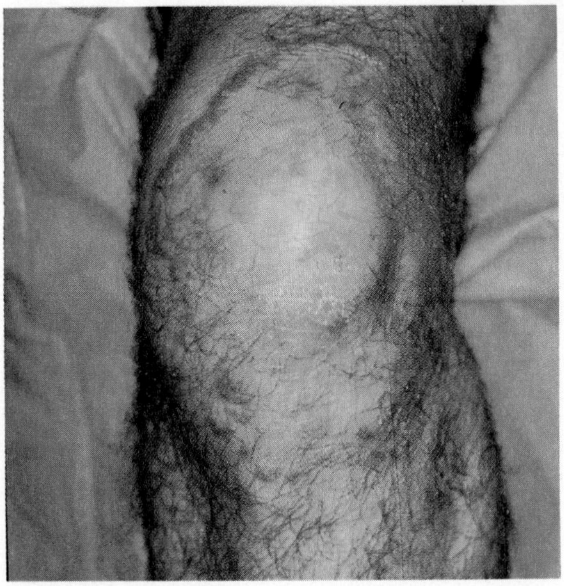

Figure 32. Tinea corporis, or ringworm, classically presents with geographic ringlike plaques with scaling and central clearing.

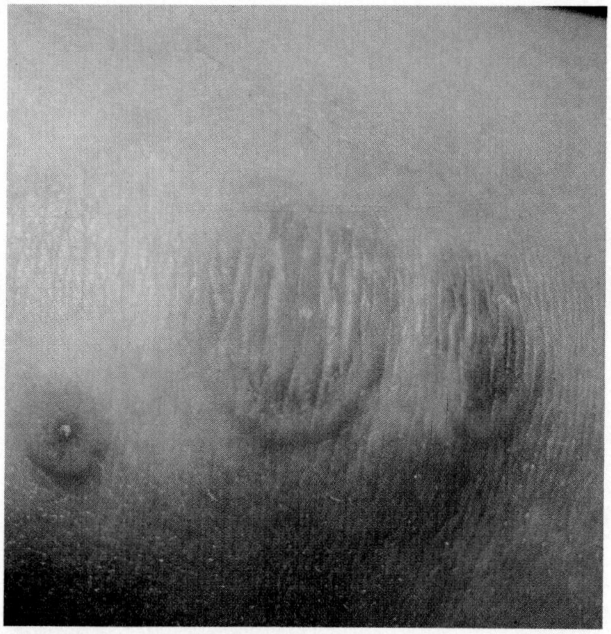

Figure 33. Persistent plaques of erythema multiforme are appropriately named "target lesions," as demonstrated by this patient.

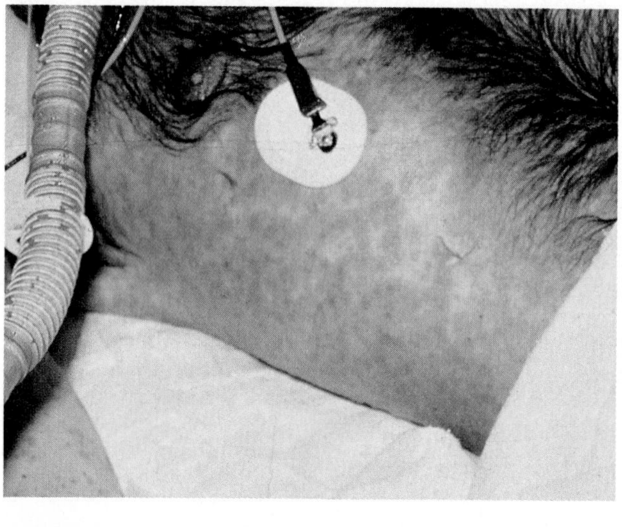

Figure 34. Note the diffuse, confluent, dusky, violaceous appearance of the chest and abdomen with two small areas of early epidermal exfoliation in this patient with toxic epidermal necrolysis.

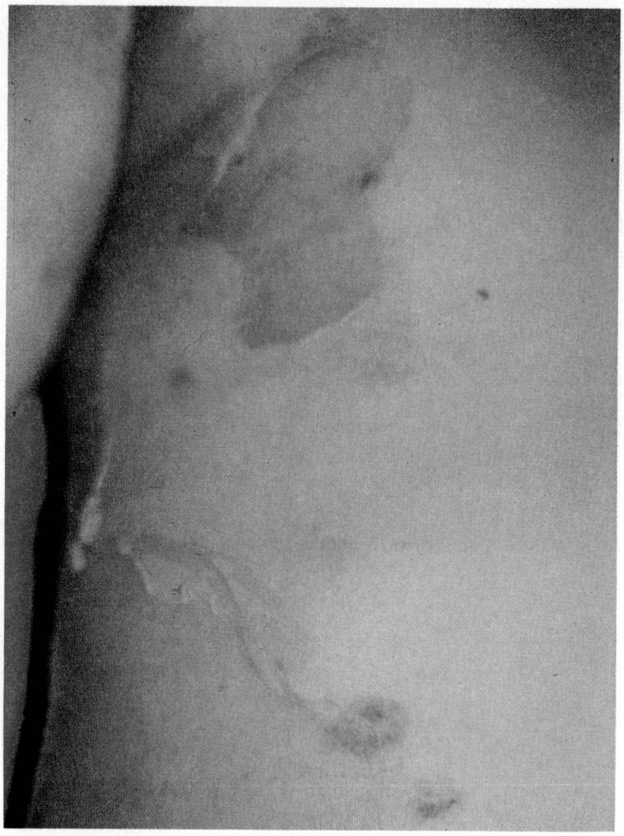

Figure 35. The subcorneal exfoliative blisters in this case of staphylococcal scalded skin syndrome must be distinguished from those of toxic epidermal necrolysis by biopsy or by frozen section analysis of the blister roof.

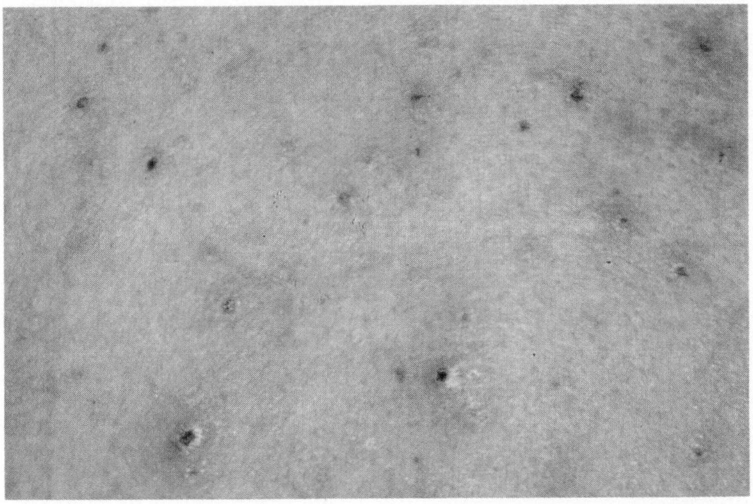

Figure 36. This patient's acne consists primarily of comedones.

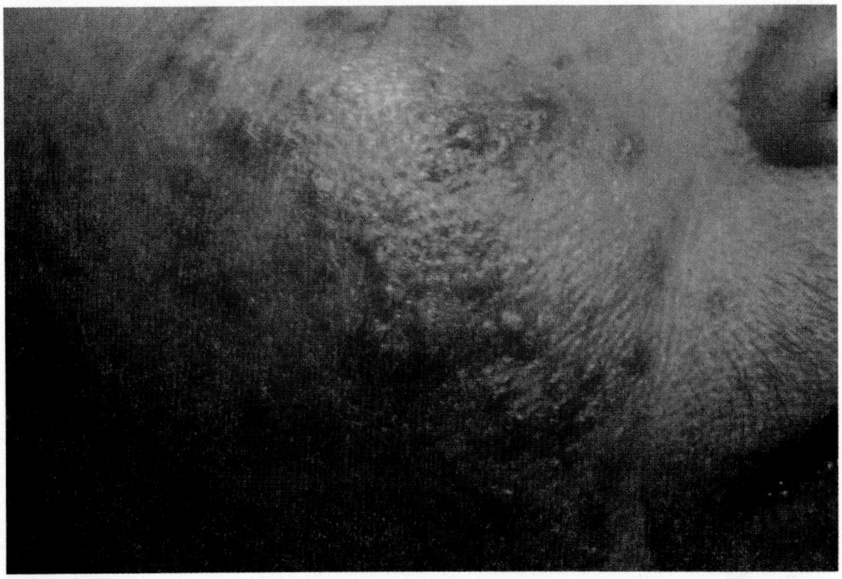

Figure 37. Erythematous papules and pustules with telangiectasia on the face are signs of acne rosacea.

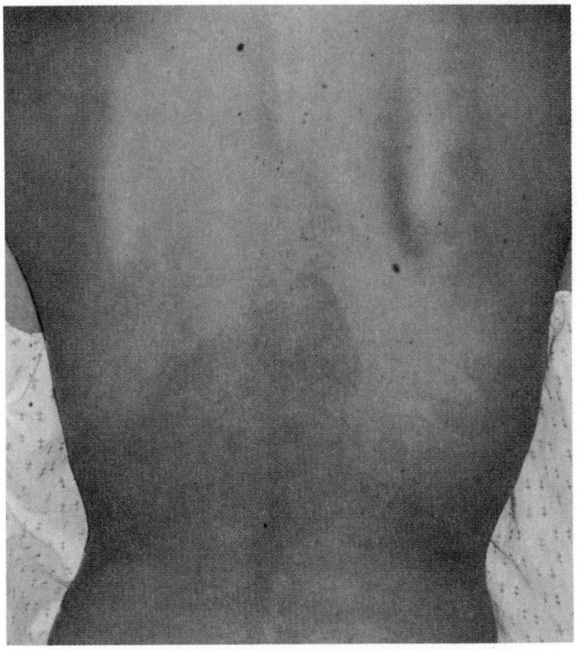

Figure 38. A large expanding dermal plaque with erythematous borders and central clearing is suggestive of erythema chronica migrans in this patient with Lyme disease.

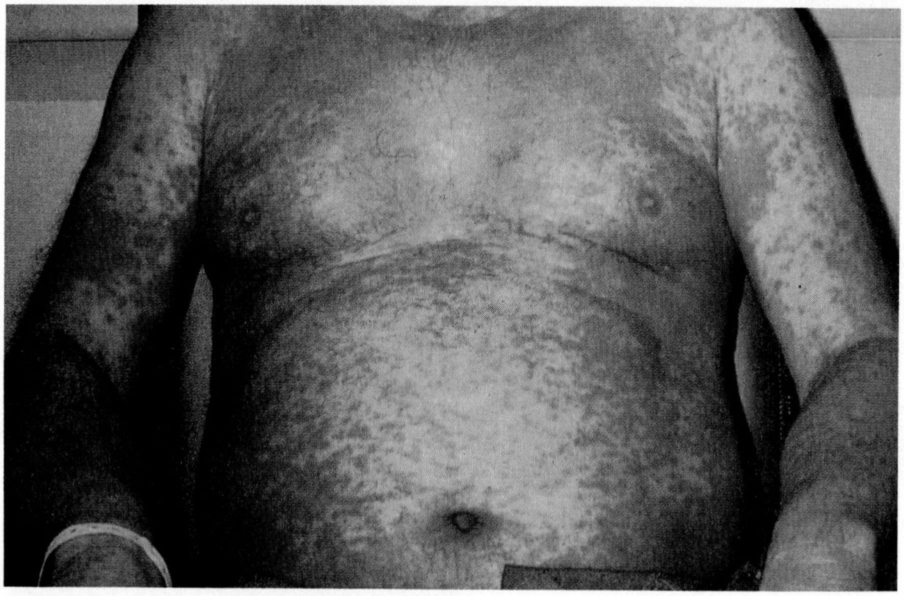

Figure 39. This patient illustrates a classic example of a morbilliform drug eruption, which in this case was due to ampicillin.

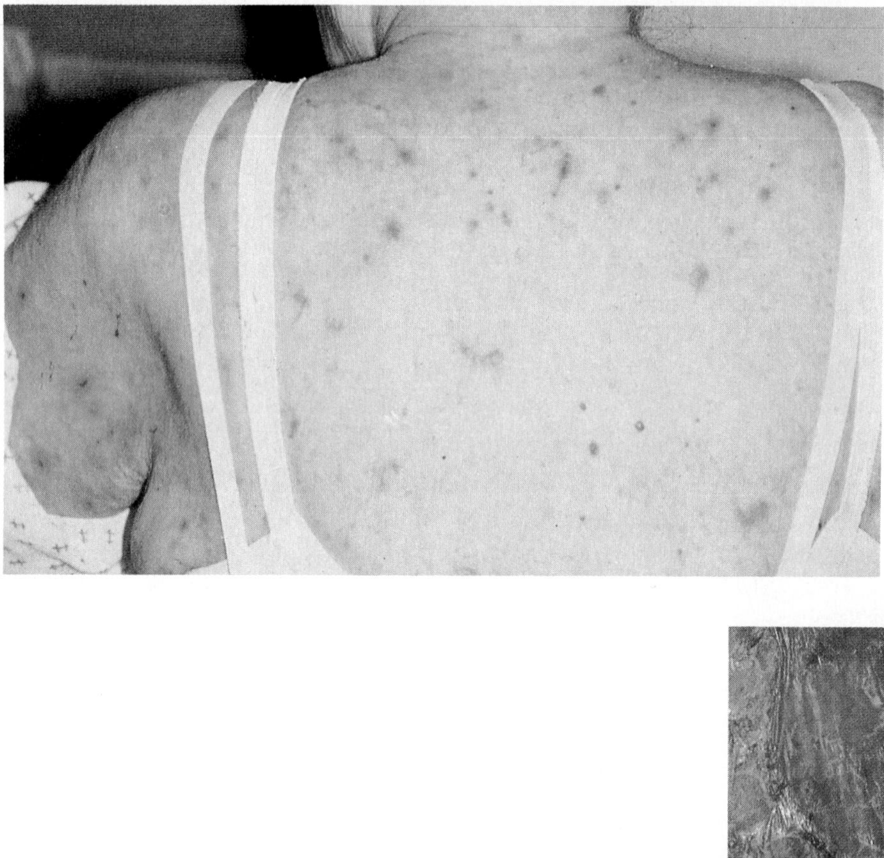

Figure 40. Widespread excoriations and papulovesicles in a severe case of scabies in a nursing home patient. Scrapings from several burrows were positive for scabies mites, ova, and feces.

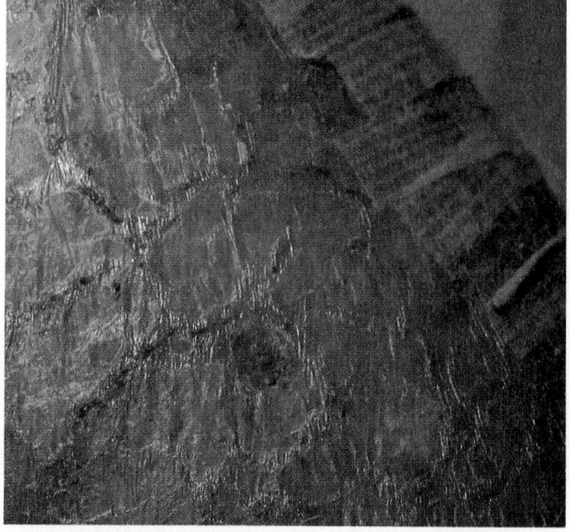

Figure 41. Extremely dry skin may be quite pruritic and can develop erythematous superficial splits or fissures. This condition is called eczema craquelé.

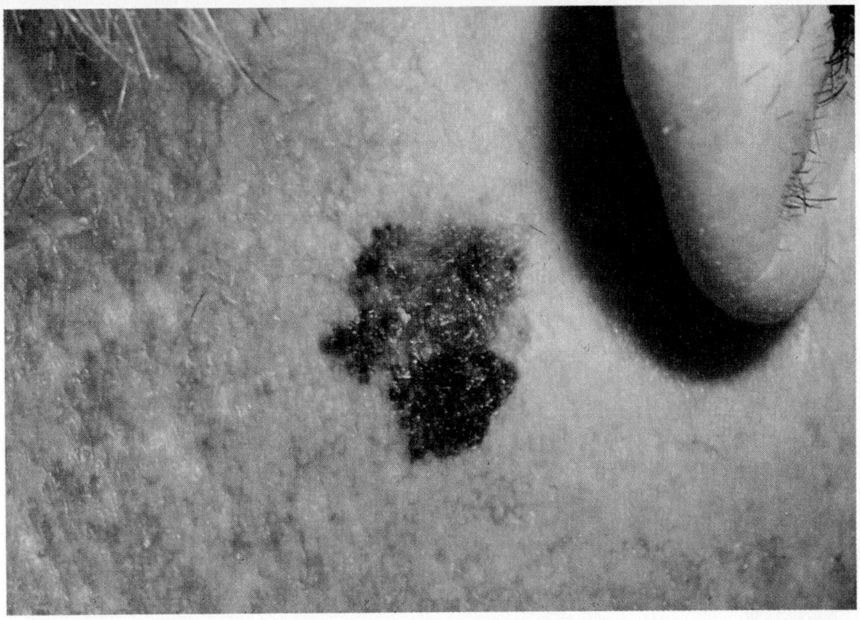

Figure 42. Note the various hues and dark color along with the irregular border in this case of superficial spreading malignant melanoma.

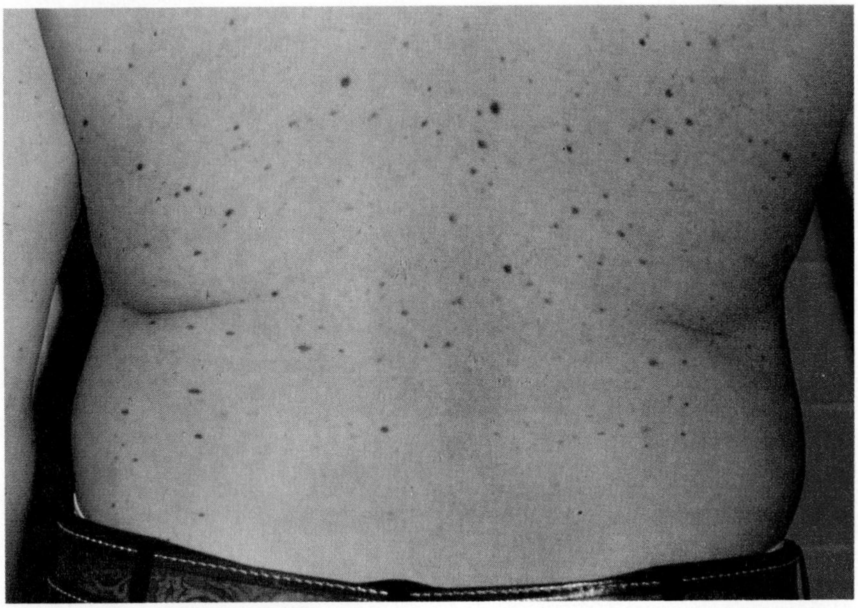

Figure 43. This patient has numerous large, irregular dysplastic nevi.

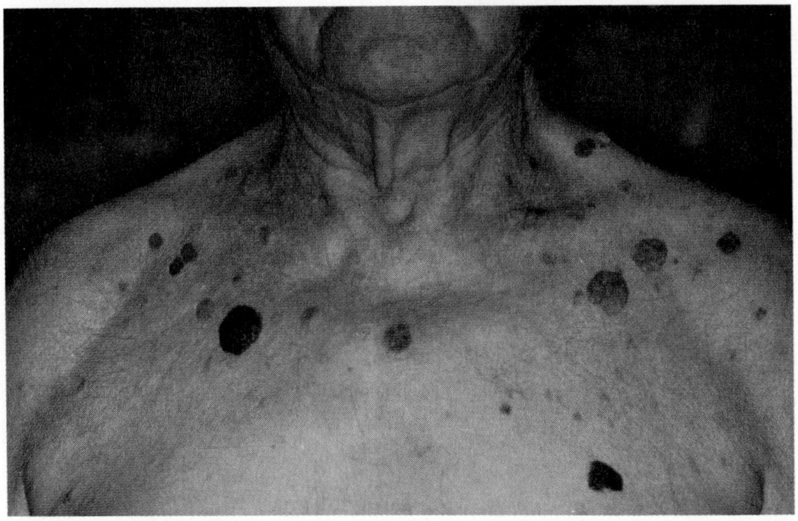

Figure 44. Large, waxy seborrheic keratoses on the chest are common in older patients.

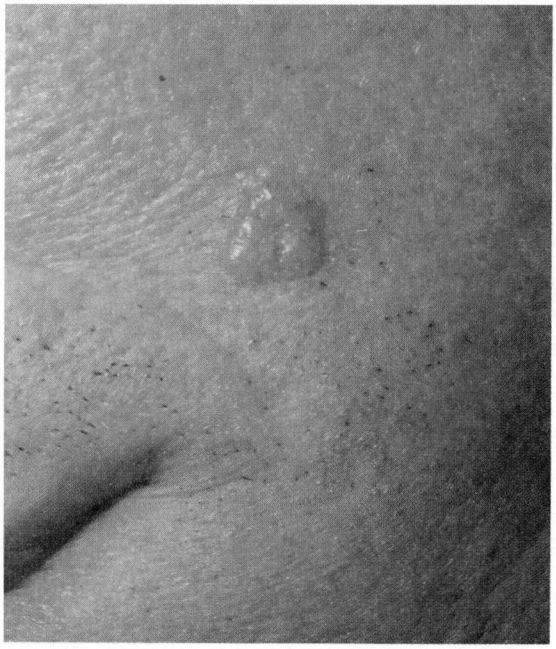

Figure 45. This waxy, translucent telangiectatic papule should prompt a biopsy to make the diagnosis of a basal cell carcinoma.

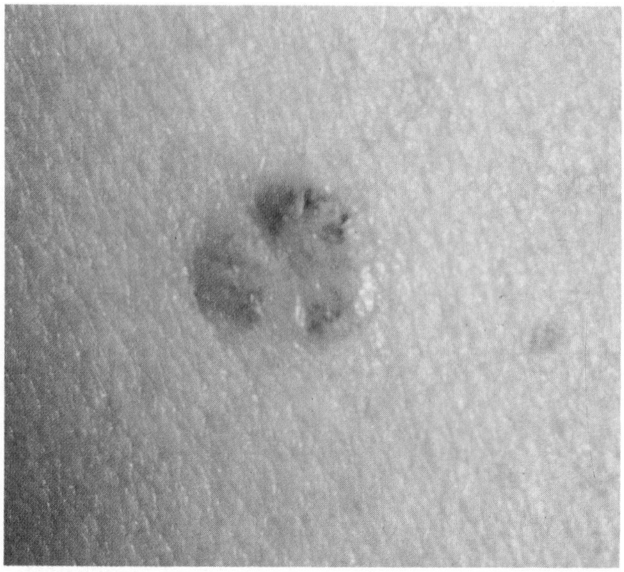

Figure 46. This waxy pink papule is pigmented and proved to be a pigmented basal cell carcinoma.

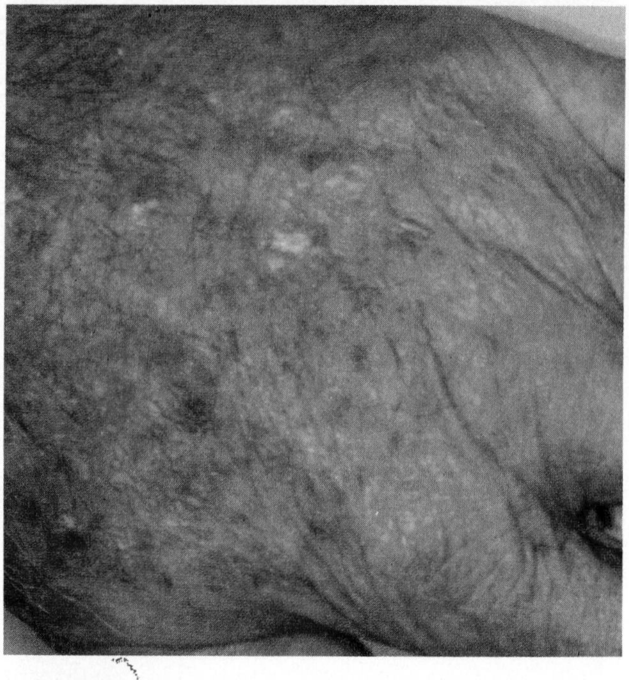

Figure 47. The rough scaly papules on the dorsum of this patient's hand are typical of actinic keratoses. Actinic keratoses are precancerous lesions that in some cases can give rise to squamous cell carcinomas.

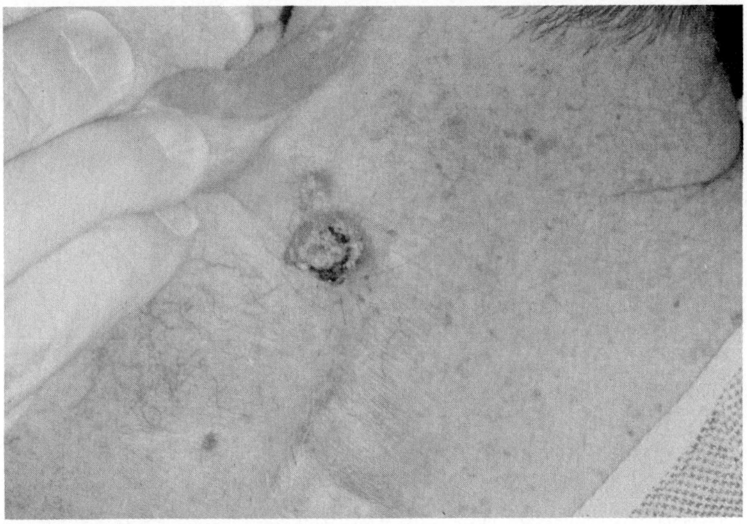

Figure 48. A crusted verrucous nodule on an erythematous base proved to be an invasive squamous cell carcinoma.

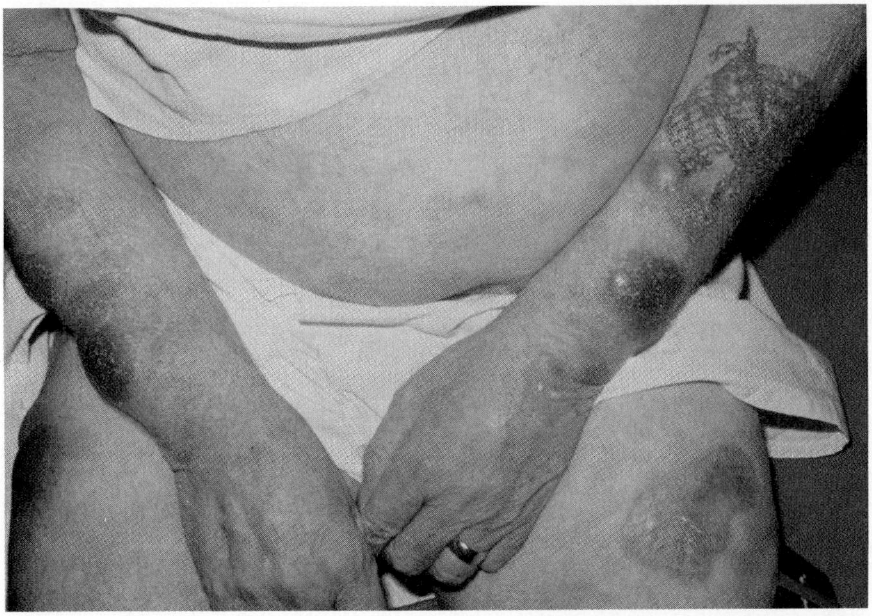

Figure 49. Skin biopsy of one of these plum-colored tumors made the diagnosis of cutaneous non-Hodgkin's lymphoma.

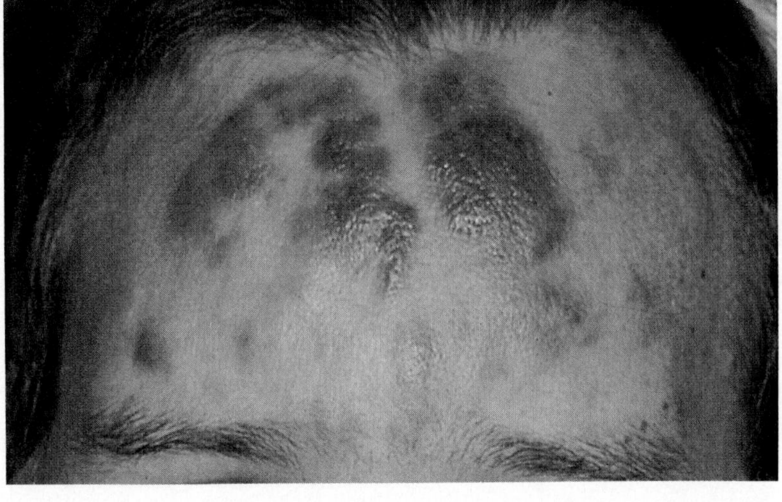

Figure 50. Kaposi's sarcoma is demonstrated by these purple dermal plaques and nodules in this patient with the acquired immunodeficiency syndrome.

Endocrinology

Amenorrhea

Christopher Longcope, MD

Thomas A. Johnson, MD

37

Definition

Although there is some variation in the temporal relationships, amenorrhea can be defined as the failure to establish vaginal bleeding (menarche) by the age of 16 or the failure to menstruate for 3 months in women with previously established episodes of vaginal bleeding.

Although in the past these categories have been approached separately as primary and secondary amenorrhea, respectively, there is a growing tendency to discard these latter subclassifications. In the normal woman, cyclic menstruation is a result of the carefully integrated activities of the hypothalamus, the pituitary gland, the ovary, and the outflow tract (uterus, cervix, and vagina). Perturbation of any of these areas can interfere with their activity and result in amenorrhea. The problem of amenorrhea should be approached with this in mind.

For menstruation to occur, gonadotropin-releasing hormone must be secreted in pulsatile fashion and stimulate the pituitary to secrete the gonadotropins—luteinizing hormone (LH) and follicle-stimulating hormone (FSH)—in an appropriate pulsatile fashion. LH and FSH stimulate ovarian follicular development, estrogen synthesis and secretion, ovulation, and subsequent progesterone secretion from the corpus luteum. The endometrium is stimulated by estrogen and progesterone, and when hormone stimulation becomes insufficient, the endometrium sloughs and exits the uterus through the cervix and vagina as the menstrual flow.

The work-up and diagnosis of amenorrhea are based on finding an abnormality in one or more of these areas.

Etiologies and Characteristics

Hypothalamic-Pituitary Dysfunction

With one exception, women with all of the following conditions have low or low-normal LH and FSH levels and, if progesterone is administered, no menses will occur after the progesterone is stopped. The one exception is polycystic ovary disease, in which there is usually a slightly elevated LH level and low FSH, resulting in an abnormally high LH : FSH ratio. Gonadotropin assays are required in all patients.

Common Causes

Prolactinoma. As awareness increases and diagnostic tools improve, this condition is being recognized with increasing frequency. It is generally associated with galactorrhea but should be considered in any woman with amenorrhea. Prolactin levels are elevated and visual field defects are present with larger tumors (macroadenomas). However, the majority of patients present with small tumors (microadenomas) that do not produce visual field defects. Headache, however, may be present with either micro- or macroadenomas. Hirsutism is occasionally present. Laboratory diagnosis rests on elevated serum prolactin levels and evidence of a pituitary tumor on computed tomography (CT) scans or magnetic resonance imaging (MRI).

Hypothalamic-Pituitary Space-Occupying or Infiltrating Lesions (Other than Prolactinoma). Any lesion that encroaches on a critical area of the hypothalamus, pituitary, or pituitary stalk, interfering with the secretion of gonadotropin-releasing hormone or acting directly on the gonadotropins, can result in amenorrhea. Tumors interfering with certain critical hypothalamic nuclei can block release or transport of prolactin-inhibitory factor, causing hyperprolactinemia and a resultant decrease in gonadotropin secretion. If a functioning pituitary tumor is the cause, there will be signs and symptoms resulting from overproduction of hormone produced by the tumor. The most common functioning pituitary macroadenomas are prolactinomas and growth hormone–producing tumors.

In the case of Cushing's disease, the tumor itself may not interfere with gonadotropin secretion; rather, the excess production of adrenal androgen suppresses gonadotropin release.

Hypothalamic Amenorrhea. This includes several entities that influence hypothalamic function through obscure mechanisms but probably involves excess endorphin activity. These entities include stress, marked weight loss (including anorexia nervosa), and strenuous exercise. Diagnosis rests, in part, on the history and the finding of normal prolactin levels. Imaging of the skull, by either CT or MRI, may be required to rule out tumors or other space-occupying lesions.

Less Common Causes

Amenorrhea with Anosmia (Kallman's Syndrome). Midline defects frequently result in cleft lip and cleft palate. Some of these patients also have anosmia and amenorrhea. The latter problems are due to a hypothalamic rather than a pituitary defect, because these patients usually respond to the administration of synthetic LH-releasing hormone (LRH). Many of these patients do not have clinically apparent midline defects. Amenorrhea in the presence of anosmia does not require an extensive laboratory work-up. In some individuals, the loss of gonadotropin function is incomplete, with only LH or FSH present. Nevertheless, amenorrhea will also occur in these patients.

Morbid Obesity. Although the correlation between obesity and amenorrhea is not as good as that between an underweight state and amenorrhea, women who are very obese are likely to have amenorrhea. The diagnosis of obesity-associated amenorrhea can be made only after other causes of amenorrhea are excluded by laboratory and radiographic testing.

Delayed Puberty. Chronic systemic diseases cause a functional form of hypothalamic amenorrhea. If this occurs during the adolescent years, it is also associated with delayed puberty. Organic lesions of the hypothalamus or pituitary can produce a similar picture, and they must be ruled out, particularly when there is no evidence of systemic disease. This is essentially a diagnosis of exclusion.

Sheehan Syndrome. This syndrome, secondary to postpartum uterine hemorrhage with hypotension, is usually associated with general pituitary failure. The classic history is one of gradual onset of symptoms, including inability to lactate following delivery. The work-up requires that the function of all the pituitary polypeptide hormones be evaluated.

Rare Causes

Laurence-Moon-Biedl Syndrome. This is associated with retinitis pigmentosa, mental retardation, obesity, polydactyly, and other congenital defects. Interestingly, these individuals may have either primary gonadal failure or difficulties with gonadotropin secretion.

Amenorrhea After Oral Contraceptive Use. The incidence of amenorrhea after use of oral contraceptives is about 2.2 per 1,000 users. This is not much greater than the incidence of amenorrhea in nonusers and thus may not be directly related to pill use. Prolactin measurements are essential because, in some cases, prolactinomas become evident after oral contraceptive use is discontinued.

Ovarian Dysfunction

In patients with ovarian dysfunction, serum gonadotropin levels may be normal or high and the progesterone withdrawal test may be positive or negative.

Common Causes

Menopause. Menopause, the age-related loss of ovarian function, is the most common cause of amenorrhea. The median age at which menopause occurs in the United States is 51.4 years, and most women experience it between 48 and 55 years of age. The years just before menopause may be associated with anovulatory, irregular cycles. These cause hot flashes, atrophic vaginitis, and loss of bone mass leading to osteoporosis. Premature menopause, with menses ceasing in the teens or twenties owing to ovarian failure, is uncommon. Although this can represent an extreme of the "normal" processes that lead to menopause, it may also result from autoimmune disease, chemotherapy, or radiation exposure.

Pregnancy. Pregnancy should be considered in any woman of reproductive age who is sexually active and experiences amenorrhea. A pregnancy test should be done as part of the work-up of such individuals. The associated signs and symptoms of pregnancy, including nausea, breast fullness, and uterine enlargement, may not be present at the time of the visit.

Chromosomal Defects. These include XO gonadal dysgenesis (Turner's syndrome) as well as mosaicism. Short stature, shield chest, lymphedema (at birth), skeletal anomalies, coarctation of the aorta, and pterygia may occur in varying frequency. Individuals with XO mosaicism may show few associated features, and some may experience a few bleeding episodes; rarely, pregnancies have been reported. The work-up need not be extensive in subjects with classic findings, but it would include determination of Barr-body presence. Karyotyping may be necessary. The association of hirsutism or other masculinizing features indicates the probable presence of a Y chromosome and the need for removal of gonadal tissue because of its malignant potential.

Polycystic Ovary Disease. Some individuals with amenorrhea, hirsutism, and large ovaries have normal LH and FSH levels and ratio. In some of these patients, an isolated ovarian defect may be the cause. The work-up should include evaluation of androgen levels to rule out an ovarian tumor (patients with the latter usually have testosterone levels greater than 2.5 ng/ml), measurement of serum gonadotropins, and pelvic ultrasonography.

Less Common Causes

Ovarian Androgen-Secreting Tumors. These tumors result in varying degrees of virilization; arrhenoblastomas, lipoid cell, and hilar cell are the more common types of tumor. The amenorrhea that accompanies these tumors is due to suppression of gonadotropins by the circulating androgen.

Syndromes Associated with Androgen Resistance (Testicular Feminization, Lubs and Gilbert-Dreyfus Syndromes). These disorders consist of varying degrees of peripheral resistance to circulating androgens. The individuals are actually genetic males, i.e., XY with testes. Depending on the degree of peripheral resistance, the external phenotype will range from that of a normal woman who lacks sexual and ambosexual hair to that of a masculinized woman; however, the internal organs of reproduction are absent, and the vagina consists of a blind pouch or little more than a dimple. Usually, there is a defect in the binding of androgen to its cytosol receptor, although other mechanisms have been reported. Subjects generally have normal male testosterone levels and slightly elevated levels of estrogen and gonadotropin.

Rare Causes

Asherman's Syndrome. Asherman's syndrome results from destruction of the endometrium, usually from infection or overzealous curettage. These subjects will not have menses after progesterone withdrawal or even after combined estrogen-progesterone stimulation.

Mullerian Abnormalities. This group includes imperforate hymen and obliteration or discontinuities of the vaginal orifice or canal. This form of amenorrhea cannot be ruled out without an adequate gynecologic exam. Absence of the cervix or uterus may also occur in some individuals with a normal vagina.

Work-up of Amenorrhea

As can be appreciated from the previous section, a thorough history and physical examination can, in many cases, pinpoint the diagnosis precisely; e.g., a 16-year-old girl who has had no menses, has no secondary sexual development, has eunuchoid features, and is anosmic needs very little laboratory testing for a diagnosis of Kallman's syndrome to be reached. On the other hand, a 16-year-old girl who has had no menses, has no secondary sexual characteristics, and is relatively short may require karyotyping and even laparotomy in order to be diagnosed as a mosaic with gonadal dysgenesis in whom a portion of the Y chromosome is present.

If the diagnosis is not readily apparent from the initial visit, a progesterone withdrawal test can be done. In a sexually active woman this should be done only after pregnancy is ruled out by appropriate physical examination and laboratory testing. The progesterone withdrawal test involves the intramuscular administration of 100 mg of progesterone-in-oil or the oral administration of a progestin, preferably medroxyprogesterone acetate, 10 mg a day for 7 days. In addition, the serum prolactin level should be measured.

Subjects with at least minimal function of the hypothalamic-pituitary-ovarian axis and a normal outflow tract will have withdrawal bleeding within 2 to 7 days after administration of the progesterone. The amount of bleeding depends, in part, on the levels of circulating estrogen; the more estrogen, the heavier the bleeding. Minimal spotting implies minimal estrogen activity.

If there is bleeding, the likely cause is chronic anovulation secondary to polycystic ovary disease, and the work-up should aim to establish this diagnosis with assessment of gonadotropin levels and pelvic ultrasonography.

If there is no bleeding and the prolactin level is normal, gonadotropin measurements should be made to localize the problem to the hypothalamic-pituitary area (low LH and FSH) or to the ovary (high LH and FSH). If gonadotropins are low, skull radiographs, a CT scan, or a pituitary MRI study may be necessary.

If there is no bleeding and the prolactin level is elevated, CT or MRI of the pituitary should be done.

It should be stressed that a good history and physical can often lead to an immediate diagnosis, and only minimal laboratory testing need be done for confirmation. Pregnancy should always be considered in any sexually active woman of reproductive age who presents with amenorrhea. For most subjects, testing with LRH to distinguish between pituitary or hypothalamic disease is not necessary. Furthermore, LRH tests are difficult to interpret because not all individuals with LRH deficiency respond the first time they are tested with LRH.

Primary Amenorrhea (Fig. 37-1)

Women without the development of secondary sexual characteristics by age 15 should also be included in this category. It is important to rule out historical factors, e.g., systemic illness, endocrine disturbance (other), emotional insult, or weight loss, but physical examination is of particular importance. It may reveal an obstructive pelvic anatomic anomaly and allows classification into four separate diagnostic groups according to the presence or absence of breasts and uterus.

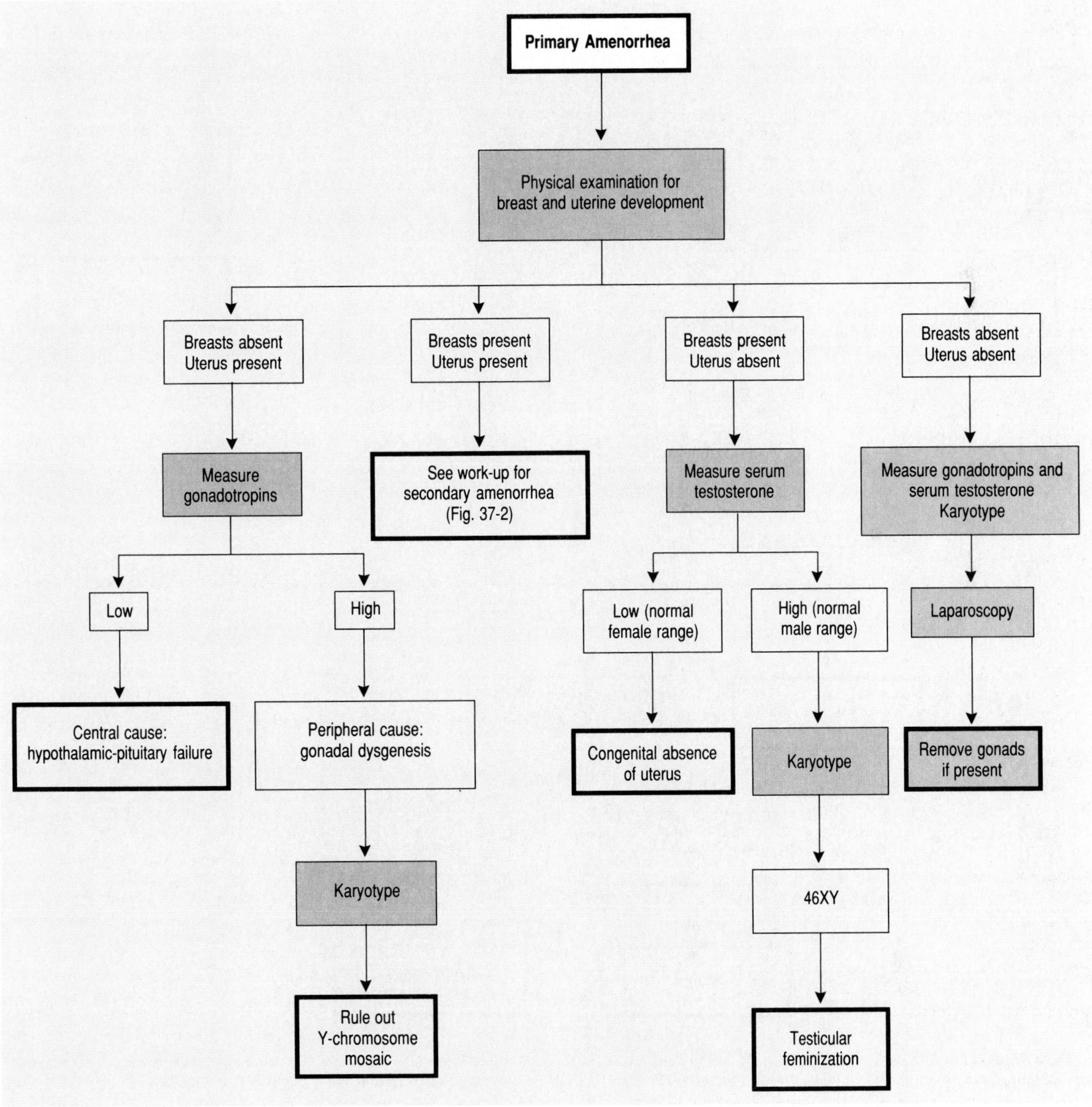

Figure 37-1 Algorithm for the evaluation of primary amenorrhea.

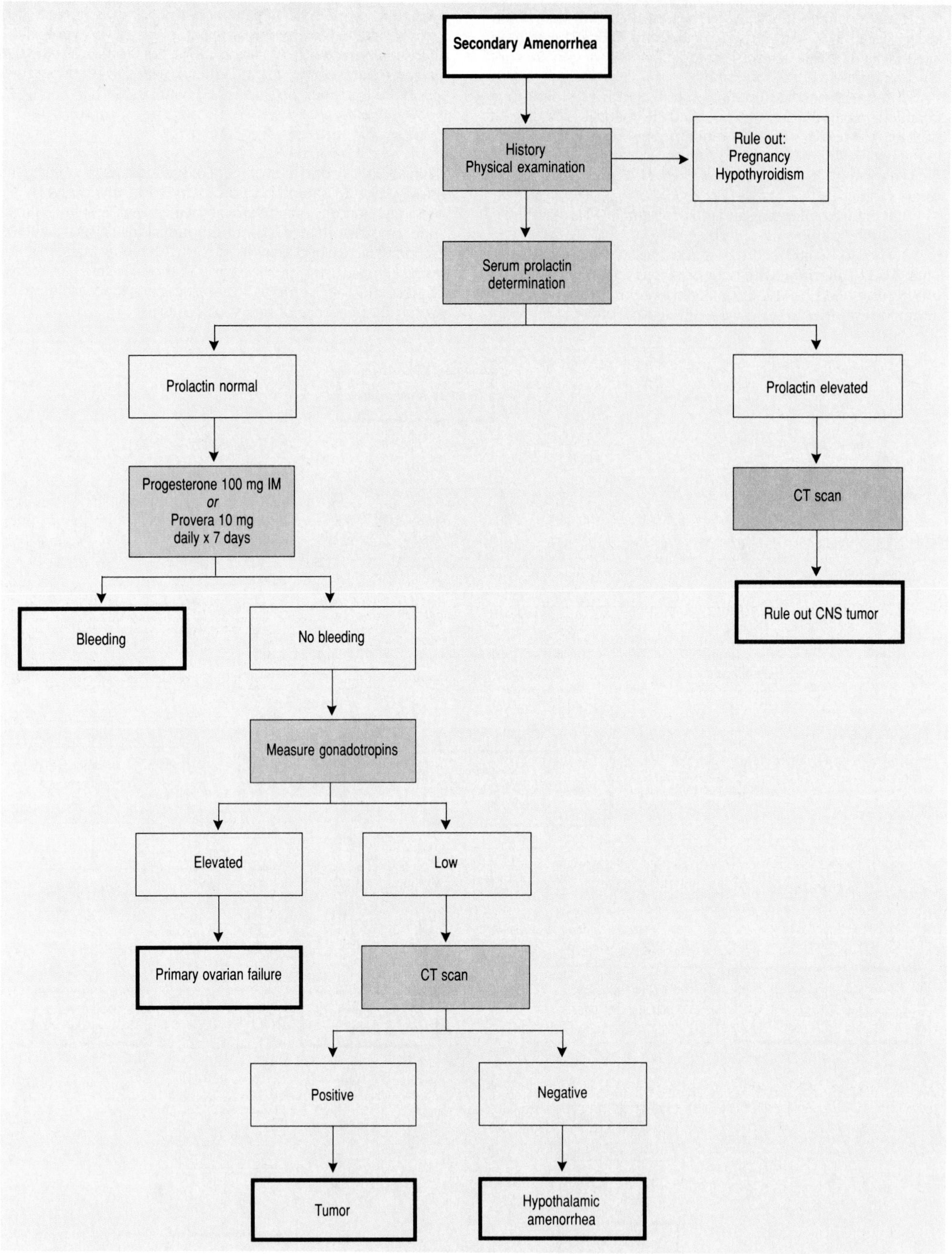

Figure 37-2 Algorithm for the evaluation of secondary amenorrhea. CNS = central nervous system, CT = computed tomography.

Table 37-1 Response to Progesterone Challenge

Progesterone challenge	LH or FSH	Diagnosis
Positive response (withdrawal bleeding)	LH elevated approximately 3/1 compared with FSH	These patients are likely to have polycystic ovary disease
Positive response	LH normal	These patients are likely to have hypothalamic-pituitary dysfunction*
Negative response (no withdrawal bleeding)	FSH normal	History suggestive of Asherman's syndrome (e.g., destruction of endometrium by surgical trauma or infection); perform hysterography or hysteroscopy
Negative response	FSH low or normal	These patients have hypothalamic-pituitary failure; perform serum prolactin and pituitary evaluation
Negative response	FSH elevated	These patients have ovarian failure or gonadotropin-resistant ovarian syndrome (rare)

Abbreviations: FSH = follicle-stimulating hormone, LH = luteinizing hormone.

* Some authorities suggest a serum prolactin determination to rule out hyperprolactinemia, even in the absence of galactorrhea. If galactorrhea is present or the serum prolactin level is elevated, a pituitary work-up should be performed.

Breasts Absent and Uterus Present. This not uncommon finding in patients with primary amenorrhea speaks for failure of estrogen production, which may be of central (hypothalamic-pituitary failure) or peripheral (gonadal dysgenesis) origin. FSH (and LH) will differentiate a central cause (low levels of FSH and LH) from a peripheral cause (invariably, an elevated level of FSH). A Y-chromosome mosaic state must be ruled out because gonadectomy would be indicated in that instance. These patients are sterile.

Breasts and Uterus Present. This group of patients, taken collectively with those in whom breasts are absent and a uterus is present, represents the largest number of patients with primary amenorrhea (see the section on secondary amenorrhea).

Breasts Present and Uterus Absent. Two subgroups may be identified by serum testosterone (free). If there is testicular feminization, serum testosterone is in the normal male range and karyotype reveals 46 XY. If there is congenital absence of the uterus, serum testosterone is in the normal female range.

Breasts and Uterus Absent. This is a rare category of patients. Diagnosis may be confirmed by findings of elevated FSH, male karyotype, and normal female testosterone level. A determination of presence or absence of gonadal tissue must be made (laparoscopy); if present, gonads would be prophylactically removed. The etiology of this disorder is uncertain.

Secondary Amenorrhea (Fig. 37-2)

Historical data are important in establishing a differential diagnosis, especially to aid in ruling out pregnancy, one of the most common conditions in this group, and pregnancy-related trauma or dilatation and curettage.

Physical examination is important to detect significant weight loss, hirsutism, galactorrhea, or evidence of pregnancy or estrogen deprivation. The major diagnostic technique is that of challenging these patients with progesterone. This can be done only after pregnancy is ruled out by appropriate physical examination and laboratory testing. Other laboratory testing should be directed to investigate clinical evidence of excess cortisol or androgen production. These studies should be performed prior to the progesterone challenge. Some physicians also advocate a serum thyroid-stimulating hormone test and 2-hour postprandial glucose test to rule out hypothyroidism and diabetes mellitus. If endogenous estrogen levels are normal and the end organ is intact, administration of progesterone-in-oil, 100 mg intramuscularly, should produce some withdrawal bleeding in 2 weeks. Alternatively, oral Provera (medroxyprogesterone acetate), 10 mg a day for up to 7 days, may be used. Note that pregnancy must be ruled out *prior* to the challenge. This testing identifies five groups of patients (Table 37-1).

References

Fries H, Nillius SJ, Petersson F. Epidemiology of secondary amenorrhea. Am J Obstet Gynecol 1974; 118:473.

Kallio H. Cytogenetic and clinical study on 100 cases of primary amenorrhea. Acta Obstet Gynecol Scand 1973; 24:1.

Lachelin GCL, Yen SSC. Hypothalamic chronic anovulation. Am J Obstet Gynecol 1978; 130:825.

McDonough PG. Amenorrhea—etiologic approach to diagnosis. Fertil Steril 1978; 30:1.

Speroff L, Glass RH, Kase NG. Amenorrhea. In: Clinical gynecologic endocrinology and infertility. 4th ed. Baltimore: Williams & Wilkins, 1989:165.

Vaitukaitis JL. Clinical reproductive neuroendocrinology. New York: Elsevier Biomedical, 1983.

Yen SSC. Chronic anovulation: Due to CNS-hypothalamic-pituitary dysfunction. In: Yen SSC, Jaffe RB, eds. Reproductive endocrinology. Philadelphia: WB Saunders, 1986:500.

Galactorrhea

Neil Aronin, MD

38

Definition

Galactorrhea is the inappropriate production of milk, i.e., lactation outside of the peripartum period.

Physiology

Galactorrhea is dependent on the presence of a mature tubular ductal system in the mammary gland and a sufficient concentration of prolactin to initiate lactation. Numerous hormones are likely to contribute to the normal development of the tubular ducts, including estrogens, growth hormone (and somatomedin), insulin, thyroxine, and glucocorticoids. Post partum, increased plasma prolactin and oxytocin concentrations initiate milk production. Maintenance of lactation is associated with adequate nipple stimulation, which may act in part to stimulate prolactin secretion via the pathways in the central nervous system.

Appropriate prolactin secretion depends on the presence of anterior pituitary cells (lactotrophs) capable of synthesizing and releasing prolactin and an intact hypothalamic-posterior pituitary axis. The lactotrophs frequently are found in the lateral aspects of the anterior pituitary and increase in number in the presence of elevated estrogens, whether from pregnancy or exogenous administration. The central regulation of prolactin secretion is most closely associated with dopamine, which inhibits prolactin release. The axons of many aminergic neurons in the hypothalamus terminate on a dense capillary network in the median eminence, from which dopamine reaches the lactotroph via the hypothalamic–anterior pituitary portal system. The precise roles of other candidate prolactin-inhibitory factors or prolactin-releasing factors are still unclear.

Etiology

Galactorrhea is frequently associated with elevated serum levels of prolactin. Hyperprolactinemia results from either a primary overproduction of hormone by autonomous lactotrophic cells or from a primary failure of dopamine-mediated inhibition of normal lactotrophic tissue. The former is commonly the result of a pituitary tumor comprising lactotrophic cells, referred to as a prolactinoma. The latter may be caused by agents such as certain drugs or hormones that directly inhibit dopamine release or by any lesion that interrupts the flow of dopamine from hypothalamus to anterior pituitary. Table 38-1 outlines some of the factors affecting prolactin secretion.

Because elevated levels of prolactin can disrupt normal menstrual function through a number of endocrine mechanisms, it is common for galactorrhea to coexist with amenorrhea or oligomenorrhea. To some degree, the level of prolactin measured in the blood is helpful in defining the etiology of galactorrhea in a given patient. The most common cause of galactorrhea with amenorrhea or oligomenorrhea, in combination with a serum prolactin concentration greater than 300 ng/ml, is a radiologically detectable prolactin-secreting pituitary tumor. When the prolactin level is greater than 100 ng/ml, galactorrhea with amenorrhea principally results from a prolactinoma and occasionally is associated with another etiology, most likely dopamine antagonism.

Drugs that commonly produce hyperprolactinemia are dopamine antagonists (phenothiazines, metoclopramide). These drugs may act at a hypothalamic or a pituitary site, or both. Interruption of dopamine flow to the pituitary by a mass lesion (craniopharyngioma, meningioma, glioma, aneurysm, macroadenoma of the pituitary impinging on the portal supply) is most often associated with moderate elevations of plasma prolactin (30 to 100 ng/ml).

Other causes of galactorrhea with hyperprolactinemia include section of the pituitary stalk, depletion of hypothalamic dopamine stores (reserpine, alpha-methyldopa), stimulation of lactotrophs (estrogen, birth control pills, polycystic ovary), cannabinoids (marijuana), association with endocrine hypofunction (hypothyroidism, Addison's disease), decreased clearance of prolactin (renal disease), and untoward stimulation of the breast (mechanical, trauma, inflammation). Interestingly, very high levels of circulating estrogens, as found during pregnancy, actually inhibit lactation despite the increase in prolactin levels.

A substantial number of patients have galactorrhea, normal menses, and normal prolactin levels. The etiology of galactorrhea in these women is not known.

Clinical Evaluation

The history should focus on those elements that provide information as to etiology: menstrual history, medications, disturbances in hypothalamic function (temperature, polyuria, thirst, appetite), symptoms of sellar mass (visual field deficits, headaches), symptoms of pituitary hypofunction or hyperfunction (especially acromegaly), and hypothyroidism.

The physical examination should be directed to document the galactorrhea. This is done by gently, but firmly, applying

Table 38-1 Factors Affecting Prolactin Secretion

Physiologic	**Nonpituitary Disorders**
Pregnancy	Chronic renal failure
Estrogens	Polycystic ovary disease
Neurogenic	Hypothyroidism
Breast stimulation	Hypothalamic disease (craniopharyngioma)
Chest wall lesions	Sarcoidosis
Spinal cord lesions	
Sleep	**Pituitary Disorders**
Stress	Prolactinomas
Exercise	Acromegaly
Hypoglycemia	Pituitary stalk section
Pharmacologic Agents	Empty sella syndrome, often with microadenoma
Neuroleptics	
Phenothiazines	
Butyrophenones	
Metoclopramide	
Alpha-methyldopa	
Reserpine	
Cimetidine (intravenous)	
Opiates	

pressure to the breast, particularly the subareolar area. The color and consistency of any expressed fluid are noted. Visual fields should be assessed by the confrontation method. Pituitary function should be evaluated. Findings suggestive of hypothyroidism (coarse hair, dry skin, hoarse voice, "hung up" reflexes) and hypogonadism (sparse axillary and pubic hair, atrophy of breasts and genitalia) should be sought. In addition, note features of acromegaly (coarsening of facial features, enlargement of hands, feet, and jaw) and Cushing's syndrome ("buffalo hump," "moon facies," violaceous abdominal striae, acne, hirsutism, proximal muscle weakness).

Laboratory Evaluation

Measurement of serum prolactin levels is absolutely necessary, and a thyroid index is generally done. Additional studies will depend on the history and physical examination. When pituitary tumor is suspected, an evaluation of the sella turcica, performed either by computed tomography (CT) or magnetic resonance imaging (MRI), is essential. In addition, in cases in which tumor is suspected, formal measurement of visual fields by perimetry and a thorough evaluation of pituitary function may be valuable. For a discussion of pituitary function testing, the reader is referred to one of the sources in the reference list.

References

Frantz AG, Wilson JD. Endocrine disorders of the breast. In: Wilson JD, Foster DW, eds. Williams' textbook of endocrinology. Philadelphia: WB Saunders, 1985:402.

Kleinberg DL, Noel GL, Frantz AA. Galactorrhea: A study of 235 cases, including 48 with pituitary tumors. N Engl J Med 1977; 296:589.

Koppelman MCS, et al. Hyperprolactinemia, amenorrhea, and galactorrhea. A retrospective assessment of 25 cases. Ann Intern Med 1984; 100:115.

Gynecomastia

Neil Aronin, MD

39

Endocrinology

Definition

Gynecomastia is the development of an increased amount of breast tissue in men. Tissues of the breast can be divided into glandular (or ductal) and fibrous (or stromal) types. Hyperplasia of either of these tissues can result in gynecomastia; often the growth of one breast is disproportionate.

Etiology

Gynecomastia can be considered a consequence of increased estrogen effect. In men, circulating estrogens can be produced from secretion of estrogen or increased peripheral conversion of androgens to estrogens (aromatization). Increased estrogen effect is also evident in disorders with decreased serum testosterone levels and unaltered estrogen concentrations.

The conditions associated with gynecomastia are widely varied (Table 39-1), to the extent that the etiology of the increased estrogen effect is sometimes uncertain. In the gynecomastia of puberty, which occurs transiently in the majority of male teenagers, there is evidence of increased peripheral conversion of androgens to estrogens. It is speculated that enhanced peripheral aromatization may also occur in obesity and may in part explain the gynecomastia of some liver disorders, improved nutritional state following starvation, and hyperthyroidism, particularly with Graves' disease.

Increased estrogen secretion can occur in hypergonadotropic hypogonadal states, tumors of the Leydig cell, and tumors of the adrenal cortex. The most common cause of hypergonadotropic hypogonadism in men is Klinefelter's syndrome, which is found in approximately 1 in 600 men and is classically characterized by small testes, gynecomastia, azoospermia, and an XXY chromosomal pattern (chromatin-positive buccal smear). It appears that mental retardation is more frequent in Klinefelter's syndrome. As in most cases of gynecomastia, the breast enlarge-

Table 39-1 Classification of Gynecomastia

Physiologic
- Newborn
- Adolescence
- Aging

Pathologic
- Testosterone Deficiency (diminished testosterone synthesis or action with or without elevated testicular synthesis of estradiol)
  - *Primary*
    - Congenital anorchia
    - Klinefelter's syndrome
    - Androgen resistance (testicular feminization and Reifenstein's syndrome)
    - Defects in testosterone synthesis
  - *Secondary*
    - Viral orchitis
    - Trauma
    - Castration
    - Neurologic disease
    - Granulomatous disease
    - Renal failure
- Increased Estrogen Production
  - Testicular (testicular tumors, hCG-producing tumors, i.e., bronchogenic carcinoma)
  - Adrenal estrogen production (feminizing tumors)
  - Peripheral estrogen production (idiopathic, liver disease, starvation and refeeding, thyrotoxicosis)
- Drugs
  - Inhibitors of testosterone synthesis and action (cimetidine, flutamide, spironolactone, ketoconazole)
  - Estrogens (stilbestrol, birth control pills, digitalis)
  - Gonadotropin administration
  - Unknown mechanisms (cyproheptadine, busulfan, ethionamide, isoniazid, tricyclic antidepressants, marijuana, heroin)

Abbreviation: hCG = human chorionic gonadotropin.

ment is generally bilateral overall, but it may be asymmetric. Pathologically, hyperplasia of stromal tissue is present. In Reifenstein's syndrome, there is a partial insensitivity to androgens, increased circulating gonadotropins (especially luteinizing hormone), and increased production of androgens and estrogens. As in testicular feminization (complete insensitivity of androgens), the increased estrogen effect on the breast likely results in part from the androgen insensitivity. Hypergonadotropic hypogonadism with increased estrogen production also may occur in testicular atrophy from inflammatory or infectious disease.

Tumors, including choriocarcinoma and bronchogenic carcinoma, that produce gonadotropins are associated with gynecomastia. The most common gonadotropin is chorionic gonadotropin.

The etiology of the gynecomastia of hypothyroidism, pulmonary tuberculosis, diabetes mellitus, heart failure, renal failure, and nonhormonal tumors is less well understood. That associated with hyperprolactinemia may result from diminished testosterone production.

Drugs that promote breast growth act by a variety of mechanisms. Exogenous administration of estrogens, androgens, and human chorionic gonadotropin increase the concentration of circulating estrogens. Cimetidine, spironolactone, digitalis, progestogens, and marijuana interfere with the binding or action of androgens. Medications that block dopamine effects or decrease dopamine content in the hypothalamus increase prolactin secretion, which in turn may produce a hypogonadal state.

Diagnostic Approach

The development of gynecomastia is often slow and may be unnoticed by the patient. Breasts that enlarge rapidly, as sometimes occurs in association with hormone-producing tumors, can be painful and tender. Systemic disorders in which bilateral gynecomastia prevails occasionally present as unilateral breast enlargement. Palpation of glandular tissue is therefore essential in the diagnosis of gynecomastia, but should there be doubt

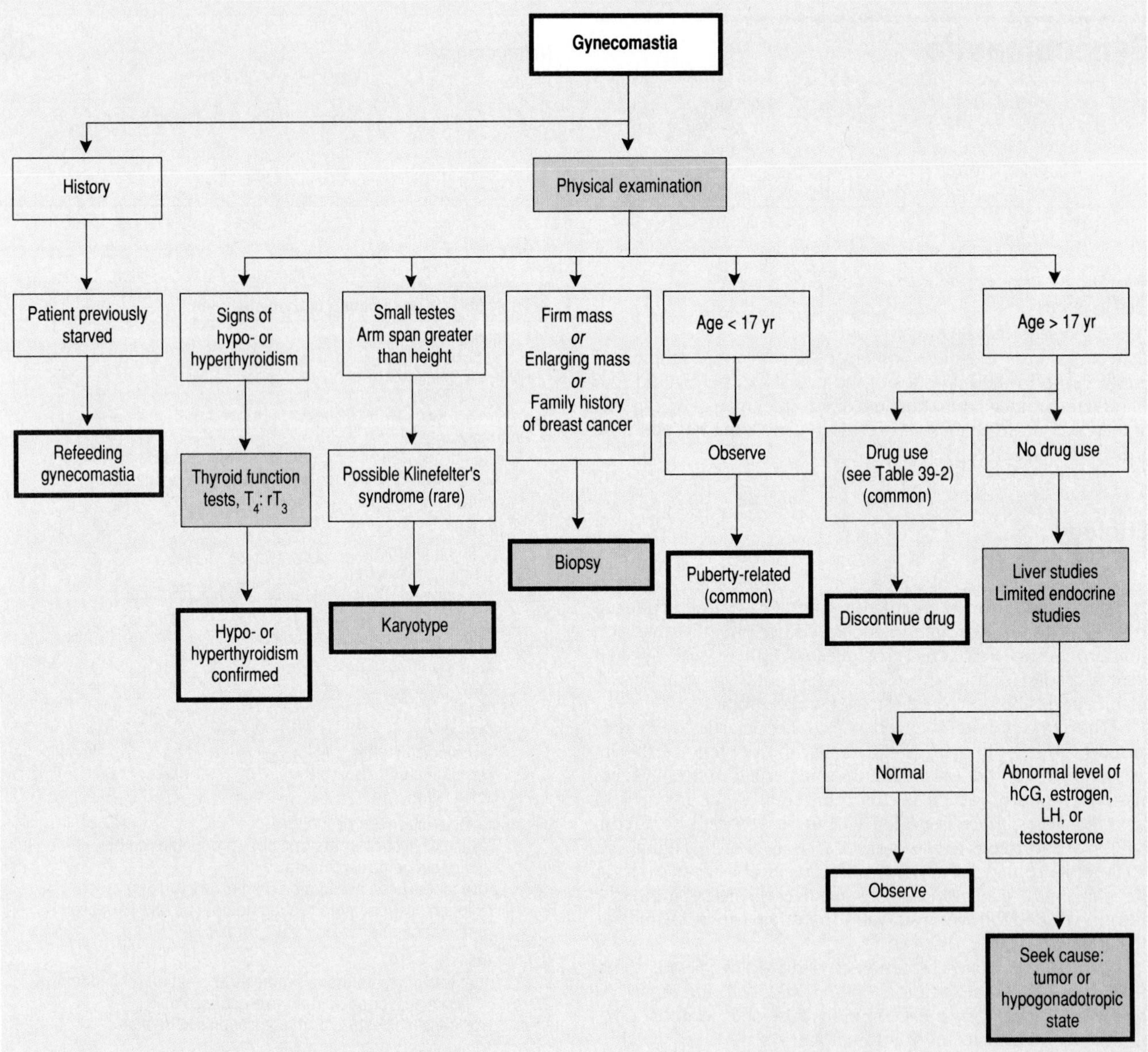

Figure 39-1 Algorithm for the evaluation of gynecomastia. hCG = human chorionic gonadotropin, LH = luteinizing hormone, rT_3 = reverse triiodothyronine, T_4 = thyroxine.

Table 39-2 Drugs Associated with Gynecomastia

Alcohol	Imipramine
Estrogen	Phenytoin
Androgen	Heroin
Spironolactone	Cimetidine
Digitalis	Marijuana
Phenothiazines	Diazepam
Amphetamines	Busulfan
Reserpine	Vincristine
Methyldopa	Nitrosoureas
Isoniazid	D-Penicillamine

about the presence of unilateral gynecomastia or an unexplained breast mass, an excisional biopsy is mandatory.

The history and physical examination are directed toward the possible etiology of gynecomastia. A careful drug history is essential (Table 39-2). In the male pubertal adolescent, mild gynecomastia is common, and in the absence of signs of thyroid disease, testicular masses, increased human chorionic gonadotropin plasma levels, and signs of chronic disease need not require an extensive evaluation. When the gynecomastia persists or develops in a mature male, necessary examination includes assessment for testicular masses (hormone-producing tumors), testicular atrophy (Klinefelter's or idiopathic atrophy), and signs of hyper- or hypothyroidism and liver disease. Essential laboratory tests include serum human chorionic gonadotropin (hCG) concentrations (or its beta subunit), serum estrogen (estrone, estradiol) and androgen (androstenedione, testosterone) levels, serum prolactin concentrations, and studies of liver function. When Klinefelter's syndrome is strongly considered, chromosomal karyotyping is performed. Gonadotropin levels are measured when there is suspicion of hypogonadism of any cause. Increased serum concentration of hCG may indicate the presence of germinal cell, bronchogenic, gastrointestinal, or liver carcinomas, and appropriate studies of these systems should be considered (examination of the chest and abdomen by computed tomography [CT] is recommended in some centers). High levels of estrogens are consistent with adrenal or testicular carcinoma, and radiologic examination of these organs (ultrasonography or CT prior to invasive studies) is appropriate. Increased serum prolactin may require study of sellar size and visual field examination. For further information on the evaluation of elevated serum prolactin levels, see Chapter 38, "Galactorrhea."

A flow diagram for evaluating gynecomastia is provided in Figure 39-1.

References

Carlson HE, Gynecomastia. N Engl J Med 1980; 303:795.

Wilson JD, Airnan J, MacDonald P. The pathogenesis of gynecomastia. Adv Intern Med 1980; 25:1.

Endocrinology

Disorders of Serum Divalent Cations, Calcium and Magnesium

John L. Stock, MD

40

Definitions

The divalent cations, calcium and magnesium, are essential for life. Calcium is a primary structural component of the skeleton, and more than 95 percent of the total body stores are in bone. Despite small circulating and intracellular components, calcium is important to basic biologic processes at the cellular level. The skeletal stores of magnesium are large, and magnesium is also important in multiple cellular functions, including DNA transcription and degradation, protein synthesis, and oxidative phosphorylation.

Total circulating calcium is commonly measured by atomic absorption or colorimetric methods and maintained in the range of 8.5 to 10.5 mg/dl. Of the total calcium measured, approximately 50 percent is free (or ionized) and active physiologically. The remainder is bound to proteins (mostly albumin) and anions such as phosphate and citrate. Although ionized calcium can be measured directly, this method is not widely available. The total calcium can be corrected for the serum albumin to better reflect the ionized calcium, using the following formula:

$$\text{Corrected total calcium (mg/dl)} = \text{measured total calcium (mg/dl)} + 0.8\ \text{mg/dl for each gram of albumin} < 4.5\ \text{g/dl}$$

The pH also affects ionization of calcium, with acidosis favoring increased, and alkalosis decreased, ionization.

The average adult consumes 500 to 1,000 mg of calcium daily and absorbs 25 to 70 percent of this by active transport and passive diffusion. Net calcium absorption is controlled by 1,25-dihydroxyvitamin D via synthesis of calcium-binding proteins in the small gut. Calcium is excreted by the kidney, and approximately two-thirds of filtered calcium is resorbed in the proximal tubule and one-third in the distal tubule. Proximal tubular calcium handling is linked to that of sodium. Pharmacologic intervention at this site is used in treatment of hypercalcemia. Distal tubular resorption of calcium is promoted by parathyroid hormone (PTH) and may also be affected by drugs such as thiazide diuretics. The overall equilibrium of serum calcium is determined by the net influx into bone, gut absorption, and renal (and gut) excretion.

The normal total serum magnesium is 1.5 to 2.0 mEq/L (1.8 to 3.6 mg/dl). Of this, 65 to 75 percent is free or ionized and 25 to 35 percent is bound, mainly to albumin. Total magnesium is measured by methods similar to those used to measure calcium, but there are no routine methods for measuring ionized magnesium.

Approximately 10 to 40 percent of the ingested magnesium is absorbed, mostly in the distal small bowel. Magnesium may be secreted in bile, pancreatic, and intestinal juices. The kidneys are involved with fine regulation of magnesium levels, and the majority of filtered magnesium is resorbed in the thick ascending limb. Diuretics of all types increase magnesium excretion, and the effects of PTH are variable. The tubular resorption of magnesium may be decreased by extracellular fluid volume expansion, renal vasodilatation, drugs, or hormones. In states of severe magnesium depletion, the kidneys are able to conserve almost 100 percent of the filtered load. In renal failure, serum magnesium may increase, but not usually until glomerular filtration is less than 15 ml per minute.

Etiologies of Disorders of Serum Divalent Cations

Hypercalcemia

Primary hyperparathyroidism is the most frequent cause of hypercalcemia in an outpatient. The excess PTH secretion is usually due to a single parathyroid adenoma; less often, four-gland hyperplasia; and rarely, parathyroid carcinoma. This is a common disease, with an estimated annual incidence of almost 200 per 100,000 in women older than 60 years of age. It is somewhat less frequent in younger persons and men.

In the sick, hospitalized patient, malignancy is the usual cause of hypercalcemia. Patients may have skeletal involvement, as commonly found in multiple myeloma or breast carcinoma, or may display no evidence of skeletal metastases. Humoral substances secreted by tumors mediate the hypercalcemia. These factors are not PTH; however, certain malignant tumors may produce polypeptides that are similar in structure to PTH. These PTH-like factors have some of the biologic effects of PTH but are structurally different enough that they are not detected by sensitive PTH radioimmunoassays.

Immobilization is often a contributing factor to hypercalcemia. Alterations in gravitational forces alter the balance between bone formation and resorption. Any patient with underlying bone disease will be subject to increased bone turnover when immobilized. This might lead to hypercalciuria and hypercalcemia. A classic example is Paget's disease. Most patients with Paget's disease are normocalcemic. However, they are prone to hypercalcemia if they become immobilized.

Thiazide diuretics can be a contributing factor to hypercalcemia, partly owing to their ability to decrease renal excretion of calcium.

Vitamin D intoxication is a less common, but important, cause of hypercalcemia. Persons consuming excessive amounts of the fat-soluble vitamin D develop increased stored levels of 25-hydroxyvitamin D, which, although less potent than the active 1,25-dihydroxyvitamin D metabolite, may cause increased absorption of calcium as well as have direct effects in mobilizing calcium from bone. Patients with sarcoidosis or other granulomatous diseases may develop hypercalcemia as a result of increased formation of the active metabolite 1,25-dihydroxyvitamin D. These patients are particularly susceptible to hypercalcemia if their vitamin D intake is high or if their sun exposure is increased. Hyperthyroidism, adrenal insufficiency, vitamin A toxicity, and excessive consumption of dairy products and calcium-containing antacids are less common causes of hypercalcemia.

Hypocalcemia

This disorder is relatively uncommon compared with hypercalcemia. In otherwise healthy outpatients, hypocalcemia is most often due to hypoparathyroidism resulting from previous thyroid or parathyroid surgery during which the parathyroid glands were inadvertently removed or had their blood supply compromised. Less commonly, hypoparathyroidism is due to a congenital lack of parathyroid glands, autoimmune failure of the parathyroids, or hereditary resistance to the actions of PTH (pseudohypoparathyroidism). This latter disorder may be associated with somatic abnormalities such as short stature, round facies, and short fourth metacarpals or with other endocrine disorders such as hypothyroidism.

Sick, hospitalized patients may have a number of metabolic disturbances causing hypocalcemia. Many have a decrease in serum albumin that causes a low total calcium level, but the corrected ionized fraction is normal. Patients with acute renal failure tend to be hypocalcemic owing to relative hyperphosphatemia, defects in vitamin D metabolism, and resistance to PTH. Hypomagnesemia can cause hypocalcemia owing to decreased PTH secretion as well as a resistance to its action. Vitamin D deficiency due to such problems as dietary insufficiency or malabsorption also may cause hypocalcemia. Patients with acute pancreatitis may rapidly develop hypocalcemia as a result of precipitation of calcium soaps in the peripancreatic area.

Hypomagnesemia

Hypomagnesemia is most commonly noted in ill, hospitalized patients and is usually due to increased renal losses of magnesium. This may be caused by intravenous fluid therapy; diuretics; other drugs, such as aminoglycoside antibiotics or cisplatin chemotherapy, which cause renal wasting of magnesium; or any intrinsic renal disease. Other mechanisms include decreased gastrointestinal absorption or increased gastrointestinal loss due to such disorders as malabsorption, chronic gastrointestinal suction, or diarrhea. Less frequently, hyper- or hypoparathyroidism, phosphate deficiency, primary hyperaldosteronism, and acute pancreatitis have been implicated in causing hypomagnesemia.

Hypermagnesemia

Hypermagnesemia is relatively unusual, except in patients with significant renal impairment who receive either magnesium-containing antacids or excessive parenteral magnesium supplementation.

Clinical Manifestations

Hypercalcemia

Routine screening of healthy asymptomatic outpatients or sick in-patients may reveal elevations in the total serum calcium level. Hypercalcemia may also be suspected in patients with the symptoms listed below, or in those with associated diseases such as malignancy or sarcoidosis. Because of the universal role of calcium in physiologic processes at the cellular level, hypercalcemia affects many organ systems and causes similar signs and symptoms independent of etiology. Neuropsychiatric and musculoskeletal symptoms such as lethargy, weakness, and achiness are common and may progress to confusion and coma in severe cases. Effects on the gastrointestinal tract, including anorexia and constipation, also occur frequently. Some patients complain of burning epigastric pain relieved by food or antacids or may even manifest gastrointestinal bleeding owing to peptic ulcer disease. Acute pancreatitis may result from hypercalcemia and presents as severe abdominal pain radiating to the back, nausea, vomiting, and fever. Renal effects of hypercalcemia include decreased glomerular filtration and concentrating ability, hypercalciuria, and deposition of calcium phosphate in the renal tubules. The inability to concentrate the urine may lead to symptoms of polyuria and may predispose to dehydration. Colicky back or flank pain, hematuria, or calcifications on abdominal radiographs may suggest the presence of renal stones. In severe and chronic hypercalcemia, other areas may demonstrate calcification, including the eye, skin, and blood vessels. Band keratopathy is corneal calcification at the limbus (the margin of the cornea overlapped by the sclera), usually at the 3 and 9 o'clock positions. Deposition of calcium salts in the skin may cause pruritus. Finally, hypercalcemia may affect the cardiovascular system. Hypercalcemic patients are prone to hypertension. Review of the electrocardiogram may demonstrate a shortening of the Q-T interval, and in patients taking digitalis, a potentiation of the inotropic and toxic effects of this drug may be noted.

Hypocalcemia

This diagnosis may be suggested by associated findings such as a history of neck surgery, the presence of other autoimmune endocrine deficiencies, or somatic abnormalities or family history suggestive of pseudohypoparathyroidism. Hypocalcemia of any etiology has protean manifestations due to increased neuromuscular irritability. The level of symptoms may depend on the rapidity in fall of serum calcium. Severe but chronic hypocalcemia may be asymptomatic except for nonspecific malaise. More commonly and in the acute setting, tingling, paresthesias, and even seizures and tetany may follow as the serum calcium falls. A positive Chvostek's sign is suggestive of hypocalcemia and is elicited by gentle tapping over the facial nerve in front of the ear, with a resultant reflex contraction of the facial muscles. Trousseau's sign is elicited by obstructing arterial flow to the arm for several minutes by means of a blood pressure cuff or tourniquet, which causes carpopedal spasm. In hypocalcemic patients, the Q-T interval may be long on the electrocardiogram and there may be a predisposition to cardiac arrhythmias. Basal ganglia calcification is sometimes seen in the skull films of patients with chronic hypocalcemia. They are also predisposed to the development of cataracts.

Hypomagnesemia

The serum magnesium is not routinely ordered as a screening laboratory test. Hypomagnesemia should be suspected in hospitalized patients when hypocalcemia or hypokalemia becomes refractory to supplementation. Hypomagnesemia may also cause cardiac arrhythmias. Prime candidates are patients receiving cisplatin therapy for malignant tumors, those treated with aminoglycoside antibiotics, patients with malabsorption, or those undergoing prolonged diuresis. Hypomagnesemia resembles hypocalcemia clinically. Neuromuscular irritability, including weakness, muscle cramps, tremor, and in severe cases, tetany, have been reported. A feeling of internal movement and total tremulousness is often described. Chvostek's and Trousseau's signs may be positive because of hypomagnesemia alone. In addition to arrhythmias, the electrocardiogram may demonstrate prolonged P-R and Q-T intervals and broad, flat T waves. There may be an increased susceptibility to digitalis toxicity. Other more unusual symptoms include dysphagia and hemolytic anemia.

Hypermagnesemia

Hypermagnesemia is uncommon, except in patients with significantly impaired renal function who are given supplemental magnesium. Neuromuscular function is commonly impaired, with increasing inhibition as magnesium levels rise. Mild hypermagnesemia might cause a decrease in deep tendon reflexes, whereas higher levels lead to somnolence and even paralysis or apnea. In severe cases, cardiovascular function is also affected with bradycardia and orthostatic hypotension. The electrocardiogram may show multiple abnormalities. Nausea, vomiting, flushing, and an impairment in hemostasis have also been described.

Diagnostic Approach

Hypercalcemia

The history of patients with hypercalcemia may be very helpful in a differential diagnosis. A chronically elevated calcium level usually implies a benign process such as primary hyperparathyroidism, whereas recent onset is more consistent with a rapidly growing tumor, immobilization, or institution of drug therapy. The drug history is critical. It is important to inquire specifically about use of thiazides, vitamin D, and calcium-containing antacids. The review of systems might uncover other clues to a malignancy such as weight loss, anorexia, or bleeding. A family history of hypercalcemia suggests one of the familial forms of hyperparathyroidism.

The physical examination is less useful. The parathyroids are rarely large enough to be palpable in primary hyperparathyroidism. Evidence of a malignancy such as a breast mass may occasionally be helpful. Patients with severe and chronic hypercalcemia may have visible band keratopathy. This is more commonly found when the serum phosphorus level is also elevated in patients with non–parathyroid-mediated hypercalcemia or renal insufficiency.

Laboratory studies may allow a definitive diagnosis. The serum albumin should be checked to give a better indication of the level of ionized calcium. Because of the effects of PTH on tubular resorption of phosphate, a low serum phosphorus level or increased tubular resorption of phosphate suggests hyperparathyroidism, whereas the reverse findings are more consistent with parathyroid suppression. PTH also causes a tubular loss of bicarbonate that might be denoted by a mild hyperchloremic acidosis. The alkaline phosphatase tends to be elevated in any form of hypercalcemia mediated by increased bone turnover. The most useful laboratory test is often the serum PTH. An elevated serum PTH in the face of hypercalcemia in a patient with normal renal function is virtually diagnostic of primary hyperparathyroidism. Serum PTH is low in patients with malignancy, as the humoral substances mediating the hypercalcemia are not recognized by the PTH radioimmunoassay and the hypercalcemia tends to suppress normal parathyroid function. Increased levels of PTH are also found in patients with impaired renal function because of an appropriate secondary hyperparathyroidism as well as the inability to clear fragments of the hormone. These inactive fragments are recognized by carboxy-terminal and midregion PTH radioimmunoassays. In the next few years, it is likely that improved assays for PTH and assays for hypercalcemic factors produced by tumors will become available.

In unusual instances, other tests may be necessary, such as further malignancy work-up, 25-hydroxyvitamin D levels, or thyroid function tests. The urinary excretion of cyclic AMP will be increased in some malignancies and primary hyperparathyroidism but decreased in other forms of hypercalcemia, so that this test is occasionally useful. A course of glucocorticoids may suppress the hypercalcemia of sarcoidosis, vitamin D toxicity, and some malignancies, but not primary hyperparathyroidism. This test may have diagnostic as well as therapeutic utility.

Hypocalcemia

The most common pertinent historical detail in a patient with hypocalcemia is frequently a history of previous thyroid or parathyroid surgery. A history of other endocrine disorders such as hypothyroidism, adrenal insufficiency, or pernicious anemia suggests the possibility of autoimmune-mediated hypoparathyroidism. Pseudohypoparathyroidism may be suggested by a family history of hypocalcemia, short stature, or skeletal defects. Recent fluid therapy, diuretic use, or a history of diarrhea, bulky stools, or gastrointestinal surgery raises the possibility of magnesium or vitamin D deficiencies.

Physical examination is less useful. A positive Chvostek's or Trousseau's sign, when it had been negative before, makes the drop in calcium more clinically significant. Obviously, a neck scar, skeletal deformities such as a short fourth metacarpal, and abdominal pain suggest certain diagnoses.

Screening laboratory studies should include serum albumin, creatinine, amylase, and phosphorus. A normal serum magnesium or vitamin D will rule out these deficiencies. The serum PTH is again very useful in differential diagnoses, being low or undetectable in patients with hypoparathyroidism, markedly elevated in those with pseudohypoparathyroidism, and mildly elevated in states of secondary hyperparathyroidism such as vitamin D deficiency.

Hypomagnesemia and Hypermagnesemia

As stated previously, these disorders are seen in certain clinical settings and are documented by measuring the serum magnesium. The history may be helpful, but physical examination or other laboratory studies are rarely useful.

References

Aurbach GD, Marx SJ, Spiegel AM. Parathyroid hormone, calcitonin, and the calciferols. In: Wilson JB, Foster DW, eds. Williams' textbook of endocrinology. 7th ed. Philadelphia: WB Saunders, 1985:1137.

Broadus AE, Rasmussen H. Clinical evaluation of parathyroid function. Am J Med 1981; 70:475.

Fisken RA, Heath DA, Somers S. Hypercalcemia in hospital patients: Clinical and diagnostic aspects. Lancet 1981; i:202.

Rude RK, Singer FR. Magnesium deficiency and excess. Ann Rev Med 1981; 32:245.

Schneider AB, Sherwood LM. Pathogenesis and management of hypoparathyroidism and other hypocalcemic disorders. Metabolism 1975; 24:871.

Whang R. Magnesium deficiency: Pathogenesis, prevalence, and clinical implication. Am J Med 1987; 82(suppl 3A):24.

Zaloga GP, Chernow B. Hypocalcemia in critical illness. JAMA 1986; 256:1924.

Disorders of Phosphorus Metabolism

Robert M. Black, MD

41

Phosphorus is a principal component of all cell membranes and organelles. It is an essential intermediate in enzyme function and is involved in multiple transport processes (such as those requiring energy in the form of ATP). It should not be surprising, therefore, that derangements in phosphorus metabolism can result in a number of abnormalities ranging from subclinical biochemical findings to potentially lethal conditions. Before proceeding to the diagnosis and management of these clinical disorders, it is helpful to review the physiology of normal phosphorus metabolism.

Normal Phosphorus Metabolism

Approximately 1,000 g of phosphorus is present in a 70-kg adult, principally in bone (85 percent) and in cells (14 percent). In comparison, less than 1 percent (under 60 mg) circulates in the extracellular fluid. However, it is the phosphorus in this compartment (approximately 2.5 to 4.5 mg/dl of plasma) that is measured in the laboratory as the plasma inorganic phosphorus concentration. The latter is completely ionized, circulating primarily as HPO_4^{2-} or $H_2PO_4^-$.

Daily phosphorus intake averages about 1,200 mg in a healthy adult. Of this, 800 mg is absorbed (mainly in the jejunum) and 400 mg is excreted in the feces. Under normal circumstances, intestinal phosphorus absorption is probably accomplished almost entirely by a diffusional process that depends primarily on dietary intake. Although there is convincing evidence for the existence of an active phosphorus absorptive process that is sensitive to 1,25 $(OH)_2D_3$, the active component probably becomes important only under unusual conditions such as an extremely low dietary phosphorus intake that stimulates 1,25 $(OH)_2D_3$ synthesis (Lee, Kurokawa, 1987).

Absorbed phosphorus enters the circulating pool in the extracellular fluid, where most of it remains bound to lipids and proteins. Plasma phosphate refers to the unbound, inorganic portion that comprises the remaining 30 percent.

Approximately 7,200 mg of plasma phosphate is filtered at the glomerulus each day.* Under normal circumstances, most filtered phosphate (about 85 percent) is then reabsorbed primarily in the proximal convoluted tubule. That portion of the filtered phosphate load that escapes reabsorption (approximately 800 mg per day) is excreted in the urine. Under circumstances of dietary phosphorus depletion, the fraction of filtered phosphate reabsorbed increases and the urinary excretion of phosphate becomes almost undetectable. This effect is independent of parathyroid hormone (PTH), which inhibits the proximal reabsorptive process, thereby increasing the percent of filtered phosphate excreted in the urine.

Plasma Phosphorus

The normal plasma phosphate concentration is 2.5 to 4.5 mg/dl. Plasma inorganic phosphate is completely ionized and circulates as HPO_4^{2-} and $H_2PO_4^-$.

$$HPO_4^{2-} + H^+ \leftrightarrow H_2PO_4^-$$

The plasma phosphate concentration is measured in terms of the elemental *phosphorus* contained in the *phosphate* molecules.

The usual ratio of HPO_4^{2-} to $H_2PO_4^-$ is 4 : 1. It is extremely important to be aware that this ratio can be altered both in vivo

*The daily filtered phosphate load can be calculated by multiplying the normal glomerular filtration rate (180 L per day) by the plasma phosphate concentration (4 mg/dl).

and in administered solutions by changes in pH. These potential alterations can be shown using the Henderson-Hasselbalch equation for phosphoric acid:

$$pH = 6.8 + \log HPO_4^{2-}/H_2PO_4^-$$

Because phosphorus is contained in both inorganic phosphate species, an increase in pH, as occurs, for example, with alkalosis, would increase the ratio of HPO_4^{2-} to $H_2PO_4^-$. Therefore, alkalemia would raise the total milliequivalents (mEq) of phosphate (because milliequivalents are determined by valence), whereas total *milligrams* of phosphate would not be changed. As a result, the plasma phosphate concentration is measured in terms of the elemental phosphorus contained in the phosphate molecules, usually in milligrams per deciliter or in millimoles per liter. The significance of this finding can be seen in the following example.

Assuming a normal 4:1 ratio of circulating HPO_4^{2-} to $H_2PO_4^-$, 5 mmol of phosphate contains 4 mmol HPO_4^{2-} and 1 mmol $H_2PO_4^-$. Because there are 8 negative charges in 4 mmol HPO_4^{2-} and 1 negative charge in 1 mmol of $H_2PO_4^-$, a total of 9 negative charges is normally distributed among 5 mmol of circulating phosphate, resulting in 1.8 negative charges per millimole.

As can be seen, the number of milliequivalents per liter can be altered by a deviation in blood pH. In contrast, there is approximately 1 mmol/L of phosphorus at a plasma concentration of 3.1 mg/dl,* regardless of blood pH, because millimoles per liter are not influenced by changes in valence. Consequently, the plasma phosphate concentration can be reported as milligrams per deciliter or millimoles per liter, but it should not be expressed in terms of milliequivalents per liter.

Hyperphosphatemia

Definition

Hyperphosphatemia is present when the plasma phosphorus concentration exceeds 4.5 mg/dl. This disorder can be caused by either an increased phosphate load (exogenous or endogenous) or a reduced renal phosphate excretion.†

Pathophysiology and Clinical Manifestations

Hyperphosphatemia exerts its effects in part by affecting calcium metabolism. Therefore, it is necessary to review briefly some of the relevant aspects of calcium homeostasis.

The plasma calcium concentration is controlled by a number of endocrine systems, with PTH and vitamin D_3 being the most important. Vitamin D_3 is the inactive form of the vitamin; it enters the body in the diet or by conversion from 7-dehydrocholesterol by sunlight in the skin. Activation requires transport first to the liver, where a 25-hydroxylation forms 25 $(OH)D_3$, and subsequently to the kidney, where a 1-hydroxylation results in the most active form of the vitamin, 1,25 $(OH)_2D_3$.

The synthesis of 1,25 $(OH)_2D_3$ is affected by a number of factors, including phosphorus intake, the plasma phosphate concentration, and the functional renal mass available for 1-hydroxylation. Hyperphosphatemia, for example, suppresses renal activation of 25 $(OH)D_3$, thereby reducing the plasma concentration of 1,25 $(OH)_2D_3$.

Once formed, 1,25 $(OH)_2D_3$ has several important actions on mineral metabolism that affect the intestine, bone, and probably the kidney. One of the most important is to enhance intestinal calcium absorption, principally in, but not limited to, the duodenum. In the absence of adequate calcium absorption, hypocalcemia may develop, stimulating PTH synthesis and release. Recent studies also have noted the presence of 1,25 $(OH)_2D_3$ receptors capable of directly inhibiting PTH release in parathyroid glands (Slatopolsky et al, 1984). Low levels of 1,25 $(OH)_2D_3$ can adversely affect bone because PTH (released in response to hypocalcemia and low 1,25 $(OH)_2D_3$ concentrations) attempts to restore the plasma calcium concentration to normal, but does this at the expense of bone integrity by stimulating bone resorption.

The symptoms associated with hyperphosphatemia are usually due to metabolic bone disease (particularly in patients with chronic renal failure) and tend to appear over many years. This may be manifested by bone pain or pathologic fractures, although many patients with end-stage renal disease are asymptomatic, offering no musculoskeletal complaints.

In comparison, patients with more acute increases in the plasma phosphorus concentration that develop over hours or days may exhibit more dramatic findings. These signs and symptoms (referred to as the "phosphate excess" syndrome) are due to the combination of hypocalcemia (that may result in the neuromuscular manifestations of tetany) as well as the deposition of calcium phosphate salts in almost any tissue, including the cornea (band keratopathy), skin, kidneys (nephrocalcinosis), cardiac conduction system, and small blood vessels. In its most dramatic form, vascular calcification may cause the rare syndrome of calciphylaxis, which leads to extensive ischemic necrosis, particularly in diabetic patients on dialysis and less commonly in renal transplant patients. PTH appears to be important in the development of this potentially fatal disorder, because rapid resolution has been reported in some patients following parathyroidectomy (Fox et al, 1983).

In addition to the adverse effects of hyperphosphatemia on bone and calcium metabolism, it has been suggested that renal phosphate deposition may accelerate the rate of progression of chronic renal failure to end-stage renal disease. The deposition of calcium phosphate in the renal interstitium (due to a high calcium-phosphate product) may initiate an inflammatory reaction that contributes to tubulointerstitial damage. Increased renal calcium content has been demonstrated in humans relatively early in the course of renal disease, even before the plasma creatinine is above 1.5 mg/dl (Gimenez et al, 1987). A potentially deleterious role for these deposits is suggested by the experimental observation that dietary phosphorus restriction is associated with decreased renal calcium deposition and slower disease progression (Lumbertgul et al, 1986).

Etiology

Hyperphosphatemia is always caused by an increased phosphate load or a reduction in the ability of the kidneys to excrete this mineral (Table 41-1). Even a normal phosphorus intake may produce hyperphosphatemia in patients with moderate renal failure.

Increased Phosphate Load

An increase in dietary phosphorus is normally excreted rapidly in the urine because the renal tubular phosphate reabsorptive system is almost always saturated. Moreover, elevations in the plasma phosphate concentration lead to depressed synthesis of 1,25 $(OH)_2D_3$, reducing phosphorus absorption from the gastrointestinal tract. Consequently, a sustained elevation of plasma phosphate level is rarely produced by diet alone, even in patients who develop hypercalcemia as a result of excessive intake of vitamin D.

In contrast to oral ingestion, phosphorus loads may be administered by other means. Intravenous phosphate infusions,

* The molecular weight of phosphorus is approximately 31. Millimoles are determined by dividing milligrams of phosphorus contained in 1 L of plasma by its molecular weight.

† Rarely, hyperglobulinemia, as in multiple myeloma, may spuriously increase the plasma phosphate concentration (pseudohyperphosphatemia) by interfering with automated measurement (Adler et al, 1988).

Endocrinology

Table 41-1 Major Causes of Hyperphosphatemia

Increased Phosphate Load	
Exogenous	Diet and vitamin D (rare) Phosphate infusions Phosphate-containing laxatives and enemas
Endogenous	Cytolytic therapy Rhabdomyolysis or other tissue breakdown Lactic and ketoacidosis (before therapy)
Decreased Renal Phosphate Excretion	
Decreased filtered load	Renal insufficiency (GFR < 30 ml/min)
Increased tubular reabsorption of phosphate	Hypoparathyroidism

Abbreviation: GFR = glomerular filtration rate.

which are used in some patients to treat hypercalcemia, may cause severe hyperphosphatemia, in part because of the rapid infusion rate, but also because reduced renal phosphate excretion (due to hypercalcemia-induced renal failure) is often present concomitantly. Hyperalimentation solutions also can cause this problem, especially if they contain large quantities of phospholipids. Phosphate-containing laxatives (laxative abuse) and phosphate-containing enemas (usually in children) may raise the plasma phosphorus concentration as well, if renal phosphate excretion is impaired.

Phosphorus may also be added to the plasma endogenously when intracellular phosphate is released into the extracellular space. Cell integrity may be lost, as occurs in patients with extensive rhabdomyolysis or in patients with cell breakdown following cytolytic therapy for leukemia or lymphoma. Because both of these conditions are frequently associated with concurrent acute renal failure, the phosphorus released from damaged cells may not be excreted in the urine, and severe hyperphosphatemia may ensue. This explains why acute and chronic renal failure cannot be differentiated on the basis of hyperphosphatemia alone.

Intracellular phosphorus may be released into the circulation, with resulting hyperphosphatemia but without complete loss of cell integrity. The most common disorders identified in this setting are lactic and ketoacidosis (before therapy). Metabolic acidosis directly reduces tubular reabsorption of phosphate leading to increased urinary phosphorus excretion. Early in these organic acidoses, however, phosphorus is released from cells both as a result of protein and phospholipid catabolism and of blunted cellular phosphate uptake due to impaired carbohydrate metabolism (Lumbertgul et al, 1986). In the presence of superimposed renal insufficiency (frequently due to reduced renal perfusion or acute tubular necrosis), mild to moderate hyperphosphatemia may be observed. It should be emphasized that although pretreatment plasma phosphate levels may be elevated in ketoacidosis, total body stores are below normal owing to ongoing urinary losses. As a result, subsequent *hypo*phosphatemia is not uncommon; it usually occurs within 12 to 24 hours after fluid and insulin replacement has begun (see the section on hypophosphatemia).

Reduced Renal Phosphate Excretion

The most common causes of sustained hyperphosphatemia are a decreased filtered load of phosphate (usually due to acute or chronic renal failure) and enhanced tubular reabsorption of phosphate (usually from hypoparathyroidism). The plasma phosphorus level remains normal in chronic renal failure until the glomerular filtration rate (GFR) falls to about 30 percent of normal (Pcr approximately 3.0 mg/dl). Until this point, both secondary hyperparathyroidism and impaired synthesis of 1,25 $(OH)_2D_3$ are able to compensate for the reduction in filtered phosphate. As the GFR decreases further, dietary phosphorus intake exceeds the ability of these hormones to maintain phosphate balance. In patients with severe hyperparathyroidism, extensive bone resorption also contributes to high plasma phosphate concentrations, explaining in part why restriction of dietary phosphate and phosphate binding medications (see the section on treatment of hyperphosphatemia) are not always successful in restoring phosphate levels to normal.

Hypoparathyroidism is the most frequent cause of chronic hyperphosphatemia in patients with normal renal function. In the absence of PTH, tubular reabsorption of phosphate increases, leading to elevated plasma phosphorus levels despite a normal filtered phosphate load. The concomitant presence of hyperphosphatemia and hypocalcemia in a patient with normal renal function should suggest this diagnosis.

Treatment of Hyperphosphatemia

In most acute settings, high phosphate levels will resolve spontaneously as the phosphate load is reduced and as renal function improves. Efforts to maintain a normal plasma phosphorus concentration, therefore, should be reserved for patients with chronically elevated levels, almost all of whom will have chronic renal failure. Treatment is important to prevent and treat the metabolic bone disease of renal failure (renal osteodystrophy), and restriction of phosphorus intake also may slow the progression of renal disease in some patients.

Two means (other than dialysis) can be used to lower phosphate levels in renal insufficiency: reduce phosphorus intake or administer phosphate-binding antacids. Dietary phosphorus restriction can prevent hyperphosphatemia in experimental animals. In some studies, however, marked phosphorus depletion was induced by severely limiting intake (Rose, Black, 1988). It seems reasonable, therefore, to institute a moderate phosphorus restriction (800 mg per day) in most patients with moderate or severe renal insufficiency. Frequently, however, dietary phosphate restriction is difficult to maintain or cannot restore the plasma phosphate concentration to normal. Phosphate binders that reduce phosphorus absorption from the gastrointestinal tract are usually administered when this occurs.

The most commonly used phosphate-binding antacids are aluminum hydroxide and calcium carbonate. Magnesium-containing antacids generally should be avoided because of the impaired ability to excrete this cation in renal failure. The administration of aluminum hydroxide has been criticized because it can contribute to the aluminum burden normally present in chronic renal failure. Aluminum appears to be important in the pathogenesis of both the bone disease (Hercz et al, 1988) and the anemia (Altmann et al, 1988) observed in this setting. Recent studies indicate that calcium carbonate is an effective alternative (Slatopolsky et al, 1986). It is important to remember that all phosphate-binding antacids are most effective when given with meals.

Patients who have severe secondary hyperparathyroidism from chronic renal failure may have hyperphosphatemia that is unresponsive to even large doses of phosphate-binding antacids and dietary phosphate restriction. In this setting, persistently high plasma phosphorus levels are maintained in part by PTH-induced resorption of bone (Farrington et al, 1982). In rare circumstances, parathyroidectomy may be indicated in symptomatic patients.

Hypophosphatemia

Definition

Hypophosphatemia is present when the plasma phosphate concentration is below 2.5 mg/dl. Severe hypophosphatemia refers to a level less than 1.0 mg/dl.

Phosphate depletion may be caused by renal phosphate wasting or extrarenal phosphate losses. Consequently, these disorders are discussed separately.

Hypophosphatemia Associated with Renal Phosphate Wasting

The urine normally becomes almost completely free of phosphate (less than 100 mg per day) when body stores are depleted. In contrast, certain disorders are caused by renal phosphate losses, and these losses continue despite a reduction in the plasma phosphate concentration. Plasma phosphate levels range between 1.5 and 2.5 mg/dl in most individuals when renal losses account for the hypophosphatemia.

Signs and Symptoms

Renal phosphate wasting is frequently chronic, but rarely leads to plasma levels below 1.2 mg/dl. Abnormalities in bone metabolism are the principal findings in these individuals: osteomalacia (adults) or rickets (children) is observed when vitamin D deficiency occurs (see the following section on etiology and pathogenesis), and subperiosteal bone resorption may be seen when hyperparathyroidism is present. Extraskeletal manifestations are typically due to the underlying disease that is causing renal phosphate wasting rather than the hypophosphatemia per se.

Etiology and Pathogenesis

The disorders causing renal hypophosphatemia are listed in Table 41-2. Hyperparathyroidism is associated with high PTH levels and often with hypercalcemia. Similar findings may be observed in patients with humoral hypercalcemia of malignancy (HHM), most commonly caused by squamous carcinoma of the lung. HHM appears to be caused by a peptide that shares some identity with the normal circulating PTH molecule, but that lacks sufficient immunogenic similarity to be detected by the PTH assay (Mangin et al, 1988). In both conditions, proximal tubular reabsorption of phosphate is reduced. Renal transplant patients commonly exhibit mild to moderate hypophosphatemia that may result from persistent hyperparathyroidism, although a primary renal tubular phosphate leak also has been proposed (Rosenbaum et al, 1981).

The Fanconi syndrome describes a generalized defect in proximal tubular reabsorptive function that causes glycosuria, uricosuria, aminoaciduria, bicarbonaturia, and phosphaturia. This disorder is rare but should be considered whenever hypophosphatemia is associated with hypouricemia and a non–anion gap metabolic acidosis. When the Fanconi syndrome is observed in adults, it is important to exclude the presence of multiple myeloma, in which toxic light chains damage the renal tubular transport mechanisms. The absence of proteinuria by dipstick (which detects only albumin), but its identification by the addition of sulfosalicylic acid (which detects all proteins) to the urine, should suggest this diagnosis.

Hypophosphatemia may be observed in association with other tumors as well. This entity, which is referred to as *oncogenic osteomalacia,* is usually seen with mesenchymal tumors. The cause of the disorder is not known, but studies have suggested that altered vitamin D metabolism, possibly leading to reduced 1,25 $(OH)_2D_3$ levels, may be important (Drezner, Feinglos, 1977).

Vitamin D deficiency or resistance also may be associated with persistent renal phosphate losses despite concomitant hypophosphatemia. In this setting, the low plasma phosphorus level is multifactoral. Reduced intestinal phosphorus absorption is generally present as a result of malabsorption (which also causes vitamin D deficiency), and the resultant hypocalcemia due to impaired gastrointestinal calcium absorption leads to secondary hyperparathyroidism, thereby decreasing renal tubular phosphate reabsorption.

Table 41-2 Major Causes of Hypophosphatemia

Renal phosphate wasting	Renal phosphate conservation*
Hyperparathyroidism (primary or secondary)	Hyperalimentation
Humoral hypercalcemia of malignancy	Recovery after severe burns
After renal transplantation	Refeeding (alcoholism, ketoacidosis, starvation)
Fanconi syndrome (myeloma, malabsorption, vitamin D deficiency)	Acute respiratory alkalosis
Vitamin D–resistant and –dependent rickets	Chronic use of phosphate-binding antacids
Oncogenic osteomalacia	

* May cause severe hypophosphatemia (plasma phosphate < 1.0 mg/dl).

Treatment

The approach to individuals with mild hypophosphatemia due to renal phosphate wasting is aimed at correction of the underlying disorder. For example, hypophosphatemia caused by malabsorption of calcium and vitamin D should be repaired by measures that reduce diarrhea and by vitamin D and calcium supplementation. Phosphorus replacement can be given, but this form of therapy remains controversial because carefully controlled studies showing a benefit have not been performed in this setting (Lee, Kurokawa, 1987).

Hypophosphatemia with Low Urinary Phosphate Excretion (Phosphate Depletion Syndrome)

Individuals with *hypophosphatemia and hypophosphaturia* exhibit several features that distinguish them from phosphaturic patients. The hypophosphatemia tends to be more severe (plasma phosphorus concentration frequently below 1.2 mg/dl), and it tends to develop more acutely, characteristically *after* admission to the hospital, primarily as a result of a rapid shift of phosphate from the plasma into cells (Knochel, 1985).

Clinical Manifestations

Severe hypophosphatemia is manifested clinically by changes in the neuromuscular, cardiovascular, and hematopoietic systems (Table 41-3). The pathogenesis of these findings is complex and includes abnormalities of ATP generation (leading to impaired formation of cell proteins and structures), reduced 2,3 diphosphoglycerate levels in red blood cells (causing a leftward shift of the hemoglobin-oxygen dissociation curve, which decreases the Po_2 at which hemoglobin releases oxygen to tissues), and altered intracellular H^+ and calcium ion concentrations. It should be emphasized that symptoms of phosphate depletion do not usually develop until the plasma phosphate concentration falls below 1.0 mg/dl. In comparison, hypophosphatemia that is associated with normal body phosphorus stores (as with hyperventilation) is typically asymptomatic.

Table 41-3 Clinical Manifestations of Severe, Acute Hypophosphatemia

Neuromuscular	Cardiovascular	Hematologic
Ptosis, dysarthria, dysphagia, ileus, proximal muscle weakness	Arrhythmias	Decreased oxygen release to tissues (decreased 2,3-diphosphoglycerate levels)
Confusion, coma	Cardiomyopathy?	Hemolysis
Respiratory failure (occasionally hyperventilation)		Impaired leukocyte function
Rhabdomyolysis		Decreased platelet function and number

Etiology and Pathogenesis

Severe hypophosphatemia develops primarily in four clinical settings: hyperalimentation, recovery from severe burns, refeeding of malnourished or alcoholic individuals or treatment of diabetic ketoacidosis, and respiratory alkalosis (Knochel, 1985). A shift of phosphate from the plasma into cells is common to each of these disorders. Less commonly, chronic use of phosphate-binding antacids may result in phosphate depletion (Insogna et al, 1980).

Hyperalimentation was a common cause of hypophosphatemia prior to the addition of adequate phosphate to feeding solutions. Because synthesis of phosphorylated proteins and lipids requires phosphorus, administration of phosphate-deficient solutions impairs cell structure and function and may ultimately deplete body phosphorus needed for energy (e.g., ATP) requirements as well. Hypophosphatemia is typically delayed until after the first week of hyperalimentation, the time required to deplete phosphorus stores in a previously replete individual (Fig. 41-1).

Large fluid and protein losses through the skin are characteristically present during the acute phase of *extensive burns*. Maintenance of adequate intra- and extracellular fluid stores requires a substantial intake that commonly leads to the development of edema. With recovery, there is a salt and water diuresis as this "third-spaced" fluid is mobilized, a process that increases urinary phosphate excretion. Hypophosphatemia will ensue if the quantity of phosphorus in intravenous and oral feedings is inadequate to replenish these continuing urinary losses. In general, it takes at least 1 week for hypophosphatemia to be detected because these patients are not usually phosphate depleted before admission to the hospital (see Fig. 41-1).

Refeeding hypophosphatemia refers to the fall in plasma phosphate that occurs when body stores are low *before* normal or even low caloric feedings (usually in the form of carbohydrate) are begun. Hypophosphatemia in this setting results from the transfer of phosphorus from the extracellular fluid into cells. Stimulation of intracellular processes requiring phosphate (such as glycolysis, which is activated by insulin release in response to a carbohydrate load) appears to be particularly important in promoting this transcellular phosphorus shift. The caloric intake required to precipitate this disorder is quite low in susceptible individuals (e.g., an intravenous solution of 5 percent dextrose), and its onset is more rapid than the hypophosphatemia observed with hyperalimentation or recovery from burns (see Fig. 41-1).

The conditions associated with refeeding hypophosphatemia are alcoholism, diabetic ketoacidosis, and starvation. In each of these conditions, body phosphate stores are depleted before admission to the hospital, either by reduced intake or by large urinary losses (as in ketoacidosis due to the osmotic diuresis and metabolic acidosis or alcoholism due to malabsorption with vitamin D deficiency or hypomagnesemia*). In comparison, plasma phosphate levels are usually normal or even increased before refeeding (or insulin therapy) is initiated.

Refeeding hypophosphatemia also may be observed in the postoperative surgical patient. In this setting, increased tissue metabolism and consequent shifts of phosphate from the blood into cells as well as diuretic-induced renal phosphate losses appear to be important. As a result, phosphate stores may become rapidly depleted, although body stores are frequently normal on admission.

Acute hyperventilation that results in a *respiratory alkalosis* is another cause of profound hypophosphatemia.* In contrast to these other disorders, clinical manifestations of the phosphate depletion syndrome are absent if phosphorus stores are normal. For example, acute respiratory alkalosis can cause severe hypophosphatemia in normal individuals. The mechanism appears to involve stimulation of the glycolytic enzyme phosphofructokinase by the increased intracellular pH. This enzyme catalyzes the conversion of fructose-1-phosphate to fructose-1,6-diphosphate, causing a shift of phosphorus intracellularly for use in this and other related processes. Despite these changes that can decrease the plasma phosphorus concentration below 1.0 mg/dl, symptomatic hypophosphatemia does not develop. Although it is possible that sustained hyperventilation in a phosphorus-replete individual might provoke clinical manifestations of hypophosphatemia, most studies suggest that symptomatic hypophosphatemia is rare in the absence of depleted body stores of phosphorus.

The use of phosphate-binding antacids (principally aluminum hydroxide) can, in rare circumstances, produce profound hypophosphatemia by reducing intestinal phosphate absorption (Shields, 1978). This is most likely to occur when these compounds are administered in excess to individuals with normal renal function.

Treatment

Most cases of severe hypophosphatemia occur in the hospital hours or days after admission (see Fig. 41-1); therefore, the best treatment is prevention. Patients likely to develop this complication should be followed closely for signs and symptoms of hypophosphatemia and should have serial measurements of their plasma phosphate levels, particularly when insulin or intravenous solutions containing dextrose are being administered. The use of *prophylactic* phosphate-containing solutions in patients at risk for refeeding hypophosphatemia (as in diabetic ketoacidosis) does not appear to affect the clinical outcome (Krane, 1987). It should be emphasized, however, that individuals with diabetic ketoacidosis who have hypophosphatemia at the time of presentation should probably receive phosphate salts (Knochel, 1985).

Once severe hypophosphatemia (plasma phosphate concentration $\leq$1.0 mg/dl) is manifest, prompt phosphorus replacement should be considered. This is especially important

* In rats, magnesium depletion causes phosphaturia; in contrast, urinary phosphate losses may not be increased by hypomagnesemia in humans (Lee, Kurokawa, 1987).

* Metabolic alkalosis does not significantly alter the plasma phosphate concentration (Knochel, 1977).

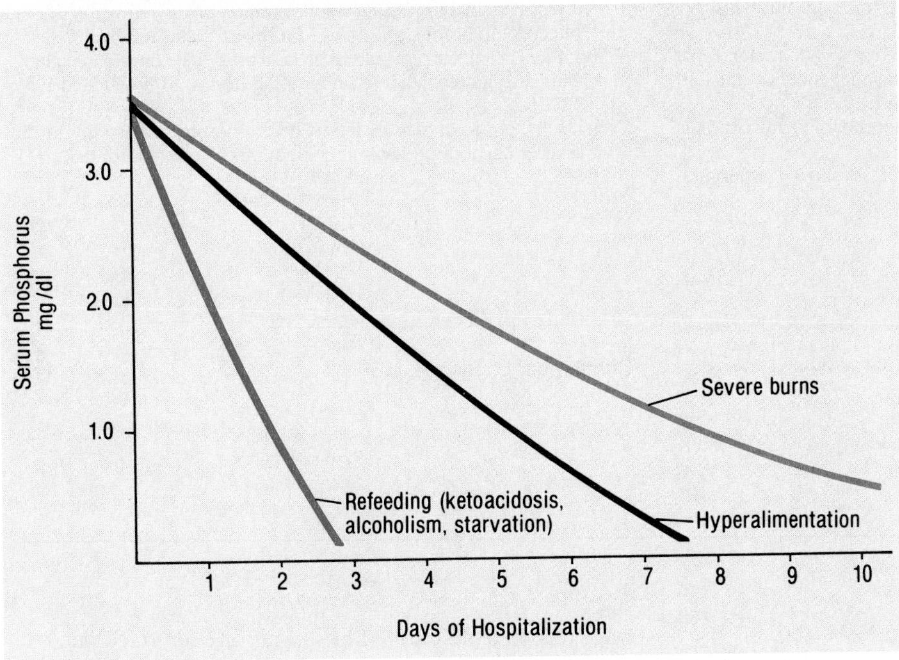

Figure 41-1 Development of the phosphate depletion syndrome.

in patients with otherwise unexplained symptoms. Treatment can be administered orally or intravenously, the former route being less likely to cause complications such as hyperphosphatemia, hypocalcemia, and metastatic calcification. Thus, oral replacement is the preferred route of administration whenever feasible.

Oral Phosphorus Treatment. Oral phosphorus replacement doses are generally between 25 and 75 mmol/day. Solutions that contain either sodium phosphate or potassium phosphate are available; the proper solution is determined on the basis of potassium or sodium requirements. Each milliliter of sodium phosphate ($NaH_2PO_4 \cdot Na_2HPO_4$) contains approximately 1.6 mmol of phosphate (Knochel, 1977). Approximately 30 ml can be given orally in divided doses to replenish phosphorus stores. Diarrhea appears to occur infrequently until body stores are normal. Alternatively, administration of potassium phosphate (Neutra-Phos) is appropriate for hypokalemic individuals. The capsules are not swallowed, but must first be dissolved in water. Each capsule contains approximately 8 mmol of phosphate and 7 mEq of potassium.

An alternative that may avoid the potential for hypocalcemia is the use of skim or low-fat milk.* There are approximately 33 mmol of phosphorus and 1,000 mg of calcium in each quart. Two quarts of milk daily will replenish depleted phosphorus stores in most patients.

Intravenous Phosphorus Replacement. Parenteral phosphate should be reserved for patients who cannot tolerate oral feedings or who are severely symptomatic, and it should be administered at a rate of less than 10 mmol per 12 hours (Vannatta et al, 1981). Because hypophosphaturia characteristically persists during the early phase of phosphate replacement, a more rapid infusion rate can transform a state of hypophosphatemia into one of extreme hyperphosphatemia. This is particularly important because the distribution of administered phosphate is uncertain in any patient; phosphorus may remain in the extracellular space or be transferred intracellularly, depending on the blood pH, glucose concentration, and insulin activity. As a result, soft-tissue calcification, hypocalcemia, and hyperkalemia (with potassium phosphate) are more likely to be seen with parenteral administration.

* Whole milk may be poorly tolerated in certain individuals, causing diarrhea that may exacerbate hypophosphatemia.

References

Adler SG, et al. Hyperglobulinemia may spuriously elevate measured serum inorganic phosphate levels. Am J Kidney Dis 1988; 11:260.

Altmann P, et al. Aluminium chelation therapy in dialysis patients: Evidence for inhibition of haemoblogin synthesis by low levels of aluminium. Lancet 1988; 1:1012.

Drezner MK, Feinglos MN. Osteomalacia due to 1-alpha-25-dihydroxy cholecalciferol deficiency: Association with a giant cell tumor of bone. J Clin Invest 1977; 60:1046.

Farrington K, et al. Hypophosphatemia after parathyroidectomy in chronic renal failure. Br Med J 1982; 284:856.

Fox R, Banowsky LH, Cruz AB. Post-renal transplant calciphylaxis: Successful treatment with parathyroidectomy. J Urol 1983; 129:362.

Gimenez LF, Solez K, Walker WG. Relation between renal calcium content and renal impairment in 246 human renal biopsies. Kidney Int 1987; 31:93.

Hercz G, et al. Reversal of aluminum-related bone disease after substituting calcium carbonate for aluminum hydroxide. Am J Kidney Dis 1988; 11:70.

Insogna KL, et al. Osteomalacia and weakness from excessive antacid ingestion. JAMA 1980; 244:2544.

Knochel JP. The clinical status of hypophosphatemia: An update. N Engl J Med 1985; 313:447.

Knochel JP. The pathophysiology and clinical characteristics of severe hypophosphatemia. Arch Int Med 1977; 137:203.

Krane EJ. Diabetic ketoacidosis: Biochemistry, physiology, treatment, and prevention. Pediatr Clin North Am 1987; 34:935.

Lee DB, Kurokawa K. Physiology of phosphorus metabolism. In: Maxwell MH, Kleeman CR, Narins RG, eds. Clinical disorders of fluid and electrolyte metabolism. 4th ed. New York: McGraw-Hill, 1987.

Lumbertgul D, et al. Phosphate depletion arrests progression of chronic renal failure independent of protein intake. Kidney Int 1986; 29:658.

Mangin M, et al. Identification of a cDNA encoding a parathyroid hormone-like material from a human tumor associated with humoral hypercalcemia of malignancy. Proc Natl Acad Sci 1988; 85:597.

Rose BD, Black RM. Manual of clinical problems in nephrology. Boston: Little, Brown, 1988.
Rosenbaum RW, et al. Decreased phosphate reabsorption after renal transplantation: Evidence for a mechanism independent of calcium and parathyroid hormone. Kidney Int 1981; 19:568.
Shields HS. Rapid fall of serum phosphorus secondary to antacid therapy. Gastroenterology 1978; 75:1137.
Slatopolsky E, et al. Marked suppression of secondary hyperparathyroidism by intravenous administration of 1,25-dihydroxycholecalciferol in uremic patients. J Clin Invest 1984; 74:2138.
Slatopolsky E, et al. Calcium carbonate as a phosphate binder in patients with chronic renal failure undergoing dialysis. N Engl J Med 1986; 315:157.
Vannatta JB, et al. Efficacy of intravenous phosphorus therapy in the severely hypophosphatemic patient. Arch Intern Med 1981; 141:885.

Hirsutism

Christopher Longcope, MD

42

Definition

Excessive growth of hair or the growth of hair in unusual places is a dictionary conception of hirsutism. For the purposes of this chapter, however, hirsutism should be defined physiologically.

There are three general types of hair follicles: (1) the nonhormonally dependent hair follicles consist of eyebrows, eyelashes, and the hair on the forearms and lower lip; (2) ambosexual hair follicles are present in the axilla and lower pubic regions of both men and women and are stimulated by low levels of androgens; and (3) sexual hair follicles, which depend on high concentrations of androgens, are present in the beard, ear, trunk, and upper pubic regions. Hirsutism, as discussed later, is characterized by excessive growth of sexual hair.

Although it has not been rigorously proven, it is probable that the androgens that stimulate ambosexual and sexual hair growth are the 5α-reduced androgens dihydrotestosterone and the androstanediols. These steroids are made primarily in the hair follicle from precursors, dehydroepiandrosterone, androstenedione, and testosterone, which in women arise from the adrenal glands and ovaries.

Hirsutism is a manifestation of increased androgen activity at the level of the hair follicle. Although hirsutism could theoretically occur as a result of increased sensitivity of the receptor or the genome to normal levels of circulating androgen or an increase in the activity of the 5α-reductase enzyme (the enzyme responsible for the formation of dihydrotestosterone and androstanediols from precursor androgens), these conditions have not yet been identified clinically. However, recent work by Horton et al (1982, 1986) suggests that increased 5α-reductase activity may occur and be more common than expected.

A major stimulus to the hair follicle could result from an increase in the amounts of androgen precursor reaching the 5α-reductase enzyme. This increase could be brought about from either exogenous sources (i.e., drugs) or endogenous sources (i.e., the adrenals or ovaries).

Drugs causing hirsutism include the androgens, adrenocorticotropic hormone (ACTH), high doses of glucocorticoids, and some of the synthetic progestins. Dilantin and diazoxide can cause hypertrichosis, and certain systemic diseases, e.g., anorexia nervosa, porphyria, and dermatomyositis, may cause excessive generalized or local hair growth but not hirsutism as it is defined here.

A careful history of possible hormone use should be taken. Once this possible cause of hirsutism has been ruled out, one should consider the endogenous causes of hirsutism.

Etiology and Clinical Characteristics

Common Causes

Polycystic Ovary Disease

Individuals with this disorder are usually obese, amenorrheic, and infertile. The ovaries are enlarged and cystic and thought by some endocrinologists to be the main source of the excess circulating androgen. Others, however, believe that there is a combined adrenal ovarian defect and that both glands can be involved in the excess androgen production. The circulating luteinizing hormone (LH) level is elevated, and the circulating follicle-stimulating hormone (FSH) level is decreased, resulting in an abnormally high LH : FSH ratio, which is a hallmark of the disorder. The degree of hair growth that occurs is variable, ranging from a few chin hairs to a marked increase of all sexual hair. The disorder can appear throughout the reproductive years and in previously fertile women. Circulating levels of testosterone, dehydroepiandrosterone (DHEA), and dehydroepiandrosterone sulfate (DHAS) may be in the upper normal range or slightly increased, and free testosterone is often increased. Pelvic ultrasonography is useful in evaluating ovarian size and the number and size of ovarian cysts.

Postpubertal Adrenal Hyperplasia (Nonclassic Congenital Adrenal Hyperplasia)

Differentiating this condition from polycystic ovary disease can be difficult, but circulating LH and FSH levels and the LH : FSH ratio are normal in postpubertal adrenal hyperplasia, and as noted later, the response of 17α-hydroxyprogesterone to ACTH is abnormal. The frequency of this syndrome is not well established, but according to some researchers, it may be common. A minor defect in one of several enzymes (e.g., 21-hydroxylase or 3β-hydroxysteroid dehydrogenase) involved in the biosynthesis of glucocorticoids can result in an excess production of androgen precursors (e.g., Δ^4-androstenedione and DHEA/DHAS). The androgen precursors are then converted to the active androgens in peripheral tissues, including the hair follicle. The enzyme block appears to be a low-grade one that is clinically manifest after puberty and does not involve symptoms of cortisol or mineralocorticoid deficiency. In the case of a defect of the 21-hydroxylase enzyme, androstenedione and 17α-hydroxyprogesterone (or its metabolite pregnanetriol) will be elevated, often only after ACTH administration. In subjects with a defect in 3β-hydroxysteroid dehydrogenase, the elevations will be noted in the Δ^5-steroids, 17β-hydroxypregnenolone, and DHEA.

Hirsutism is variable in extent, and acne is usually present, but clitoromegaly and other signs of virilization are generally absent. The subjects are often obese. Irregularities of menstrual cycle, oligo- or amenorrhea, are less common than with polycystic ovary disease and result from gonadotropin suppression by the excess adrenal androgens.

The exact diagnosis depends on demonstrating an enzyme block with high levels of 17α-hydroxyprogesterone, 17α-hydroxypregnenolone, or Δ^4-androstenedione and DHEA in the plasma, or pregnanetriol in the urine after adrenal stimulation with ACTH.

Idiopathic Hirsutism

Individuals who fall into this category have hirsutism with normal ovaries and normal adrenal testing. As the latter testing becomes more sophisticated with ACTH stimulation and extensive plasma steroid measurements, the incidence of this diagnosis is decreasing. There are, however, a number of women with hirsutism with normal menstrual cycles and normal steroid measurements. It is possible that these women have an intracellular defect in the expression of androgen biologic activity that is not demonstrable by current techniques.

The diagnosis is essentially one of exclusion, but the finding of an elevation in circulating levels of 5α-androstanediol glucuronide is often helpful in making the diagnosis.

Less Common Causes

Adrenal Tumors

Both adrenal carcinomas and adenomas can produce high levels of androgen precursors Δ^4-androstenedione and DHEA/DHAS, which will result in hirsutism. Carcinomas usually produce signs of glucocorticoid excess, such as diabetes, or abnormal fat distribution in addition to hirsutism. With adenomas, however, signs of androgen excess such as hirsutism, temporal baldness, clito-

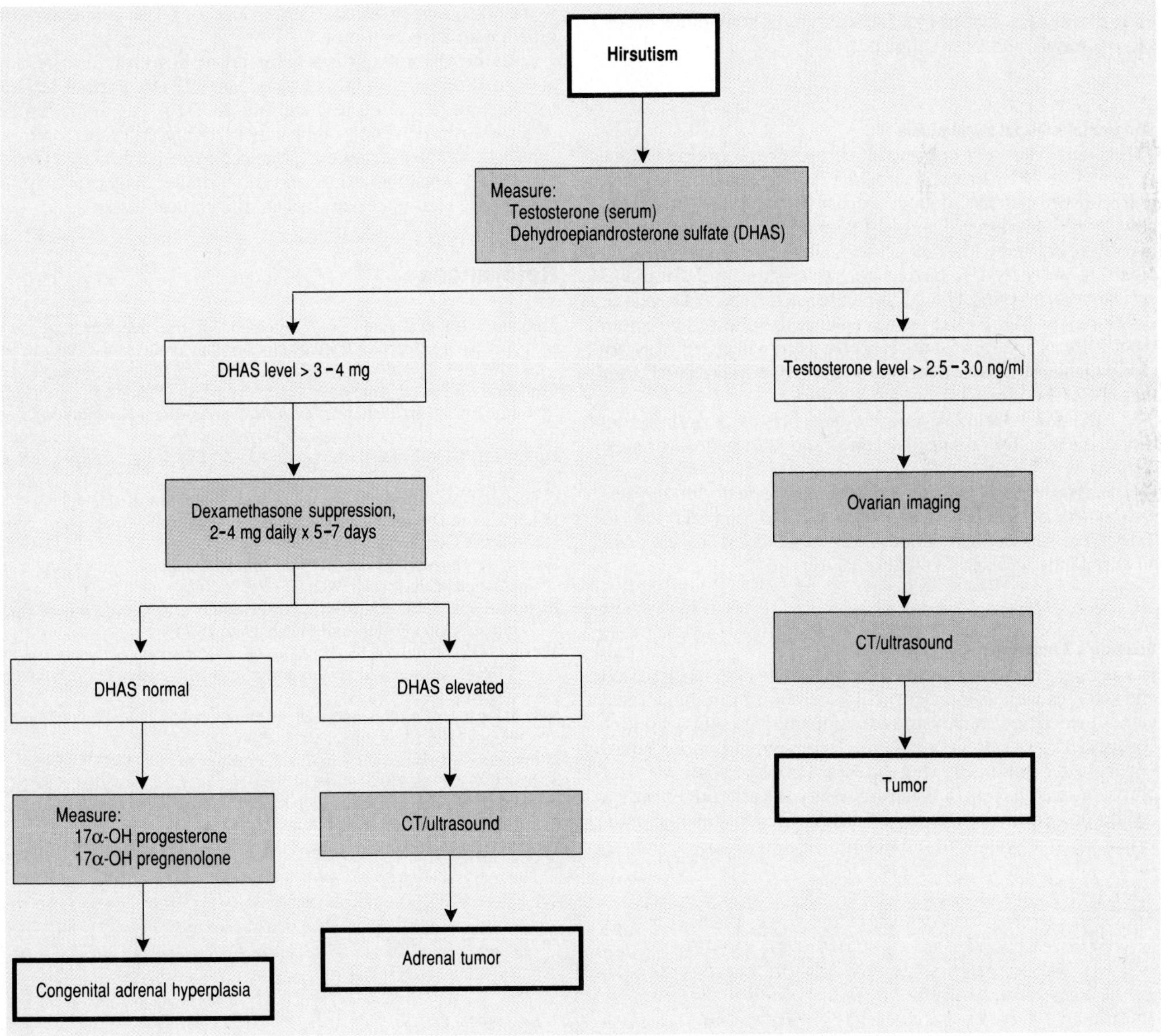

Figure 42-1 Algorithm for the evaluation of hirsutism. CT = computed tomography.

romegaly, and menstrual disturbances occur without evidence of glucocorticoid excess.

Blood levels of Δ^4-androstenedione and DHEA are above normal. The high levels of blood steroids do not suppress to normal with dexamethasone (2 to 4 mg per day for 5 to 7 days). Computed tomographic (CT) scanning or ultrasonography should be done to locate the tumor.

In rare cases, the tumor will secrete primarily testosterone, which will circulate at levels greater than 2.5 ng/ml. Although these tumors are located in the adrenal area, they have biochemical characteristics that suggest that they are of ovarian origin because they respond to human chorionic gonadotropin.

Ovarian Tumors

Certain ovarian tumors such as arrhenoblastoma, lipoid cell tumors, hilar cell tumors, and thecomas are androgen, primarily testosterone, secreting. Patients who have these tumors present with hirsutism, varying degrees of virilization, and amenorrhea. Obesity is frequently seen in women with lipoid cell tumors.

Laboratory testing shows a testosterone level of more than 2.5 to 3.0 ng/ml and normal to slightly elevated levels of plasma DHEA and DHAS. Physical examination usually reveals the tumor, but ultrasonography or CT scanning is sometimes necessary, especially in obese subjects.

Congenital Adrenal Hyperplasia

This is due to a severe enzyme block, the most common being a defect of the 21-hydroxylase, but defects of the 11β-hydroxylase and 3β-hydroxysteroid dehydrogenase do occur, the latter probably more commonly than once thought. These disorders are usually associated with some abnormalities in the external genitalia that are noted at birth. Otherwise, signs and symptoms appear prior to puberty, with hirsutism, acne, and male muscle development. There is early skeletal growth, followed by epiphyseal closure, and short stature, so that a girl will give the history of being taller than her peers early in life but eventually shorter than they. There may be a familial history.

Laboratory testing reveals elevated plasma Δ^4-androstenedione, DHEA, DHAS, testosterone, and 17α-hydroxyprogesterone.

Diagnosis depends on the preceding coupled with suppression to near normal with dexamethasone, 2 to 4 mg a day for 5 to 7 days. The suppressibility of the adrenal differentiates congenital adrenal hyperplasia from adrenal tumors.

Cushing's Syndrome

In Cushing's syndrome, the excess ACTH results in increased androgen as well as glucocorticoid secretion from the adrenal gland. Evidence of hirsutism is accompanied by signs of glucocorticoid excess, and generally the latter signs are more apparent than the hirsutism. Thus, unless there are some signs of glucocorticoid excess, it is not necessary to carry out extensive testing procedures to diagnose Cushing's syndrome in an individual who presents with hirsutism.

Rare Causes

Pituitary tumors are a rare cause of hirsutism. Acromegaly can cause some degree of hirsutism, but it need not be considered unless signs of excess growth hormone are present. Some prolactinomas may be associated with hirsutism. Thus, a prolactin level should be obtained in all subjects with hirsutism.

Work-Up

In the evaluation of a patient with hirsutism, the initial laboratory testing should include the measurement of circulating testosterone and DHAS levels (Fig. 42-1). The finding of a circulating testosterone level greater than 2.5 to 3.0 ng/ml should be followed immediately by a search for an ovarian tumor using ultrasound or CT. The finding of a DHAS level above 3 to 4 mg or urinary 17-ketosteroids above 25 mg/ml should be followed by dexamethasone suppression testing, 2 to 4 mg per day for 5 to 7 days, to see if the elevated values return to normal. If they do, further measurements of 17α-hydroxyprogesterone and 17α-hydroxypregnenolone should be done to establish the diagnosis of congenital adrenal hyperplasia. If the levels do not suppress, work-up should proceed to ultrasound or CT scanning to demonstrate an adrenal tumor.

In the majority of cases of hirsutism, however, testosterone is normal or only slightly elevated, as is DHAS. Further laboratory testing (e.g., free testosterone, ACTH stimulation) can be done as desired. In view of the general benignity of the common causes of hirsutism, however, one can proceed directly to treatment with dexamethasone, and the ultimate diagnosis may remain somewhat uncertain despite the clinical response.

References

Abraham GE. Evaluation and treatment of the hyperandrogenized woman. In: Scholler R, ed. Endocrinology of the ovary. Paris: Sepe, 1976:395.

Chrousos GP, et al. Late-onset 21-hydroxylase deficiency mimicking idiopathic hirsutism or polycystic ovarian disease. Ann Intern Med 1982; 96:143.

Futterweit W. Polycystic ovarian disease. New York: Springer-Verlag, 1984.

Goldzieher JW. Polycystic ovarian disease. Fertil Steril 1981; 35:371.

Hatch R, et al Hirsutism: Implications, etiology and management. Am J Obstet Gynecol 1981; 140:819.

Horton R, Hawks D, Lobo R. 3α-17β-Androstanediol glucuronide in plasma. J Clin Invest 1982; 69:1203.

Horton R, Lobo RA, eds. Androgen metabolism in hirsute and normal females. Clin Endocrinol Metab 1986; 15:213.

Maroulis GB, Manlimos FS, Abraham GE. Comparison between urinary 17-ketosteroids and serum androgens in hirsute patients. Obstet Gynecol 1977; 49:454.

New MI. Clinical and endocrinological aspects of 21-hydroxylase deficiency. Ann NY Acad Sci 1985; 458:1.

Rittmaster RS, Loriaux DL. Hirsutism. Ann Intern Med 1987; 106:95.

Speroff L, Glass RH, Kase NG. Hirsutism. In: Speroff L, Glass RH, Kase NG, eds. Clinical gynecologic endocrinology and infertility. 4th ed. Baltimore: Williams & Wilkins, 1989:233.

Yen SSC. The polycystic ovary syndrome. Clin Endocrinol 1980; 12:177.

Thyroid Function Testing

Marjorie Safran, MD

43

In order to understand thyroid function tests, a brief review of the physiology of the hypothalamic-pituitary-thyroid axis is useful. The thyroid gland secretes two important hormones—thyroxine (T_4), which contains four iodine molecules in a double-ringed structure, and triiodothyronine (T_3), which contains three iodine molecules. All of the T_4 in the circulation is produced by the thyroid gland. However, only 20 percent of the circulating T_3, the active form of thyroid hormone, is secreted by the thyroid. The remaining 80 percent is produced by conversion of T_4 to T_3 in organs such as liver, kidney, muscle, and brain, which contain T_4 outer-ring deiodinase enzymes. Many of these tissues also contain inner-ring deiodinase enzymes. These convert T_4 to reverse T_3 (rT_3). Five percent of circulating rT_3 is secreted by the thyroid. The remainder is generated from peripheral conversion of T_4 to rT_3.

As noted, T_3 has greater thyromimetic effects than T_4 and is probably the active form of thyroid hormone. In contrast, rT_3 is almost entirely devoid of thyroid hormone activity. The peripheral conversion of T_4 to T_3 or rT_3 is altered by drugs, illness, and physiologic status (Table 43-1). Thus, in starvation, during severe illness, or when drugs such as prednisone are administered, there is decreased production of T_3. In summary, T_4 is a prohormone, and its hormonal action is influenced by factors that affect conversion of T_4 to T_3.

The production of T_4 and T_3 by the thyroid gland is under the control of thyrotropin (TSH). Pituitary TSH secretion is dependent on the hypothalamic production of thyrotropin-releasing hormone (TRH). A finely tuned negative-feedback system also regulates TSH secretion. Increases in serum T_4 or T_3 suppress TSH secretion; when thyroid hormone production is decreased, TSH secretion is enhanced.

Most of the circulating T_4 and T_3 is bound to specific carrier proteins in serum. Only 0.03 percent of circulating T_4 and 0.3 percent of T_3 is in the free or unbound state. The free levels of these hormones determine their activity both in the peripheral tissues and in the brain and pituitary. The most important thyroid hormone binding serum protein is thyroxine-binding globulin (TBG). It binds between 70 and 75 percent of bound T_4 and T_3. Changes in the serum TBG concentration will alter the total serum T_4 and T_3 concentration without changing the free concentration. The remainder of bound hormone is bound to thyroxine-binding prealbumin (TBPA) and albumin. Changes in the serum concentrations of these proteins have far less effect on total serum thyroid hormone concentrations.

Iodide is necessary for thyroid hormone production. The thyroid is able to transport iodide actively from the extracellular fluid in order to obtain sufficient iodide for thyroid hormone synthesis. It also has the ability to autoregulate iodine uptake. When the serum iodide concentration is low, a high percentage of iodide is trapped and organified. The converse is also true. Very high concentrations of intrathyroidal iodide inhibit not only iodide uptake by the thyroid but also thyroid hormone synthesis and release (Wolff-Chaikoff effect). This would eventually lead to subnormal circulating thyroid hormone concentrations, except that with continued iodide exposure, the thyroid normally escapes from this effect. Some patients with Hashimoto's thyroiditis and other thyroid disorders develop hypothyroidism when exposed to pharmacologic amounts of iodine. These patients are unable to escape from the Wolff-Chaikoff effect. The other major factor that influences iodide uptake is the circulating TSH level. If the plasma TSH concentration is elevated, iodide uptake will be enhanced. When TSH is suppressed, there is little active uptake of iodide by the thyroid.

Serum T_4, Resin T_3 Uptake, and Free Thyroxine Index

The most frequently performed test of thyroid function is the measurement of the serum T_4 concentration by radioimmunoassay. This test measures both the bound and free hormone. However, because so little hormone is free, the test actually provides an index of the bound T_4. In most situations, the T_4 usually reflects the patient's thyroid status. With a few exceptions, which are detailed later, the serum T_4 concentration is elevated in hyperthyroidism and low or low normal in hypothyroidism. However, an abnormal serum TBG concentration will also be associated with a serum T_4 that is abnormal despite the fact that the patient is euthyroid. Table 43-2 lists the situations in which abnormal serum TBG concentrations are found.

Because of these factors, further tests are required to distinguish changes in serum T_4 that are secondary to thyroid dysfunction from those due to alterations in thyroid hormone binding proteins. One approach is to measure the free concentration of T_4 in serum. The free T_4 concentration can be measured by a dialysis technique. However, this is time consuming and expensive. The more usual practice is to estimate the free T_4 concentration by combining the T_4 test with a test called the resin T_3 uptake. This test does not measure the serum T_3; rather, it is

Table 43-1 Clinical Settings for Impaired Peripheral Conversion of T_4 to T_3*

Nonthyroidal acute and chronic illness
Starvation
Fetus and newborn
Drugs: Oragrafin, Telepaque, propranolol, glucocorticoids

* In these patients, the serum T_3 is low; therefore, it is usually not worthwhile to order the test if a patient fits into one of these categories.

Table 43-2 Factors That Alter Serum TBG Concentrations

TBG decreased	TBG increased
Androgens	Estrogens
High-dose corticosteroids	Heroin
L-Asparaginase	Methadone
Inherited trait	Inherited trait

Abbreviation: TBG = thyroxine-binding globulin.

influenced by the serum TBG concentration and the serum T_4 concentration itself. In the way it is usually reported, the result is inversely proportional to the TBG concentration. Thus, an elevated resin uptake often indicates a low TBG concentration, whereas a low resin uptake may reflect an increased TBG concentration. If the resin T_3 uptake is expressed relative to a value obtained for a pool of normal serum, it is called the resin T_3 uptake ratio. Thus, the "average" normal subject has a resin T_3 uptake ratio of 1.00.

Multiplying the value for the serum T_4 concentration by the resin T_3 uptake ratio generates the free thyroxine index (FTI), which usually reflects the underlying thyroid status. Thus, in a euthyroid patient with an elevated TBG concentration, the total T_4 concentration is increased. However, the resin T_3 uptake ratio is decreased. The high T_4 combined with a low resin T_3 uptake ratio yields a normal FTI. The converse is true in patients with low serum TBG concentrations. In these patients, the T_4 is subnormal and the resin T_3 uptake ratio is elevated. The FTI may still be somewhat low, however, because the elevation in the resin T_3 uptake ratio is often not sufficient to compensate completely for the decrease in serum T_4. A useful feature of the resin T_3 uptake ratio test is that, although it is inversely proportional to the serum TBG concentration, it changes in direct proportion to the serum T_4 concentration. Thus, in true hyperthyroidism, not only the serum T_4 but also the resin T_3 uptake ratio tends to be elevated. Consequently, the FTI is usually increased. Conversely, the FTI is usually decreased in hypothyroidism unless it is mild.

Serum T_3 Measurement

The serum T_3, like serum T_4, is measured by a specific radioimmunoassay. Measurement of the serum T_3 concentration is invaluable in the work-up of hyperthyroidism (Fig. 43-1). In Graves' disease the thyroid gland secretes a relatively high proportion of T_3 in comparison to T_4. This is true for all situations in which thyroid stimulators circulate in high concentration. In some hyperthyroid patients, the serum T_3 concentration is markedly elevated, whereas the serum T_4 concentration is only slightly above normal or even within the normal range. This is called T_3 toxicosis. T_3 toxicosis is more common in patients with early Graves' disease. It is also seen in hyperthyroid patients with autonomous thyroid nodules. Measurement of the serum T_3 concentration, in addition to being the specific test for T_3 toxicosis, is also useful in judging the severity of hyperthyroidism. By contrast, measurement of serum T_3 is of no value in the diagnosis of hypothyroidism. Many euthyroid patients with systemic illness have diminished T_3 concentrations secondary to decreased T_4 to T_3 conversion. In addition, the failing thyroid gland will preferentially produce T_3 under TSH stimulation.

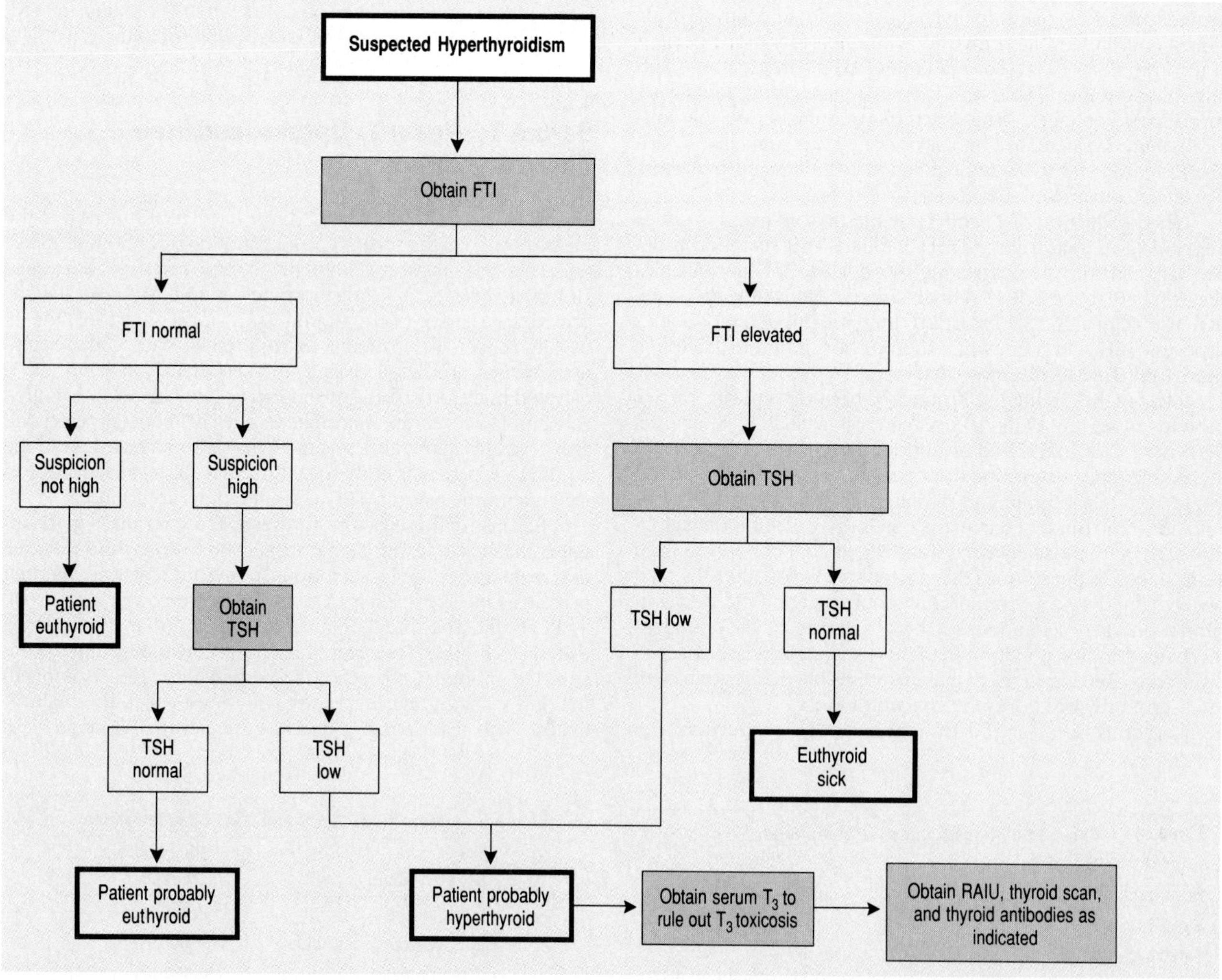

Figure 43-1 Algorithm for the evaluation of suspected hyperthyroidism. Note that serum thyrotropin (TSH) must be measured using an ultrasensitive TSH assay. FTI = free thyroxine index, RAIU = radioactive iodine uptake, T_3 = triiodothyronine.

Therefore, in mild hypothyroidism, the serum T_3 concentration may be normal, and other tests are required to establish the diagnosis of hypothyroidism.

Thyroid Stimulating Hormone

The serum TSH is measured by radioimmunoassay. As noted previously, the pituitary is very sensitive to changes in circulating thyroid hormone concentrations. Even mild thyroid failure, a situation in which the serum T_4 concentration may still be within normal range, will cause the serum TSH to be elevated. If the serum T_4 concentration is in the low-normal range and hypothyroidism is suspected, TSH measurement is indicated (Fig. 43-2). These patients are said to have "subclinical hypothyroidism." This is often seen in patients with Hashimoto's thyroiditis or those with a previous history of ablative treatment for hyperthyroidism (such as surgery or radioactive iodine). With the availability of ultrasensitive TSH assays, the converse is also true. Thus, in even mild primary hyperthyroidism (Graves' disease, toxic multinodular goiter and other entities), the serum TSH concentration is reduced to hyperthyroid or undetectable ranges.

Theoretically, serum TSH determinations should be able to distinguish between primary and secondary hypothyroidism. In some patients with pituitary disorders, however, the serum TSH concentration is normal or even mildly elevated despite the fact that the patient is hypothyroid. These patients produce a TSH that is biologically less active but is still measured by the TSH radioimmunoassay.

TRH Testing

The serum TSH response to the intravenous administration of TRH can be used to determine the thyroid status of a patient in difficult situations. It is of interest for historical reasons and because it illustrates pituitary thyroid physiology; however, it is rarely used now that ultrasensitive serum TSH assays have become available. TRH normally causes the pituitary to increase TSH secretion; however, when serum thyroid hormone concentrations are increased even slightly, the effect of TRH on TSH release is markedly inhibited. Thus, in patients with slightly elevated T_4 or T_3 concentrations in whom the diagnosis of hyperthyroidism is questionable, 200 to 500 μg of TRH can be administered intravenously and serum TSH concentrations measured. An increase in TSH of at least 3 $\mu U/ml$ rules out all but a few very unusual forms of hyperthyroidism. The absence of a response is not always as helpful. This is seen in some elderly men and in patients with acute psychiatric or severe medical illness.

The TRH test should be useful in the work-up of secondary hypothyroidism. That is, TSH deficiency could be due to either disease of the pituitary or TRH deficiency resulting from hypothalamic disease. In hypothalamic hypothyroidism, TRH administration should elicit a TSH response; with intrinsic pituitary

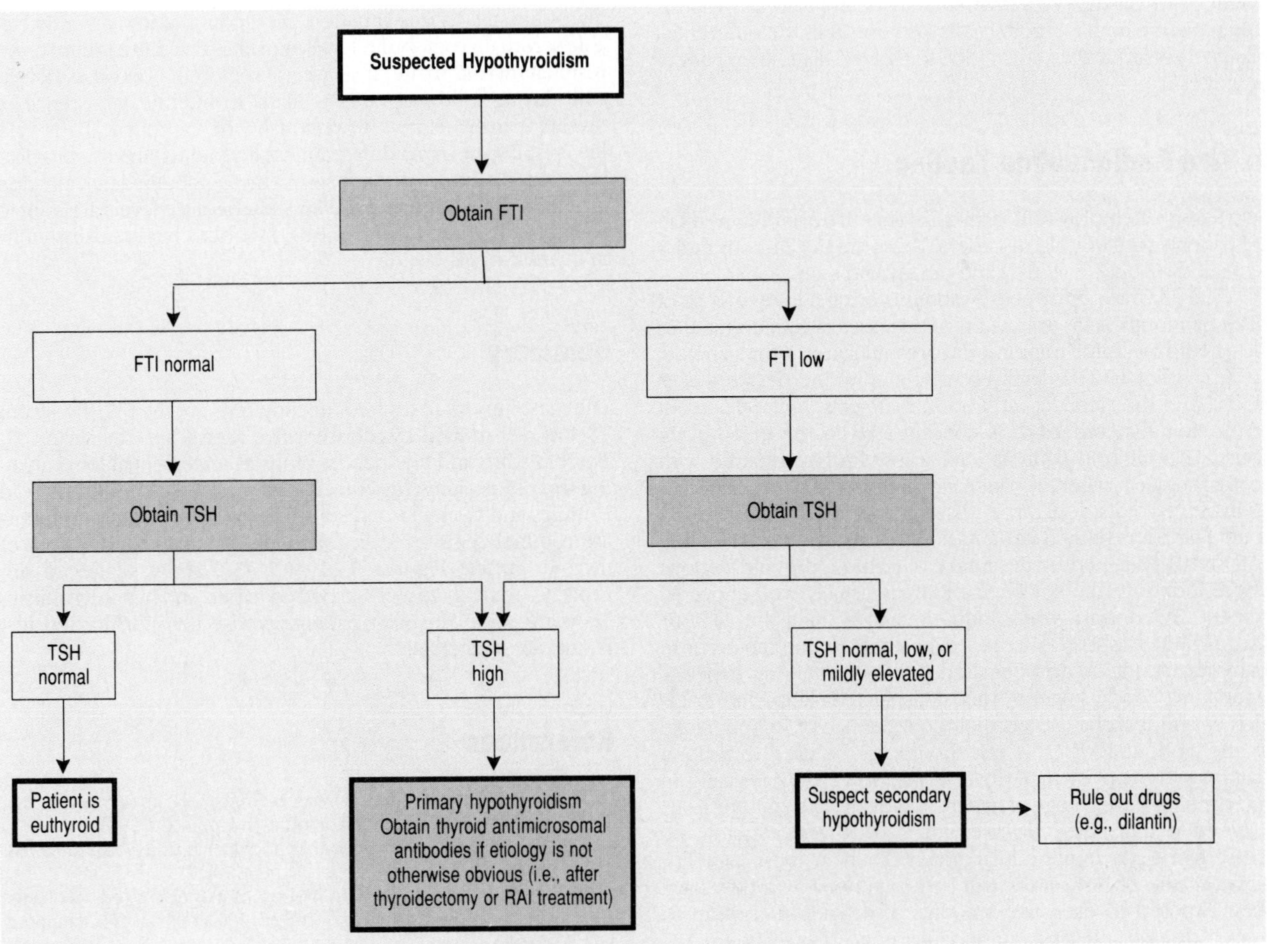

Figure 43-2 Algorithm for the evaluation of suspected hypothyroidism. FTI = free thyroxine index, RAI = radioactive iodine, TSH = thyrotropin.

disease, TRH should not be capable of eliciting a TSH response. Unfortunately, in actual studies the TRH test has often failed to distinguish between patients with pituitary disease and those with hypothalamic lesions.

Thyroid Antibodies

Autoantibodies to thyroid antigens are present in the serum of many patients with thyroid diseases. These antibodies can be classified in two groups. In the first are antibodies directed against the TSH receptor on the surface of thyroid follicular cells. These antibodies stimulate the receptor and mediate the hyperthyroidism of Graves' disease. They have been given various names, including the long-acting thyroid stimulator (LATS) and thyroid-stimulating immunoglobulins (TSI). TSI-positive serum is usually confined to patients with Graves' disease. High titers are said to indicate a decreased probability that the disease will go into remission. Unfortunately, these assays are not standardized, and their usefulness in clinical practice is not well established.

The second group of antibodies are those directed against thyroglobulin or follicular cell microsomes (antithyroglobulin and antimicrosomal antibodies, respectively). These antibodies are found in the serum of many patients with a variety of thyroid disorders. They are present in high titer in most patients with Hashimoto's thyroiditis and in lower titer in many patients with Graves' disease. Antithyroglobulin and antimicrosomal antibodies are sometimes found, usually in low titer, in patients with nodular goiter, subacute thyroiditis, or thyroid carcinoma. The measurement of these antibodies is helpful in confirming the diagnosis of Hashimoto's thyroiditis in a euthyroid or hypothyroid patient who has a goiter. It is also useful in the differential diagnosis of hyperthyroidism due to Graves' disease and nodular goiter.

In Vivo Radionuclide Testing

Two tests that employ radioactive isotopes are useful in evaluating patients with thyroid disorders. These are the 24-hour radioactive iodine uptake (RAIU) and the thyroid scan.

The RAIU is performed by administering a known dose of I-123 by mouth. A large fraction of this dose is concentrated in the thyroid by iodide trapping and organification. After 24 hours, the uptake of I-123 is measured by a counting device that is placed over the gland. In most normal subjects, 10 to 30 percent of the administered I-123 is concentrated in the gland at 24 hours. Hypothyroid patients have a low RAIU compared with normal subjects, whereas patients with the most common forms of hyperthyroidism (Graves' disease and toxic multinodular goiter) have an elevated RAIU. As noted previously, however, the RAIU is also affected by the intake of stable iodine. In regions where iodine intake is low, the RAIU is usually well above 30 percent. By contrast, when iodine intake is high, the 24-hour RAIU is quite low. Exposure to excess stable iodine can occur in many forms, including potassium iodide–containing expectorants, x-ray contrast agents, foodstuffs such as kelp, and drugs such as amiodarone. Because of the influence of iodine intake on the 24-hour RAIU, this test should not be used to make a diagnosis of hypo- or hyperthyroidism. However, it is useful in determining the etiology of hyperthyroidism. The 24-hour RAIU is elevated in Graves' disease and is usually moderately increased in toxic multinodular goiter. Even in these patients, however, the 24-hour RAIU will be normal or low if they have been exposed to excessive amounts of iodine. In contrast to Graves' disease and toxic multinodular goiter, the 24-hour RAIU is low when hyperthyroidism is due to subacute thyroiditis or to silent thyroiditis (painless thyroiditis, spontaneously resolving thyroiditis). The 24-hour RAIU is also very low in thyrotoxicosis factitia. In subacute or silent thyroiditis, the disruption of follicular cells leads to leakage of thyroid hormones into the circulation that is sufficient to suppress TSH secretion and secondarily decrease RAIU. In addition, the iodine-concentrating mechanism of the cells is also disrupted. In thyrotoxicosis factitia, the ingestion of thyroid hormones suppresses TSH secretion; this results in a low RAIU.

Thyroid scans are used to determine the size and shape of the thyroid and to localize areas of increased or decreased function. Scans are also used to localize the thyroid tissue in conditions in which it is found outside the neck (e.g., substernal goiter, metastatic thyroid cancer). The most common reason for ordering a thyroid scan is to evaluate the function of palpable thyroid nodule(s). (Examples of thyroid scans are shown in Figure 17-6, page 87.)

Thyroglobulin

Thyroglobulin can be detected in the circulation in almost all individuals. Serum thyroglobulin concentrations are elevated in patients with most forms of hyperthyroidism, multinodular goiter, and benign and malignant neoplasms of the thyroid; therefore, the finding of elevated serum thyroglobulin does not indicate a specific diagnosis. Serum thyroglobulin concentrations are most commonly ordered in the follow-up of patients with thyroid cancer, particularly when surgery and radioactive iodine have been used in an attempt to achieve total ablation of thyroid tissue. In this situation, the finding of low or undetectable serum thyroglobulin levels indicates that there is little or no residual thyroid tissue. If serum thyroglobulin becomes detectable during follow-up, this is likely to indicate recurrence of thyroid cancer. As noted previously, the 24-hour RAIU is very low in subacute thyroiditis, painless thyroiditis, and thyrotoxicosis factitia. In this situation, a serum thyroglobulin determination is helpful in the differential diagnosis, because levels are high in subacute thyroiditis and painless thyroiditis but are usually low in thyrotoxicosis factitia.

Summary

The most important thyroid function tests are the FTI, the serum TSH as determined by ultrasensitive assays, and the serum T_3. Thyroid scans and fine-needle biopsies are essential for evaluating thyroid nodules (discussed further in Chapter 44, "Thyroid Nodules and Goiter"), and serum thyroglobulin measurements are routinely employed in following patients with a history of thyroid cancer. Figures 43-1 and 43-2 show suggested approaches to patients with suspected hyper- and hypothyroidism. They are useful in most patients whose thyroid function test results are abnormal.

References

Cavalieri RR. Quantitative in vivo tests. In: Ingbar SH, Braverman LE, eds. Werner's the thyroid. Philadelphia: JB Lippincott, 1986.

Hay ID, et al. Thyroid dysfunction. Endocr Metab Clin North Am 1988; 17:473.

Ingbar SH. The thyroid gland. In: Wilson JB, Foster DW, eds. Williams' textbook of endocrinology. 7th ed. Philadelphia: WB Saunders, 1985:682.

Thyroid Nodules and Goiter

Charles H. Emerson, MD

44

In the United States, where current levels of iodine intake are adequate, the prevalence of goiter (thyromegaly) ranges from 0.5 to 7 percent. The solitary thyroid nodule, a variant of goiter, is also common. However, when a single nodule is noted on physical examination, there is a 50 percent chance that additional nodules can be found at surgery or autopsy. When large populations in the United States are followed with physical exams, the incidence of new nodules is about 0.1 percent per year.

Patients with small goiters are usually asymptomatic if thyroid hormone secretion is normal. At this stage, the goiter is typically detected only if a physical examination is performed. If the goiter becomes larger, the patient or a friend is apt to notice it. A few patients complain of a choking sensation, but this is an unusual presenting symptom. This symptom is more common in patients who are being followed for a goiter. The choking sensation tends to wax and wane without apparent reason and differs from dysphagia due to esophageal obstruction because it occurs both with and without ingestion of food or liquids. The choking sensation can progress to frank dyspnea, particularly on assumption of the supine position. Even when this occurs, upper airway flow as assessed by pulmonary function studies is frequently normal. Some patients with goiter have tracheal deviation or compression. This is seen on chest radiograph, but it may not be associated with pressure symptoms.

Goiters and thyroid nodules are occasionally painful. Pain tends to radiate to the ear, jaw, or temporomandibular joint. The involved portion of the thyroid is tender, but the patient may not perceive pain in the thyroid. The diagnostic significance of thyroid pain is discussed in a subsequent section.

Thyroid function is disturbed in a minority (approximately 10 percent) of patients with goiter or solitary nodule, giving rise to protean signs and symptoms.

Etiology

On a functional basis, thyroid enlargement can be divided into three basic categories: (1) primary goiter due to a benign or malignant lesion that arises de novo in the gland; (2) thyroinvasive secondary goiter due to invasion of the thyroid by a malignant, infectious, or fibrous process; and (3) thyrostimulatory goiter due to circulating substances that promote thyroid growth. The common causes of these forms of goiter are outlined in Table 44-1. Table 44-1 also presents an estimate of the relative incidence of goiter based on a review of the literature and the author's experience. (These data apply only to regions where iodine intake is normal.)

Simple goiter accounts for about three-quarters of all goiters. There is a diffuse and a multinodular variant. With time, the diffuse variant tends to become nodular. These nodules may calcify, resulting in a hard texture that can suggest carcinoma. The adenomatous nodules of simple goiter have varying degrees of autonomous (thyrotropin-independent) function. In a small percentage of patients, this may eventually result in hyperthyroidism (toxic multinodular goiter). Toxic multinodular goiter is usually seen in elderly individuals. However, all individuals with multinodular goiter who ingest pharmacologic doses of iodine are susceptible to hyperthyroidism. Symptoms develop insidiously and occur in the weeks after, rather than during the time of, iodine exposure. Common sources of excess dietary iodine are cough medications and kelp. The latter is widely available in health food stores. Radiographic contrast agents are also a source of iodine and have been known to precipitate hyperthyroidism in euthyroid patients with multinodular goiter.

Most forms of thyroid cancer present as a solitary nodule, but goiter formation does not rule out thyroid cancer. Familial medullary carcinoma and the papillary-follicular carcinoma that follows head and neck irradiation have a tendency to be multicentric, simulating other forms of goiter. With the exception of sporadic medullary carcinoma and undifferentiated carcinoma, most forms of thyroid cancer are relatively indolent neoplasms. Therefore, systemic symptoms are usually not the presenting complaints. Painless cervical adenopathy occurs in papillary-follicular carcinoma; pulmonary metastases are a late event. Pure follicular carcinoma eventually metastasizes to lung and bone, resulting in dyspnea and bone pain. Undifferentiated carcinoma is a locally invasive, virulent tumor that is seen almost exclusively after the fifth decade of life. Survival of more than 1 to 2 years is rare.

Hashimoto's thyroiditis is both a thyroinvasive and thyrostimulatory form of secondary goiter. The thyroid enlarges because of infiltration by lymphocytes and stimulation by high levels of circulating thyrotropin (TSH). Hypothyroidism is the outcome of most cases, but many patients are euthyroid when first seen. Most glands are diffusely enlarged, nontender, firm, and lobulated. Some have a pebbly feel. Rarely, a single nodule is felt. There is often a family history of goiter or hypothyroidism. In addition, the patient may have associated autoimmune disorders such as Addison's disease, rheumatoid arthritis, or alopecia areata.

The goiter of Graves' disease is caused by circulating thyroid-stimulating antibodies that activate the TSH receptor. The presenting complaint is usually one or more of the symptoms of hyperthyroidism. Occasionally, patients seek medical attention because of neck swelling, but careful evaluation is

Table 44-1 Important Causes of Goiter*

Type of goiter	Relative frequency
Primary Goiter	
Simple goiter	Very common
Thyroid cancer	Infrequent
Thyrostimulatory Secondary Goiter	
Graves' disease	Infrequent
Hashimoto's thyroiditis	Common
Congenital hereditary goiter	Rare
Thyroinvasive Secondary Goiter	
Hashimoto's thyroiditis	Common
Subacute thyroiditis	Infrequent
Reidel's thyroiditis	Rare
Metastatic tumors to the thyroid	Rare

* This table applies to regions of normal iodine intake.

likely to elicit subtle signs or symptoms of hyperthyroidism. The thyroid is diffusely enlarged, and if a bruit is present, it establishes the diagnosis. Because the bruit is due to venous blood flow, it extends through diastole. Thyroid bruits should be distinguished from cervical venous hums, carotid bruits, and referred cardiac murmurs.

Hereditary goiters are rare causes of thyromegaly. They are usually noted in infancy or childhood. There is a discrete defect in thyroid hormone production that augments TSH secretion. This in turn promotes thyroid growth. In common with other forms of thyrostimulatory goiter, diffuse thyroid enlargement is characteristic of the early stage. With prolonged stimulation, there is a tendency for nodules to develop. The defect in thyroid hormone secretion is often mild and compensated by increased TSH; therefore, patients are not necessarily hypothyroid. A strong family history of similar goiters is characteristic. Some patients' family members have other phenotypic abnormalities such as deafness.

Subacute thyroiditis is an important form of thyroinvasive secondary goiter. The syndrome is probably due to infection of the thyroid with a viral, or rarely, bacterial, agent. Systemic symptoms such as malaise, low-grade fever, and mild sore throat frequently herald the disorder. The involved portion of the thyroid swells, becomes tender and painful, and discharges thyroid hormone. Therefore, a transient period of hyperthyroidism is common. Symptoms resolve over a period of several weeks. Because this disorder has a distinctive clinical course, the cause of thyroid enlargement is straightforward.

Reidel's thyroiditis is an invasive fibrosis of the thyroid. It is very rare, and the cause is unknown. Some patients have fibrosis in other tissues such as the mediastinal region, the retroperitoneal fascia, and the retro-ocular space. Metastatic tumors to the thyroid are another rare cause of thyroid enlargement. Both Reidel's thyroiditis and intrathyroidal metastasis are usually painless. The diagnosis must be made by biopsy.

The Solitary Thyroid Nodule

The concept of the solitary thyroid nodule implies that the remainder of the gland is normal. Benign follicular adenomas account for most solitary thyroid nodules. Occasionally, they hypersecrete thyroid hormone and cause clinical hyperthyroidism. Many histologic features of the follicular adenoma and the nodules of simple goiter are similar, suggesting that the lesions are variants of the same process. A small number of apparently solitary thyroid nodules are due to Hashimoto's thyroiditis or, rarely, to a painless form of subacute thyroiditis. Another small

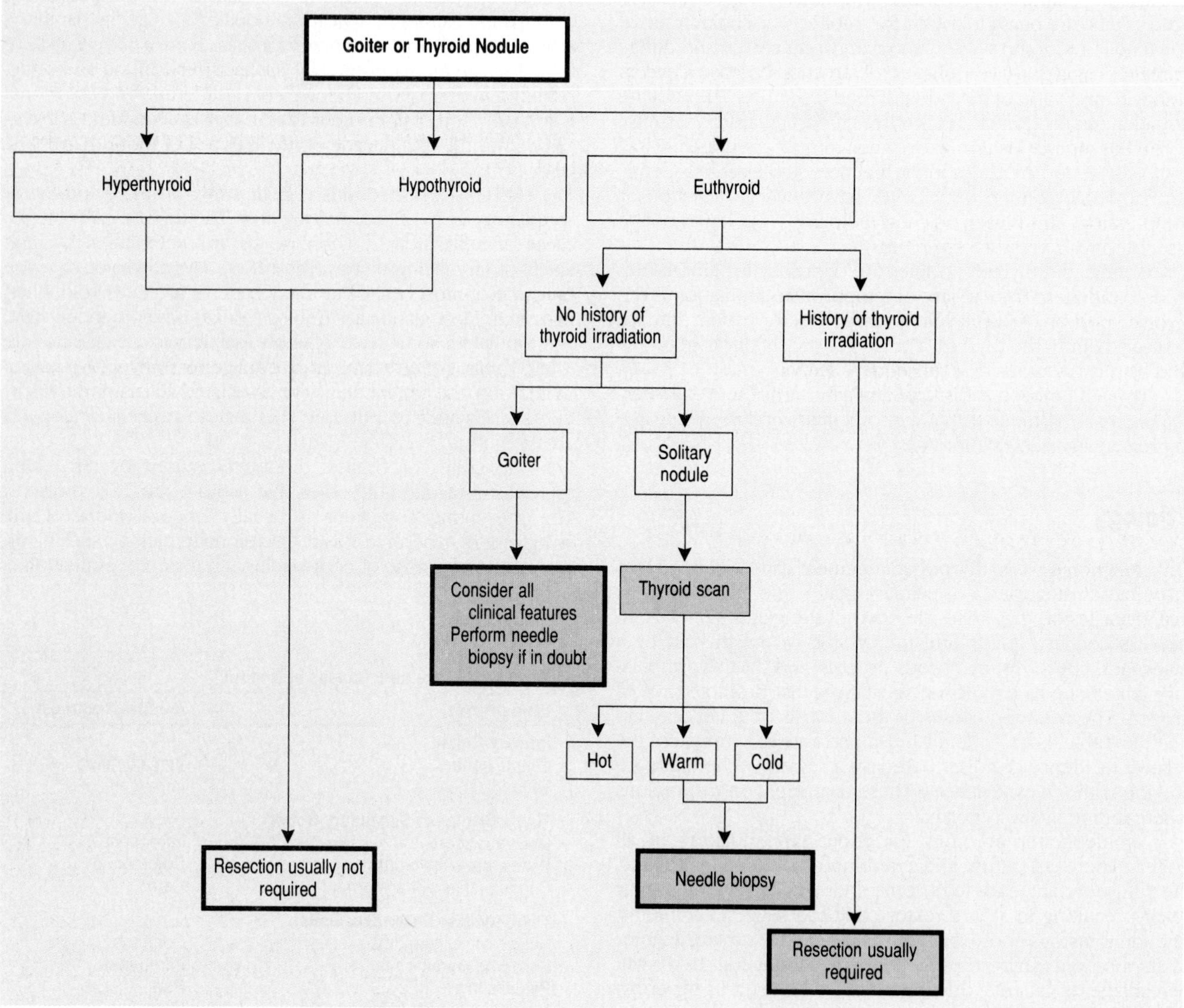

Figure 44-1 A decision-making scheme for diagnostic thyroid biopsy or resection.

percentage are purely cystic. Pure cystic lesions are almost always benign. This is not the case, however, for partially cystic nodules.

Thyroid cancer is found in 8 to 20 percent of surgically removed thyroid nodules. The prevalence is much lower, about 3 percent, in autopsy series. When normal populations in the United States are screened, the prevalence is perhaps even lower. These differences in the prevalence of thyroid cancer are due to the fact that preoperative evaluation is able to identify, in part, those patients who are most likely to have thyroid cancer.

Diagnostic Approach

As noted previously, goiters are usually uncovered because the patient sees or feels neck enlargement or are found during a physical examination for unrelated problems. Other structures in the neck such as lymph nodes (adenopathy) and blood vessels (aneurysms) can enlarge. However, the characteristic location of the thyroid and its movement with deglutition make palpation a reliable method of identifying a goiter or thyroid nodule. In patients with thick necks, a thyroid scan or ultrasound examination is sometimes necessary for positive identification. A thyroid scan is essential if the goiter is substernal.

Clinicians consider two questions in evaluating thyroid enlargement: whether the goiter harbors a malignancy and whether it is associated with thyroid dysfunction. This section deals with the former question. Resection of the goiter or thyroid nodule is the most reliable means of diagnosing thyroid cancer; however, this approach is not warranted for all nodules and goiter because the ratio of benign to malignant thyroid growths is high, and most thyroid cancers are slow growing and associated with less morbidity and mortality than other malignant neoplasms. Fortunately, the most common form of thyroid cancer, papillary follicular carcinoma, often responds well to treatment, even when regional lymph node metastases are present.

A simplified scheme to help one decide if there is a need for diagnostic thyroid biopsy or resection is presented in Figure 44-1. Exceptions to this general approach are sometimes required. As Figure 44-1 indicates, if the patient has hyper- or hypothyroidism, the chances of malignancy are low; therefore, thyroid surgery for diagnostic purposes is rarely indicated. On the other hand, most patients with a history of irradiation to the thyroid area should have thyroid surgery if a thyroid nodule or asymmetric enlargement of the thyroid is noted. Patients with a history of thyroid irradiation and no palpable thyroid abnormalities should have yearly neck examinations. Surgery is indicated in most euthyroid subjects with goiter if there is a family history of thyroid tumors or if recent growth is rapid. Patients with a family history of thyroid tumors should also undergo calcium or pentagastrin infusion tests to diagnose medullary thyroid carcinoma. A thyroid scan should be performed in the patient with a solitary thyroid nodule. A hyperfunctioning nodule that suppresses uptake in the remainder of the gland or an autonomous nodule that continues to concentrate iodine when thyroid hormone is administered generally does not require diagnostic resection. Warm and cold nodules and suspicious goiters should be evaluated by aspiration needle biopsy. If palpation suggests a cyst, some authorities suggest an echographic exam. Complete cysts are rarely malignant; however, if the lesion is partially cystic by echographic exam, this provides little useful information.

Needle biopsy is the most useful guide for determining whether excisional biopsy is required. This requires expertise, both in obtaining the sample and in the cytopathologic interpretation. The patient's age and sex, the palpatory character of the nodule, and the response to thyroid hormone administration are lesser factors that influence the decision. For example, surgery is more frequently recommended for men with thyroid nodules than for women with similar physical findings, because the ratio of malignant to benign thyroid nodules is higher in men than in women. Thyroid nodules that shrink after thyroid hormone treatment are more likely to be benign. It is clear that the decision regarding surgery is a matter of clinical judgment. However, needle biopsy is the most important study in arriving at this decision. Even if the needle biopsy is consistent with a benign process, the patient should be followed and re-evaluated as necessary.

References

Gharib H, et al. Fine-needle aspiration biopsy of the thyroid. The problem of suspicious cytologic findings. Ann Intern Med 1984; 101:25.

Rojeski MT, Gharib H. Nodular thyroid disease. N Engl J Med 1985; 313:428.

45 Obesity

Katherine L. Kahn, MD

Judith K. Ockene, PhD

Jean L. Kristeller, PhD

The conventional definition of obesity is body weight in excess of 20 percent of "ideal," as determined by actuarial tables based on life expectancy and dependent on height, gender, and body frame. Mild obesity is 20 to 40 percent excess weight; moderate obesity is 41 to 100 percent over ideal weight; morbid obesity is more than 100 percent over ideal weight.

A more biologically based definition involves measurement of excess adipose tissue in the range of 10 to 20 percent. In the laboratory, fat tissue is determined by body-density determination or isotope dilution studies. In the clinical setting, however, the physician must be careful not to inappropriately label as obese those who are overweight because of excess body fluid or because of a well-developed muscular structure. A gross objective measure of the body's subcutaneous fat stores may be obtained by the skin-pinch test. Excessive fat stores are defined as a skinfold measurement in excess of 1 inch when the skin is pinched in the midtriceps or subscapular region.

The efficiency of fat in conserving food energy has been an evolutionary advantage. A healthy adult of normal weight can live without food intake for approximately 8 weeks by consuming stored fat. In today's American society, however, a relative excess intake of food in combination with a sedentary lifestyle has been a problem for many, with approximately 20 to 30 percent of men and 30 to 40 percent of women classified as obese. Women, particularly those of lower socioeconomic status and those who are recent immigrants, have the highest prevalence of obesity. In some cultures, obesity in older women (and men) is the norm; treatment in such a sociologic milieu may be especially difficult. In all cases, the excess accumulation of adipose tissue results from caloric intake exceeding caloric utilization.

Differential Diagnosis

A small proportion of obese patients, possibly less than 10 percent, have endocrine, neurologic, or genetic disorders underlying their obesity. Table 45-1 lists the medical conditions associated with obesity.

For the patient with no underlying medical problems causing obesity, an assessment is needed to determine the age of onset of the condition and the behavioral and psychosocial factors contributing to its development and maintenance. Obese individuals often use overeating as a coping strategy in response to stress or negative emotional feelings. In many instances, they have learned that food is a source of pleasure or relief. They generally have other coping mechanisms available to them in their repertoires of behavior but, in many cases, have not learned how to utilize these in place of food. In these patients some new learning may need to take place. In other cases, especially those with early-onset problems, obesity is often related to personality and developmental disturbances or to problems in learning. The psychological factors that seem to relate directly to obesity are lack of hunger awareness, with eating precipitated by external rather than internal stimuli, and a distorted body image. Both of these disturbances are more prevalent in patients who developed obesity in childhood. Obesity occurring in adulthood is sometimes a reaction to a traumatic event, including loss of a loved one, a job, or status. However, a major factor in adult-onset obesity may be a progressive change in metabolic rate, accompanied by a decrease in activity level and gradual changes in eating habits. Obesity occurring in adulthood is generally easier to treat than childhood-onset obesity. However, treatment of obesity in which significant components of compulsive eating or emotionally triggered food intake exist requires attention to these components, regardless of weight history.

The role of the physician in assisting patients with weight loss depends somewhat on the nature and extent of the underlying behavioral or psychological problems. Short-term dieting efforts, without changes in eating or activity patterns, not only are ineffective and frustrating in the long run but also may lead to increased weight for both physiologic and psychological reasons.

Table 45-1 Organic Causes of Obesity

Hypothyroidism
Destructive lesions of the ventromedial nucleus
Trauma
Encephalitis
Craniopharyngioma
Genetic conditions
von Gierke's disease
Laurence-Moon-Biedl syndrome
Cushing's syndrome
Hyperinsulin states
Medications
Corticosteroids
Antidepressants (amitriptyline)
Antipsychotics (chlorpromazine, haloperidol)
Antipruritics (cyproheptadine)

Diagnostic Approach

The three major diagnostic questions for the clinician working with the obese patient are as follows: Is there evidence for an underlying organic etiology for the obesity? Is there evidence for pathologic consequences of the obesity? To what extent are psychological factors involved in maintaining the obesity? Is the patient looking for a "quick fix," or does he or she understand the need to change underlying behavior patterns? What resources is the patient able or willing to commit to the problem?

Organic Causes of Obesity

Most organic causes of obesity offer clues that raise suspicions about the underlying etiology. Destructive lesions of the ventromedial nucleus from trauma, encephalitis, or craniopharyngiomas may stimulate the appetite, with resultant obesity. However, these lesions are usually apparent from neurologic or ophthalmologic signs. Occasionally, genetic syndromes are associated with obesity, but this is usually apparent from the family history and other characteristics of the syndrome. Von Gierke's disease, a glycogen storage disease appearing shortly after birth, and Laurence-Moon-Biedl syndrome, a rare recessive condition, are examples of genetic syndromes associated with obesity. Although endocrine pathology is an uncommon cause of obesity, it is the most common organic cause. A small percentage of obese patients are hypothyroid, whereas 60 percent of hypothyroid patients gain weight. Rarely, obesity occurs in a hyperthyroid patient whose appetite has been stimulated. Thyroid function screening tests should be performed in the obese patient if a careful history and physical examination suggest thyroid pathology (see Chapter 43, "Thyroid Function Testing").

A rare but distinctive cause of obesity is Cushing's syndrome, which is characterized by a central truncal obesity, moon facies, and cervical or supraclavicular fat deposits. The combination of obesity, hypertension, and diabetes should prompt consideration of Cushing's syndrome. Although a 24-hour urine sample for 17-hydroxycorticoids is a useful screening test for the obese patient, the 24-hour urine tests may be elevated simply on the basis of obesity. A dexamethasone suppression test has the best predictive value in the obese patient, but both the low-dose and high-dose suppression tests may be falsely abnormal in the obese patient.

Antidepressant medications (amitriptyline), antipsychotic agents (chlorpromazine, haloperidol), and other drugs (corticosteroids, cyproheptadine) have been associated with appetite stimulation and resultant obesity, sometimes becoming apparent months after treatment was begun. Fluoxetine, an antidepressant that inhibits serotonin uptake, shows some indication of decreasing appetite, leading to weight loss.

Complications of Obesity

Pathologic consequences of obesity are important when deciding on the priority for treatment. Mortality rates for obese patients more than 30 percent above normal weight are higher than for nonobese age- and sex-matched controls. This increase in mortality is largely due to the increased incidence of coronary artery and cerebrovascular disease noted in obese patients. Although obesity itself is an independent risk factor, it is also associated with higher incidences of diabetes, hypertension, and hyperlipidemia. Upper-body (abdominal) obesity is more highly associated with morbidity than is lower-body obesity. Other vascular sequelae of obesity include varicose veins and thromboembolic disease.

Blood-pressure readings may be falsely elevated in the obese patient when a standard sphygmomanometer cuff is used; therefore, blood-pressure measurements should be done with the large-size cuff if the width of the standard blood-pressure cuff is not greater than two-thirds of the arm's diameter or if the length of the inflatable section is not greater than two-thirds of the arm's circumference. A reduction in weight is frequently associated with a reduction in blood pressure.

Diabetes often complicates obesity because obesity is associated with insulin resistance, even in the presence of hyperinsulinemia. Approximately 80 percent of adult-onset diabetic patients are obese. Most of these obese diabetic patients will have their diabetes controlled by weight reduction because this improves the responsiveness of peripheral insulin receptors to endogenous insulin. Hyperlipidemia is also a common accompaniment of obesity. Total body cholesterol, cholesterol turnover, and hepatic production of very low density lipoprotein (VLDL) are increased in obesity. There may be an association between the increased removal of cholesterol from the biliary circulation and the increased incidence of cholelithiasis in obesity.

The markedly obese patient is prone to the hypersomnolence syndrome, with subsequent respiratory difficulty. Obesity may cause upper airway obstruction followed by episodes of hypoxemia, hypercapnia, and daytime somnolence. This sequence may result in inadequate nocturnal sleep, daytime fatigue, arrhythmias associated with the hypoxemia, or even polycythemia, pulmonary hypertension, and cor pulmonale. Weight reduction can reverse the hypersomnolence syndrome. Unfortunately, if the problem has been long-standing, as it frequently is, the resultant cardiac pathology may be irreversible.

Obesity alters at least three hormonal systems. The obese individual typically shows greater insulin production than the nonobese individual, but he or she also shows insulin resistance. The degree of insulin resistance correlates with the level of obesity. In contrast, the release of growth hormone with stimulation by hypoglycemia or exercise is reduced in the obese patient. The urinary 17-hydroxycorticoid levels may be high, as noted previously.

Degenerative joint disease is another common accompaniment of obesity because of long-standing stress on the weight-bearing joints. The joints most commonly affected are the hips and knees, often in a symmetric fashion. Table 45-2 summarizes the major sequelae of obesity.

Behavioral and Psychosocial Factors

The clinician dealing with the obese patient must evaluate the behavioral and psychosocial factors associated with the obese condition and explore with the patient whether weight reduction is realistic. If weight reduction is realistic, an individualized plan must be developed, even in those patients in whom a metabolic component contributes to the obesity.

The determination of whether the obesity is of juvenile onset or adult onset is a very important piece of history. The approach to the patient who has been obese since childhood is different from one directed at a patient who became obese as an adult. The physician should be cognizant of the need to refer these patients in order to provide help with the underlying problems that may have precipitated the weight gain. The individual who has been obese since childhood is likely to have a difficult time maintaining weight loss unless he or she makes a lifelong commitment to severe dietary restriction. Setting goals in increments of 10 to 15 percent of weight may help maintain motivation; even this limited weight loss may ameliorate some physical symptoms, such as high blood pressure or poor control of diabetes. Lifelong obesity may have become an important stable factor in the patient's life, so that changing it can be distressing. If this possibility is evident, a referral for psychological evaluation in conjunction with a weight-loss program may be indicated.

After understanding the history of the patient's weight problem, the next step is the determination of the patient's awareness of the effects of obesity on his or her health. If the patient lacks information about the possible consequences of obesity, such information can be provided. Enough time should be allowed for the patient to ask questions and assimilate the information. During this process, informing the patient about the value of weight reduction is important. The scientific evidence implicating obesity as a risk factor is not as strong as the evidence for other risk factors such as smoking and hypertension. As a result, patients sometimes have a more difficult time using health as a motivation for weight reduction and may benefit from assessment of other motivating factors for weight loss. Prevention of physical illness is not a common motivation for weight loss, although aesthetics and social circumstances often provide the necessary stimulus. The physician must be careful, however, not to impose on the patient cultural biases against the obese. The goal is to empower the patient toward change, not to humiliate and shame.

If the physician is to provide the primary intervention rather than referral, support, and follow-up, the next step is an adequate assessment of the patient's daily food intake and exercise program. Obese individuals often underestimate the amount of food they eat and are also unlikely to exercise to any extent. An accurate measurement of intake and output can be accomplished by having the patient keep records of eating and exercise behavior. Keeping these records also facilitates examination of the circumstances and feeling surrounding eating (Fig. 45-1). The amount of food eaten is recorded, as well as information about when, why, and how much the individual felt a need to eat.

Recording not only gives the patient and physician a more accurate picture of the behavior but also demands that the patient become more aware of it. This awareness facilitates change and helps in the development of a weight-reduction program. It is not unusual for a patient to lose weight once he or she begins using behavioral records. Patients can be asked to keep these records for a negotiated number of days in preparation for the next visit, which should be scheduled as a follow-up for obesity. Such a follow-up visit will also permit feedback on any tests that were done and collaboration between the patient and physician in developing a plan for weight reduction.

An assessment of whether the patient believes that he or she is capable of weight loss is necessary. If an individual does not believe that he or she can lose weight, there is little value in attempting the change. Many obese individuals, especially women, have tried many methods of weight loss and are familiar with the benefits and problems of available techniques. The physician can help the patient focus on what has occurred in the past, what the problems have been, and whether success is possible. Questions similar to those used for smokers (see Chapter 147, "Cigarette Smoking") can be used to assess the obese patient's beliefs and past experiences. This problem also lends itself to the approach described in Chapter 149, "Principles of Behavioral Change."

Table 45-2 Major Medical Sequelae of Obesity

Coronary artery disease*	Hypersomnolence syndrome*
Cerebrovascular disease*	Insulin resistance, hyperinsulinemia
Hypertension*	Increased urine 17-hydroxycorticoid
Thromboembolism*	Blunted growth hormone response
Varicose veins	Degenerative joint disease
Diabetes mellitus*	
Hyperlipidemia*	
Cholelithiasis	

* Associated with increased mortality.

Endocrinology

Name ______________________________ Date ____________

Time		Place	Need	Alone, or with whom	Associated activity	Food and amount	Mood/Reason
Start	End						

Need Rating:
1 = Extremely important (can't function without it)
2 = Important (would be difficult to do without it)
3 = Uncertain about importance (not sure if necessary)
4 = Not important (wouldn't miss it)

Figure 45-1 Sample record of food intake and associated activities.

Summary

The physician's diagnostic approach with obese patients requires an assessment of the possible organic causes, the pathologic consequences of the obesity, and the extent of psychological, social, and behavioral factors affecting the eating behavior. By understanding and determining each of the clinical concerns as well as being aware of the available weight-reduction methods and community resources, the physician is in a more favorable position to help the patient determine if weight reduction is feasible and, if it is realistic, which method would most likely be successful. The information that is gathered can also aid the physician in deciding whether he or she can intervene adequately or whether a referral for weight loss is indicated.

References

Bouchard C, Tremblay A, Depres J-P. The response to long-term overfeeding in identical twins. N Engl J Med 1990; 322:1477.

Bray GA. Obesity: Basic aspects and clinical applications. Med Clin North Am 1989; 73:1.

Brownell KD, Stunkard AJ. Exercise in the development and control of obesity. In: Stunkard AJ, ed. Obesity. Philadelphia: WB Saunders, 1980.

Hafen BQ. Overweight and obesity: Causes, fallacies, treatment. Provo, UT: Brigham Young University Press, 1975.

Health implications of obesity. Ann Intern Med 1985; 103:1073.

James WPT. Research on obesity. A report of the DHSS/MRC Group. London: Department of Health and Social Security Medical Research Council, 1976.

Stunkard AJ. Obesity. In: Cavenar JO Jr, et al, eds. Psychiatry. New York: Basic Books, 1987.

Belching

Gregory L. Eastwood, MD

Definition

Belching, burping, and eructation have roughly the same meaning and refer to the passage of gas from the stomach or esophagus through the mouth. In some patients, belching is the only symptom. In others, belching may be accompanied by abdominal discomfort, chest pain, or the passage of excess flatus. An approach to the evaluation is shown in Figure 46-1.

Etiology

All people normally belch from time to time. Because several milliliters of ambient air may accompany each normal swallow,

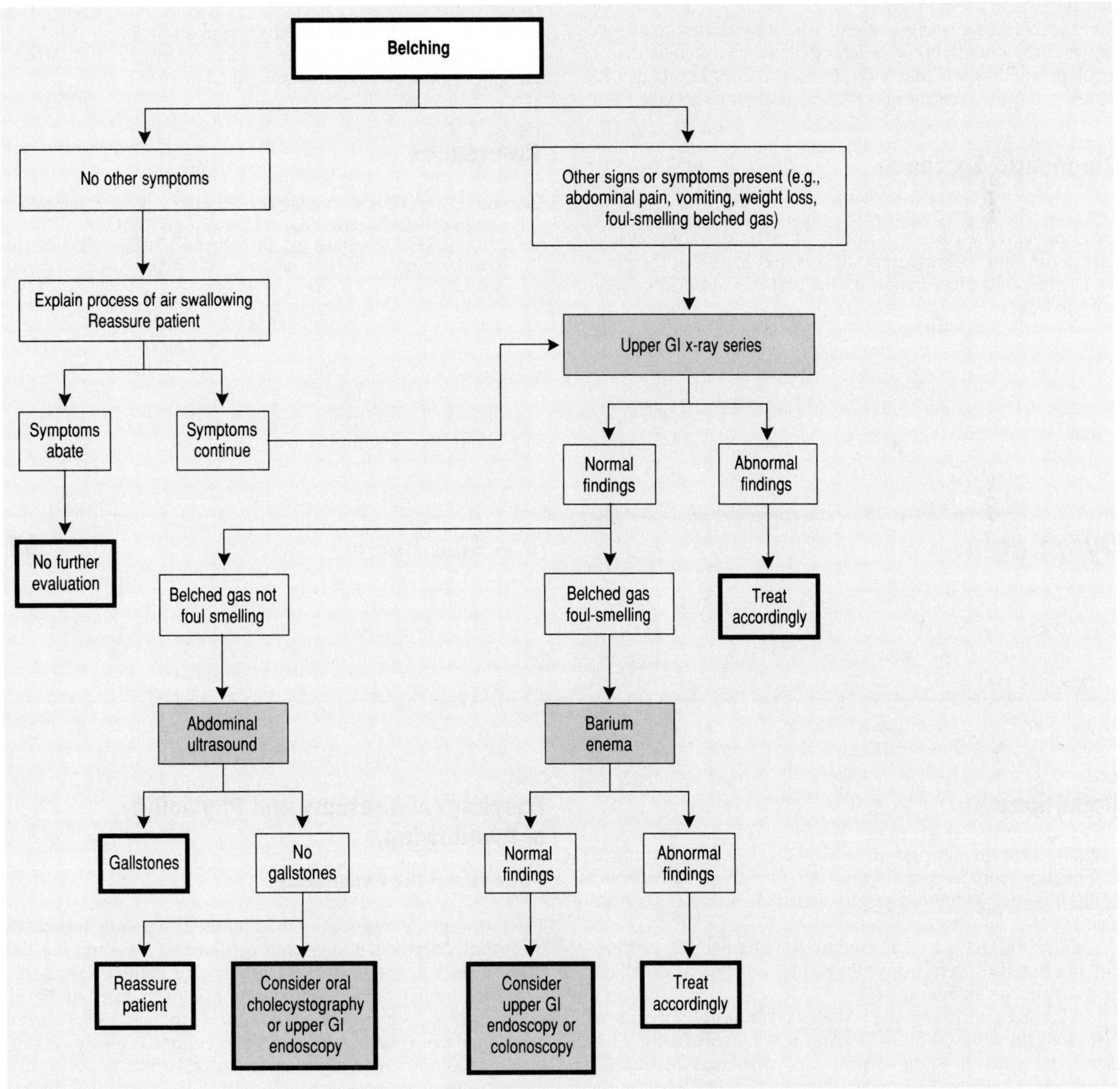

Figure 46-1 Algorithm for the evaluation of belching. GI = gastrointestinal.

air may accumulate in the stomach, particularly after a meal and when gum is chewed. Although much of the air passes into the intestines and contributes to normal flatus, some of the intragastric air may be belched. The belching of carbon dioxide and air after drinking carbonated beverages is also a universally recognized phenomenon.

Symptomatic belching usually is not associated with demonstrable organic disease. Most patients who complain of belching can be shown to swallow excess amounts of air. In fact, they may unwittingly take air into the esophagus before each belch that never reaches the stomach and that then is eructated. This practice may be associated with psychological stress or is thought by some patients to relieve other abdominal symptoms. Often a physician's explanation of the cause of belching and reassurance that there is no serious disease results in an improvement in symptoms or at least allows the patient to tolerate the belching.

Occasionally, belching is a sign of organic disease. If the gastric outlet is obstructed partially by peptic disease or carcinoma, swallowed air cannot pass into the bowel and patients may develop eructation. These patients also may have vomiting. For unexplained reasons, patients who have symptomatic gallstones may complain of belching. Finally, the belching of feculent-smelling gas may indicate a gastrocolic fistula that has developed from a carcinoma of the stomach or transverse colon.

Diagnostic Approach

The diagnosis of psychogenic belching is usually apparent after speaking with the patient. A history of carbonated-beverage ingestion or gum chewing may support the diagnosis. If patients do not respond to alteration in diet and reassurance, or if another sign or symptom is present in addition to belching, such as abdominal pain, vomiting, or weight loss, a search for organic disease should be carried out.

Upper gastrointestinal (GI) x-ray series or upper GI endoscopy will evaluate the stomach for partial outlet obstruction and rarely may indicate a gastrocolic fistula complicating a gastric carcinoma. In general, because gastric outlet obstruction or a gastric carcinoma that is large enough to erode into the colon is likely to be diagnosed by the upper GI x-ray series, that study would be the appropriate first step in the diagnostic evaluation of belching. However, some patients with peptic disease who do not have a discrete ulcer may complain of belching. In these patients, if the upper GI x-ray series is nondiagnostic, an upper GI endoscopy may be required in order to make the diagnosis. If the patient belches foul-smelling gas and the question of a gastrocolic fistula remains after a nondiagnostic upper GI x-ray series, a barium enema should be performed.

The diagnosis of gallstones can be made either by ultrasonography of the upper abdomen or by oral cholecystography. The ultrasound study is more convenient for the patient, costs roughly the same as oral cholecystography, and is said to be more accurate. However, if the clinical suspicion of gallstones remains high after the negative ultrasound examination, an oral cholecystogram should be obtained.

References

Eastwood GL, Avunduk C. Intestinal gas. In: Manual of gastroenterology: Diagnosis and therapy. Boston: Little, Brown, 1988:177.

Levitt MD, Bond JH. Intestinal gas. In: Sleisenger MH, Fordtran JS, eds. Gastrointestinal disease. 4th ed. Philadelphia: WB Saunders, 1989:257.

Dysphagia

Canan Avunduk, MD, PhD

47

Definitions

Dysphagia means difficulty in swallowing. It refers clinically to the inability to initiate swallowing or to the sensation that solids or liquids stick in the esophagus after a swallow has been initiated.

Odynophagia is a term used to describe pain on swallowing. In some disorders, odynophagia may accompany dysphagia or it may occur independently.

Globus hystericus is the sensation of a lump in the throat that is usually relieved by swallowing. It is a manifestation of an emotional state. It is the converse of dysphagia in that the symptoms are relieved momentarily by swallowing, whereas the symptoms of dysphagia are brought on by swallowing.

Esophageal Anatomy and Physiology of Swallowing

Structure of the Esophagus

The esophagus is a muscular tube about 25 cm long. It extends from the pharynx at the cricoid cartilage to the cardia of the stomach after it passes through the left crus of the diaphragm.

The luminal surface of the esophagus is lined by stratified, nonkeratinized squamous epithelium. At the gastroesophageal junction, there is an abrupt change to columnar glandular mucosa. The submucosa contains an extensive lymphatic plexus in a loose connective-tissue network, which accounts for the early and extensive submucosal spread of esophageal cancer. The muscle layer of the esophagus consists of an inner circular and an outer longitudinal coat. The musculature of the pharynx, upper esophageal sphincter, and upper one-third of the esophagus is striated. Striated and smooth muscle intermingle below the upper third until the muscle coat becomes entirely smooth muscle in the lower half of the esophagus. In between the muscle layers is a myenteric plexus of nerves.

Before the esophagus joins the stomach, the smooth muscle is specialized for a distance of 2 to 4 cm in the distal esophagus to form a zone of increased resting pressure. This area is called the lower esophageal sphincter (LES). The LES is both physiologically and pharmacologically distinct from the esophageal smooth muscle immediately adjacent to it. Basal LES pressure is normally 10 to 25 mm Hg higher than intragastric pressure and drops promptly with swallowing. The control of the LES remains poorly understood, but it is thought to involve the complex interaction of neural, hormonal, and myogenic activities.

Physiology of Swallowing

The function of the esophagus is to transport food and secretions from the mouth to the stomach. This coordinated process delivers a liquid or solid bolus to the stomach irrespective of the force of gravity.

Swallowing begins as a bolus is propelled to the back of the mouth by the tongue into the pharynx. The upper esophageal sphincter (UES, the cricopharyngeus muscle), which is just below the pharynx, relaxes, allowing the bolus to pass into the upper esophagus. Next, a primary peristaltic contraction propels the bolus down the esophagus. Secondary peristaltic contractions are initiated when the esophagus is distended by the bolus. When the food reaches the mid to lower esophagus, the LES relaxes to allow the passage of the bolus into the stomach.

The relaxation of the UES and peristalsis in the upper esophagus are initiated by the voluntary act of swallowing, which is controlled by the swallowing center in the brain stem through cranial nerves V, VII, IX, X, XI, and XII. These nerves coordinate movements of the bolus to the hypopharynx, closure of the epiglottis, relaxation of the UES, and contraction of the striated muscle in the upper esophagus. The sequential nature of this function is due to progressive activation of nerve fibers carried in the vagi through a central mechanism. However, the peristalsis in the smooth muscle portion of the esophagus is regulated by activation of adjacent neurons located within the muscle coats in the myenteric plexus by cholinergic nerves. The vagi innervate the upper esophagus in its striated muscle portion only. If the vagi are cut below this level, peristalsis in the lower half of the esophagus and the function of the LES remain intact.

Etiology and Pathophysiology

Dysphagia may be divided into two categories: pre-esophageal (or oropharyngeal) and esophageal dysphagia.

Pre-esophageal Dysphagia

Patients who have pre-esophageal dysphagia have problems with the initial steps of swallowing. They may have difficulty in propelling food to the hypopharynx, or once the food is in the hypopharynx, pain, a mass lesion, or a neuromuscular disorder may interfere with the orderly sequence of pharyngeal contraction, closure of the epiglottis, UES relaxation, and initiation of peristalsis by contraction of the striated muscle in the upper esophagus. These patients cough, sputter, expel ingested material through the mouth and nose, or aspirate when they attempt to swallow. Pre-esophageal dysphagia results from either a neural defect caused by cerebral vascular disease, bulbar or pseudobulbar palsy, and other central nervous system disorders or diseases affecting the striated muscle, including myasthenia gravis, poliomyelitis, muscular dystrophy, dermatomyositis, and amyloidosis. Mucosal lesions of the pharynx, such as pharyngitis, candidiasis, and herpetic esophagitis, may also cause pharyngeal dysphagia associated with pain on swallowing. Space-occupying lesions that may obstruct the oropharynx, hypopharynx, or upper esophagus, e.g., tumor, abscess, or a Zenker's diverticulum, must also be included in the differential diagnosis.

Esophageal Dysphagia

Esophageal dysphagia is produced by defective transport of the bolus within the esophagus and is usually described by the patient as food sticking behind the sternum. It occurs when there is a lesion in the body of the esophagus, the LES, or the esophagogastric junction. The causes of esophageal dysphagia may be divided into structural disorders resulting in mechanical obstruction and motility disorders arising from neuromuscular defects affecting the esophageal motor function.

Patients who have diseases affecting the striated muscle usually also have pre-esophageal dysphagia. On the other hand, diseases that affect smooth muscle involve the mid and lower esophagus and the LES.

A structural disorder is usually a discrete lesion, such as a neoplasm, a stricture, or an extrinsic compression, that interferes with the passage of the swallowed bolus. Motility disorders alter the esophageal motor function and cause dysphagia or odynophagia because peristalsis is absent or inadequate, contractions are uncoordinated or too forceful, or the LES fails to relax adequately or is incompetent, allowing reflux of gastric contents.

Clinically, the diagnosis of a motility disorder versus a structural disorder often can be made on the basis of history alone. If the patient recalls that the difficulty of swallowing initially occurred while ingesting both solids and liquids, a motility disorder is suggested. However, if the patient has experienced progressive dysphagia, initially with solids, later with liquids, the disorder is most likely a structural one.

Infections, e.g., with *Candida* or herpesvirus, or esophageal inflammation resulting from radiation therapy of the thorax may also cause dysphagia, but in such cases, dysphagia is also accompanied by odynophagia.

Primary Motility Disorders

Achalasia. Achalasia is a disorder of the smooth muscle portion of the esophagus, resulting from either a lack of or a dysfunction in the postganglionic parasympathetic neurons in the myenteric plexus. It is characterized by two major motility defects: a loss or disorder of peristalsis in the lower two-thirds of the esophagus and abnormal LES function. The resting pressure of the LES is either elevated or normal, but characteristically, it fails to relax completely with swallowing. The consequence of poor peristalsis and inability of the LES to relax is that food and secretions build up in the body of the esophagus and pass through the LES only when the hydrostatic pressure exceeds the LES tone. This results in dilatation of the esophagus and regurgitation and aspiration of esophageal contents, which may lead to aspiration pneumonitis or pulmonary abscess formation (Fig. 47-1).

Achalasia is usually idiopathic. It affects all age groups but is more common in middle age. An achalasia-like syndrome has been described in association with malignancy in the gastroesophageal region or elsewhere, e.g., oat cell carcinoma of the lung and pancreatic carcinoma.

Esophageal Spasm. The disorder of esophageal motility classified under diffuse esophageal spasm (DES) constitutes a hetero-

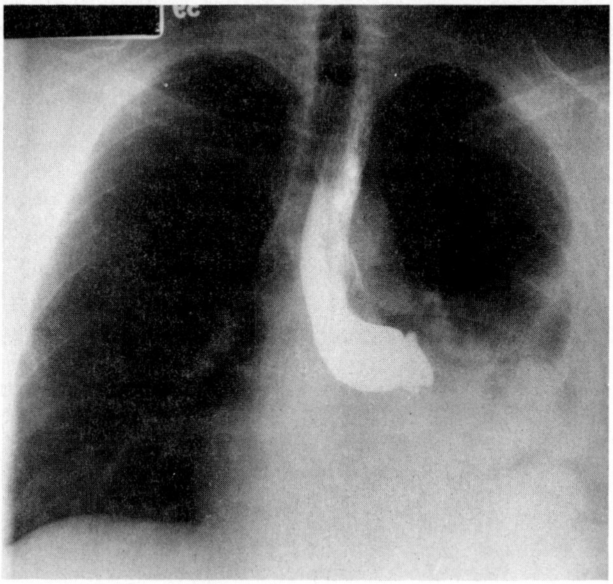

Figure 47-1 Chest radiograph of a patient with achalasia, demonstrating the dilated esophagus with its characteristic beak-like distal portion.

geneous group. These patients have various degrees of excessive motility in the body of the esophagus. The motility pattern may include repetitive contraction waves (more than two peaks), simultaneous (nonperistaltic) contractions, contractions with long duration (longer than 5 seconds), and high-amplitude waves (above 120 mm Hg) intermixed with normal peristalsis. In up to one-third of these patients, the resting pressure of the LES is elevated and may not completely relax with swallowing.

Dysphagia is intermittent. It occurs with both liquids and solids. Sometimes it is exacerbated with hot or cold foods, and it may cause chest pain. In fact, the chest pain of DES is often confused with chest pain of cardiac origin because it also may be relieved with smooth muscle relaxants, such as nitroglycerin and calcium-channel blocking agents given for angina pectoris.

Achalasia and DES may represent two extremes in a spectrum of primary esophageal motility disorders. There are patients who may present initially with symptoms of DES and progress to achalasia over time. Some patients may have only a "hypertensive LES," with normal peristalsis in the body of the esophagus. Others may have "nutcracker esophagus," with high-amplitude peristaltic contractions. In "vigorous achalasia" relaxation of the LES is incomplete, and patients also have simultaneous contractions in the lower esophagus. Dysphagia in all such patients typically is to both liquids and solids and is usually accompanied by chest pain.

Secondary Motility Disorders

Some systemic disorders that affect multiple organs in the human body also cause esophageal dysfunction that may present as dysphagia. These include connective tissue diseases, especially progressive systemic sclerosis (scleroderma), diabetes mellitus, Chagas' disease, and chronic idiopathic intestinal obstruction.

In scleroderma patients with esophageal involvement, there is atrophy of the smooth muscle of the esophagus and replacement by collagen. This leads to decreased LES pressure and weak contractions in the smooth muscle portion of the esophagus, resulting in defective peristalsis and poor esophageal clearing. These patients are particularly at risk of developing esophagitis and peptic strictures of the esophagus. Thus, they often complain of heartburn and dysphagia; the latter may be on the basis of the motility disorder as well as stricture formation.

Diabetes mellitus and chronic alcohol consumption, which may cause neuropathy, often affect esophageal motor function. Most commonly, there is a decrease in the force of peristalsis. Sometimes the motility abnormality may resemble diffuse esophageal spasm.

Nonspecific motility abnormalities are seen frequently with aging. The amplitude of esophageal contractions may be decreased, leading to less effective peristalsis. However, these patients are rarely symptomatic unless some other motor abnormality is present in addition to age.

In certain areas of the world, Chagas' disease, caused by infection with *Trypanosoma cruzi,* results in destruction of the myenteric plexus in many portions of the gastrointestinal tract. This leads to such disorders as megacolon and esophageal motility defects resembling achalasia. It differs from idiopathic achalasia in that the esophagus is never the only organ involved.

Some patients with idiopathic intestinal pseudo-obstruction may also have abnormal esophageal peristalsis.

Structural Disorders

Structural disorders produce dysphagia by causing mechanical obstruction to the passage of food. Initially, dysphagia is noted when solids are ingested. Later, as the esophageal lumen narrows, ingestion of liquids may also become difficult.

Tumors. Squamous carcinoma accounts for 95 percent or more of esophageal cancers. Excessive alcohol intake and cigarette smoking seem to increase the risk. Other predisposing factors include head and neck cancer, Plummer-Vinson syndrome (anemia and esophageal web), tylosis, achalasia, and lye stricture.

Adenocarcinomas of the esophagus constitute 1 to 5 percent of esophageal cancers and are thought to arise from extension of gastric carcinoma; from malignant transformation of esophageal glands that lie beneath the squamous epithelium of the esophagus; or from the columnar metaplasia of the squamous epithelium (Barrett's epithelium), which is associated with chronic gastroesophageal reflux.

The rich submucosal lymphatic network allows early spread of esophageal carcinoma within and outside of the esophagus. Mediastinal extension of the tumor is also facilitated by the lack of serosal covering of the esophagus. The 5-year survival rate for esophageal carcinoma unfortunately remains below 5 percent.

Benign tumors of the esophagus are rare and account for less than 10 percent of esophageal tumors. Leiomyomas that arise from within the wall of the esophagus are the most common. These tumors are covered by normal squamous epithelium of the esophagus and protrude into the esophageal lumen. Fibroadenomas may become very long and may cause obstruction.

Strictures. Most benign esophageal strictures are found in the distal or mid esophagus. They are the result of chronic inflammation caused by chronic reflux into the esophagus of stomach and duodenal contents, e.g., acid, pepsin, and bile. Strictures associated with Barrett's epithelium may harbor malignancy.

Esophageal burns caused by ingestion of corrosive substances, e.g., strong alkali and acids, may result in esophageal stricture in one or more locations of the esophagus.

Rings and Webs. These are usually thin, circumferential mucosal shelves that protrude into the esophageal lumen and cause intermittent dysphagia, especially with large pieces of food, such as poorly chewed meat. Webs occur in the upper and mid esophagus, and rings most often are found at the esophagogastric junction. The latter are also called Schatzki's rings. Rarely, a more substantial ring, which is due to thickened esophageal muscle, may occur just above the esophagogastric junction. The pathogenesis of these lesions is unknown.

Extrinsic Compression. The esophageal lumen may be narrowed from compression by an external lesion. These lesions include primary or metastatic mediastinal tumors, aberrant subclavian artery, and enlargement of the aortic arch or cardiac chambers, especially the left atrium.

Esophageal diverticula are common and may cause dysphagia by externally compressing the esophageal lumen when they become large and distended with food and secretions. Zenker's diverticulum is the most common and originates just above the UES from the posterior hypopharyngeal wall. Mid-esophageal diverticula are called traction diverticula. They are thought to be caused by hilar or mediastinal scarring and traction of the esophageal wall. Epiphrenic diverticula are found in the lower esophagus. Most of these diverticula are associated with some esophageal motor abnormality.

Gastroesophageal Reflux

The reflux of gastric or duodenal contents into the esophagus may cause patients to experience heartburn after eating and on recumbency. Esophagitis caused by gastroesophageal reflux of acid, pepsin, and bile may cause dysphagia in some patients, especially if they develop esophageal ulceration or stricture.

Diagnostic Approach

An algorithm that outlines the evaluation of dysphagia is shown in Figure 47-2.

History

Differentiation of the major causes of dysphagia can be facilitated by eliciting the history on three critical points: (1) the type of food causing dysphagia (solids or liquids), (2) the presence of intermittent or progressive symptoms, and (3) the presence or absence of heartburn.

As mentioned before, a motility disorder usually causes dysphagia to both solids and liquids from the onset of symptoms, whereas a structural disorder causes dysphagia to solids first, then semisolids, and finally, liquids.

The duration and constancy of the symptoms are also diagnostically pertinent. Intermittent dysphagia for solid food only is typical of a lower esophageal (Schatzki's) ring. A patient with a long history of heartburn may notice the disappearance of his or her symptoms of heartburn when a stricture develops. The stricture may prevent clinically significant reflux but may now cause dysphagia, especially to solids. The patient with esophageal cancer typically has a more accelerated course of dysphagia over several months.

The history of neurologic, muscular, connective tissue, or systemic disorders and the use of certain drugs that may affect the esophageal function should also be obtained from the patient.

Physical Examination

The physical examination is helpful only in the diagnosis of secondary dysphagia, i.e., dysphagia due to other systemic disorders, as mentioned previously. Demonstration of the presence of a mass in the neck, a deviated trachea, or an epigastric mass may also be helpful.

Diagnostic Tests

Chest Radiograph

The chest radiograph may be helpful indirectly in the diagnosis of dysphagia. In advanced achalasia with dilatation of the esophagus, a widened mediastinal shadow with an air-fluid level consisting of food and secretions may be apparent. Mediastinal masses or cardiomegaly with chamber enlargement as a cause of extrinsic compression on the esophagus may also be evident on the chest radiograph.

Barium Swallow and Upper Gastrointestinal Series

This is usually the first diagnostic study in the evaluation of dysphagia. The patient is asked to swallow liquid barium, and the movement of the barium bolus is observed by the radiologist fluoroscopically and recorded on the x-ray film or videotape. In this manner, the course of the bolus is followed from the mouth to the stomach, providing information about pre-esophageal swallowing function, the nature of the peristaltic activity, the presence of gastroesophageal reflux, and the anatomy of the esophagus with respect to structural disorders such as carcinoma, stricture, esophageal ring, and extrinsic compression.

The barium study is less helpful in the diagnosis of motility disorders than of structural disorders. In achalasia, however, one may see a dilated esophagus with a "parrot-beak" narrowing at the esophagogastric junction (see Fig. 47-1). Tertiary or corkscrew contractions may suggest the diagnosis of diffuse esophageal spasm. However, this may be a normal finding, especially in elderly patients.

Esophageal Manometry

Esophageal manometry records intraesophageal pressures and peristaltic activity after wet and dry swallows. It is useful in the diagnosis of motility disorders and gives some information about the activity and pressure of the LES and the UES.

The typical manometry tube is a thin, soft, flexible tube that has three recording sensors arranged linearly in a spiral fashion 5 cm apart from one another at the distal end. The patient is asked to swallow the tube, which is advanced into the stomach and then slowly pulled upward. Initially, all three sensors pass sequentially through the lower esophageal sphincter and measure its pressure. In the body of the esophagus, peristaltic contractions are recorded in a sequential manner as they pass down the esophagus, first with the proximal sensor, next with the middle, and last with the distal. If peristalsis is progressive, normal function is observed. However, if the contractions occur simultaneously or are repetitive, of abnormally high amplitude, or absent, an esophageal motor abnormality may be present. When the middle or distal sensor lies within the LES, the relationship between esophageal peristaltic contractions and sphincter relaxation can be observed. Similarly, when the upper sensor is in the pharynx and the middle one lies in the UES, the relationship between pharyngeal contractions and upper sphincter relaxation can be recorded.

Upper Gastrointestinal Endoscopy

The flexible fiberoptic panendoscopes allow direct visual examination of the esophagus, stomach, and proximal duodenum. The patient is asked to swallow the endoscopic tube after proper local anesthesia of the pharynx and general sedation. The endoscope is advanced gradually, and the esophageal, gastric, and duodenal mucosae are examined carefully. Endoscopic biopsy and cytologic specimens may be obtained if lesions are observed or suspected.

Upper gastrointestinal endoscopy is helpful in evaluating patients with structural as well as inflammatory disorders. It can also help in the diagnosis of gastroduodenal disorders such as peptic ulcer disease, which may coexist with or give symptoms that may be confused with esophageal disorders.

Tests Useful in Diagnosis of Gastroesophageal Reflux

Prolonged monitoring of the pH of the lower esophagus over 12 to 24 hours in an ambulatory setting gives the clinician an accurate assessment of the frequency, duration, and severity of the gastroesophageal acid reflux and its relationship to the patient's symptoms.

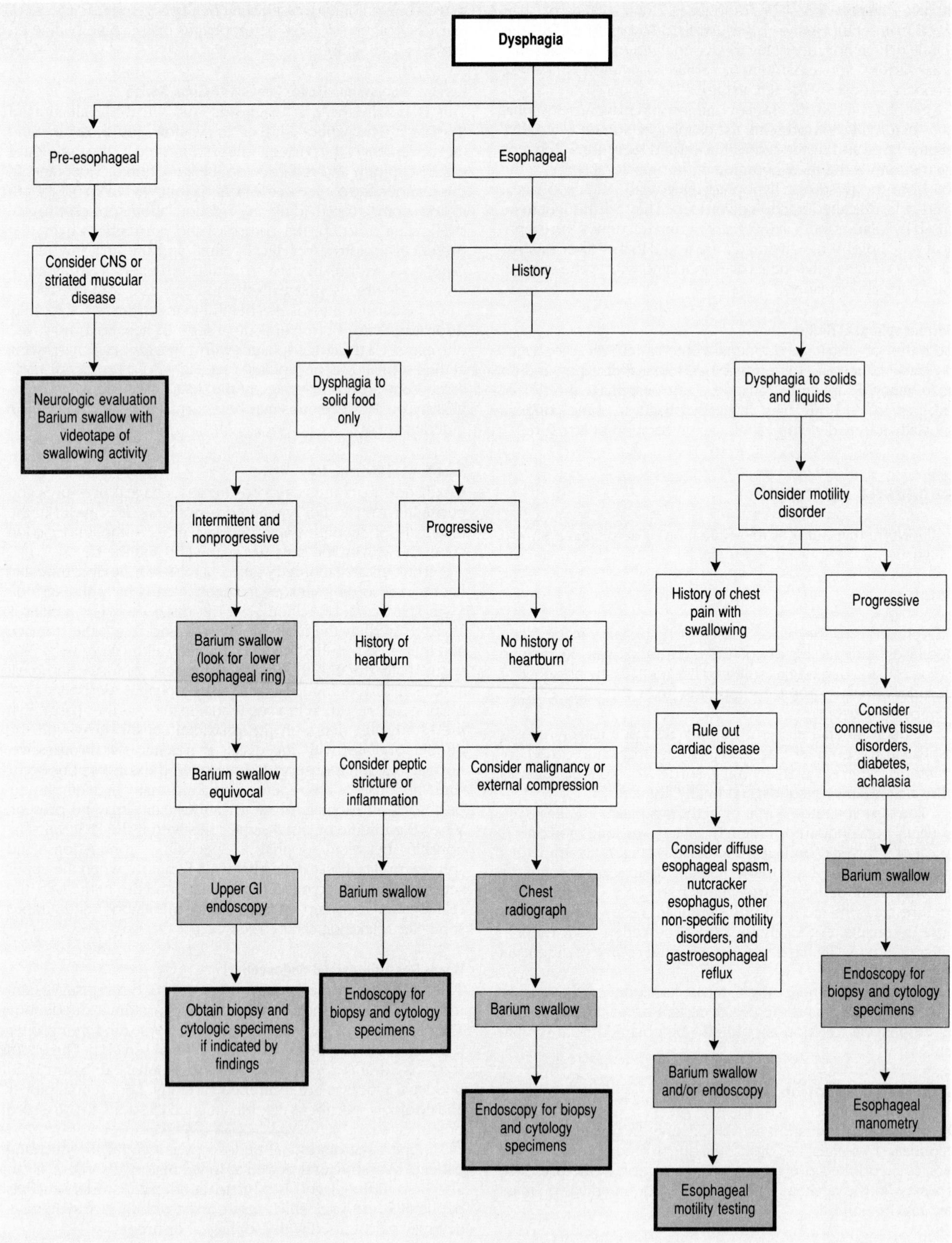

Figure 47-2 Algorithm for the evaluation of dysphagia. CNS = central nervous system, GI = gastrointestinal.

The Bernstein (acid perfusion) test is performed while the patient sits upright with a nasogastric tube passed to the mid esophagus. Normal saline and 0.1 N hydrogen chloride are infused alternately for 15 minutes to detect whether the patient's symptoms of heartburn or chest pain can be reproduced with acid infusion. The test is considered positive when the patient's symptoms are reproduced twice and relieved with normal saline infusion. A negative test does not rule out gastroesophageal reflux disease or esophagitis.

References

Avunduk C, Eastwood GL. Dysphagia. In: Manual of gastroenterology: Diagnosis and therapy. Boston: Little, Brown, 1988.

Burns TW. Motor disorders of the esophagus: Diagnosis and treatment. South Med J 1984; 77:956.

Castell DO. Esophageal motility disorders: The specter of the spectrum. Dig Dis Sci 1985; 30:2.

Pope CE II. Heartburn, dysphagia, and other esophageal symptoms. In: Sleisenger MH, Fordtran JS, eds. Gastrointestinal disease. 4th ed. Philadelphia: WB Saunders, 1989:200.

Richter JE, et al. Nutcracker esophagus. Dig Dis Sci 1985; 30:188.

Tucker HJ, Snape WJ Jr, Cohen S. Achalasia secondary to carcinoma: Manometric and clinical features. Ann Intern Med 1978; 89:315.

Van Trappen G, et al. Achalasia, diffuse esophageal spasm, and related motility disorders. Gastroenterology 1979; 76:450.

Heartburn, Peptic Symptoms, and Indigestion

Gregory L. Eastwood, MD

48

Definition

Patients use a number of terms to describe various symptoms that are thought to arise from the upper gastrointestinal tract. An understanding of the relationship between the patient's vocabulary and medical terminology will allow us to categorize better our patients' symptoms.

Heartburn is what patients say they feel when irritating gastric substances reflux into the esophagus. Patients with gastroesophageal reflux typically complain of substernal burning pain after meals or upon recumbency. Often the pain awakens the patient from sleep. A nocturnal cough suggests that the patient is aspirating refluxed material into the upper airways or the lungs. The substernal burning sensation may radiate to the neck, back, or arms, often making it difficult to distinguish the pain of reflux from the pain of cardiac origin. In some patients the gastric contents may actually reflux up into the mouth, creating a sour or bitter taste, or may stimulate the overflow of copious amounts of salivary secretions, which is called water brash. A history describing the effect that position has on symptoms is helpful; some patients have to expectorate refluxed material when they stoop over in the garden or to tie their shoes.

Peptic ulcer disease may cause pain that is described by patients as burning or boring, usually in the epigastrium, sometimes radiating to the back. The pain typically occurs on an empty stomach and thus is evident before meals and several hours after meals. It may awaken the patient from sleep in the early morning hours. The pain will be relieved temporarily by food or antacids. Peptic disease encompasses a spectrum of signs and symptoms. Some patients have the typical symptoms of peptic ulcer and, on diagnostic evaluation, indeed are found to have an ulcer. Other patients have severe symptoms, but instead of an ulcer, inflammation of the stomach (gastritis) or duodenum (duodenitis) or no lesion at all is found. Still other patients have a discrete ulcer that is asymptomatic. The term *peptic ulcer* refers to the injury resulting from the action of acid, pepsin, and other irritants on the mucosa of the esophagus, stomach, duodenum, or jejunum to form an ulcer. However, because a discrete ulcer is not necessary for patients to have symptoms, a better term may be *peptic disease*.

Patients vary in what they mean by indigestion. *Indigestion* is a word patients often use to describe a vague postprandial abdominal discomfort, a transient stomach ache, or many other symptoms associated with eating. Some patients interpret the pain of gastroesophageal reflux, peptic disease, gallbladder disease, or pancreatitis as indigestion.

Etiology

Heartburn

Heartburn results from the action of irritating substances on the mucosa of the lower esophagus. The majority of irritating substances reflux from the stomach and thus may include not only hydrochloric acid, pepsin, and food but also bile, pancreatic juice, and other duodenal contents that have refluxed from the duodenum into the stomach. Some irritating substances, such as citrus juices, are ingested and cause symptoms when they come into contact with an inflamed esophagus.

In normal individuals, two factors are important in the prevention of gastroesophageal reflux symptoms. First, a competent lower esophageal sphincter (LES), which is located at the esophagogastric junction, lessens the likelihood of reflux of gastric contents into the esophagus. Second, clearing of the lower esophagus by primary and secondary peristalsis and clearance of any material that is refluxed decreases the chance of mucosal injury. If a patient develops an incompetent LES, inadequate esophageal clearing of the refluxed material, or both, symptoms of gastroesophageal reflux may occur.

Gastroesophageal reflux is usually idiopathic. Certain substances are known to decrease the pressure of the LES and thus contribute to the development of symptoms in susceptible individuals (Table 48-1). These substances should be avoided by patients with gastroesophageal reflux. In a minority of patients, an intrinsic muscle disorder is responsible for a weakened LES and hypoperistalsis of the lower esophagus. Such a muscle dis-

Table 48-1 Substances That Weaken the Lower Esophageal Sphincter

Fatty meat	Chocolate
Smoking	Theophylline-containing medications
Alcoholic beverages	Anticholinergic medications

order may be associated with scleroderma (progressive systemic sclerosis), other connective tissue disorders, Raynaud's disease, or diabetes mellitus.

For many years, a hiatal hernia was held responsible for the symptoms of gastroesophageal reflux, simply because a hiatal hernia is a protrusion of the upper portion of the stomach through the diaphragmatic hiatus into the chest. Hiatal hernia probably is not a primary cause of gastroesophageal reflux, but it may contribute to reflux symptoms in susceptible individuals by providing a reservoir at the esophagogastric junction for material that can be readily refluxed into the esophagus. When hiatal hernias themselves are symptomatic, the symptoms are not usually those of gastroesophageal reflux; rather, they are due to torsion of a large hernia or distention of the hernia sac by food and secretions.

Peptic Disease

Peptic disease occurs as a result of the injurious action of acid and pepsin on the mucosa of the upper gastrointestinal tract. Because pepsin is active only at pH 1 to 4, neutralization of acid or inhibition of acid production eliminates the harmful effects of pepsin. A number of agents damage the gastric or duodenal mucosa directly and thus augment the injurious effects of acid and pepsin. These agents include aspirin, ethanol, most nonsteroidal anti-inflammatory drugs, and bile acids. Corticosteroids also appear to predispose to ulcer formation, although they do not damage the mucosa directly. Some evidence indicates that corticosteroids inhibit the process of epithelial renewal, which could lead to ulcer formation because of a failure to heal existing lesions.

In the absence of exposure to one of the "ulcerogens" just indicated, it is not understood why certain individuals develop peptic disease and others do not. Environmental influences may play a role. For example, before 1850, duodenal ulcer was a rare occurrence. By 1900, numerous reports of duodenal ulcer had appeared. The incidence of the disease peaked about 1960 in Western society and has declined subsequently. These observations raise the possibility that dietary factors, psychological stress, or other accompaniments of progressive civilization may predispose to ulcer formation. Why the incidence of duodenal ulcer has decreased recently remains unknown.

In rare patients, peptic disease is due to abnormally high serum levels of the acid secretory hormone gastrin. Hypergastrinemia in association with acid hypersecretion occurs in the Zollinger-Ellison syndrome (gastrinoma), antral G-cell hyperplasia (increased numbers of gastrin-producing cells in the antrum of the stomach), the retained antrum syndrome, and gastric outlet obstruction. Hypergastrinemic conditions should be considered when a patient has peptic disease that is refractory to conventional medical or surgical treatment. However, the retained antrum syndrome is a consideration only if the patient has undergone antrectomy and gastrojejunostomy (Billroth II). This condition is a rare consequence of Billroth II surgery in which a small amount of gastrin-containing antral mucosa is retained

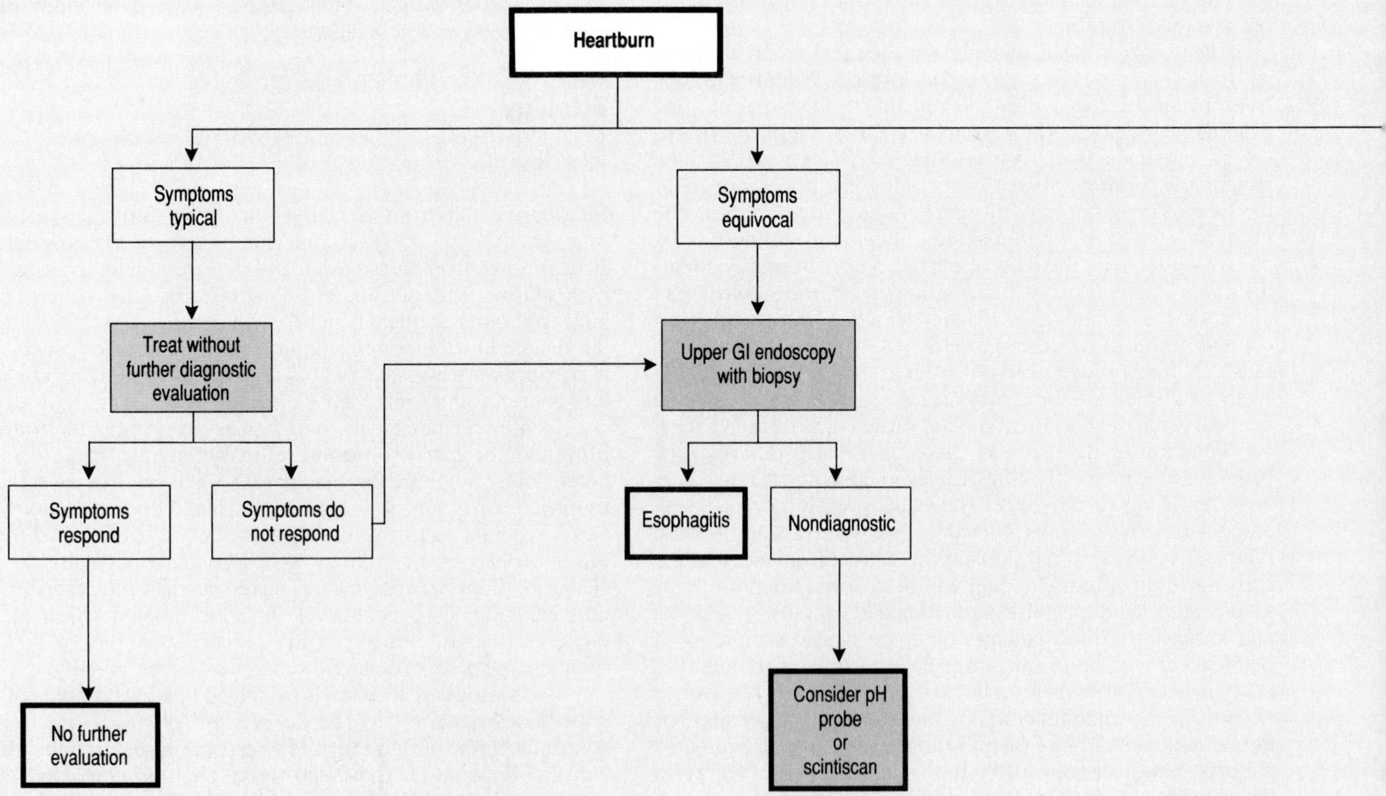

Figure 48-1 Algorithm for the evaluation of heartburn. GI = gastrointestinal.

Table 48-2 Differential Diagnosis of Indigestion

Peptic disease	Malabsorptive diseases
Gastroesophageal reflux	Irritable bowel syndrome
Esophagitis	Motility disorders
Gallbladder disease	Inflammatory bowel disease
Pancreatitis	Abdominal angina

inadvertently in the proximal duodenal cuff and continues to secrete large amounts of gastrin.

Indigestion

Symptoms attributed to indigestion are usually caused by gastroesophageal reflux or peptic disease. However, many other disorders may also cause abdominal discomfort after eating. The differential diagnosis of indigestion is listed in Table 48-2.

Diagnostic Approach

Heartburn

If a patient complains of postprandial or nocturnal heartburn, no further diagnostic evaluation usually is necessary before initiating therapy with antacids or histamine-2 antagonists. However, patients with heartburn who do not respond to treatment, who freely regurgitate gastric material, or who experience dysphagia should undergo diagnostic testing. Also, patients with chest discomfort in whom the clinical diagnosis of gastroesophageal reflux is not clear may require studies to establish the diagnosis of reflux or an alternative cause of their symptoms.

A description of some of the diagnostic tests that may be considered in the further evaluation of a patient with heartburn follows. An algorithm that outlines the use of the tests appears in Figure 48-1.

An upper gastrointestinal (GI) radiographic series is of little use in making the diagnosis of gastroesophageal reflux. Many normal people will be seen to reflux variable amounts of barium from the stomach into the esophagus. If large amounts of barium reflux to the upper esophagus or pharynx under x-ray examination, the clinical diagnosis of gastroesophageal reflux usually has already been made in those patients without the aid of x-ray studies. If dysphagia is present, however, barium contrast studies may be useful in identifying the cause. Benign strictures that are secondary to chronic reflux, malignant neoplasms, and benign rings of the lower esophagus may be identified radiographically.

Upper GI endoscopy is diagnostically superior to barium contrast studies. By means of flexible fiberoptic endoscopes, which are well tolerated by most patients, the mucosa of the esophagus can be inspected directly and, if necessary, small biopsy specimens can be taken. The diagnosis of esophagitis can be made when biopsies show the typical signs of inflammation, such as edema or infiltration with neutrophils and lymphocytes. However, there is poor correlation between reflux symptoms, the endoscopic appearance of mucosal inflammation, and the histologic signs of esophagitis. Frequently, mucosal biopsy samples of the lower esophagus from symptomatic patients do not contain inflammatory cells or edema.

Three histologic findings do appear to correlate well with symptomatic reflux in the absence of mucosal inflammation. First, the basal cell layer of the epithelium increases in reflux

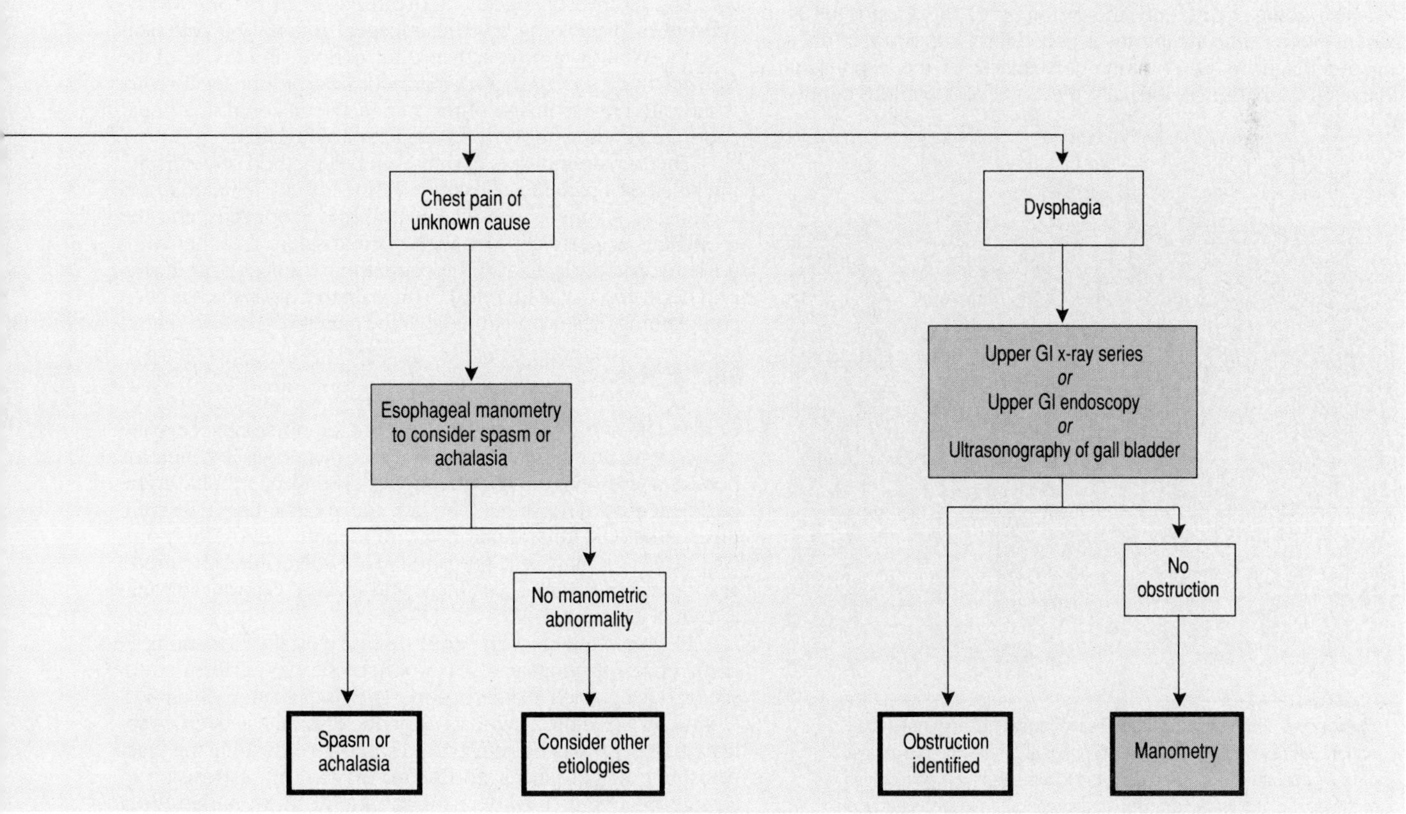

Figure 48-1 *Continued*

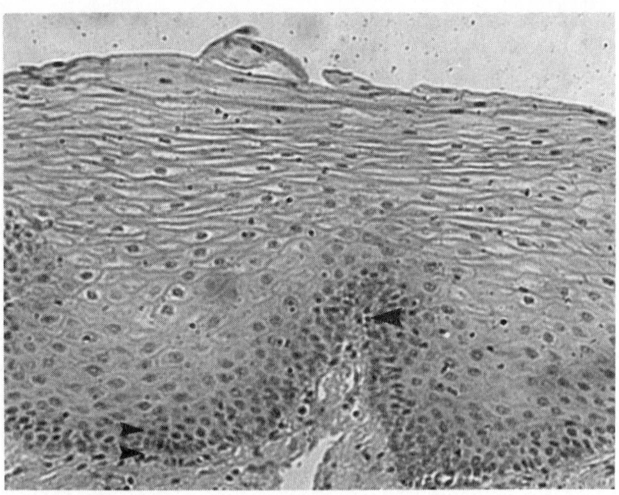

Figure 48-2 Photomicrograph of normal human esophageal epithelium. The basal layer of polygonal cells comprises less than 15 percent of the total thickness of the stratified squamous epithelium (*small arrows*). A papilla projects into the epithelium but extends less than two-thirds of the total thickness of the epithelium (*large arrow*).

patients to greater than 15 percent of the total thickness of the epithelium (Figs. 48-2 and 48-3). The second histologic finding is a relative lengthening of the papillary projections of the lamina propria into the epithelium to a distance greater than two-thirds the thickness of the epithelium (see Figs. 48-2 and 48-3). Third, increased numbers of eosinophils in the epithelium in the absence of other inflammatory cells may signify gastroesophageal reflux.

The ability to identify the histology of the esophagus in patients with reflux symptoms is particularly important in making the diagnosis of columnar metaplasia of the esophagus (Barrett's epithelium). Normally, the stratified squamous epithelial lining of the esophagus ends abruptly at the esophagogastric junction, where the columnar-glandular epithelium of the stomach begins. In Barrett's epithelium, the epithelium of the lower esophagus becomes columnar-glandular for a variable extent, presumably in response to the injurious effects of chronically refluxed material. Barrett's epithelium itself is a benign condition, but it predisposes to the development of adenocarcinoma of the esophagus. Thus, it is important to identify Barrett's epithelium and follow such patients closely for symptoms that might suggest carcinoma.

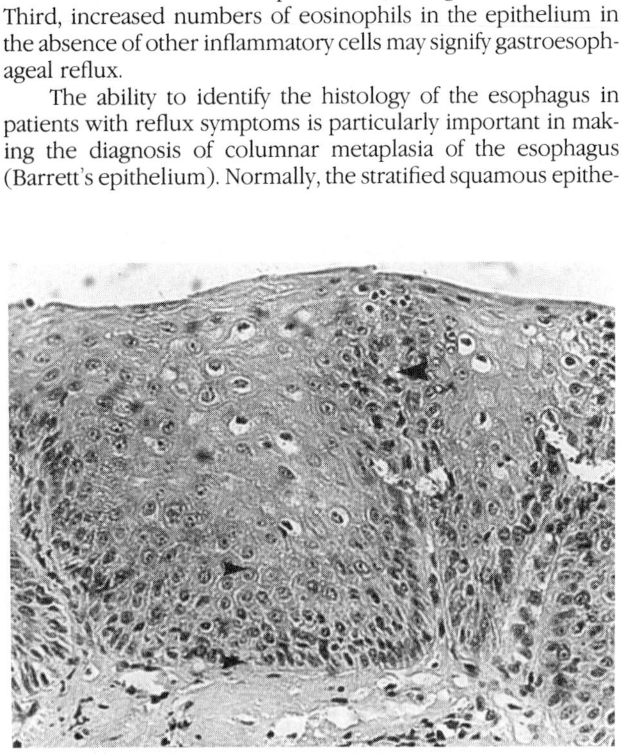

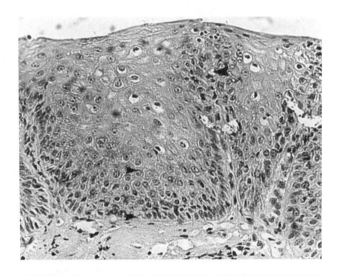

Figure 48-3 Photomicrograph of esophageal epithelium from a patient with symptoms of gastroesophageal reflux. The basal layer of polygonal cells occupies more than 15 percent of the thickness of the epithelium (*small arrows*), and the papillae extend nearly to the epithelial surface to occupy more than two-thirds of the total thickness of the epithelium (*large arrow*).

Esophageal manometry provides information about the function of the upper and lower esophageal sphincters as well as peristaltic activity in the body of the esophagus. Most patients with severe reflux symptoms have a decreased LES pressure, which may predispose to reflux of gastric contents. Some patients have impaired peristalsis, which may interfere with esophageal clearing of the refluxed material. However, many patients with reflux symptoms have normal esophageal motility tracings. Thus, the value of esophageal manometry in the diagnosis of gastroesophageal reflux is limited, and the test usually is not indicated in most patients with reflux symptoms.

The real value of esophageal manometry is in evaluating esophageal function in patients with unexplained chest pain or with dysphagia due to a suspected esophageal motility disorder. If esophageal manometry indicates high-amplitude, sustained, simultaneous, or nonperistaltic contractions, the diagnosis of diffuse esophageal spasm or another motility disorder can be made.

Prolonged pH monitoring of the lower esophagus is one of the few tests that actually measure gastroesophageal reflux. If a pH probe is positioned 5 cm above the LES, the measured pH should be above 6 in normal persons. In a patient who has reflux, the lower esophageal pH may remain low or may drop in certain positions or for prolonged periods of time postprandially. Some studies have indicated that 12- or 24-hour pH monitoring is an accurate indicator of gastroesophageal reflux.

The gastroesophageal scintiscan has been reported to be reliable in diagnosing gastroesophageal reflux. The patient is asked to swallow a radioactive sulfur colloid, and a scan of the stomach and esophagus is performed. Gastroesophageal reflux is indicated by an image of the radioactive material in a linear pattern extending above the stomach into the chest.

The Bernstein test is a time-honored method of determining whether a patient's chest pain is due to acid irritation of the esophagus. A tube is passed into the mid esophagus, and the esophagus is perfused first with normal saline and then with 0.1 N hydrochloric acid. If the patient experiences pain during acid perfusion that is identical to the pain that he or she has been complaining of, it is presumed that the pain is due to acid reflux.

Peptic Disease

Complaints of mild epigastric pain on an empty stomach may be treated with antacids without a specific diagnosis. If symptoms persist or are severe, however, upper GI endoscopy should be performed to determine whether the patient has a discrete ulcer, erosions, inflammation, or no identifiable lesion. A precise diagnosis may help the physician to determine the mode and duration of initial treatment and may be relevant to long-term management.

Because patients with peptic disease typically have multiple recurrences of symptoms, it is not necessary to perform endoscopy during each exacerbation. This is a matter of clinical judgment. Once the diagnosis of peptic disease has been established, therapy may be reinstituted without reaffirming the diagnosis. In other instances, endoscopy may aid in the decision to change treatment (e.g., determining the need for surgery in a patient whose ulcer does not heal on medical therapy).

Although upper GI endoscopy is diagnostically superior to

an upper GI radiographic series, the question of cost effectiveness is raised when the two studies are compared for the diagnosis of peptic disease. In general, endoscopy is 1.5 to 2 times more expensive than the x-ray study. The added expense of endoscopy must be balanced against the fact that some small ulcers, most erosions, and all mucosal erythema will be missed by upper GI x-ray series. Many physicians will choose to order an x-ray study as the first diagnostic test. If an ulcer is identified, they have a diagnosis. If the study is nondiagnostic, they may decide to treat the patient empirically for peptic disease. Eventually, if symptoms persist or recur, endoscopy should be performed.

The diagnosis of gastric ulcer deserves special mention. Although malignant duodenal ulcers have been reported, patients with this disorder are rare. Thus, for practical purposes, malignancy is not a consideration when the diagnosis is duodenal ulcer. If the duodenal ulcer patient responds symptomatically to treatment, documentation of ulcer healing usually is not required. However, because carcinomas of the stomach may present as a gastric ulceration, the evaluation of the patient who has a gastric ulcer is influenced by the possibility that the ulcer may be malignant. Several considerations make the diagnosis of gastric cancer more likely. One is the age of the patient. Malignant gastric ulcers occur most frequently after middle age and are encountered rarely in patients less than 35 years old. Further, several conditions may predispose to the development of gastric carcinoma, such as gastric atrophy and other chronic inflammatory lesions of the gastric mucosa.

Most gastric cancers arise in stomachs that are capable of secreting acid. However, about 25 percent of gastric cancers are associated with achlorhydria. Because acid is necessary for the development of a benign ulcer, the occurrence of a gastric ulcer in the absence of acid is strong evidence in favor of malignancy.

A reasonable approach to patients who have had a gastric ulcer diagnosed by upper GI x-ray series is to perform upper GI endoscopy on all such patients over age 35. At endoscopy, the appearance of the ulcer, biopsy specimens of the ulcer edges and center, cytologic samples, and pH of the gastric juice can all be assessed. If there is no evidence of malignancy, the patient should be treated for benign peptic ulcer. The endoscopy should be repeated after 6 to 8 weeks and, if necessary, after an

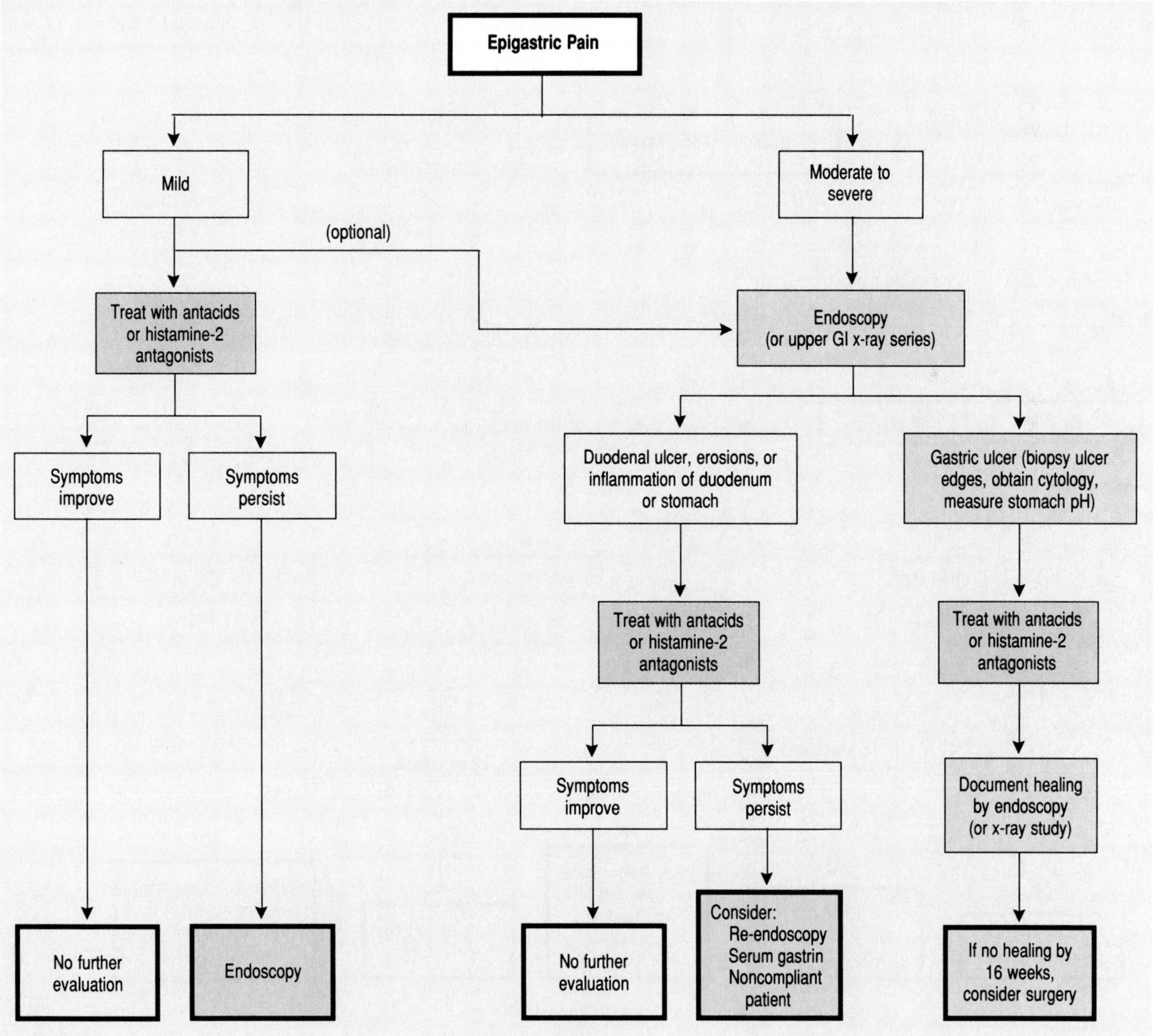

Figure 48-4 Algorithm for the evaluation of peptic disease. GI = gastrointestinal.

additional 4 to 8 weeks to demonstrate complete healing. If cancer is demonstrated or if the ulcer fails to heal after 16 weeks, surgical treatment should be considered.

If the patient is under age 35, initial endoscopy is not necessary if the diagnosis of gastric ulcer has been made by an upper GI x-ray series. Healing of the ulcer can be monitored by radiologic means, and endoscopy can be performed only if healing is delayed or if the patient's symptoms fail to respond to therapy.

Some gastric ulcers will be diagnosed initially by endoscopy. In such cases, endoscopy should be the method of documenting healing of the ulcer.

A serum gastrin determination will aid in the diagnosis of Zollinger-Ellison syndrome and related conditions. Serum gastrin values have little or no role in the initial evaluation of most patients who have peptic disease. However, if ulcers are recurrent, if they occur in unusual locations, if the patient is young or has a strong family history of ulcer disease, or if the ulcer disease is refractory to medical or surgical treatment, assessment of the serum gastrin level is indicated. The serum gastrin level should be determined in a fasted patient who has not taken antacids or other drugs for ulcer treatment for at least 24 hours. The normal fasting serum gastrin level is below 150 pg/ml. Serum gastrin levels above 500 pg/ml are strongly suggestive of a hypergastrinemic state.

In making the diagnosis of the Zollinger-Ellison syndrome, the secretin stimulation test may be helpful. This test takes advantage of the unique response of the gastrinoma to secretin, which is a potent stimulant of gastrin release from the tumor. In normal individuals, secretin inhibits the release of gastrin from the gastric antrum. Thus, after intravenous secretin, serum gastrin normally decreases or remains unchanged. In patients with gastrinomas, serum gastrin levels should rise promptly within 5 to 10 minutes after secretin injection to over 400 pg/ml above preinjection values. In ordinary ulcer disease, antral G-cell hyperplasia, or the retained antrum syndrome, the serum gastrin should decrease or remain unchanged. An algorithm that outlines the evaluation of a patient with peptic disease appears in Figure 48-4.

Indigestion

Disorders other than gastroesophageal reflux and peptic disease may cause postprandial discomfort and be interpreted as indigestion. If the evaluation for gastroesophageal reflux and peptic disease is nondiagnostic, several further diagnostic studies may be warranted.

Abdominal ultrasound examination has high sensitivity and specificity in the diagnosis of gallbladder stones. However, if the sonogram is nondiagnostic and the clinical impression of gall-

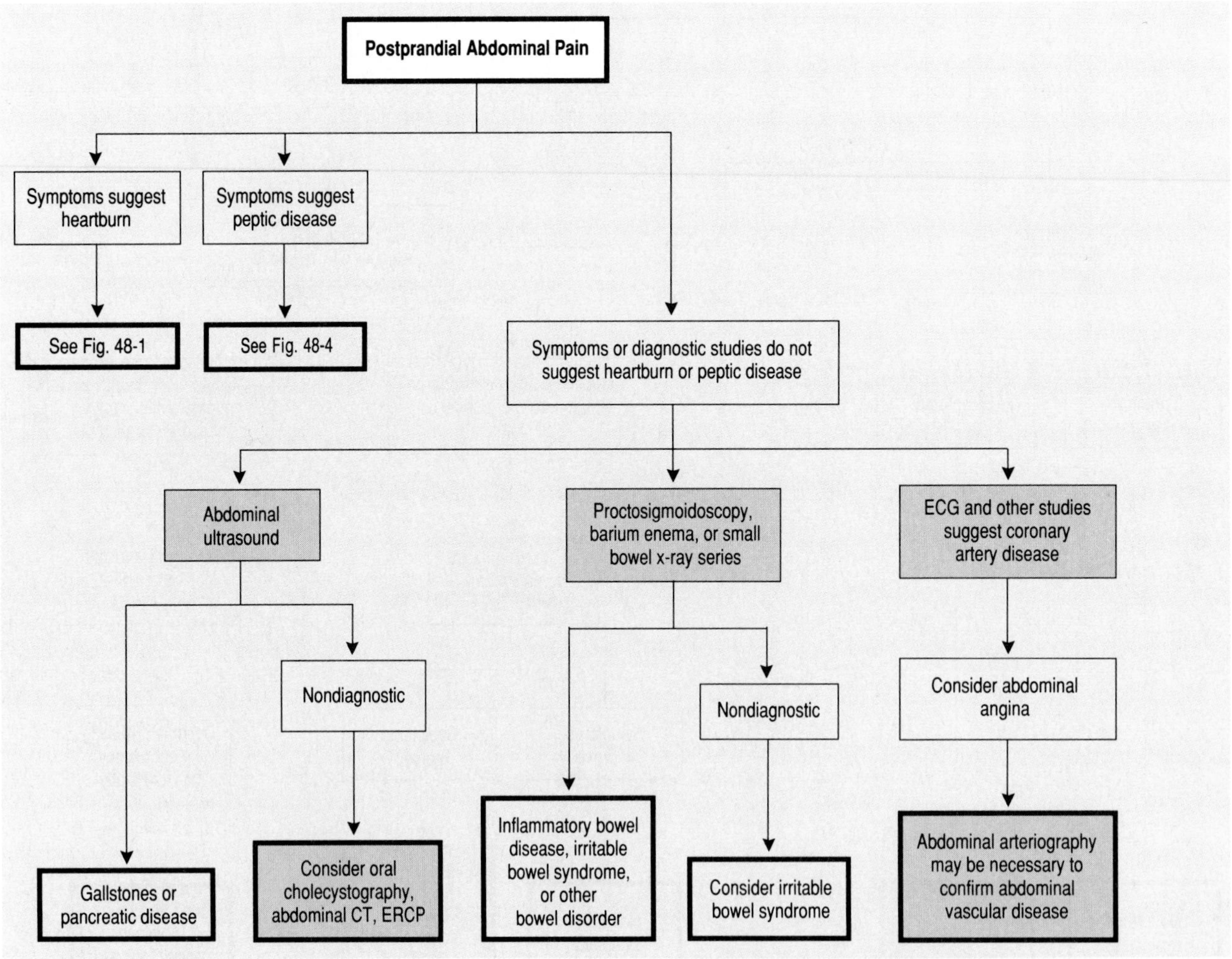

Figure 48-5 Algorithm for the evaluation of indigestion. CT = computed tomography, ECG = electrocardiography, ERCP = endoscopic retrograde cholangiopancreatography.

stones is high, an oral cholecystogram should be obtained. Ultrasonography of the abdomen also can provide information about the size and shape of the pancreas and thus may suggest the diagnosis of pancreatitis, pancreatic pseudocyst, or pancreaticobiliary carcinoma.

Computed tomography (CT) scanning and endoscopic retrograde cholangiopancreatography (ERCP) are specialized studies that can aid in the diagnosis of chronic pancreatitis, pancreatic pseudocyst, or pancreaticobiliary carcinoma.

Crohn's disease of the bowel is a diagnosis that usually is made by barium contrast studies of the bowel, although rectal involvement can be diagnosed readily by proctosigmoidoscopy. Because the majority of patients with Crohn's disease have involvement at least of the terminal ileum, a barium enema with reflux into the terminal ileum or a small bowel x-ray series will provide the diagnosis.

Diseases of the small intestine that result in malabsorption, such as celiac sprue, lymphoma, and bacterial overgrowth syndrome, may also be diagnosed with small bowel x-ray series. The irritable bowel syndrome is suggested by fluctuating abdominal complaints, such as alternating diarrhea and constipation, sometimes related to psychological stress. Other motiilty disorders of the intestines, such as pseudo-obstruction, may mimic some forms of irritable bowel syndrome. Patients with the irritable bowel syndrome typically have normal diagnostic studies of the upper and lower GI tract.

Abdominal angina is often a difficult diagnosis to make. It is suspected when abdominal pain occurs in a patient with atherosclerotic heart or vascular disease in the absence of another identifiable cause. Occasionally, abdominal arteriography is necessary to identify vascular insufficiency.

An algorithm that outlines the evaluation of the patient with indigestion appears in Figure 48-5.

References

Eastwood GL, Avunduk C, eds. Gastroesophageal reflux disease. In: Manual of gastroenterology: Diagnosis and therapy. Boston: Little, Brown, 1988:104.

Eastwood GL, Avunduk C, eds. Noncardiac chest pain. In: Manual of gastroenterology: Diagnosis and therapy. Boston: Little, Brown, 1988:123.

Eastwood GL, Avunduk C, eds. Peptic disease. In: Manual of gastroenterology: Diagnosis and therapy. Boston: Little, Brown, 1988:128.

Pope CE II. Heartburn, dysphagia, and other esophageal symptoms. In: Sleisenger MH, Fordtran JS, eds. Gastrointestinal disease. 4th ed. Philadelphia: WB Saunders, 1989:200.

Spechler SJ, Goyal RK. Barrett's esophagus. N Engl J Med 1986; 315:362.

Nausea and Vomiting

John F. Erkkinen, MD

49

Definition

Vomiting is the act of forceful expulsion of gastric and intestinal contents through the mouth. Nausea is a vague, unpleasant sensation, usually felt in the throat or epigastrium, representing an awareness in anticipation of vomiting. Because nausea and vomiting are symptoms and not diseases, appropriate management depends on an accurate assessment of their cause.

Physiology

The act of vomiting is a complicated one that involves the coordinated activities of the somatic (abdominal and thoracic) musculature and autonomic (sympathetic and parasympathetic) nervous system. Vomiting, usually preceded by nausea and retching, occurs while abdominal and gastric musculature contract during inspiration, forcing gastric and intestinal contents into the esophagus. Relaxation of the diaphragm and the pharyngoesophageal sphincter, followed by abdominal contractions, forces the contents through the mouth.

Initiation and control of vomiting take place in the "vomiting center" in the lateral reticular formation of the medulla in the brain stem (Fig. 49-1). The medulla receives afferent impulses peripherally from the gastrointestinal tract, the middle ear labyrinth, and the central nervous system. It receives impulses centrally from the chemoreceptor trigger zone near the fourth ventricle, which may be stimulated by apomorphine, other drugs, and toxins.

Diagnostic Approach

History

An accurate history of the nature, frequency, and physical characteristics of the patient's vomiting may provide valuable information regarding its cause (Table 49-1). Irritative vomiting occurring shortly after eating is characteristic of gastritis, peptic ulcer disease, or other inflammatory processes of the gastrointestinal tract, but it can be psychogenic. Vomiting that relieves abdominal pain may be a clue to pyloric edema or spasm associated with pyloric channel ulcer. Obstructive-type vomiting, which occurs 1 to 2 hours after eating (perhaps once or twice a day) and often contains undigested food, results from gastric-outlet obstruction from carcinoma, peptic ulcer, postsurgical scarring, or a motility disorder from diabetic gastroparetic neuropathy or postvagotomy states.

A description of the character of the vomitus may help identify the cause. Bloody vomitus, often with a coffee-ground appearance, is associated with mucosal injury of the upper gastrointestinal tract, which may occur in conditions such as peptic disease, radiation injury, or malignancy. Putrid or foul-smelling

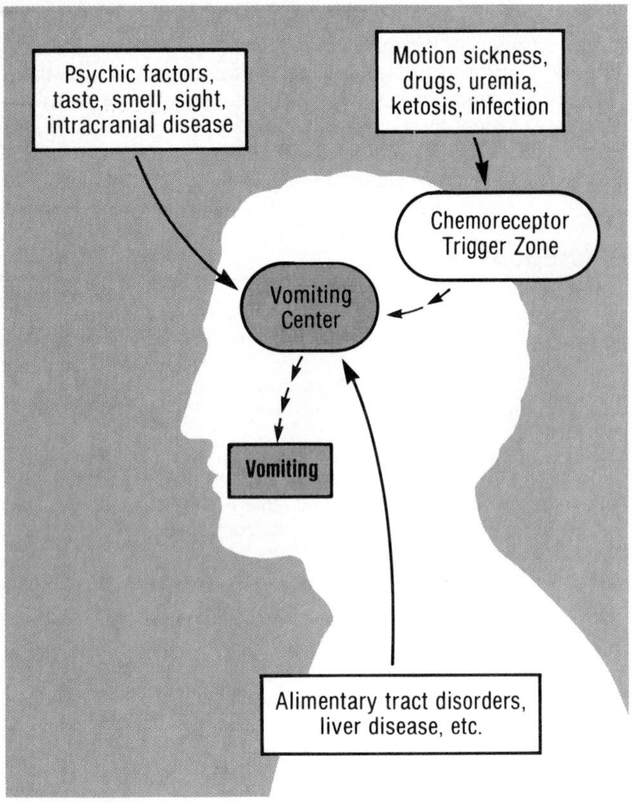

Figure 49-1 Mechanisms of vomiting. (*From* Biggs JSG. Vomiting in pregnancy. Drugs 1975; 9:299; with permission.)

vomitus results from bacterial overgrowth or fistulous communication with the lower gastrointestinal tract. A large amount of bilious drainage (most vomitus has some bile staining) usually results from obstruction distal to the papilla of Vater.

Consideration of past medical conditions and associated symptoms may be helpful (Table 49-2). A history of abdominal pain, alcohol use, recent abdominal surgery, or a cluster of vomiting among contacts suggests pathology in the gastrointestinal tract. Jaundice and epigastric or right upper quadrant pain often accompanies hepatitis or gallbladder disease. Vomiting associated with neurologic symptoms or vomiting without nausea may be seen in conditions associated with increased intracranial pressure. The acute onset of nausea and vomiting in a patient with chest pain or coronary risk factors suggests acute myocardial infarction. Early-morning nausea and vomiting are common "physiologic" accompaniments of early pregnancy. The onset of vomiting in late pregnancy suggests a "pathologic" cause such as cholecystitis, pyelonephritis, or toxemia. Chronic unexplained vomiting, a family history of vomiting, or a hostile home environment may indicate a psychogenic basis. The use of all prescription and nonprescription drugs should be documented, because nausea and vomiting are common side effects of many drugs, including digoxin, aminophylline, antibiotics, narcotics, and chemotherapeutic agents. Because hypercalcemia, hyponatremia, and uremia may present with nausea, a metabolic abnormality should also be considered in patients with unexplained vomiting.

Physical Examination

The physical examination allows the physician to distinguish those patients who need immediate and urgent attention from those in whom a more gradual approach may be taken. The patient who appears acutely ill requires the physician to rule in or out rapidly those causes of vomiting that require emergency treatment. Examples include bowel obstruction, acute myocardial infarction, acute neurologic catastrophe, and metabolic abnormalities, including drug toxicity. It is helpful to remember that on early inspection, some patients will look seriously ill from nausea and vomiting, even when the etiology is physiologic or benign, such as early pregnancy or uncomplicated gastroenteritis. Once the truly urgent conditions have been ruled out by history, physical examination, and appropriate laboratory studies, the physician may evaluate the patient less urgently while considering the extensive list of differential diagnoses outlined in Table 49-1.

The physical examination should focus on clues about the possible causes of vomiting. Fluid status is assessed by measuring skin turgor and the patient's orthostatic blood pressure and pulse. This will help the clinician determine whether the vomiting is associated with volume depletion. Abdominal distention, tenderness, or hypoactive bowel sounds suggest an intra-abdominal inflammatory process such as appendicitis, cholecystitis, or pancreatitis. Succussion splash may be noted when fluid is sequestered in a dilated stomach, as in gastric outlet obstruction. When present, a "splash" will be heard if the stethoscope is placed below the left costal margin while the abdomen is gently shaken. A distended abdomen, high-pitched

Table 49-1 Causes of Nausea and Vomiting

Abdominal pain					
Acute illness	*Persistent symptoms*	**Drug-induced**	**Hormonal**	**Neurologic**	**Psychogenic**
Gastroenteritis	Gastric outlet obstruction	Digitalis toxicity	Early pregnancy	Intracranial pressure	Anorexia nervosa
Gastritis	Intestinal obstruction	Narcotic use	Ketoacidosis	Midline cerebellar hemorrhage	Self-induced
Food poisoning	Bile reflux after gastric surgery	Chemotherapy	Hypercalcemia	Vestibular disease	Acute pain
Peptic ulcer disease	Cholelithiasis	Antibiotics	Adrenal insufficiency	Migraine headaches	Acute intense emotions
Acute pancreatitis, appendicitis, cholecystitis, cholangitis, pyelonephritis	Pancreatitis	Aminophylline			
Myocardial infarction (usually inferior)		Ethyl alcohol (binges)			
Perforated viscus					
Peritonitis					

Table 49-2 Differential Diagnosis of Nausea and Vomiting

Associated abdominal pain	Associated neurologic signs	Predominant symptoms	
		Acute	*Recurrent or chronic*
Viral gastroenteritis	Increased intracranial pressure	Digitalis toxicity	Psychogenic vomiting
Acute gastritis	Midline cerebellar hemorrhage	Ketoacidosis	Metabolic disturbances
Food poisoning	Vestibular disturbances	Opiate use	Gastric retention
Peptic ulcer disease	Migraine headaches	Cancer chemotherapeutic agents	Bile reflux after gastric surgery
Acute pancreatitis		Early pregnancy	Pregnancy
Small bowel obstruction		Inferior myocardial infarction	
Acute appendicitis		Drug withdrawal	
Acute cholecystitis		Binge drinking	
Acute cholangitis		Hepatitis	
Acute pyelonephritis			
Inferior myocardial infarction			

Adapted from Gorrol AH, May LS, Mulley AG. Primary care medicine. Philadelphia: JB Lippincott, 1981:239; with permission.

"tinkling" bowel sounds, and occasionally, visible peristalsis often accompany bowel obstruction. Jaundice, hepatomegaly, or right upper quadrant tenderness focuses on the hepatobiliary system as the cause of the emesis. Hepatitis, liver metastases, and cholecystitis are examples.

Vomiting associated with focal neurologic signs, a stiff neck, ataxia, papilledema, or seizure is characteristic of increased intracranial pressure. A patient with vomiting and nystagmus, tinnitus, or a hearing impairment may have a labyrinthine disorder or, rarely, a cerebellar or eighth cranial nerve lesion. A normal examination may be seen with metabolic abnormalities such as drug toxicity, uremia, electrolyte imbalance, psychogenic vomiting, or with any of the causes of vomiting.

Laboratory Studies

The laboratory assessment is dictated by the history and physical examination. In the setting of vomiting associated with abdominal pain, gastroenteritis is common, and observation and reassurance may be all that is required if a patient is not volume depleted or severely ill. If the symptoms are persistent, medications should be withheld, if possible, as they may be a contributory factor. When nausea, vomiting, and abdominal pain occur in a patient who looks ill, surgical conditions such as appendicitis, bowel obstruction, cholecystitis, or cholangitis must be considered. A kidneys, ureters, and bladder film, complete blood count, serum amylase determination, and urinalysis are important in the initial assessment. If cholelithiasis is considered, an abdominal ultrasound study or oral cholecystography will be helpful. Vomiting, with or without nausea, with new focal or neurologic signs requires careful neurologic examination and usually emergency computed tomographic examination. Severe nausea without focal signs or abdominal pain should prompt the clinician to check serum electrolytes, glucose, blood urea nitrogen, and transaminase and perform a pregnancy test and a drug screen to rule out a metabolic abnormality.

References

Davenport HW. Physiology of the digestive tract. 5th ed. Chicago: Year Book Medical Publishers, 1982:98.

Feldman M. Nausea and vomiting. In: Gastrointestinal disease. 4th ed. Sleisenger MH, Fordtran JS, eds. Philadelphia: WB Saunders, 1989:222.

Frytak S, Moertel CG. Management of nausea and vomiting in the cancer patient. JAMA 1981; 245:393.

Siegel LJ, Longo DL. The control of chemotherapy-induced emesis. Ann Intern Med 1981; 95:352.

Wyman JB, Wick MR. The vomiting patient. Am Fed Proc 1980; 21:139.

Abdominal Distention 50

Elise Jacques, MD

Definition

Any swelling or relative increase in girth of the abdomen constitutes abdominal distention. Increase in girth may occur rapidly over minutes or hours or may develop insidiously over months or years. Abdominal distention may result from accumulation of fat, gas, fluid, or solid tissue (tumor mass) within the abdominal cavity. Distention may be diffuse and symmetric or localized.

Fluid, gas, or solid (tumor mass) may accumulate within the bowel lumen, in the bowel wall, the mesentery, or other tissue spaces (e.g., pancreas, liver), or freely in the abdominal or

Table 50-1 Etiologies of Abdominal Distention

Fluid Causes
Free fluid
Ascites*
Peritonitis (spontaneous due to ruptured viscus)
Bleeding (arterial, aneurysm, or splenic rupture)
Loculated fluid
Cysts
Pancreatic pseudocysts
Abscesses
Bowel wall edema
Intraluminal fluid
Gastric dilatation
Bowel obstruction
Bladder distention
Gaseous Causes
Free (perforated viscus)
Intramural (pneumatosis cystoides intestinalis)
Intraluminal
Obstruction
Ileus
Solid Causes
Organomegaly
Liver
Spleen
Kidney
Tumor mass (benign or malignant)
Fecal retention
Pregnancy
Normal abdomen accentuated by lordosis

* Occasionally ascites is *chylous* owing to the presence of thoracic or intestinal lymph or, rarely, *bilious* as a result of a bile leakage.

Table 50-2 Mechanisms and Causes of Ascites

Mechanism	Cause
Increased venous or portal pressure	Cirrhosis, acute liver injury, congestive heart failure, hepatic venous thrombosis (benign or malignant)
Decreased oncotic pressure	Hypoalbuminemia
Increased hepatic lymph formation	Active inflammatory liver disease, cirrhosis
Increased renal retention of sodium	Cirrhosis
Decreased splanchnic lymphatic drainage	Tumor, lymphoma
Increased peritoneal capillary permeability	Infection, especially tuberculosis; tumor

peritoneal cavity (Table 50-1). When free fluid accumulates in the peritoneal cavity, it is called ascites, which is the major subject of discussion in this chapter.

Differential Diagnosis and Pathophysiology of Ascites

More than 90 percent of patients with ascites have cirrhosis, neoplasia, congestive heart failure, or tuberculosis as the etiology. The ascites in cirrhosis results from a combination of portal hypertension, hypoalbuminemia, abnormal lymphatic flow, redistribution of renal blood flow, hormonal factors, and renal retention of salt and water. Congestive heart failure, constrictive pericarditis, inferior vena cava obstruction, and hepatic vein obstruction (Budd-Chiari syndrome) occur as a result of mechanical or functional impairment of portal blood flow. Hypoalbuminemia causes ascites from decreased oncotic pressure when serum albumin is less than 2.5 g/dl, but it is most common with albumin less than 1.5 g/dl. Less common causes of ascites include myxedema, ovarian disease (Meigs' syndrome), protein-losing enteropathy, malnutrition, and pancreatic, bile, and chylous ascites.

Table 50-2 lists the mechanisms and causes of ascites.

Diagnostic Approach

Medical History

An increase in abdominal girth with ascites is a slow process. It commonly develops over months in the cirrhotic patient or over weeks in the patient with viral or alcoholic hepatitis. The patient or a family member may first notice the need to switch to a larger belt or pants size. When transient and noted only by the patient, abdominal distention usually does not represent ascites, but it may signify a functional gastrointestinal disorder. When distention is persistent, the patient may ignore it, believing the abdomen is merely becoming obese. With significant distention, however, the patient may note a pulling or stretching feeling in the groin, flanks, or lower back. Pain is not a common accompaniment of mild or moderate ascites, so when present, it should be explained. Pancreatitis, hepatitis, hepatoma, and peritonitis should be considered. If the ascites becomes tense, the patient may experience increased intra-abdominal pressure and complain of dyspeptic symptoms. Abdominal distention, secondary to ascites, may cause secondary problems from hernia development (especially umbilical) or respiratory distress from diaphragmatic elevation or coexistent pleural effusion.

Because cirrhosis is the most common cause of ascites in the United States, the medical history should include careful inquiry for a history of alcohol abuse or prior liver disease. The physical examination may show a firm enlargement of the liver and spleen, or this may be obscured by massive ascites. The presence of stigmata of liver disease, including palmar erythema, spider angiomata, small testicles, or asterixis (the latter suggesting hepatic encephalopathy), supports the chronicity of the liver disease.

A history or signs of cardiopulmonary failure suggest congestive heart failure as an etiology. The physical examination may show evidence of pericardial disease. Weight loss or anorexia is often associated with neoplasia, cardiac cachexia, malnutrition, and protein-losing enteropathy. A careful search for lymph nodes should be performed. The presence of Virchow's node in the left supraclavicular fossa suggests gastrointestinal malignancy. The rare myxedematous patient presenting with ascites will have classic findings of weight gain (may be slight), hoarseness, psychomotor slowing, cold sensitivity, bradycardia, or constipation. On occasion the patient will give a history of prior tuberculous infection or exposure.

Physical Examination

An algorithm for the evaluation of possible ascites is shown in Figure 50-1.

On inspection, the abdomen may be minimally distended or tense, depending on the degree of fluid accumulation. The venous pattern may be prominent, particularly in inferior vena caval or hepatic venous obstruction. The flow of blood in the dilated veins is usually cephalad. Dilatation of the paraumbilical vein, called caput medusae, may accompany hepatic or portal vein obstruction. Abdominal distention resulting from ascites is

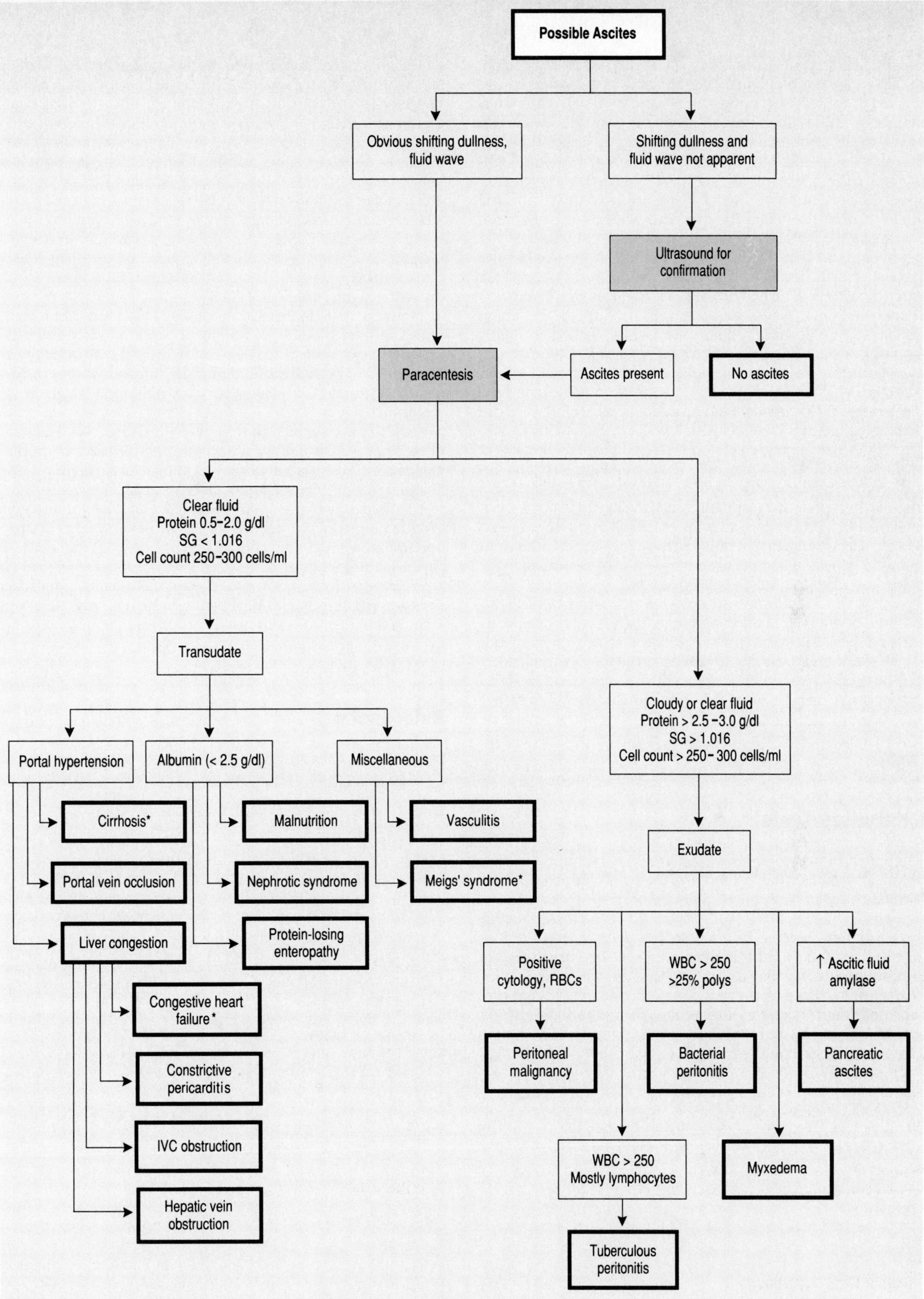

Figure 50-1 Algorithm for the evaluation of possible ascites. Conditions marked with an asterisk may present as exudates. IVC = inferior vena cava, polys = polymorphonuclear leukocytes, RBCs = red blood cells, SG = specific gravity, WBC = white blood cell count.

usually symmetric from xiphoid to pubis. In the supine position, the flanks are often bulging. The umbilicus may be everted and pushed downward. In contrast, in pregnancy or with large ovarian cysts, the umbilicus is usually displaced upward. Obstruction as the cause of distention may be apparent if visible ridges of intestine are noted. On auscultation, one may hear the high-pitched rushing sounds of intestinal obstruction. Succussion splash is present when fluid and gas are present in a dilated viscus. A bruit may mark the presence of a vascular neoplasm (hepatoma). A friction rub may accompany liver metastasis. On percussion, an area of dullness is located in the flanks with resonance in the midline. The area of resonance shifts to the left when the patient is turned on the right side. This is referred to as shifting dullness. Fat in the mesentery may also give shifting dullness. On palpation, a fluid wave can be elicited by lightly tapping one flank and palpating for the sensation of fluid against the opposite flank. Because motion of fat may mimic a fluid wave, an assistant placing a hand over the midline may help differentiate fat from fluid. Shifting dullness and a fluid wave can be overlooked in the patient with less than 1 L of ascitic fluid.

With tense ascites, palpation is often difficult. Ballottement of the liver and spleen may help in judging their size. Splenomegaly may accompany cirrhosis or lymphoma, whereas a hard, nodular liver may suggest malignancy. An erythematous, periumbilical induration known as Sister Joseph's nodule may also be seen with malignancy. A pulsatile liver, jugular venous distention, and hepatojugular reflux in a patient with ascites are likely to be secondary to tricuspid insufficiency.

Abdominal tenderness suggests infected ascitic fluid. Rigidity and rebound may herald a perforated viscus, but spontaneous bacterial peritonitis may present with the same dramatic findings. Free air under the diaphragm on upright x-ray examination may be useful in differentiating these two entities. Encapsulated ovarian cysts may be movable or asymmetric and should not have demonstrable shifting dullness. When very large, they may be indistinguishable from free tense ascites by physical examination.

Laboratory Tests

Abdominal ultrasonography or computed tomography (CT) is useful to establish the presence of free fluid and should be obtained prior to paracentesis if history or physical examination suggests loculated fluid (i.e., pancreatic pseudocyst, ovarian cyst). A kidneys, ureters, bladder film may show haziness or loss of psoas shadows, but this finding is not specific. Paracentesis is important in establishing the etiology of ascites. A small amount (20 to 100 cc) of the ascitic fluid should be analyzed for appearance; cell count and differential; protein concentration; amylase; and, *if indicated*, Gram and acid-fast stain; routine, mycobacterial, and fungal cultures; and cytologic study. Transudates, which are characteristic of cirrhosis, congestive heart failure, and nephrosis, typically have a clear appearance, protein content of 0.5 to 2.0 g/dl, specific gravity less than 1.016, and cell count usually less than 300 cells per cubic milliliter (predominantly mononuclear and mesothelial cells). Exudative fluid is characteristic of neoplasia, tuberculosis, purulent bacterial peritonitis, inflammatory process, Budd-Chiari syndrome, and myxedema. The exudate generally has protein content greater than 2.5 g/dl. A bacterial peritonitis is suggested by total ascitic fluid white cell count greater than 25 percent polymorphonuclear leukocytes. Cloudy fluid with predominantly polymorphonuclear leukocytes is consistent with bacterial infection. Blood-tinged exudative fluid with lymphocytes predominant is seen with neoplastic or tuberculous ascites. Other causes of bloody ascites include intraperitoneal bleed from trauma or ruptured varix, and hemorrhagic pancreatitis. The latter condition is also associated with high levels of peritoneal fluid amylase. Chylous ascites in lymphatic obstruction is associated with milky fluid high in triglyceride content.

Cytologic examination may detect malignancy—metastatic disease, most commonly, or occasionally primary peritoneal malignancy (i.e., mesothelioma). Cytologic findings are positive in approximately 60 percent of cases of malignant ascites.

Venography of the inferior vena cava and the portal system may be necessary to establish the diagnosis of venous obstruction. Lymphangiography should be considered if the ascites is chylous. If tuberculous peritonitis is suspected, acid-fast stain is only occasionally diagnostic, and even cultures may be falsely negative. Highest diagnostic yield comes from peritoneoscopy with directed peritoneal biopsy. Peritoneoscopy may be useful in diagnosing carcinomatosis or underlying liver disease as the cause of the ascites.

References

Bender MD, Ockner RK. Ascites. In: Sleisenger MH, Fordtran JS, eds. Gastrointestinal disease. 4th ed. Philadelphia: WB Saunders, 1989:428.

Boyer TD, Kahn AM, Reynolds TB. Diagnostic value of ascitic fluid lactic dehydrogenase, protein, and WBC levels. Arch Intern Med 1978; 138:1103.

Correia JP, Conn HP. Spontaneous bacterial peritonitis in cirrhosis: Endemic or epidemic? Med Clin North Am 1975; 59:963.

Kline MM, McCallum RIO, Guth PH. The clinical value of ascites fluid culture and leukocyte count studies in alcoholic cirrhosis. Gastroenterology 1976; 70:408.

Luberman FL, Denison EK, Reynolds TB. The relationship of plasma volume, portal hypertension, ascites, and renal sodium retention in cirrhosis: The overflow theory of ascites formation. Ann NY Acad Sci 1970; 170:202.

Schiff L, Schiff E, eds. Diseases of the liver. 6th ed. Philadelphia: JB Lippincott, 1987.

Wolfe JHN, Behn AR, Jackson BT. Tuberculous peritonitis and role of diagnostic laparoscopy. Lancet April 21, 1979.

Abdominal Pain

John F. Erkkinen, MD

51

Etiology

Abdominal pain is a frequent complaint of patients visiting a physician's office. Table 51-1 lists the causes of abdominal pain, which may result from pathology in virtually every organ system in the body (vascular, neurologic, urologic, gynecologic, gastrointestinal, and so forth). The most common causes of abdominal pain, however, relate to the gastrointestinal system, and this chapter emphasizes pain of gastrointestinal origin.

Pain originating from a hollow viscus, such as the stomach, intestine, or gallbladder, is different from that originating from somatic structures such as the skin or parietal peritoneum. Visceral pain is not affected by cutting, burning, needling, or chemical injury, but it is exquisitely sensitive to tension, twisting, distending, or traction of the organs involved. Pain originating from a hollow viscus is often vague, crampy, or of a colicky nature, whereas pain originating from a somatic structure is steady and well localized.

Diagnostic Approach

In the early assessment of a patient presenting with abdominal pain, it is important to differentiate the patient with an acute condition that requires urgent evaluation and treatment from the patient with a more subacute or chronic problem. In general, the patient with acute abdominal pain (Table 51-2) associated with acute obstruction or metabolic or cardiopulmonary disease will need to be evaluated further in the hospital. Patients with non–life-threatening subacute or chronic abdominal pain (Fig. 51-1) can generally be evaluated in the outpatient setting. Because abdominal pain may result from disease in any organ system, the history, physical examination, and laboratory studies must include the entire patient.

Table 51-1 Principal Mechanisms of Abdominal Pain

Obstruction	**Metabolic Disturbance**
Gastric outlet	Diabetic ketoacidosis
Small bowel	Porphyria
Large bowel	Lead poisoning
Biliary tract	**Nerve Injury**
Urinary tract	Herpes zoster
Peritoneal Irritation	Root compression
Infection	**Muscle Wall Disease**
Chemical irritation (blood, bile, gastric acid)	Trauma
Systemic inflammatory process	Myositis
Spread from a local inflammatory process	Hematoma
Vascular Insufficiency	**Referred Pain**
Embolization	Pneumonia (lower lobes)
Atherosclerotic narrowing	Inferior myocardial infarction
Hypotension	Pulmonary infarction
Aortic aneurysm dissection	**Psychological Stress**
Mucosal Injury	Depression
Peptic ulcer disease	Situational stress
Gastric cancer	Intrapsychic conflict
Altered Motility	
Gastroenteritis	
Inflammatory bowel disease	
Irritable colon	
Diverticular disease	

History

The history should include questions regarding family history of abdominal pain, prior episodes of abdominal pain, gastrointestinal disease, or abdominal surgery. In addition, a history of alcohol use, medications, and allergies should be documented. All previously diagnosed medical conditions must be considered. In women it is essential to obtain a careful gynecologic history. A history of a change in menstrual cycle, postmenopausal bleeding, vaginal discharge, or dyspareunia may help localize the source of pain. Flank pain, dysuria, or hematuria is often associated with abdominal pain originating from the kidneys, ureters, or bladder. Patients with poor cardiac output or known vascular disease may have mesenteric ischemia. Patients with atrial fibrillation may develop mesenteric ischemia from embolization to the mesenteric vessels.

As part of this detailed systemic history, the physician should also consider other gastrointestinal symptoms. The presence of anorexia, belching, abdominal bloating, nausea, vomiting, or hematemesis or a change in bowel habits suggests a problem originating in the gastrointestinal tract. When melena or hematochezia accompanies the abdominal pain, it is usually related to mucosal disease of the gastrointestinal tract. Pre- or postprandial pain that is relieved by antacids suggests acid-peptic disease of the esophagus, stomach, or duodenum. Pain

Table 51-2 Acute Abdominal Pain: Diagnostic Clues and Associated Characteristics

Clue	Diagnosis
Peritoneal signs	Surgical abdomen
Dysuria/hematuria	Pyelonephritis Ureteral obstruction
History of cardiovascular disease	Abdominal aortic aneurysm Mesenteric ischemia Myocardial infarction Intestinal infarction
Alcoholism	Pancreatitis Hepatitis Gastritis
Altered menses	Ruptured ectopic pregnancy Pelvic inflammatory disease Ruptured ovarian cyst
No fever Mild or moderate pain No peritoneal signs	Peptic ulcer disease (see Chapter 48)

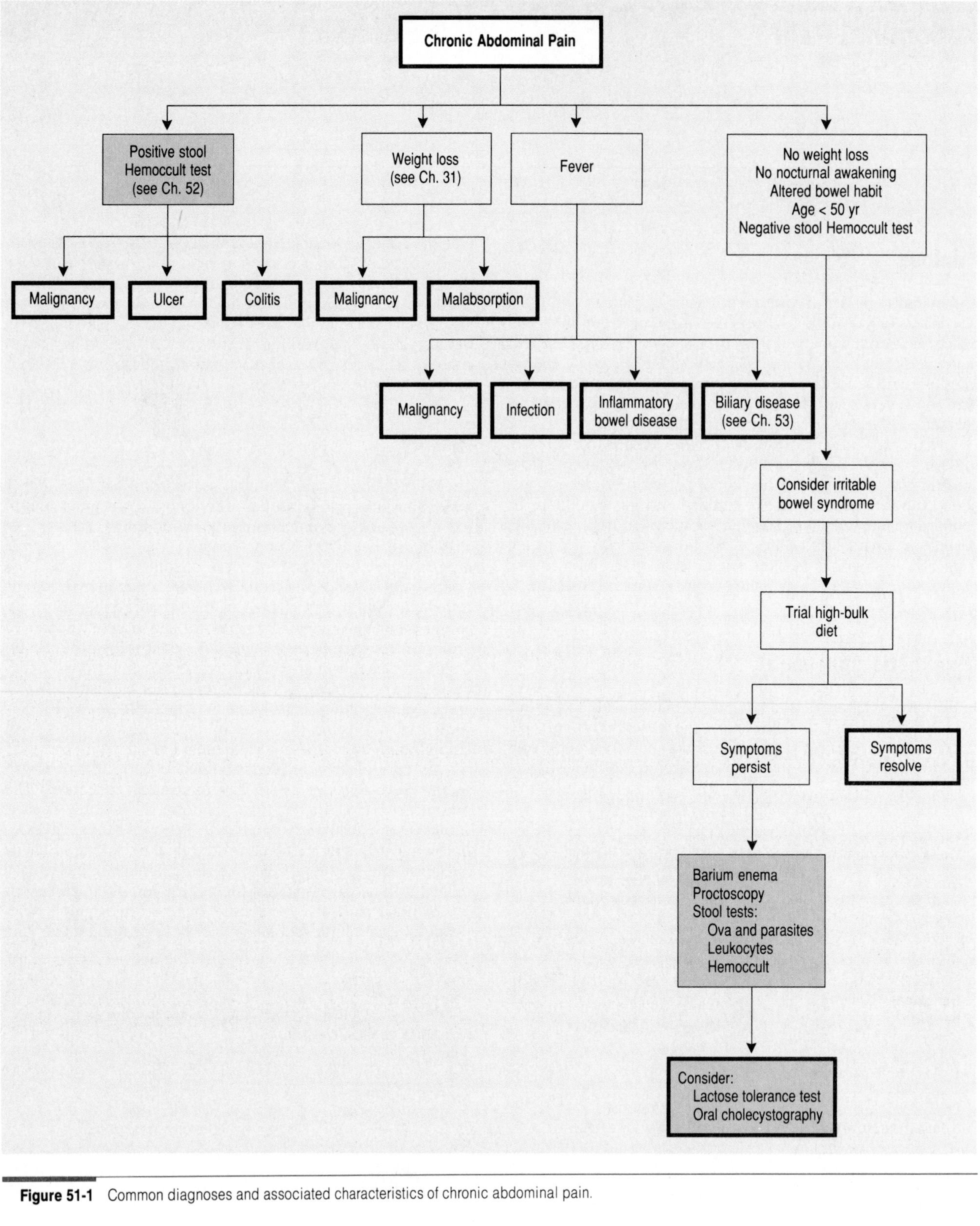

Figure 51-1 Common diagnoses and associated characteristics of chronic abdominal pain.

exacerbated or relieved by a bowel movement or flatus suggests a colonic or rectal origin.

The perception of pain, including abdominal pain, is the result of a physiologic stimulus and the patient's reaction to that stimulus. Because a patient's description of the quality and severity of pain is in large part a subjective assessment, more objective criteria for the pain should be sought, including the location and timing of the pain.

Early in embryologic development, the gastrointestinal tract, including the pancreas and biliary tree, is a midline structure. After fetal development, it retains its bilateral midline innervation. Thus, most gastrointestinal pain is felt in the midline. As an example, pain of early appendicitis starts in the midline. Later, as inflammation involves contiguous somatic structures, the pain localizes, usually to the right lower quadrant (Fig. 51-2). Pain of the upper gastrointestinal tract is usually referred to the

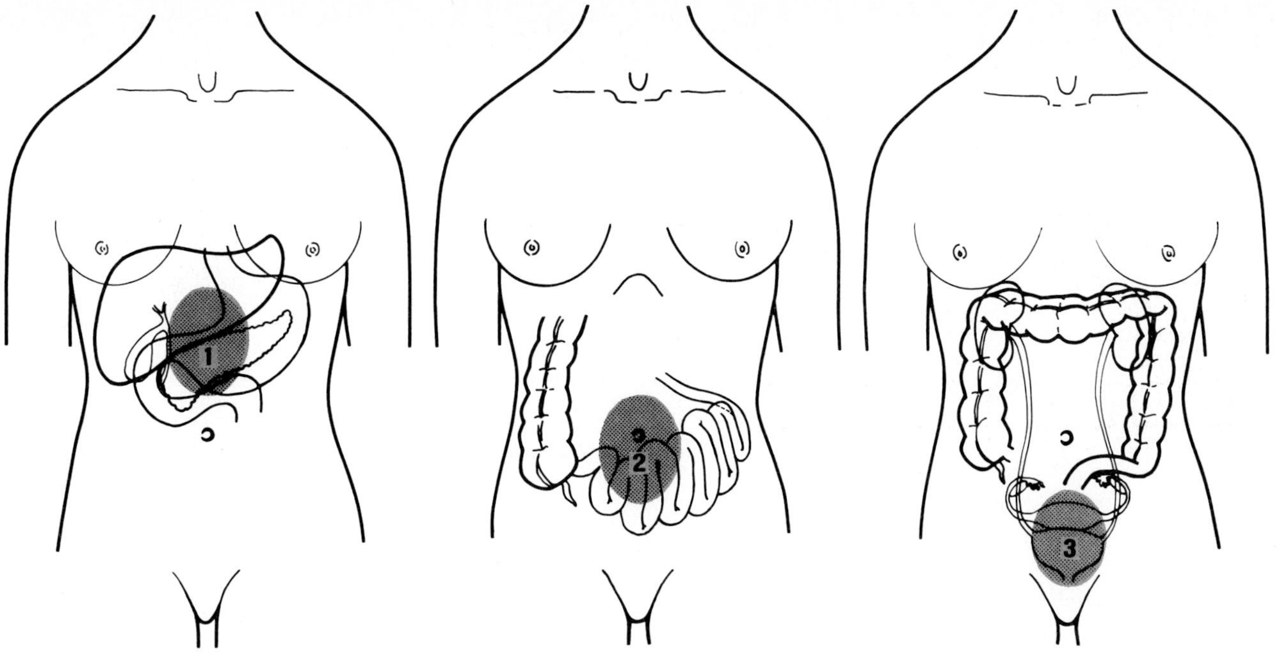

Figure 51-2 Referred abdominal pain. Pain of the upper gastrointestinal tract is usually referred to the epigastrium (*1*); pain from the midgut is referred to the periumbilical area (*2*); and pain in the colon is referred to the suprapubic midline (*3*).

epigastrium; pain from the midgut, to the periumbilical area; and colonic pain, to the suprapubic midline.

The temporal quality of pain may also provide important information. Pain with an instantaneous onset suggests a ruptured organ (e.g., perforated ulcer, pneumothorax, dissecting aneurysm), whereas a more gradual onset suggests an inflammatory process (e.g., pancreatitis, abscess, regional enteritis). Accurate assessment of the duration and frequency of the pain may also be helpful (Fig. 51-3). The pain of a peptic ulcer is intermittent and of short duration, whereas biliary colic has an abrupt onset and typically lasts 6 to 12 hours, with recurrent episodes of pain separated by weeks or months. The pain of pancreatitis usually has a gradual onset. It may last days to weeks, and attacks often may be separated by months or years.

Abdominal pain may be caused by alterations in bowel motility. These patients may complain of constipation alternating with diarrhea. The large bowel may develop spasms and nonpropulsive contractions that result in high intraluminal pressure and abdominal cramps. The most common gastrointestinal motility disorder is the so-called functional or irritable bowel syndrome. Patients with this problem generally complain of abdominal pain and varied bowel habits ranging from constipation to diarrhea.

An important task for the physician in assessing a patient with abdominal pain is distinguishing those patients who have organic disease from those who have functional or psychogenic abdominal pain. The presence of abdominal pain associated with fever, nocturnal awakening, blood per rectum, weight loss, or onset after the age of 50 makes the diagnosis of irritable bowel syndrome unlikely and should alert the physician to consider other causes.

Physical Examination

The physical examination should be complete and thorough; the entire patient should be examined, not simply the abdomen. Begin with the assessment of the patient's general appearance and position. If the patient repeatedly assumes a certain position because it decreases the abdominal pain, this should be noted, as it may offer an important diagnostic clue. Patients with visceral pain (e.g., biliary colic, early bowel obstruction) frequently pace

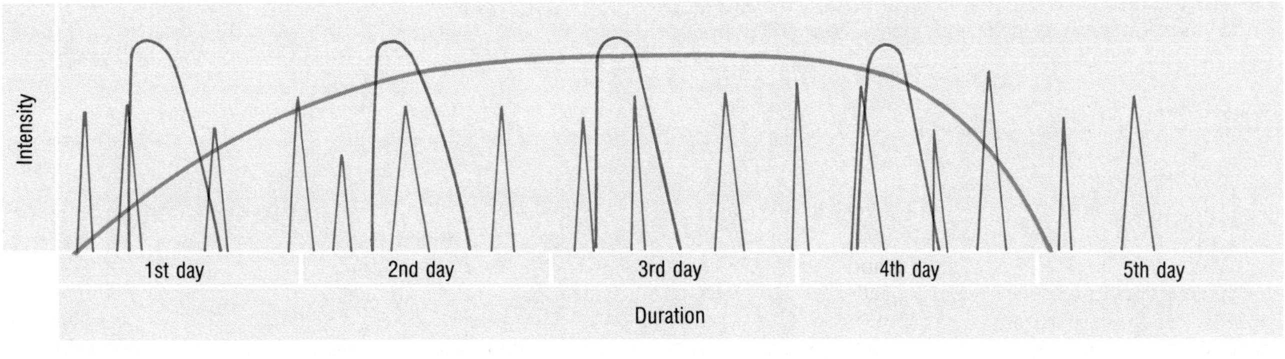

Figure 51-3 Characteristics of abdominal pain. Duodenal ulcer (*blue*), biliary colic (*red*), pancreatitis (*green*).

the floor or change their position to try to alleviate the discomfort, whereas patients with somatic pain (e.g., peritonitis, pancreatitis) usually remain motionless because irritation of the somatic structures enhances their pain.

The presence of fever suggests an inflammatory or infectious process. Orthostatic changes in the blood pressure and pulse, defined as a drop of more than 10 mm Hg in the systolic blood pressure and an increase in the heart rate of more than 20 per minute, when the patient changes from a supine to upright position, suggest a greater than 20 percent loss in intravascular volume. The presence of an irregular pulse raises the possibility that the patient may have had an embolus to the mesenteric vessels. Assess the patient's sclera and skin for evidence of icterus, implying obstruction or disease of the hepatobiliary system. Search for lymphadenopathy. Specifically, inspect the left supraclavicular fossa for Virchow's node, which may be associated with malignancy of the gastrointestinal tract. Assess the cardiorespiratory system for chest splinting, pleural or pericardial disease, lung consolidation, congestive heart failure, or atrial fibrillation. The vascular examination should include palpation for an abdominal aortic aneurysm. Percussion or "punch" tenderness in the flank region may be elicited in patients with renal inflammation or ureteral obstruction.

The abdomen should be assessed first by inspection. Abdominal distention may be due to obesity, gaseous distention, ascites, or tumor. Flank or umbilical discoloration may result from retro- or intraperitoneal hemorrhage. Dilated superficial abdominal veins may result from portal hypertension. An abdominal scar may provide a clue to previous injury or surgery. Auscultation of the abdomen may reveal absence of bowel sounds, as in peritonitis. Intermittent high-pitched "rushes" of peristaltic activity (borborygmi), coinciding with episodes of colicky abdominal pain, suggest mechanical small bowel obstruction. An abdominal bruit may be associated with ischemic bowel disease. A friction rub heard over the liver may accompany hepatic malignancy. Abdominal palpation may detect abdominal masses, fluid, hernia, or tenderness. Rebound tenderness is elicited by suddenly releasing pressure on the palpated abdomen, which produces exquisite pain and is indicative of peritoneal irritation. A palpable enlarged gallbladder indicates biliary obstruction from malignancy or stone. Tenderness occurring under the right costal margin with inspiration (Murphy's sign) is a helpful sign in acute cholecystitis. A psoas sign (exacerbation of pain with hyperextensions of the thigh while the patient lies on the left side) may be noted in a patient with an inflamed retrocecal appendix.

Laboratory Tests

Laboratory assessment of the acutely ill patient is dictated by the history and physical examination.

Complete Blood Count with Differential. An elevated white blood cell count or left shift may be a clue to an active infectious or inflammatory process in the abdomen. A normal blood count does not rule out disease.

Urinalysis. This test may provide information regarding a urinary or pararenal/ureteral process such as infection or stones.

Amylase. The amylase level is usually elevated in pancreatitis, but it may be abnormal in other conditions such as biliary tract disease, peptic ulcer disease, or salpingitis (see Chapter 54, "Increased Serum Amylase").

Serum Electrolytes. Serum electrolytes may be abnormal as a result of a variety of metabolic disturbances (e.g., decreased serum bicarbonate associated with sepsis or diarrhea, hypokalemia associated with vomiting or diarrhea, hypernatremia associated with dehydration).

Radiography of the Chest. Chest radiographs may give clues to an intra-abdominal process (pleural effusion, atelectasis, or air under the diaphragm) or a pulmonary process (pneumonia, malignancy, embolus, or pleurisy).

Radiographs of the Abdomen. Flat plate and upright radiographs often are extremely helpful in the assessment of abdominal pain (e.g., ileus, obstruction, ascites, bowel edema). This is particularly true of acute abdominal pain. The plain film of the abdomen should be obtained in a patient with acute abdominal pain when bowel obstruction, renal or ureteral calculi, gallbladder disease, trauma, or mesenteric ischemia are considered or the physical examination reveals moderate to severe abdominal tenderness. The plain film of the abdomen is less helpful in chronic abdominal pain, although in certain circumstances, it may provide clues about the diagnosis, e.g., calcifications of pancreas in chronic pancreatitis.

After the history and physical and laboratory assessment are completed, observing a patient over a period of time may be helpful in determining the cause and the course of the abdominal pain. This is true whether the patient has acute or chronic abdominal pain. For patients with acute onset of abdominal pain, serial abdominal examinations may be repeated over intervals of minutes to hours. In patients with more subacute or chronic abdominal pain, the interval may be days or weeks.

References

Beal JM, Raffensperger JG. Diagnosis of acute abdominal disease. Philadelphia: Lea & Febiger, 1979.

Eisenberg RL, et al. Evaluation of plain abdominal radiographs in the diagnosis of abdominal pain. Ann Intern Med 1982; 97:257.

Silen W, ed. Cope's early diagnosis of the acute abdomen. 17th ed. New York: Oxford University Press, 1987.

Sreenivas VI. Acute disorders of the abdomen. New York: Springer-Verlag, 1980.

Way LW. Abdominal pain. In: Sleisenger MH, Fordtran JS, eds. Gastrointestinal disease. 4th ed. Philadelphia: WB Saunders, 1989:238.

Gastrointestinal Bleeding

Gregory L. Eastwood, MD

52

Definition

All people normally lose 1 to 3 ml of blood a day from the gastrointestinal (GI) tract as a result of transudation of red blood cells across the mucosa and small amounts of bleeding from tiny abrasions. Strictly speaking, loss of blood in excess of this amount can be regarded as GI bleeding. However, clinical manifestations of GI bleeding usually require rates of blood loss that are far in excess of the normal amount.

Occult blood in the stool may be noted with as little as 15 to 20 ml of blood per day. Melena, which is black stool, may develop with loss of 50 ml or more of blood per day. However, these figures should not be regarded as absolute because the volume and rate of passage of stool will affect the concentration of blood in the stool.

More brisk rates of bleeding may manifest as red blood per rectum (hematochezia) or vomiting of blood (hematemesis). If gastric acid acts on fresh blood, the vomitus becomes dark and resembles coffee grounds. Hematemesis usually signifies an upper GI source, whereas hematochezia is usually a sign of lower GI bleeding. However, profuse bleeding from the upper GI tract, such as from a bleeding duodenal ulcer or from esophageal varices, may also result in hematochezia.

In addition to direct evidence of GI bleeding, acute blood loss may be manifested by a drop in blood pressure and a rise in pulse rate. If the pulse rate increases by more than 20 beats per minute and the systolic blood pressure drops more than 10 mm Hg after the patient sits upright from a supine position, it is likely that the blood loss has exceeded 1 L. Other manifestations of GI bleeding include coolness of the extremities secondary to vasoconstriction and pallor of the conjunctivae, mucous membranes, nailbeds, and palmar creases.

Etiology

Gastrointestinal bleeding generally is classified as either upper or lower in origin because the presenting signs and symptoms usually are characteristic for either an upper or lower GI source and because the source rarely is found to be in the jejunum or ileum. Anatomically, the boundary of differentiation is the ligament of Treitz. Gastrointestinal bleeding also may be divided into acute and chronic bleeding. The etiologic possibilities of GI bleeding are numerous. They may be divided into sources from the upper (Table 52-1) and lower (Table 52-2) GI tracts.

Some aspects of the history or presenting signs may favor one diagnosis over another. Vigorous upper GI bleeding is often associated with peptic ulcer disease or esophageal varices. The recent ingestion of aspirin, alcohol, or another ulcerogenic drug raises the possibility that erosive gastritis may be the cause of bleeding. A history of a known lesion that could bleed, such as peptic ulcer disease, ulcerative colitis, diverticulosis, and polyposis, may suggest the diagnosis. Historical information sometimes is misleading, however. For example, over half of bleeding patients with known esophageal varices will have another lesion of the upper GI tract that could account for the bleeding.

With respect to lower GI bleeding, the patient's age makes certain diagnoses more or less likely. In young people, acute bleeding per rectum is commonly due to colonic polyps, ulcerative colitis, or enteric bacterial or parasitic diseases. The most common causes of lower GI bleeding in patients over 60 years old are diverticulosis, ischemic bowel disease, angiodysplastic lesions of the colon, and carcinoma. In patients of all ages, the most common cause of rectal bleeding, hemorrhoids, must be considered.

Diagnostic Approach

In acute GI bleeding, the orderly sequence of history taking, physical examination, diagnostic evaluation, and treatment often is altered to meet the immediate demands, and the important aspects of each are carried out in the first critical moments of managing the patient (Fig. 52-1). After an intravenous catheter has been placed and saline or Ringer's lactate has been infused in anticipation of blood transfusions, the diagnostic evaluation may begin.

Table 52-1 Diagnostic Considerations in Upper Gastrointestinal Bleeding

Nose or pharyngeal bleeding	Leaking aortic aneurysm or vascular graft (usually in duodenum)
Hemoptysis	Hematobilia
Esophageal rupture (Boerhaave's syndrome)	Neoplasms
Esophagitis	Arterial-enteric fistulas
Esophageal ulcer	Vascular anomalies
Esophageal varices	Angiodysplasia
Esophageal carcinoma	Arteriovenous malformations
Esophagogastric mucosal tear (Mallory-Weiss syndrome)	Elastic tissue diseases
Gastritis	Pseudoxanthoma elasticum
Gastric ulcer	Ehlers-Danlos syndrome
Gastric varices	Vasculitis syndrome
Gastric carcinomas	Diverticulosis
Leiomyoma	Intussusception
Duodenitis	
Duodenal ulcer	
Duodenal varices	
Anastomotic ulcer (after gastroduodenostomy or gastrojejunostomy)	

Table 52-2 Diagnostic Considerations in Lower Gastrointestinal Bleeding

Hemorrhoids	Leaking aneurysm or vascular graft
Anal fissure or fistula	Brisk bleeding from an upper gastrointestinal source
Proctitis	Neoplasms
Inflammatory bowel disease (ulcerative colitis or Crohn's disease)	Arterial-enteric fistulas
Carcinoma of the rectum or colon	Vascular anomalies
Rectal or colonic polyps	Angiodysplasia
Diverticulosis	Arteriovenous malformations
Ischemic colitis	Elastic tissue diseases
Radiation colitis	Pseudoxanthoma elasticum
Antibiotic-associated colitis	Ehlers-Danlos syndrome
Amyloidosis	Vasculitis syndrome
Meckel's diverticulum	Diverticulosis
Intussusception	Solitary colonic ulcer

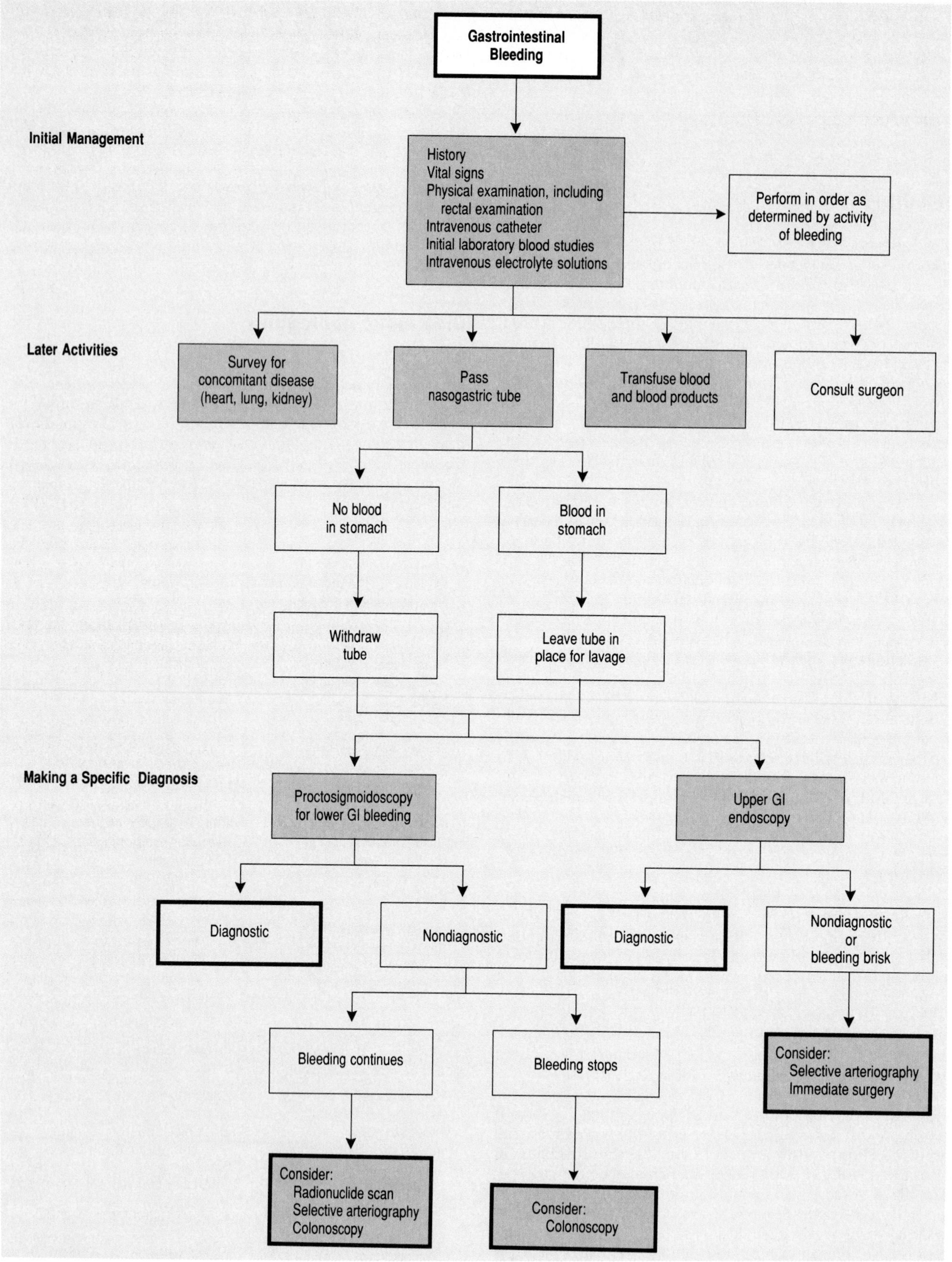

Figure 52-1 Algorithm for evaluation of gastrointestinal bleeding. GI = gastrointestinal.

Although acute GI bleeding is dramatic and is discussed in detail later, most of the diagnostic studies used in the evaluation of acute bleeding apply also to the evaluation of chronic bleeding, but in a less urgent manner.

Nonspecific Diagnostic Studies

The rectal examination provides direct access to the GI tract and should not be omitted in instances of seemingly obvious upper GI bleeding. Aside from information about the anus, perianal area, and possible rectal masses, the character of the stool can be confirmed. If the patient has vomited blood or coffee-ground material, yet the stool is brown or even negative for occult blood, that may indicate that the bleeding has been of brief duration.

A nasogastric tube should be passed and the patient placed in the left lateral decubitus position in all instances of acute GI bleeding, unless the patient has only passed small quantities of bright red blood per rectum, raising the good possibility of hemorrhoids or a rectal lesion. If the nasogastric aspirate is clear or clears readily with lavage, the tube may be removed. If there is fresh blood or a large amount of old blood or retained material, the stomach should be lavaged by means of a larger tube. Removal of as much clot and intragastric material as possible is important to allow the stomach walls to collapse and contribute to hemostasis. Moreover, a clean stomach facilitates subsequent endoscopy or barium swallow radiography.

Certain laboratory studies may help in the diagnosis of GI bleeding. The level of hemoglobin and hematocrit may have some relation to the degree of blood loss. However, the hemoglobin and hematocrit may be normal or only slightly reduced in patients who bleed so rapidly that there is not sufficient time for the blood volume to equilibrate. A low mean cell volume may suggest that the patient is iron deficient and the duration of blood loss has been prolonged. An elevated mean cell volume may indicate folate or vitamin B_{12} deficiency and raises the possibility of ethanol abuse, chronic liver disease, gastric cancer in association with pernicious anemia, or regional enteritis involving the terminal ileum. Clotting status should be assessed with platelet count, prothrombin time, and partial thromboplastin time. A moderate leukocytosis is sometimes associated with acute GI bleeding but usually does not exceed $15{,}000/mm^3$. However, leukocytosis should not be attributed to acute bleeding without first seeking sources of infection. Because blood in the upper GI tract may be digested and absorbed in the small intestine, an elevated blood urea nitrogen (BUN) in a patient who has recently had a normal BUN or who remains with a normal serum creatinine can be used as supportive evidence for an upper GI source for the bleeding. Finally, because body fluids and electrolytes are affected by GI bleeding and the infusion of blood and other fluids, frequent assessment of serum electrolytes, hemoglobin, and hematocrit is necessary.

Specific Diagnostic Studies

Endoscopy

Although upper GI endoscopy is diagnostically superior to upper GI x-ray studies, there is no good evidence that early endoscopy of patients who are acutely bleeding results in reduced morbidity or mortality. Nevertheless, most physicians agree that endoscopy should be the first specific diagnostic study in patients who appear to be bleeding from the upper GI tract. Certainly, knowledge of the bleeding lesion may dictate specific therapy. For example, the treatment of bleeding esophageal varices is different from the treatment for peptic ulcer disease. Further, the endoscopic identification of the so-called stigmata of recent hemorrhage within an ulcer crater may have some prognostic and therapeutic significance. Stigmata include a protruding visible vessel, an adherent clot, a black eschar, and actual oozing or spurting of blood. Patients with these stigmata are more likely to have uncontrolled bleeding or recurrent bleeding and to require intervention by therapeutic endoscopy or surgery. Finally, if the patient bleeds sufficiently to require surgical treatment, a precise diagnosis often will aid the surgeon in determining the most effective operation.

Numerous endoscopic methods have been used to treat GI bleeding, including laser photocoagulation, thermal electrocoagulation, and injection of epinephrine, ethanol, hypertonic solutions, or sclerosing agents. Currently, the strongest enthusiasm is for endoscopic injection sclerosis of bleeding esophageal varices.

The initial specific diagnostic procedure for acute lower GI bleeding is proctosigmoidoscopy. The role of fiberoptic colonoscopy in lower GI bleeding is still somewhat controversial, as blood and stool tend to obscure visibility. Recently, osmotically balanced electrolyte solutions, administered orally or by nasogastric tube, have been used to lavage the colon in preparation for colonoscopy.

Selective Arteriography

Extravasation of dye at the bleeding site may be visualized by selective arteriography of the celiac axis, superior mesenteric artery, inferior mesenteric artery, or their branches. In order for the dye to be visualized, the rate of bleeding must be on the order of 0.5 to 1.0 ml per minute. A focal collection of extravasated dye indicates a bleeding arterial lesion. A diffuse blush in the region of the stomach may indicate hemorrhagic gastritis. During the venous phase, gastric or esophageal varices may be seen, although actual bleeding from the varices usually is not apparent.

When a bleeding lesion is identified by arteriography, infusion of vasopressin to constrict arterioles or injection of autologous clot or small pieces of Gelfoam to embolize arteries that supply the bleeding sites may control the bleeding.

Radionuclide Scanning

If a patient's red blood cells or other blood components are labeled with a radionuclide marker, scanning of the abdomen may indicate the site of bleeding. The rate of blood loss required to make a diagnosis is much less than that for selective arteriography, on the order of 0.1 ml/mm. The value of the radionuclide scan is not in making a specific diagnosis but in indicating the site of bleeding in order to apply other diagnostic studies.

Barium Contrast Radiography

Upper GI x-ray series and barium enema usually provide a lower diagnostic yield than endoscopic methods. Further, if one contemplates using either endoscopy, arteriography, or radionuclide scanning during the early evaluation of the bleeding patient, barium within the GI tract may render these studies uninterpretable. For these reasons, barium contrast radiography usually is not the initial diagnostic procedure in patients with active bleeding. After a patient has been stabilized, however, an upper GI x-ray series or barium enema may be indicated in the further evaluation of the patient.

References

Alavi A. Detection of gastrointestinal bleeding with ^{99m}Tc-sulfur colloid. Semin Nucl Med 1982; 12:126.

Athanasoulis CA. Therapeutic applications of angiography. N Engl J Med 1980; 302:1117.

Caos A, et al. Colonoscopy after Golytely preparation in acute rectal bleeding. J Clin Gastroenterol 1986; 8:46.

Eastwood GL. Gastrointestinal bleeding. In: Stein JH, et al, eds. Internal medicine: A systematic approach. 3rd ed. Boston: Little, Brown, 1990:299.

Eastwood GL, Avunduk C. Gastrointestinal bleeding. In: Manual of gastroenterology: Diagnosis and therapy. Boston: Little, Brown, 1988.

Storey DW, et al. Endoscopic prediction of recurrent bleeding in peptic ulcers. N Engl J Med 1981; 305:915.

Jaundice

John K. Zawacki, MD

53

Definition

Jaundice may be defined as the yellowing of the skin or sclera in association with an elevation in serum bilirubin. Jaundice is clinically apparent when the serum bilirubin level is 2.0 to 3.0 mg/dl.

Etiology

The causes of jaundice and hyperbilirubinemia are many. Any disorder that affects bilirubin production or the uptake, conjugation, and secretion of bilirubin by the hepatocyte may result in hyperbilirubinemia. If the abnormality occurs prior to the conjugation of bilirubin with glucuronic acid, an *unconjugated* hyperbilirubinemia results that is reflected by an increase in the *indirect* fraction of the serum bilirubin. Impairment of either the secretion of conjugated bilirubin into the canalicular lumen of the hepatocyte or the flow of bile within the biliary tree results in a *conjugated* hyperbilirubinemia, which is reflected by an elevation of the *direct* fraction of the serum bilirubin. Causes of unconjugated and conjugated hyperbilirubinemia are listed in Table 53-1.

It is customary and clinically useful to characterize jaundice as being hemolytic, hepatocellular, or cholestatic. It is also helpful to categorize hepatocellular jaundice as being either acute or chronic and cholestatic jaundice as being either intrahepatic or extrahepatic.

Hemolytic jaundice is characterized by unconjugated hyperbilirubinemia, whereas hepatocellular and cholestatic jaundice are characterized by conjugated hyperbilirubinemia; i.e., the direct fraction of bilirubin equals or exceeds the indirect fraction.

Unconjugated hyperbilirubinemia characterizes all the entities listed in the left-hand column of Table 53-1. These disorders are grouped under the hemolytic pattern of liver function test abnormalities (see Chapter 55, "Abnormal Liver Function Tests"). The most important cause of unconjugated hyperbilirubinemia is overproduction, most commonly caused by hemolysis, both intra- and extravascular. Other listed causes of increased unconjugated hyperbilirubinemia include nonhemolytic mechanisms such as competition with bilirubin for albumin transport within the serum, impaired bilirubin uptake, and diminished bilirubin conjugation by the hepatocyte. The disorders listed in the right-hand column of Table 53-1 may present as an isolated bilirubin elevation, such as Dubin-Johnson and Rotor's syndromes, or more commonly, with liver function test abnormalities that reflect either an acute or a chronic hepatocellular process or a cholestatic pattern of liver injury (see Chapter 55).

A variety of agents, including viruses, ethanol, and drugs, may injure the hepatocyte and result in impaired secretion of conjugated bilirubin into the canalicular lumen. In these patients, a conjugated hyperbilirubinemia and leakage of mitochondrial and cytosol enzymes into the serum occurs and results in a hepatocellular pattern of liver injury (see Chapter 55 and Table 53-2).

Diagnostic Approach

The jaundiced patient represents a diagnostic challenge that is best approached with a careful history, physical examination, and appropriate laboratory testing. The accuracy of differentiating the various causes of jaundice by this approach is 70 to 90 percent. This section focuses on the history and physical examination as well as on how to utilize the many diagnostic tests and procedures available to the physician to make a specific diagnosis.

Jaundice usually connotes hepatobiliary disease; however, jaundice may reflect an increased bilirubin load from such sources as hemolysis, multiple blood transfusions, or ineffective erythropoiesis. A history of familial jaundice, gallstones, or anemia, together with the absence of dark urine, i.e., bilirubinuria, increases the probability of a hemolytic type of jaundice.

A history of sporadic jaundice occurring in a young adult in association with stress, fasting, or viral illness suggests a diagnosis of Gilbert's syndrome. A diagnosis of this familial defect in bilirubin uptake and conjugation is made by demonstrating an unconjugated hyperbilirubinemia in conjunction with normal

Table 53-1 Causes of Hyperbilirubinemia

Unconjugated	Conjugated
Hemolytic anemia* (hemoglobinopathies, enzyme deficiencies, autoimmune)	Viral hepatitis (hep A,* B,* C,* delta)
Gilbert's syndrome*	Chronic hepatitis*
Crigler-Najjar syndrome	Drug-induced liver injury*
Ineffective erythropoiesis (megaloblastic anemia, thalassemia)	Alcohol-induced liver injury (fatty liver, hepatitis, cirrhosis)
Chronic persistent hepatitis	Cholecystitis*
Blood transfusion	Choledocholithiasis*
Fasting	Cirrhosis*
Drugs (rifampin, gallbladder dye)	Dubin-Johnson syndrome
Neonatal	Rotor's syndrome
Hematoma	Sepsis
	Postoperative jaundice
	Parenteral nutrition

* Indicates the most common causes.

Table 53-2 Causes of Cholestasis

Extrahepatic	Intrahepatic
Biliary Tree	Drugs
Gallstone	Hormones
Stricture	Pregnancy
Cyst	Viral hepatitis
Carcinoma	Alcoholic hepatitis
Bile duct	Hodgkin's disease
Ampulla of Vater	Sarcoidosis
Lymph node involvement	Primary biliary cirrhosis
	Sepsis
Pancreas	Parenteral nutrition
Carcinoma	Postoperative
Pseudocyst	
Chronic pancreatitis	

liver function tests and the absence of laboratory evidence for hemolysis, e.g., anemia, reticulocytosis, and decreased serum hepatoglobin. A significant rise, i.e., doubling, in unconjugated bilirubin with fasting helps to confirm the diagnosis.

A familial defect in bilirubin transport and secretion, such as the Dubin-Johnson syndrome or Rotor's syndrome, is suggested by a family history of jaundice, a conjugated hyperbilirubinemia, and otherwise normal liver function tests. Differentiation between the two entities is made by a rise in the bromsulphalein (BSP) dye test between 45 and 90 minutes in the Dubin-Johnson syndrome and an increase in the 24-hour urine total coproporphyrin level in Rotor's syndrome.

A history of ethanol usage, drug abuse, prior blood or blood-product transfusions, known exposure to viral hepatitis, or the recent development of hypotension or congestive failure in a recently jaundiced patient argues for an acute hepatocellular process. A history of long-term ethanol abuse or the demonstration of an enlarged spleen, spider angiomata, gynecomastia, ascites, or a prominent abdominal venous pattern strongly suggests a chronic hepatocellular injury.

Weight loss in association with an enlarged liver would suggest an infiltrative disorder such as a metastatic cancer.

Perhaps the primary goal when evaluating a jaundiced patient is to differentiate "surgical" jaundice from "medical" jaundice or, stated more physiologically, to differentiate extrahepatic cholestasis from intrahepatic cholestasis. This differentiation is very important, for although surgery is curative or palliative in the former, it may be a source of increased morbidity and mortality in the latter.

Historical facts favoring an extrahepatic process include older age, abdominal pain, chills and fever, clay-colored stools, and prior biliary tract surgery. A history favoring an intrahepatic cholestatic process includes younger age, anorexia, use or abuse of drugs, and exposure to viral hepatitis.

The single most helpful physical sign of extrahepatic cholestasis is a palpable gallbladder. This results in a certain diagnosis of "surgical" jaundice. Physical signs favoring an intrahepatic cholestasis include stigmata of chronic liver disease, xanthelasma or xanthomata, a markedly enlarged liver, splenomegaly, and a friction rub or bruit over the liver.

Physicians rely heavily on liver function testing when evaluating a jaundiced patient (see Chapter 55, "Abnormal Liver Function Tests"). Whether history and physical examination are performed before, during, or after obtaining routine liver function tests is not as important as interpreting these tests within the context of a good history and physical exam. Integration of these three components maximizes the physician's chance of correctly identifying the cause of a patient's jaundice. For example, a young male health care worker with a liver function test pattern for acute hepatocellular injury and a positive hepatitis B surface antigen and anti-hepatitis B core antigen has an acute type B viral hepatitis to explain his recent onset of jaundice. A liver biopsy would confirm the clinical impression, but it is not indicated in this setting.

Frequently, proper integration of the history, physical examination, and pattern of liver cell dysfunction results in the identification of a particular type of jaundice but fails to establish a specific cause for the jaundice. For example, a jaundiced, middle-aged woman with recent weight loss, a history of cholecystectomy, and a liver alkaline phosphatase more than four times normal has a cholestatic type of jaundice. Possible causes for her cholestatic jaundice include choledocholithiasis, a biliary stricture, biliary tract neoplasm, primary biliary cirrhosis, and metastatic liver injury.

Figure 53-1 summarizes an approach to the jaundiced patient in whom a specific cause is lacking after the proper performance of a history, physical examination, and routine liver function testing. A detailed discussion of these multiple tests and procedures is beyond the scope of this chapter, but the following statements regarding each of these modalities are appropriate.

Ultrasonography

Ultrasonography is noninvasive, relatively inexpensive, and especially sensitive (85 percent) in detecting ductal dilatation associated with biliary tract obstruction. It is the initial diagnostic test in the evaluation of a patient with cholestatic jaundice. Ultrasonography is a sensitive test (90 percent) for detecting cholelithiasis and can also be employed to direct a needle biopsy of an intra-abdominal mass. The limiting factor of this test is the experience of the ultrasonographer. It is important to remember that extrahepatic biliary obstruction may occur in the presence of ultrasonically demonstrated normal-sized bile ducts.

Computed Tomography

The sensitivity of computed tomography (CT) is comparable to that of ultrasonography in demonstrating the dilated bile ducts associated with extrahepatic cholestasis; however, its greater expense and associated radiation exposure make it a less desirable procedure than ultrasonography for the evaluation of a patient with cholestatic jaundice. CT is a good test for pancreatic cancer and other abdominal masses. It is more sensitive than radionuclide scanning in demonstrating hepatic tumors or metastasis.

Magnetic Resonance Imaging

Magnetic resonance imaging (MRI) may be more sensitive than CT scanning in the differentiation of metastasis, hemangiomas, and other liver lesions from the liver parenchyma. It does not expose the patient to x-radiation; however, the procedure is lengthy and requires the patient to stay motionless for a prolonged period.

Percutaneous Transhepatic Cholangiography

Percutaneous transhepatic cholangiography (PTC) is accomplished by inserting a 23-gauge needle into the liver under fluoroscopic guidance. Aspiration is performed during needle withdrawal and a dye is injected once bile is aspirated. This test is 90 to 100 percent effective in demonstrating the biliary tree in the presence of dilated intrahepatic bile ducts. The success rate is reduced to 50 to 70 percent with nondilated intrahepatic bile ducts. PTC is relatively inexpensive and has a false positivity of 1 percent and a false negativity of 5 percent. Morbidity and mortality from this procedure are acceptable at 5 percent and 0.5 percent, respectively. PTC is the procedure of choice in visualizing the biliary tree in a patient with cholestatic jaundice and dilated intrahepatic bile ducts by ultrasonography. This same technique can be utilized in selected patients with jaundice to perform a therapeutic maneuver such as placement of a biliary stent for drainage in a patient with malignant obstruction of the biliary tree.

Endoscopic Retrograde Cholangiopancreatography

Endoscopic retrograde cholangiopancreatography (ERCP) is accomplished by endoscopically visualizing the ampulla of Vater and injecting a radiopaque dye through a catheter that has been advanced into the ampulla. Both the pancreatic and common bile ducts can be visualized successfully. In experienced hands, this can be accomplished 80 to 90 percent of the time. ERCP is especially helpful in a patient with cholestatic jaundice and normal-sized intrahepatic bile ducts, as detected by ultrasonography. Although complications occur less frequently and are less severe than with PTC, ERCP is a more expensive test. Following ERCP, a therapeutic manipulation may also be accomplished in selected patients, e.g., endoscopic sphincterotomy to allow passage of a stone obstructing the common bile duct.

Radionuclide Scanning

Technetium-99m Sulfur Colloid

Tc-99m sulfur colloid scanning depends on the uptake of Tc-99m sulfur colloid by the Kupffer cells of the liver. Space-occupying lesions such as liver abscesses, cysts, and primary and metastatic tumors appear as filling defects, whereas chronic hepatocellular disease with portal hypertension is associated with patchy uptake of the nuclide and increased uptake by the spleen and bone marrow. This test is limited by its ineffectiveness in demonstrating small space-occupying lesions (those less than 2 cm) and by its moderate expense. It is most helpful in estimating liver size and in implicating the presence of cirrhosis in a patient with normal or abnormal liver function tests.

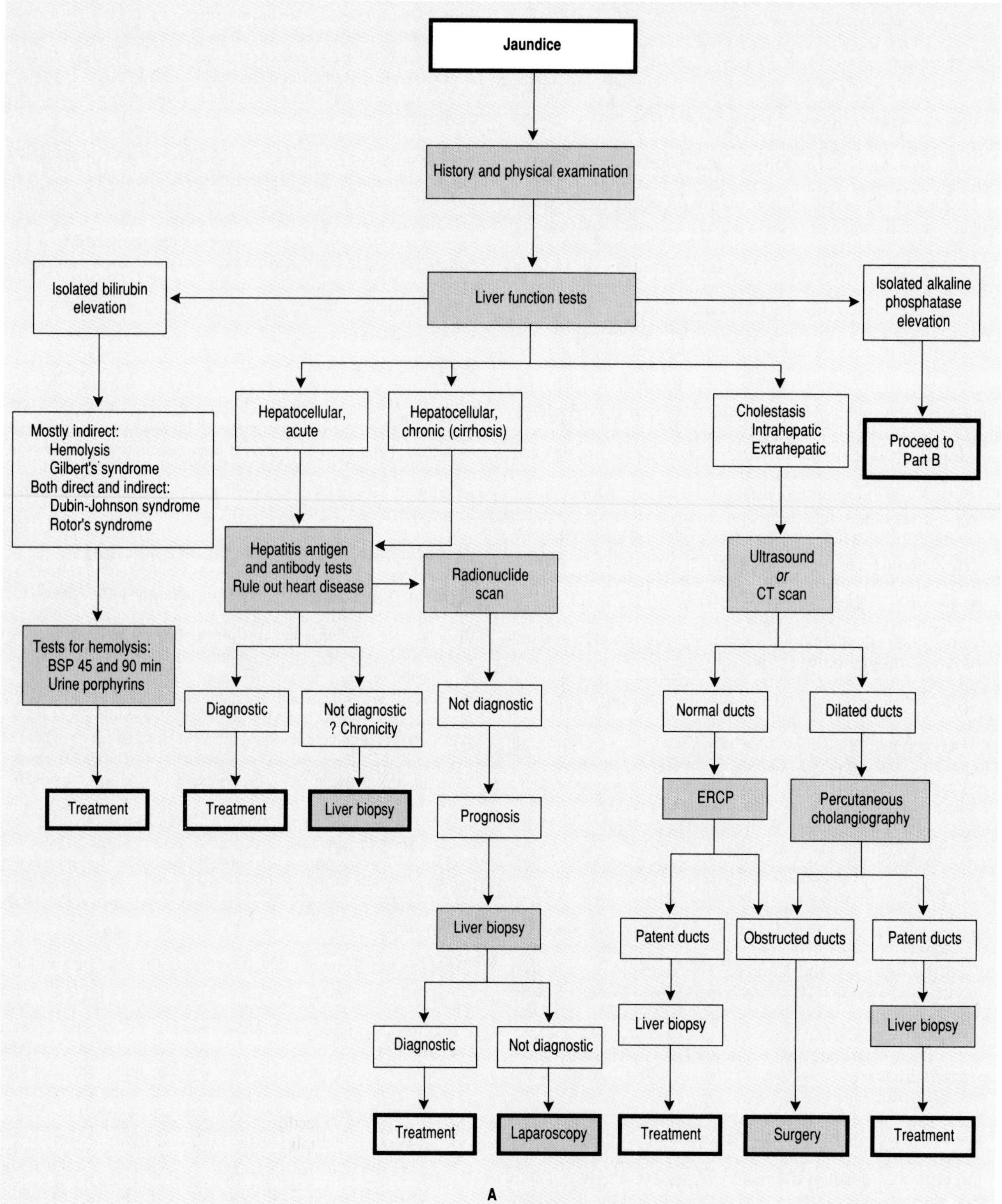

A

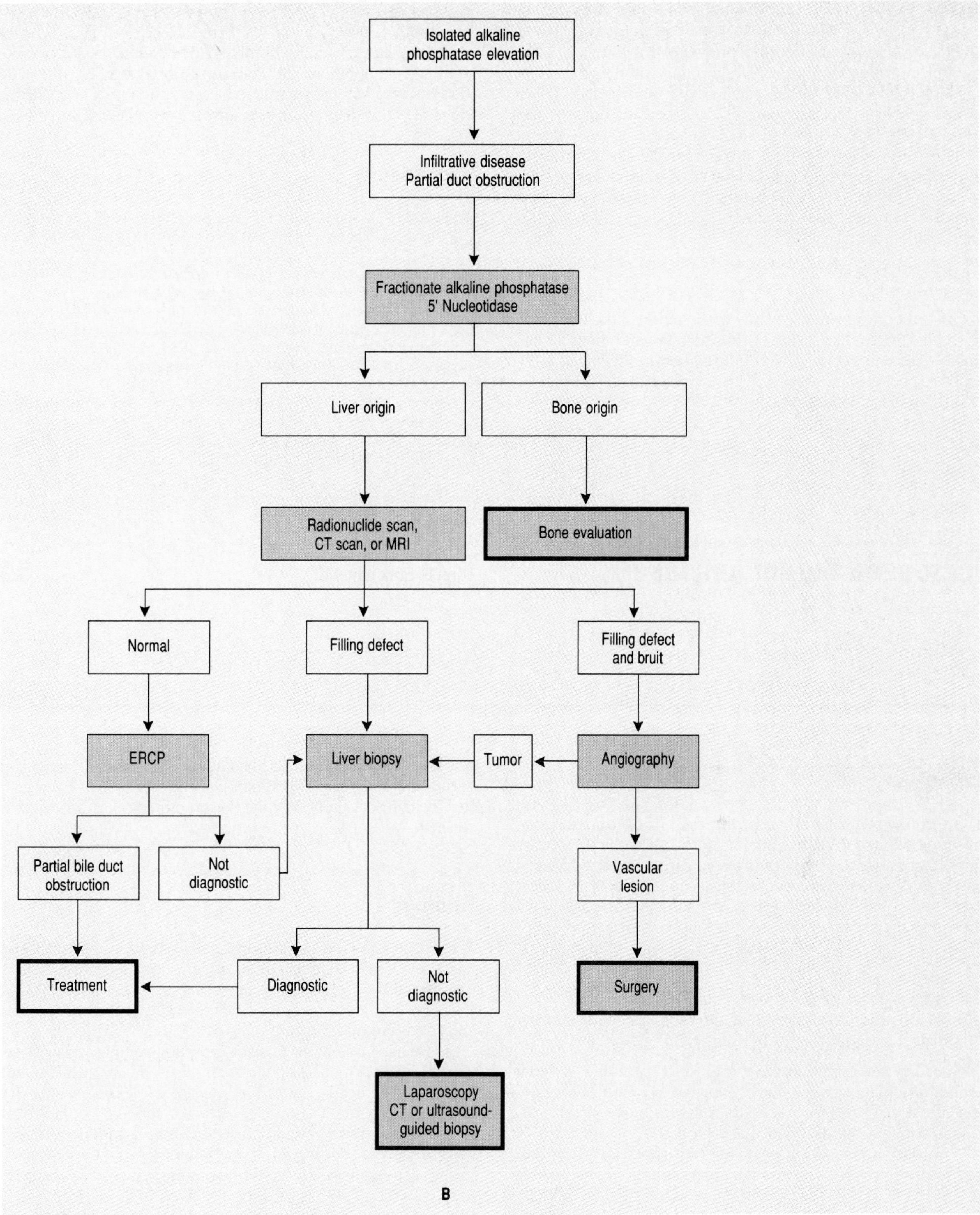

Figure 53-1 Algorithms for the clinical approach to the patient with jaundice. BSP = bromsulphalein dye test, CT = computed tomography, ERCP = endoscopic retrograde cholangiopancreatography, MRI = magnetic resonance imaging.

Technetium-99m HIDA Scan

Tc-99m–labeled diethyl acetanilid iminodiacetic acid (HIDA) is a substance that can undergo rapid uptake and secretion by the hepatocyte, even in the presence of an elevated bilirubin level. This nuclide normally enters the gallbladder within 45 minutes after intravenous injection. Failure to visualize the gallbladder within 45 minutes implies complete or partial obstruction of the cystic duct, a condition associated with acute or chronic cholecystitis. However, the test is of no value in differentiating intrahepatic from extrahepatic cholestasis.

Gastroenterology

Liver Biopsy

Liver biopsy is a safe bedside procedure of low cost that is helpful in evaluating hepatocellular injury of unknown cause, hepatomegaly, fever of unknown origin, and hepatic defects demonstrable by ultrasonography, CT, or radionuclide scanning. A 2-cm piece of liver tissue is needed to ensure accurate diagnosis; however, a sampling error can be expected 10 percent of the time, despite an adequate amount of tissue. Liver biopsy is very helpful in evaluating the patient with cholestatic jaundice, but only after extrahepatic bile duct obstruction has been ruled out.

Peritoneoscopy

Peritoneoscopy permits accurate visualization of the liver and is most effective in diagnosing cirrhosis when other methods have failed. Peritoneoscopy is also utilized when other tests fail to make a specific diagnosis for the cause of a patient's jaundice or abnormal liver function tests.

Angiography

Portal angiography is rarely utilized in seeking a specific cause of jaundice. It is helpful in evaluating portal hypertension and determining whether a vascular lesion such as a neoplasm is present within the liver and is surgically resectable.

References

Eastwood GL, Avunduk C. Jaundice and interpretation of laboratory liver tests. In: Manual of gastroenterology: Diagnosis and therapy. Boston: Little, Brown, 1988:253.

Kaplan MM. Evaluation of hepatobiliary disease. In: Stein JH, ed. Internal medicine. 2nd ed. Boston: Little, Brown, 1987.

O'Connor KW, et al. A blinded prospective study comparing four current non-invasive approaches in the differential diagnosis of medical vs. surgical jaundice. Gastroenterology 1983; 84:1498.

Scharschmidt BF, Goldberg HI, Schmid R. Approach to the patient with cholestatic jaundice. N Engl J Med 1983; 308:1515.

Schenker S, Balint J, Schiff L. Differential diagnosis of jaundice: Report of a prospective study of 61 proved cases. Am J Dig Dis 1962; 7:449.

Schiff ER. Jaundice: A clinical approach. In: Schiff L, Schiff ER. Diseases of the liver. 6th ed. Philadelphia: JB Lippincott, 1987.

Increased Serum Amylase

John F. Erkkinen, MD

54

Definition

The term *amylase* is derived from the Greek word *amylon*, meaning starch. Amylase, which is produced by the pancreas, is important in the digestion of ingested carbohydrates. Although amylase is normally present in the serum (and urine), an elevated serum amylase level represents a diagnostic challenge to the clinician, who must address the following questions:

1. Is the elevated serum amylase associated with disease or a normal variant?
2. What is the anatomic source of the amylase?
3. What is the pathophysiologic process causing this abnormality?

An elevated serum amylase level is not harmful; it is significant in providing a clue to the presence of a variety of illnesses. In general, a serum amylase reading should be obtained in any patient with abdominal pain of unclear cause.

Amylase in the serum exists in two forms; a P-type amylase derived exclusively from the pancreas, and an S-type amylase derived from a variety of other organs (salivary glands, fallopian tubes, ovary, lung, prostate, and possibly liver). In a normal, healthy person, the majority of circulating amylase is of the S type, although the proportion of P-type and S-type amylase varies from person to person. S-type amylase is metabolized predominantly by the reticuloendothelial system, whereas the majority of P-type amylase is excreted via the kidneys. Both are cleared rapidly, with a half-life of approximately 130 minutes.

The serum amylase is most helpful in the evaluation of a patient with suspected pancreatitis. Although usually elevated early in its course, false-negative values (e.g., normal serum amylase in a patient with pancreatitis) may occur, because P-type amylase is cleared quickly through the kidneys. Concomitant serum lipase determination may clarify the diagnosis because it may remain elevated after the serum amylase has returned to normal.

Etiology

The causes of an elevated serum amylase level are many (Table 54-1) and must be interpreted along with the entire clinical picture (history, physical examination, other laboratory tests). Only the most common causes of increased serum amylase are considered in this chapter.

The most common cause of hyperamylasemia is pancreatitis, which is most often due to alcoholism, biliary tract disease, and drugs. Typically, the serum amylase is elevated within the first 2 to 12 hours and remains elevated for 6 to 10 days. The height of the amylase rise in acute pancreatitis does not seem to carry any prognostic significance.

Gallstone disease is the most common cause of pancreatitis in middle-aged women and may be associated with very high levels of serum amylase. Biliary colic due to gallbladder disease may be associated with hyperamylasemia in the absence of pancreatitis. The explanation for this phenomenon is unknown.

Drugs have been implicated as an etiology of pancreatitis. Although many have been associated with pancreatitis, only a few have been unequivocally established as a cause. These include azathioprine, thiazide diuretics, estrogens, furosemide, sulfonamides, and tetracycline.

Surgical and nonsurgical (blunt and penetrating) abdominal trauma are other common causes of pancreatitis. Postoperative pancreatitis most often follows surgery involving the stom-

Table 54-1 Causes of Hyperamylasemia or Hyperamylasuria

Pancreatic Disease

- Pancreatitis
  - Acute
    - Common causes (alcoholism, gallbladder disease, etc.)
    - Uncommon (vasculitis, uremia, etc.)
    - Drug induced
    - Viral (hepatitis vs. other)
    - Postendoscopy
    - Postoperative
    - Renal transplantation
  - Chronic
  - Complications
    - Pseudocyst
    - Ascites
    - Abscess
- Pancreatic carcinoma
- Pancreatic trauma

Disorders of Nonpancreatic Origin (Mechanism Known)

- Renal insufficiency
- Salivary-type hyperamylasemia
- "Tumor" hyperamylasemia
- Salivary gland lesions
  - Mumps
  - Calculus
  - Irradiation sialadenitis
  - Maxillofacial surgery
- Macroamylasemia

Disorders of Complex Origin (Mechanism Unknown or Uncertain)

- Biliary tract disease
- Intra-abdominal disease other than pancreatitis
  - Perforated peptic ulcer
  - Intestinal obstruction
  - Ruptured ectopic pregnancy
  - Mesenteric infarction
  - Afferent loop syndrome
  - Aortic aneurysm with dissection
  - Peritonitis
  - Acute appendicitis
- Cerebral trauma
- Burns and traumatic shock
- Postoperative hyperamylasemia
- Diabetic ketoacidosis
- Renal transplantation
- Pneumonia
- Prostatic disease
- Pregnancy

From Salt WB, Schenker S. Amylase—its clinical significance: A review of the literature. Medicine 1976; 55:273; © by Williams & Wilkins; with permission.)

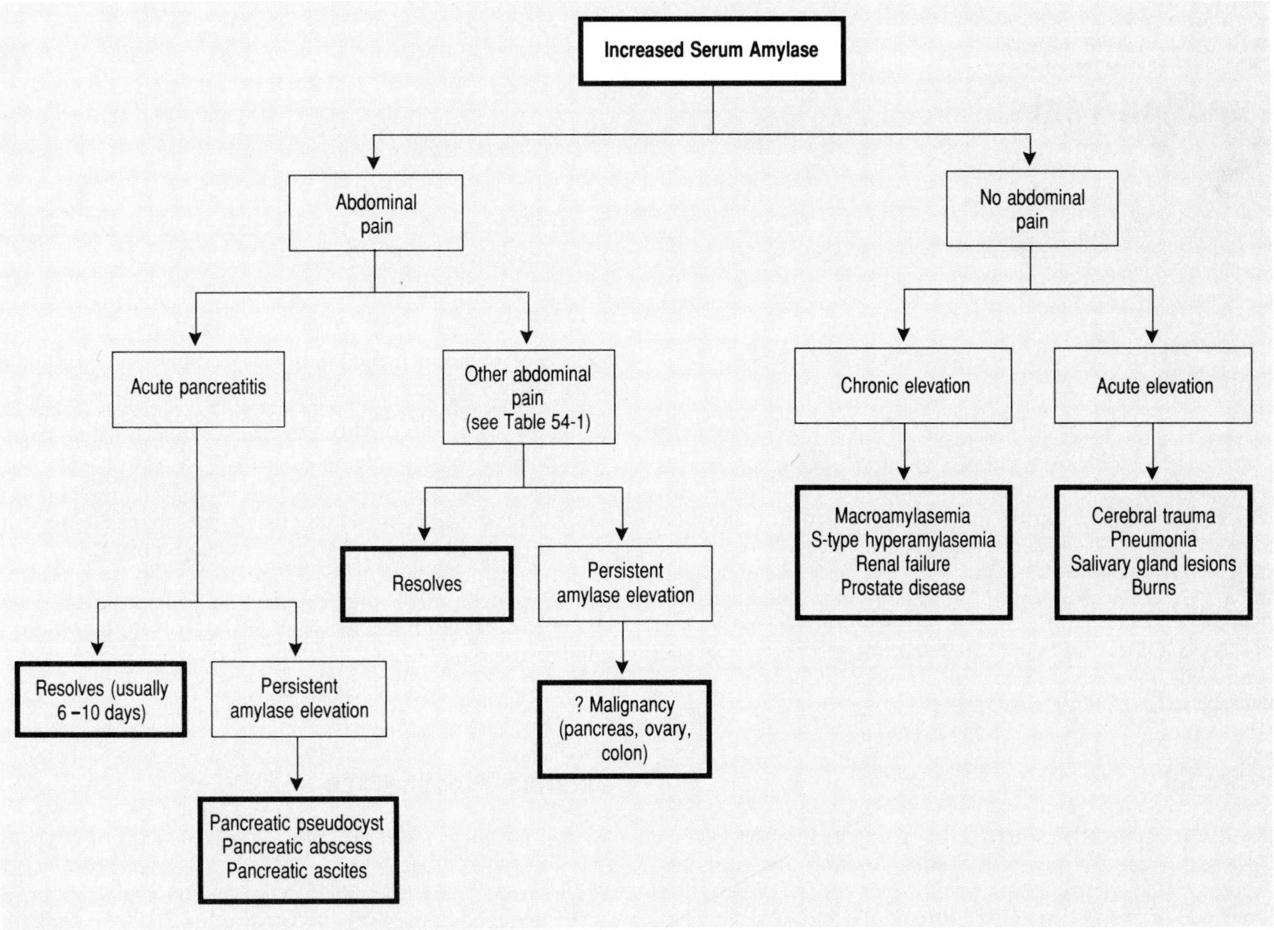

Figure 54-1 Algorithm for a diagnostic approach to increased serum amylase.

ach, duodenum, or biliary tract. Penetrating trauma (gunshot, stab wounds, and so forth) is frequently associated with injury to other internal organs. Automobile accidents and contact sports (e.g., hockey, football) are common causes of blunt trauma–induced pancreatitis.

A persistently elevated amylase level following an episode of pancreatitis may be a clue to the development of pancreatic pseudocyst, pancreatic abscess, or pancreatic ascites.

It is important to be aware of the other causes of an elevated amylase level listed in Table 54-1. The list is extensive, so only a few salient points are emphasized here.

The discovery of an elevated serum amylase level in an asymptomatic patient or in a patient in whom more usual causes of pancreatitis seem unlikely should suggest the possibility of "macroamylasemia" (Fig. 54-1). Macroamylasemia is a usually chronic benign elevation of serum amylase; it is found in approximately 1 to 2 percent of apparently healthy adults. The serum amylase increases because it is bound to circulating globulin complexes that are too large to be easily excreted. In an asymptomatic person with hyperamylasemia, a low urinary amylase level should suggest this entity, which can be confirmed with a serum macroamylase determination. In addition, a few patients with asymptomatic S-type (no macroamylase) hyperamylasemia have been identified.

Another cause of false-positive hyperamylasemia is renal failure. A modest elevation of serum amylase may result from inadequate renal clearance of amylase due to a decreased glomerular filtration rate. Hyperamylasemia in this setting is invariably less than twice the upper limits of normal.

Summary

An elevated serum amylase level occurs in a variety of circumstances. In the setting of abdominal pain, hyperamylasemia should suggest pancreatitis, but other abdominal conditions (e.g., cholangitis, mesenteric infarction, perforated ulcer) may also be implicated. In the patient without abdominal pain or with chronic hyperamylasemia, nonabdominal causes (e.g., renal failure, diseases of the salivary glands, macroamylasemia) should be considered (see Fig. 54-1). Specific measurement of serum lipase, serum pancreatic isoenzymes (P-type versus S-type urinary amylase), or serum macroamylase determination may help in making this distinction.

References

Berk JE. Amylase in diagnosis of pancreatic disease. Ann Intern Med 1978; 88:838.

Levitt MD, Ellis CJ, Meier PB. Extrapancreatic origin of chronic unexplained hyperamylase. N Engl J Med 1980; 302:670.

Salt WB, Schenker S. Amylase—its clinical significance: A review of the literature. Medicine 1976; 55:269.

Soergel KH. Acute pancreatitis. In: Sleisenger MH, Fordtran JS, eds. Gastrointestinal disease. 4th ed. Philadelphia: WB Saunders, 1989:1814.

55 Abnormal Liver Function Tests

John K. Zawacki, MD

Definition

An abnormal liver function test may be defined as an elevation or a decrease in the serum concentration of a substance that is associated with liver cell function or injury. This chapter discusses abnormalities of the routinely measured liver function tests—bilirubin, alkaline phosphatase, aminotransferase, lactic dehydrogenase, and albumin. Hepatitis B surface antigen (HBsAg), cholesterol, and prothrombin time, although frequently obtained in the evaluation of a jaundiced patient, are not discussed. Of the routinely ordered laboratory tests, only the serum bilirubin and albumin actually measure functions of the liver, namely, excretion and synthesis, respectively.

Bilirubin

Normal bilirubin values are 0.2 to 1.2 mg/dl (total) and 0 to 0.4 mg/dl (direct). The total serum bilirubin value routinely reported by a hospital or commercial laboratory is composed of *direct* and *indirect* fractions that correspond to *conjugated* and *unconjugated* bilirubin, respectively (see Chapter 53, "Jaundice"). An elevation of total serum bilirubin is indication for fractionation into its two components. If the indirect fraction is more than 85 percent of the total bilirubin, one should suspect hemolysis or another cause of unconjugated hyperbilirubinemia. Predominance of the direct fraction suggests hepatobiliary disease. In the presence of known hepatobiliary disease, fractionation of the total serum bilirubin is seldom a helpful test, because most hepatobiliary diseases result in an elevation in both direct and indirect fractions. A persistently rising total serum bilirubin signifies moderate to severe liver disease. However, significant liver disease may still exist in the presence of a normal serum bilirubin. Neither the total serum bilirubin nor its fractionation into its direct and indirect components results in a specific diagnosis.

Alkaline Phosphatase

Normal alkaline phosphatase values are 40 to 200 IU/L (15 to 20 years) and 35 to 125 IU/L (20 to 101 years). Alkaline phosphatase (ALP) is an enzyme present in high concentration in or about the canalicular membrane of the hepatocyte and the cell membrane of biliary cells. ALP is also present in bone. An ALP elevation more than four times normal is an excellent indicator of chole-

Table 55-1 Causes of an Isolated Alkaline Phosphatase Elevation

Primary or metastatic tumor of liver or bone	Hepatic abscess
Hepatic granuloma	Congestive heart failure
Hodgkin's disease	Hyperthyroidism
Inflammatory bowel disease	Diabetes
Primary biliary cirrhosis	Any bone disease with rapid turnover

stasis of either the intrahepatic or extrahepatic type (see Chapter 53, "Jaundice"), but it may also occur in bone disease. Fractionation of ALP into its bone and hepatic components helps identify the source of an elevated serum level. A concomitantly elevated 5′ nucleotidase or a gamma glutamyl transpeptidase (GGT) determination is also helpful in identifying the origin of an elevated serum ALP. An elevation of either of these two enzymes indicates a hepatic origin. An ALP elevation is most commonly associated with other abnormalities in liver function tests. An isolated ALP elevation may be seen in a variety of disorders (Table 55-1).

Aminotransferases

Aspartate aminotransferase (normal value: 7 to 40 U/L) and alanine aminotransferase (normal value: 7 to 40 U/L) are two of many hepatocellular enzymes that are often elevated in patients with hepatobiliary disease. Aspartate aminotransferase (AST) is also found in a variety of muscles (skeletal, heart) and is elevated with muscle injury. Alanine aminotransferase (ALT), unlike AST, is found almost exclusively in the liver and is therefore a more specific indicator of liver cell injury. When confronted with an elevation in serum AST, it is customary to repeat the AST determination together with a simultaneous ALT determination in an attempt to establish a hepatic origin of the AST rise. Serum elevation of both these enzymes reflects leakage from injured hepatocytes and is a sensitive indicator of liver cell injury.

Aminotransferases are most helpful in differentiating hepatocellular injury from cholestasis. Persistently high serum levels of greater than 400 U/L favor generalized hepatocellular injury, such as acute viral hepatitis, even though these high serum levels do not correlate well with the degree of liver cell death. Aminotransferase levels in the thousands may be associated with hypotension, acute heart failure, drug or viral hepatitis, exposure to hepatotoxins, and chronic active hepatitis. Cholestasis is ordinarily associated with aminotransferase values of less than 400 U/L; however, if there is an extrahepatic cause for cholestasis, such as acute biliary obstruction, transient elevations of both AST and ALT to levels greater than 400 U/L may occur. Aminotransferase levels of less than 400 U/L may be seen in a variety of mild hepatocellular injuries resulting from various causes, including virus, drug, alcohol, cirrhosis, and primary or metastatic tumor. An AST/ALT ratio greater than 2 favors diagnosis of alcohol-induced hepatitis or cirrhosis.

Lactate Dehydrogenase

The normal value of lactate dehydrogenase (LDH) is 20 to 225 U/L. LDH may be found in heart muscle, skeletal muscle, red blood cells, and hepatocytes. An LDH elevation is therefore nonspecific and may reflect injury to any of these tissues. A marked rise in LDH, with or without other liver function test abnormalities, may reflect metastatic liver disease.

Albumin

The normal albumin value is 3.5 to 5.0 g/dl. Approximately 10 g of albumin is formed each day by the liver. The half-life of serum albumin is 20 days. This latter fact explains a normal serum albumin level during a severe acute hepatocellular liver injury such as viral hepatitis. Although the serum albumin may be normal with inactive cirrhosis, chronic hepatocellular injury diminishes the liver's capacity to synthesize albumin. Thus, a low serum albumin value may reflect chronic hepatocellular injury; however, hypoalbuminemia may also occur because of protein loss through the intestinal and urinary tracts or through inadequate dietary intake of protein. This explains the hypoalbuminemia associated with inflammatory bowel disease, nephrotic syndrome, and malnutrition. Serum albumin level is neither a sensitive nor a specific test of liver function. Its primary value is in connoting chronicity to clinically evident hepatobiliary disease.

Diagnostic Approach

When confronted with an abnormality in one or several liver function tests, it is helpful to do the following:

1. Identify a particular pattern of liver injury (Table 55-2).
2. Obtain serial laboratory determinations of several liver function tests (e.g., bilirubin, alkaline phosphatase, and

Table 55-2 Patterns of Liver Function Test Abnormalities

Pattern	Bilirubin	Alkaline phosphatase	Aminotransferase	Albumin
Hemolysis	Usually elevated (mostly indirect fraction)	Normal	Normal	Normal
Acute hepatocellular	± elevation (both fractions)	Normal or <3x normal	Usually >400 U/L ALT > AST	Normal
Chronic hepatocellular	± elevation (both fractions)	Normal or <3x normal	Usually <300 U/L AST > ALT	May be decreased
Cholestasis	Usually elevated (both fractions)	≥4x normal	Usually <300 U/L	Usually normal
Infiltrative	Usually normal	Elevated often >4x normal; elevated 5′ nucleotidase	<300 U/L	Usually normal

Abbreviations: ALT = alanine aminotransferase, AST = aspartate aminotransferase.

AST) over several days, because a recognizable liver injury pattern may only develop with time.
3. Interpret the liver function test within the context of the patient's presenting symptoms and physical findings (see Chapter 53, "Jaundice").

Table 55-2 summarizes the liver function test patterns that occur with hepatobiliary disease.

Biochemical patterns of liver cell dysfunction often can overlap (e.g., a cholestatic and an infiltrative pattern). When patterns of liver injury overlap or when a specific cause cannot be identified, despite recognition of a particular pattern, a variety of tests and procedures are available to help clarify and identify the source of liver function abnormalities. These tests include further blood and urine testing, ultrasonography, computed tomography, magnetic resonance imaging, radionuclide scanning, cholangiography (percutaneous transhepatic or endoscopic retrograde), liver biopsy, angiography, and peritoneoscopy (please refer to Chapter 53 for a suggested approach in utilizing these tests and procedures). It is important to remember that abnormalities in liver function testing are not necessarily specific or sensitive; i.e., they may be abnormal in diseases not primarily affecting the liver, or they may be normal in the presence of significant liver disease. However, recognition of a pattern within the routine liver function tests, together with the patient's history and physical examination, allows the physician to make a specific diagnosis or, at the least, guides the physician in selecting other tests and procedures that will result in identifying a specific cause for the abnormal liver function tests.

References

Eastwood GL, Avunduk C. Jaundice and interpretation of laboratory liver tests. In: Manual of gastroenterology: Diagnosis and therapy. Boston: Little, Brown, 1988:253.

Kaplan MM. Evaluation of hepatobiliary disease. In: Stein JH, ed. Internal medicine. 2nd ed. Boston: Little, Brown, 1987:54.

Sherlock S, Biochemical assessment of liver function. In: Diseases of the liver and biliary system. 7th ed. Oxford: Blackwell Scientific Publications, 1985.

Diarrhea

56

Canan A. Avunduk, MD, PhD

Katherine L. Kahn, MD

Rashmi V. Patwardhan, MD

Definition

Diarrhea is a change in the normal bowel habits with an increase in the frequency, fluidity, looseness, and volume of feces expelled per day relative to the usual fecal output of the individual. In the normal adult, average daily stool weight is less than 200 g. Diarrhea always implies an increase in the quantity of water in the stool.

The diagnostic and therapeutic approaches to diarrhea depend on the severity and duration of symptoms. Diarrhea is defined as *acute* when the duration is less than 2 weeks or *chronic* when the duration is greater than 2 weeks or recurrent. In addition, diarrhea is frequently categorized as *bloody* or *nonbloody*.

Differential Diagnosis

The differential diagnosis for diarrhea encompasses a broad spectrum of conditions that are usually categorized according to the history, which provides the most revealing diagnostic information. Common etiologies of acute and chronic diarrhea are listed in Table 56-1. Careful history taking must distinguish new-onset diarrhea from acute exacerbation of chronic, recurrent diarrhea because the latter represents a different group of etiologies.

Diagnostic Approach

The diagnostic approach to the patient with diarrhea focuses on the duration of symptoms, the nature of the presenting complaint, the presence of coexistent illnesses, and prior evaluation for similar problems. Information regarding the chronicity of symptoms provides diagnostic clues because most new-onset diarrhea resolves within 2 weeks and is self-limited. A description of the character of the stool, the frequency of movements, and the presence of associated symptoms helps distinguish the etiology of the diarrhea, although there may be overlap between syndromes. Pathology of the small bowel or proximal colon generally produces large, watery, nonbloody stool that may be accompanied by pain referred to the periumbilical region or to the right lower quadrant of the abdomen. The stool may contain nondigested food or may be foul smelling or greasy. Pathology of the left colon and rectum is generally characterized by frequent passage of small volumes of stool, flatus, or mucus. Disorders of this distal segment of bowel activate the defecation reflex despite the presence of less fecal material than is usually required for defecation. The resultant stool is usually soft and non–foul smelling, but it may contain blood or mucus. Pain referred from the left colon and rectum may be referred to the lower abdomen or sacrum. The pain is frequently relieved for a brief period by passage of the stool.

The presence of blood mixed with stool suggests infection, inflammation, or neoplasia, whereas blood coating the stool or bleeding after evacuation of the stool is more likely to result from local perianal irritation and friability. Occasionally, the patient may describe passage of blood from the rectum or vagina as bloody diarrhea, despite the absence of stool. Careful history taking, examination of the patient, and inspection of the stool will clarify whether the blood is from the anus or vagina, and whether the discharge is stool, blood, or both. Frequent stools mixed with mucus without blood are suggestive of the irritable bowel syndrome, as are complaints of diarrhea alternating with

Table 56-1 Common Etiologies of Diarrhea

Viral	Norwalk agent Rotavirus Enteric adenovirus
Bacterial toxin	*Staphylococcus* *Clostridium perfringens* *Clostridium difficile* *Clostridium botulinum* *Bacillus cereus* Toxigenic *Escherichia coli*
Bacterial invasion	*Shigella* Invasive *E. coli* *Salmonella* Gonorrhea *Yersinia enterocolitica* *Vibrio parahaemolyticus* *Campylobacter fetus* and *jejuni*
Parasites	*Giardia lamblia* *Cryptosporidium* *Entamoeba histolytica*
After infection	Lactase deficiency Bacterial overgrowth
Drugs	Laxatives Antacids with magnesium (See text for other drugs)
Food toxins	Ciguatoxin, scombroid, pufferfish
Metabolic	Hyperthyroidism Adrenal insufficiency Hyperparathyroidism Diabetes mellitus
Chronic illness	Inflammatory bowel disease Ischemic colitis Malabsorption Irritable bowel syndrome

Table 56-2 Causes of Secretory Diarrhea

Organism or disorder	Secretory stimulus
Vibrio cholerae *Escherichia coli* *Staphylococcus aureus* *Bacillus cereus*	Bacterial enterotoxins that stimulate cyclic AMP
Islet cell tumors (pancreatic cholera)	Vasoactive intestinal polypeptide (VIP)
Medullary thyroid cancer	Calcitonin
Steatorrhea/malabsorption	Hydroxylated long-chain fatty acids
Ileal resection	Bile salts and fatty acids
Laxative abuse Phenolphthalein Ricinoleic acid (castor oil) Bisacodyl Diactyl sulfosuccinate Danthron Senna	Anthraquinone cathartics
Carcinoid	Serotonin
Intestinal obstruction	Prostaglandins, prostonoids
Zollinger-Ellison syndrome	Gastrin and gastric acid hypersecretion (multifactoral diarrhea)

constipation. The latter, however, is also characteristic of diabetic autonomic neuropathy or early colonic neoplasia.

Diarrhea that awakens the patient at night, is truly of large volume, and is associated with systemic signs and symptoms is likely to be organic in origin. Stool mixed with pus should suggest an infectious or inflammatory lesion. Patients with perianal Crohn's disease, a history of perianal pathology, or anorectal surgery frequently have fecal soilage or incontinence that may be described as diarrhea.

Normally, the bowel is responsible for balancing the absorption and secretion of fluids that are ingested or secreted by the bowel. *Secretory diarrhea* occurs when the bowel secretion overwhelms the absorptive mechanisms, resulting in the leak of electrolytes and water into the bowel and causing a very large volume of diarrhea, usually of 1 to 2 L daily. Common mechanisms include bacterial toxins, viral agents, and hormones. Table 56-2 lists some conditions that cause secretory diarrhea. Secretory diarrhea will persist while the patient fasts because the mechanism for the diarrhea is independent of food ingestion in most cases.

Osmotic diarrhea results when an excess of osmotically active, nonabsorbable molecules are present in the bowel lumen. A common cause is the ingestion of laxatives or antacids containing magnesium, sulfate, or phosphate. At times, laxative ingestion is surreptitious and can be a difficult diagnostic problem. Ingestion of lactose in milk and milk products produces an osmotic load within the bowel that is usually digested by lactase, an enzyme located on the luminal surface of the small bowel epithelial cells. However, following infectious gastroenteritis and with other inflammatory disorders of the small intestine, lactase may be deficient. The result is a nonabsorbable lactose load and osmotic diarrhea. Frequently, blacks, American Indians, Asians, and some northern Europeans describe diarrhea after ingestion of milk products as a consequence of primary deficiency of lactase. Resolution of the diarrhea after a lactose-free diet offers good support for the diagnosis. The clinically distinguishing feature of osmotic diarrhea is that the diarrhea improves when the patient ceases ingestion of the nonabsorbable molecules or fasts for 24 to 48 hours.

Exudative diarrhea, caused by inflammatory, ulcerative, or infiltrative lesions of the bowel, is characterized by the leakage of proteins, blood, mucus, or pus from the damaged bowel. This is usually a small-volume diarrhea. If large volumes are present, there is likely a secretory component as well. Neoplastic lesions, such as villous adenoma, may result in the exudation of mucus, fluid, and electrolytes. Infections with invasive bacteria such as *Shigella* and *Salmonella* are characterized by intestinal mucosal ulceration, invasion, exudation, and bleeding. Also, parasites such as *Entamoeba histolytica* cause exudative diarrheal illness by invasion.

A less common cause of diarrhea occurs secondary to *motility and transit disorders,* in which the contact time between the intestinal mucosa and luminal contents is inadequate for complete absorption. Rapid transit time may occur after gastric surgery, vagotomy, or intestinal bypass operations. Hyperthyroidism, hypergastrinemia, and some primary motility disorders are other causes of diarrhea. Intestinal stasis due to blind loops or sluggish motility causes bacterial overgrowth, with resultant malabsorption and diarrhea.

Malabsorption causes diarrhea by a number of mechanisms. Unabsorbed long-chain fatty acids are hydroxylated by bacteria and stimulate fluid secretion in the large bowel, thus causing diarrhea. Carbohydrate malabsorption results in osmotic diarrhea. Malabsorbed bile acids enter the colon and act as endogenous cathartics that induce mucosal secretion, resulting in diarrhea. Clinically, the patient with malabsorption usually describes the passage of large amounts of bulky stool, which may be greasy or foul smelling. The high gas content of the stool frequently, although not always, causes the stool to float. With time, the patient usually suffers from weight loss and eventually may present with signs of anemia, malnutrition, and deficiency of the fat-soluble vitamins A, D, E, and K.

Metabolic causes of diarrhea include hyperthyroidism, adrenal insufficiency, hyperparathyroidism, diabetes mellitus, and medullary carcinoma of the thyroid. *Drugs* may cause diarrhea as a consequence of osmotic load (some laxatives), mucosal injury (antibiotic-associated pseudomembranous colitis), stimulation of secretion, or malabsorption. Because so many medications may provoke diarrhea, a careful history is essential in the patient with acute, chronic, or recurrent diarrhea.

Magnesium-containing drugs, laxatives, antibiotics, antacids, digitalis, quinidine sulfate, colchicine, cholestyramine, chemotherapeutic agents, and propranolol, as well as many other drugs, are known to cause diarrhea. Medication should be considered as a potential cause for the diarrhea when its onset occurred shortly after the drug therapy was begun. Although drug-induced diarrhea may be dose related, it is not necessarily so. Resolution of the diarrhea soon after the withdrawal of the drug verifies the diagnosis.

The use of many antibiotics and occasional chemotherapeutic agents may result in "pseudomembranous" colitis. During the use of or within weeks after the discontinuation of the antimicrobial agent, patients experience fever, abdominal discomfort, and a diarrheal syndrome that may range from a mild illness to serious toxicity. The diarrhea is caused by a necrotizing toxin elaborated by *Clostridium difficile*, which overgrows in the bowel as a consequence of antibiotic usage.

Clinical Classification

A clinical classification of diarrhea evolves if diarrhea is categorized according to chronicity, the presence of bleeding, or the presence of systemic illness. Although syndromes overlap, the following clinical scenarios describe the common diagnostic characteristics.

The presence of acute diarrhea with neither bleeding nor systemic illness should cause the clinician to think of functional or drug-related illnesses. Diarrhea alternating with normal stool or constipation is suggestive of irritable bowel syndrome, particularly in a patient who describes psychosocial stresses and is not awakened at night with diarrhea. A drug history should focus on the use of new drugs, antibiotics, heavy lactose ingestion, or excess alcohol use.

The acute onset of diarrhea with systemic illness in a previously well individual suggests an infectious or inflammatory etiology. Viruses are the most common organisms causing infectious gastroenteritis in this country. Incidence is highest among children, and the illness most commonly occurs in the autumn or winter. The illness, which usually has its onset 48 to 72 hours after exposure, is characterized not only by gastrointestinal signs of nausea, vomiting, and diarrhea, but also by systemic complaints of headache, fever, diffuse abdominal discomfort, and tenderness. The abdomen is without guarding, the bowel sounds are hyperactive, and the patient's white blood cell count is normal. The diarrhea generally resolves spontaneously within 48 hours, although xylose malabsorption, fat malabsorption, or lactase deficiency may occur transiently.

Bacterial causes of diarrhea occur owing to ingestion of a preformed bacterial toxin, bacteria that will release a toxin in the bowel lumen, or bacteria that will invade the bowel mucosa. Staphylococci produce a toxin that contaminates mayonnaise, milk products, custard-filled pastries, or processed meats. The patient typically becomes ill with watery diarrhea, vomiting, and abdominal pain 3 to 8 hours after the ingestion. The symptoms improve spontaneously within 24 to 36 hours. *Clostridium perfringens* produces a toxin found in meats, poultry, dairy products, or cooked vegetables kept under inadequate refrigeration. Diarrhea and cramps, usually without vomiting, begin 8 to 24 hours after ingestion and last about a full day. *Bacillus cereus*, with its incubation period of 10 to 12 hours, causes watery diarrhea, nausea, and abdominal discomfort when meat or vegetables are contaminated by the heat-labile toxin. Toxigenic *Escherichia coli*, a very common cause of epidemic diarrhea in this country and of traveler's diarrhea elsewhere, is also a toxin-induced diarrhea that typically lasts no longer than 1 week. The major historical clue to the presence of the toxin-induced diarrhea is the ingestion of a common food by patients who develop the diarrhea. *Salmonella* invades the bowel wall and causes diarrhea that is characteristically watery and greenish, and may be associated with fever, vomiting, and cramps. Infection usually results from ingestion of unpasteurized milk, shellfish, eggs, or poultry, but occasionally has been transmitted by dogs, cats, or pet turtles. *Campylobacter* is a frequent cause of infectious diarrhea in children and adults. The illness may range from mild diarrhea to systemic illness with grossly bloody stool. *Yersinia, Vibrio parahaemolyticus*, and a series of parasites are not uncommon causes of diarrhea in the United States.

Two protozoa are important infectious sources of diarrhea in the United States in the population at large, with even greater prevalence in the homosexual population. These are *Giardia lamblia* and *Entamoeba histolytica* (amebiasis). *Giardia*, with its incubation period of 7 to 21 days, causes diarrhea that may be acute, chronic, or recurrent. Nausea, flatulence, crampy abdominal pain, or malabsorption commonly accompanies the diarrhea. *Giardia* is a water-borne organism that may be transmitted via tap water, ponds, or streams. It has especially been a cause of diarrhea to travelers and hikers. *Entamoeba histolytica* spreads via the fecal-oral route or, less commonly, venereally. Outbreaks occur in the United States, although a number of patients have described a history of recent travel to Mexico.

When the diarrhea is acute and bloody but the patient is otherwise healthy, one must consider enteric infections, particularly with *Shigella* or *Campylobacter*, in the new onset or relapse of inflammatory bowel disease. When abdominal pain and tenesmus are associated with acute bloody diarrhea, the differential diagnoses should include diverticulitis, ischemic colitis, ulcerative colitis, and carcinoma. Although carcinomas are not a common cause of acute bloody diarrhea, if there is a concomitant change in the frequency, caliber, or consistency of bowel movements, this diagnosis must be considered. The prevalence of each of these conditions increases with age, particularly after the fifth decade. Angiodysplasia, a vascular malformation of the colon that may cause bloody diarrhea, has also been associated with aortic stenosis in retrospective studies. Thus, the presence of such heart disease may provide a clue to the etiology of the bleeding. A rare cause of bloody diarrhea is endometriosis, which is suggested in a female patient who has the diarrhea concomitant with menses.

Acute bloody diarrhea in a systemically ill patient is usually associated with a more serious illness, i.e., an illness that is unlikely to be self-limited and more likely to provoke anemia or electrolyte abnormalities. This symptom complex is typical of infectious or inflammatory colitis, antibiotic-associated colitis, uremic colitis, or ischemic colitis. The history must carefully document episodes of recent travel to areas endemic for amebiasis, shigellosis, or salmonellosis. A history of drug ingestion and clues to an underlying systemic illness must also be carefully sought. Rarely, leukemia or renal failure will present with diarrhea.

When evaluating chronic diarrhea, defined by duration longer than 2 weeks, it is important but sometimes difficult to distinguish organic from functional disease. Table 56-3 lists some discriminating features of organic and functional diarrhea.

Chronic nonbloody diarrhea in a patient without systemic illness should raise suspicion of functional bowel disease, sequelae of prior gastrointestinal surgery, secretory diarrhea, laxative abuse, or giardiasis. When chronic diarrhea occurs in conjunction with systemic signs or symptoms, particularly weight loss or fatigue, the possibility of infectious, inflammatory, or neoplastic disease must be considered. Mass lesions typically

Table 56-3 Organic Versus Functional Diarrhea: Points in History

History of diarrhea	Organic diarrhea	Functional diarrhea
Duration	Variable (weeks to months)	Long (6 months to years)
Stool volume	Variable, but usually large; <200 g in weight	Usually small; may alternate with periods of normality or even constipation
Blood in stools	May be present	Never (unless from hemorrhoids, fissures, or new disease)
Time when diarrhea occurs	No special pattern	Usually morning; does not awake the patient
Urgency/ incontinence	May be present	Rare
Cramping abdominal pain	Often present	Usually present
Weight loss	Often present	May occasionally be present secondary to depression and diet restrictions
Systemic illness (e.g., fever, arthritis, skin lesions, hepatic lesions, eye lesions, oral cavity lesions)	May be present	Unrelated
Emotional stress	No regular relation to symptoms	Usually precedes, coincides with, or precipitates symptoms
Patient's age	Any age	Any age

produce diarrhea as a result of liquid stool leaking around a partially obstructing lesion. Villous adenomas cause diarrhea via the secretory mechanism.

Chronic bloody diarrhea either with or without systemic illness should alert the physician to the possibility of inflammatory bowel disease, particularly in those less than 50 years old. In people more than 50 years old, one should suspect polyps, carcinoma, or ischemic bowel disease.

History

Because diarrhea, particularly chronic diarrhea, may reflect illness of such varied systems, a complete history and physical examination in which one searches for concurrent signs and symptoms is important. Certain physical findings, when present in conjunction with diarrhea, should provoke consideration of the diseases listed in the following section. Although the prevalence of some of the following diseases is low in the general population, especially in relation to the high prevalence of diarrhea, the combination of diarrhea with the described characteristics raises the possibility of the named disease.

A history of diarrhea with recurrent peptic ulcers suggests the possibility of Zollinger-Ellison syndrome. Recurrent respiratory illnesses raise the possibility of cystic fibrosis, and recurrent infections suggest the diagnosis of immunoglobulin deficiency. When a patient with collagen vascular disease presents with diarrhea, mesenteric vasculitis should be considered. Weight loss or muscle wasting is characteristic of an organic etiology for the diarrhea such as malabsorption, inflammatory bowel disease, cancer, or hyperthyroidism. Fever with chronic diarrhea raises the possibility of ulcerative colitis, Crohn's disease, amebiasis, lymphoma, tuberculosis, or Whipple's disease. Postural hypotension with diarrhea should suggest diabetic neuropathy or Addison's disease. Flushing is seen with the carcinoid syndrome and pancreatic cholera. Arthritis in association with diarrhea should provoke consideration of ulcerative colitis, Crohn's disease, Whipple's disease, gonorrheal proctitis, or infection with *Yersinia enterocolitica.* The association of liver disease and diarrhea should suggest ulcerative colitis, Crohn's disease, or bowel cancer metastatic to the liver. Diarrhea with lymphadenopathy suggests Whipple's disease or lymphoma. Neuropathy with diarrhea is seen with diabetic autonomic neuropathy and amyloidosis. A physical examination showing hyperpigmentation should provoke consideration of Whipple's disease, celiac disease, and Addison's disease.

Physical Examination

The physical examination in the patient with acute diarrhea focuses on evidence for volume depletion by evaluating skin turgor and orthostatic signs. Abdominal examination must rule out a surgical abdomen. The rectal examination looks for evidence of anal pathology, particularly a fissure or mass. Presence of a purulent discharge from the anus suggests gonococcal proctitis. In the patient with chronic diarrhea, the physical examination may reveal evidence for malnutrition or clues to a systemic illness that may be the cause of the diarrhea.

Laboratory Studies

The following is a discussion of how to use laboratory aids in the patient with diarrhea. Multiple samples of fresh stool should be examined for blood. If the diarrhea is severe, persistent, or bloody, the stool should be stained with Gram stain or methylene blue to search for the presence of polymorphonuclear leukocytes (PMNs). Their presence suggests inflammation with invasion of the colonic mucosa. Because diarrhea caused by viruses and bacterial toxins does not disrupt the colonic mucosa by invasion, a fecal leukocyte study will be negative in these instances. *Shigella, E. coli, Yersinia, Vibrio parahaemolyticus*, and *Campylobacter* characteristically produce many fecal leukocytes. *Salmonella* infection and amoebae may not result in PMNs in the stool.

If the patient is not systemically ill, and the stool is negative for blood and leukocytes, no further immediate work-up is necessary because, in most cases, the disease is self-limited. Stool positive for blood or fecal leukocytes should be further examined by stool cultures. When the laboratory is geared to culture stool on the necessary media, the offending organism can usually be identified. However, three consecutive fecal samples may be needed, because some of the bacteria, particularly *Shigella*, are difficult to isolate. It is useful to alert the laboratory to the suspected organism(s). If pseudomembranous colitis is suspected, the laboratory should be alerted. *Clostridium difficile*, the offending agent, may be cultured in an anaerobic chamber or its toxin may be documented using a tissue-culture medium.

The trophozoites of *Entamoeba histolytica* are difficult to identify, especially if the patient has had barium studies, antibiotics, kaolin, laxatives, or enemas. Although in all cases of diarrhea it is preferable for the stool to be examined fresh, it is especially critical when searching for amoebae that the stool be examined within 1 hour of being passed. If this prompt evaluation is not possible, the best alternative is to store the stool at

4°C. A serologic study may also be useful in diagnosing active infection with *Entamoeba histolytica*.

The identification of *Giardia lamblia* depends upon recognition by well-trained laboratory personnel of the *Giardia* cysts in the stool. Because the false-negative rate for locating the cysts in the stool is significant, duodenal aspiration or biopsy may be required for diagnosis. Some have advocated a therapeutic trial with metronidazole for the patient suspected of having *Giardia* infection.

When diarrhea is voluminous or persistent, sodium and potassium levels should be checked for abnormalities resulting from loss of electrolytes. Striking or persistent hypokalemia should suggest a villous adenoma, which frequently secretes large amounts of mucus and potassium into the stool. When the etiology of diarrhea is uncertain, a complete blood count, blood urea nitrogen, sedimentation rate, and urinalysis may provide helpful clues. In the febrile, systemically ill patient, blood cultures should be obtained prior to treatment with antibiotics. Infection with *Shigella* and *Salmonella* frequently results in positive blood cultures.

Proctosigmoidoscopy should be performed if there is blood in the stool or if there is suspicion that the patient has pseudomembranous colitis. A normal sigmoidoscopic examination in a patient with chronic diarrhea that is thought to be organic in etiology should suggest small bowel disease, Crohn's disease, or ischemic colitis. Sigmoidoscopic findings of bleeding and ulceration are characteristic of ulcerative colitis, Crohn's disease, infectious colitis, and pseudomembranous colitis. The latter is named for the raised yellow pseudomembranous plaques that form on an erythematous, edematous, friable background mucosa in many, but not all, patients with the disease. Biopsy is often helpful in confirming the etiology of the inflamed mucosa.

When diarrhea persists and no infectious etiology has become apparent, it is appropriate to repeat the stool exams. Before barium studies are ordered, at least three stools should be examined for ova and parasites, because the barium interferes with recognition of the pathogens. Barium enema is usually indicated in patients with severe persistent diarrhea to search for masses or inflammatory diseases, especially in the patient who is more than 40 years old. An upper gastrointestinal series with a small bowel follow-through or an enteroclysis is indicated to search for Crohn's diseases, fistula, or blind-loop syndrome in a patient with persistent unexplained diarrhea.

A 72-hour stool collection in a patient with malabsorption will produce more than 7 g of fat daily. The D-xylose test will be abnormal if the small bowel mucosa is diffusely abnormal, as in untreated celiac sprue, Whipple's disease, immunodeficiency syndrome, or a betalipoproteinemia. The abnormal D-xylose test should be followed by a small bowel biopsy, which will distinguish the diffuse lesions noted above from lesions associated with sprue, lymphoma, amyloid, Crohn's disease, parasitic infection, or other lesions of the small bowel.

References

Avunduk C, Eastwood GL. Diarrhea. In: Manual of gastroenterology: Diagnosis and treatment. Boston: Little, Brown, 1988.

Blacklow NR. Massachusetts General Hospital case records (case 39-1985). N Engl J Med 1985; 313:805.

Falchuk ZM. Massachusetts General Hospital case records (case 47-1985). N Engl J Med 1985; 313:1341.

Guerrant RL, et al. Evaluation and diagnosis of acute infectious diarrhea. Am J Med 1985; 78(suppl 6B):91.

Olsen WA. A pathophysiologic approach to diagnosis of malabsorption. Am J Med 1979; 67:1007.

Constipation

Perry A. Gotsis, MD

57

Definition

A concise definition of constipation, based on objective criteria, is difficult to formulate because most descriptions of bowel habits are based on subjective feelings and societal bias. Parameters such as the feeling of incomplete evacuation, size, difficulty of expulsion, and stool consistency show a wide range of subjective ratings in normal individuals. Most population studies have shown that more than 90 percent of normal subjects have a bowel habit of between three bowel movements per day and three bowel movements per week. In a given patient, stool frequency should be measured over a period of several weeks. Daily stool weight is highly variable within individuals, varying between 35 and 250 g per day.

Etiology

The pathophysiologic mechanisms underlying constipation may be grouped as follows: (1) failure of propulsion along the colon (colonic inertia), or (2) failure of passage through the anorectum (outflow obstruction). The etiologies of constipation may be grouped according to underlying mechanism and are listed in Table 57-1.

The most common cause of constipation as an isolated symptom in the United States is low fiber intake. People who take in less fiber have fewer and smaller bowel movements as well as a delay in the time it takes food to reach the anus. Because exercise contributes to the peristalsis of the bowel, constipation is a common condition in sedentary individuals. Frustration and discomfort associated with constipation have caused many patients to enter a vicious cycle of chronic laxative use, decreasing effectiveness of the laxative, increasing laxative use, more slowly contracting bowel, and further constipation.

Drugs, even in low doses, may cause severe constipation, particularly in the elderly. The constipating effect of drugs is often, but not always, mediated through an anticholinergic or opiate effect. Opiate receptors have been noted throughout the gastrointestinal tract.

Abuse of laxatives such as anthraquinones (senna and cascara) may result in an acquired megacolon and unresponsive

Table 57-1 Conditions Associated with Constipation

Lifestyle Alterations	**Local Anorectal Pathology: Decreased Rectal Emptying**
Low dietary bulk-fiber	Hemorrhoid
Immobility, sedentary life	Fissure
Laxative abuse	Stricture
Drugs	Abscess
Analgesics, opiates	Proctitis
Antacids (calcium- and aluminum-containing)	Rectocele
Anticholinergics	**Bowel Obstruction**
Anticonvulsants	Tumor
Antihistamines	Stricture
Antidepressants	Sigmoid volvulus
Antiparkinsonian	Rectal prolapse
Calcium-channel blockers	**Endocrine, Metabolic**
Opiates	Hypothyroidism
Tranquilizers	Diabetes
Diuretics	Amyloid
Ganglionic blockers	Hypokalemia
Neurologic Disorders	Hypercalcemia
Spinal cord lesion	Pheochromocytoma
Multiple sclerosis	Pregnancy
Cerebral palsy	
Depression, anxiety	
Hirschsprung's disease	
Chagas' disease	
Muscular Disease	
Irritable bowel	
Progressive systemic sclerosis	
Diverticular disease	

constipation. This may result from actual damage to the intramural nerve plexuses, an observation made on both light and electron microscopy. Chronic use of the anthraquinones also leads to a condition known as melanosis coli, a characteristic dark pigmented discoloration found throughout the colon that may result from the presence of melanin pigment deposition within the colonic mucosa.

In hypothyroidism, constipation may precede or dominate other symptoms. A number of motility abnormalities have been observed in the colon and esophagus of hypothyroid patients. The pathogenesis of constipation in myxedema seems to be altered impulse transmission at neuronal synapses, caused by the myxedematous mucopolysaccharide infiltration of the submucosa and smooth muscle.

Constipation is often a problem in diabetic patients, likely secondary to autonomic neurodysfunction. The normal increase in motor activity seen in the colon shortly after a meal is absent in diabetics with severe constipation. Motor abnormalities of the esophagus and stomach are also noted in diabetes.

Hypokalemia, common with diuretic use, and hypercalcemia (Ca $\geq$ 12 mg/dl) are metabolic causes of constipation that are most prominent in the hospitalized patient.

Many of the structural disorders of the large bowel that are associated with constipation compromise the luminal diameter of the colon. Neoplasms causing constipation are usually in the rectosigmoid area. A number of inflammatory disorders may lead to stricture formation, on the basis of either active inflammation or chronic fibrosis. These inflammatory disorders include diverticulosis/diverticulitis, acute or chronic ischemic colitis, and inflammatory bowel disease, such as ulcerative colitis and Crohn's colitis. Chronic intermittent colonic volvulus, usually in the sigmoid colon, may lead to chronic constipation. Some consider that volvulus may be a complication of chronic constipation. Chronic volvulus has been noted in patients with hypothyroidism. Rectal prolapse is an obstructing cause of constipation that results from failure of the stool to pass through the anorectum.

Patients with irritable bowel syndrome may have constipation, either chronically or intermittently. It is often associated with left lower quadrant abdominal pain, the so-called spastic type of irritable bowel syndrome. The onset of symptoms is usually in the second or third decade. Colonic myoelectric studies in patients with irritable bowel syndrome have revealed a number of characteristic patterns, suggesting that the colonic smooth muscle has enhanced responsiveness to a number of stimuli. When considering the diagnosis of irritable bowel syndrome, one should be aware that the syndrome may represent a learned visceral response, or coping behavior, to life's stressful situations. Patients are frequently tense and anxious, upset, angry, and demanding. Unfortunately, the diagnosis of irritable bowel syndrome is often one of exclusion. Frequently, patients are evaluated on multiple occasions by multiple physicians and, in more extreme situations, have multiple inappropriate surgical procedures.

Progressive systemic sclerosis (PSS) frequently presents with a variety of motility disturbances of the gastrointestinal tract, with a 10 to 20 percent incidence of colonic distention and severe constipation. The pathogenesis of the motility disturbances in PSS appears to be smooth muscle atrophy and replacement by connective tissue.

Patients with diverticular disease of the colon are frequently noted to be constipated. It should be noted that the constipation is not due to the diverticulosis, per se, but to the factors that have given rise to the diverticulosis, e.g., underlying motility disturbance or dietary factors.

Constipation may result from a number of other abnormalities of the central nervous system and spinal cord. A normal defecation mechanism requires the integrity of the rectal mucosa, lumbar spinal cord, and pelvic nerves. Thus, traumatic injury to the lower spine may lead to neurogenic constipation. Also, lesions involving the sacral cord segments, the cauda, or the pelvic plexuses result in constipation.

A number of disorders of the anorectum may be associated with constipation. Anal stenosis, both congenital and acquired, may lead to difficult passage of stool. Anal fissure, perianal inflammatory disease, sometimes seen in Crohn's disease, and perirectal abscess may also be associated with constipation.

Ulcerative proctitis, a limited form of ulcerative colitis, may give rise to constipation and rectal bleeding, characteristically with blood-coated stools. Constipation in this disorder may arise from a disturbance of colonic motility, causing the fecal bolus to be held up proximal to the area of the disease.

Constipation in the elderly age group is a common phenomenon that has many factors contributing to its pathogenesis: dietary factors, lack of exercise, recumbent posture in the bedridden patient, chronic intestinal ischemia, multiple medications, and coexisting depression.

Psychogenic constipation is more frequent in children but can occur in adults. The urge to defecate is perceived only when the stools have been reduced to a smaller size and firmer consistency. Defecation is then accompanied by much pain, and the patient begins to hold back stool voluntarily to avoid pain. As the intervals between stools become longer and as the rectal vault becomes more patulous to accommodate larger volumes, the stretch mechanism that usually initiates the defecation response becomes less pronounced. As the situation progresses, overflow incontinence, known as encopresis or paradoxic soiling, occurs.

Constipation frequently occurs among psychotic patients, especially among schizophrenics and patients with severe depression. Inactivity and various psychotherapeutic drugs may contribute to this. It is also tempting to postulate that a biochemical abnormality in the central nervous system in these patients may underlie the constipation. For example, elevated levels of beta-endorphins, endogenous opiates that have been found in the cerebrospinal fluid of schizophrenic patients, may induce constipation via a separate action in the opiate receptors within the gut.

Diagnostic Approach

History

The diagnostic approach to the patient with constipation is aimed at identifying those patients who have an underlying cause for their constipation that must be addressed further. In general, patients whose constipation is benign in origin describe their constipation as chronic and without other associated complaints. However, constipation of recent origin should suggest some organic lesion within the colon. The history should search for evidence of weight loss, nausea, vomiting, melena, or hematochezia, which suggests illness rather than "normal variant" as the cause of the constipation. Clues about hypothyroidism, systemic sclerosis, neurologic disease, or other systemic illnesses (listed in Table 57-1) that cause constipation should be sought. A careful medication history should be obtained, specific questions being asked about over-the-counter, prescription, and illicit drugs.

Physical Examination

The physical examination should seek evidence to support a systemic illness that could be causing the constipation. Examination of the lymph nodes should include a careful search for the Virchow's left supraclavicular node, which may be palpable in metastatic colon cancer. In the abdominal examination, masses, distention, or hypoactive bowel sounds should be noted. Rectal examination is performed to search for a mass, guaiac-positive stools, or anorectal pathology. A pelvic examination should be performed in women to document that no mass is obstructing stool passage through the bowel. Neurologic examination will identify the delayed relaxation phase of hypothyroidism or focal neurologic deficits that may explain the constipation.

Laboratory Tests

The laboratory work-up is generally most helpful when the history and physical examination suggest systemic or organic disease. The work-up should consist of stool screening for blood, proctosigmoidoscopy, and barium enema. Metabolic work-up should be undertaken if the history offers clues suggesting a metabolic or endocrine problem.

If the constipation has occurred intermittently for many years or has been chronic, and there has been no evidence of bleeding, the patient can be observed on a controlled high-fiber diet. Dietary fiber, because of its water-holding physical properties, has been shown to shorten colonic transit time. Dietary fiber results in increased stool weight and increased water content, thus promoting the formation of a softer stool.

In those patients with chronic constipation who do not respond to a high-fiber diet, colonic transit time may be measured by using ingested radiopaque markers; the progress of the markers in the gastrointestinal tract is then followed by daily abdominal films. This examination may be useful in distinguishing the two major pathogenic mechanisms of constipation: colonic inertia and outflow obstruction.

References

Battle WM, et al. Colonic dysfunction in diabetes mellitus. Gastroenterology 1980; 79:1217.

Cummings JH, Jenkins DJA, Wiggins HS. Measurement of the mean transit time of dietary residue through the human gut. Gut 1974; 17:210.

Devroede G. Constipation. In: Sleisenger MH, Fordtran JS, eds. Gastrointestinal disease. 4th ed. Philadelphia: WB Saunders, 1989:331.

JeeJeebhoy KN. Gastrointestinal diseases: Focus on clinical diagnosis. Garden City, NY: Medical Examination Publishing Co., 1980:284.

Flatulence

Gregory L. Eastwood, MD

58

Definition

Flatus is intestinal gas that is passed through the rectum and anus. Flatulence refers to the symptom of passage of excess flatus or to the feeling that excessive gas is in the intestines. Many patients complain of bloating, meaning that the abdomen becomes uncomfortably distended, usually after eating. These patients typically attribute their bloating to excessive intestinal gas.

Etiology

Normal intestinal gas is derived from four sources: (1) ingestion of nitrogen and oxygen in swallowed air; (2) liberation of carbon dioxide from neutralization of acids in the gut; (3) formation of carbon dioxide, hydrogen, and methane from the action of bacteria on intestinal contents; and (4) diffusion of nitrogen and oxygen into the gut from the bloodstream. Thus, five odorless gases, nitrogen, oxygen, carbon dioxide, hydrogen, and methane, make up more than 99 percent of the total volume of intestinal gas. The gases that impart the characteristic olfactory qualities to flatus are present in only trace amounts. These gases include ammonia, hydrogen sulfide, and volatile short-chain fatty acids and amino acids.

The perception by patients that the amount of intestinal gas or the passage of flatus is excessive may not actually reflect an abnormal amount of intestinal gas or flatus. Although methods exist for quantifying the volume of rectal gas, they generally are not available to most practicing physicians. The semiquantitative method of counting the number of passages of flatus per day gives little information about the presence or character of a pathologic condition, although that practice may be useful in documenting improvement in various treatment regimens.

Patients who experience recurrent abdominal pain or bloating often attribute these symptoms to excess gas. However, a comparison of patients who complained of flatulence versus asymptomatic volunteers demonstrated no difference in fasting and postprandial volume and composition of intestinal gas. Despite the normal volume and composition of intestinal gas, the patients with abdominal pain and flatulence did have more reflux of gas from the intestine back into the stomach, and they tended to experience more abdominal pain after infusion of volumes of gas that were well tolerated by control subjects. These observations suggest that "gaseous" abdominal pain and bloating may not be due to excessive amounts of intestinal gas but rather to a defect in gut motility and a heightened pain response to normal volumes of gas. The bowel disorder and clinical symptoms of these individuals may be similar to those that are observed in some patients with the irritable bowel syndrome.

Some patients who complain of abdominal pain and bloating do have demonstrable organic disease, such as peptic disease, gallbladder disease, Crohn's disease, or recurrent bowel obstruction. Often considerable clinical judgment is required to differentiate patients with functional complaints from those whose symptoms are due to a specific disorder. If, in addition to complaints of gaseousness the patient has loss of weight, localized abdominal pain, vomiting, or blood in the stool, the suspicion of organic disease is increased.

Increased amounts of flatus usually result from gas that is produced by bacterial action on dietary substrates. Some patients are able to identify certain foods that aggravate their symptoms. One common offender is milk lactose, which results in excess intestinal gas production, cramps, and diarrhea in lactase-deficient individuals.

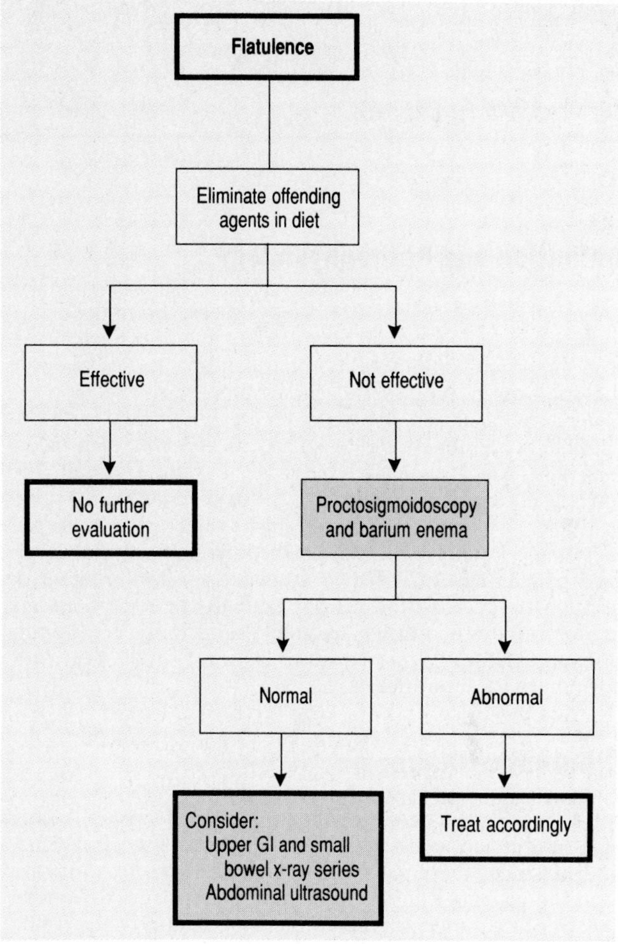

Figure 58-1 Algorithm for a diagnostic approach to flatulence. GI = gastrointestinal.

Diagnostic Approach

The evaluation of patients who complain of excess gas is often difficult and unrewarding (Fig. 58-1). Some patients need only an accurate history and physical examination plus the application of gentle reassurance. Other patients, particularly those who also have weight loss, blood in the stool, or other organic signs or symptoms, may require an extensive evaluation to rule out organic disease. A careful history may indicate certain foods that cause the patient's symptoms, and simple avoidance of those foods may bring relief. More often, however, symptoms cannot be attributed to particular foods. If they can, the reaction to those foods may be variable; sometimes ingestion of these suspected foods produces symptoms, other times not.

The physical examination usually is not helpful. The stool should be examined for gross or occult blood. If localized abdominal tenderness or a mass exists, that may lead to further diagnostic studies.

The initial evaluation of patients who complain of persistent abdominal gas or flatus should include a proctosigmoidoscopy and barium enema to rule out anorectal disease and colonic disorders. Reflux of the barium into the terminal ileum will allow evaluation for Crohn's disease. If symptoms persist despite reassurance or if they suggest organic disease, further evaluation should include an upper gastrointestinal and small bowel radiographic series or enteroclysis and abdominal ultrasonography. If the latter study is done, it should not be confined to the examination of the gallbladder and pancreas, but should include views of the mid and lower abdomen and pelvis to rule out extraintestinal masses that may be causing the patient's symptoms.

References

Eastwood GL, Avunduk C. Intestinal gas. In: Manual of gastroenterology: Diagnosis and therapy. Boston: Little, Brown, 1988:177.

Lasser RB, Bond JH, Levitt MD. The role of intestinal gas in functional abdominal pain. N Engl J Med 1975; 293:524.

Levitt MD. Volume and composition of human intestinal gas determined by means of an intestinal washout technic. N Engl J Med 1971; 284:1394.

Levitt MD, Bond JH. Intestinal gas. In: Sleisenger MH, Fordtran JS, eds. Gastrointestinal disease. 4th ed. Philadelphia: WB Saunders, 1989: 257.

Levitt MD, et al. Studies of a flatulent patient. N Engl J Med 1976; 295:260.

Anorectal Pain

Wayne E. Silva, MD

Definition and Pathophysiology

Anorectal pain is usually described as a severe, burning discomfort that may be initiated or made worse with bowel movements. In some patients, stimulation of the anal canal causes spasm of the sphincteric muscles and causes more pain. Because the lower anal canal and perianal area are lined with squamous epithelium and innervated by somatic nerves with pain receptors, this area is particularly sensitive to painful stimuli. The lower anal canal is separated from the upper canal by the pectinate line. The upper anal canal, which is lined with a mucous membrane, is innervated by sympathetic nerve fibers that do not carry pain impulses. Thus, the rectum is insensitive to cutting or burning, but rectal lesions usually cause discomfort by distending the rectal wall, causing spasm of the rectum, or by putting pressure on nearby musculature. Figure 59-1 illustrates the anatomy of the anorectal region.

Differential Diagnosis

Ninety-five percent of anorectal pain is caused by complications of fissure in ano, hemorrhoids, or perirectal abscesses. Figure 59-2 illustrates these pathologies. Anorectal pain is commonly found in patients with acquired immunodeficiency syndrome. One-third of these patients have evidence of abscess, fistula, proctitis, fissures, or condylomata.

Anal fissures are the most common cause of anorectal pain. They are cracks in the anal mucosa that may result in ulcers in the anorectal region. The posterior midline of the anal canal is a common site for the development of fissures because it has few muscular fibers to resist the high pressures generated for the passage of stool. The most common causes of anal fissures are the passage of hard stool, inflammation of the anal crypt (cryptitis), and ulceration over a thrombosed hemorrhoid. The pain resulting from the fissure usually causes sphincter spasm, further pain, and constipation. The spasm, then, helps sustain an anal fissure. Acute fissures are superficial breaks in the skin that usually heal rapidly. Chronic fissures are deeper and may extend even to the level of the internal sphincter muscle. They are characterized by cycles of healing by scar formation, followed by recurrent breakdown, followed by healing again. Proctitis, acute diarrhea, Crohn's disease, and ulcerative colitis are associated with a high incidence of anal fissures, which may be the first evidence of inflammatory bowel disease.

Hemorrhoids (piles) are dilatations or varicosities of the normal hemorrhoidal plexus of veins that occur in the region of the dentate (pectinate) line. Hemorrhoids are described as internal when they are above the dentate line and covered with the mucous membrane, and external when they are beneath the dentate line and covered by squamous epithelium. Internal and external hemorrhoids communicate with each other. Hemorrhoids occur commonly, and they are usually associated with the following predisposing factors: heredity, advancing age (70 percent of people over 50 years of age have hemorrhoids), or any cause that increases the pressure in the hemorrhoidal venous system. Thus, the presence of anal discomfort in a patient with constipation, straining at stool, pregnancy, prolonged upright position, abdominal or pelvic tumor, or portal hypertension suggests hemorrhoids. Hemorrhoids, especially external hemorrhoids, may cause a low-grade ache or burning because of the inflammation or ulceration of the surrounding area. External

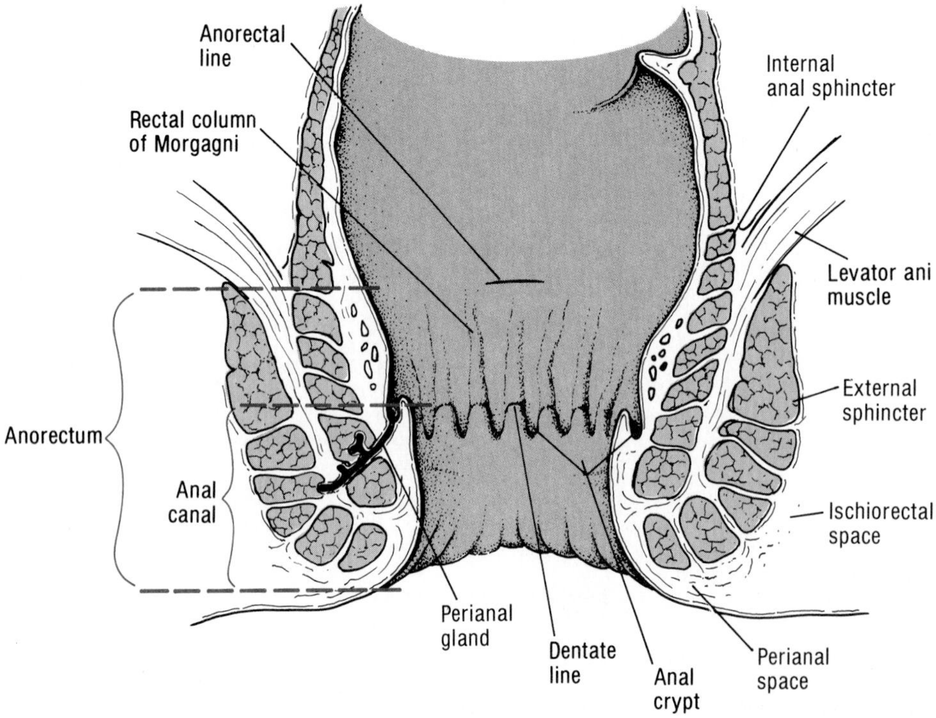

Figure 59-1 Anorectal anatomy.

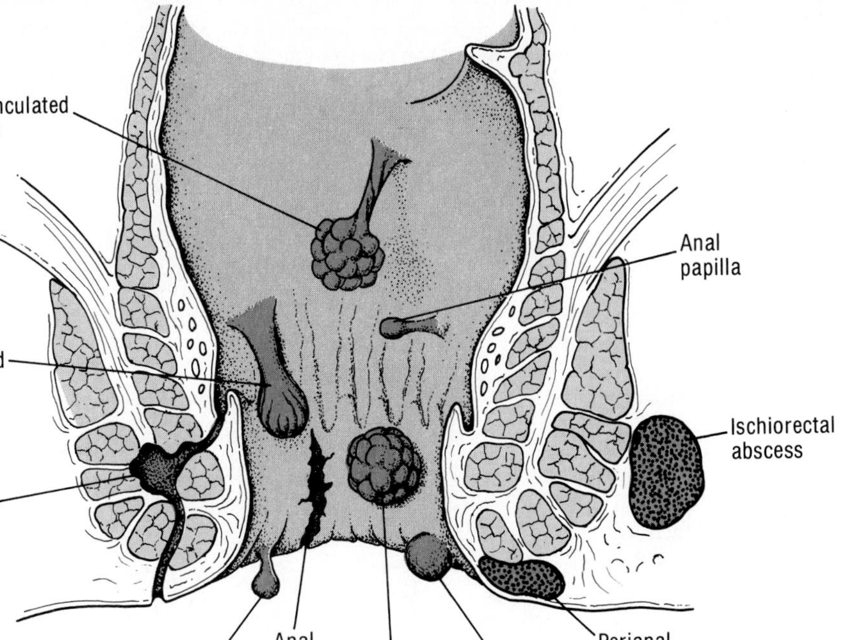

Figure 59-2 Anorectal pathology.

hemorrhoids may become acutely painful with the development of thrombosis and associated tissue swelling and inflammation. Internal hemorrhoids are less likely to become severely painful because of the lack of sensory innervation. However, they may become severely painful if they are complicated by strangulation by the anal sphincter.

Anorectal abscesses, a common cause of severe anorectal pain, develop from infection in the anorectal region that spreads to the ischiorectal or perirectal spaces, which contain large fatty deposits. The infection usually begins in one of the anal glands and spreads via the intersphincteric plane (plane between the internal and external sphincters) in several directions, resulting in the different presentations of anal abscesses.

1. Perianal abscess represents 80 percent of anorectal abscesses and is a result of downward extension of infection from the intersphincteric space.
2. Intersphincteric or submucous abscesses are rare and are a result of upward extension of the intersphincteric infection.
3. Ischiorectal abscesses represent 15 percent of anorectal abscesses and are a result of the infection crossing through the sphincter into the ischiorectal space.
4. Supralevator abscesses extend into the pelvis above the levator muscles. They are very uncommon.

Although most anal abscesses result from infections of the anal glands, other known causes include anal fissures, infected anal hematoma, infected complicated hemorrhoids, and any injury to the anal lining, particularly injuries due to instrumental manipulation. Approximately 75 percent of patients with perianal abscesses will have further problems in the form of recurrent abscess or fistulas. Anorectal abscesses should be treated with surgery.

Proctalgias are a group of symptom complexes that have pain as the predominant characteristic. Proctalgias probably arise from ligaments of the pelvic floor. The conditions of levator spasm syndrome, proctalgia fugax, and coccygodynia are poorly understood entities and are frequently diagnoses of exclusion.

Proctitis is a general term covering any inflammation within the rectal ampulla. The chief symptoms are bleeding, mucous discharge, and tenesmus (severe urge to defecate). The differential diagnosis includes ulcerative colitis, Crohn's disease, radiation proctitis, and specific infections or infestations such as shigellosis or amebiasis.

Anal papillitis is inflammation of the anal papillae, which are the small nubbins of tissue at the ends of the anal valves, near the dentate line. The papillae become inflamed and painful if they prolapse within or even outside the canal. With such prolapse, the inflammation is repeatedly worsened by even simple hygienic measures, such as use of toilet tissue.

Anal cryptitis is an inflammation at the dentate line where folds of ectoderm create anal valves and crypts. These may occasionally become inflamed and cause rectal pain. *Rectal gonorrhea* and infection with *herpes simplex virus* are the most common causes of pain in male homosexuals.

Diagnostic Approach

History

A carefully taken history can do much to elucidate the cause of anorectal pain. Pain associated with bowel movements is usually caused by an anal fissure or ulcer. Thrombosed external hemorrhoids are characterized by constant pain of recent onset. Thrombosed hemorrhoidal pain is characteristically maximal at the outset and then subsides. Pain due to rectal abscess is continuous and constantly increases in severity. Levator syndrome and proctalgia fugax are described as a sensation of pain, pressure, or discomfort in the rectum associated with a sensation of relief following a bowel movement or passage of flatus. Characteristically, the levator syndrome occurs intermittently and awakens patients from sleep. The pain is brief, lasting seconds to several minutes. Rarely, it may last hours. Pain may be induced by sexual orgasm, may increase with sitting, and may be associated with low back, gluteal, or thigh pain.

Physical Examination

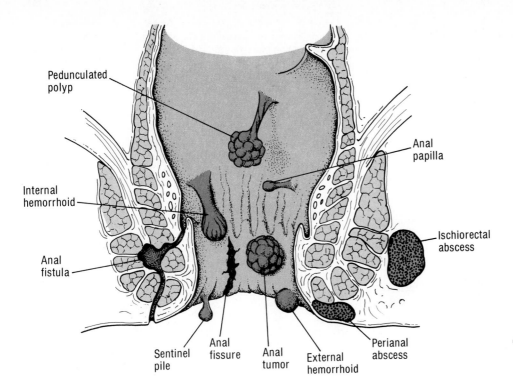

Examination of the patient with anorectal pain should be done with special care because digital probing or instrumentation can cause severe discomfort. The diagnosis can usually be made by visual inspection. A painful thrombosed hemorrhoid is visible and presents as a violaceous mass at the anal opening. Gentle retraction of the buttocks at the anterior and posterior ends of the anus allows the demonstration of an anal fissure. Most fissures are located posteriorly, and only about 10 percent, particularly in women, are found in the anterior midline. A "sentinel pile," or hypertrophic anal papilla, is frequently identified at the site of the fissure. An abscess is not always easily identified on examination. The soft tissues around the anus may be erythematous and swollen, but in many cases no signs of inflammation are present. Perirectal tissue may be tender, particularly with a perianal abscess. An ischiorectal abscess is found in the tissues of the buttock, somewhat lateral to the anus. Tenderness is usually present. Intermuscular abscesses show no visible signs on the anal skin, but a gentle rectal examination may elicit tenderness. A foreign body may be the cause of anorectal pain, particularly in a patient with a psychiatric problem.

In order to examine a patient in the presence of anorectal pain, the topical or subcutaneous placement of several milliliters of lidocaine into the anal canal is usually helpful. After waiting a few minutes, gently insert a well-lubricated index finger, with its widest aspect parallel to the anteroposterior axis of the anal canal. Exert pressure away from the area of expected tenderness. One should feel for the irregularity of an anal fissure or the tender mass of a strangulated internal hemorrhoid, a tender anal papilla, or an intermuscular abscess. A small anoscope can be inserted in exactly the same manner. In the presence of pain, it is important to avoid rotating the finger or anoscope in the anal canal. In order to examine all surfaces, the finger or the anoscope should be removed and then re-placed in the desired direction. In the presence of acute anorectal pain, sigmoidoscopic examination can usually be deferred until the acute problem (if fissure) has resolved. If sigmoidoscopy must be performed, it is best done under anesthesia.

References

Kirsner JB, Shorter G, eds. Diseases of the colon, rectum and anal canal. Baltimore: Williams & Wilkins, 1988:573.

Sleisenger MH, Fordtran JS, eds. Gastrointestinal disease. 4th ed. Philadelphia: WB Saunders, 1989:1570.

Sohn N, Weinstein MA, Rabbins RD. Anorectal disorders. Curr Probl Surg 1983; 20(1).

Anal Mass

Wayne E. Silva, MD

60

Definition and Pathophysiology

A patient may complain of having an anal mass or the sensation of a mass being present and describe it as a protrusion, a pressure, or a sense of incomplete evacuation. Anal mass may develop as a result of infection, inflammation, or neoplasia. The venous system of the anal region drains to the inferior vena cava, and the lymphatic system drains to the inguinal lymph nodes. Thus, the spread of infections or malignancy may follow these routes.

Differential Diagnosis

The most common causes of anal masses are hemorrhoids, condylomata acuminata, rectal prolapse, rectal abscess, fecal impaction, and neoplasia.

Hemorrhoids, which are dilated veins, are discussed in Chapter 59, "Anorectal Pain." They may present as an anal mass because of prolapsing of an internal hemorrhoid or as skin tags that are in fact old, scarred external hemorrhoids.

Rectal prolapse is a condition that may present as a mass. It is the protrusion of some or all layers of the rectum through the anus. Severity ranges from simple mucosal prolapse to full-thickness prolapse, called rectal procidentia. Prolapse results from diminished anal sphincter tone and the loss of pelvic support of the anorectum. It commonly occurs in women over age 60 and in patients with decreased anal sphincter tone.

Hypertrophied anal papillae also may present as a rectal mass. Anal papillae are located at the pectinate or dentate line, which divides the mucous membrane–lined portion of the rectum from the squamous epithelium–lined lower portion. With chronic irritation from poor anal hygiene, local disease, or bowel dysfunction, the anal papillae may hypertrophy, become red, swollen, painful, and feel like a mass.

Condylomata acuminata (venereal warts) are caused by a virus and occur in heterosexual men and women as well as in male homosexuals. Besides presenting as a mass, they are frequently painful. Venereal warts appear as multiple small excrescences on the perianal skin and within the anal canal or as large masses with multiple villi and fronds.

Fecal impaction may give the patient the sensation of an anal mass. There is often an associated history of chronic constipation or laxative use.

Neoplasias and *abscesses* of the anus and pelvis may cause anal masses. Abscesses are discussed in Chapter 59, "Anorectal Pain." Cancers of the anorectal region are very rare. In order of frequency, the following tumors occur in the perianal region: epidermoid carcinoma, malignant melanoma, Bowen's disease, Paget's disease, and basal cell carcinoma. Despite the infrequency of anal cancers, a high index of suspicion must be maintained in order to make an early diagnosis and begin appropriate management.

On occasion, female patients complain of a sensation of something "dropping" in the perianal region. A *rectocele,* which is the anterior protrusion of the rectum into the vagina, results from weakening of the posterior vaginal wall. Although the mass is actually the protruded rectum, the finding will be noted on pelvic examination.

Diagnostic Approach

History

Ask the patient about the duration of the symptoms and the presence of bleeding or mucus. A patient may describe the mass as being protruding, pruritic, or feeling like a pressure sensation or like incomplete evacuation. In male homosexuals, condylomata acuminata and Bowen's disease are especially common. A history of constipation may suggest the presence of fecal impaction. A long history of straining at stool may suggest the possibility of a rectal prolapse. A history of leukoplakia, chronic hemorrhoids, anal fissure, lymphogranuloma venereum, chronic fistulas, previously irradiated anal skin, and anal condyloma have all been considered to be potential predisposing causes to the development of cancer in this area.

Physical Examination

Inspection of a perianal mass can usually lead to the correct diagnosis. The characteristic picture of a large wet condyloma acuminatum is not quickly forgotten. Large edematous hemorrhoids and a hypertrophied anal papilla appear as soft bluish masses. A mass visible within the perianal region should be biopsied; malignant lesions can be mistaken for hemorrhoids and vice versa. A polypoid adenocarcinoma can appear as a hypertrophied anal papilla. Condyloma acuminata may very well contain an element of carcinoma. Bowen's disease, a premalignant condition, appears as a simple dermatologic problem. Rectal examination will help in differentiating among fecal impaction, rectal lesion, pelvic tumor, and abscess. Rectovaginal examination may reveal a rectocele. The diagnosis of rectal prolapse may not be particularly obvious, but it can be easily demonstrated by having the patient perform the Valsalva maneuver or sit on a toilet exerting pressure as though having a bowel movement. The prolapse will quickly develop. In the case of a villous adenoma of the rectum, rectal examination must be done slowly, carefully, and with much concentration, because the tumor is quite soft and difficult to feel with the examining finger. Because lymphatic drainage from the lower portion of the rectum and the anus is to the inguinal lymph nodes, palpation of that area is also indicated when malignancy is suspected.

Laboratory Studies

Anoscopic and sigmoidoscopic examinations are indicated in most conditions, both to document the extent of perianal disease and to identify other possible masses. For example, condylomata acuminata may extend into the anal canal. Biopsy and histologic examination are indicated because one cannot rely entirely on the gross morphologic features to make the diagnosis. Work-up of condylomata acuminata should include evaluation of the patient for forms of sexually transmitted diseases, including serologic tests for syphilis, cultures for gonorrhea, and testing for infection with human immunodeficiency virus.

Management

The management of anal masses should be individualized. Acute edematous hemorrhoids can be managed conservatively by recumbency, preferably in a Trendelenburg position, with the patient's head 30 degrees down; with astringents; and by daily use of stool softeners. In the mild forms of rectal prolapse, perineal strengthening exercises may be helpful, or the patient may be taught to replace the prolapse himself. Extensive prolapse requires surgical correction. The treatment of a rectocele is also surgical. Condylomata acuminata, when large, should be treated by excision, laser coagulation, electrocoagulation, or cryosurgery. Conservative treatment consists of applying 25 percent podophyllin. Other treatments include application of trichloroacetic acid, topical 5-fluorouracil cream, and antiviral immunizations.

References

Corman ML. Colon and rectal surgery. 2nd ed. Philadelphia: JB Lippincott, 1989:49.

Quan SH. Anal and para-anal tumors. Surg Clin North Am 1978; 58:591.

Sleisenger MH, Fordtran JS, eds. Gastrointestinal disease. 4th ed. Philadelphia: WB Saunders, 1989:1570.

Gastroenterology

Pruritus Ani

Wayne E. Silva, MD

61

Definition and Pathophysiology

Pruritus ani is a common symptom and not a disease. It is an unpleasant cutaneous sensation causing an intense desire to scratch. Anal skin is extremely sensitive and susceptible to varying degrees of injury. Therefore, the symptoms of pruritus ani may vary from itching to burning or soreness, depending upon the amount of injury and the presence of excoriation and secondary infection. It is common for patients to complain of the symptoms more intensely at night, when external stimuli of the day have decreased or are absent. Fecal soiling, leakage, and moisture are the primary irritants in most patients.

Differential Diagnosis

The numerous causes of pruritus ani are listed in Table 61-1. An approach to the differential diagnosis is shown in Figure 61-1. By the time the patient is first seen by the physician, the original initiating cause has often been complicated by secondary problems. The problem often becomes a self-perpetuating one in that the already damaged skin initiates itching and scratching, which causes further irritation and further symptoms, resulting in further scratching, further damage, and so forth. Eighty-five percent of cases of pruritus ani are the result of local anorectal problems and overzealous cleansing of this area by the patient.

Overzealous cleansing involves vigorous rubbing, which irritates the perianal skin and causes inflammation and pruritus. Local anorectal and vaginal pathology, including hemorrhoids, fissures, fistulas, polyps, proctitis, prolapse, or neoplasm, cause excessive chronic moisture to the anorectal region. The persistent presence of excess mucus, stool, urine, vaginal discharge, or perspiration in the anorectal area predisposes to skin irritation, infection, or inflammation as causes of pruritus. Dermatologic disorders are the cause of pruritus ani in approximately 15 percent of patients. Candidiasis in the patient using antibiotics, contact dermatitis, psoriasis, and syphilis are the most common skin lesions that cause anal itching. Laundry detergents, sprays, douches, deodorants, sanitary napkins, and toilet tissue can all be allergenic. Certain foods have been identified as causes of pruritus ani. The symptoms may result from the food causing a change in stool pH or from particular foods causing diarrhea. Acidic foods such as tomatoes, citrus fruits and juices, chocolate, coffee, beer and alcoholic beverages, nuts, spices, and even milk have been cited as being responsible for pruritus ani. Drugs that commonly cause diarrhea, including quinidine, colchicine, and mineral oil, often cause anal itching. Ironically, patients' itching may be exacerbated by the very drugs they apply locally to treat pruritus ani. On occasion, anal itching can be the initial or major complaint of the patient with a systemic illness such as obstructive jaundice, diabetes mellitus, lymphoma, or leukemia. Parasites (such as pinworm and ascariasis) should also be considered.

Psychoemotional factors have been cited as a cause of pruritus ani, particularly in very tense and anxious individuals. Despite a thorough history and physical examination, the inciting cause of pruritus ani often cannot be found. If the clinician is convinced that there is no serious underlying pathology, reassurance, symptomatic therapy, and careful follow-up are usually sufficient to deintensify or totally relieve the symptoms.

Diagnostic Approach

History

Most patients complaining of pruritus ani are men, in a ratio of about 4 : 1. These patients are frequently overweight, hairy, and perspire a great deal. Tight-fitting clothes may result in friction and increased moisture, which may damage the perianal skin. Red-haired and fair-skinned individuals tend to have more sensitive skin and an increased risk of damage. A history of any of the conditions listed in the differential diagnosis should be sought, along with a history of bowel complaints. A careful review should be conducted of the patient's bowel habits, stool consistency, and specific circumstances surrounding the symptoms of pruritus ani. Symptoms frequently recur around times of stress, such as income tax time. A detailed description of use of toilet tissue for wiping should be obtained because many patients believe that harder wiping will make the anus cleaner and therefore prevent the itch. This, in fact, simply produces more skin damage. Pruritus ani caused by pinworms (enterobiasis) frequently occurs in school-age children and institutionalized patients. The symptom is most prevalent at night because that is when the gravid female worms migrate.

Physical Examination

Acute pruritus ani is characterized by a red weeping perianum, occasionally with petechiae. When chronic, the skin is thickened and frequently erythematous, with deep furrows and excoriations. Lichenification occasionally occurs and presents as white patches on the chronically irritated perianal skin. The presence of a local condition such as a prolapsed hemorrhoid, fissure, fistula, or neoplasm is usually obvious on examination and can be identified as an inciting cause. Patients with a dermatologic problem usually, but not always, have evidence of the condition elsewhere (i.e., the characteristic lesions of psoriasis or seborrheic dermatitis). The presence of a systemic disease is usually marked by characteristic findings elsewhere, such as the diffuse adenopathy of a lymphoma. Rectal examination may demonstrate the presence of a condition not initially obvious on inspection, such as the presence of a prolapsing internal hemorrhoid, anal papillitis, minimal rectal prolapse, anal fissure, polyp, or rectal neoplasm. Villous adenomas produce large amounts of mucus that seep through the anus. Although difficult to feel, they can be palpated during rectal examination.

Laboratory Studies

The largest proportion of cases of pruritus ani are caused by very obvious local anorectal abnormalities. A standard initial management plan that does not include extensive or expensive instrumentation or laboratory studies is advised for virtually all patients. It includes local therapy aimed at symptom control as a diagnostic trial. Should the patient not respond to these initial simple management methods, further work-up may be indicated.

Evaluation for systemic disease in the patient without local anal pathology, but with persistent symptoms, should include a glucose determination to rule out diabetes and other appropriate tests for other systemic diseases.

In children or institutionalized patients, a search for pinworms should be done. A diagnosis of pinworms can often be made at the bedside using a cellophane tape swab. The cellophane tape, arranged with the sticky side out, is placed over a tongue depressor blade and pressed firmly against the perianal region. The tape is then spread on a glass slide and examined under the microscope at low power. The patient may bring the swabs in from home and have them examined in the laboratory for ova. With three such consecutive preparations made before bathing or defecation, the diagnosis can be established in approximately 90 percent of cases. Stool evaluation for eggs is seldom helpful, although on occasion they may be found in stool after laxative or enema use. A potassium hydroxide (KOH) prep-

Table 61-1 Factors Associated with Pruritus Ani

Overzealous Cleansing	**Foods**
Vigorous rubbing	Tomatoes
Local Anorectal Pathology	Hot peppers
Hemorrhoids	Citrus fruits and juices
Anal fissure	Chocolate
Fistula in ano	Coffee
Anal polyp	Alcoholic beverages
Rectal prolapse	Nuts
Neoplasm	Spices
Excess perspiration	Milk
Chronic vaginal discharge	**Systemic Diseases**
Urinary incontinence	Obstructive jaundice
Fecal incontinence	Diabetes mellitus
Dermatologic Conditions	Lymphoma, leukemia
Psoriasis	**Parasites**
Contact dermatitis	Pinworm
Syphilis	*Ascaris*
Candidiasis	**Drugs**
Condylomata acuminata	Local anorectal treatments
Allergic Reactions	Quinidine
Anorectal treatments	Colchicine
Laundry detergents	Mineral oil
Sprays, douches	**Psychoemotional**
Deodorants	
Sanitary napkins	**Idiopathic**
Toilet tissues	

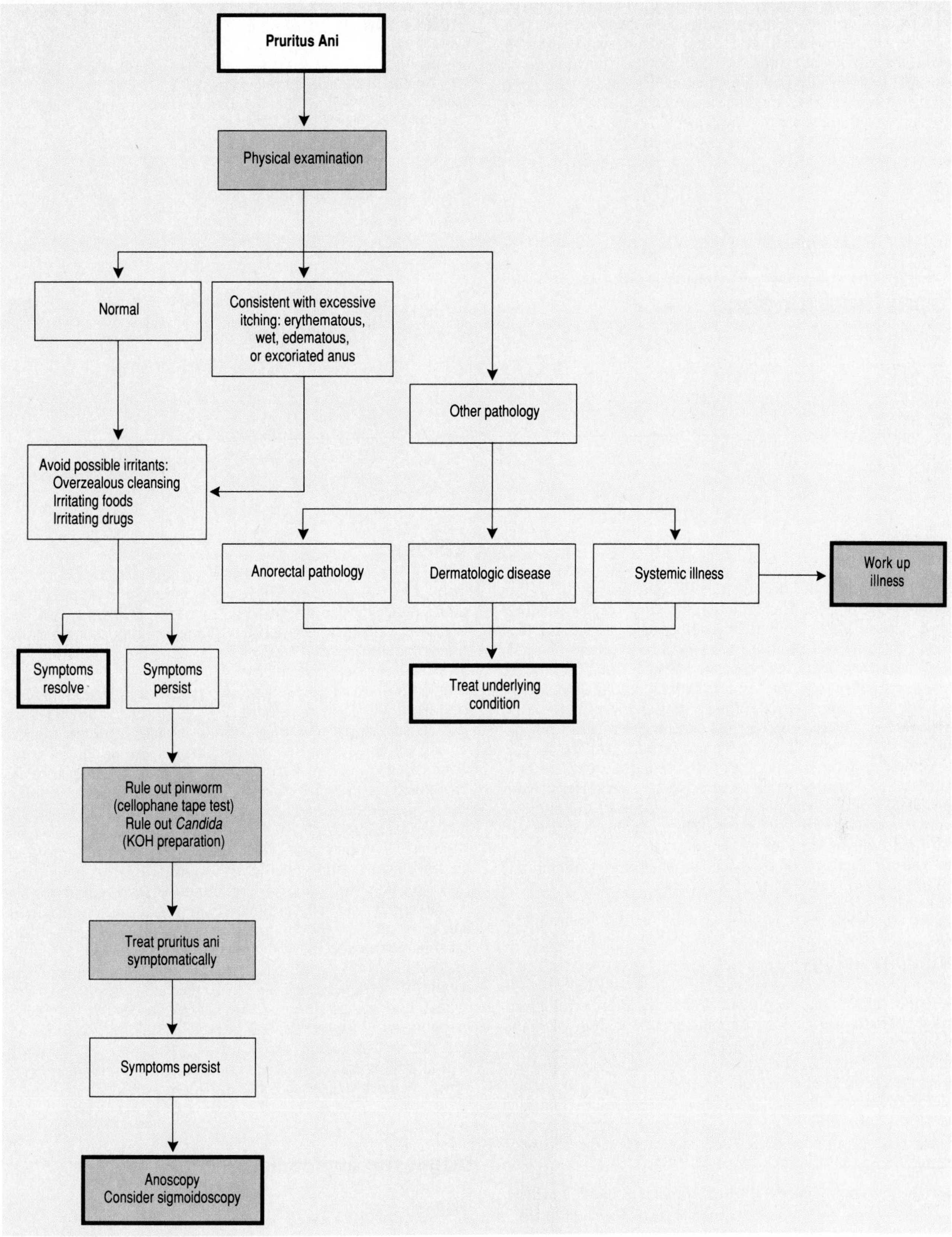

Figure 61-1 Algorithm for a diagnostic approach to pruritus ani.

aration of anal skin scrapings looking for the branching hyphae of *Candida* may document the presence of *Candida* infection. In the male homosexual, gonococcal cultures and serologic testing for syphilis are indicated. With persistent symptoms or signs suggesting more pathology than is evident by inspection and palpation, anoscopy or sigmoidoscopy may reveal proctitis, a tumor, or the presence of pinworms.

References

Kirsner JB, Shorter G, eds. Diseases of the colon, rectum and anal canal. Baltimore: Williams & Wilkins, 1988:692.

Sleisenger MH, Fordtran JS, eds. Gastrointestinal disease. 4th ed. Philadelphia: WB Saunders, 1989.

Fecal Incontinence

Wayne E. Silva, MD

62

Definition

The definition of fecal incontinence depends greatly upon the patient's point of view. The definition will vary with the patient's fastidiousness: minor soiling or inability to control flatus is a disaster to some, but a minor inconvenience to others.

Partial fecal incontinence, defined as intermittent soiling or involuntary passage of flatus, occurs with pathology of the internal sphincter or the external sphincter muscle. Total anal incontinence, secondary to complete loss of sphincter muscle control, results from a physical loss of muscle tone, damage to the sensory innervation, or pathology of the central nervous system. Overflow anal incontinence occurs when a large fecal load stretches the rectal ampulla, causing relaxation of the internal sphincter and loss of the defecation reflex, despite the presence of normal sphincter muscle mechanism.

The mechanisms of fecal incontinence are shown in algorithm form in Figure 62-1.

Pathophysiology

The spectrum of fecal incontinence extends from involuntary passage of flatus to total loss of sphincter tone, with involuntary passage of formed stool. Some patients with fecal incontinence will describe only "diarrhea" to the physician for fear of embarrassment. The anal canal has an external sphincter that is controlled voluntarily after toilet training. The internal sphincter, made of rectal smooth muscle, is controlled autonomically. It relaxes as feces push against it. Fecal continence depends upon several factors:

1. Effective contraction of the anal sphincter complex, which depends upon the consistency of the rectal contents and the presence of sensory receptors in the rectum and anal canal to appreciate the presence of rectal contents.
2. Maintenance of the normal acute angulation of the anorectum.
3. An intact perineal body.

This combination of physiologic and anatomic factors results in normal continence. Interruptions of all or some of the factors may result in fecal incontinence.

Etiology

The most common cause of fecal incontinence is anorectal pathology that may interfere with any of the mechanisms noted previously. Surgical trauma due to anal operations such as fistulectomy and hemorrhoidectomy is a common precursor to fecal incontinence, particularly in the patient who has had recurrent surgical procedures. Extensive perirectal infection or scarring from abscesses or fistulas disrupts normal sphincter tone and sensory appreciation of rectal contents. Obstetric trauma during childbirth, most commonly due to a third-degree laceration or episiotomy, may cause transient postoperative or more prolonged incontinence. Low rectal resections and anastomoses that are performed as an attempt to spare the patient a colostomy may also cause incontinence. Rectal prolapse results from weakened anal sphincter tone and the loss of pelvic support in the anorectum. Although this is a gradual process, when the prolapse is chronic, fecal incontinence is a common accompaniment. Chronic laxative abuse results in an atrophied and lax sphincter, which allows stool leakage. Fecal impaction causing obstruction may be complicated by diarrhea surrounding the impaction. Obstipation may become apparent when the patient has fecal soilage. Spinal cord disease, cauda equina syndrome, and diabetic neuropathy may be associated with fecal incontinence. Diseases affecting muscle, such as scleroderma and polymyositis, may also cause the symptom. Psychogenic soiling, called encopresis, is a common cause of fecal incontinence, especially on psychiatric in-patient wards.

Diagnostic Approach

History

A careful history of anorectal surgery, obstetric trauma, or chronic perirectal infection is important to obtain, because most cases of true incontinence are the result of one of these factors. A careful search in the history for psychiatric problems and laxative abuse is necessary. A long history of chronic constipation may suggest the presence of fecal impaction or a rectal prolapse. A good review of systems is necessary when the possibility of a neuromuscular deficit is considered.

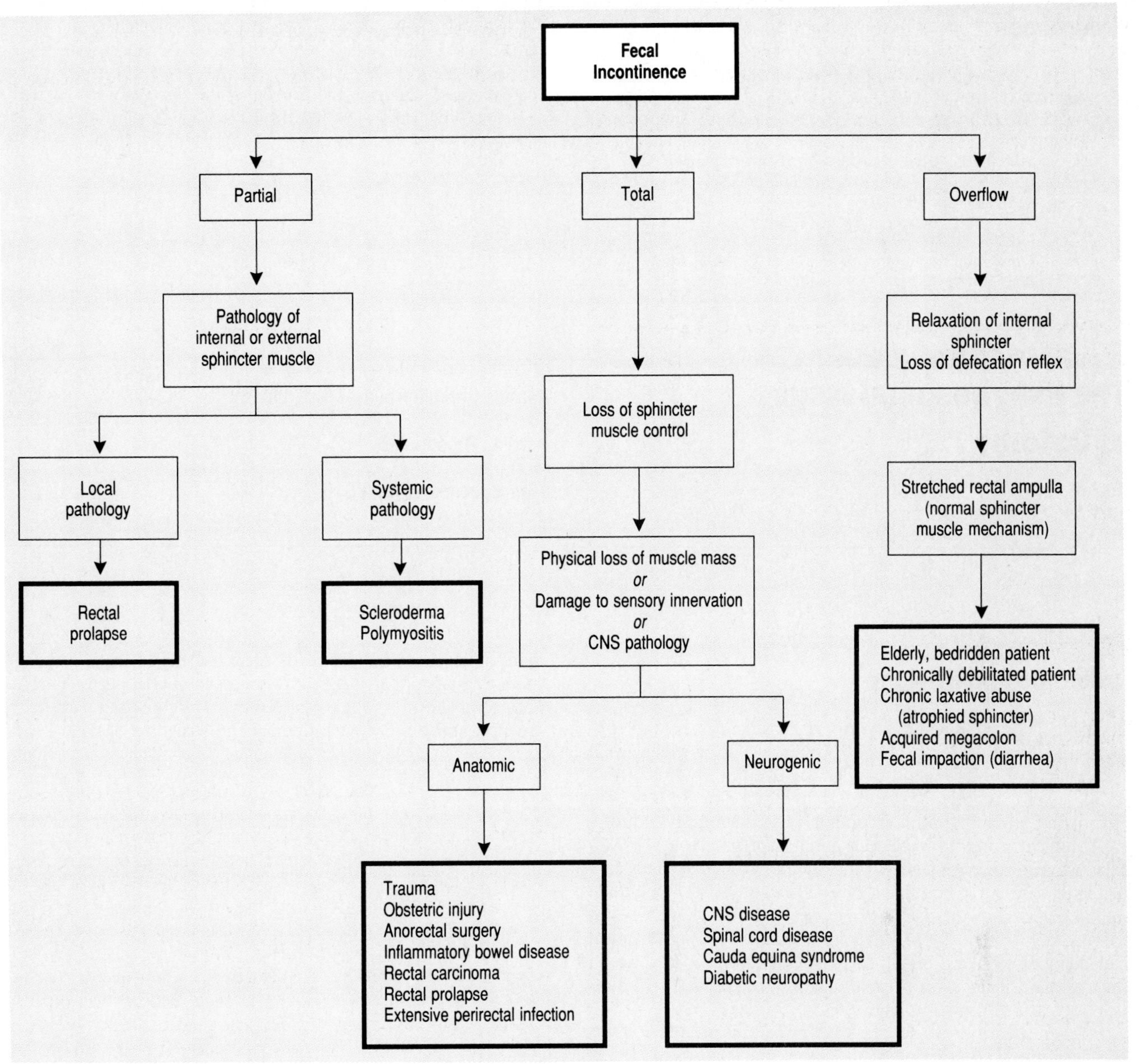

Figure 62-1 Mechanisms of fecal incontinence. CNS = central nervous system.

Physical Examination

Inspection may result in some clues to the etiology of the incontinence by identifying evidence of surgical or obstetric trauma or a perirectal infection. A rectal prolapse may be especially obvious after coughing. Digital examination may identify the presence of fecal impaction, but particularly important is confirmation of normal sphincter muscle tone. With the examining finger placed gently into the rectum, a normal sphincter should exert a constant firm and steady encircling pressure on the examining finger when the patient tries to bear down. The normal sphincter responds to gentle touching of the perianal skin by contracting. With the examining finger, anatomic defects or breaks within the sphincter mechanism should be sought.

The identification of a break or defect in the normal sphincter suggests local anorectal pathology as the cause of the leakage. A lax, but uninterrupted sphincter (no defect on palpation, but inadequate contraction around the finger on command) is most commonly the result of a chronically distended and relaxed ampulla. This is usually secondary to chronic constipation and laxative abuse. The absence of a palpable sphincter defect in association with a lax sphincter, but an empty ampulla, should raise the possibility of a more unusual cause of incontinence. In such a situation, if there is no obvious anorectal local pathology such as hemorrhoids, prior obstetric or anal trauma, laxative abuse, chronic constipation, or abscess, then neurologic pathology should be considered. An extensive neurologic history and physical should be performed, and an electromyographic (EMG) study should be considered.

Laboratory Studies

Most causes of fecal incontinence require no diagnostic laboratory evaluation because the history and physical examination provide the diagnosis. Occasionally, anoscopy and sigmoidoscopy may demonstrate scars or destructive lesions within the anal canal. EMG is occasionally necessary to assess the degree of sphincter function. Anorectal manometry studies can be helpful. Often, a trial of conservative management including sphincter strengthening exercises, the use of bulk preparation in the diet, and drugs to decrease intestinal motility may provide diagnostic clues.

References

Corman ML. Colon and rectal surgery. 2nd ed. Philadelphia: JB Lippincott, 1989:171.
Corman ML. The management of anal incontinence. Surg Clin North Am 1983; 63:177.
Fry RD, Gardner IJ. Anorectal disorders. Clin Symp 1985; 37(6).
Hoexter B, Labow SB. Office diagnosis of common anorectal problems. Hosp Med, February 1981:41.
Kirsner JB, Shorter G, eds. Diseases of the colon, rectum and anal canal. Baltimore: Williams & Wilkins, 1988:693.
MacLeod JH. A method of proctology. Hagerstown, MD: Harper & Row, 1979:85.
Shackelford RT, Zuidema GD. Surgery of the alimentary tract. 2nd ed. Philadelphia: WB Saunders, 1982:327, 381, 630.
Sohn N, Weinstein MA, Rabbins RD. Anorectal disorders. Curr Probl Surg 1983; 20(1).

The Psychosocial Issues of Ostomy

63

Patricia Gamble-Hovey, MSW, LICSW
Harry L. Greene, MD
Jean Boucher, RNC, MS, ET

Definition and Etiology

The psychosocial issues of ostomy are those concerns and conflicts produced as the result of surgery to alter the normal elimination of body wastes through the urethra or anus (Table 63-1). A stoma is created on the abdomen to restore the person to function and health. It is frequently a life-saving procedure.

Medical conditions necessitating approximately 110,000 new ostomy surgeries per year include (1) acute bowel abscess or fistula formation, requiring diversion of stool; (2) long-term inflammatory bowel disease; (3) obstruction that may result from tumor or adhesions from prior operations; (4) perforation caused by disease or trauma; and (5) congenital abnormalities in the case of infants. The normal anatomy of the digestive and urinary tracts is shown in Figure 63-1.

Essentially, there are three kinds of ostomies. Colostomy is most common, comprising 65 to 75 percent of all ostomies. In colostomy the stoma empties from the large intestine. There are several forms of colostomy, which may be permanent or temporary (Fig. 63-2). Ileostomy diverts wastes from the small intestine along the ileum (Fig. 63-3). Urostomy bypasses the bladder, allowing drainage of urine directly from the kidneys (Fig. 63-4).

Each kind of ostomy is performed for precise medical or surgical indications, and each may have its own unique management or psychosocial concerns. Most ostomy patients, however, share a set of concerns. Ostomy necessitates changes in lifestyle. The ostomate must "let go" and reorganize life-long patterns of function and belief that influence the structure of daily living.

Table 63-1 Psychosocial Issues Affecting the Ostomate

Concerns of life and death	Relational/social acceptance by: Partner Family Significant others
Loss of body parts	Educational systems and vocational systems
Altered body function	Sexuality as concern of special need
Stoma management Leakage of wastes Odor Gas Audible noises	Loss process across all psychosocial concerns
Altered self-perceptions Self-image Self-esteem Body image Sexuality	

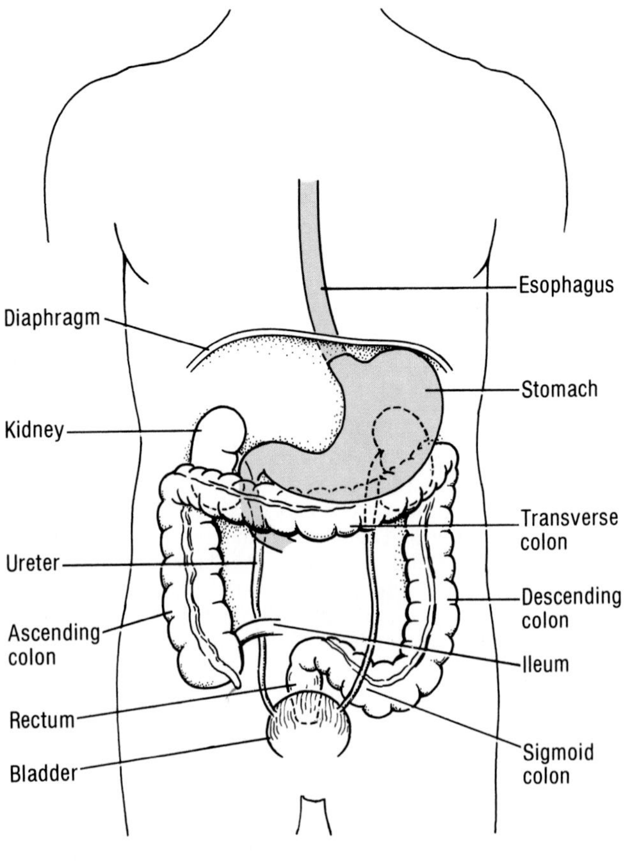

Figure 63-1 Normal anatomy of the digestive and urinary tracts.

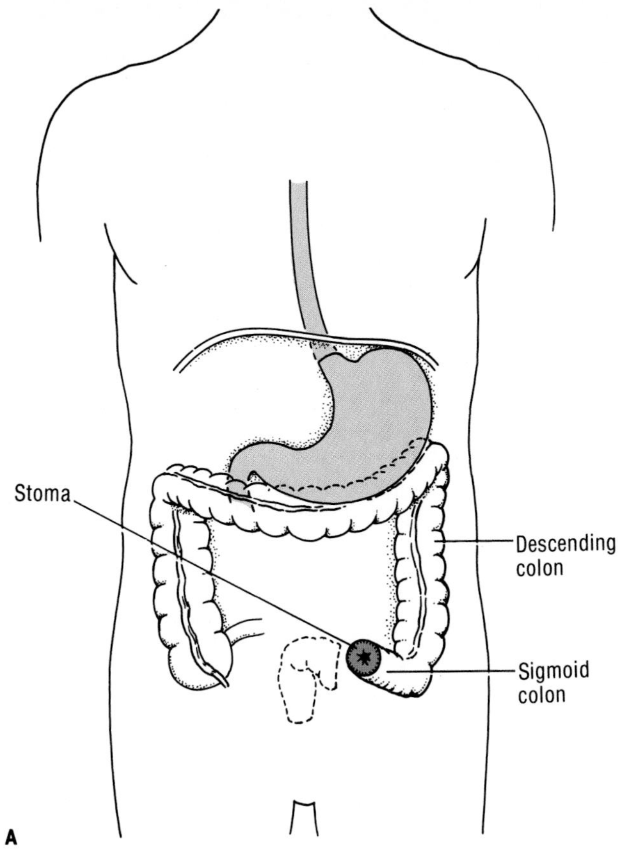

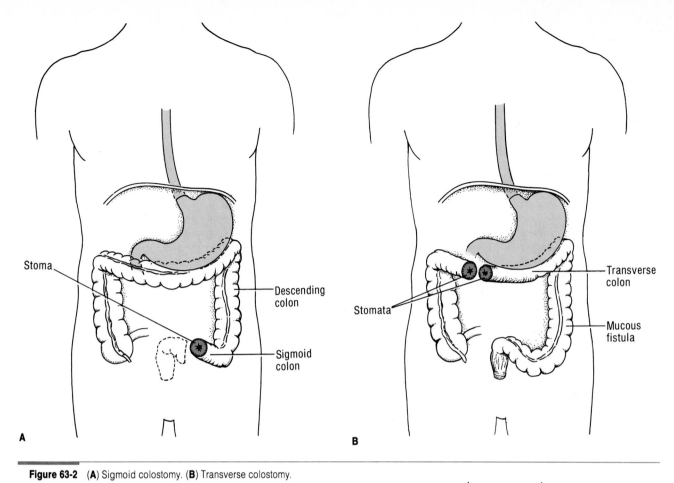

Figure 63-2 (**A**) Sigmoid colostomy. (**B**) Transverse colostomy.

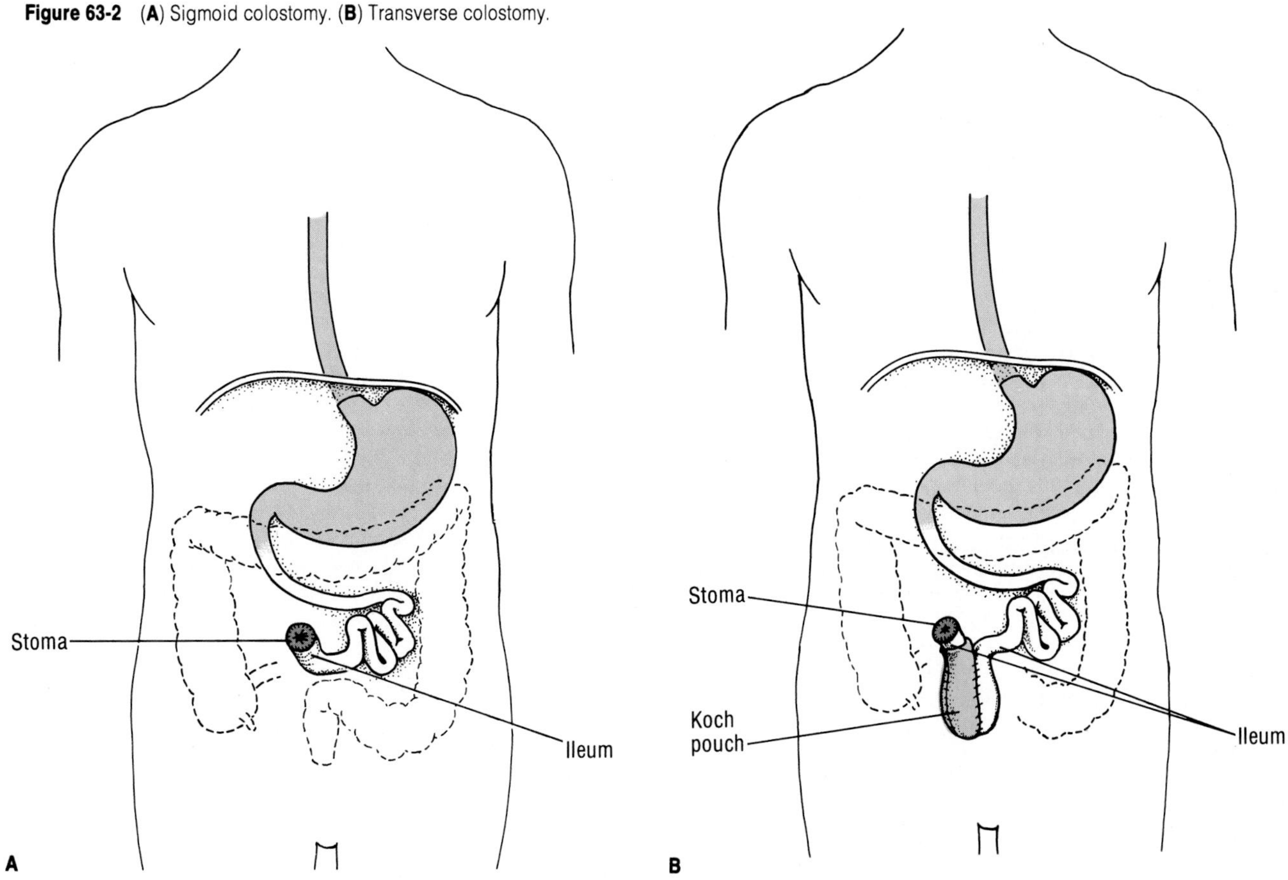

Figure 63-3 (**A**) Ileostomy. (**B**) Continent ileostomy.

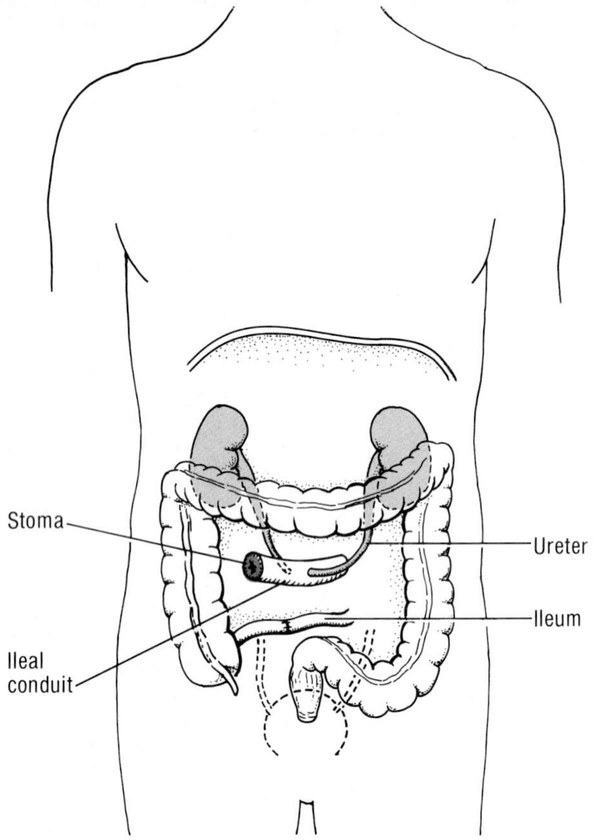

Figure 63-4 Urostomy.

The results of ostomy force an individual to alter body function, which threatens the area of social demand for control and conformity of the earliest developmental stages. The loss of body parts requires appropriate grieving and demands acceptance and resolution of fundamental personal perceptions. The individual's self-esteem, body image, and sexuality are altered and must be helpfully reconstructed. Acceptance and positive inclusion by the patient's friends and family are critical. Maslow's theory of a hierarchy of needs applies to the ostomate. Saving the patient's life is the first issue. This is followed by the ability to manage the new pattern of waste elimination in a manner that is both personally and socially acceptable. Continuance of gratification and maintaining quality of living in the community with others is the third level of need, but it cannot be separated out. The three elements of acceptable life enmesh in an interdependent pattern. Therefore, the goal of the health care team responsible for a person who is about to become a new ostomate is to facilitate the patient's process of loss and acceptance, management of altered body function, and development of new concepts of self that enable him or her to enjoy a positive, meaningful life.

The Ostomy Care Team

It is the responsibility of the ostomy care team to initiate psychosocial assessment and diagnosis and to provide rehabilitative care to the ostomy patient. The team should include the following personnel: (1) the patient's primary care physician; (2) the surgeon; (3) the staff nurse; (4) an enterostomal therapist (a certified registered nurse) trained in stoma management, appliance variations, and psychosocial ostomy issues); (5) a United Ostomy Association (UOA) volunteer visitor, a trained person who has experienced similar circumstances; and (6) a social worker who may help with organization of needed home care or other services.

It is unusual for all of these persons to be found in any single hospital or medical center. It is the responsibility of the primary care physician to provide assessment and diagnosis for psychosocial concerns in consultation and collaboration with other health care personnel. Most hospitals do have registered nurses who are known for skill and sensitivity with ostomy patients. Failure to prepare the patient adequately for ostomy and educate him or her about its use may permanently impair or markedly increase problems. The UOA is a resource available across the country, with approximately 600 chapters in the United States. This group of patient-peers provides leadership in all aspects of ostomy care. It is the optimal source of personal knowledge regarding management, supplies, and current technology to facilitate living with a stoma. The wise physician, anticipating an ostomy surgery, immediately consults and collaborates with as many of these persons as are needed. The telephone number to call to reach a UOA volunteer is (714) 660–8624. The staff at this number will identify a local chapter in your area.

Diagnostic Approach

Definitive Periods of Care for the Ostomate

Prior exposure of the patient to ostomy can set the tone for acceptance. This can be easily accomplished by asking if the patient knows someone with an ostomy and what that person's experience has been. This contact and information provide an opportunity to dispel myths and correct misconceptions.

There are three definitive periods of time in which the ostomate struggles with the preceding concerns: (1) the preoperative period, (2) the postoperative, early recovery period, and (3) the post-discharge, follow-up period. Developmental stage, age, and required life tasks of the individual will influence the person's unique response to ostomy surgery and necessary psychosocial adjustment. For example, the life tasks that shape personal identity and intimate relationships in the young adult will involve different psychosocial issues for resolution than those of the middle-aged person who may be in the midst of meeting the heavy economic demands of college-age children or the increasing needs of aging parents. Also, in the middle-aged person, the ostomy may necessitate a major shift of family roles; at a time when careers are often peaking, this adds special stresses.

Preoperative Period

It is optimal to begin rehabilitative measures before surgery whenever medical circumstances allow the time. Assessment and diagnosis of patient concerns begins when the surgeon defines the need for surgery, its expected procedure, and the location, where possible, of the best stoma site. This early preoperative period is the ideal time to involve the enterostomal therapist. Although most surgeons performing this procedure are aware of the importance of proper location, the enterostomal therapist can be consulted for stoma marking.

Symptoms of psychosocial concerns are listed in Table 63-2. Development of a trusted working relationship, honest answers and information, and reassurance that the team will be there to assist the person throughout the recovery process will enable the patient to express these symptoms of psychosocial need directly or indirectly.

Postsurgical Period

In the first several days following surgery, the bodily demands of surgery, including the management of pain and the wound itself,

Table 63-2 Symptoms and Concerns Suggesting Inadequate Adjustment in the Ostomate

Open questions about value of life	Oversimplified behavior
Anger	Acting out
Fear	Increased demands on staff
Depression	Increased dependence
Altered mood	Unrealistic independence
Shift in behavioral patterns	Irritability with significant others
Withdrawal	Reluctance or refusal to begin stomal management
Isolation	Reluctance or inability to share with members of care team or support system
Silence	
Mania	

divert the attention of the patient and provide a transition period before he or she begins to form new life patterns and attitudes. Symptoms of conflict and resolution overlap and evolve across periods. As the reality of the ostomy begins to affect the patient, observable or elicited symptoms of stress may include the following:

1. Double strain of diagnosis and prognosis coupled with the impact of the stoma.
2. Repugnance toward stoma function, and fear that others will find them repugnant.
3. Reluctance or refusal to look at or to touch the stoma.
4. Reluctance or refusal to begin learning stoma management.
5. Fear of waste leakage, odor, audible noise, gurgling, or gas.
6. Fear that the stoma and/or appliance will be visible to others with certain clothing and activity.
7. Withdrawal, anger, anxiety, depression, and sadness.
8. Overly enthusiastic, manic posture, or denying behaviors.
9. Fear that their partner will find them unattractive and sexually unacceptable.
10. Fear of social isolation or isolation of self to avoid embarrassment or possibility of fears being realized.
11. Questions regarding ability to return to school or work with normal function.
12. Questions regarding economic impact on family and support system.
13. Costs of management supplies.
14. Sense of being less whole as a man or woman.
15. Questions like "Who am I?" "Who am I in relation to you?" "How will this affect our lives together?"
16. Increased anxiety as discharge from the hospital approaches.

The steady presence and personal support of the physician, enterostomal therapist, nurses, and the social worker will allow the health care team to focus on support and essential rehabilitative teaching of the stoma management throughout these postoperative days. A prime objective of the enterostomal therapist is to provide sufficient time for the patient's partner, family, and friends to share their feelings and fears in careful therapeutic conversations. The direction of this intervention will be toward open communication, acceptance, and resolution of fears and problems. The UOA visitor is invaluable in providing a model for return to normal living by one who has experienced similar circumstances.

Special attention needs to be given to the impact on sexuality during this postoperative period. The reality of human physiology and anatomy is such that a person's elimination and sexual functions are interdependent. Waste elimination and personal sexual patterns are taboo subjects of conversation in our culture. We use intricate vocabulary of innuendo when alluding to these subjects with anyone. The variations of patterns and need in these areas are as individual as people are unique, and it is important to allow adequate time to deal with individual needs.

According to older UOA members, it was a rare person in the past who had discussed implications for sexuality before or after ostomy surgery. The response to this vacuum ranges from irritation to rage. It is hoped that we are doing better in modern times. The percentages of sexual impairment for men with colostomies and urostomies may be high. Even limited potency may require as long as 2½ years to return. The responses of partners may range from total support of the ostomate to complete rejection. Consideration of developmental stage and life tasks of the ostomate is critical in professional assessment of sexual implications. The choice of penile implants, pharmacologic erectile therapy, vacuum devices, or prosthetic devices may be part of counseling. It should be assumed that sexual concerns are primary for all persons facing ostomy surgery, whether the concerns are articulated or not. It is the responsibility of the physician and the team to initiate communication and facilitate treatment of these sexual problems.

Post-Discharge Follow-up Period

Regular post-discharge appointments in the ostomy outpatient clinic maintain the bridge of interdependence with the care team that enables the new ostomate to rehabilitate. In the process of evaluating stoma care concerns, the enterostomal therapist is sensitive to the symptoms described previously and evaluates them with the patient in collaboration with the primary physician and social worker. It becomes increasingly important to assess whether presenting problems are primary or secondary. Relational problems of long standing may now surface and no longer be tolerable in view of the new life circumstances. Ongoing counseling may be needed to facilitate the sorting-out process and find options for resolution. Participation in the regular meetings of the local UOA may prevent the new ostomate's temptation to avoid social activity and adopt reclusive patterns.

The degree of life-coping skills the person has demonstrated in relationship with others in the past will indicate the degree of help the ostomate will need to develop new self-perceptions and life patterns.

The radical life-shaping implications of ostomy, colostomy, ileostomy, and urostomy surgeries for altered body function and perceptions of self in relation to others indicate the critical need for assessment and diagnosis of psychosocial issues of the ostomate and their support systems. The goals for these patients are acceptance of their situation; coping with altered body function and management, relational/role shifts, and changing perceptions of self; and reintegration into the social system. As Adlai Stevenson has said, "Understanding human needs is half the job of meeting them." This is nowhere more true than in dealing with the new ostomate.

References

Abrams JS. Abdominal stomas. Boston: John Wright, PSG Inc, 1984.

Burroughs ML. Enterostomal therapy in the Canadian health care system. In: Broadwell DC, Jackson BS, eds. Principles of ostomy care. St. Louis: CV Mosby, 1982.

Hughes SW. Establishing an outpatient clinic. In: Broadwell DC, Jackson BS, eds. Principles of ostomy care. St. Louis: CV Mosby, 1982.

Jeter KF. These special children: The ostomy book for parents of children with colostomies, ileostomies and urostomies. Palo Alto, CA: Bull Publishing, 1982.

Liss JL. Psychiatric issues in ostomy management. In: Broadwell DC, Jackson BS, eds. Principles of ostomy care. St. Louis: CV Mosby, 1982.

Mahoney JM. Rehabilitation. In: Guide to ostomy nursing care. Boston: Little, Brown, 1976:177–190.

Mikolon S. Economic facilitators and barriers to living with an ostomy. In: Broadwell DC, Jackson BS, eds. Principles of ostomy care. St. Louis: CV Mosby, 1982.
Mikolon S. Psychosocial issues in ostomy management. In: Broadwell DC, Jackson BS, eds. Principles of ostomy care. St. Louis: CV Mosby, 1982.
Mullen BD, McGinn KA. The ostomy book: Living comfortably with colostomies, ileostomies, and urostomies. Palo Alto, CA: Bull Publishing, 1980.
Negata FK. Human sexuality. In: Broadwell DC, Jackson BS, eds. Principles of ostomy care. St. Louis: CV Mosby, 1982.
Ostomy quarterly. Los Angeles: United Ostomy Association.
Steele G, Osteen RT. Colorectal cancer: Current concepts in diagnosis and treatment. New York: Marcel Dekker, 1986.
Sultenfuss SR. Psychosocial issues and therapeutic intervention. In: Broadwell DC, Jackson BS, eds. Principles of ostomy care. St. Louis: CV Mosby, 1982.

Urethral Discharge

Nelson M. Gantz, MD

Definition

Urethral discharge refers to secretions passed through the urethral meatus at times other than voiding. The secretions may be described as clear, purulent, or bloody. The complaint of urethral discharge is generally found only in men and is rarely noted in women. The problem of urethral discharge is the most frequent complaint reported by men with a sexually transmitted disease. The discharge arises from the urethral glands and less often represents prostatic secretions.

Etiology

The causes of urethral discharge include both noninfectious and infectious etiologies. The discharge that occurs immediately after ejaculation is normal and consists of semen or seminal components. Other noninfectious causes of urethral discharge include mechanical or chemical irritation, urethral stricture, nonbacterial prostatitis, urethral diverticula, urethral caruncle, and phimosis. In the majority of patients, the urethral discharge has an infectious etiology. Infectious causes of urethral discharge may be classified as gonococcal urethritis, if caused by *Neisseria gonorrhoeae*, or nongonococcal urethritis (NGU), if not caused by *N. gonorrhoeae*. There is increasing evidence that NGU is more frequent than gonorrhea and is the most common sexually transmitted disorder in men. It should be noted that the two forms of urethritis are not mutually exclusive, as mixed infections (15 to 25 percent) may be present in the same patient.

Gonorrhea is caused by *N. gonorrhoeae,* a relatively fastidious gram-negative diplococcus that is distinguished from other *Neisseria* species by sugar-fermentation reactions. Several agents have been implicated as causes of NGU. Studies show that *Chlamydia trachomatis*, an obligate intracellular organism, can be isolated from about 40 to 50 percent of patients with NGU. Chlamydial serotypes D, E, F, G, H, I, J, and K have been associated with urethral, cervical, and ocular infections and pelvic inflammatory disease. Other organisms responsible for a small percentage of cases of NGU include *Ureaplasma urealyticum*, or T-strain (tiny) mycoplasma, *Trichomonas vaginalis,* and herpes simplex virus. *C. trachomatis* also causes about 80 percent of cases of postgonococcal urethritis (PGU), a disorder that occurs in men following treatment of gonococcal urethritis with penicillin. These men have a mixed infection with *N. gonorrhoeae* and *C. trachomatis.*

Diagnostic Approach

Table 64-1 compares the clinical features in patients with gonococcal urethritis with those seen in patients with NGU, and Table 64-2 lists the costs of evaluating a patient with a urethral discharge. Although the clinical picture of NGU is different from that seen in patients with gonococcal urethritis, there is sufficient overlap between the symptoms of the two entities that a Gram stain and culture of the discharge are essential for diagnosis.

A flow chart for diagnosing gonococcal urethritis and NGU is presented in Figure 64-1. When a man presents with a discharge or dysuria, or both, material should be obtained for Gram stain and culture by stripping or "milking" the distal urethra. If no discharge is obtained, insert a calcium alginate nasopharyngeal swab into the urethra for a distance of 2 cm to obtain material for a gonococcal culture. Material should also be obtained in this manner for a Gram stain to look for neutrophils and intracellular gram-negative diplococci.

Because recent voiding may decrease the amount of discharge and interfere with obtaining a specimen for Gram stain, the urethral specimen should be collected at least 3 hours after voiding.

A presumptive diagnosis of gonococcal urethritis can be made if the Gram stain of the material shows typical gram-negative intracellular diplococci. The sensitivity of the Gram stain of urethral discharge exceeds 95 percent in men with gonococcal urethritis. The urethral culture for gonococcal ure-

Table 64-1 Clinical Distinction Between Gonococcal and Nongonococcal Urethritis

Manifestation	Gonococcal	Nongonococcal
Incubation period	2–7 days	10–21 days
Onset	Abrupt	Gradual
Discharge	Yellow, profuse	Thin, clear, watery
Dysuria	Moderate	Mild

Table 64-2 Costs of Evaluating a Patient with a Urethral Discharge

Test	Cost ($)
Gram-stained smear	12.00
Culture for gonococcal urethritis	23.00
Serologic test for syphilis	17.00
Calcium alginate swab	0.25

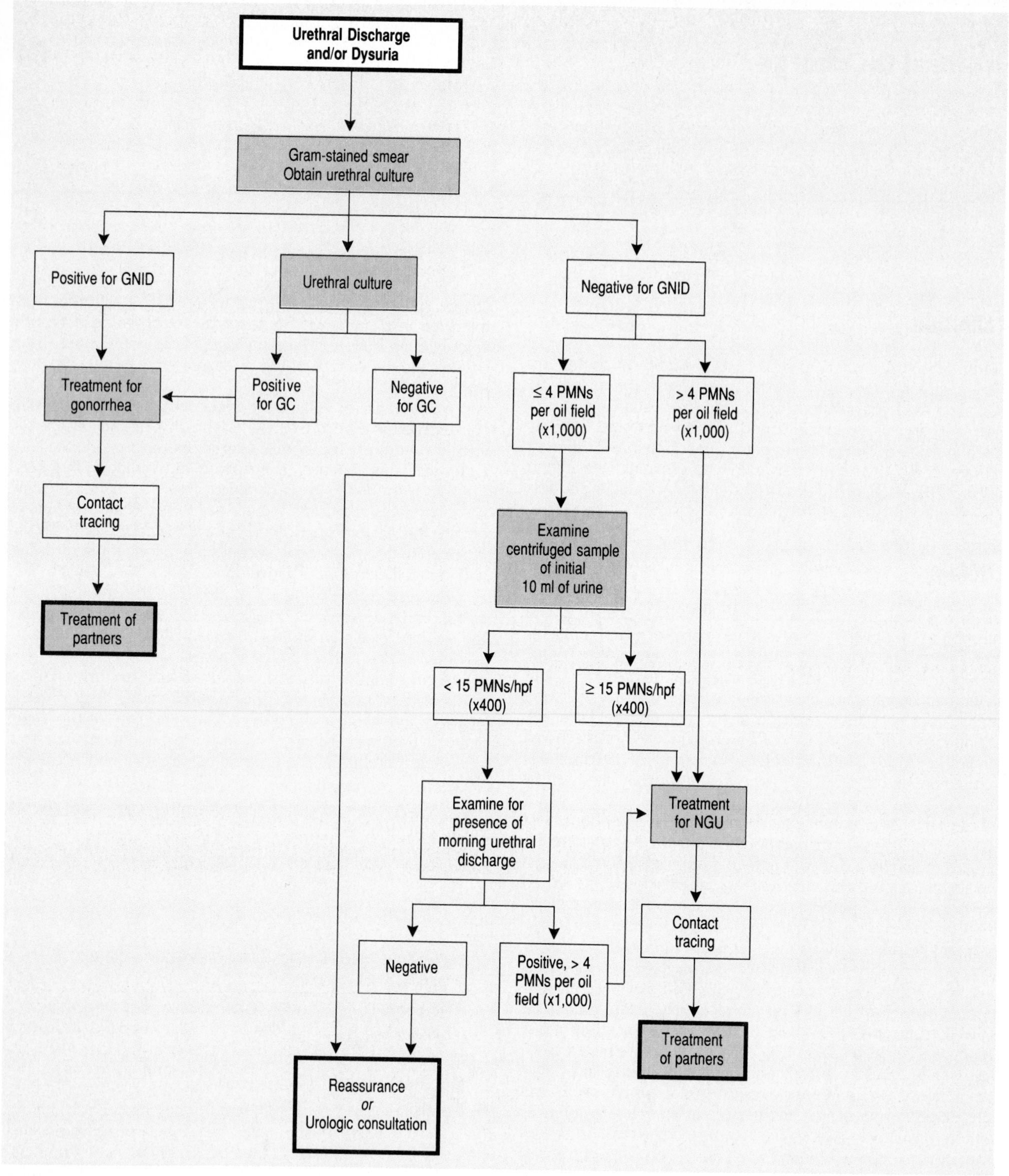

Figure 64-1 Algorithm for the diagnosis of gonococcal and nongonococcal urethritis. GC = gonococcal urethritis, GNID = gram-negative intracellular diplococci, NGU = nongonococcal urethritis, PMNs = polymorphonuclear leukocytes.

thritis will confirm the diagnosis and detect an additional 5 percent of smear-negative cases. If the urethral smear reveals only extracellular or atypical gram-negative diplococci, the diagnosis depends on the culture results. Cultures of the anal canal and pharynx are also essential in male homosexuals with suspected gonorrhea. For patients from whom material cannot be obtained for examination, the first 10 drops of urine can be obtained for Gram smear and culture. Material for gonococcal culture should be inoculated onto modified Thayer-Martin medium or collected and transported on swabs placed in modified Stuart's or Amies plus charcoal transport medium. Plates should be incubated in an atmosphere of 3 to 5 percent carbon dioxide (candle jar or incubator) at 35°C to 37°C for 48 hours. Beta-lactamase tests should be performed on all isolates of *N. gonorrhoeae.* A serologic test for syphilis should also be obtained in all patients with suspected gonococcal arthritis or NGU, because a patient may have more than one sexually transmitted disease.

The diagnosis of NGU is usually one of exclusion. Because laboratory facilities to culture chlamydial and ureaplasmal organisms are not readily available to clinicians, the diagnosis of NGU is established by demonstrating urethral inflammation (>4 polymorphonuclear leukocytes per high power field) with no evidence of *N. gonorrhoeae*, by Gram-stained smear or urethral culture. Noncultural methods to detect chlamydial antigen are available, but those tests lack the sensitivity of a culture. In patients with NGU who have a persistent urethral discharge after treatment with tetracycline, one must consider medication-compliance problems, failure to treat sexual partners, reinfection, an uncommon cause of NGU such as *Trichomonas* infection, or tetracycline-resistant *U. urealyticum.* A wet preparation of the urethral discharge should be examined for the presence of *T. vaginalis.* The female sexual partner should also be examined for *Trichomonas* organisms, which may be easier to detect in a woman.

Herpesvirus may also cause NGU, but skin lesions are usually present that help to establish the diagnosis. Reiter's syndrome, a disorder of unknown etiology, should also be considered in a patient with NGU who fails to respond to treatment. Patients with Reiter's syndrome note a urethral discharge that usually begins 1 to 2 weeks after sexual intercourse. Other features of the syndrome that often appear 1 to 5 weeks after the onset of the urethral discharge include an arthritis, mucocutaneous skin lesions called keratosis blennorrhagica and balanitis circinata sicca, and conjunctivitis. The findings may not be present all at once, and there is no diagnostic laboratory test. Patients with Reiter's syndrome are often positive for HLA-B27 histocompatibility antigen.

References

Centers for Disease Control. 1989 STD treatment guidelines. MMWR 1989; 38(No. S-8).

Slamm WE, et al. *Chlamydia trachomatis* urethral infections in men: Prevalence, risk factors, and clinical manifestations. Ann Intern Med 1984; 100:47.

Swartz SL, et al. Diagnosis and etiology of nongonococcal urethritis. J Infect Dis 1978; 138:445.

Impotence

Charles H. Emerson, MD

65

Genitourinary

Definition

Impotence is an inability to maintain an erection suitable for vaginal penetration or an inability to ejaculate. Male infertility means that the patient is unable to impregnate a normal woman. Impotence is one cause of male infertility, but not all infertile men are impotent. For example, patients with a block of the testicular excretory system or with primary disorders of the seminiferous epithelium are infertile; however, they have normal erectile and ejaculatory function. Libido refers to the desire for sexual intercourse. Complete loss of libido will result in impotence, but the converse is not true. In certain forms of impotence, there may be only a marginal decline in libido.

The most frequent complaint is an inability to achieve a satisfactory erection. A small number of patients are able to maintain an erection but cannot ejaculate. Inability to ejaculate with completely normal erectile function is unusual and tends to occur in men who are taking drugs that antagonize the sympathetic nervous system. In normal men, orgasm and ejaculation occur simultaneously. Rarely, patients describe orgasm without ejaculation. This history indicates retrograde ejaculation and is not necessarily a feature of impotence. However, because of its neurologic basis, it is frequently seen in men with some degree of erectile dysfunction.

Etiology

Clinically, it is useful to classify impotence under several categories: neurologic, endocrine, drug-induced, psychogenic, primary penile, and miscellaneous (Table 65-1). Erection and ejaculation are controlled by neurogenic mechanisms. Sensory and psychic stimuli are integrated in the cerebral cortex and flow throughout the limbic system to the lumbar spinal cord. At this level, a sympathetic outflow and a parasympathetic outflow through S2-S4 control the vasculature in the corpus cavernosum that regulates penile blood flow. Relaxation of the afferent arteries and constriction of the efferent arteries lead to penile vascular engorgement and subsequent erection. Tonic contraction of the transverse perineal, bulbocavernosus, and ischiocavernosus muscles also helps to maintain erection. In addition to the neurogenic outflow originating in the cerebral cortex, parasympathetic outflow from S2-S4 is reflexively triggered by tactile stimulus of the genital and perineal regions, and by bowel and bladder distention. This also results in erection. Ejaculation is controlled predominantly by sympathetic outflow from the spinal cord. A lesion in any of these neurologic pathways can cause impotence.

Almost all forms of endocrine impotence are due to low plasma testosterone or elevated plasma estrogen concentra-

Table 65-1 Classification of Impotence*

Endocrine
Primary testicular insufficiency
Hypopituitarism
Pituitary tumors, prolactinoma
Estrogen-producing neoplasms (adrenal, testes)

Drugs and Toxins
Alcohol
Estrogen
Narcotics
Antiestrogens (spironolactone, cimetidine)
Beta-adrenergic blockers
Anticholinergic agents
Sympatholytics (guanethidine, reserpine, alpha-methyldopa)
Antipsychotics (phenothiazines, thioxanthenes)
Antidepressants (tricyclics, monoamine oxidase inhibitors)

Neurologic
Diabetic peripheral and autonomic neuropathy
Spinal cord trauma
Multiple sclerosis

Psychogenic

Penile
Priapism (also a component of neurologic dysfunction)
Peyronie's disease
Penile trauma

Miscellaneous
Vascular disease of the lower aorta, iliac arteries

* This list is partial. In particular, there are many more neurologic diseases that cause impotence.

tions. Testosterone is necessary for normal penile growth and stimulates the cortical outflow pathway controlling erection. Estrogen, in amounts greater than those produced by the normal man, antagonizes the actions of testosterone. Primary disorders of the endocrine glands are the major cause of endocrine impotence. However, hepatic and renal disease can alter the plasma testosterone : estrogen ratio. Drugs produce impotence by several mechanisms. They can alter testosterone-estrogen balance or produce neurologic blockage in pathways controlling erectile function. Alcohol produces impotence by two mechanisms. High blood alcohol levels produce neurologic blockage, whereas chronic ethanol exposure lowers the plasma testosterone : estrogen ratio by a toxic action on the liver and testes.

Psychic and physical stress, particularly that associated with severe illness, decreases libido. This in turn decreases cortical outflow, a prime regulator of erectile function (psychogenic impotence). Psychic stress is so important and common that almost all men experience, at some time in their lives, the inability to have or maintain an erection. Because erectile dysfunction is, in itself, a form of stress, there is a definite tendency for impotence to be self-reinforcing.

In addition to diseases of the penis itself, there are miscellaneous causes of impotence. The most important of these is atherosclerotic disease of the lower abdominal aorta or iliac arteries. This causes impotence by reducing blood flow to the penis.

The exact incidence of the various forms of impotence is difficult to gauge. Lesions of the penis that impair coital function are rare. In these patients, the diagnosis is obvious if a careful history and physical examination are performed. Drugs are an important cause of impotence, and almost all patients taking certain kinds of medications experience some degree of erectile or ejaculatory dysfunction. Endocrine disorders, a classic cause of impotence, are less common, but they are not rare. These disorders are being diagnosed with increased frequency with better testing procedures. Impotence is common in patients with spinal cord trauma. This is a significant problem in countries like the United States, where the incidence of motor-vehicle accidents is high. Impotence is not uncommon in long-standing diabetic neuropathy; therefore, a relatively large percentage of impotence patients are diabetics.

Diagnostic Approach

History

As in all areas of clinical medicine, the work-up begins with the history. The time of onset, frequency, severity, and other attributes of the patient's erectile dysfunction should, like any other symptom, be determined. Acquired endocrine disorders and neuropathies generally produce slow, insidious loss of erectile dysfunction. Abrupt onset is characteristic of drug-induced impotence and, in some cases, psychic stress. The importance of a comprehensive history of drug or toxin exposure cannot be overemphasized. The physician should inquire about alcohol, narcotics, marijuana, prescription drugs, over-the-counter preparations, and industrial toxin exposure.

For purposes of both diagnosis and management, it is necessary to determine the state of the libido. This may be difficult, because sexual function is an intensely personal and ego-supportive aspect of life. Anxiety, evasiveness, and denial are frequently encountered when this question is explored. In most cases, the history should also be taken from the patient's sexual partner. Caution and understanding are required because this is likely to increase the patient's anxiety. In most cases a decreased libido is associated with psychogenic or physical stress. Lesions of the spinal cord and peripheral nerves, vascular insufficiency, and primary penile lesions do not directly reduce libido; however, the stress associated with these disorders can be a secondary cause of decreased libido. A gradual loss of libido in the absence of obvious psychic or physical stress suggests insidious failure of testosterone secretion. However, sexual behavior is strongly ingrained, and many men with failing testosterone secretion deny loss of libido.

One should determine whether the patient continues to experience nocturnal erections or awakens with an erection. In normal men, erections occur during the rapid eye movement (REM) stage of sleep and with bladder distention. In organic impotence the loss of erectile function is as great during REM sleep as it is during erotic stimuli. This is not the case in psychogenic impotence. Other questions can provide clues that help identify the specific cause of impotence. If there has been a loss of testicular and adrenal androgens, the patient will have decreased frequency of shaving and loss of pubic and axillary hair. There may also be symptoms of hypothyroidism or adrenal insufficiency. This suggests pituitary disease. Headache is a common problem in many individuals, but in a patient with the insidious development of impotence, it raises the possibility of a pituitary tumor. Question the patient thoroughly about paresthesia, paralysis, decreased sensation, and symptoms of autonomic nervous system dysfunction. The neurologic control of erectile function is closely associated with bowel and bladder innervation. Patients with neurogenic impotence frequently have symptoms of bowel or bladder dysfunction, such as incontinence or retention. A characteristic of impotence associated with diabetic neuropathy is the absence of testicular pain after firm palpation or blows to the testes. A history of claudication in the buttocks or lower extremities raises the possibility of disease of the lower abdominal aorta or iliac arteries.

Physical Examination

Certain parts of the physical examination deserve emphasis. A careful neurologic examination is essential. Sensation in the

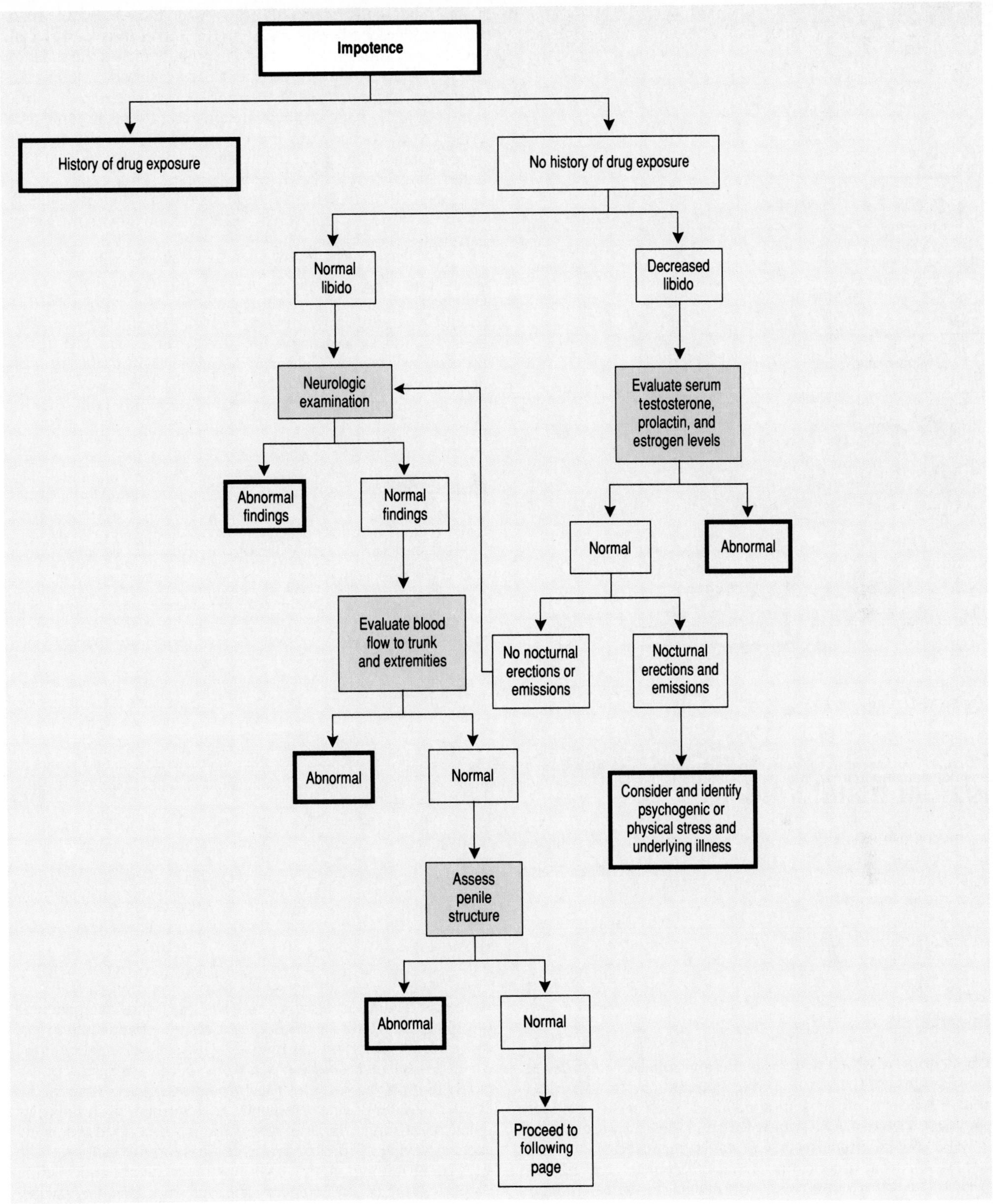

Figure 65-1 Algorithm for the diagnostic evaluation of impotence.

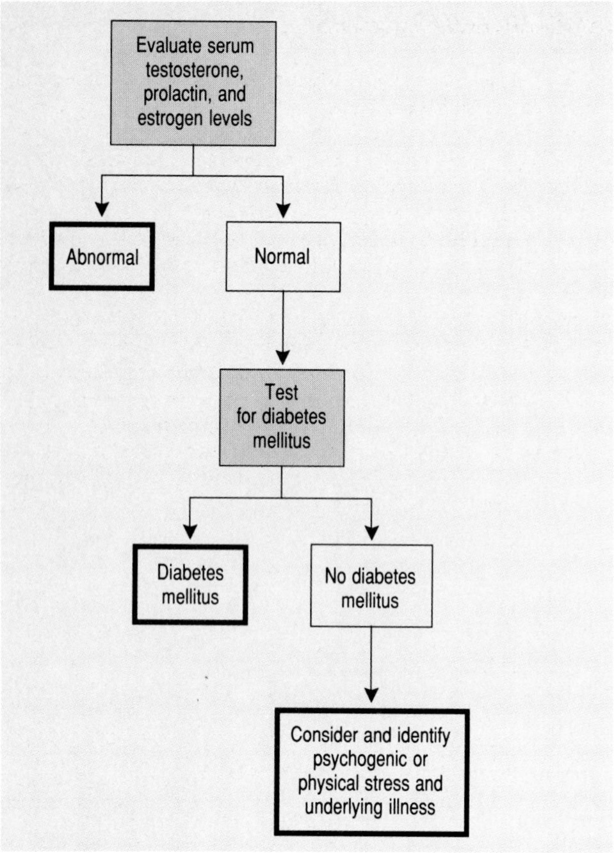

Figure 65-1 *Continued*

genital and perineal regions and the bulbocavernosus reflex (during the rectal examination, contraction of the external anal sphincter occurs after the physician gently pinches the dorsum of the glans penis) must be specifically checked. Evidence of decreased testosterone secretion or increased estrogen secretion should be sought. Physical signs are a loss of pubic and axillary hair, a change in the voice, and the development of gynecomastia. The size and consistency of the testes should be noted. A testicle less than 4 cm in diameter is frequently associated with decreased testosterone secretion. The visual fields should be tested by confrontation, and blood flow in the lower extremities should be evaluated.

The causes of impotence are so numerous that a detailed discussion of each entity is beyond the scope of this book. However, Figure 65-1 outlines a conceptual approach that should be useful in narrowing the differential diagnosis. The figure cannot be taken too literally because, as noted in the preceding discussion, a number of caveats apply to these guidelines. Moreover, even in certain patients with diseases that produce organic impotence, the major basis for impotence may be psychogenic.

References

Fisher C, et al. Evaluation of nocturnal penile tumescence in the differential diagnosis of sexual impotence. Arch Gen Psychiatry 1979; 36:431.

Krane RJ, et al. Impotence. N Engl J Med 1989; 321:1648.

Levine SB. Marital sexual dysfunction: Introductory concepts. Ann Intern Med 1976; 84:448.

Masters WH, Johnson VE. Human sexual inadequacy. Boston: Little, Brown, 1970.

Dysfunctional Voiding

Timothy B. Hopkins, MD

66

Definitions

Dysfunctional voiding symptoms are abnormal or disordered characteristics of urination. The symptoms may be separated into irritative bladder symptoms and obstructive bladder symptoms. There may be some overlap in these two categories.

The *irritative bladder syndrome* is characterized by frequency, nocturia, urgency, or dysuria. Frequency can be described as voiding more often than normal for that particular individual, or repeated voidings in short intervals. Nocturia means awakening at night (or after going to sleep) to urinate. Urgency indicates a sudden strong urge to urinate or a sensation of bladder fullness. Dysuria is defined as pain or discomfort associated with or immediately following urination. In men, this may be felt in the distal urethra or in the glans penis. In women, this generally feels as if it occurs in the tip of the urethra.

Several symptoms should be distinguished from irritative bladder syndrome. *Polyuria* is an abnormally increased volume of urinary output or frequent voiding in large amounts. *Nycturia* is the passage of larger quantities of urine at night (when the patient is recumbent) than during the day (when the patient is upright). *Strangury* is defined as difficult painful passage of urine accompanied by spasms.

The *obstructive bladder syndrome* is characterized by hesitancy, diminished force of the urine stream, dribbling, or increased residual urine. Hesitancy is described as straining or delay in initiating urination. Loss of force is described as slowing and narrowing of the stream or decrease in the caliber of the stream. Dribbling is the inability to terminate micturition abruptly at the end of urination; it is often manifested by starting and stopping of the stream at the end of urination. Intermittency is characterized by interruption of the stream. Residual urine can be described as the feeling or sensation of incomplete bladder emptying. Normally, after voiding, less than 100 cc should remain within the bladder.

Etiology

Understanding the innervation of the bladder and urethra is fundamental to establishing the etiology of voiding dysfunction.

The body of the bladder is primarily innervated by the parasympathetic nervous system (cholinergic). Cholinergic stimulation causes bladder contraction; conversely, cholinergic suppression or inhibition causes bladder relaxation. Some beta-adrenergic receptors in the body of the bladder act similarly to cholinergic fibers. The bladder neck is richly innervated by noradrenergic (alpha-sympathetic) nerve terminals. Stimulation of these fibers causes bladder neck contraction, whereas inhibition causes relaxation. The bladder neck acts as a proximal (internal) urethral sphincter. The brain acts primarily as an inhibitory factor to voiding.

In searching for the etiology of voiding dysfunction, remember that certain physiologic changes accompany normal aging. Bladder capacity, bladder and urethral elasticity (compliance), ability to postpone voiding, and urinary flow rate are reduced in the elderly. Uninhibited bladder contractions and postvoid residual volumes are increased. Younger people excrete most of their daily ingested fluids by 9 PM, but the elderly excrete more of theirs after 9 PM.

Irritative Bladder Symptoms

The symptoms of an irritative bladder (Fig. 66-1) generally occur concomitantly, although frequency, urgency, and dysuria each can occur as an isolated symptom. The etiology of irritative symptoms, for the most part, can be separated into local pathology, with decreased bladder capacity, or neurologic pathology, with cortical or upper spinal cord pathology.

Decreased bladder capacity may be secondary to bladder inflammation (most common etiology) or fibrosis. Inflammation of the mucosa, submucosa, or muscularis causes edema, which results in decreased functional bladder capacity. Bladder neck inflammation may result in premature afferent stimulation prior to complete filling of the bladder, with subsequent decreased bladder capacity. Bladder inflammation may be caused by infectious agents such as bacteria, viruses, *Chlamydia*, fungi, or noninfectious conditions such as foreign body, stone, or tumor. Bladder fibrosis occurs secondary to radiation injury, chronic infection, chronic obstruction, tuberculosis, cyclophosphamide

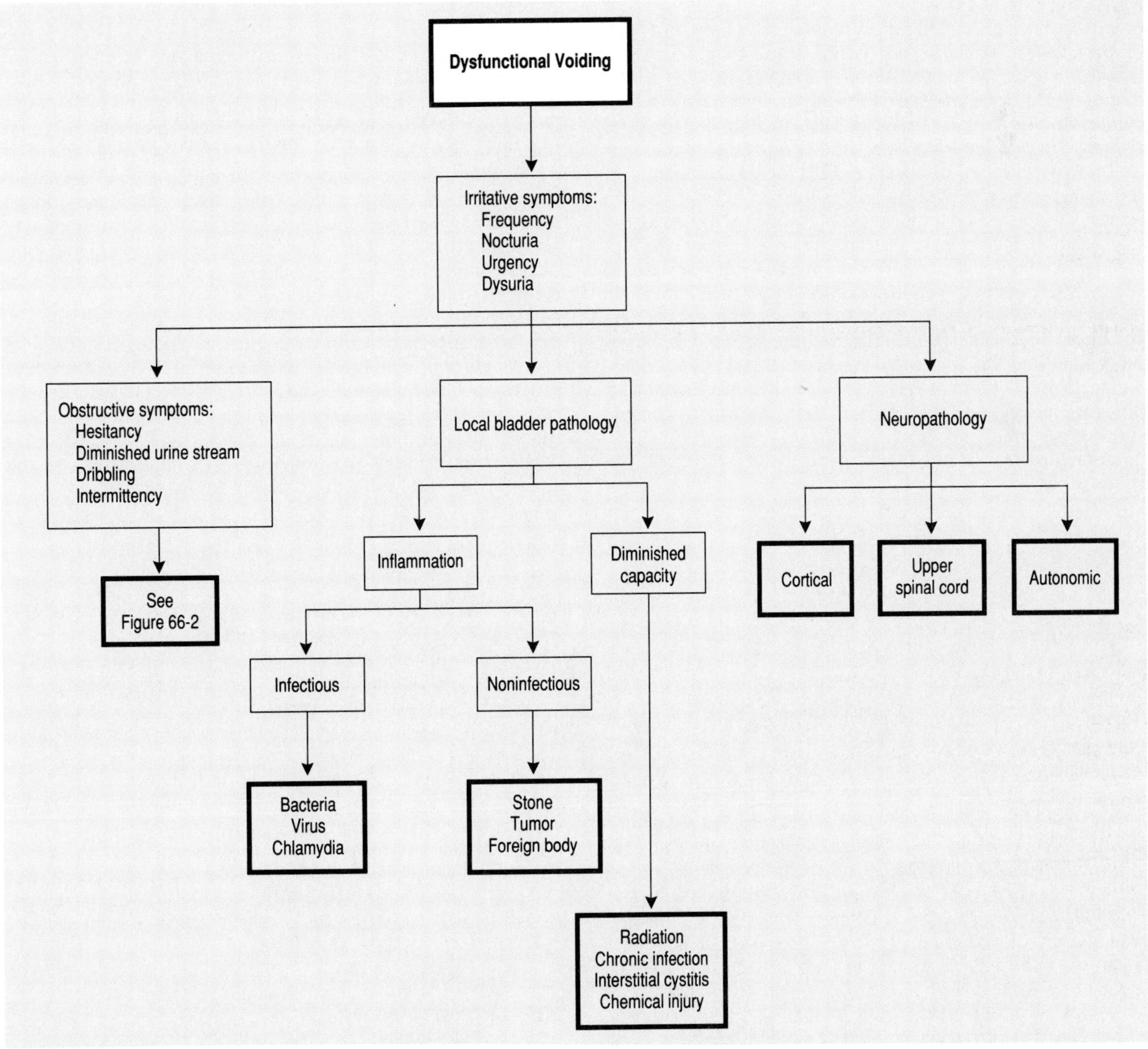

Figure 66-1 Algorithm for the evaluation of irritative bladder symptoms in dysfunctional voiding.

Genitourinary

use, or long-standing interstitial cystitis. Atrophic vaginitis contributes to reduced urethral tone and increased bladder neck sensitivity, which leads to frequency and urgency.

Neurologic disorders are frequently responsible for the patient's complaints of irritative bladder symptoms. Upper cortical centers normally have an inhibitory influence on voiding. Interruption of this inhibition by stroke, cerebral atrophy, or neurologic disease, such as multiple sclerosis, results in irritative symptoms or incontinence. Upper spinal cord injury or other neurologic disease affecting the upper spinal cord may also lead to a reflex uninhibited detrusor (spastic bladder). However, lower lesions involving the conus medullaris or peripheral nerves generally result in a flaccid bladder, not irritative symptoms. Anxiety associated with increased autonomic nervous system discharge may also lead to irritative symptoms.

Infection or inflammation of the urethra, urethral meatus, or the surrounding structures, such as the vagina and vulva, may also cause dysuria without frequency and urgency. Urethral obstruction may also lead to progressive irritative symptoms.

Symptoms to Be Distinguished from Irritative Symptoms

Polyuria, Nycturia, and Strangury

Polyuria and nycturia often reflect systemic problems, not bladder dysfunction. Polyuria, one of the earliest signs of renal disease, is a decrease in concentrating ability and an increase in urine output; it is seen most notably with diabetes insipidus. The osmotic diuresis of glucosuria in diabetes mellitus and the large oral intake in a compulsive water drinker or coffee drinker may also cause polyuria in the absence of bladder dysfunction.

An increased rate of urine production secondary to use of a diuretic, the decreased antidiuretic hormone (ADH) effect following alcohol ingestion, or the diuretic and stimulant effects of xanthine following coffee, tea, or soda ingestion also may lead to frequency or nocturia, even in the otherwise normal individual.

Nycturia, which implies improved renal perfusion with recumbency, is a manifestation related to the systemic mobilization of fluid into the intravascular space that had been sequestered in the interstitium of the lower extremities in a patient with right-sided congestive heart failure, liver disease, or chronic venous stasis.

Strangury may result from severe cystitis, prostatitis, or bladder stone.

Obstructive Bladder Symptoms

Obstructive bladder symptoms (Figs. 66-2 and 66-3) may be either congenital or acquired and acute or chronic. The group of obstructive symptoms generally occur simultaneously, although hesitancy, diminished stream, dribbling, intermittency, or a sensation of a residual urine may occur as an isolated symptom. Congenital lesions are more common in children, whereas acquired lesions are far more common in the adult. Common causes of obstructive bladder symptoms are as follows:

1. Benign prostatic hypertrophy or carcinoma of the prostate
2. Urethral stricture secondary to infection or injury
3. Neurogenic dysfunction
4. Acute infection of the urethra or prostate
5. Bladder stone
6. Bladder tumor involving the bladder neck
7. Severe constipation
8. Medication
9. Postoperative retention
10. Altered mental status

The bladder works much like the heart in that it reacts to an increasing workload by passing through successive phases of compensation and, finally, decompensation. In the early stages of obstruction, the bladder musculature hypertrophies to overcome the resistance imposed by obstruction. The bladder may develop pressures of 60 to 100 cm of water rather than its normal 30 to 50 cm of water with voiding. Because the bladder becomes more sensitive to filling as it hypertrophies, irritative symptoms of urgency and frequency are sometimes superimposed upon the classic obstructive symptoms. Hesitancy eventually occurs as the bladder develops contractions strong enough to overcome the obstruction. The stream, however, may gradually slow down, especially toward the end of voiding, as the detrusor muscle becomes exhausted. The detrusor muscle contraction that stimulates voiding may not be sustained, eventually leading to incomplete voiding and a residual urine. A progressive imbalance between the strength of the detrusor contraction and the urethral resistance may lead to a gradual increasing residual and, finally, chronic retention. Complications of the obstructive process include infection of the residual urine and acute urinary retention. Acute retention occurs as rapid filling of the bladder (due to a large fluid intake, especially alcohol, or use of a diuretic), or delay in voiding leads to overstretching of the already compromised hypertrophied detrusor.

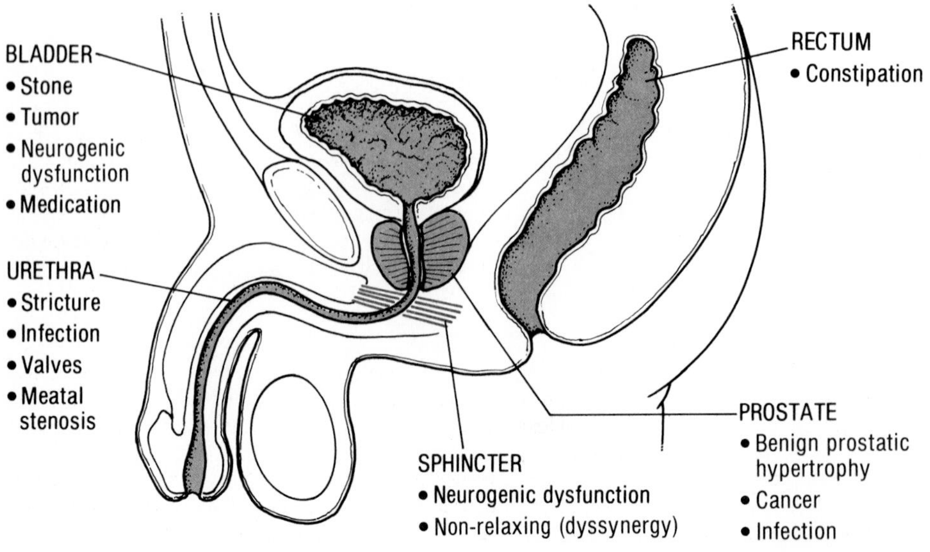

Figure 66-2 Causes of bladder obstructive symptoms.

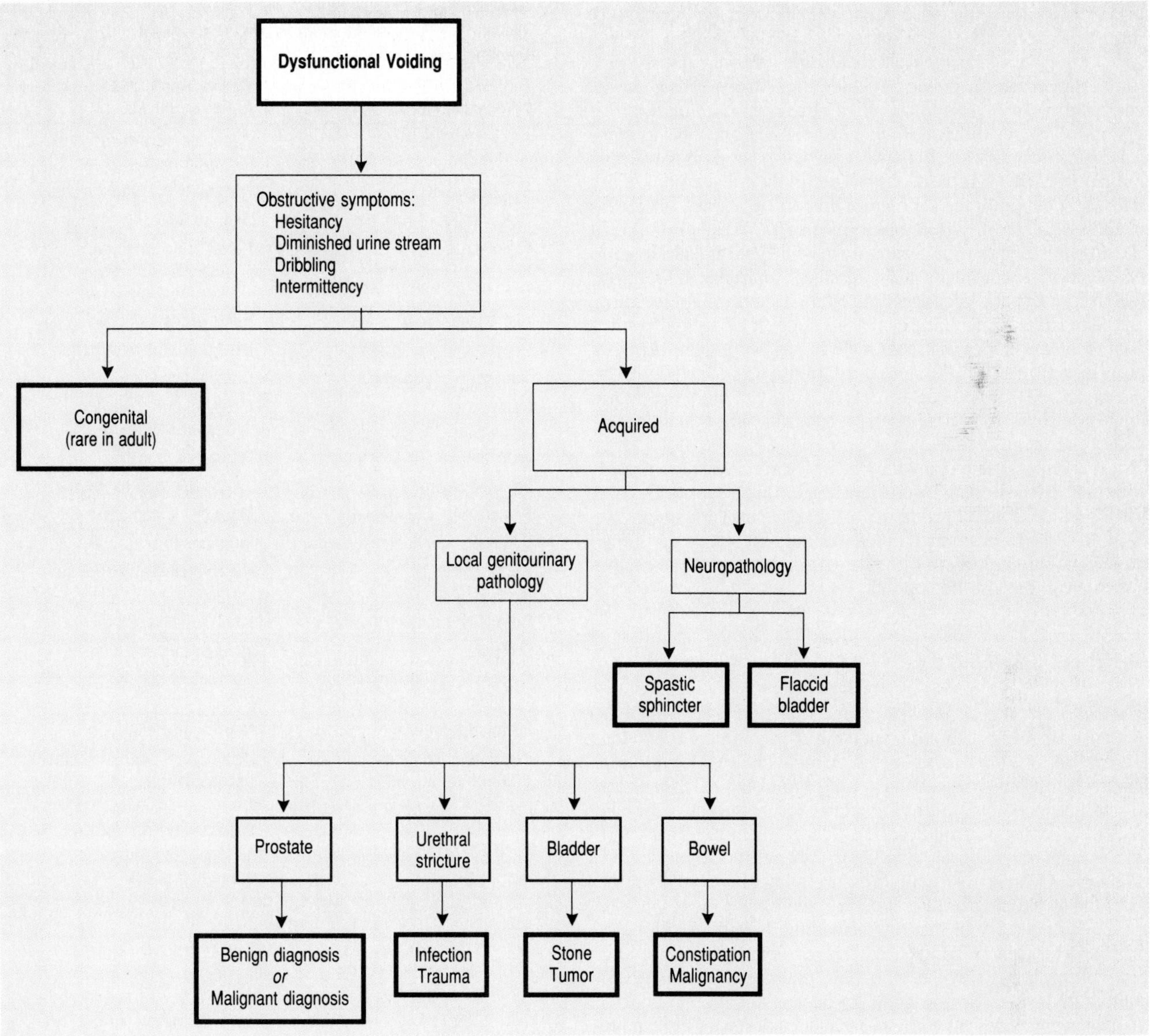

Figure 66-3 Algorithm for the evaluation of obstructive bladder symptoms in dysfunctional voiding.

Acute urinary retention may also be precipitated by infection or medications such as anticholinergics, antidepressants, tranquilizers, or calcium-channel blockers that decrease bladder tone or cloud the sensorium. Decongestants or adrenergic agonists may increase bladder neck tone and resistance.

Urinary retention in the early postoperative period may have been precipitated by bladder overdistention (while the patient was anesthetized), clouded sensorium and anticholinergic effect of pain medication, and recumbency.

Diagnostic Approach

An understanding of the patient's past and present symptoms often leads to the correct diagnosis and avoids the many pitfalls of rushing to a diagnosis. A clear understanding of how long each complaint has been present, how it has changed, what circumstances make it better or worse, and its relation to other symptoms is important. A history of similar symptoms in the past, the diagnosis of those symptoms, and treatment may significantly shorten the work-up. The history and physical examination are directed along the lines of the common etiology of each complaint.

Irritative Symptoms

When the irritative symptoms (see Fig. 66-1) of frequency, nocturia, urgency, and dysuria have an acute onset, search for other symptoms suggestive of urinary or prostate infection, because infection is the most common cause of irritative symptoms. The sudden onset of irritative symptoms, especially in a patient with fever or a history of past urinary tract infection, suggests infection as the principal cause of the patient's symptoms. If intermittent or colicky flank pain accompanies fever and irritative symptoms, consider the diagnosis of a kidney stone with infection, which would require prompt urologic intervention. A history of recent sexual contact or urethral or vaginal discharge or genital lesions should prompt consideration of venereal disease as the cause of infection.

Chronic or persistent symptoms after treatment of an acute urinary tract infection suggest a nonspecific urethritis, trigonitis, urethral diverticulum, or tuberculosis. However, if the initial and subsequent urine cultures show no growth, the diagnosis of interstitial cystitis or painful bladder syndrome is likely.

Inquire about prior pelvic radiation, chronic cystitis, urethral catheterization, pelvic or bladder operations, foreign body, chemical injury (including chemotherapy, e.g., cyclophosphamide), or recent viral illness. Associated symptoms of painless hematuria, passage of tissue, weight loss, or pain may imply tumor. Irritative symptoms associated with colicky flank pain, nausea and vomiting, a previous history of stone, or recent passage of gravel or blood may imply that a low ureteral stone is causing these symptoms. Strangury may indicate a bladder stone or infection. A complaint of increasing suprapubic discomfort, with frequency and urgency relieved for a short time by voiding, and a negative urine culture strongly suggest interstitial cystitis. Recurrent frequency that lasts a few hours without nocturia or other symptoms implies nervous tension. Frequency should be distinguished from polyuria. Nocturia (frequent night-time voiding) should be distinguished from nycturia (large quantities of night-time urine).

It is important to consider a neurologic etiology in a patient with a previously diagnosed neurologic disease or with fecal incontinence, spinal cord injury, or other complaint suggestive of neurologic disease, such as leg weakness or spasticity, numbness, visual difficulties, or radicular pain. A history of obstructive symptoms must also be sought.

Obstructive Symptoms

In addition to the classic symptoms of obstruction (hesitancy, decreased stream, dribbling, a feeling of incomplete emptying, increase in frequency, and nocturia), renal failure with minimal urinary symptoms may also be a presenting sign of obstruction in rare instances. Symptoms are often exacerbated by the intake of alcohol, coffee, or medications such as anticholinergics, antidepressants, decongestants, calcium-channel blockers, or tranquilizers. Obstructive symptoms are generally worse upon morning awakening or after a delay in voiding.

A prior history of spraying urination; difficult, multiple, or prolonged catheterization; urethritis; or venereal disease suggests urethral stricture as a possible diagnosis. Recent sexual contact or lesions on the genitalia or vagina suggest venereal disease (i.e., herpes). Weight loss in association with bony pains and urinary obstructive symptoms suggests advanced metastatic prostate cancer as the cause of the obstruction.

A thorough neurologic history in search of radicular pain suggestive of a lumbar herniated disk or tumor must be obtained. A history of a recent operation should be obvious.

Physical Examination

The physical examination should begin with a general assessment of the patient's reliability and mental status (Table 66-1). A general examination should search for clues of infection, prostatic cancer, or endocrine or metabolic abnormalities. In both men and women, attempt to observe the patient voiding to get an accurate assessment of the urinary stream, straining, or dribbling. Perform a careful abdominal examination to search for evidence of a flank mass or tenderness. Palpate and percuss the suprapubic area, looking for a distended or tender bladder. The epididymis and spermatic cord should be distinguished from the body of the testicle. Examine the inguinal region for lymphadenopathy and hernia.

In women, a pelvic examination must be done to look for cervical or vaginal discharge and tenderness or mass of the bladder, urethra, cervix, or adnexa. Vaginal mucosal friability and punctate hemorrhages or a urethral polyp may indicate atrophic vaginitis. Suprapubic tenderness without a mass would most likely be the result of an infection or inflammation. A suprapubic mass would imply retention or, rarely, a tumor.

Table 66-1 Physical Examination in the Evaluation of Dysfunctional Voiding

Physical examination	Clinical information to be sought
General appearance	Cachexia, severity of symptoms
Mental status	Reliability of history, anxiety
Observation of voiding	Description of symptoms
Flank mass	Renal cell carcinoma, polycystic kidney, hydronephrosis
Flank tenderness	Renal stone, infection
Suprapubic distention	Bladder-outlet obstruction
Suprapubic tenderness	Bladder irritation
Penis	Mass, anatomic variant, meatus adequacy
Scrotum	Mass, infection
Inguinal region	Lymphadenopathy, hernia
Female pelvic tenderness	Mass or inflammation
Vaginal or cervical discharge	Inflammation
Rectal tone	Neurologic dysfunction or mass
Bulbocavernosus reflex	Intact lower reflex arch
Prostate	Mass or inflammation
Genital sensation, perianal reflex	Neurologic deficit
Peripheral reflex	Neurologic deficit
Leg spasticity, exaggerated DTR	Often corresponds to bladder spasticity
Leg flaccidity, diminished DTR	Often corresponds to bladder flaccidity
Postvoid residual greater than 100 cc	Obstruction or diminished bladder tone

Abbreviation: DTR = deep tendon reflexes.

A rectal examination should be done in both men and women; assess rectal tone, feel for a rectal mass, and perform a bulbocavernosus reflex test (feeling for rectal sphincter contraction when the glans penis or clitoris is squeezed), which implies an intact lower reflex arch.

The prostatic contour, consistency, and tenderness must be assessed in men. An area of hardness in the prostate may imply tumor, stone, or chronic prostatitis. A boggy, hot, and tender prostate suggests infection.

Carefully check genital sensation, perianal reflexes, and peripheral reflexes and sensations for any neurologic deficit. If the legs are spastic, the bladder is often spastic as well; if the legs are flaccid, the bladder is often flaccid. A very active bulbocavernosus reflex may imply some spasticity of the urethral sphincter. Its absence may be related to sensory or motor denervation of the bladder.

If there is a suggestion of retention of urine and no prostatic or urethral infection, pass a urethral catheter to measure the residual urine. If this is greater than 100 cc, an obstructive lesion is likely. If the catheter meets obstruction distal to the prostate or sphincter in men or is difficult to pass in women, a stricture is likely. If obstruction is at the sphincter level, ask the patient to try to void, as this may relax a tight external urethral sphincter and allow passage of the catheter.

Laboratory Evaluation

A urinalysis should be done on every patient because it provides important information about the etiology of dysfunctional symptoms. A first-morning specimen should have a specific gravity greater than 1.020. If not, there may be a lack of renal concentrating ability. Proteinuria may imply renal disease. Glucosuria could implicate diabetes mellitus. A pH greater than 7 may be associated with a urea-splitting bacteria, such as *Proteus*, that is causing a urinary tract infection. Microhematuria and pyuria may be seen with infection, tumor, or stone. Bacteriuria is much more significant in implicating a urinary infection than is pyuria. There need not be pyuria at all in the presence of a urinary infection. Pyuria without bacteriuria is suggestive of vaginal contamination, a treated urinary tract infection, *Chlamydia*, viral infection, or tuberculosis. If the urinalysis is nearly normal in a man, a second urine sample should be taken after gentle massage of the prostate. The presence of multiple white cells in the postmassage specimen implies prostatitis. If a urinary tract infection is suspected, urine must be sent for culture. In the presence of microhematuria alone, three urine cytologic studies should be performed.

Blood tests would include a blood urea nitrogen and creatinine to evaluate renal function, complete blood count with differential for anemia or infection, an acid phosphatase, and prostatic-specific antigen if any prostatic irregularity or hardness is noted to check for prostatic carcinoma. A prostatic nodule necessitates urologic consultation for consideration of biopsy. An intravenous pyelogram with a postvoid film should be done if there is any question about upper urinary tract pathology or microhematuria without infection, or in the presence of significant unexplained obstructive or irritative symptoms.

An understanding of the pathophysiology of dysfunctional voiding should lead to the appropriate therapeutic intervention. Urologic consultation should be obtained if the appropriate diagnostic tests have not determined the patient's specific problem or if surgical treatment or further diagnostic evaluation, such as urodynamic evaluation or cystoscopy, is necessary.

References

Carlton CE, Scardino PT. Initial evaluation. In: Walsh PC, et al, eds. Campbell's urology. Philadelphia: WB Saunders, 1986:276.

Tanagho EA. Urinary obstruction and stasis. In: Smith DR, ed. General urology. 11th ed. Norwalk, CT: Appleton & Lange, 1988.

Wein AJ. Classification of voiding dysfunction. AUA Update Series. Lesson 4. Vol. 6. 1987.

67 Urinary Incontinence

Timothy B. Hopkins, MD

Definitions

Urinary incontinence is the involuntary urethral or extraurethral loss of urine. This occurs more frequently in women than in men, particularly in older women. The severity of urinary incontinence should be graded from mild to severe.

Stress incontinence is the involuntary loss of urine associated with any activity that causes an increase in intra-abdominal pressure, e.g., Valsalva maneuver, cough, strain. It is also called sphincter insufficiency, because this incontinence occurs when intraurethral pressure involuntarily falls below bladder pressure. *Urgency incontinence* is the involuntary loss of urine shortly after a sensation of bladder fullness or the urge to void is noted. It is also called detrusor instability. *Overflow incontinence* (also called paradoxical incontinence) is the involuntary loss of urine from an overdistended bladder, which occurs when bladder pressure temporarily exceeds intraurethral pressure. *Total incontinence* is the continuous loss of urine unassociated with activity or the feeling of a need to urinate. In *reflex incontinence,* no stress or warning precedes periodic involuntary voiding. *Functional incontinence* is described as wetting because severe cognitive impairment or mobility limitations prevent toileting. *Mixed incontinence* involves more than one type of wetting, especially in the elderly. *Nocturnal enuresis* is bedwetting.

Etiology

A basic understanding of bladder and urethral innervation as outlined in Chapter 66, "Dysfunctional Voiding," will help one classify incontinence and facilitate understanding and management of incontinence. The two basic stages of the normal micturition cycle are filling–storage and emptying–expulsion. Normally, the detrusor muscle and bladder outlet act as a coordinated unit. Storage of urine is mediated by detrusor relaxation, closure of the bladder outlet, and absence of involuntary bladder contractions. Bladder emptying involves a detrusor contraction coordinated with sphincter relaxation in the absence of anatomic obstruction.

Stress incontinence (sphincter insufficiency) occurs when bladder neck and external urethral sphincter incompetence produce pressures within the urethra that are lower than pressures within the bladder. Normally, increased intra-abdominal pressure is transmitted equally to the bladder and urethra when the urethra is in normal position. With pelvic floor laxity, however, the proximal urethra and bladder neck herniate through the pelvic floor with increased intra-abdominal pressure. Therefore, pressure is unequally transmitted to the urethra, and incontinence occurs. Most commonly, this is secondary to urethral hypermobility from weakening of the supporting muscles and ligament structures, which occurs during childbirth. These same supporting structures may lose tissue tone and elasticity as a result of hormone changes at menopause, psychotropic drugs, severe chronic coughing, or marked obesity. A nulliparous woman may have stress incontinence secondary to an inherent weakness of the bladder neck or a short urethra. Surgery involving the urethra or prostate may cause external sphincter damage or weakness.

Urgency incontinence (detrusor instability) is most commonly caused by inflammation or infection of the lower urinary tract. Bladder hyperreflexia with normal or impaired detrusor contractility is the most common cause of incontinence in the elderly. About one-third of patients have more than one potentially contributing cause. Neurologic disease such as stroke, Parkinson's disease, Alzheimer's disease, or brain tumor and old age can cause a loss of cerebral inhibition of voiding, which may also produce urgency incontinence. Interference with spinal inhibitory pathways by a tumor or herniated disk might also be implicated. A foreign body, a low urethral or bladder stone, or urethritis is a less common cause of detrusor overactivity. Bladder hypersensitivity may also occur with benign prostatic hypertrophy and obstruction. Loop diuretics may provoke leakage by inducing a brisk diuresis and sudden overload of the bladder. A cough or sneeze (stress) may precipitate an uninhibited bladder contraction.

Overflow incontinence occurs when the weight or pressure in a distended bladder intermittently overcomes outlet resistance. This is caused by outlet obstruction, an underactive detrusor muscle, or a combination of the two. In men, an enlarged prostate (benign or malignant) is the most common etiology. Bladder neck stricture, fecal impaction, urethral stricture, and alpha-adrenergic agonists (prescribed or over-the-counter medicine) may also cause obstruction. Intra- or postoperative overdistention, anticholinergics, calcium-channel blockers, sedatives, bladder denervation following radical pelvic surgery, genital herpes infection, diabetes mellitus, or neurogenic dysfunction may lead to decreased bladder tone and detrusor decompensation. The bladder may be replaced by fibrous and connective tissue in chronic obstruction and thus be unable to contract adequately.

Total incontinence in the adult is either congenital or secondary to common problems or diseases such as paraplegia, multiple sclerosis, and spina bifida. Trauma (external or iatrogenic) to both the external sphincter and bladder neck in men or the perineal muscles in women may also result in total incontinence. A fistula from the bladder or ureter secondary to surgery, radiation, tumor, invasive carcinoma of the cervix in women, or obstetric injury may also cause total incontinence.

Reflex incontinence is classically due to suprasacral spinal cord lesions such as tumor, spondylosis, or trauma. This interferes with cortical inhibition as well as pathways that coordinate detrusor contraction and outlet relaxation. Severe cerebral cortical damage may also cause this.

Functional incontinence occurs when the patient is unable to reach the toilet because of difficulty ambulating or undressing, the inability to manipulate a urinal or bedpan, or because facilities are unavailable. Prescribed medication may diminish sensory awareness and worsen this problem.

Mixed incontinence is often seen in the elderly. More than one type of incontinence may be seen at the same time, secondary to a combination of the etiologies described previously.

Nocturnal enuresis may be primary (occurring since birth) or of adult onset. Seventy percent of adults with persistent primary enuresis have uninhibited bladder activity, usually without an organic process. Urinary infection, neurologic disease, or obstruction may occasionally be implicated. Adult-onset enuresis usually occurs with other symptoms, but it may be a sign of obstruction or neurologic disease. Absence of the normal nocturnal rise in plasma vasopressin has also been postulated as a cause.

Diagnostic Approach

The diagnostic approach to the patient with urinary incontinence relies on a combination of historical, physical, and laboratory findings (Fig. 67-1). It is important to understand the precise nature of the symptoms, precipitating events, severity, duration, and significance the patient places on the symptoms. A baseline voiding record by the patient or nursing personnel that indicates the frequency, timing, and severity of incontinence may be of great help. Have these symptoms occurred before? How were they treated? Does anything make the symptoms better or make them worse? Does the incontinence occur in different positions? Does the patient have a diagnosis or symptoms of neurologic disease or diabetes mellitus? What medicines is the patient taking, including over-the-counter medication, and how long has he or she been taking them? Has the patient ever had genitourinary tract or pelvic surgery or radiation? These considerations are important in whatever type of incontinence the patient has. Laboratory test results, as described later in this chapter, should be checked. Urinary tract infection, fecal impaction, acute illness, and atrophic vaginitis must be treated primarily. Catheterization for residual urine immediately after voiding will help stratify further evaluation. Classification into a specific type of incontinence will facilitate understanding and management and further direct the investigation.

Stress Incontinence

A history of leakage of urine associated with coughing, sneezing, laughing, walking, stepping off a curb, running, or other exertion in the absence of previous desire to void is pathognomonic. Stress incontinence is usually associated with the loss of only small amounts of urine. Try to date the onset of these symptoms and delineate a precipitating event such as genitourinary surgery, childbirth, or menopause. It is also important to evaluate how extensively these symptoms affect the patient's lifestyle, because minimal stress incontinence is "tolerable" for many patients. Once the diagnosis is confirmed, it may require no further intervention. Search diligently for associated symptoms such as dysuria, urgency, or urgency incontinence, which would imply more than simple stress incontinence. *An important clue to the presence of stress incontinence is the inability to stop the urinary stream while voiding.* A smoking history, pulmonary diseases associated with chronic coughing, or obesity can increase intra-abdominal pressure and worsen stress incontinence.

Urgency Incontinence

The history usually reveals incontinence occurring soon after a strong urge to void is noted, but before the patient is able to make it to the toilet. Frequency, urgency, and nocturia often accompany urgency incontinence. Ask about dysuria, suprapubic discomfort, vaginal or urethral discharge, and a feeling of incomplete emptying to rule out an infectious etiology. Leg spasticity, weakness, numbness, or loss of rectal sphincter control implies a neurologic etiology for the detrusor instability. A history of prior catheterization, frequent bubble baths, or vaginal douching suggests irritation or inflammation of the bladder or urethra. Hematuria, dysuria, or passage of tissue may implicate a bladder tumor. Urgency incontinence is frequently a complaint in elderly patients because of loss of the cerebral inhibition of voiding. Be careful to rule out more readily treatable causes of incontinence in these patients. Wetting after a 5- to 15-second delay following stress suggests stress-induced bladder instability.

Overflow Incontinence

The history in cases of overflow incontinence often reveals the unexpected loss of urine associated with prior obstructive symptoms of hesitancy, decreased urinary stream, frequency, and nocturia, thereby implicating prostatic obstruction. A patient who recently has undergone major pelvic surgery (such as an anterior-posterior resection for bowel cancer) may be incontinent from a hypotonic overdistended bladder and may have no

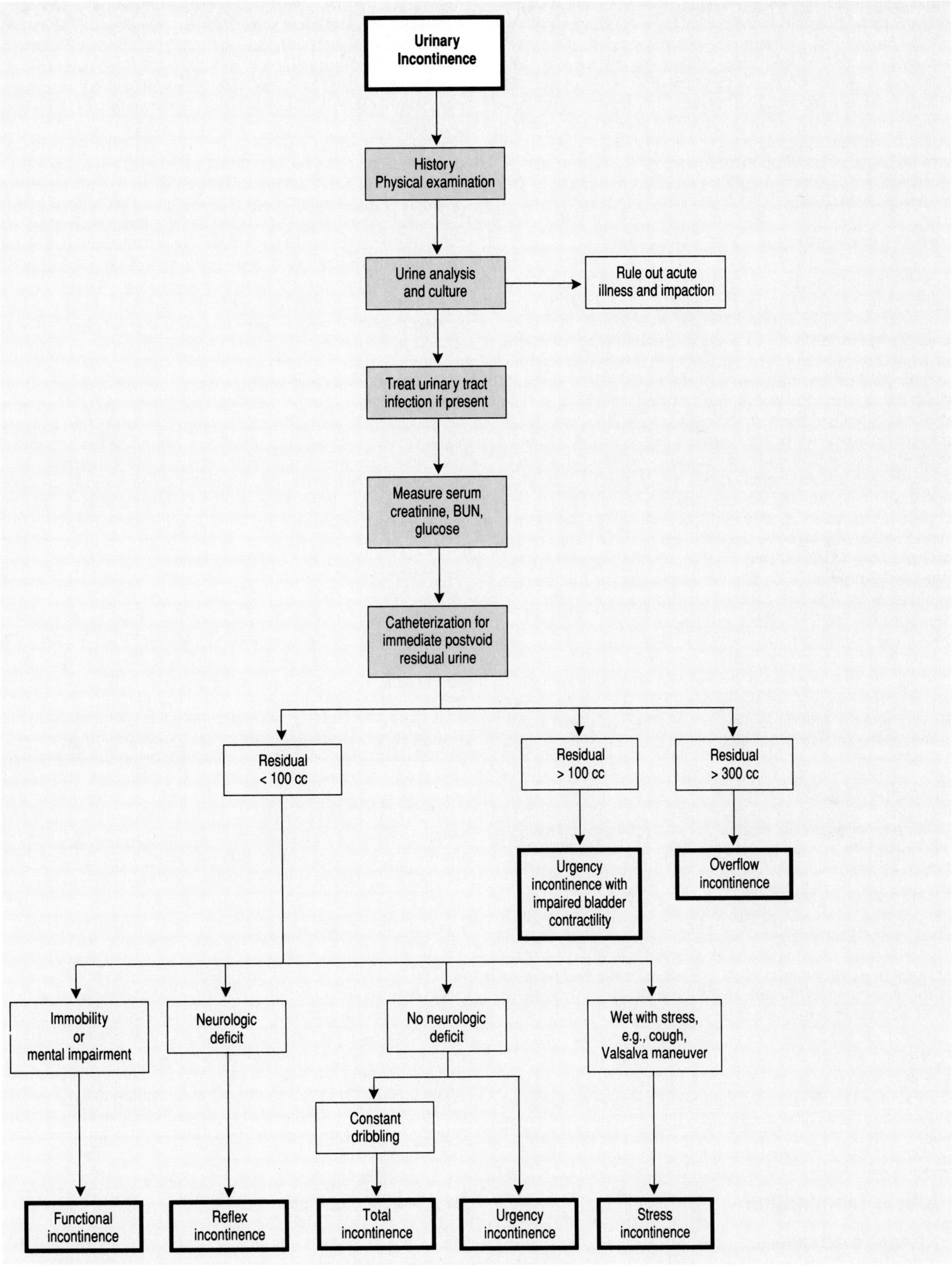

Figure 67-1 Algorithm for the evaluation of urinary incontinence. BUN = blood urea nitrogen.

urge at all to void. Following prolonged anesthesia with a large fluid-volume replacement, the patient may have lower abdominal discomfort and incontinence from a temporarily decompensated overdistended bladder. Symptoms of neurologic disease must also be sought. Occasionally, a history of herpetic lesions of the genitalia may be obtained, implicating neurologic dysfunction secondary to herpes infection. A history of diabetes mellitus, with its associated hypotonic bladder, is important. Recent change in medication or ingestion of "cold medicine," especially in an older man, may precipitate retention, as can excessive alcohol intake.

Total Incontinence

A careful neurologic history, with special attention paid to leg spasticity or flaccidity and poor bowel control, will usually elucidate a neurologic causation. A young woman who has never been dry in her life but frequently voids with a normal stream most likely has an ectopic ureteral opening. This situation must be distinguished from the normal variant of female anatomy, in which the urethral meatus is more posterior than usual. This results in partial voiding into the vagina, which may cause leaking of the vaginal urine when the patient stands. Continuous leaking without an awareness of an urge to void following recent obstetric or gynecologic procedures, pelvic surgery, radiation, pelvic cancer, or drainage of perirectal abscess implies a fistula. A history of recent onset of incontinence following transurethral surgery implicates injury to the sphincter as the etiology of this incontinence. Advanced pelvic or cervical cancer usually has associated symptoms such as pain, weight loss, or spotting and would presumably be discovered on physical examination.

Reflex Incontinence

A history of spinal cord injury, sciatic-type symptoms, or neurologic leg deficit often suggests this diagnosis. The patient's alertness and orientation to time, place, and person may delineate severe cerebral cortical loss.

Functional Incontinence

A baseline record may be of great help here. Can the patient get to the bathroom without assistance? Is he or she mentally alert enough to appreciate the urge to void? Is a bedpan or urinal available, and did the patient, by chance, spill it?

Mixed Incontinence

A history of a combination of the previously described types of wetting is sometimes elicited. There is certainly some overlap in any classification of incontinence.

Enuresis

In an adult with enuresis, symptoms of obstruction, infection, detrusor instability, or neurologic dysfunction must be carefully sought.

Physical Examination

A thorough, careful anatomic and neurologic examination must be performed on all incontinent patients. This begins with a general evaluation of the patient, including vital signs, general appearance, evidence of systemic illness, and assessment of the patient's reliability and orientation. It is useful to watch a man void to assess hesitancy, strength of stream, ability to stop his stream, and dribbling (signs of obstruction). In both sexes, the observation of incontinence may define the problem. Obvious neurologic disease such as spina bifida, paraplegia, spasticity of multiple sclerosis, the tremor and rigidity of Parkinson's disease, or dementia must be noted.

Inspect the back for deformities, dimples (indicating defective closure of the bony spinal canal), and evidence of operation or trauma.

Percuss and palpate the abdomen and flank for masses, organomegaly, tenderness, or a distended bladder. A low suprapubic, tender abdominal mass may well imply an overdistended bladder, whereas tenderness alone might imply infection. Inspect the genitalia carefully for herpetic lesions, urethral or vaginal discharge, erythema, or obvious inflammation. A rectal examination and bimanual examination must be done in both men and women. Assess anal tone. Any rectal mass must be described carefully and fecal impaction ruled out. Prostatic size, tenderness, and firmness must be noted. In men, the foreskin should be inspected for balanitis (frequently seen in diabetes mellitus).

Further neurologic examination should be done by noting perianal reflexes (performed by stroking the perianal area, with the result being contraction of the anus, the "anal wink"). Check for peripheral sensations and reflexes while looking for neurologic abnormalities. Ankle tendon reflexes must be checked.

Residual urine should be measured in almost all cases (except in a man with suspected acute prostatic infection). Normally, urine residual volume should be less than 100 cc.

Stress Incontinence

A pelvic examination with a speculum must be done in women. The pelvic musculature should be evaluated for evidence of a urethrocele (bulging of the urethra and bladder neck with stress). The most specific finding is the demonstration of loss of urine when the patient coughs with a full bladder. The patient may need to be in a standing position to demonstrate this. During the physical examination, one should be able to demonstrate cessation of incontinence by improving the supporting structure. For purposes of this test, the physician may use a cotton swab, or even the fingers, to support each side of the urethra, being careful not to compress the urethra. If incontinence is stopped with a cotton swab, this implies that surgery should correct the problem. (This is called a positive Marshall test.) The urinary residual is usually less than 100 cc.

Urgency Incontinence

Marked prostatic, urethral, or bladder tenderness, warmth, or bogginess implies infection. Overactive bulbocavernosus reflex or tendon reflexes suggest detrusor instability on a neurologic basis. Dementia or obvious neurologic disease should be readily apparent. The periurethral and vaginal mucosa must be inspected for atrophic vaginitis. An enlarged, firm prostate may suggest that prostatic obstruction is contributing to the urgency incontinence. The residual urine is usually slight. However, in patients with impaired detrusor (bladder) contractility, it may be more than 100 cc.

Overflow Incontinence

At least 300 cc of postvoid residual urine is to be expected if the patient has voided just prior to catheterization. Palpation should reveal a suprapubic mass or fullness. Bimanual examination should demonstrate a full bladder. A hard or indurated prostate may imply carcinoma or chronic infection. Decreased anal tone may be seen with a lower motor neuron lesion, and the bulbocavernosus reflex may be weak. Balanitis may be a clue that occult diabetes mellitus is contributing to bladder hypertonicity and overflow. Obvious abdominal or back surgery may implicate postoperative urinary retention.

Total Incontinence

Look for an ectopic orifice or a fistula. Careful observation around the urethral meatus and in the vestibular and anterior vagina may reveal an ectopic opening. Urologic consultation may suggest instillation of methylene blue into the bladder to search for a fistula. If no methylene blue is seen leaking, place a sponge in the vagina and inspect it a few minutes later for blue dye. If no drainage is seen, methylene blue may be injected intravenously, and one can look for external leakage. Continuous dripping of urine from the urethra or vagina may reveal the source.

Reflex Incontinence

Paraplegia or lower leg neurologic deficit may be obvious or subtle. A very active bulbocavernosus reflex or spastic lower extremities with overactive tendon reflexes may be suggestive. Dementia or cerebral central nervous system disorder should be obvious.

Functional Incontinence

A general assessment of the patient's mobility and mental alertness is imperative for this diagnosis.

Enuresis

Signs of infection and neurologic deficit should be excluded.

Laboratory Evaluation

A routine urinalysis is imperative in all patients with incontinence. Examine a first morning urine for specific gravity, which should be greater than 1.020 to rule out a concentrating defect, especially in enuresis and diabetes mellitus. Obvious abnormalities such as glucosuria, as seen in diabetes mellitus, or proteinuria, as seen in renal failure, must be excluded. A microscopic examination is imperative; look for pyuria and, more specifically, bacteriuria. If more than three white cells or any bacteria are seen on urinalysis, a specimen must be sent for culture and sensitivity testing. Note cells in the spun sediment, as they may be enlarged or abnormal in the presence of tumors. Microhematuria in the absence of infection must be further evaluated with three urine cytologic studies and intravenous pyelography and cystoscopy. Serum creatinine and blood urea nitrogen must be checked to rule out secondary renal failure in overflow incontinence. Blood glucose is measured to rule out diabetes mellitus. Cystoscopy is required in most cases of incontinence to rule out other relevant abnormalities, such as trigonitis, chronic cystitis, tumor, stone, or urethral abnormality, and to evaluate bladder trabeculation, which may possibly indicate a neurologic etiology. If the cause and treatment of incontinence are not delineated definitely, a urodynamic evaluation (study of the dynamic activity and function of the bladder, urethra, and related strictures) is indicated. Intravenous pyelography should be done in the presence of microhematuria or overflow incontinence, or if the primary etiology of incontinence is not perfectly clear. A voiding cystourethrogram with a lateral view has been suggested in the work-up of stress incontinence, but in most urologic settings, it has not been found to be a cost-effective test (cost is $48.00). Enuresis rarely requires radiographic study, unless daytime dribbling, urgency incontinence, or other unexplained symptoms are encountered, especially in the adult.

References

Hadley HR, Zimmern PE, Raz S. The treatment of male urinary incontinence. In: Walsh PC, et al, eds. Campbell's urology. Philadelphia: WB Saunders, 1986:2658.

Resnick NM, Yalla SV, Laurino E. The pathophysiology of incontinence among institutionalized elderly persons. N Engl J Med 1989; 320:1.

Shortliffe LM, Stamey TA. Urinary incontinence in the female. In: Walsh PC, et al, eds. Campbell's urology. Philadelphia: WB Saunders, 1986:2680.

Sier H, Onslander J, Orzeck S. Urinary incontinence among geriatric patients in an acute care hospital. JAMA 1987; 257:1767.

Exposure to Sexually Acquired Disease

Nelson M. Gantz, MD

68

Definition

Many individuals present to clinicians with a history of sexual contact or exposure and a "concern" that a sexually transmitted disease may have been acquired. Often, the person has no symptoms or signs of a sexually acquired disease (SAD), but considerable anxiety and fear are usually visible. Sympathetic questioning as to why he or she believes that a SAD may have been contracted is critical to sorting out the problem. Tact and a nonjudgmental approach to the situation are important.

Etiology

The number of SADs that may be acquired as a result of a contact has expanded considerably in recent years. The list includes the classic venereal diseases, such as gonorrhea and syphilis; other diseases such as nongonococcal urethritis (NGU), trichomoniasis, herpes, and pediculosis; and enteric pathogens such as giardiasis, shigellosis, and amebiasis; as well as acquired immunodeficiency syndrome (AIDS; discussed in detail in Chapter 80). Each year, the list expands and includes both common pathogens, such as hepatitis viruses and cytomegaloviruses, and uncommon organisms, like *Cryptosporidium* and *Isospora*.

Diagnostic Approach

The history is key to determining the etiology of a possible SAD (Fig. 68-1). Ask the person if there was an exposure, when the exposure occurred, and what type of contact occurred (genital, oral, or anal sexual activity). Occasionally, patients deny any sexual contact but are concerned about fomite transmission. Reassurance to the individual that fomites such as toilet seats, doorknobs, towels, and whirlpools are unlikely sources of a SAD helps relieve anxiety and establishes a relationship for future visits. Educational efforts stressing how SADs are acquired should also occur at this time.

The incubation period can be estimated by obtaining a history of a single sexual contact or exposure to a new partner. Table 68-1 lists some common SADs and their incubation periods, which provide diagnostic clues. A genital ulcer that develops within hours to 1 day after contact suggests trauma, not primary syphilis. However, reactivation of genital herpes can occur within 12 hours after coitus. Urethral discharge that develops 1 week after sex with a new partner should suggest that NGU is more likely than gonococcal urethritis. Sexual contact while traveling in the Far East should raise the possibility of penicillinase-resistant strains of *Neisseria gonorrhoeae,* chancroid, lymphogranuloma venereum, and donovanosis. A history of multiple exposures increases the risk of a SAD. The sites of sexual activity determine where one should obtain cultures; activities such as anal intercourse and anilingus raise the possibility of sexually transmitted enteric disease. Sexual preferences such as male homosexuality expand greatly the list of possible pathogens that can be acquired after sexual contact.

Attempt to determine what disease(s) the patient suspects he or she may have acquired. Determination of the symptoms, signs, and diagnosis of the sexual contact are helpful. Sometimes, a call to the consort's physician will simplify matters

Table 68-1 Some Common Sexually Acquired Diseases and Their Incubation Periods

	Incubation period	
Disease	*Range*	*Usual*
Gonorrhea	1–14 days	3–5 days
Nongonococcal urethritis	2–23 days	7–14 days
Primary syphilis	10–90 days	21 days
Herpes simplex	2–12 days	3–7 days
Lymphogranuloma venereum	7–84 days	7–21 days
Trichomoniasis	4–28 days	—
Venereal warts	28–42 days	—
Pediculosis	28 days	—
Papillomavirus	21–240 days	84 days
AIDS	4.2–15 yr	7.8 yr

Abbreviation: AIDS = acquired immunodeficiency syndrome.

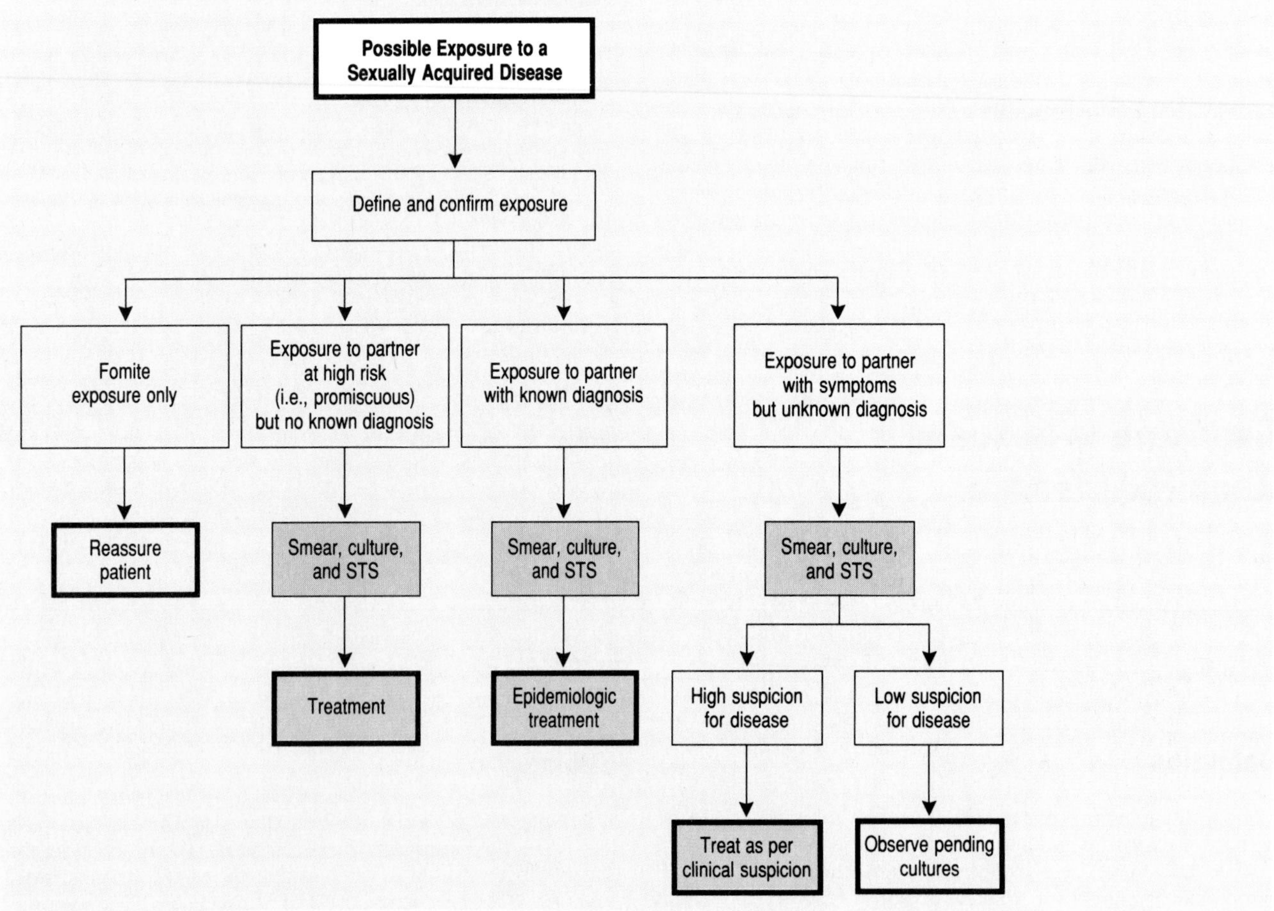

Figure 68-1 Diagnostic approach to an asymptomatic patient who may have been exposed to a sexually acquired disease. STS = serologic test for syphillis.

Table 68-2 Serologic Testing for Syphilis

Test	Use	Method	Accuracy (true-positive percentage)	Conditions producing a false-positive test
Nontreponemal Venereal Disease Research Laboratory (VDRL) *or*	Screening and case finding	Measure IgG, IgM antibody to antigen	Primary (77%) Secondary (98%)	Malaria Leprosy
Rapid plasma reagin–circle card test (RPR-CT)	Screening and case finding	Cardiolipin/lecithin	Early latent (95%) Late latent (73%)	Systemic lupus erythematosus Vaccinia virus Lymphogranuloma venereum Hepatitis Rheumatoid arthritis Rheumatic fever Polyarteritis nodosa *Streptococcus pneumoniae* pneumonia
Treponemal Fluorescent treponemal absorbed (FTA-ABS)	Confirm VDRL or RPR-CT Diagnose late latent syphilis and neurosyphilis	Serum is allowed to react with nonpathogenic treponemes (absorption) and is then placed over *Treponema pallidum* (syphilis). A fluorescent-labeled antihuman globulin is added, and fluorescence is quantitated.	Primary (86%) Secondary (100%) Early latent (96%)	Infectious mononucleosis Pregnancy (repeat after delivery)

considerably. If it is possible to establish a diagnosis in the consort, epidemiologic therapy based on history of exposure, not laboratory confirmation, should be given to the exposed person after appropriate cultures have been obtained. The advantage of epidemiologic, or "epi," treatment is that it allows treatment to be given to a person who is suspected of or known to have been exposed to an infectious disease, especially gonorrhea, syphilis, or NGU, before symptoms occur, a period in which the untreated person could infect several others. A full therapeutic dose of whatever antibiotic is used for that particular infection is given, even though the person is asymptomatic. All sites of sexual contact should be cultured for *Neisseria gonorrhoeae,* and a serologic test for syphilis (STS) obtained (Table 68-2). It is important to inquire about any treatment the person took and other sexual contacts that occurred subsequent to the possible exposure. Furthermore, a small dose of antibiotic taken at the time of exposure may result in a person's being asymptomatic, but uncured.

Frequently, it is impossible to determine the etiology, or even the presence, of a disease in the sexual consort. The patient should be examined at all sites of sexual exposure. Cultures for *Neisseria gonorrhoeae* should be obtained from the appropriate sites of sexual contact. Also, an STS should be obtained; however, the STS will be negative before the appearance of the primary lesion, and in up to 30 percent of patients with a new chancre, the STS will be nonreactive. If herpes is suspected, and an ulcer is present that is not crusted over, a viral culture for herpes is the best test to establish the diagnosis. Vaginal discharge should be examined for possible sexually transmitted

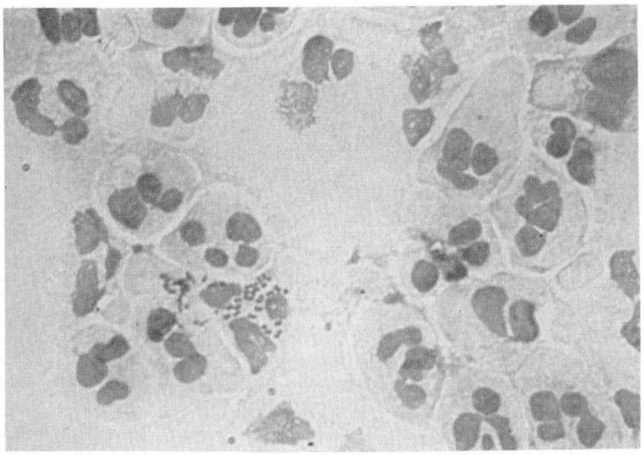

Figure 68-2 Gram-stained smear of a sample of endocervical discharge showing gram-negative intracellular diplococci, which indicates an infection caused by *Neisseria gonorrhoeae*.

Table 68-3 Risks of Transmitting Some Common Sexually Acquired Diseases

Index case	Contacts positive (%)
Gonococcus (man)	36–92
Gonococcus (woman)	40–90
Chlamydia (man)	60–75
Chlamydia (woman)	25–50
Papillomavirus (venereal warts)	60–76
Trichomonas (man)	100
Trichomonas (woman)	30–70
Syphilis	10–90

pathogens with a saline wet preparation for trichomonads and a Gram stain of the endocervical discharge for gram-negative intracellular diplococci (Fig. 68-2).

Table 68-3 lists some common SADs and the risks of acquiring these diseases following intercourse with a person known to be positive. Generally, a venereal disease contact is treated epidemiologically for the suspected offending pathogen. Optimal management depends on determining what disease, if any, the consort had and may have transmitted to the exposed individual.

References

Hart G. Epidemiologic treatment for syphilis and gonorrhea. Sex Transm Dis 1980; 7:149.

Johnson RE, et al. Seroepidemiologic survey of the prevalence of herpes simplex virus type 2 infection in the United States. N Engl J Med 1989; 321:7.

Judson FN, Wolf FC. Tracing and treating contacts of gonorrhea patients in a clinic for sexually transmitted diseases. Public Health Rep 1978; 93:460.

Scrotal Masses

Robert D. Blute, Jr., MD

69

Palpation of an abnormal mass within the scrotal cavity occurs frequently during a careful examination of the male external genitalia. The importance of this finding depends on the establishment of an accurate diagnosis. Most often, an accurate history and physical examination are all that is required to establish a diagnosis and determine subsequent management. Discovery and diagnosis of a scrotal mass will rely on the examiner's familiarity with the anatomy involved and experience gained from consistently examining the "normal" intrascrotal contents of many patients (Fig. 69-1). It is important to be able to ascertain the absence of normal structures (i.e., undescended testicle [Fig. 69-2], absence of the vas deferens or epididymis), as well as the presence of abnormal ones.

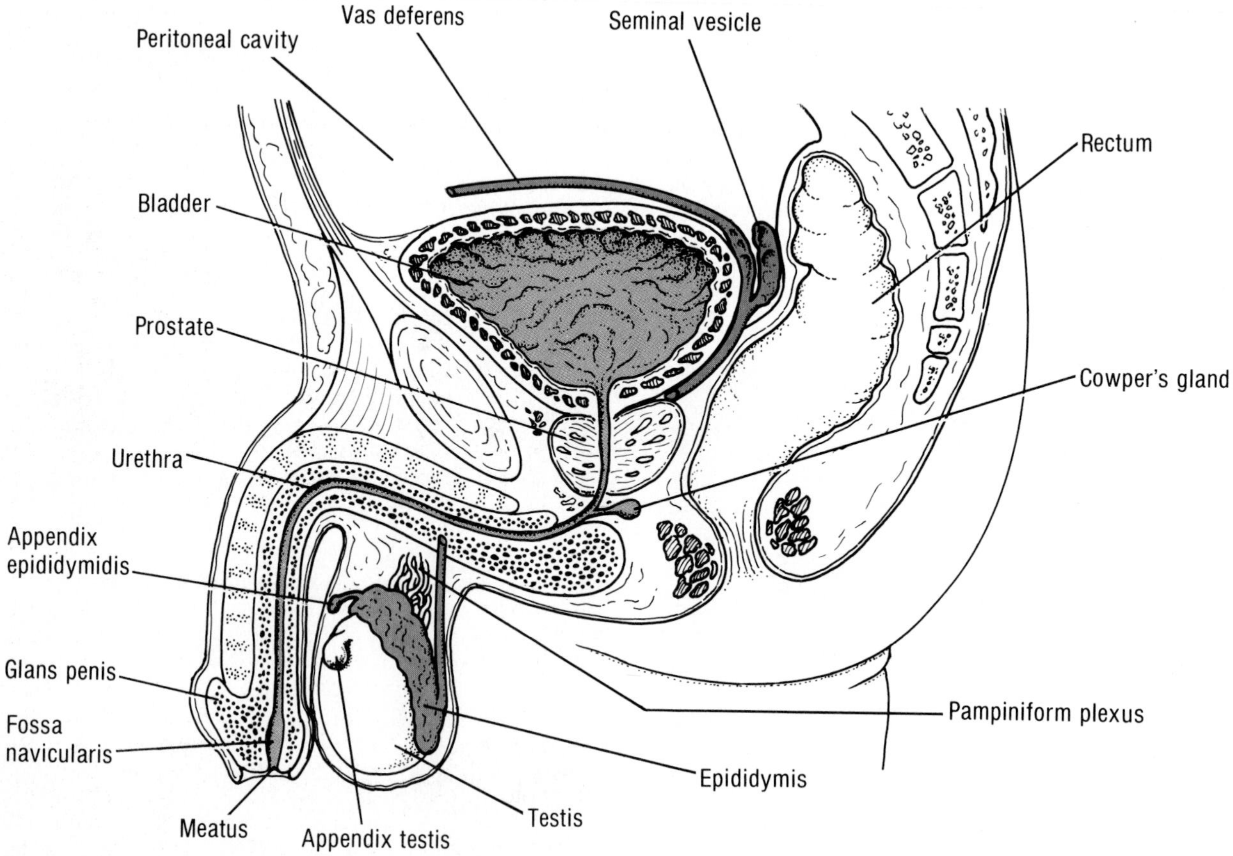

Figure 69-1 Normal male anatomy.

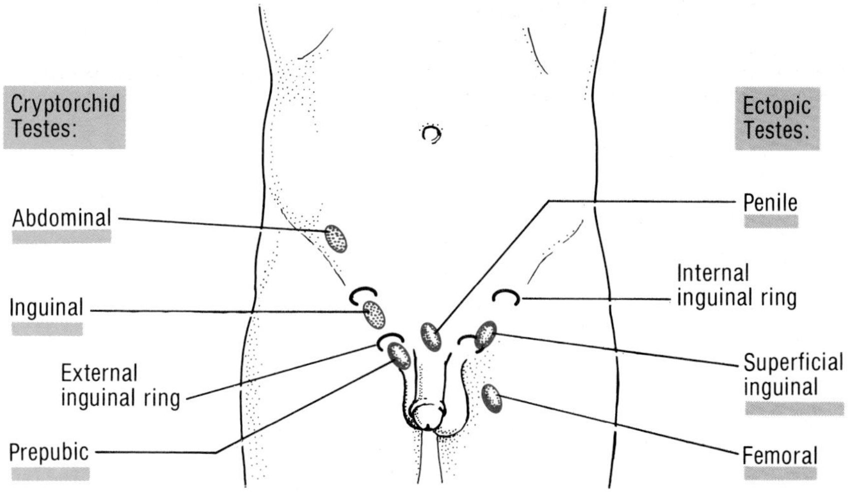

Figure 69-2 Cryptorchid and ectopic undescended testes.

Etiology

Scrotal masses usually arise in the structures within the scrotal contents, but they may originate from the intra-abdominal cavity or the retroperitoneum. Inguinal hernias often allow the presence of small bowel, colon, or even bladder in the scrotum. Retroperitoneal abscesses, hemorrhage, or lymphedema may dissect loose tissue planes and allow scrotal involvement. Retroperitoneal masses, renal vein thrombosis, vena cava obstruction, or renal carcinoma may be manifested by a scrotal varicocele.

The etiology of intrascrotal masses depends on the structure of origin. They are divided into (1) testicular masses, (2) epididymal masses, and (3) spermatic cord masses. Some of the more common scrotal masses are listed in Table 69-1.

In general, the underlying etiology of a scrotal mass may be structural, infectious, neoplastic, vascular, traumatic, or the result of obstruction of the lower reproductive tract.

Diagnostic Approach

Once a scrotal mass has been discovered, certain historical features should be ascertained. The age of the patient is of extreme importance because there are underlying etiologies of certain scrotal masses that occur most frequently in a specific age distribution. The presence or absence of pain must be elicited. The patient should be questioned as to how long he has been aware of the mass, whether or not it has increased in size, and how it was discovered. A history of drugs, medications, prior operative procedures, and the presence or absence of voiding symptoms should be sought.

During physical examination of the mass, its size, location, and consistency are precisely documented. The patient *must* be examined in both supine and erect positions. Finally, the physical examination must include the determination of whether or not the mass transilluminates (allows the passage of light). Almost all scrotal masses that are benign transilluminate easily, whereas tumors do not. One notable benign exception is a hematocele (hemorrhage into a hydrocele).

If the etiology of the lesion remains in doubt, scrotal ultrasonography has been found to be an effective means of differentiating intrascrotal masses. In cases in which differentiation between epididymitis and testicular torsion arises, use of the Doppler or technetium-99 scan has been advocated. If tumor or torsion cannot be excluded, scrotal exploration is mandatory; watchful waiting is condemned. Patients can sustain damage in only a few hours if torsion is the problem. It is a true emergency!

Table 69-1 Intrascrotal Masses Grouped According to Their Structure

Testicular Masses	**Spermatic Cord Masses**
Hydrocele	Varicocele
Torsion	Spermatocele
Testicular	Sperm granuloma
Appendage	Neonatal torsion
Orchitis	Hydrocele
Testicular tumors	Spermatic cord tumors
Masses of the tunica albuginea	
Traumatic	
Epididymal Masses	
Epididymitis	
Acute	
Chronic	
Spermatoceles	
Epididymal cysts	
Torsion of the epididymal appendages	

Common Scrotal Masses

Testicle

Hydrocele

A hydrocele is a scrotal mass of varying size that is ventral, superior, and anterior to the testicle (Fig. 69-3). It is nontender and transilluminates easily. Hydroceles may be congenital or acquired. In the child, they are a result of incomplete obliteration of the processus vaginalis and are often associated with an inguinal hernia. In the adult, hydroceles result from decreased absorption by the tunica vaginalis. This is the result of serous effusion as a consequence of epididymitis, tuberculosis, or other inflammatory processes. Hydroceles vary in size, but they may reach up to 25 cm in diameter; they are benign and require no treatment unless they are a source of discomfort to the patient. Because 10 percent of testicular tumors are associated with a hydrocele, aspiration should be performed if the testicle is not palpable.

Genitourinary

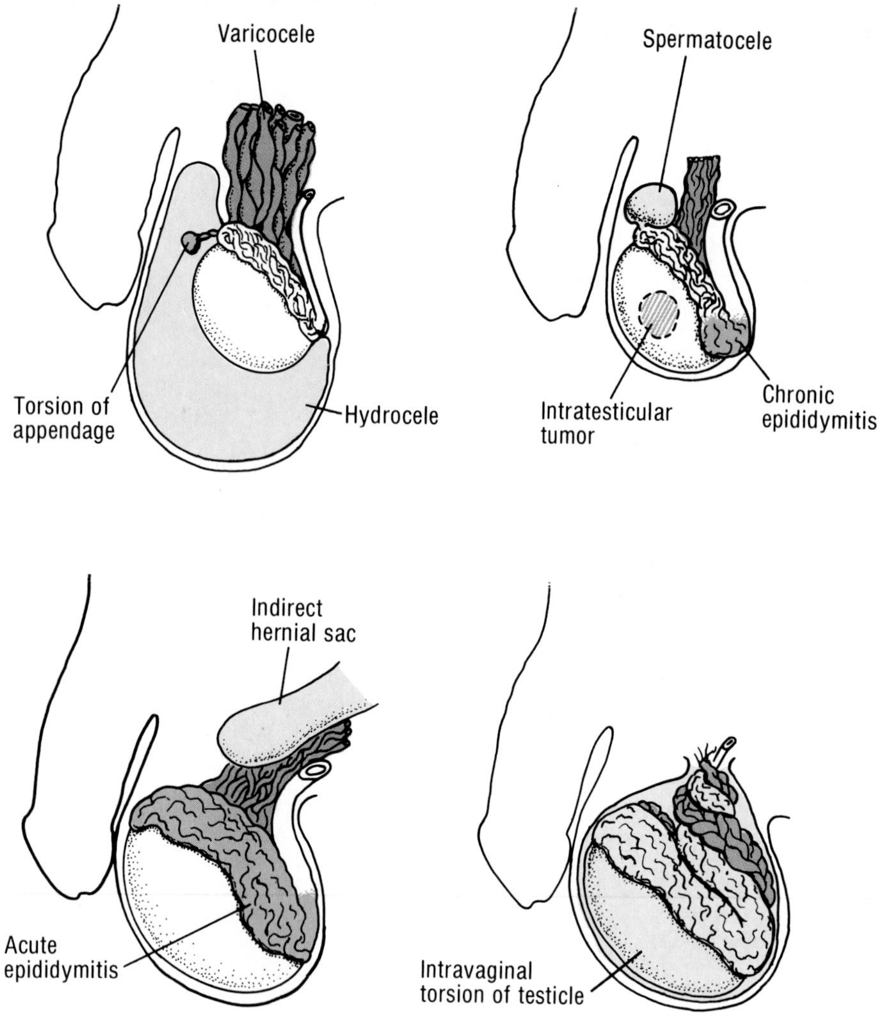

Figure 69-3 Disorders of the testes.

Testicular Tumors

Testicular neoplasms are the most common solid tumor in the 20- to 39-year age group. Although there is an increasing incidence of testicular tumors in the United States, they are rare and represent only 1 to 2 percent of all malignant neoplasms. These patients usually present with a mass *within* the substance of the testes (see Fig. 69-3). Patients often discover a "lump" while bathing. The mass is either smooth or nodular, rock-hard, and painless. The patient may note a dull ache or heavy sensation in the scrotum or inguinal region. Occasionally, pain may be part of the clinical picture because of tumor necrosis, hemorrhage, or an epididymo-orchitis. Less commonly, older patients with seminoma may present with a large, nontender scrotal mass. These masses do not transilluminate, and all such masses should be promptly explored through an inguinal incision.

Torsion of the Testicle

Patients with torsion of the testicle usually present with *acute* onset of severe scrotal pain with edema and cellulitis. Torsion of the testicle occurs as a result of a congenital deficiency in the attachment of the testicle and epididymis to the scrotal wall. Thus, these two structures are suspended from the spermatic cord within the tunica vaginalis, creating the so-called bell clapper deformity. The propensity for "intravaginal" torsion increases just before puberty, presumably as a result of testicular enlargement; it may occur, however, at any age (see Fig. 69-3). At the time, differentiation from acute epididymitis may be extremely difficult. In children younger than 12 years of age, acute epididymitis is exceedingly rare, and the diagnosis should be made at the operating room table. Doppler techniques and technetium-99 studies have been advocated as diagnostic aids to demonstrate decreased blood flow to the testicle. Because irreversible damage presumably occurs within less than 6 hours, exploration with these techniques should not be delayed if the index of suspicion is high.

Torsion of Appendix Testes

Torsion of the appendix testes also presents with *acute* onset of pain, scrotal mass, and cellulitis (see Fig. 69-3). Usually, the epididymis and testes are palpable and are not as exquisitely tender as a small mass located on the ventral superior aspect of the testicle. Transillumination may demonstrate a "dot" in this location that is accentuated by a small amount of reactive hydrocele. A small, tender pedunculated mass may be palpated. The degree of pain (often associated with nausea and vomiting) is out of proportion to the physical findings and may radiate to the ipsilateral inguinal region. The absence of voiding symptoms and benign urinalysis findings help in differentiating this entity from acute epididymitis.

Mumps Orchitis

Testicular swelling with malaise, fever, and acute parotitis without scrotal cellulitis or edema is a hallmark of mumps orchitis. It usually occurs in postpubertal men with a history of recent acute parotitis. Testicular atrophy may result from this viral illness.

Adenomatoid Tumors

These scrotal masses represent a benign tumor of the tunica albuginea of the testicles. They are firm, nontender, occasionally plaquelike masses that arise from the *surface* of the testicle. There is no intraparenchymal mass. Exploration may be required to differentiate them from a testicular tumor.

Trauma

Traumatic injury resulting in a scrotal mass is a common clinical entity. The diagnosis is often evident from the history and physical findings. A clear cause-and-effect relationship must be sought. Furthermore, the *degree* of the traumatic blow must correlate with the *extent* of injury. The presence of ecchymosis in addition to pain and swelling is certainly helpful in assuring a correct diagnosis. The caveat in this clinical situation is that any scrotal mass, especially an asymptomatic testicular tumor, will "predispose" this area to trauma and allow the patient and examiner the comfort of ascribing the mass to injury. Ultrasonography is of particular help in this instance, not only in determining the correct diagnosis but also in ascertaining whether immediate operative intervention for repair of a testicular rupture is warranted.

The integrity of the penile urethra must be determined. If the patient can void and the urine is clear, no further evaluation is in order. If the patient cannot void or is found to have microscopic or gross hematuria, retrograde urethrography should be performed. Do not attempt to pass a catheter without establishing the integrity of the urethra following a traumatic injury.

Finally, all open scrotal wounds or penetrating injuries should be explored for removal of foreign body, debridement, drainage, and so forth.

Epididymal Masses

Acute Epididymitis

Acute epididymitis is a common clinical entity in postpubertal adult men (see Fig. 69-3). It is characterized by the *gradual* onset of pain, swelling, cellulitis, and a scrotal mass that is exquisitely tender. In adults less than 40 years of age, *Chlamydia trachomatis* is often the initiating organism; in older men, gram-negative bacteria are likely to be the cause. Associated urinary tract infection may or may not be present. This entity is thought to result from retrograde ascension of the inciting organism from the vas deferens and prostate gland. The patient may be afebrile and have leukocytosis. Examination is difficult, and differentiation from testicular torsions is often impossible. If epididymo-orchitis is present, the acutely inflamed epididymis may be rock-hard and larger than the testicle itself. If torsion can be safely excluded, treatment consists of bed rest, elevation, ice, antibiotics, and pain control. Follow-up examination must be stressed to the patient to ensure that an underlying testicular tumor is not present after the acute inflammatory response has subsided.

Chronic Epididymitis

Chronic epididymitis is an extremely common entity found in elderly men (see Fig. 69-3). It is usually the result of low-grade inflammation in the head of the epididymis or a resolving acute epididymitis. Classically, the patient is unaware that he has any scrotal pathology. On physical examination, tenderness is elicited when the caput or the cauda epididymis is palpated. The epididymis may be somewhat inflamed, indurated, and thickened. This condition requires no treatment unless an acute flare-up is experienced.

Spermatocele

This nontender, transilluminating mass arises in the head of the epididymis as a result of inflammatory obstruction of the efferent ductules (see Fig. 69-3). The mass contains a thin, milky fluid in which sperm are present. Spermatoceles may reach 3 to 4 cm in diameter, but they are usually not greater than 1 cm in diameter. They require no treatment unless they are tender or cause discomfort for the patient.

Epididymal Cysts

These small, firm masses are located within the body or the head of the epididymis and are clearly separated from the testicle. They are asymptomatic and require no treatment.

Spermatic Cord Masses

Varicocele

Scrotal varicoceles are very common, being present in 10 to 15 percent of the normal male population (see Fig. 69-3). This scrotal mass represents a dilated pampiniform plexus of the spermatic cord that is a result of an incompetent venous valve mechanism. The left spermatic vein enters the left renal vein 10 cm higher than the right spermatic vein enters the vena cava. The pooling of blood in the pampiniform plexus results in a left scrotal mass of varying size that, in the erect position, has the consistency of a "bag of worms." Usually, varicoceles are asymptomatic, but they may reach a large size, resulting in a "dragging" sensation in the scrotum, with discomfort radiating to the left inguinal region. They are important for two reasons: (1) The finding of a varicocele that does not decompress in the supine position should prompt evaluation of the retroperitoneum for a cause of spermatic vein obstruction. This is especially true if the varicocele is of acute onset. (2) In many patients, the presence of an acute varicocele is associated with oligospermia. Fertility may be improved if these patients undergo ligation of the spermatic vein.

Sperm Granuloma

Sperm granuloma is perhaps the most frequently encountered mass in the spermatic cord in men who have undergone a vasectomy. This is a foreign-body reaction to the leakage of sperm at the site of the transection of the vas deferens. Occasionally, this mass may give rise to discomfort and require excision, but it is usually asymptomatic. Sperm granuloma may be located anywhere from the tail of the epididymis to the high scrotal region, depending on the site of the vasectomy. Antisperm antibodies have been detected in many patients after vasectomy. Recent data from studies of Rhesus monkeys have suggested an increase in arteriosclerotic disease in vasectomized animals; however, this has not been documented in man.

Other

Tumors of the spermatic cord are extremely rare; however, lipomas, liposarcomas, and rhabdomyosarcomas have been reported. Genitourinary tuberculosis may result in an indurated, "beaded" vas deferens and epididymis. Lesions of the cord should be suspected when a hard mass is palpated superior to the epididymis and testicle. In addition, these lesions should be differentiated from an incarcerated inguinal hernia or other mass originating from the inguinal or retroperitoneal region. Biopsy of the mass may be required to determine its nature.

References

Beccia DJ, Krane RJ, Olsson CA. Clinical management of nontesticular intrascrotal tumor. J Urol 1976; 116:476.

Essenhigh DM. Scrotal swelling. Practitioner 1974; 212:216.

Gatt LJ. Common scrotal pathology. Am Fam Phys 1977; 15:165.

Goodson JD. Evaluation of scrotal pain, masses and swelling. In: Goroll AH, May LA, Mulley AG, eds. Primary care medicine. 2nd ed. Philadelphia: JB Lippincott, 1981:507.

Hematology

Abnormal Peripheral Blood Smear

Laszlo Leb, MD

L. Michael Snyder, MD

70

Definition

Three types of formed elements are routinely examined in the peripheral blood smear: erythrocytes, leukocytes, and platelets. An examination of these elements can yield important diagnostic information. For an accurate assessment, the peripheral blood must be spread thinly on a glass slide or coverslip and, after air-drying, stained with either Wright or Giemsa stain. In order to evaluate the various formed elements in the peripheral blood, a thin area of the slide is examined under the low power of the microscope. This ensures that the red blood cells are neither distorted nor overcrowded and present a well-defined central pallor. A more detailed analysis of the formed blood elements is obtained by looking under oil immersion.

Erythrocytes

The erythrocytes or red blood cells should be examined for size, hemoglobin content and distribution, shape, and inclusions. The mean size of a red blood cell is about 7.5 ± 1.5 μm in diameter. Each cell has an area of central pallor covering approximately one-third of the total diameter of the cell. The size can be evaluated by comparing the red cell with the size of the polymorphonuclear granulocytes (approximately half of the diameter of the granulocyte) or with a small lymphocyte (approximately the same size). When red cells are normal in size and central pallor, their morphology is described as *normocytic* and *normochromic*. Large red cells are called *macrocytes,* and small ones, *microcytes.* Cells with a larger central pallor are called *hypochromic cells.* Cells with no central pallor are often called *spherocytes* rather than hyperchromic cells. Variability in size is termed *anisocytosis* (Fig. 70-1).

The normal erythrocyte is round, but even in normal conditions a mild variation in shape can be seen. *Poikilocytosis* is the term used when variations in shape are marked (Fig. 70-2). *Spherocytes* are small, round, densely stained cells with virtually absent central pallor. *Echinocytes* (from the sea urchin or echinoderm; also called crenated cells or burr cells) are erythrocytes with multiple spiny projections or a scalloped edge that is regularly distributed over the cell surface, and *acanthocytes* (spur cells) are red cells with multiple spicules of uneven length that are irregularly distributed over the cell surface. *Elliptocytes* (ovalocytes) are oval-shaped red cells, whereas *stomatocytes* (mouth cells) are normal-shaped red cells with a narrow, elongated central pallor. *Teardrop cells,* as the name implies, have the shape of a teardrop or pear. *Schistocytes* are fragmented erythrocytes that appear in a variety of sizes and shapes, from small triangular forms to normal-sized cells with grossly irregular outlines. *Sickle cells* have the appearance of elongated crescents because of the formation of rodlike polymers of abnormal hemoglobin S.

In certain conditions, red cells may contain inclusion bodies, such as Howell-Jolly bodies, which are small spherical blue bodies that represent nuclear debris. Cabot's rings, remnants of fused microtubules, are blue-stained threadlike inclusions, and basophilic stippling consists of coarse or fine punctate bluish inclusions that are the remnants of ribosomal RNA.

Occasionally, red cells may be stacked on one another, forming rouleaux that must be distinguished from irregularly agglutinated red cells.

Significance

Changes in Size (Anisocytosis)

Macrocytes are typically found in megaloblastic anemias due to vitamin B_{12} or folic acid deficiency when DNA synthesis is impaired. Macrocytes can also be found in liver disease, "occult alcoholism," aplastic anemia, scurvy, myxedema, myelodysplastic syndromes, and the postsplenectomy state. Red cells are usually round in the latter conditions; oval macrocytes are seen in megaloblastic anemias. Reticulocytes may also appear as large bluish erythrocytes and are increased after brisk hemolysis or hemorrhage. The microcytic red cell is characteristic of conditions with decreased hemoglobin concentration, such as iron deficiency anemia, thalassemia syndromes, sideroblastic anemia, lead poisoning, simple anemia of chronic disease, and hereditary spherocytosis. Unlike other microcytes that are hypochromic, the red cells in hereditary spherocytosis lack the central pallor.

Changes in Shape (Poikilocytosis)

Echinocytes may be due to artifacts of preparation, pathologic conditions such as uremia, or, in certain congenital hemolytic anemias, lowering of intraerythrocytic potassium and unstable ATP levels (pyruvate-kinase deficiency). Acanthocytes are seen in large numbers in a rare hereditary abnormality of lipid metabolism (abetalipoproteinemia), in patients with severe end-stage liver disease associated with cirrhosis or hepatitis, and occasionally after splenectomy. Stomatocytes are found in the rare condition of hereditary stomatocytosis, a congenital red cell membrane abnormality; more commonly, they are found in liver cirrhosis, obstructive liver disease, acquired erythrocyte sodium-potassium pump defects, and hereditary spherocytosis. Elliptocytes are seen in very small numbers (less than 1 percent) on normal smears and in larger numbers (up to 10 percent) in anemias of almost any type. In hereditary elliptocytosis, a higher percentage of elliptocytes is usually seen. The presence of spherocytes almost always indicates a hemolytic process, most commonly, hereditary spherocytosis. Smaller numbers of spherocytes are seen in other hemolytic processes such as autoimmune or isoimmune hemolytic anemias. Teardrop cells occur in agnogenic myeloid metaplasia, cancer metastatic to the bone marrow, tuberculosis involving the bone marrow, Heinz body formation, and thalassemia. Schistocytes occur in conditions in which the red cells are destroyed mechanically in the circulation (i.e., intravascular coagulation, prosthetic heart valves, vasculitis, thrombotic thrombocytopenic purpura, hemolytic-uremic syndrome). In uremia and severe burns, schistocytes may also be present in the peripheral blood smear. The occurrence of sickle cells is pathognomonic for the homozygous form of hemoglobin S disease, whereas in the heterozygous or carrier state, the

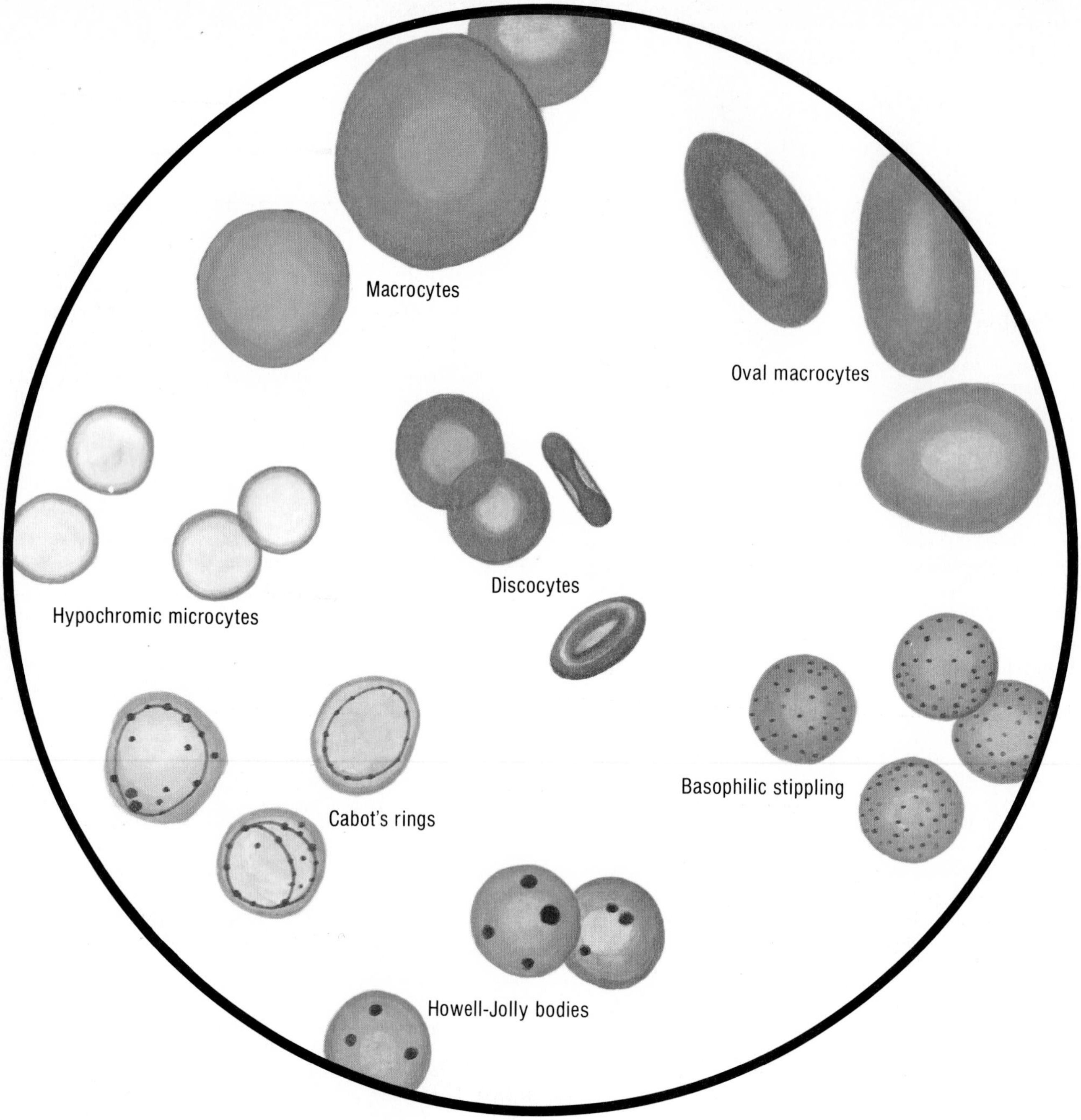

Figure 70-1 Changes in size of erythrocytes (anisocytosis) and their inclusion bodies.

formation of sickle cells is rare and restricted to hypoxic episodes only. Target cells can be artifacts or are present in pathologic conditions such as thalassemia and other hemoglobinopathies (C-C, SC, S-Thal, C-Thal, SS), rarely in iron deficiency anemia, and after splenectomy. In obstructive jaundice and liver disease, they may represent 75 percent of all the red cells. In the rare congenital deficiency of lecithin-cholesterol acetyltransferase (LCAT), target cells are also seen.

In pathologic conditions involving invasion of the bone marrow, nucleated red cells may be present in the peripheral blood. Thus, they are noticed in leukemias or other myeloproliferative syndromes, myelophthisic anemia, multiple myeloma, extramedullary hematopoiesis, megaloblastic anemias, and any severe anemia, particularly when it is associated with hemolysis. Sometimes they occur after a sudden extreme marrow stimulation, like acute hemorrhage or acute hypoxemia. Numerous Howell-Jolly bodies are seen in hyposplenism, megaloblastic anemia, or after splenectomy, whereas Cabot's rings occur only occasionally in megaloblastic anemia and lead poisoning. Basophilic stippling is a common occurrence in hemolytic anemias, thalassemias, uremia, or lead poisoning, or after blood loss. In malaria, parasites can be seen in the red cells associated sometimes with Schüffner's dots, which look like red-staining multiple inclusions.

Rouleaux formation can be seen in multiple myeloma, Waldenström's macroglobulinemia, hypergammaglobulinemia, hyperfibrinogenemia, cold agglutinin disease, viral infections, malignancy, and rarely in pregnancy.

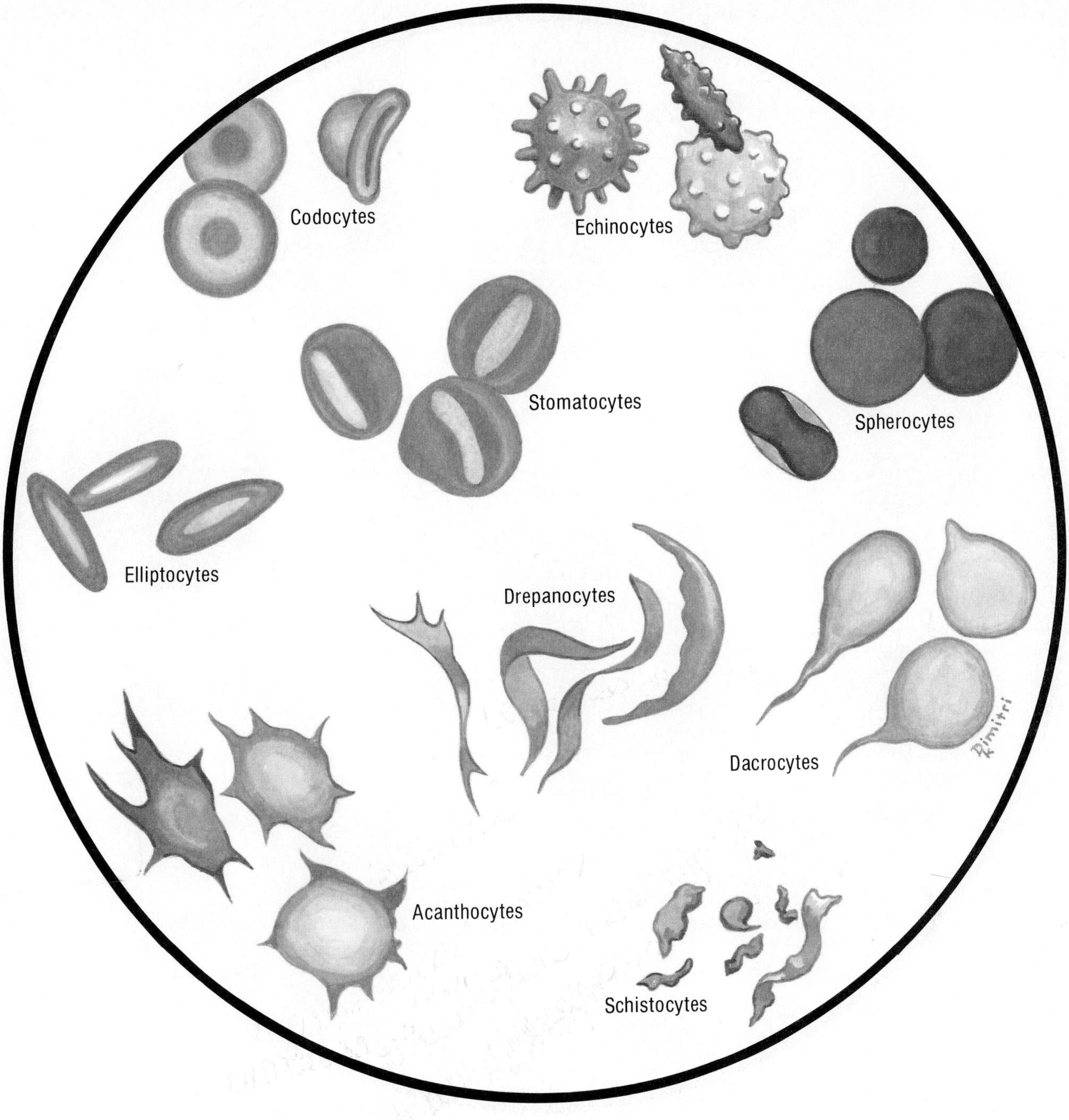

Figure 70-2 Changes in shape of erythrocytes (poikilocytosis).

Leukocytes

Leukocytes normally present in the peripheral blood smear are polymorphonuclear leukocytes of the neutrophilic, eosinophilic, and basophilic types as well as lymphocytes and monocytes (Fig. 70-3). The polymorphonuclear leukocyte precursors (myeloblasts, promyelocytes, myelocytes, metamyelocytes, and band forms) are not found in the normal peripheral blood smear, with the exception of an occasional band form. *Neutrophilic polymorphonuclear leukocytes* have a lobulated nucleus (two to five lobes), and the degree of segmentation probably corresponds to the age of the granulocyte. The nuclear chromatin is dense, with dark blocks separated by a clear network of lighter-stained bands. The nucleus of approximately 10 percent of the neutrophils in women may have an appendage shaped like a drumstick (Barr body) that represents the randomly inactivated X chromosome. The cytoplasm of the neutrophil is pink and contains many small purple granules distributed evenly throughout the cells. The less mature neutrophils (band or stab forms) are identical to the mature polymorphonuclear leukocytes, except that the nucleus is U-shaped or has only rudimentary lobes connected by a thick band rather than a thread, as can be seen in mature neutrophils. *Eosinophils* are the same size as neutrophils, but the nucleus has only two lobes, and their cytoplasm characteristically contains many refractile, orange-red granules. *Basophils* are similar to other polymorphonuclear leu-

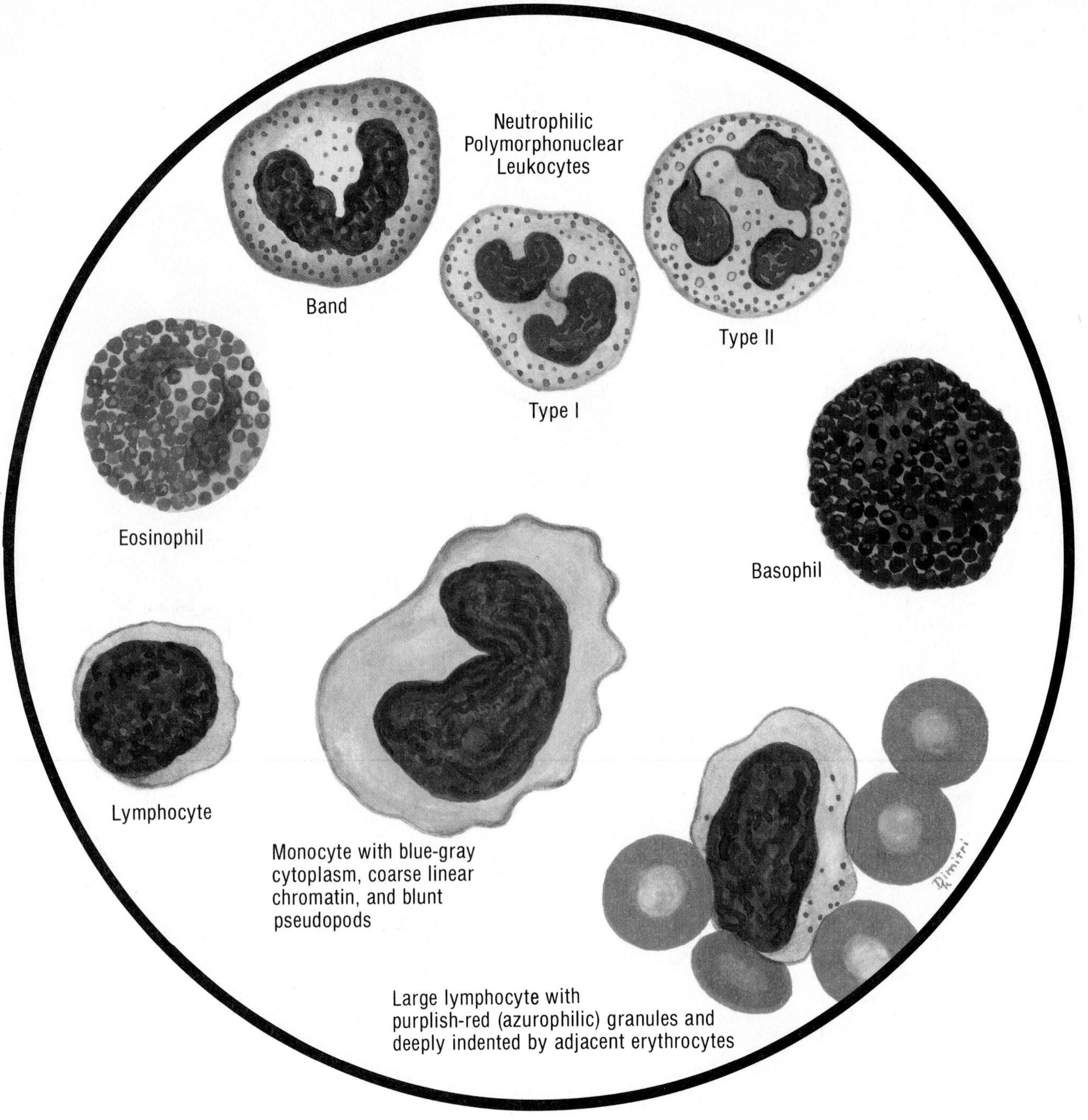

Figure 70-3 Normal leukocytes found in peripheral blood.

kocytes, but their granules are dark violet or purple and are fewer in number.

Lymphocytes include a large number of cells with various functions that often do not have a morphologic counterpart. The immature form, the lymphoblast, is normally not seen in the peripheral blood smear. The peripheral blood lymphocytes are arbitrarily divided into large and small lymphocytes, although intermediate-size cells are also recognized. Large lymphocytes measure approximately 9.0 to 15 μm, and they have a central or slightly eccentrically located nucleus, with chromatin arranged in compact blocks separated by lighter zones without sharp demarcation; nucleoli are rarely seen. The scanty light-blue cytoplasm contains few azurophilic granules in approximately 5 to 30 percent of these lymphocytes. The small lymphocyte has a diameter of 6.0 to 9.0 μm, its nucleus is round or slightly oval, and the nuclear chromatin is dense and dark violet. The cytoplasm surrounding the nucleus may appear only as a small bluish rim or may be barely visible.

Monocytes are the largest leukocytes normally seen in the peripheral blood, measuring 25 to 30 μm in diameter. The nucleus has various shapes: round, kidney shaped, oval, lobulated, or folded. The chromatin is pale and has a lacelike or reticular appearance without compact chromatin blocks. The cytoplasm is abundant, grayish-blue, with occasional numerous fine purple granules. Cytoplasmic vacuoles are quite common. Some monocytes are smaller (15 to 25 μm in diameter), and their nucleus is round or oval shaped, with a pale and floccular chromatin. The cytoplasm is dusky blue, and the cell is sometimes difficult to distinguish from a large lymphocyte.

In technically poor smears the leukocytes may be arti-

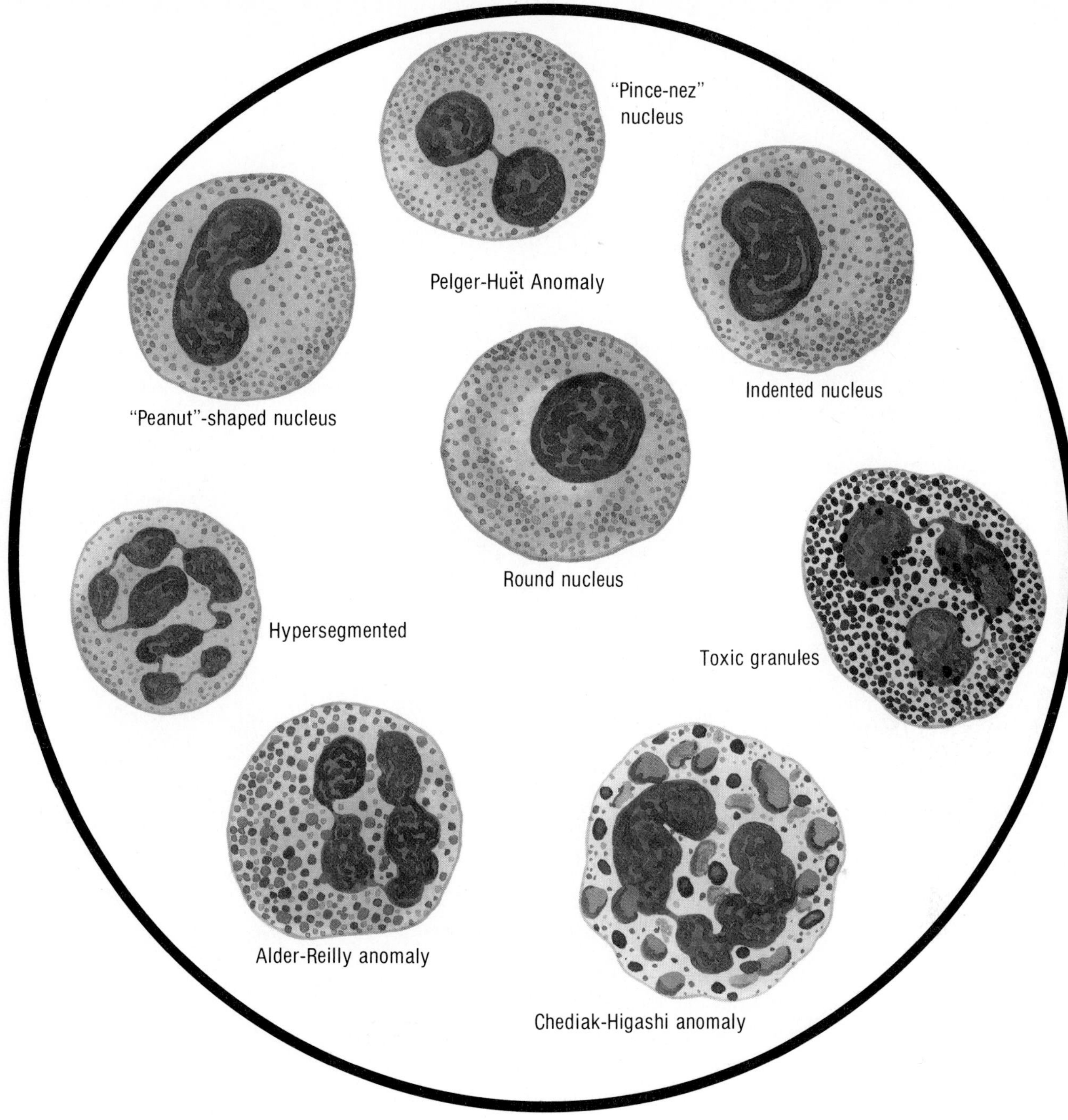

Figure 70-4 Abnormal leukocytes.

factually distorted; therefore, it is important that a proper area of the smear be surveyed. In the thick part of the blood film, white cells appear small and may be compressed by surrounding erythrocytes, thus distorting the characteristics of the nucleus and cytoplasm. In some damaged leukocytes, the nucleus appears enlarged, with altered chromatin structure and a prominent blue nucleus that resembles the structure of reticulum cells (basket or smudged cells).

Significance

Quantitative changes are more important than morphologic alterations of leukocytes. An increased number of neutrophils is found in bacterial infections, inflammations, neoplasms, myeloproliferative disorders, or hemolysis. It also may be drug related (e.g., corticosteroids, lithium, epinephrine), and sometimes is seen in certain physiologic conditions, i.e., after physical activity. A decreased number of neutrophils may represent a bone marrow derangement, i.e., hypoplasia or aplasia, which occurs after the administration of certain drugs (antineoplastic agents) or after radiotherapy, myelophthisis, marrow invasion (e.g., by cancer, fibrosis), megaloblastic anemia, or in ill-defined conditions like inherited or cyclic neutropenia. Significant neutropenia may also occur in conditions with increased destruction or sequestration of circulating neutrophils, such as hypersplenism, viral and bacterial infections, leukocyte antigen-antibody reactions, and drug-induced, antibody-mediated destruction.

Increased numbers of eosinophils are a common finding in allergic disorders, connective tissue diseases, and parasitic infections. They are also increased in Hodgkin's disease, chronic

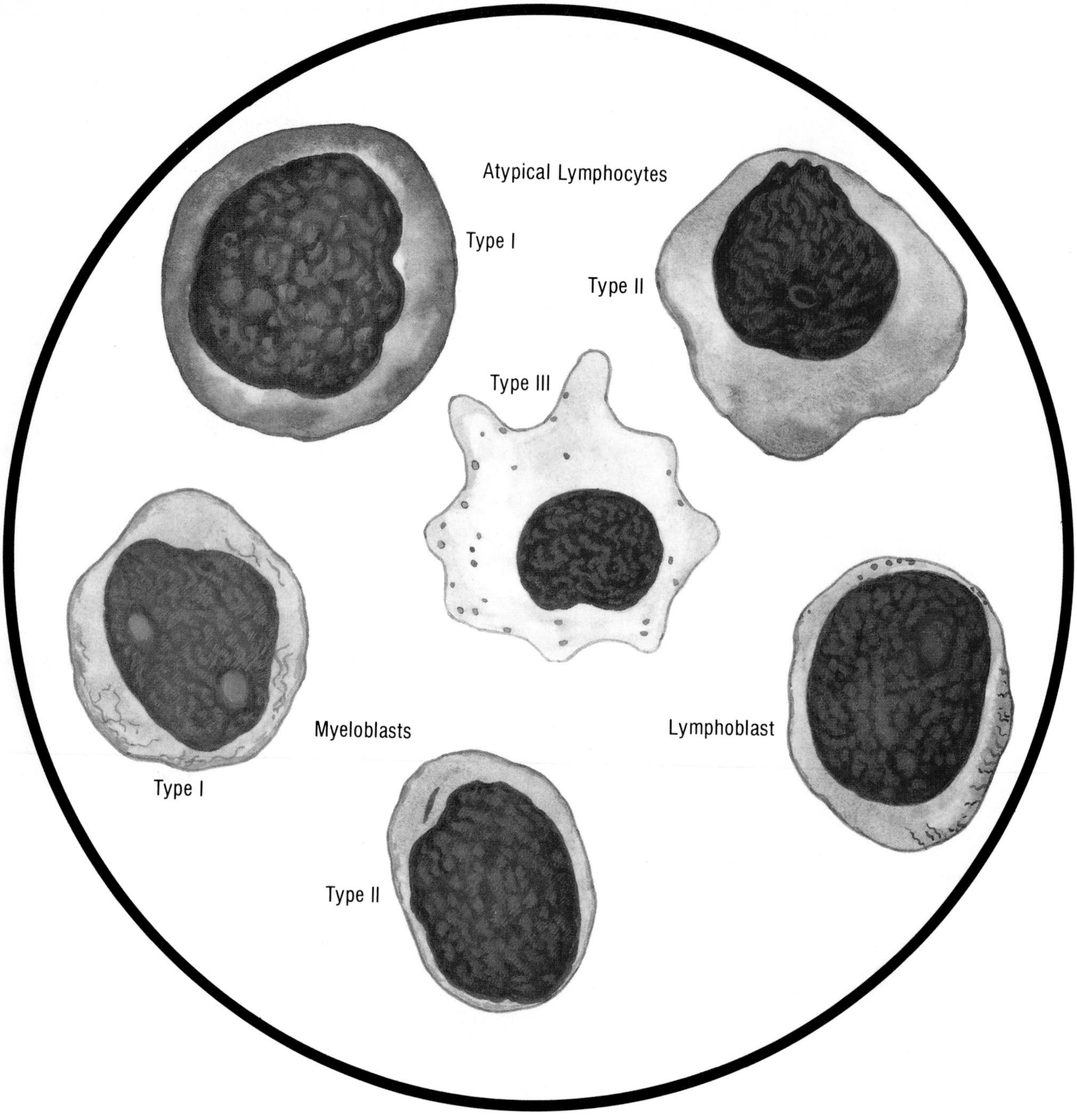

Figure 70-5 Pathologic leukocytes.

myelocytic leukemia and other malignant conditions, tissue necrosis (e.g., after radiation), sarcoidosis, tuberculosis, chronic skin diseases, and eosinophilic leukemia.

Increased basophils are found in conditions in which blood eosinophilia is present as well. They are particularly characteristic of chronic myelocytic leukemia or other myeloproliferative syndromes.

In certain pathologic conditions immature leukocytes, including bands, metamyelocytes, myelocytes, and promyelocytes, may be seen in the peripheral blood. Many such immature cells are present in severe infections and intoxications, extensive tissue necrosis, myeloproliferative syndromes, leukemia (chronic myelocytic), and hyposplenism. The presence of immature leukocytes (termed a shift to the left in maturation), often with an increase in total number of leukocytes, is called a leukemoid reaction. Morphologic changes of leukocytes are less well characterized than those of erythrocytes (Fig. 70-4). The Pelger-Huët anomaly is an abnormality of the neutrophil nucleus, either inherited or acquired. The inherited abnormality is benign and may manifest either as a heterozygous form, with a bilobed nucleus mistaken for a band granulocyte, or as a homozygous condition, with a peanut-shaped nucleus. The acquired form of the Pelger-Huët anomaly may occur in the early phase of myeloproliferative or myelodysplastic syndromes. It can also occur in severe infections and cancer metastatic to the bones, and can be induced by certain drugs (colchicine, sulfonamides, alkylating agents). Sometimes the neutrophils contain more than five lobes (*hypersegmented neutrophils*). Hypersegmentation of neutrophils is seen predominantly in megaloblastic anemia, but occasionally in infections or malignancy.

In "toxic" states, the granules of the neutrophils are larger and stain violet-purple with Giemsa (toxic granulation). Such granules are seen in severe infections, poisoning, inflammations, and malignancy and after chemotherapy. The Alder-Reilly anomaly presents leukocytes with large granules, which are indicators of a metabolic disorder (mucopolysaccharidosis). Large misshapen granules are found in the polymorphonuclear leukocytes, and giant azurophilic granules are sometimes seen in lymphocytes of patients who have the Chediak-Higashi anomaly, a syndrome with generalized alteration of the cell membrane fluidity. Small (1 to 2 μm) blue cytoplasmic inclusions (Dohle bodies) located near the periphery of the neutrophil cytoplasm that represent aggregates of rough endoplasmic reticulum are seen in infections, inflammations, burns, and myeloid leukemia or other myeloproliferative syndromes. Similar inclusions are seen in the May-Hegglin anomaly, an autosomal dominant condition in which thrombocytopenia and giant poorly granulated platelets are present. Auer rods are sharply outlined red-staining rods found in the cytoplasm of immature cells in acute myelogenous leukemia, for which they are pathognomonic.

Increased numbers of monocytes are observed in infections and inflammatory diseases (tuberculosis, bacterial endocarditis), leukemias, lymphomas, solid tumors, myelodysplasia, after bone marrow suppression, and secondary to certain drugs. Histiocytes (macrophages) derived from mature monocytes are not seen in the peripheral blood under normal conditions; however, they may occur in small numbers in severe infections, inflammatory diseases, leukemias, lymphomas, malignant histiocytosis or other malignancies, hemolytic anemias, and agranulocytosis.

Lymphocytes are increased in infections such as acute infectious lymphocytosis, *Bordetella pertussis* infection, subacute and chronic infections, brucellosis, tuberculosis, and secondary syphilis. Moderate lymphocytosis, with atypical morphology of the cells, which have large, irregularly scalloped, basophilic cytoplasm and a lobulated nucleus with a nucleolus, is seen in infectious mononucleosis, cytomegalovirus infection, viral hepatitis and other viral infections, toxoplasmosis, and drug reactions (penicillin sensitivity, after transfusion). In chronic lymphocytic leukemia, the lymphocytes may disintegrate and appear as smudged cells in the peripheral smear.

Normally, plasma cells are not seen in the peripheral blood; however, in multiple myeloma, plasma cell leukemia, malignancy, aplastic anemia, chronic renal disease, tuberculosis, and any severe infectious or inflammatory condition, a few plasma cells may be observed in the peripheral blood smear.

Leukemic cells (lymphoblasts, myeloblasts) that have a large nucleus and a fine chromatin network containing one or two nucleoli and a small rim of bluish cytoplasm are seen mostly in leukemias (Fig. 70-5). A few immature blast cells, however, may be seen in myeloproliferative syndromes and, rarely, in severe infections or inflammations, poisoning, myelophthisis, or recovery after severe marrow suppression.

Platelets

Platelets appear in the peripheral blood smear as small round or oval blue bodies with red or purple granules. Normally, they have a diameter of about 2 to 5 μm and are evenly distributed on the smear. When the platelet count is normal, 10 to 20 platelets should be visible in each oil immersion field (one platelet represents approximately 15,000 platelets per microliter). Even under normal conditions the platelets vary considerably in size, and a few larger platelets are not uncommon. Sometimes giant platelets, *megathrombocytes,* with a diameter of up to 20 μm, are seen even in normal conditions.

Significance

Platelets with a very large diameter, megathrombocytes or giant platelets, are mostly indicative of myeloproliferative disorders, absence of the spleen, or increased peripheral destruction, which is seen in immune or nonimmune thrombocytopenias; they may be pathognomonic for May-Hegglin anomaly. Occasionally, giant granules can be identified in platelets, and this should alert the clinician for the presence of a myelodysplastic syndrome.

Rarely, for unknown reasons, platelets may adhere to the membrane of neutrophils (platelet satellitism). Sometimes, mostly resulting from in vitro aggregation, platelets form clumps on the peripheral smear and the platelet count may appear spuriously decreased (pseudothrombocytopenia).

References

Lee GR, et al, eds. Wintrobe's clinical hematology. 9th ed. Philadelphia: Lea & Febiger, 1990.

Platt WR. Color atlas and textbook of hematology. Philadelphia: JB Lippincott, 1979:23–156.

Anemia

Jack E. Ansell, MD

71

Definition

Anemia is best defined as a reduction in hemoglobin that leads to a reduction in oxygen supply to peripheral tissues. Alternative definitions include a reduction in red blood cell (RBC) count or a reduction in hematocrit (volume of packed RBCs). Anemia is not a disease but a manifestation of an underlying illness. The discovery of anemia should automatically lead to a search for its etiology.

Etiology

Anemia may be classified according to pathophysiologic mechanism, morphologic appearance of the red cells, or etiology. It is most beneficial to classify anemias according to the pathophysiologic mechanism and the red cell morphology. Such an approach will lead to an understanding of the etiology, as demonstrated in the algorithm presented in Figure 71-1.

According to this approach, the pathophysiologic mecha-

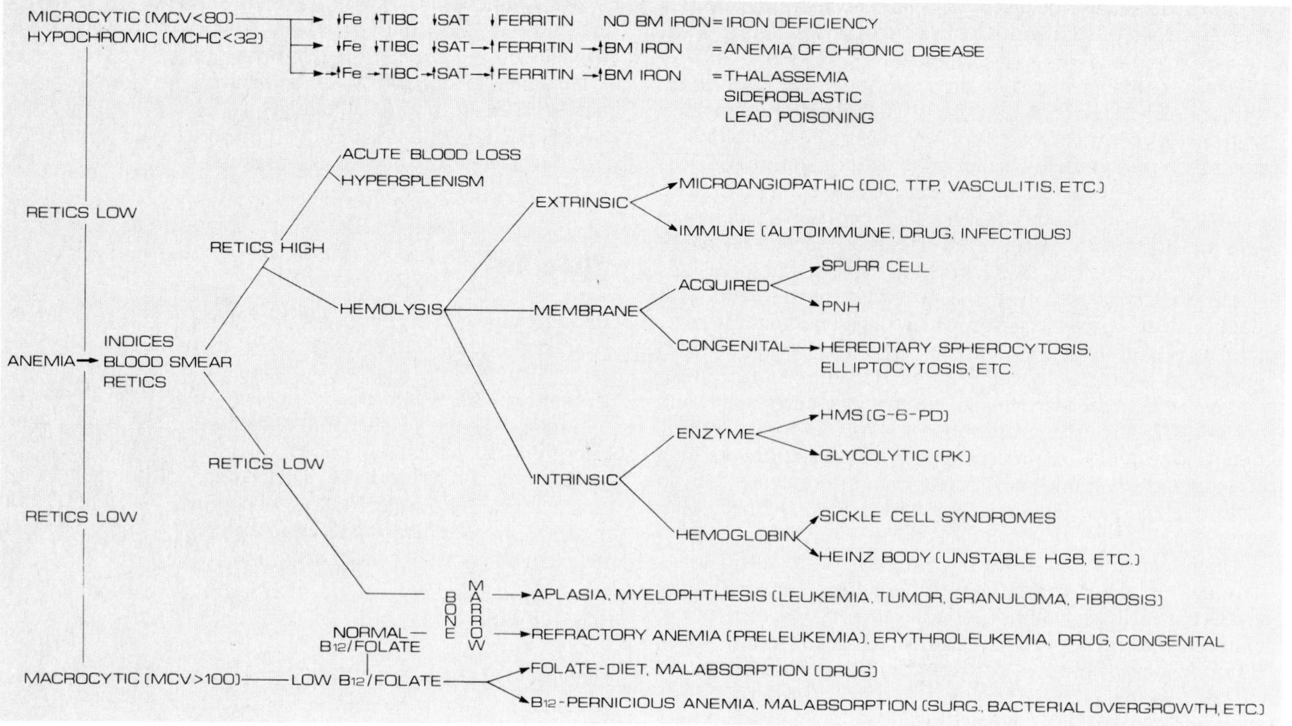

Figure 71-1 Systematic laboratory approach to the patient with anemia. BM = bone marrow, DIC = disseminated intravascular coagulation, Fe = iron, HGB = hemoglobin, HMS = hexose monophosphate shunt, MCHC = mean cell hemoglobin concentration, MCV = mean cell volume, PK = pyruvate kinase, PHN = paroxysmal nocturnal hemoglobinuria, SAT = saturation, TIBC = total iron-binding capacity, TTP = thrombotic thrombocytopenic purpura.

nism of anemia is either failure of the bone marrow to produce enough RBCs (hypoproliferative anemia) or excessive and premature destruction of RBCs in the circulation (hemolytic anemia). The former category also includes anemias due to red cell maturation abnormalities, and the latter includes anemias due to excessive loss of RBCs (i.e., bleeding). Morphologically, anemias can be characterized by RBCs that are large, normal, or small (macrocytic, normocytic, or microcytic) and normal colored or pale (normochromic, hypochromic). Densely colored cells are referred to as spherocytes.

The most common cause of anemia in the United States is iron deficiency. It results in a maturation abnormality, with decreased hemoglobin and red cell production, and it represents one-quarter of anemias seen in a population of hospitalized patients. Anemias due to acute blood loss represent another 25 percent of cases in hospitalized patients, and anemias due to certain chronic inflammatory diseases represent a further 25 percent of cases. The remaining 25 percent of patients suffer from all other causes of anemia. For the non–hospital-based practitioner, the first three categories probably account for 90 percent or more of cases of anemia seen in the office.

Diagnostic Approach

Anemia produces symptoms depending upon its duration, the pathophysiologic mechanism, and the specific etiology. Anemias that develop acutely over hours or a few days are usually due to blood loss. They produce symptoms of intravascular volume depletion, including postural lightheadedness (hypotension), weakness, cardiac strain, and shock. Such rapidly developing anemias may also be caused by fulminant hemolysis, but in that situation symptoms are primarily attributable to the deleterious effects of hemoglobin metabolites. For any level of hematocrit or hemoglobin, those anemias that develop slowly will be better tolerated because of a compensatory increase in plasma volume. Symptoms are primarily related to tissue hypoxia and cardiac strain. They include fatigue, irritability, headache, dyspnea, orthopnea, palpitations, and angina. Chronically developing anemias are frequently due to decreased or abnormal erythropoiesis, as seen in anemia of chronic disease, iron deficiency, and folic acid or vitamin B_{12} deficiency. Mild ongoing hemolysis or gradual blood loss, however, may produce similar symptoms.

The specific etiology of an anemia is also important in understanding the symptoms and physical findings. For example, iron deficiency leads to atrophic and inflammatory changes in the oral mucosa, occasional dysplasia of the esophageal mucosa (esophageal web), a peculiar concavity or spooning of the fingernails (koilonychia), and cravings for unusual substances (pica), such as ice (pagophagia). Vitamin B_{12} deficiency causes changes in the oral mucosa and tongue (glossitis), a neurologic disorder characterized primarily by sensory changes in the lower extremities (subacute combined systems disease), and occasionally a change in mental status referred to as "megaloblastic madness." It is important to keep in mind that many mild anemias produce no symptoms at all, and only laboratory testing will indicate the presence of a reduced hemoglobin.

Final conclusions regarding the etiology of anemia cannot be made until specific laboratory tests are performed. Anemia can be suspected on clinical grounds, but confirmation by hemoglobin, RBC count, or hematocrit must be obtained. Most blood counts today are performed by electronic particle counters and are exceedingly accurate. A complete blood count (CBC) includes a white blood cell (WBC) count, RBC count, hemoglobin, hematocrit (Hct), red cell indices, and differential count of the WBCs (Table 71-1). Red blood cells can be morphologically categorized by examining the peripheral blood smear under a microscope as well as by calculating the red cell indices, which denote average cell size, hemoglobin content, and hemoglobin concentration. The mean cell volume (MCV), mean cell hemoglobin (MCH), and mean cell hemoglobin concentration (MCHC) are determined by the following formulas:

Table 71-1 Complete Blood Count: Normal Adult Values

	Male	Female
Hemoglobin (g/dl)	13.5–17.5	12.5–15.5
Hematocrit (%)	40–52	36–48
Red cell count (× 10^{12}/L)	4.5–6.5	3.9–5.6
Mean cell hemoglobin (pg)	27–34	27–34
Mean cell volume (fl)	80–95	80–95
Mean cell hemoglobin concentration (g/dl)	30–35	30–35
White blood cell count (× 10^9/L)	4–11	4–11
Platelet count (× 10^9/L)	150–450	150–450
Reticulocyte count (%)	0.5–1.5	0.5–1.5

$$\text{MCV} = \frac{\text{Hct (L/L)}}{\text{RBC count } (\times 10^{12}/\text{L})} \times 1{,}000 \qquad 80\text{–}100 \text{ fl } (10^{-15}\text{ L})$$

$$\text{MCH} = \frac{\text{Hemoglobin (g/dl)}}{\text{RBC count } (\times 10^{12}/\text{L})} \qquad 27\text{–}32 \text{ pg } (10^{-12}\text{ g})$$

$$\text{MCHC} = \frac{\text{Hemoglobin (g/dl)}}{\text{Hct (L/L)}} \qquad 32\text{–}36 \text{ g/dl}$$

One must interpret indices obtained by an electronic counter with care, because some counters report an average cell size (MCV) that can obscure the presence of a dimorphic anemia (i.e., large cells and small cells giving a normal average cell size). Microscopic examination of the peripheral blood smear is essential. It serves as a double check on the red cell indices and provides additional information, as discussed later. Knowledge of the red cell morphology, especially size and hemoglobin concentration, provides important information about which pathway of investigation to pursue for further evaluation of the anemia.

A reticulocyte count (RC) should always be determined when anemia is present. The reticulocyte percentage gives an indication of the bone marrow's capacity to respond to anemia by increased production. The average normal RC is 1 percent (range 0.5 to 2 percent), meaning that approximately 1 percent of a given population of red cells contain reticulum and are young cells. Reticulocyte counts are performed by incubating blood with a supravital stain, new methylene blue, which precipitates and stains the remaining ribosomal RNA in young cells. A smear is made, a count of 1,000 red cells is performed, and the percentage of reticulocytes calculated. An RC is a relative number and should be corrected by multiplying it by the patient's Hct divided by the normal Hct (corrected reticulocyte count), or by determining the absolute number of reticulocytes per microliter of blood by multiplying the RC by the RBC count (absolute reticulocyte count). Two examples follow:

Patient A: Hct, 20%; RBC count, 1.5 × $10^6/\mu$l; RC, 4%

Corrected reticulocyte count

$$4 \times \frac{20}{45} = 1.8\%$$

Absolute reticulocyte count

$$(0.04) \times (1.5 \times 10^6) = 60{,}000 \text{ reticulocytes}/\mu\text{l}$$

Patient B: Hct, 20%; RBC count, 1.5 × $10^6/\mu$l; RC, 15%

Corrected reticulocyte count

$$15 \times \frac{20}{45} = 6.6\%$$

Absolute reticulocyte count

$$(0.15) \times (1.5 \times 10^6) = 225{,}000 \text{ reticulocytes}/\mu\text{l}$$

Even though the RC is elevated in both patients, patient A clearly has an inadequate response, with a corrected RC of 1.8 percent, suggesting that the bone marrow is not responding to the anemia and that deficient or defective RBC production may be the cause or is contributing to the anemia. Patient B has a good response to the anemia, suggesting that the bone marrow is normal and that the cause may be hemolysis or blood loss. A normal bone marrow is able to increase erythroid production six- to eightfold. If the average absolute RC is 50,000/μl (1 percent of 5 million RBCs), the maximum increase in RC in response to hemolysis or blood loss should range between 250,000 and 400,000 reticulocytes/μl.

A reticulocyte production index (RPI) has also been formulated to provide additional insight into bone marrow function. The RPI is calculated by dividing the corrected RC by a maturation factor that varies with the degree of anemia and takes into account the earlier release of reticulocytes from the bone marrow and a longer period of maturation in the circulating blood when erythropoiesis is increased. An RPI of less than two times normal suggests an inadequate bone marrow response. An index should be at least 2 for an Hct of 35 percent, and 3 or better for an Hct of 25 percent or less if the bone marrow is functioning normally. Utilizing the examples given previously,

Patient A

$$\text{RPI} = \frac{4 \times \frac{20}{45}}{2} = 0.8$$

Patient B

$$\text{RPI} = \frac{15 \times \frac{20}{45}}{2} = 3.3$$

Maturation factor for Hct

36–45 = 1
26–35 = 1.5
16–25 = 2
<16 = 2.5

In general, these corrections are not necessary when the RC is markedly elevated or low in the setting of significant anemia.

Examination of the peripheral blood smear to assess morphologic abnormalities of RBCs is imperative in the evaluation of anemias. Simple observation of the blood smear may lead directly to the diagnosis, avoiding the cost and time of various diagnostic tests. Table 71-2 lists the commonly seen abnormalities in RBC shape and their pathophysiologic significance. Included in this table are various red cell inclusions and their clinical significance. These abnormalities are illustrated in Figures 70-1 and 70-2 (see pages 300 and 301).

On the basis of the results of these preliminary studies, an anemia can usually be categorized and attributed to defective RBC production or increased RBC destruction (hemolysis) or loss. Additional testing is then required to identify the specific etiology.

Diagnostic and Therapeutic Guidelines

Figure 71-1 outlines the systematic laboratory approach to the patient with anemia. It is based on pathophysiologic and morphologic criteria and takes into consideration cost-effectiveness. Results of a CBC, red cell indices, RC, and blood smear should indicate which pathway of analysis to pursue. Remember that patients may have combined defects and that disease processes do not always adhere to their textbook descriptions.

Table 71-3 provides a summary of the approximate costs of commonly requested tests for the evaluation of anemias. A disheartening observation is the all-too-frequent request for a CBC, serum iron, total iron-binding capacity, serum ferritin, B_{12}, and folate level. This "shotgun" approach to the initial evaluation of anemia must be avoided. Therapy of iron deficiency, the most common cause of anemia, is similarly subject to costly abuses. Table 71-4 summarizes approximate costs of various iron-

Table 71-2 Common Abnormalities in Red Blood Cell Shape or Inclusions Seen in the Wright-Stained Blood Smear

Shape/inclusion abnormality	Description	Associated diseases
Target cell	Circular mid-zone of pallor, with peripheral and central color	Liver disease, hemoglobinopathy, thalassemia, after splenectomy
Spherocyte	Round, frequently small, with no central pallor	Hereditary spherocytosis, acquired autoimmune hemolytic anemia
Schistocyte	Helmet or triangular-shaped cell; fragmented RBC	Microangiopathic hemolytic anemias (e.g., disseminated intravascular coagulation)
Burr cell	Scalloped perimeter, echinocyte, crenated	Uremia
Spur cell	Acanthocyte, spiculated	Advanced liver disease, abetalipoproteinemia
Teardrop cell	Pear or teardrop shaped	Myelofibrosis and other myeloproliferative diseases, thalassemia major, severe iron deficiency
Macro-ovalocyte	Large, egg shaped	B_{12} or folate deficiency
Howell-Jolly body	Dark purple, dotlike inclusions, often at the periphery of cell; represents nuclear remnant	After splenectomy or splenic dysfunction, severe megaloblastic anemia
Heinz body	Dark purple, irregularly shaped inclusions seen by supravital stain (crystal violet); represents denatured hemoglobin	G-6-PD deficiency, unstable hemoglobins, thalassemia
Basophilic stippling	Dark purple, pinpoint stippling in RBC on Wright stain; represents polyribosomes	Beta-thalassemia, lead poisoning, and many toxic states
Siderocyte	Dark cluster of three to four granules in RBC; represents iron granules	After splenectomy
Normoblast	Nucleated RBC	After splenectomy, leukoerythroblastic anemia (myelophthisis), tumor and other infiltrative disease in bone marrow

Abbreviations: G-6-PD = glucose-6-phosphate dehydrogenase, RBC = red blood cells.

Table 71-3 Approximate Costs of Commonly Requested Tests for the Evaluation of Anemia (circa 1990)*

Test	Price ($)
White blood cell count	4.22
Differential	4.22
Hemoglobin/hematocrit	5.59
Complete blood count (includes all above)	7.31
Reticulocyte count	6.93
Platelet count	7.31
Serum iron/total iron-binding capacity	14.83
Serum ferritin	31.37
B_{12}	21.36
Folate	21.36
Hemoglobin electrophoresis	22.53

* From commercial laboratory in northeastern United States.

Table 71-4 Approximate Costs of Various Iron Preparations (circa 1990)

Name	Elemental iron content/pill (mg)	Generic price/100 ($)	Brand name price/100 ($)
Ferrous sulfate	60	3.79	6.59 (Feosol)
Ferrous gluconate	37	2.99	5.79 (Fergon)
Fero-Gradumet	105	—	17.63
Fero-Grad 500	105 (+ vitamin C)	—	19.16
Fero-Folic	105 (+ vitamin C/folate)	—	22.65
Fero-Sequels	50 (+ stool softener)	—	19.99
Simron	10	—	30.58
Geritol	50	6.73	14.18

containing medications. In the overwhelming majority of cases, ferrous sulfate tablets will suffice for the successful treatment of iron deficiency.

References

Beutler E. The common anemias. JAMA 1988; 259:2433.

Crosby WH. Reticulocyte counts. Arch Intern Med 1981; 141:1747.

Strobach RS, et al. The value of the physical examination in the diagnosis of anemia. Arch Intern Med 1988; 148:831.

Ward PCJ. Red cell indices revisited. Postgrad Med 1979; 65:282.

Ward PCJ. Investigation of poikilocytic normochromic normocytic anemia. Postgrad Med 1979; 65:215.

Wheby MS. Using a clinical laboratory in the diagnosis of anemia. Med Clin North Am 1966; 50:1689.

Erythrocytosis

Andrew I. Cederbaum, MD

Harry L. Greene, MD

72

Definition

Erythrocytosis is an absolute increase in the red blood cell mass. It is most often noted from the finding of an elevated red blood cell count, an elevated hemoglobin concentration, or an elevated hematocrit. A synonym for erythrocytosis is polycythemia. Like anemia, it is not a disease but a manifestation of an underlying illness. The presence of erythrocytosis should prompt an evaluation for its etiology.

Etiology

The modern classification of erythrocytosis can be based on the knowledge of the important roles of erythropoietin and hypoxia as the normal controlling mechanisms of red blood cell production. If one uses this approach, a primary or autonomous marrow proliferation is characterized by a decreased erythropoietin concentration. This situation is seen in polycythemia rubra vera and occasionally in other myeloproliferative disorders. If the erythropoietin level is elevated, a secondary polycythemia is present. This may be the result of hypoxia produced by high altitude, chronic severe pulmonary disease, cardiac disease with right-to-left shunt, hemoglobins that have a decreased oxygen-carrying capacity, i.e., methemoglobin or carboxyhemoglobin, or an abnormal structural hemoglobin that leads to an increased oxygen affinity.

There are also situations in which the erythropoietin level is elevated but hypoxia is not the provoking factor. These conditions cause an increased secretion or the spurious production of erythropoietin, and include tumors, renal lesions producing elevated renal parenchymal pressure, i.e., cysts or hydronephrosis, Cushing's syndrome, and androgens. Lastly, polycythemia may be relative or spurious. In this situation, erythropoietin is normal and the red blood cell mass is normal as well. It is attributable to a reduction in plasma volume and is seen in situations in which the plasma volume is reduced with a normal red blood cell mass, such as occurs in dehydration.

Diagnostic Approach

An algorithm for the evaluation of polycythemia is shown in Figure 72-1.

The finding of an elevated hematocrit, hemoglobin, or red cell count prompts an evaluation for erythrocytosis. One should undertake a screening evaluation when the red blood cell count is above $6 \times 10^6/\mu l$, when the hemoglobin is above 18.0 g/dl in a man or above 16.0 g/dl in a woman, or when the hematocrit is above 52 percent in a man or above 47 percent in a woman. Screening is performed by initially repeating the study that raised the question of polycythemia to be certain of its accuracy, and then, if the value is still elevated, measuring the red blood cell mass to be certain that true polycythemia exists and not simply a decrease in plasma volume. A red blood cell mass is determined by labeling a sample of the patient's red cells with radioactive phosphorus (^{32}P), reinjecting the sample, and then measuring its hemodilution. A previously established formula can be used to calculate the red cell mass. A normal red cell mass suggests the presence of a relative or spurious polycythemia (decreased plasma volume), whereas an elevated value confirms real or absolute polycythemia, which requires further differentiation of primary versus secondary causes. A white blood cell count, differential, and platelet count are done to look for primary erythrocytosis, i.e., polycythemia rubra vera or a myeloproliferative disease, because in polycythemia rubra vera, granulocytes and megakaryocytes may be elevated as well.

A physical examination is performed to search for hepatomegaly or splenomegaly, which might indicate polycythemia vera. An arterial blood gas reading is made to evaluate the arterial Po_2 and directly measure oxygen saturation. If Po_2 and oxygen saturation are low (less than 92 percent), attention should be directed toward a cardiopulmonary cause for erythrocytosis. If the oxygen saturation is normal and there is no evidence of polycythemia rubra vera or other myeloproliferative diseases, a renal or malignant lesion should be considered as the possible cause.

Renal tumors or lesions, including cysts, hydronephrosis, renal cell cancer, and in some patients, polycystic kidney disease, may be associated with erythrocytosis. In these situations, erythropoietin production is increased and may come from the lesion itself or from compressed renal tissue. Intravenous pyelography has been the traditional screening test for nonhypoxic secondary polycythemia, although ultrasonography or computed tomography (CT) can be used. The nonrenal tumors that produce secondary erythrocytosis include cerebellar hemangioblastomas, uterine myomas, and hepatomas. These can often be excluded by a review of symptoms; careful neurologic, liver, and pelvic examination; and appropriate scans, if indicated.

Much less frequent than the aforementioned causes is the presence of abnormal hemoglobins. These may produce familial erythrocytosis, in which an abnormal hemoglobin has an increased affinity for oxygen. Thus, tissue hypoxia develops, which leads to increased erythropoietin production. The affected heterozygotes are normal in all other respects. Most of these hemoglobins have a normal electrophoretic pattern. The Po_2 and the calculated oxygen saturation are normal, and an oxygen dissociation curve must be determined for diagnosis. The hemolysate of these red cells will show an oxygen dissociation curve that is shifted to the left with a low P50. Erythropoietin levels appear to be normal in these compensated polycythemic states.

In the case of nonfunctional hemoglobins, i.e., hemoglobins such as methemoglobin that do not carry oxygen, they may produce a compensatory polycythemia in two ways. First, the resulting tissue hypoxia may lead to increased erythropoietin production. Secondly, the presence of these hemoglobins confers a left-shifted oxygen dissociation curve on the remaining normal hemoglobin, which further increases hypoxia. Drugs, particularly androgenic steroids, may cause erythrocytosis. In many cases of erythrocytosis the cause is never diagnosed, but some will eventually meet the criteria for a myeloproliferative disease or polycythemia rubra vera.

Polycythemia rubra vera serves as a prototype of the myeloproliferative diseases in that there is an apparent unregulated proliferation of red blood cells, white blood cells, and platelets. Despite a marked elevation of the red blood cell mass, erythropoietin is low, indicating that the marrow is intrinsically abnormal or is responding to an abnormal stimulus.

At present, our knowledge of the natural history of this disease exceeds our understanding of its basic pathophysiology.

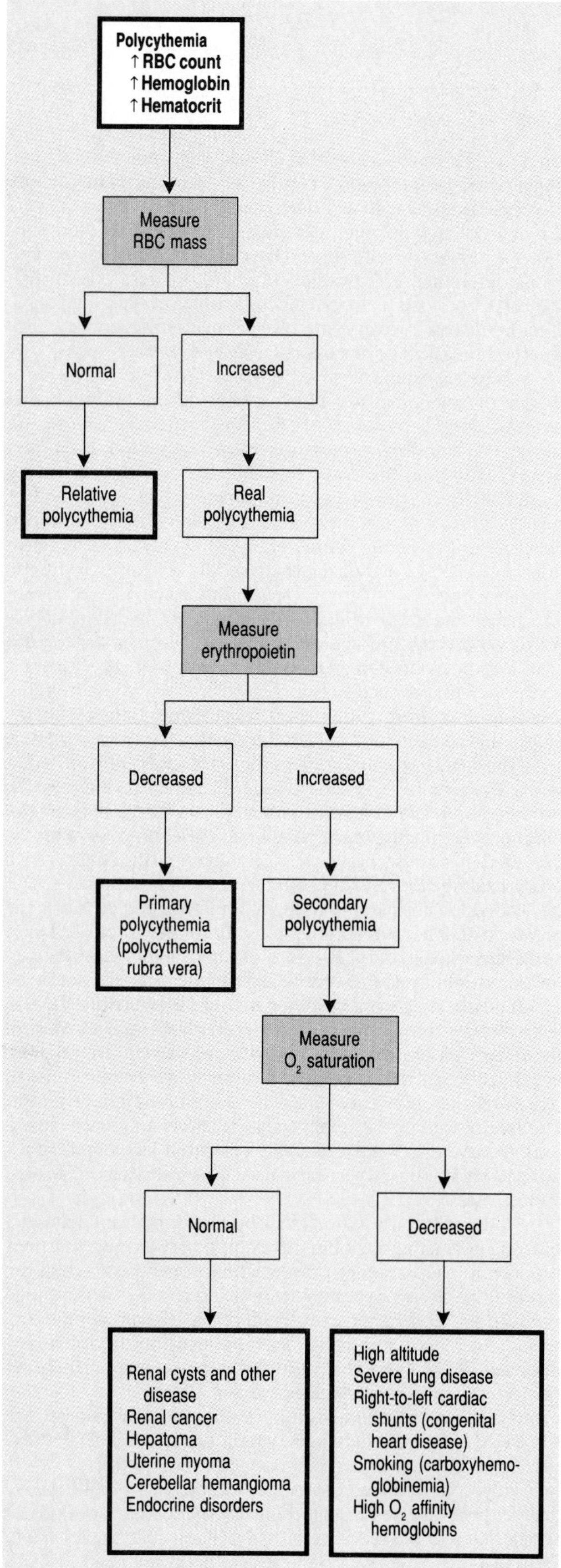

Figure 72-1 Algorithm for the evaluation of polycythemia. Because of variabilities in erythropoietin (EPO) assays and difficulties of interpretation, EPO is not routinely measured. Rather, primary and secondary polycythemia are most often distinguished on the basis of the presence of associated findings in patients with polycythemia rubra vera, the results of an arterial blood gas determination, and the presence or absence of other obvious causes of secondary polycythemia. The O_2 saturation will appear normal in patients with high O_2 affinity hemoglobins, and an O_2 dissociation curve must be determined. In heavy smokers, carboxyhemoglobin must be measured directly. RBC = red blood cell.

The laboratory evaluation for polycythemia rubra vera is easy when there is an unexplained leukocytosis, basophilia, thrombocytosis, and splenomegaly with a relatively normal oxygen saturation. In early cases, however, only one of these findings may be present, and other studies should be done, including a bone marrow biopsy to look for hypercellularity of all cell lines and a determination of leukocyte alkaline phosphatase, which should be elevated in polycythemia rubra vera.

During the course of polycythemia vera, it is not unusual for the marrow to fail and for the patient to become anemic. At this stage the marrow may be fibrotic, and the spleen may achieve enormous dimensions. This phase of the disease may then be indistinguishable from myelofibrosis with myeloid metaplasia. The clinical problem now becomes refractory anemia and not polycythemia. The huge spleen may lead to a high transfusion requirement, and splenectomy may be helpful in those cases in which the platelet count is not elevated.

In some cases of polycythemia vera, the white blood cell count may rise to levels that suggest the diagnosis of chronic myelogenous leukemia; however, the leukocyte alkaline phosphatase level remains high and the Philadelphia chromosome is not found. Another group of patients may develop extremely high platelet counts and mimic the disease essential thrombocythemia.

A small proportion of cases terminate in acute myeloblastic leukemia. This complication appears to be greater in patients who are treated with ^{32}P.

Symptoms

An increased blood volume leading to greater blood viscosity that impairs blood flow may give the sensation of fullness in the head, dizziness, headache, and visual irregularities, and may produce weakness and fatigue. Bleeding or thrombotic episodes may occur because of abnormal platelet function. Elevated blood histamine levels may lead to pruritus, which is classically increased following a warm bath. Increased uric acid production may lead to gouty arthritis and nephropathy. On physical examination these patients have plethoric facies, distention of veins on funduscopic exam, rarely papilledema, splenomegaly, hepatomegaly, and excoriations due to scratching. The complications of polycythemia rubra vera can be divided into early and late. Early manifestations include venous thrombosis, especially in unusual locations such as the portal, hepatic, mesenteric, or dural sinuses. This is preventable if the red blood cell mass and hyperviscosity are controlled. Bleeding (frequently from the gastrointestinal tract) is another early complication. Peptic ulcers are also noted and have been attributed to elevated histamine levels. Hyperuricemia and secondary gout, pruritus, or excoriations with secondary infection may also occur.

Late manifestations of polycythemia vera include "spent" polycythemia, with the development of anemia that is often associated with myelofibrosis and myeloid metaplasia. This may be accompanied by splenic infarction, hypersplenism, portal hypertension, and severe hypermetabolism, and it is extremely difficult to treat. Finally, polycythemia vera may evolve into an acute myeloblastic leukemia.

The treatment of polycythemia vera is generally gratifying. Early deaths from thrombosis and hemorrhage can be prevented. The survival of patients with this disorder who are treated with phlebotomy or ^{32}P is as long as a median of 13 years in some series. Where this information is available, the untreated patient lives only 1 to 4 years.

Phlebotomy remains an effective form of treatment in patients whose platelet count and spleen size do not show progressive increments. The production of iron deficiency by phlebotomy is probably responsible for slowing erythropoiesis sufficiently to keep the frequency of phlebotomy at a minimum. On the other hand, the development of severe iron deficiency with markedly hypochromic cells may be undesirable, even in polycythemia.

The development of dangerous thrombocytosis (over $1 \times 10^6/\mu l$), progressive splenomegaly, hypermetabolism, or a very high phlebotomy requirement is an indication for the use of radiation (^{32}P) or chemotherapy. The long-term unknown risk of producing leukemia is definitely less than the short-term morbidity and mortality resulting from uncontrolled disease. Many patients can be controlled with phlebotomy and the judicious administration of ^{32}P. The use of allopurinol may be helpful in controlling hyperuricemia until the cell proliferation is controlled.

References

Balcerzak SP, Bromberg PA. Secondary polycythemia. Semin Hematol 1975; 12:353.

Berlin NI. Diagnosis and classification of polycythemias. Semin Hematol 1975; 12:339.

Golde DW. Polycythemia: Mechanisms and management. Ann Intern Med 1981; 95:71.

Koeffler HP,Goldwasser E. Erythropoietin radioimmune assay in evaluation of patients with polycythemia. Ann Intern Med 1981; 94:44.

Wasserman LR. The treatment of polycythemia vera. Semin Hematol 1976; 13:57.

Waterbury L. Hematology for the house officer. Baltimore: Williams & Wilkins, 1988.

73 Leukocytosis and Leukopenia

John A. Merritt, MD

Definition

Leukocyte is the term used to define all white blood cells. Leukocytosis is present when the total white cell count is greater than 10,000 per microliter and leukopenia is defined as a white cell count that is less than 4,300 per microliter. Clinically, it is of greater importance to determine the specific type or types of leukocytes responsible for the change. In making this determination, the absolute count of the cells that are involved should be calculated, because the percent of each cell type that is present in the differential count is not sufficient to make an accurate estimate. It is obtained by multiplying the total leukocyte count by the percent of the particular cell that is being assessed. For example, a patient whose leukocyte count is 2,500 per microliter, with 70 percent lymphocytes and 30 percent neutrophils in the differential count, has 1,750 lymphocytes per microliter, which is normal, but only 750 neutrophils per microliter, which is reduced below the normal value. Furthermore, it is important to recognize that significant changes may occur in the absolute numbers of the less numerous types of leukocytes in the peripheral blood in the presence of a total leukocyte count that is normal.

Pathophysiology

An increase in the absolute number of leukocytes in the peripheral blood may be the result of an increase in the rate of entry of cells into the circulation, a decrease in the number of cells that are normally marginated along blood vessel walls, or a reduction in the rate of egress of cells from blood vessels. A decline in the number of circulating leukocytes occurs when there is diminished production, increased margination, or an augmentation in the rate of exodus of leukocytes out of blood vessels. More than one of these changes may be found simultaneously in the same patient.

The kinetics of the neutrophil have been studied more extensively than the other leukocyte populations. The half-life of these cells in the circulation is 7 hours, and the actual numbers of neutrophils that are measured in the peripheral blood under normal conditions represent only 50 percent of the cells that are actually present within the blood vessels. The remaining cells are "marginated" along the walls of blood vessels, and they are not recorded in the blood leukocyte count. When levels of epinephrine are increased by either injection or increased endogenous synthesis, these cells are rapidly demarginated into the circulating white cell pool, and this causes an elevation in the leukocyte count that disappears within 30 minutes after epinephrine levels return to normal. In addition, there are approximately 10 times more mature neutrophils stored in the bone marrow than are found in the blood. Administration of adrenal corticosteroids releases many of these cells in the circulation, resulting in the appearance of a polymorphonuclear leukocytosis without an increase in band forms; either acute or chronic administration of adrenal corticosteroids will bring about a neutrophilia. An increase of 2,000 neutrophils per microliter 5 hours after the oral administration of 40 mg of prednisone indicates good marrow function, and it is a more sensitive method for determining cellularity than marrow biopsy.

Monocytes arise in the bone marrow and circulate in the blood, with a half-life of 8 hours. After leaving the circulation, they become incorporated into exudates or they enter various tissues where they develop into macrophages.

Blood lymphocytes are composed of a variety of subpopulations that vary in site of origin, length of time in the blood and lymphatic circulations, and function. The subpopulations cannot be specifically identified on Wright-stained smears of blood.

Technical difficulties have limited the studies of eosinophil and basophil kinetics.

Leukocytosis

Polymorphonuclear Leukocytosis (>7,500 per Microliter)

Etiology

Elevation of circulating neutrophils, known as polymorphonuclear leukocytosis or neutrophilia, accompanies a wide variety of disorders, the most common of which are enumerated in Table 73-1.

During the course of bacterial infection, the neutrophil count usually increases, but the degree of elevation is not a good indication of severity or prognosis. If neutrophilia develops during an obvious viral illness, it should suggest the possibility of a secondary bacterial infection.

The chronic myeloproliferative disorders, which include chronic myelogenous leukemia, polycythemia rubra vera, and myelofibrosis with myeloid metaplasia, usually are associated with neutrophilia and the presence of immature forms in the peripheral blood. Similar findings occurring with nonhematologic malignancies may be a source of confusion. Neutrophilia commonly occurs with acute hemorrhage or hemolysis as well as with acute infarction of any tissue, but it is not found with ischemic chest pain in the absence of infarction.

Diagnostic Approach

Evidence obtained by history and physical examination should help to narrow the number of diagnostic possibilities that may account for the patient's neutrophilia. If infection is suspected, cultures and Gram stains of exudates and blood are indicated. If tuberculosis or fungal or parasitic infections are suspected, appropriate stains, cultures, and serologic studies are ordered in accordance with impressions, which should be based on the existing data. The presence of many neutrophils with toxic granulation (prominent deep blue granules in the cytoplasm) or cytoplasmic vacuoles usually is associated with systemic infections. Dohle bodies are blue-gray cytoplasmic inclusions that are found in severe infection, but they may be present with cancer, burns, or myeloproliferative disorders as well.

The neutrophilia present with acute infection is accompanied by increased band forms and, occasionally, more immature cells (leukemoid reaction). In most instances, chronic infection, inflammatory disorders, and physical and emotional stress are not associated with an increase in immature forms.

It may be difficult to differentiate the nonhematologic malignancies from the chronic myeloproliferative disorders. The latter are usually associated with splenomegaly. Furthermore, an elevation in hemoglobin suggests polycythemia vera. A low leukocyte alkaline phosphatase, basophilia, and a Philadelphia chromosome in bone marrow cells are usually found in chronic myelogenous leukemia. Teardrop-shaped erythrocytes and the presence of fibrosis on examination of a bone marrow biopsy support the diagnosis of myelofibrosis. Characteristics of the chronic myeloproliferative syndromes are summarized in Table 73-2. The leukemoid and leukoerythroblastic blood pictures are discussed later in this chapter.

Eosinophilia (>700 per Microliter)

Etiology

An elevation in the eosinophil count accompanies a variety of allergic reactions, dermatologic disorders, parasitic infections, and reversible obstructive pulmonary disease. Certain drugs such as sulfonamides, para-aminosalicylic acid, and nitrofurantoin may give rise to eosinophilia. An elevation in the eosinophil count with transient pulmonary infiltrates should lead one to consider Loeffler's syndrome, a benign condition that may be associated with a variety of infections or may occur in the absence of any identifiable cause. Eosinophilic leukemia is extremely rare, and all other sources of an elevated eosinophil count should be carefully ruled out before this possibility is considered.

Diagnostic Approach

If the history and physical examination do not identify the cause, occult parasitic infection should be considered. Examinations for ova and parasites in stool samples may prove diagnostic.

Basophilia (>150 per Microliter)

Etiology

An absolute increase in basophils is an uncommon finding, but it may be very useful in differentiating chronic myelogenous leukemia, with which it is almost always found, from nonhematologic neoplasms and benign conditions accompanied by an elevation in the blood neutrophil count. It is less consistently present with polycythemia vera, myelofibrosis, hypothyroidism, and ulcerative colitis, and following injection of foreign proteins.

Table 73-1 Common Causes of Leukocytosis

Neutrophilia (>7.5 × 10^9/L)	Monocytosis (>1 × 10^9/L)	Eosinophilia (>0.035 × 10^9/L)	Lymphocytosis (>4 × 10^9/L)
Physiologic (adrenocorticosteroids and epinephrine)	Chronic infections	Allergic	Acute viral infections
Infections	With neutropenia	Dermatologic	Chronic infections
Inflammatory disorders	Inflammatory disorders	Parasitic	Lymphocytic leukemias
Acute hemorrhage, hemolysis	Myeloproliferative disorders (chronic myelogenous leukemia, polycythemia rubra vera, myelofibrosis)	Periarteritis nodosa	Non-Hodgkin's lymphoma
Tissue infarction	Monocytic leukemia	Myeloproliferative disorders (chronic myelogenous leukemia, polycythemia rubra vera, myelofibrosis)	
Myeloproliferative disorders (chronic myelogenous leukemia, polycythemia rubra vera, myelofibrosis)	Other malignancies	Other malignancies	
Other malignancies			

Table 73-2 Characteristics of Chronic Myeloproliferative Syndromes

Disease	Predominant cell type	Manifestations	Laboratory results	Therapy	Course
Chronic myelogenous leukemia	Granulocytes	Age: 30–50 years Hypermetabolic symptoms; ± bruises; symptoms of anemia; moderately enlarged spleen	WBC: 30,000–300,000/μl; left shifted; <15% blasts; promyelocytes; basophilia RBC: high, normal, or decreased; occasionally nucleated PLT: high, normal, or decreased LAP: very low; vitamin B_{12} TCI high; Philadelphia chromosome positive in >90%; if negative, poorer prognosis BM: hypercellular; little fat; ± increased reticulin	Busulfan or hydroxyurea Bone marrow transplant	Mean survival 3.5 yr; transformation to acute leukemia almost uniform Currently being defined
Agnogenic myeloid metaplasia	All three cell lines (granulocytic, erythrocytic, megakaryocytic)	Age: >60 yr ± Hypermetabolic symptoms; ± bruises; symptoms of anemia common; markedly enlarged spleen; moderately enlarged liver	WBC: <50,000/μl; left shifted; occasionally basophilia, blasts, promyelocytes RBC: decreased; teardrop forms; nucleated RBCs common PLT: high, normal, or decreased; dysfunctional LAP: high; vitamin B_{12}/TCI high BM: dry tap common; marked increase in reticulin count on biopsy	Transfusion for anemia; busulfan when counts are high or there is severe hypersplenism; ?splenectomy or irradiation	Mean survival 5–7 yr; transforms to AML, CML, polycythemia rubra vera
Polycythemia rubra vera	RBC	Age: >50 yr Hyperviscosity; plethora; pruritus; enlarged spleen; thrombosis/hemorrhagic problems	WBC: normal to increased; ± basophilia, eosinophilia RBC: increased mass; decreased erythropoietin PLT: normal to increased; dysfunctional LAP: increased BM: panhypercellularity	Phlebotomy, especially if platelets normal; busulfan or ^{32}P	Mean survival 9–10 yr; transforms to AMM, AML, CML
Essential thrombocythemia	Platelets	Age: >50 yr Thrombosis/hemorrhagic problems; peptic ulcer; enlarged spleen	WBC: normal; ± increased RBC: decreased secondary to bleeding with iron deficiency PLT: markedly elevated (>1 million); dysfunctional LAP: normal to increased BM: panhypercellularity with marked increase in megakaryocytes with dysplasia	Busulfan or ^{32}P	Mean survival long; transforms to polycythemia vera, AML

Abbreviations: AML = acute myeloblastic leukemia, AMM = agnogenic myeloid metaplasia, BM = bone marrow, CML = chronic myelogenous leukemia, LAP = leukocyte alkaline phosphatase, ^{32}P = radioactive phosphorus, PLT = platelets, RBC = red blood cells, TCI = transcobalamin I.

Diagnostic Approach
The diagnosis of chronic myeloproliferative disorders was discussed briefly in the section on neutrophilia. Serum thyrotropin (TSH) levels, barium enema, and sigmoidoscopy may be useful when the other diagnostic possibilities are considered.

Monocytosis (>1,000 per Microliter)

Etiology
A wide variety of bacterial, protozoal, and rickettsial infections are associated with an increase in blood monocytes. This increase is common in active tuberculosis, a disorder in which any of the leukocyte types may be increased or decreased. A transient elevation of the monocyte count during recovery from bacterial infections is common; however, if it continues for several days, persistence of the infection is likely. Granulomatous diseases such as ulcerative colitis, regional enteritis, and sarcoidosis, as well as the connective tissue disorders, are frequently accompanied by monocytosis. In addition, most patients with disseminated malignancies, including the lymphomas, have increased monocyte counts. Monocytic leukemia is another relatively rare form of leukemia, and one should exclude other causes before accepting that possibility.

Diagnostic Approach
Diagnostically useful procedures may include a skin test for tuberculosis as well as a chest radiograph, which may be abnormal in sarcoidosis and cancer as well. Rheumatoid factor and antinuclear antibodies are useful when connective tissue disorders are considered. Biopsies of lymph nodes or other possible areas of involvement are required to confirm the presence of lymphomas and other malignancies.

Lymphocytosis (>4,000 per Microliter)

Etiology
Lymphocytosis with splenomegaly and lymphadenopathy is usually noted with infectious mononucleosis, the acute and chronic lymphocytic leukemias, and the "leukemic" phase of non-Hodgkin's lymphoma. Furthermore, the absolute lymphocyte count may be useful in helping to differentiate the infectious agent responsible for a febrile illness. Lymphocytosis usually is not found with bacterial infections in adults, except in the presence of tuberculosis or chronic brucellosis.

Diagnostic Approach
When the initial clinical and laboratory data are confusing, suggesting either infectious mononucleosis or one of the hematologic malignancies, look for the "atypical lymphocyte" that is characteristic of infectious mononucleosis and occasionally other viral illnesses. This contrasts with the more homogeneous lymphocyte morphology that is associated with hematopoietic malignancies.

The Leukemoid Blood Picture

Etiology
The term *leukemoid blood picture* is used to describe an elevation of the leukocyte count that is caused by a marked increase in the more mature granulocytic elements or by the presence of varying numbers of granulocytic precursors in the peripheral blood, which simulates leukemia. It may be seen with infections, acute severe hemolysis, gastrointestinal bleeding, or malignancy. Confusion with chronic myelogenous leukemia is the most common problem. When nucleated red blood cells are found in the peripheral smear with myeloid precursors, the term *leukoerythroblastic blood picture* is used. The majority of these patients have neoplastic disorders that are often associated with metastases to the bone marrow. Myelofibrosis with splenomegaly secondary to extramedullary hematopoiesis is the most common hematologic malignancy associated with these findings.

Diagnostic Approach
The characteristic features of the chronic myeloproliferative disorders have been discussed. Appropriate cultures and biopsy of the bone marrow or other appropriate tissues may be useful. Hemolysis and bleeding must be extensive in order to cause a leukemoid reaction, and either diagnosis should be obvious from the history, physical examination, and initial laboratory studies, which should include a reticulocyte count and serum bilirubin levels. The presence of nucleated red blood cells in the peripheral blood smear may be an early clue to the diagnosis of a hematologic malignancy or to the presence of a tumor with metastases to the bone.

Leukopenia

Neutropenia (<1,500 per Microliter)

Etiology
The disorders that are most commonly associated with leukopenia are shown in Table 73-3. In the absence of a preexisting bone marrow disorder, the presence of neutropenia suggests a viral etiology in the acutely febrile patient. However, decreased neutrophil counts may be seen with several less common bacterial and fungal infections. Combined neutropenia and lymphopenia are often seen in patients with infectious hepatitis before the onset of jaundice and abnormal liver function tests. In addition, administration of most of the antineoplastic agents regularly induces neutropenia, often with anemia and thrombocytopenia. Occasionally, a variety of other drugs cause similar abnormalities.

If physical examination reveals the presence of an enlarged spleen, increased destruction of cells in that organ must be considered. Systemic lupus erythematosus, Felty's syndrome, and portal hypertension are common examples of disorders associated with increased neutrophil destruction. Furthermore, neutropenia with or without thrombocytopenia may be seen with the myelodysplastic syndromes, vitamin B_{12} or folic acid deficiency anemias, and bone marrow replacement by fibrosis or tumor cells.

There are several familial and nonfamilial chronic neutropenias, and a cyclic form of neutropenia exists, but these disorders are quite rare.

Diagnostic Approach
In the neutropenic patient, bone marrow biopsy and aspiration are often very useful. Patients with portal hypertension, Felty's

Table 73-3 Common Causes of Leukopenia

Neutropenia ($<1.5 \times 10^9$/L)	Lymphopenia ($<1.2 \times 10^9$/L)
Severe bacterial infections	Adrenal corticosteroids
Viral infections	Acute infections
Drugs and chemicals	Active tuberculosis
Ionizing radiation	Malignancies
Hemodialysis	Renal failure
Hypersplenism	Systemic lupus erythematosus
Rheumatoid arthritis and systemic lupus erythematosus	Acquired immunodeficiency syndrome
Folate or B_{12} deficiency	
Marrow infiltration	

syndrome, or systemic lupus erythematosus usually have hyperplasia of the bone marrow. A history of alcoholism or hepatitis and abnormal liver function tests are found with portal hypertension. Longstanding physical changes of rheumatoid arthritis and a positive test for rheumatoid factor are associated with Felty's syndrome. Positive antinuclear antibody studies are helpful in the diagnosis of systemic lupus erythematosus.

In patients with neutropenia and megaloblastic anemias, determination of serum vitamin B_{12} and folate levels and a Schilling test are required to identify the specific etiology.

Replacement of bone marrow by tumor, fibrosis, or marrow aplasia is often associated with failure to obtain an adequate specimen on aspiration ("dry tap"), and biopsy is needed to confirm the diagnosis. Hypoplasia is often seen with drug-induced neutropenia as well.

Diagnosis of familial, nonfamilial, and cyclic neutropenias is suggested when there is a positive family history of low leukocyte counts and frequent severe infections. Furthermore, biweekly leukocyte counts for 3 weeks may reveal the presence of cyclic neutropenia. Bone marrow morphology is not diagnostic in these disorders.

When the absolute neutrophil count falls below 500 cells per microliter the likelihood of developing a life-threatening infection rises markedly. A count that progressively decreases with increasing numbers of circulating myelocytes and metamyelocytes may be a poor prognostic sign, indicating an inability of the bone marrow to produce adequate numbers of myeloid cells.

Monocytopenia (<200 per Microliter)

Little information relating to decreased monocyte counts is available, but it has been well documented that a diminished blood monocyte count follows the administration of adrenal corticosteroids. The mechanism of this change is not clear at present. Aplasia or infiltration of the bone marrow may also result in monocytopenia.

Eosinopenia (<50 per Microliter)

Low eosinophil counts also follow the administration of adrenal corticosteroids, and similar changes may occur early in the course of bacterial infections.

Lymphocytopenia (<1,200 per Microliter)

Diminished lymphocyte counts are common with acute infections and active tuberculosis, and are prominent in patients with acquired immunodeficiency syndrome (AIDS). In addition, patients with malnutrition or malignancy often have lymphopenia, and this finding is especially common in patients with Hodgkin's disease. Antineoplastic agents and irradiation also contribute to the cancer patient's low lymphocyte count. Furthermore, administration of corticosteroids and a variety of disorders associated with increased plasma cortisol levels are accompanied by lymphopenia.

References

Cassileth PA. Lymphocytosis. In: Williams WJ, et al, eds. Hematology. 3rd ed. New York: McGraw-Hill, 1983:950.

Dale DC, et al. Chronic neutropenia. Medicine 1979; 58:128.

Jandl JH. Blood: Textbook of hematology. Boston: Little, Brown, 1987:433.

Lee GR, et al, eds. Wintrobe's clinical hematology. 9th ed. Philadelphia: Lea & Febiger, 1990.

Strausbaugh L. Hematologic manifestations of bacterial and fungal infections. Hematol Oncol Clin North Am 1987; 1:185.

Young GAR, Vincent PC. Drug-induced agranulocytosis. Clin Haematol 1980; 9:483.

Thrombocytosis

Mary Ellen M. Rybak, MD

74

Definition

Thrombocytosis refers to the presence of an abnormally high number of platelets in the circulation. This is usually defined as an elevation of the platelet count above 400,000 per microliter. The causes of thrombocytosis can be divided into three basic mechanisms: (1) transitory or "physiologic," (2) reactive or secondary, and (3) autonomous or "primary" thrombocytosis. The basic causes of thrombocytosis are summarized in Table 74-1.

Pathophysiology

In transitory or physiologic thrombocytosis, there is mobilization of preformed platelets from an extravascular platelet pool. The available pools include the spleen and the lung; e.g., epinephrine administration induces a 20 to 50 percent rise in the platelet count. This epinephrine-induced thrombocytosis does not occur in asplenic patients; therefore, it appears that the released platelets originate from the splenic pool.

Reactive thrombocytosis frequently involves both release of preformed platelets and an increase in platelet production. It can be divided into acute and chronic forms. In acute reactive thrombocytosis, the platelet appears to act as an "acute phase reactant." This is seen in patients with acute hemorrhage, acute inflammatory disease, tissue necrosis, or recent surgery. An elevation of the platelet count from 500,000 to 600,000 per microliter is common, and platelet counts of over 1 million have been described. Patients who recover from an episode of thrombocytopenia due to bone marrow suppression or severe folate deficiency may have a period of platelet rebound after correction of the underlying disorder. The postsplenectomy period is one time in which the platelet count in acute reactive thrombocytosis commonly rises above 600,000 per microliter and may exceed 1 million per microliter. The normal spleen contains one-third of the total body platelet mass in a "pool" that is freely exchangeable with the peripheral blood. A rising platelet count is usually noted 1 to 10 days after splenectomy, and it reaches a peak 1 to 3 weeks later. Postsplenectomy thrombocytosis usually resolves over several weeks to a few months. If there is an underlying myeloproliferative disease, or ongoing hemolytic anemia, postsplenectomy thrombocytosis may persist indefinitely. Although the platelet count is often sufficiently alarming to cause the

Table 74-1 Causes of Thrombocytosis

Physiologic
Exercise
Epinephrine
Pregnancy and parturition
Reactive
Acute
Infection
Acute inflammation
Tissue necrosis
Postoperative
Chronic
Chronic infections: tuberculosis, osteomyelitis
Gastrointestinal: ulcerative colitis, sprue, regional enteritis
Chronic inflammatory diseases: rheumatoid arthritis, periarteritis nodosa, acute rheumatic fever, Wegener's granulomatosis
Sarcoidosis
Neoplasms
Hodgkin's disease and other lymphoid neoplasms
Breast cancer
Lung cancer
Any carcinoma
Accelerated hematopoiesis
Acute blood loss
Hemolysis
"Rebound" thrombocytosis
Recovery following megaloblastic anemia
Recovery following marrow suppression
Asplenic State
After splenectomy
After splenic vein thrombosis
Autonomous
Essential thrombocythemia
Polycythemia vera
Agnogenic myelofibrosis and myeloid metaplasia
Chronic myelogenous leukemia
Refractory anemia with excess blasts

physician to prescribe antithrombotic medication, thromboembolic complications are rare, occurring in less than 4 percent of hematologically normal patients.

Patients with chronic inflammatory diseases such as rheumatoid arthritis, chronic inflammatory bowel disease, chronic infections such as tuberculosis, and chronic osteomyelitis, and patients with malignant disease may have chronic reactive thrombocytosis, which often parallels the activity of the underlying disease. The platelet count usually does not exceed 1 million per microliter, but higher counts have been reported, especially with cancer. The precise pathogenesis is unknown, and clinically evident disease is usually present when thrombocytosis is noted. Occasionally, however, thrombocytosis may occur when the malignant disease is still occult.

In iron deficiency there is great variability in the platelet count, which can range from normal to strikingly elevated values. If the platelet count is elevated, it usually returns to a normal level within 1 to 2 weeks after iron replacement is initiated.

In autonomous or primary thrombocytosis, platelet production is sustained independent of normal regulatory processes. Megakaryocytes are markedly increased in number and mass; platelet production may be increased as much as 15-fold. This autonomous proliferation may be manifest only in thrombocytosis (termed thrombocythemia) or may involve other cell lines as part of a myeloproliferative disorder such as agnogenic (i.e., cause unknown) myelofibrosis and myeloid metaplasia, polycythemia vera, or chronic myelogenous leukemia. These diseases are characterized by their clinical characteristics and by the cell line most prominently involved. An increase in production that involves predominantly megakaryocytes results in essential thrombocythemia. In essential thrombocythemia, there are markedly increased platelets, normal to mildly increased white cells, and normal red cells. A predominant increase in red cells is seen in polycythemia vera, but platelets and white cells may also be elevated. An increase in all cell lines, but predominantly white blood cells, is seen in agnogenic myelofibrosis, myeloid metaplasia, and chronic myelogenous leukemia.

Diagnostic Approach

Clinical findings in reactive thrombocytosis are usually those of the underlying disorder. In general, patients are not predisposed to thrombotic or hemorrhagic complications, and no preventive antiplatelet therapy is indicated unless the patient has had evidence of thrombotic problems. In patients with essential thrombocythemia or other myeloproliferative disorders, splenomegaly is apparent in more than 80 percent of patients. Patients may describe symptoms of early satiety and abdominal fullness. Some patients with autonomous thrombocytosis may have thrombotic and hemorrhagic complications or both, including gastrointestinal hemorrhage, epistaxis, and postsurgical hemorrhage. They may also experience thrombosis of veins and arteries, including unusual sites such as the hepatic vein and mesenteric vessels. Patients with thrombocytosis and myeloproliferative disorders may also develop a syndrome called erythromelalgia. This presents as an acute, exquisitely painful, warm erythema of an extremity that is caused by intense vasodilation. It is relieved by aspirin, indomethacin, or other potent cyclooxygenase inhibitors, and it is a result of the release of vasoactive mediators from platelets.

Laboratory Studies

Platelet morphology is usually normal, and the platelet count is usually (although not always) less than 1 million per microliter in patients with reactive thrombocytosis. Platelet function studies are usually normal. Other hematologic cell lines, i.e., red cells and white cells, are usually normal unless there are changes due to the underlying disease. A bone marrow aspirate will usually be normal to hypercellular, with increased megakaryocytes that are morphologically normal. Other laboratory abnormalities may occur owing to the specific underlying disease.

Laboratory findings in essential thrombocythemia include a markedly elevated (>1 million per microliter) platelet count that is often chronic, morphologically abnormal platelets, and sometimes abnormal platelet function. Other cell lines may be affected. This may be manifested as immaturity of circulating white cells and nucleated red blood cells and teardrop red cells in the peripheral blood. Bone marrow biopsy usually shows a marked increase in number of megakaryocytes. Megakaryocytes may appear dysplastic. A summary of some distinctions between reactive thrombocytosis and essential thrombocythemia is shown in Table 74-2.

It is important to note that false elevations of some serum chemistries (e.g., potassium, acid phosphatase, lactate dehydrogenase) may be found in the setting of any thrombocytosis (usually >1 million per microliter) owing to excessive release of these substances by the markedly elevated number of platelets.

Differential Diagnosis

In the patient with a clear, recent antecedent for an acute reactive thrombocytosis, no evaluation is necessary in the acute

Table 74-2 Differentiation of Thrombocythemia and Reactive Thrombocytosis

	Reactive thrombocytosis (secondary)	Thrombocythemia (primary)
Thrombokinetic Features		
Total megakaryocyte mass	Slightly increased	Greatly increased
Megakaryocyte number	Increased	Increased
Megakaryocyte volume (mean)	Decreased	Increased
Platelet turnover or production rate	Increased	Increased
Total platelet mass	Increased	Increased
Platelet survival	Normal	Normal to slightly decreased
Clinical and Laboratory Features		
Thromboembolism and hemorrhage	Uncommon	Common
Duration	Often transitory	Usually persistent
Splenomegaly	Absent*	Present in 80% of cases
Platelet count	Usually $<1{,}000{,}000/\mu l$	Usually $>1{,}000{,}000/\mu l$
Bleeding time	Usually normal	Often prolonged
Platelet morphology and function	Usually normal	Often abnormal
Leukocyte count	Usually normal	Increased in 90% of cases

* Unless as the result of the underlying disorder.

setting. The platelet count may be observed until it returns to normal. Conversely, in patients in whom thrombocytosis can be documented for months or years, an underlying disorder should be suspected and the patient should be evaluated. When a patient presents with an unexplained elevation in the platelet count, the diagnosis may be obvious, e.g., a history strongly suggestive of malignant or inflammatory disease or of iron deficiency. Such a diagnosis must be confirmed by appropriate examinations. Correction or treatment of the underlying disorder should result in amelioration of the thrombocytosis; if improvement does not occur, further evaluation may be necessary. When a patient presents with associated abnormalities such as an elevated white cell count or abnormal platelet or red cell morphology, the diagnosis of autonomous thrombocytosis due to a myeloproliferative disorder should be suspected. This is also true if a patient with unexplained thrombocytosis is noted to have an enlarged spleen on physical examination. Appropriate laboratory evaluation includes a leukocyte alkaline phosphatase level, which is very low in chronic myelocytic leukemia but markedly elevated in essential thrombocythemia and other myeloproliferative diseases. When the diagnosis cannot be made with certainty, platelet aggregation studies may be of help. Subtle abnormalities of aggregation may be detected in myeloproliferative disorders. Occasionally, the distinction still cannot be made with certainty, so the patient must be observed or an empiric noninvasive search for underlying malignancy should be undertaken.

Treatment

Treatment must be directed toward the underlying disorder in reactive thrombocytosis (e.g., inflammatory disease, cancer). In primary thrombocytosis, treatment should be directed toward the cell line that is provoking the patient's current symptoms or may cause potential problems. In essential thrombocythemia, radioactive phosphorus therapy may reduce the platelet count and decrease the risk of thrombosis. The decision to use antiplatelet agents should be individualized, because the data suggest that the hemorrhagic tendency in myeloproliferative disorders is markedly increased with these agents.

References

Buss DH, Stuart, JJ, Lipscomb GE. The incidence of thrombotic and hemorrhagic disorders in association with extreme thrombocytosis. Am J Hematol 1955; 20:365.

Fabio F, et al. The possible value of platelet aggregation studies in patients with increased platelet number. Blut 1981; 43:279.

Hehlmann R, et al. Essential thrombocythemia: Clinical characteristics and course in 61 patients. Cancer 1988; 61:2487.

Kessler CM, Klein HG, Havlik RJ. Uncontrolled thrombocytosis in chronic myeloproliferative disorders. Br J Haematol 1982; 50:157.

Levin J, Conley CL. Thrombocytosis associated with malignant disease. Arch Intern Med 1964; 114:497.

Marchasin S, Wallerstein RO, Aggeler PM. Variations of the platelet count in disease. Calif Med 1964; 101:95.

Sedlacek SM, et al. Essential thrombocythemia and leukemic transformation. Medicine 1986; 65:353.

Selroos O. Thrombocytosis. Acta Med Scand 1973; 193:431.

Silverstein MN. Primary or hemorrhagic thrombocythemia. Arch Intern Med 1968; 122:18.

Ziegler Z, Murphy S, Gardner F. Microscopic platelet size and morphology in various hematologic disorders. Blood 1978; 51:479.

Zucker S, Mielke CH. Classification of thrombocytosis based on platelet function tests: Correlation with hemorrhagic and thrombotic complications. J Lab Clin Med 1972; 80:385.

Thrombocytopenia

Mary Ellen M. Rybak, MD

75

Definition

Thrombocytopenia is defined as a subnormal circulating platelet count, usually below 100,000 per microliter, but platelet counts between 100,000 and 150,000 per microliter may represent an underlying pathologic process.

As expected, bleeding is the principal manifestation of thrombocytopenia. Patients with platelets counts greater than 50,000 per microliter usually have minimal symptoms or manifest only post-traumatic bleeding. With platelet counts below 20,000 per microliter, spontaneous bleeding is seen and central nervous system and gastrointestinal bleeding may be life threatening. At any given platelet count, other factors that may influence bleeding, such as infection, gastritis, coagulation abnormalities, and concomitant platelet inhibitory drugs, must be considered. Hypertension may specifically predispose to central nervous system bleeds. Bleeding symptoms of thrombocytopenia usually involve mucocutaneous lesions (petechiae and purpura) and prolonged bleeding after minor trauma. Hemarthroses and deep intramuscular hematomas, which are commonly seen in hemophilia, are uncommon in patients with thrombocytopenia. These differences are summarized in Table 75-1. Retinal hemorrhages are also seen, especially in anemic patients.

Table 75-1 Clinical Bleeding in Disorders of Hemostasis

Findings	Disorders of coagulation	Disorders of platelets or vessels ("purpuric" disorders)
Petechiae	Rare	Characteristic
Deep dissecting hematomas	Characteristic	Rare
Superficial ecchymoses	Common; usually large and solitary	Characteristic; usually small and multiple
Hemarthrosis	Characteristic	Uncommon
Delayed bleeding	Common	Uncommon
Bleeding from superficial cuts and scratches	Minimal	Common
Sex of patient	80–90% of hereditary forms occur only in men	Relatively more common in women
Positive family history	Common (but not essential)	Rare

Etiology

Thrombocytopenia should be considered a symptom like anemia or back pain, and a specific etiology must be sought. The causes of thrombocytopenia can be approached clinically by dividing them into four classes (Table 75-2): decreased production, increased destruction, abnormal distribution, and dilution. Within these general classes are specific etiologic categories.

Decreased Production

Decreased platelet production can be due either to a decrease in the total number of megakaryocytes in the bone marrow or to ineffective thrombopoiesis, in which there are normal or increased megakaryocytes but inadequate production of platelets. The thrombocytopenia of decreased production may occur in combination with pancytopenia, i.e., a decrease in erythroid and myeloid elements as well as platelets, such as aplastic anemia. Decreased platelet production can also be the result of a drug effect on the bone marrow (Table 75-3). Drugs are also a major cause of secondary aplastic anemia. Some drugs, such as chemotherapeutic agents, cause a reproducible, usually dose-related, bone marrow suppression in all patients who receive them.

Myelophthisic processes, in which there is marrow infiltration by leukemia, other malignancies, or myelofibrosis, can also result in decreased megakaryocytes. Some infections, such as measles, occasionally affect megakaryocytes, producing selective thrombocytopenia. However, viral infections frequently have a multifactorial effect on the platelet count, including immune-mediated platelet destruction. Thrombocytopenia is commonly seen in the acquired immunodeficiency syndrome (AIDS), which is associated with human immunodeficiency virus (HIV) infection. A variety of mechanisms of thrombocytopenia have been described with HIV infection, including decreased platelet production and increased platelet destruction.

Ineffective thrombopoiesis can result from various nutritional disorders, such as vitamin B_{12} or folate deficiency. The deficiency is generally severe if significant thrombocytopenia occurs; therefore, changes in red cells and white cells are usually apparent. There is usually megaloblastic maturation with macro-ovalocytes, anemia, and hypersegmented polymorphonuclear leukocytes, with or without leukopenia. In hematopoietic stem cell disorders such as paroxysmal nocturnal hemoglobinuria or myelodysplastic syndromes, a combination of decreased megakaryocyte production and ineffective thrombopoiesis may be seen, although the first mechanism is much more common. In addition, there are rare congenital disorders in which megakaryocytes are seen but the infant is thrombocytopenic.

Increased Destruction

Decreased platelet survival is caused by increased platelet destruction or consumption. In most cases large platelets, megathrombocytes, are present on the peripheral smear, and megakaryocytes are increased in the bone marrow.

Immune Mechanisms

Increased destruction can result from immune mechanisms. This can occur if there are autoantibodies directed against antigens on the platelet surface, as in "idiopathic" or immune thrombocytopenic purpura (ITP) or in the immune thrombocytopenia associated with other autoimmune disorders such as systemic lupus erythematosus or with lymphoproliferative disorders such as chronic lymphocytic leukemia. Increased immunoglobulin, complement, or both can often be detected on the platelet membrane by a variety of techniques in immune thrombocytopenia. Sensitized platelets are removed by the reticuloen-

Table 75-2 Classification of Thrombocytopenia

Decreased Production
Decreased megakaryopoiesis
- Drugs
- Primary bone marrow failure
- Myelophthisic processes
- Some infections
- Congenital

Ineffective thrombopoiesis
- Nutritional disorders: B_{12} deficiency; folate deficiency
- Paroxysmal nocturnal hemoglobinuria

Miscellaneous
- Cyclic thrombocytopenia
- ? Thrombopoietin deficiency

Increased Destruction
Immune
- Autoantibodies
- Alloantibodies
  - Post-transfusion purpura
  - Isoimmune neonatal thrombocytopenia
- Immune complex disease
- Drug induced
- Infections

Nonimmune: increased consumption
- Disseminated intravascular coagulation
- Kasabach-Merritt syndrome (giant hemangioendotheliomas)
- Thrombotic thrombocytopenic purpura, hemolytic-uremic syndrome
- Extracorporeal circulation, other prosthetic surfaces
- Post-decompression sickness in divers

Abnormal Distribution
Hypersplenism
Hypothermic anesthesia

Dilutional

dothelial system, primarily in the spleen, although hepatic sequestration is important in many cases. The spleen is a major source of antibody production; therefore, therapeutic splenectomy removes the site of platelet destruction as well as a major site of antibody production. Almost all patients with ITP have increased megakaryocytes in the bone marrow, although rare cases are associated with decreased megakaryocytes. In the latter cases, suppression of megakaryopoiesis has been attributed to a humoral factor.

Two major patterns of ITP occur: an acute and a chronic form. ITP in children is of the acute form in 90 percent or more of cases. There is a peak incidence between 2 and 6 years of age, and males and females are equally affected. The problem is usually brought to the attention of a physician because of the sudden appearance of petechiae on the lower extremities. With careful questioning, a history of an antecedent infection, usually a viral infection of the upper respiratory tract, can be elicited in more than 80 percent of children. Symptoms other than petechiae or minor bleeding are usually absent, and physical examination is unremarkable. Splenomegaly is rare, but if it is found, another cause of thrombocytopenia should be strongly suspected. Major bleeding, including central nervous system hemorrhage, usually does not occur, in spite of the rather severe thrombocytopenia that is usually present. Treatment is supportive and the illness is self-limited, with symptoms in 90 percent or more of children resolving over a few months. Glucocorticosteroids may elevate the platelet count, but these drugs do not alter the natural history of the disease or improve survival in children. In the acute ITP of childhood, splenectomy is rarely indicated.

Chronic ITP occurs predominantly in adults and in 10 percent of children with immune thrombocytopenia. The onset is insidious, with a history of easy bruising or minor bleeding for

Table 75-3 Therapeutic and Chemical Agents That May Produce Thrombocytopenia

Direct Marrow Suppressants
Generalized marrow hypoplasia or aplasia
- Antimetabolites
- Antimitotic agents
- Antitumor antibiotics
- Benzenes and derivatives
- Ionizing radiation
- Nitrogen mustard and cogeners
- Azidothymidine

Occasional association with marrow hypoplasia or aplasia
- Chloramphenicol
- Gold compounds
- Methylphenylethyl hydantoin (Mesantoin), trimethadione (Tridione)
- Phenylbutazone
- Quinacrine
- Cimetidine

Selective suppression of megakaryocytes
- Chlorothiazides
- Estrogenic hormones
- Ethanol
- Tolbutamide

Production of Thrombocytopenia by an Immunologic Mechanism

Acetazolamide (Diamox)	Methyldopa
Allyl isopropyl carbamide	Novobiocin
Carbamazepine	Organic arsenicals
Centulin	Para-aminosalicylic acid (PAS)
Chlorpheniramine	Phenytoin (Dilantin)
Chlorpropamide	Quinidine
Desipramine	Quinine
Diazepam	Rifampin
Digitoxin	Sodium valproate
Gold salts	Stibophen (Fuadin)
Ethyl chlorvinyl	Sulfamethazine
Hydroxychloroquine	Sulfathiazole
Lidocaine	Sulfisoxazole

Direct Damage to Circulating Platelets and Immune Mechanisms
Heparin

Probable Immunologic Mechanism; Antibodies Not Always Demonstrated

Acetaminophen	Nitroglycerin
Aminopyrine	Paramethadione
Aspirin and sodium salicylate	Penicillin
Barbiturates	Phenacetin
Bismuth	Phenylbutazone
Carbutamide	Potassium iodide
Cephalothin	Prednisone
Chloroquine	Prochlorperazine
Chlorpheniramine maleate	Promethazine
Chlorpromazine	Propylthiouracil
Codeine	Pyrazinamide
Dextroamphetamine sulfate	Reserpine
Diazoxide	Spironolactone
Digitalis and digoxin	Streptomycin
Disulfiram (Antabuse)	Sulfonamides (sulfadiazine, sulfadimetine, sulfamerazine, sulfamethoxazole, sulfisoxazole)
Ergot	
Erythromycin	
Insecticides	
Iopanoic acid (Telepaque)	Tetracycline
Isoniazid	Tetraethylammonium
Meperidine	Thiourea
Meprobamate	Trimethadione
Mercurial diuretics	Turpentine
Organic hair dyes	

several months. Women are more commonly affected than men. Bleeding manifestations include petechiae and ecchymoses, menorrhagia, hematuria, melena, epistaxis, and gingival bleeding, although more severe gastrointestinal and central nervous system bleeding can occur. The onset is usually not associated with an identifiable antecedent infection. The physical examination is unremarkable, and splenomegaly is rarely found. Diagnosis is usually made by the clinical history, large platelets on peripheral smear with normal red and white blood cells, the presence of antiplatelet antibodies, a bone marrow with increased megakaryocytes with normal erythroid and myeloid elements, and exclusion of other disorders that cause increased platelet destruction. Corticosteroids are usually the initial treatment of choice. A favorable clinical response occurs in 70 to 90 percent of patients. A complete and sustained normalization of the platelet count, however, occurs in less than half that number, and many patients remain dependent on steroids. Splenectomy is the next treatment approach in healthy subjects who are a low surgical risk. Complete and sustained remissions are obtained in 50 to 80 percent of patients following splenectomy. Other forms of treatment include immunosuppressive agents, vincristine, plasmapheresis, and intravenous gamma globulin. After exhausting all modalities of therapy, generally a small group of 10 to 25 percent of patients remain refractory to treatment. Some of these patients may remit spontaneously over several years. Others may succumb to the illness as a result of bleeding complications.

Thrombocytopenia is often an early manifestation of exposure to HIV. This has been described in intravenous drug users, hemophiliacs, homosexuals, and heterosexual partners of individuals with HIV infection. The mechanism of platelet destruction is complex. Levels of platelet-associated IgG, C3, C4, and IgM are often elevated, as are serum immune complexes. The antibody in some patients may be directed against a 25,000-dalton antigen on the surface of the platelet, or immune complexes may become associated with the platelet. In still other patients, antibodies against $F(ab')_2$ (i.e., anti-immunoglobulins) have been implicated in thrombocytopenia.

Alloantibodies can also produce thrombocytopenia. This is seen in isoimmune neonatal purpura, in which maternal antibodies (IgG) cross the placenta and cause platelet destruction in the fetus, if the fetus and mother have different platelet surface antigens. This fetomaternal incompatibility is frequently for the PLA-1 antigen. A number of other platelet antigen systems have also been implicated in neonatal thrombocytopenia.

Alloantibodies are also involved in post-transfusion purpura. This uncommon clinical condition is usually based on recipient-donor incompatibility for the PLA-1 antigen. Routine blood typing and crossmatches before transfusions are administered do not involve screening for this antigen. In this syndrome, a patient who is PLA-1 negative (less than 3 percent of the American population) receives a blood transfusion from a PLA-1 positive donor (97 percent of the population). After this transfusion, the patient destroys not only the transfused platelets but also his or her own platelets. This clinical situation usually occurs in patients who have been sensitized by previous transfusion or pregnancy. The precise mechanism of post-transfusion purpura is unknown, although immune complexes may be involved.

Alloimmunization is also involved in the destruction of transfused platelets in the sensitized thrombocytopenic recipient; this involves HLA and platelet-specific antigen mismatches.

Drug-induced thrombocytopenia is frequently on an immune basis. The platelet as an "innocent bystander" is destroyed by antibodies that have been produced against the drug, a drug carrier complex, against drug bound to the platelet surface, or against a new platelet antigen induced by drug. The drug-protein-antibody complex may bind by the Fc portion of the antibody to the Fc receptor on the platelet surface, with subsequent complement fixation and platelet destruction, or antibody may bind by its F (ab) portion directly to the platelet. Drug-induced immune thrombocytopenia is a common cause of increased platelet destruction, and over 70 drugs have been implicated in this problem. Table 75-3 presents a partial list.

Treatment of drug-induced thrombocytopenia involves discontinuation of the offending drug. Recovery usually occurs in 1 to 2 weeks, although it may be delayed if the drug (e.g., gold salts) is excreted slowly. There is little role for corticosteroids, although their use has been recommended in cases in which drug excretion is slow.

Nonimmune Mechanisms

Increased platelet consumption is also seen in a variety of nonimmune disorders, including disseminated intravascular coagulation (DIC). Disseminated intravascular coagulation involves the pathologic activation of coagulation and fibrinolysis associated with a number of conditions, including sepsis, malignancy, trauma, and obstetric complications. This causes consumption of coagulation factors and thrombocytopenia. The diagnosis is made clinically and by the combination of thrombocytopenia and multiple abnormal coagulation studies, including prolonged prothrombin time, partial thromboplastin time, and thrombin time, decreased fibrinogen, and elevation of fibrin degradation fragments.

Thrombotic thrombocytopenic purpura (TTP) and hemolytic-uremic syndrome (HUS) are other nonimmune disorders of platelet destruction. In TTP and HUS, there are intravascular hemolysis and severe thrombocytopenia due to platelet destruction associated with fever, renal failure, and varying degrees of neurologic dysfunction. Neurologic symptoms are usually more prominent in TTP than HUS. In TTP there appears to be a plasma component that promotes spontaneous platelet aggregation in the circulation. Diagnosis includes the clinical syndrome and laboratory findings of anemia, abnormal peripheral smear showing numerous fragmented red blood cells, thrombocytopenia with large platelets, and impaired renal function. TTP has been treated successfully with plasma transfusion and plasmapheresis. Other, less successful, treatment modalities include splenectomy, corticosteroids, and antiplatelet agents. These treatments have been less helpful in HUS, in which the patient may spontaneously recover as long as temporary dialysis is used to correct metabolic abnormalities.

Abnormal Distribution

Abnormal distribution of platelets is seen in hypersplenism. In this clinical situation, the total platelet mass within the body is normal, but a significant percentage of the platelet pool is in the spleen. This is due to a prolonged transit time of platelets through the spleen, while platelet survival is normal or only minimally decreased. Splenomegaly also significantly decreases the percent recovery of the transfused platelets in patients who are thrombocytopenic from other causes. Such splenomegaly is usually apparent on physical examination.

Dilution

Massive transfusion therapy in a patient with gastrointestinal bleeding or trauma can result in a dilutional thrombocytopenia. This can be avoided by serial measurement of the platelet count and judicious use of platelet transfusions. The standard dose of platelets is 10 units of platelets per 8 to 10 units of red blood cells. In general, it is recommended that the platelet count be monitored and transfusions administered only as needed.

Diagnostic Approach

The diagnostic evaluation of the patient with thrombocytopenia should be directed in a logical fashion to determine first the mechanism of the thrombocytopenia and then the specific etiology. Diseases that require immediate or rapid treatment must be detected early. After excluding life-threatening diseases, one may proceed at a more deliberate pace. This evaluation includes history, physical examination, and laboratory evaluation.

History

All patients, especially adults, must be questioned about medications when thrombocytopenia is evaluated. When questioning an individual about drugs, specific questions should be asked, because many patients do not consider proprietary drugs purchased without a prescription to be "medications." The patient should also be questioned about his or her beverage intake. Even the small amount of quinine found in tonic water in a cocktail can produce thrombocytopenia, or "cocktail purpura." A general history of ethanol intake should be pursued, as this is a relatively common cause of mild thrombocytopenia in the adult patient. In the child with ITP, a history of recent viral infection and acute onset of purpura or "purple freckles" is often obtained. The history should also include possible symptoms of an underlying connective tissue disease; weakness, weight loss, or fatigue from an underlying malignancy; a history of infection; and a history of similar episodes in the past.

In the neonate with thrombocytopenia, a family history is important, including a history of thrombocytopenia in siblings at birth, a history of familial thrombocytopenia, a history of maternal immune thrombocytopenia, and maternal and paternal blood types.

All patients should be asked about the presence of complications of thrombocytopenia, including visual symptoms, central nervous system symptoms, hematuria, and gastrointestinal bleeding.

Physical Examination

Physical examination should include inspection of the skin for petechiae, the buccal mucosa for hemorrhagic bullae and petechiae, and the retina for retinal hemorrhages. When performing a general physical exam, pay special attention to the lymph nodes, examine the abdomen for hepatosplenomegaly, and search for signs of underlying connective tissue disease.

Laboratory Studies

All patients with thrombocytopenia must have a complete blood count and differential. The presence of thrombocytopenia should be confirmed by peripheral smear. Large platelets, or megathrombocytes, suggest a shortened platelet survival. A concomitant anemia, leukocytosis, or leukopenia may indicate that several cell lines are involved in a generalized process. The observation of abnormal circulating cells (e.g., blasts or atypical lymphocytes) may lead one to the diagnosis of acute leukemia or infectious mononucleosis. Fragmented red cells (schistocytes) suggest a microangiopathic hemolytic anemia, as in DIC or TTP; spherocytes, an autoimmune hemolytic process; and macrocytes, excessive alcohol use, liver disease, vitamin B_{12} and folic acid deficiency, or dysmyelopoietic states. Unless a specific disease is diagnosed as the definitive cause of the thrombocytopenia, a bone marrow aspirate and biopsy must be performed early in the evaluation. Bone marrow evaluation will reveal not only the adequacy of platelet production (i.e., decreased or increased production as indicated by number of megakaryocytes) but may also reveal a primary bone marrow disorder, if present, as the cause of thrombocytopenia.

Most patients should have a prothrombin time, partial thromboplastin time, and thrombin time performed early in the evaluation to help screen for acute or chronic DIC in the appropriate setting and to assess the general integrity of the humoral arm of hemostasis.

Immune-mediated thrombocytopenia can be detected in many patients by the presence of antiplatelet antibodies in the patient's plasma or on the surface of the patient's platelets, or the presence of complement on the platelet surface. Increased platelet-associated immunoglobulin may be seen in thrombocytopenia that is not based on an immune mechanism; conversely, increased platelet immunoglobulin may not be detectable in all cases that are immunologically mediated. Thus, clinical judgment must be used in the interpretation of antiplatelet-antibody testing, and no one laboratory test is definitive for ITP.

Other tests to be considered in the evaluation of thrombocytopenia include antinuclear antibodies, rheumatoid factor, complement levels, and anti-DNA antibodies. An HIV screening test should be obtained if the history is at all suggestive of exposure.

Treatment

Therapy of thrombocytopenia depends on the precise etiology, as briefly described above. In some patients, particularly if active bleeding or a local lesion is present, platelet transfusions may be helpful. If there is increased platelet destruction, these transfused platelets are usually destroyed as rapidly as the patient's own platelets; however, transfusion may still improve symptoms. All patients being evaluated for thrombocytopenia, particularly those evaluated on an outpatient basis, must be warned that absolutely no aspirin or other drugs with antiplatelet activity should be taken; in fact, all drugs should be avoided, if possible.

References

Camitta B, et al. Aplastic anemia. N Engl J Med 1982; 306:645.

Cines DB, et al. Heparin associated thrombocytopenia. N Engl J Med 1980; 303:788.

Difino SM, et al. Adult idiopathic thrombocytopenic purpura. Clinical findings and response to therapy. Am J Med 1980; 69:430.

Jackson DP. Management of thrombocytopenia in hemostasis and thrombosis. In: Colman RW, et al, eds. Hemostasis and thrombosis. 2nd ed. Philadelphia: JB Lippincott, 1987:530.

Kaplan BS, Proesmans W. The hemolytic uremic syndrome of childhood and its variants. Semin Hematol 1987; 24:148.

Karpatkin S. Immunologic thrombocytopenic purpura in HIV-seropositive homosexuals, narcotic addicts and hemophiliacs. Semin Hematol 1988; 25:219.

Kelton JG, et al. A prospective study of the usefulness of the measurement of platelet associated IgG for the diagnosis of idiopathic thrombocytopenic purpura. Blood 1982; 60:1050.

Kwaan HC. Clinicopathologic features of thrombotic thrombocytopenic purpura. Semin Hematol 1987; 24:71.

Kwaan HC. Miscellaneous secondary thrombotic microangiopathy. Semin Hematol 1987; 24:141.

Lee GR, et al, eds. Wintrobe's clinical hematology. 9th ed. Philadelphia: Lea & Febiger, 1990.

Lian E C-Y. Pathogenesis of thrombotic thrombocytopenic purpura. Semin Hematol 1987; 24:82.

McMillan R. Chronic idiopathic thrombocytopenic purpura. N Engl J Med 1981; 304:135.

Nair JMG, et al. Thrombotic thrombocytopenic purpura in patients with the acquired immunodeficiency syndrome (AIDS)-related complex. Ann Intern Med 1988; 109:299.

Parker JC, Barret DA II. Microangiopathic hemolysis and thrombocytopenia related to penicillin drugs. Arch Intern Med 1971; 127:474.

Shepard KV, Bukowski RM. The treatment of thrombotic thrombocytopenic purpura with exchange transfusions, plasma infusions and plasma exchange. Semin Hematol 1987; 24:178.

Bleeding and Bruising

Peter H. Levine, MD

76

Definitions

The most common form of "easy bruising" is seen in ambulatory well patients, especially women, and represents the presence of no disease. The bruising is real, not imagined, is common on the lower legs, and may represent estrogen-conditioned changes in subendothelium that lead to lessened platelet-plug formation. Ingestion of aspirin makes this cosmetically unpleasant problem worse.

Petechiae, which are pinpoint to less than 3-mm red cutaneous hemorrhages, are usually indicative of serious disease, either of the small blood vessels or of the platelets. Examples of diseases of vessels that cause petechiae include vasculitis (as seen in diverse diseases such as systemic lupus erythematosus, Henoch-Schönlein disease, or Rocky Mountain spotted fever), scurvy, and conditions that suddenly produce great pressure on the capillary bed and arterioles, such as with prolonged Valsalva maneuver, as seen in crying in children and infants. Examples of diseases of platelets that lead to petechiae include quantitative disorders such as immune thrombocytopenic purpura (ITP), the thrombocytopenia of aplastic anemia or of leukemia, and, paradoxically, the severe thrombocytosis of myeloproliferative disorders such as polycythemia rubra vera or myelofibrosis with myeloid metaplasia. Qualitative platelet disorders (e.g., uremia and congenital thrombocytopathy) can also cause petechiae.

Purpura are cutaneous hemorrhages that are up to 1 cm or slightly larger in diameter. They can be thought of as representing confluent petechiae, and the differential diagnosis is the same as for the presence of petechiae.

Ecchymoses are what are generally recognized as common bruises. If they are not the trivial lesions described in the first paragraph of this chapter, they could represent the vascular or platelet disorders just described; the fragile connective tissue seen in either the elderly or patients undergoing long-term corticosteroid therapy; or a disorder of fibrin clot formation, such as hemophilia, disseminated intravascular coagulation, or liver disease, or one that is associated with therapeutic anticoagulants.

Unless it is due to major trauma, bleeding into a joint space, or *hemarthrosis,* should lead one to suspect hemophilia (deficiency of factor VIII, IX, or rarely XI) or severe von Willebrand's disease.

A *hematoma* is an ecchymosis with substance, indicative of the build-up of blood in subcutaneous tissue or muscle, usually with pain. This lesion, unless it is due to local trauma, usually indicates a disorder of fibrin clot formation, such as hemophilia, liver disease, or one that is caused by use of therapeutic anticoagulants.

Bleeding of mucous membranes, such as recurrent gingival or nasal bleeding, is almost always due to local causes, such as gingivitis or nose picking. If this bleeding is unexplained and recurrent, and if it is seen in the presence of unexplained gastrointestinal bleeding or menorrhagia, von Willebrand's disease should be considered.

Etiology

The major differential diagnoses for bleeding and bruising are shown in Table 76-1. In the table, diseases are divided into hereditary and acquired, and then further subdivided into vascular disorders, platelet disorders, and disorders of fibrin clot formation. Several important coagulopathies cause disorders that are not limited to one of these three elements of the hemostatic response; e.g., liver disease can involve platelet function as well as fibrin clot formation, whereas systemic lupus erythematosus might adversely affect the microvasculature and the platelet number as well as lead to a circulating anticoagulant that inhibits (or paradoxically accelerates) fibrin clot formation.

A word of explanation is in order concerning the category of thrombocytosis. There are many etiologies of thrombocytosis other than the several listed in Table 76-1; however, only those listed generally lead to petechiae, purpura, or other hemorrhagic manifestations, possibly because there is a concomitant platelet function disorder in these diseases.

Diagnostic Approach

The differential diagnosis of the bleeding patient includes three major categories: local causes, congenital coagulopathies, and acquired defects. Unless a cut vessel in need of ligation is evident, local causes cannot be diagnosed with certainty until coagulopathy has been excluded by laboratory testing. Mild congenital coagulopathies commonly go undiagnosed until adult life, when some surgical or traumatic stress reveals their presence. A careful history may reveal bleeding episodes in the patients or their relatives. Ask specifically about dental work. Bleeding after dental extractions is a common first sign of mild hemophilia, von Willebrand's disease, and familial thrombocytopathy. The acquired coagulopathies such as disseminated intravascular coagulation (DIC), liver disease, uremia, or anticoagulant overdose come to mind when postoperative bleeding is multifocal. Nurses may be the first to note multifocal bleeding, but they may not bother to volunteer the fact that venipuncture sites bleed excessively or that vaginal bleeding has suddenly begun. Questioning the nurse may yield the first strong evidence that the patient has a hemostatic defect.

What laboratory studies should be ordered? What constitutes a minimum acceptable coagulation screen in the dead of night? The consultant should have at his or her fingertips a readily available minimum screening battery. It must be technically feasible, not horribly expensive, and possible to complete in an hour's time. This evaluation must take into account all phases of the complicated clotting cascade, and a normal result must exonerate the clotting system.

Because clotting usually begins with the platelet, a platelet count and bleeding time test must be done. These exclude quantitative and severe qualitative platelet defects. No coagulation survey is complete without three tests of fibrin clot for-

Table 76-1 Differential Diagnosis of Bleeding and Bruising

- No disease is present
- Local anatomic abnormality or injury
- Congenital disorders
  - Vascular
    - Hereditary hemorrhagic telangiectasia
    - Connective tissue disease such as Marfan's syndrome
  - Platelet quantity
    - (Rare) Congenital thrombocytopenias such as thrombocytopenia with absent radius (TAR syndrome)
  - Platelet quality
    - Congenital thrombocytopathy
    - Thrombaesthenia
  - Fibrin clot formation
    - Hemophilia A (factor VIII deficiency)
    - Hemophilia B (factor IX deficiency, Christmas disease)
    - Hemophilia C (factor XI deficiency)
    - von Willebrand's disease and its variants
    - Other isolated factor deficiencies (e.g., factors VII, X, XIII)
    - Dysfibrinogenemia
    - (Rare) Disorders of the inhibitors of fibrinolysis (antiplasmins)
    - (Rare) Disorders of the inhibitors of protein C (expressed as combined deficiency of factors V and VIII)
- Acquired disorders
  - Vascular
    - Scurvy (vitamin C deficiency)
    - Immune
      - Henoch-Schönlein disease (anaphylactoid purpura)
      - Systemic lupus erythematosus
      - Rheumatoid arthritis
    - Infectious
    - Corticosteroid therapy, Cushing's disease
    - Senile purpura
  - Platelet quantity
    - Thrombocytopenia of decreased production
      - Aplastic anemia
      - Myelophthisis (any cause)
      - Drug-induced (e.g., chloramphenicol, chemotherapy)
      - Radiation therapy
      - Deficiency state (vitamin B_{12}, folate)
    - Thrombocytopenia of increased destruction
      - Hypersplenism
      - Immune thrombocytopenic purpura
      - Thrombotic thrombocytopenic purpura
      - Disseminated intravascular coagulation
      - Drug-induced (e.g., sulfa, gold, quinidine, quinine)
      - Dilutional (massive blood transfusion)
    - Thrombocytosis
      - Polycythemia rubra vera
      - Chronic granulocytic leukemia
      - Myelofibrosis with myeloid metaplasia
      - Primary thrombocytosis
  - Platelet quality
    - Uremia
    - Severe hepatocellular disease
    - Dysproteinemia
    - Deficiency states (e.g., vitamin B_{12}, folate)
    - Myeloproliferative syndromes
    - Drug-induced
      - Aspirin
      - Nonsteroidal anti-inflammatory agents
  - Fibrin clot formation
    - Hepatocellular disease
    - Heparin therapy
    - Warfarin therapy
    - Fibrinolytic therapy
    - Circulating anticoagulant
      - Lupus-type
      - Inhibitor of factor VIII in hemophilia
      - Inhibitor of factor VIII in the elderly, or post partum
      - Other specific antibody
    - Disseminated intravascular coagulation
    - Dilutional (massive blood transfusion)
    - Acute hypocalcemia (e.g., citrate poisoning)
    - Certain snake or spider bites

mation—the prothrombin time (PT), the partial thromboplastin time (PTT), and the thrombin time (Fig. 76-1). Although the fibrin clot is always the endpoint, each of the three tests measures a different phase of the clotting cascade. The thrombin time measures the final reaction, the ability of thrombin to convert fibrinogen to fibrin. The PT measures the extrinsic system of fibrin formation, which is initiated by tissue thromboplastin. The PTT examines another route of fibrin formation—the intrinsic system. This system is accelerated by platelet phospholipid, and this route measures several factors that are not involved in the prothrombin time test. In addition to this battery of tests, a blood smear should be made in search of red cell fragmentation and as a check on the platelet count.

The platelet count must be formally performed in a counting chamber or by an electronic particle counter. Estimated counts from blood smears are useful only when the platelets are remarkably increased or decreased. The bleeding time, when prolonged, almost always indicates a platelet problem. The Ivy (forearm) method, in which one uses a standardized template technique that allows the test to be quite reproducible, is preferred. Failure to determine the bleeding time results in inability to detect severe qualitative platelet abnormalities such as are seen commonly in uremia, myeloproliferative syndromes, and hereditary thrombocytopathies. Von Willebrand's disease may also be missed if the bleeding time is not measured.

The PT simulates the tissue thromboplastin-induced (extrinsic) clotting system. Commercially obtained tissue thromboplastin and calcium are added to citrated plasma, and clot formation is timed. The sequence of activation involves factors VII, X, V, II (prothrombin), and I (fibrinogen). Significant decreases in any of these factors prolong the PT. An abnormal result of this test most often reflects acquired disease, such as liver disease, malabsorption syndrome, warfarin therapy, or DIC. A perfectly normal prothrombin time virtually excludes DIC.

The activated partial thromboplastin time (aPTT) simulates the platelet-induced (intrinsic) clotting system. Commercially

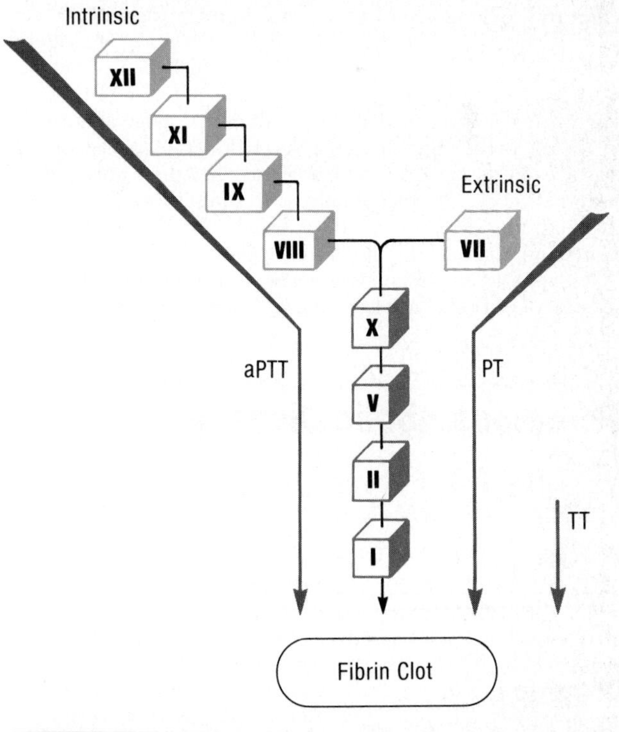

Figure 76-1 A simplified scheme of the coagulation cascade illustrating those factors assessed by the prothrombin time (PT), activated partial thromboplastin time (aPTT), and thrombin time (TT).

obtained phospholipid and calcium are added to citrated blood, and clot formation is timed. The phospholipid simulates platelet factor III. The sequence of activation involves factors XII, XI, IX, and VIII and then proceeds just as does the prothrombin time, via factors X, V, II, and I. Abnormalities of any of these factors may produce a prolonged aPTT. An isolated abnormality of the aPTT usually reflects a congenital disorder, such as hemophilia A or B (Christmas disease).

The thrombin time is one of the most neglected of the useful tests in medicine. It is an excellent, inexpensive, easy-to-do part of the coagulation screen. In this test, one adds commercially obtained thrombin to the citrated plasma and times the conversion of fibrinogen to a fibrin clot. A number of rare disorders can make the test results abnormal, but excluding these, there are only three main causes of prolonged thrombin time:

1. Severe hypofibrinogenemia, for which the thrombin time is a good rapid screening test.
2. The presence of an anticoagulant in the plasma, such as heparin, will prolong the thrombin time. Fibrin-split products, the result of fibrinolysis and themselves anticoagulants, also prolong this test.
3. Endogenous anticoagulants, as seen, for example, in systemic lupus erythematosus, can also cause an abnormal thrombin time.

The PT, aPTT, and thrombin time may all be done with a few milliliters of citrated plasma. If DIC is suspected, a fibrinogen level can be run on the same sample, but this test is not a necessary or usual part of the basic evaluation. A test for fibrin-split products is also done when DIC is suspected.

Every screening evaluation should include examination of the blood smear for three reasons. The first is to check the accuracy of the platelet count report. The second is to search for giant, bizarre platelets, which may be seen with increased platelet production. They also occur in the myeloproliferative syndromes, in which these platelets may be qualitatively abnormal. Third, the blood smear allows a search for the helmet cells and other red cell fragments that are seen in many cases of DIC.

The tests just described can detect the majority of coagulopathies. A valuable adjunct would be the inclusion of the clot solubility test, which screens for deficiency in factor XIII (fibrin-stabilizing factor). This deficiency will not produce abnormalities in any of the other clotting tests. A clot that lacks factor XIII dissolves in dilute acetic acid; a normal clot does not. Patients with a history of postoperative bleeding should have this checked; this disorder, which is usually familial, is probably more common than the literature suggests.

A test for fibrinolysis need not be done routinely. Fibrinolysis most often occurs as a facet of DIC and, as such, is a secondary phenomenon. Moreover, it may be a life-saving reaction that prevents severe intravascular clotting.

The basic screening evaluation, including platelet count, bleeding time, PT, PTT, thrombin time, blood smear, and possibly the clot solubility test, should be available day or night in any hospital that has an operating room or an emergency ward. Typical costs are shown in Table 76-2. Although the exact interpretation of various combinations of abnormal test results may require eventual hematologic consultation, the on-the-spot internist should be able to determine rapidly whether a coagulopathy is present. The confusing jargon and eponyms of the coagulationist should not deter the physician or the hospital laboratory from making an attempt at sound diagnosis. "Fresh whole blood" is never an acceptable therapeutic answer to excessive or multifocal bleeding.

Table 76-2 Typical Costs of Blood Coagulation Tests

1. Prothrombin time	$9–$20
2. Partial thromboplastin time	$9–$20
3. Thrombin time	$9–$20
4. Clot solubility test (factor XIII)	$9–$20
5. Template bleeding time	$21–$40
6. Fibrinogen level	$14–$30
7. Fibrin-split products	$20–$40
8. Euglobulin lysis time	$15–$30
9. Studies to screen for circulating anticoagulant	$20–$50
10. Specific factor assay (e.g., factor VIII)	$35–$80
11. Factor VIII antigen by radioimmunoassay	$44–$100
12. von Willebrand's factor assay	$55–$100
13. Platelet count	$8–$15
14. Platelet aggregation study	$50–$120
Minimum screening battery (tests 1–5)	$40–$120
DIC screen (tests 1–3, 6–8, and 13)	$75–$175

Abbreviation: DIC = disseminated intravascular coagulation.

References

Colman RW, et al. Hemostasis and thrombosis: Basic principles and clinical practice. 2nd ed. Philadelphia: JB Lippincott, 1987.

Thompson AR, Harker LA. Manual of hemostasis and thrombosis. 3rd ed. Philadelphia: FA Davis, 1983.

Williams WJ, et al. Hematology. 3rd ed. New York: McGraw-Hill, 1983.

77 Thromboembolic Disease

Jack E. Ansell, MD

Definition

A thrombus is an intravascular mass composed of cellular elements and other constituents of the blood. An embolus is an intravascular mass that travels from one part of the body to another. Frequently, a thrombus fragments, and parts of the thrombus move with the flowing blood to other parts of the body, creating a thromboembolus. Three types of thrombi are recognized, and their characteristics depend on blood flow characteristics at the time of thrombus formation. White thrombi form in high-flow states found in the arterial circulation and are composed of layers of platelets interposed with bands of fibrin, red cells, and white cells in a meshwork. Red thrombi form in

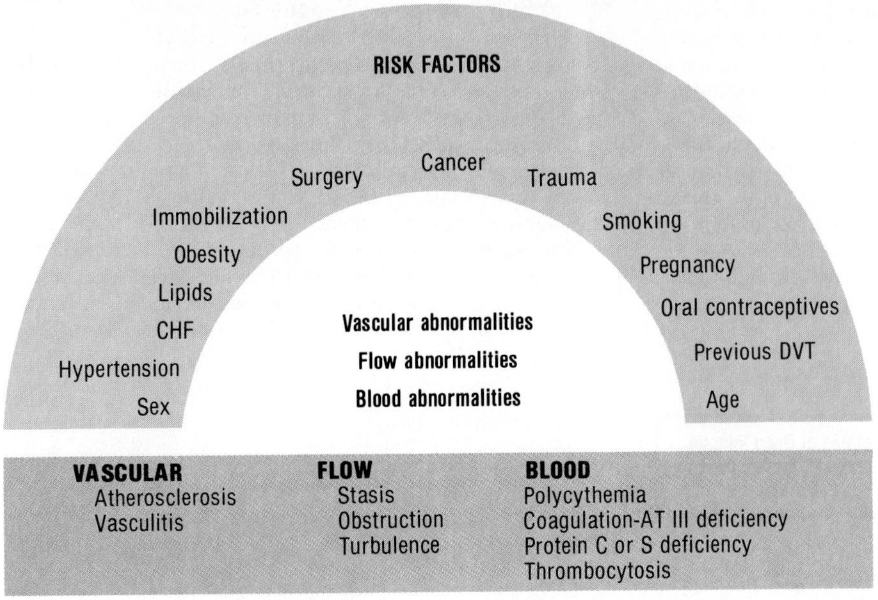

Figure 77-1 The risk factors for thrombosis mediate their effect through one of the components of Virchow's triad—blood vessels, blood flow, or blood. AT III = antithrombin III, CHF = congestive heart failure, DVT = deep venous thrombosis.

low-flow situations or in areas of stasis characteristic of the venous circulation. They are composed almost entirely of a meshwork of fibrin and red cells with randomly interspersed platelets and white cells. Mixed thrombi have features of both red and white thrombi and represent more closely the type of thrombi found clinically.

Etiology

Thromboemboli result from abnormalities of blood vessels, blood flow, or the blood itself. Accordingly, damaged endothelium may initiate thrombosis by inducing platelet activation and aggregation. Venous obstruction and stasis of blood flow may activate coagulation by contact activation of factor XII. Deficiencies of coagulation inhibitors can allow subclinical factor activation to go unopposed and result in thrombosis. Thromboemboli are also associated with various conditions or risk factors. Figure 77-1 denotes several factors that enhance the risk of thrombosis and, in a sense, create a "prethrombotic state."

Symptoms produced by thromboemboli depend on their location and the particular vascular system involved. Arterial thrombi produce signs of ischemia. Venous thrombi cause retrograde congestion and inflammation. Central nervous system thrombi produce neurologic deficits. Pulmonary emboli cause respiratory symptoms and alterations in cardiovascular hemodynamics.

Although thromboemboli occur anywhere in the body, certain regions have a predilection for involvement, and such thromboemboli lead to well-recognized clinical syndromes. These areas include the veins of the lower extremities, the pulmonary circulation, the systemic arterial system, and the central nervous system. Table 77-1 lists common symptoms produced by thromboemboli in these areas.

Diagnostic Approach

The diagnosis of thromboembolic disease begins with the clinical history. It is fairly easy to differentiate problems of the arterial

Table 77-1 Common Symptoms of Specific Thromboembolic Syndromes

Systemic arterial thromboemboli	Cerebro-vascular thromboemboli	Pulmonary emboli	Deep venous thrombosis of lower extremities
Pain Paresthesias Paralysis Pallor Pulselessness Cold	**Carotid System** Paresis Paresthesia Monocular visual defect Dysphagia Dysarthria Headache **Vertebro-basilar System** Binocular visual defect Vertigo Paresthesias Diplopia Ataxia Paresis Syncope Dizziness	Dyspnea Apprehension Tachycardia Pain (pleuritic) Hemoptysis Cyanosis Hypotension Syncope	Swelling Tenderness Pain Venous distention Discoloration Homan's sign (calf pain with dorsiflexion of foot)

system from those of the venous system, as well as the area of the body affected. However, it is more difficult to determine whether the symptom is related to thromboembolism or some other disease process. The clinical history and physical examination are often not helpful in the diagnosis of deep venous thrombosis (DVT) of the lower extremities. The symptoms caused by pulmonary embolism are often nonspecific and frequently occur with other cardiorespiratory diseases. It is sometimes impossible to differentiate among embolic, hemorrhagic, and thrombotic cerebral vascular accidents. Table 77-1 lists some of the common manifestations of lower extremity DVT and pulmonary embolism. For definitive diagnosis, however, objective tests are required.

Lower Extremity Deep Venous Thrombosis

Diagnostic tests are based on two major principles: (1) demonstration of venous outflow obstruction by either flow measurements or visualization, and (2) demonstration of thrombus by a clot-localizing substance. Ultrasonography based on the Doppler principle and impedance plethysmography both detect obstruction to venous blood flow. Contrast venography visually demonstrates the patency of veins. Radioisotope-labeled proteins such as ^{125}I-fibrinogen accumulate in clots and facilitate their detection by measurement of radioactivity over affected areas. Each of these tests has advantages and disadvantages. Ultrasound and plethysmography are noninvasive, but they are

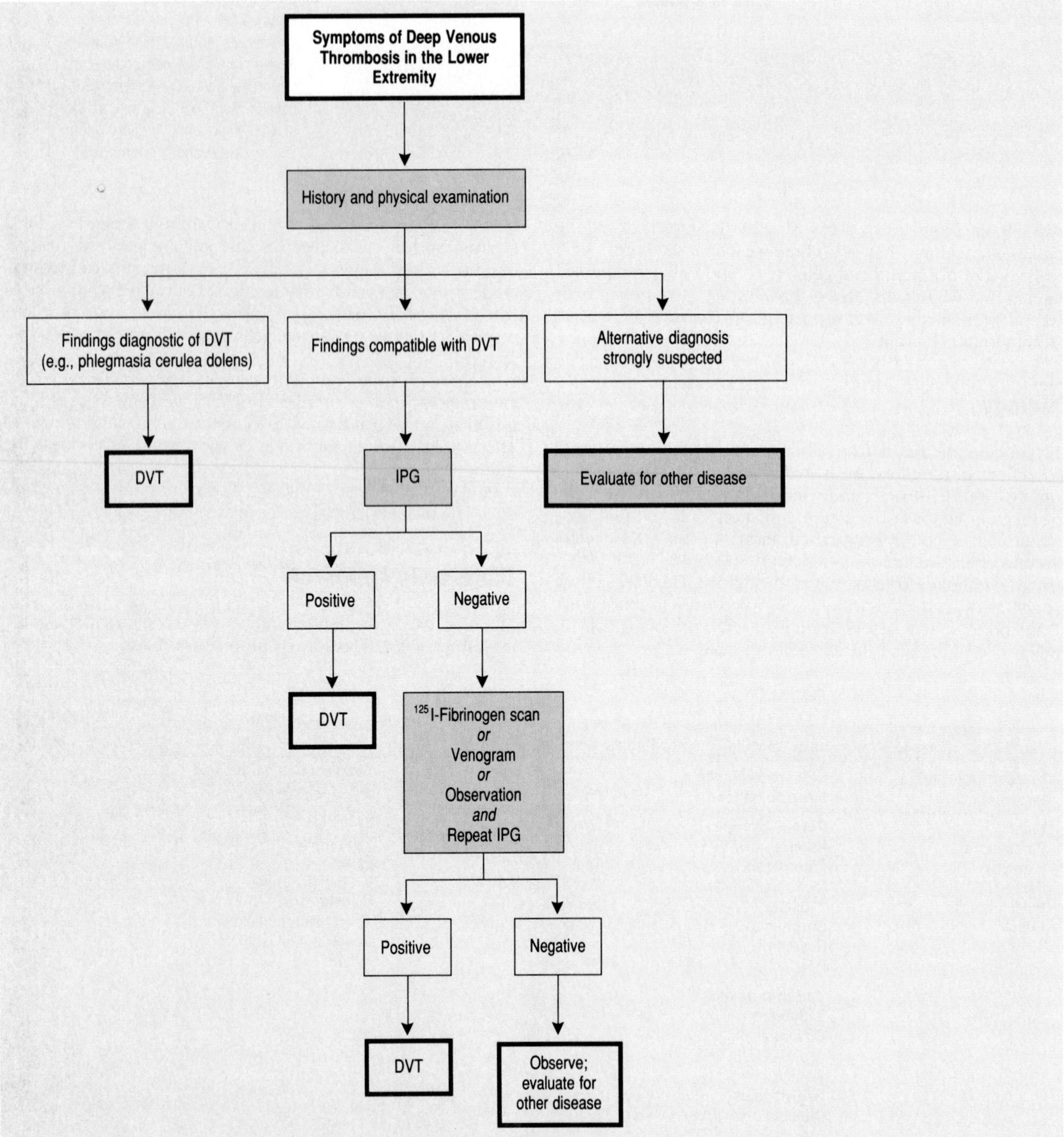

Figure 77-2 Approach to diagnosis of lower extremity deep venous thrombosis (DVT) based on impedance plethysmography (IPG). (*Modified from* Hirsh J, et al. Venous thromboembolism. New York: Grune & Stratton, 1981:78.)

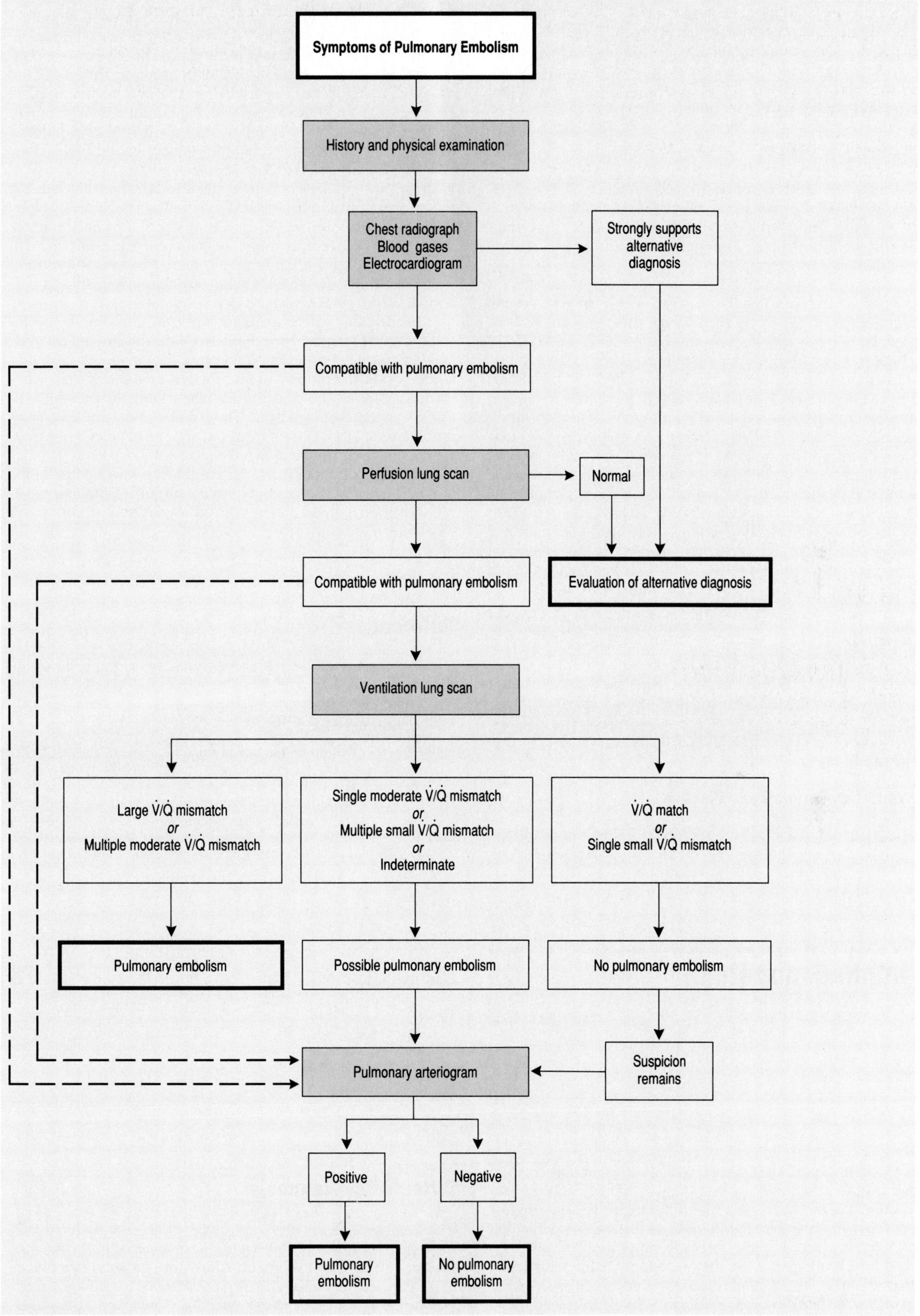

Figure 77-3 Approach to diagnosis of pulmonary embolism. $\dot{V}/\dot{Q}$ = ventilation-perfusion. (*Modified from* Hirsh J, et al. Venous thromboembolism. New York: Grune & Stratton, 1981:97.)

reliable only for thrombosis above the knee. ^{125}I-fibrinogen scans are very sensitive for calf vein thrombosis but less so for thrombosis in the upper thigh. Venography, the ultimate standard, is a costly and invasive procedure that requires great expertise. Figure 77-2 illustrates an orderly investigative approach to these problems.

Pulmonary Embolism

Pulmonary embolism, most often a consequence of DVT of the lower extremities, is even more difficult to document. Objective tests include arterial blood gas determination, chest radiography, perfusion lung scanning, ventilation lung scanning, and pulmonary arteriography.

Patients with significant pulmonary embolism often have a reduction in arterial oxygen saturation (Po_2). However, many other disorders lead to decreased Po_2; thus, this test is most beneficial when its results are normal, because this tends to exclude significant pulmonary embolism. A chest radiograph by itself is most helpful in excluding other pulmonary pathology, such as pneumonia. Pulmonary emboli frequently cause no abnormality detectable on a chest radiograph. Perfusion lung scanning provides an assessment of the pulmonary vascular system by means of a radioisotope-labeled protein that distributes itself throughout the blood. A significant embolus leads to absence of blood flow in a segment of lung. Unfortunately, chronic obstructive pulmonary disease causes many structural vascular abnormalities in the lung, as do other pathologic processes; therefore, a positive perfusion scan may be of limited value. A normal perfusion scan, on the other hand, excludes the possibility of pulmonary embolism. A ventilation lung scan (inhalation of radioactive gas) in combination with a perfusion scan is more specific. Areas of the lung that show normal ventilation and segmental perfusion defects are highly suggestive of pulmonary embolism and less likely to represent other pathologic conditions. Pulmonary arteriography is the "gold standard," but like venography, it is invasive and may be associated with morbidity.

Figure 77-3 outlines an approach to the diagnosis of pulmonary embolism.

Arterial Thromboembolic Disease

The clinical diagnosis of acute peripheral arterial thromboembolism is often less difficult than the diagnosis of venous occlusion because the symptoms, especially in an extremity, are often prominent and quite specific. It may be difficult to differentiate thrombosis from embolism, but the diagnosis of vascular occlusion can frequently be made on clinical grounds. The role of the vascular laboratory has increased dramatically in the last 10 years because of technologic advances in the noninvasive assessment of arterial blood flow. Doppler ultrasonography and plethysmography are the basic techniques for evaluating blood flow. Various modifications of these tests have been adapted to assess vascular flow in different parts of the arterial system, such as the lower extremity and the carotid vessels. Contrast arteriography is still the "gold standard" for assessing vascular patency, but like venography, it presents the risks of hemorrhage, allergic dye reactions, thrombosis, and embolization. However, these risks rarely outweigh the benefits of an accurate diagnosis and corrective surgery when such serious conditions exist.

In addition to determining the presence of vascular occlusions, careful cardiac evaluation is called for in patients with sudden-onset arterial emboli, because the heart is a common source of these emboli. Cardiac rhythm monitoring and echocardiography are the usual means of assessing the possibility of emboli arising from the heart. These emboli may originate from mural cardiac thrombi or from thrombi or platelet aggregates associated with damaged or prosthetic heart valves.

Because peripheral arterial emboli can produce ischemia and irreversible damage, and because surgery is often the treatment of choice, these patients must be evaluated promptly and efficiently if therapy is to be successful.

References

Bergan JJ. Peripheral arterial occlusive disease and thrombosis. In: Kwaan HC, Bowie EJW, eds. Thrombosis. Philadelphia: WB Saunders, 1982:132.

Gallu AS, et al. Diagnosis of venous thromboembolism. Semin Thromb Hemost 1976; 2:203.

Hull RD, et al. Diagnostic efficacy of impedance plethysmography for clinically suspected deep venous thrombosis. Ann Intern Med 1985; 102:21.

Hull RD, et al. Diagnostic value of ventilation-perfusion lung scanning in patients with suspected pulmonary embolism. Chest 1985; 88:819.

Owen CA, Bowie EJW. Predisposing factors in thrombosis. In: Kwaan HC, Bowie EJW, eds. Thrombosis. Philadelphia: WB Saunders, 1982:29.

78 Lymphadenopathy

Gary M. Strauss, MD

Enlargement of peripheral lymph nodes is a commonly encountered problem for two major reasons. Lymphadenopathy is a component of the wide spectrum of disease processes, ranging from those that are self-limited to those that are incurable and fatal. Furthermore, because of their superficial location, enlarged lymph nodes may be the presenting manifestation of a systemic illness. The patient often discovers an enlarged node and brings the mass to a physician's attention with considerable consternation because of fear that it may represent a malignancy.

Differential Diagnosis

Diseases associated with lymph node enlargement are usually classified within the broad categories of inflammatory and neoplastic. Inflammatory conditions are further subdivided into those that are infectious and those that are not, such as connective tissue diseases or drug reactions. Much less commonly, diseases that are neither inflammatory nor neoplastic may be the cause, including lipid storage diseases (such as Gaucher's disease) or certain endocrinopathies (hyperthyroidism, Addison's disease). Many manifestations of disease associated with the human immunodeficiency virus (HIV) are associated with lymphadenopathy, some of which are inflammatory, some of which represent opportunistic infections, and others of which represent neoplasms associated with the acquired immunodeficiency syndrome (AIDS).

Inflammatory Diseases

The infectious diseases associated with lymphadenopathy include those caused by bacteria, viruses, protozoa, fungi, and *Chlamydia.* Acute pyogenic bacterial infections such as those caused by streptococci and staphylococci present with tender lymphadenitis, which is often associated with other localized manifestations of infection such as a sore throat or a skin wound. However, other bacterial infections may present with generalized and nontender lymphadenopathy. These include tuberculosis, atypical mycobacterial infections, brucellosis, tularemia, and syphilis.

A variety of viral diseases have generalized lymphadenopathy as a prominent manifestation of their presentation. Young children are much more likely than adults to develop generalized lymphadenopathy in association with a wide spectrum of very minor and self-limited viral infections. In adolescents and young adults, infectious mononucleosis due to infection with the Epstein-Barr virus is perhaps the most common disease associated with lymphadenopathy. It should be recognized that about 10 to 15 percent of the time, a mononucleosis-like syndrome that involves generalized lymphadenopathy and atypical lymphocytosis may be due to infection by cytomegalovirus or by the protozoan *Toxoplasma,* rather than Epstein-Barr virus. Certain fungal infections such as histoplasmosis, coccidioidomycosis, and sporotrichosis may involve lymph nodes, and lymphogranuloma venereum, a chlamydial infection, is usually associated with inguinal adenopathy.

Many noninfectious inflammatory conditions have lymph node enlargement as a prominent manifestation of a systemic illness. Connective tissue diseases such as rheumatoid arthritis, systemic lupus erythematosus, and mixed connective tissue disease need to be prominently considered in the differential diagnosis of a patient who presents with enlarged peripheral lymph nodes.

Hypersensitivity reactions to certain drugs may produce a syndrome involving lymphadenopathy. Reactions to phenytoin are perhaps the best known, but hydralazine, para-aminosalicylic acid, and allopurinol may do the same.

A variety of diseases of unknown etiology produce lymphadenopathy. Sarcoidosis may be associated with peripheral lymphadenopathy, although hilar adenopathy is more characteristic. Whipple's disease may be associated with generalized lymphadenopathy, and cat-scratch fever with regional or, less commonly, generalized adenopathy.

Immunoblastic lymphadenopathy is a syndrome that usually occurs in elderly individuals; it involves generalized lymphadenopathy and hepatosplenomegaly, skin rash, systemic symptoms, polyclonal hypergammaglobulinemia, and autoimmune hemolytic anemia. The course of illness is usually progressively downhill; some patients develop overt malignant lymphoma, although others may have an indolent course. It is associated with a characteristic lymph node histology.

Neoplastic Diseases

Neoplastic diseases represent the other major disease category associated with lymphadenopathy. Lymphomas and leukemias are primary hematologic neoplasms that often involve peripheral lymph nodes as part of the initial expression of the malignant process. The lymphomas include Hodgkin's disease as well as the various non-Hodgkin's lymphomas. All leukemias may produce lymphadenopathy, although it is usually somewhat more prominent in the lymphocytic leukemias than in the myelocytic leukemias. Peripheral lymphadenopathy is particularly common in chronic lymphocytic leukemia.

Carcinomas commonly metastasize to lymph nodes and are a frequent cause of regional lymphadenopathy, particularly in older patients. Carcinomas are much less likely than lymphomas to produce generalized lymphadenopathy. Sarcomas usually disseminate hematogenously rather than via the lymphatic route; thus, they usually bypass the lymph nodes. In 10 percent of cases, however, they do disseminate lymphangitically and produce regional lymphadenopathy similar to carcinomas. Rhabdomyosarcoma and spindle cell sarcoma are the soft-tissue sarcomas most likely to metastasize to lymph nodes.

HIV Infection

Lymphadenopathy is a prominent feature of infection with HIV. HIV is a retrovirus that is the etiologic agent in AIDS. At present, the virus is contracted primarily by one of three major routes of transmission: sexual contact with an infected individual (most commonly by homosexual contact among gay or bisexual men, but also through heterosexual transmission); use of contaminated needles in the context of parenteral drug abuse; or transplacental transmission from an infected mother. The universal screening of donor blood for HIV has virtually eliminated currently transfused blood as a source of HIV transmission, but previously this was also a major route of transmission of infection, primarily among hemophiliacs (see Chapter 80, "Acquired Immunodeficiency Syndrome").

Persistent generalized lymphadenopathy (PGL) is recognized as a distinct syndrome by the Centers for Disease Control (CDC) in individuals who are infected by HIV. It is defined as palpable lymphadenopathy at two or more extrainguinal sites that lasts for more than 3 months in the absence of any associated condition to explain the finding. The lymphadenopathy may be the only expression of disease, or patients may have a variety of associated constitutional symptoms such as fever, weight loss, malaise, or diarrhea. Patients classified as having PGL must lack clinical features that would classify them in one of the other HIV-related disease categories (see below).

AIDS-related complex (ARC), as defined by the CDC, requires the presence of two clinical features plus two laboratory abnormalities. The clinical features may include lymphadenopathy, fever, weight loss, night sweats, fatigue, and diarrhea. The laboratory abnormalities include fewer than 400 helper T cells per microliter, a helper-to-suppressor T cell ratio of less than 1.0, blood count cytopenias, elevated serum globulin levels, or skin test anergy.

The term *AIDS* should be applied only to the individual infected with HIV who has developed at least one life-threatening opportunistic infection or neoplasm associated with this devastating illness. The most common opportunistic infection associated with AIDS is *Pneumocystis carinii* pneumonia. The most common secondary infection associated with lymphadenopathy in established AIDS is caused by the organism *Mycobacterium avium-intracellulare.*

Lymph node enlargement is an extremely common feature in several of the malignant neoplasms associated with AIDS. Generalized lymphadenopathy is observed along with cutaneous lesions in the majority of patients with Kaposi's sarcoma, the most common malignancy associated with AIDS. Lymphomas, most often high-grade B-cell lymphomas, such as Burkitt's lymphomas, and intermediate-grade non-Hodgkin's lymphomas and Hodgkin's disease are also commonly a manifestation of AIDS. These lymphomas are regularly associated with lymphadenopathy, but it should be pointed out that extranodal involvement is extremely common in AIDS-related lymphoma and frequently overshadows the lymphadenopathy as an important clinical feature.

History and Physical Examination

A carefully elicited history and physical examination will almost always provide important diagnostic clues and frequently produce a specific diagnosis. The age, sex, and race of the patient provide clues. Lymphadenopathy in older patients is likely to be secondary to an underlying malignancy, whereas inflammatory conditions predominate in young children. Certain connective tissue diseases such as systemic lupus erythematosus and rheumatoid arthritis are more common in women than in men. Sarcoidosis is more common in blacks than in whites, whereas infectious mononucleosis is more common in whites than in blacks. It is very important to note the duration of lymph node enlargement and whether the lymph nodes are producing any symptoms. Lymph nodes that appear rather suddenly and are tender are very likely to be due to an infection or other inflammatory cause, whereas those that have been present for weeks or months and are not tender are more suspect in terms of a cancer. However, it is also important to realize that malignant nodes can be tender and can wax and wane in size.

It is critical to take a careful epidemiologic history in order to focus on possible infectious causes of lymphadenopathy. Has there been any recent contact with other individuals who have been ill (HIV-related disease, infectious mononucleosis, tuberculosis)? Has there been travel to areas where certain diseases are endemic (histoplasmosis, coccidioidomycosis)? Is the patient a sexually active homosexual or bisexual, or has there been sexual exposure to a person at high risk for AIDS (HIV-related disease)? Is the patient an intravenous drug abuser, and has there been use of shared needles (HIV-related disease)? Has there been any recent contact with animals (brucellosis, tularemia, toxoplasmosis, atypical *Mycobacterium,* cat-scratch fever)?

The history should, of course, also establish what other symptoms are present that might suggest a diagnosis in which the presence of lymphadenopathy is a secondary phenomenon. For example, is there skin rash, joint symptoms, or muscle weakness that would suggest the presence of a connective tissue disease? Is there dysphagia, hoarseness, a breast symptom, or skin lesions that would suggest the existence of an occult carcinoma of the head and neck or breast or a melanoma? Is there a sore throat that would raise the possibility of a strep throat or infectious mononucleosis? Inquire about the presence of fevers, night sweats, and weight loss, which are the classic systemic "B" symptoms associated with lymphomas; however, an indistinguishable symptom complex may be seen in infectious mononucleosis, other subacute infections, or, on occasion, certain connective tissue diseases.

The importance of a complete physical examination in helping to establish the nature of lymphadenopathy should be self-evident. Pay particular attention to whether there is associated splenomegaly or hepatomegaly. Determine the distribution of the lymph nodes to ascertain whether the adenopathy is generalized, regional, or localized.

A variety of infectious diseases are associated with cervical lymphadenopathy. Bacterial infections are likely to involve anterior cervical nodes, whereas viral infections (including infectious mononucleosis) often involve the posterior cervical nodes, although there are many exceptions to this pattern. In addition, one should determine the quality of the involved nodes. Are the nodes tender, fluctuant, and warm, with overlying skin fixation, which are characteristic of infection with lymphadenitis? Are they hard and matted, with muscle fixation, which are signs of malignant lymphadenopathy? Lymphomatous lymph nodes are often described as "rubbery" in character, whereas those secondary to carcinomatous involvement are described as "rock hard." Although there may indeed be differences in character between lymphomatous and carcinomatous nodes, these differences are quite subtle, and the distinction cannot be made with any degree of certainty by physical examination alone.

Laboratory and Radiographic Studies

Many laboratory and radiographic studies and skin tests are useful in establishing the presence of diseases that can be associated with lymphadenopathy, as indicated in Table 78-1. The cost of indiscriminately performing all the studies listed in the table would be close to $2,000. Clearly, one needs to be selective in applying laboratory and radiographic tools based on the clinical leads provided by the history and physical examination. If a specific diagnosis or group of potential diagnoses is suggested by the history and physical examination, a directed work-up should be undertaken immediately by those studies suggested in the table or, if appropriate, by lymph node biopsy or biopsy of other involved organs.

Enlarged cervical lymph nodes usually should be investigated first for potential infection, particularly in younger patients. If pharyngitis exists, a throat culture should be obtained. If there is any evidence of local infection or if the nodes are quite tender, suggesting suppurative lymphadenitis, a trial of penicillin or other antibiotic is appropriate and may lead to prompt resolution of the problem.

If the clinical triad of fever, sore throat, and lymphadenopathy is present, laboratory investigation needs to focus on the possibility of infectious mononucleosis. A complete blood count with differential characteristically reveals an absolute lymphocytosis, with more than 10 percent of the total white cells being atypical lymphocytes (often 30 percent at the peak of the atypical lymphocytosis). Serologic evidence for infectious mononucleosis should be sought by performance of a heterophile antibody test or a Monospot test. If the patient is suspected of having mononucleosis but initial laboratory studies are nonconfirmatory, a policy of observation and re-evaluation after 7 to 10 days is appropriate, because the atypical lymphocytosis and positive serologic tests might not appear until the second or third week of illness. (It is a wise policy to store a frozen serum sample at the initial evaluation for possible future use in acute and convalescent serum testing.) If infectious mononucleosis is still suspected but the serologic tests remain negative, keep in mind that about 10 percent of cases due to the Epstein-Barr virus are Monospot and heterophile negative, particularly in younger children, and that cytomegalovirus may cause a mononucleosis-like syndrome. Acute toxoplasmosis may also give rise to a syndrome identical to mononucleosis, so serologic tests for this organism should also be obtained.

In patients with axillary adenopathy, the major infectious possibilities include suppurative processes caused by streptococci or staphylococci, cat-scratch fever, sporotrichosis, and tularemia. In patients with inguinal adenopathy, pyogenic processes, syphilis, and lymphogranuloma venereum need to be specifically considered. Generalized adenopathy would raise the question of an HIV-related illness, a mononucleosis-like syndrome, or brucellosis, histoplasmosis, or coccidioidomycosis. Mycobacterial infections frequently involve the lymph nodes. One of the commonest manifestations of extrapulmonary tuberculosis is tuberculous lymphadenitis. Any lymph node group can be involved, but the cervical lymph nodes are most common (scrofula). Several of the atypical mycobacteria can produce lymphadenitis. *Mycobacterium scrofulaceum* is the most common; it characteristically produces involvement of the submandibular nodes in children. Whenever any of these conditions is suspected on clinical grounds, laboratory investigation should proceed along the lines indicated in Table 78-1, although

Table 78-1 Laboratory and Radiologic Studies Helpful in Diagnosis of Disease Associated with Lymphadenopathy

Disease	Test	Cost
Infectious Diseases		
Atypical mycobacteria	Culture	$48.00
Brucellosis	Agglutinin test	$25.00
Coccidioidomycosis	Chest radiograph	$50.00
	Complement fixation test	$23.00
	Culture	$40.00
Cytomegalovirus	Complement fixation test	$50.00
	Viral culture	$50.00
Histoplasmosis	Chest radiograph	$50.00
	Complement fixation test	$25.00
	Culture	$40.00
Infectious mononucleosis	Complete blood count and differential	$28.00
	Monospot test	$11.00
	IgM antibodies to Epstein-Barr viral capsid antigen	$85.00
	Heterophile	$25.00
Lymphogranuloma venereum	Complement fixation test	$25.00
Sporotrichosis	Culture	$40.00
Streptococcal pharyngitis	Throat culture	$16.00
Syphilis		
Primary	Dark-field exam	$9.00
Secondary	VDRL	
	FTA absorption	$10.00
Toxoplasmosis	IgM-fluorescent antibody test	~$25.00
Tuberculosis	PPD skin test	$5.00
	Chest radiograph	$50.00
	Culture and smear	$48.00
Tularemia	Skin test	$5.00
	Agglutinin test	$25.00
Inflammatory Diseases		
Mixed connective tissue disease	Antinuclear antibody	$32.00
	Antiribonucleoprotein	$42.00
Rheumatoid arthritis	Rheumatoid factor	$11.00
Sarcoidosis	Chest radiograph	$50.00
	Kveim test	Unavailable
	Angiotensin converting enzyme	
Sjögren's syndrome	Rheumatoid factor	$11.00
	Schirmer's test	$10.00
Systemic lupus erythematosus	Antinuclear antibody	$32.00
	Anti–double-stranded DNA	$55.00
	Anti-Sm antigen	$33.00
Neoplastic Diseases		
Breast cancer	Mammogram (bilateral)	$83.00
Leukemia	Peripheral smear	$20.00
	Bone marrow	
Lymphomas	Chest radiograph	$50.00
	Abdominal CT scan	$350.00
	Lymphangiogram	$295.00
Lung cancer	Chest radiograph	$50.00
Thyroid cancer	Thyroid scan	$114.00
AIDS/ARC	Test for human antibody to HIV	
	Western blot	
	Enzyme-linked immunosorbent assay (ELISA)	
	Helper T-cell count	
	Helper:suppressor cell ratio	

Abbreviations: AIDS = acquired immunodeficiency syndrome, ARC = AIDS-related complex, CT = computed tomography, FTA = fluorescent treponemal antibody, HIV = human immunodeficiency virus, PPD = purified protein derivative, VDRL = Venereal Disease Research Laboratory.

many of these entities require confirmation by culturing the involved nodes. Anyone with generalized adenopathy who falls into one of the risk groups for AIDS should have an enzyme-linked immunosorbent assay (ELISA) test for HIV.

Suspicion of one of the connective tissue diseases will be raised by the presence of some of the myriad signs and symptoms characteristic of these conditions. An antinuclear antibody (ANA) test is highly sensitive for lupus and mixed connective tissue disease. Accordingly, a negative ANA would tend to exclude one of these conditions; if a positive ANA is obtained, however, the more specific test for these diseases should be ordered, as indicated in Table 78-1. If sarcoidosis is suspected, a chest radiograph should be obtained. The diagnosis of sarcoidosis often requires invasive procedures.

Lymph Node Biopsy and Other Invasive Procedures

When a specific diagnosis cannot be made by the noninvasive studies indicated in the preceding section, and the involved nodes persist for more than 2 to 4 weeks, biopsy of a lymph node (or other involved tissue) may be indicated. The biopsy should be diagnostic or highly suggestive of a wide variety of conditions. However, a high percentage of the time (up to 40 to 60 percent in various series), the biopsy will reveal only reactive hyperplasia and accordingly will be nondiagnostic.

Those conditions for which lymph node biopsy is capable of providing a specific diagnosis include most of the neoplastic diseases, including the lymphomas and carcinomas; immunoblastic lymphadenopathy; tuberculosis and the atypical mycobacterial infections; toxoplasmosis; syphilis; pyogenic lymphadenitis; cat-scratch fever; and the fungal infections. In sarcoidosis and Whipple's disease, the appearance of the involved node will usually be highly suggestive but not diagnostic. In most of the connective tissue diseases and viral diseases, the node will show reactive hyperplasia and remain nondiagnostic.

The indications for lymph node biopsy in patients who have positive antibody tests for HIV and who have generalized lymphadenopathy are unsettled. Patients with PGL who are otherwise asymptomatic, do not have laboratory abnormalities, and demonstrate stability in the size of nodes probably do not require biopsy. Patients who do have associated systemic symptoms; laboratory abnormalities such as leukopenia, thrombocytopenia, or a markedly elevated sedimentation rate; or focally enlarged lymph nodes should also undergo biopsy. It should also be noted that mediastinal adenopathy is not a feature of PGL, so biopsy should be performed in this setting as well. In addition to possibly demonstrating evidence for secondary infections or malignancies, lymph node biopsies in patients with HIV-related disease may show one of three patterns with prognostic significance. The most common pattern in PGL or ARC is nonspecific follicular hyperplasia, which is often florid. A second pattern is that of partial lymphoid depletion, and this pattern often indicates serious opportunistic infections. The third pattern is that of complete lymphoid depletion (burnout) of both B-cell and T-cell areas; this pattern is particularly ominous and heralds a poor prognosis.

There is one situation in which a lymph node biopsy may actually be harmful: the evaluation of the older adult who presents with cervical lymphadenopathy. Such a patient may have metastatic carcinoma from a primary site in the head and neck area. Such patients who have had biopsy of metastatic neck nodes have a higher incidence of distant metastases and a higher incidence of local recurrence than patients who do not have the biopsies. The proper approach would be an evaluation for an occult carcinoma in the oral cavity, nasopharynx, hypopharynx, or larynx by an otorhinolaryngologist. Removal of the nodes should be part of definitive surgical therapy, rather than node biopsy, which violates surgical planes.

Many diseases are associated with lymphadenopathy in which biopsy of organs other than the lymph nodes may be appropriate—e.g., sarcoidosis (transbronchial lung biopsy), systemic lupus erythematosus (renal biopsy), and Whipple's disease (biopsy of the proximal small intestine). In patients with suspected leukemia, bone marrow aspiration and biopsy in conjunction with examination of the peripheral smear are usually diagnostic. In patients with suspected metastatic carcinoma and a suspected primary cancer, it is usually preferable to biopsy the suspected primary lesion so that a node biopsy does not interfere with later wide excision.

The evaluation of lymphadenopathy is a challenging problem that requires considerable clinical judgment and skill on the part of the physician in synthesizing important historical and physical findings into a rational diagnostic framework and formulating a plan of investigation utilizing appropriate noninvasive and invasive diagnostic procedures. The goal is to reach a diagnosis as efficiently and cost-effectively as possible, avoiding delays that could compromise effectiveness of therapy or lead to excessive costs.

References

Armstrong D. Opportunistic infections in the acquired immune deficiency syndrome. Semin Oncol 1987; 14:40.

Centers for Disease Control. Classification system for human T-lymphotropic virus type III/lymphadenopathy-associated virus infections. Ann Intern Med 1986; 105:234.

DeVita V, Helman S, Rosenberg S, eds. AIDS: Etiology, diagnosis, treatment and prevention. Philadelphia: JB Lippincott, 1985.

Gleckman R. Prolonged fever and generalized lymphadenopathy. In: The manual of clinical problems and infectious disease. New York: Plenum, 1988.

Greenfield S, Jordan M. The clinical investigation of lymphadenopathy in primary care practice. JAMA 1978; 240:1388.

Haynes BF. Enlargements of lymph nodes and spleen. In: Braunwald E, et al, eds. Harrison's principles of internal medicine. 11th ed. New York: McGraw-Hill, 1987:273.

Knowles DM. Lymphoid neoplasms associated with the acquired immunodeficiency syndrome (AIDS). Ann Intern Med 1988; 108:744.

Lee Y, Terry R, Lukes R. Lymph node biopsy for diagnosis: A statistical study. J Surg Oncol 1980; 14:53.

Levine AM. Non-Hodgkin's lymphoma and other malignancies in the acquired immune deficiency syndrome. Semin Oncol 1987; 14:34.

Margolis I, Matteucci D, Organ C. To improve the yield of biopsy of the lymph nodes. Surg Gynecol Obstet 1978; 147:376.

McGuirt W, McCabe D. Significance of node biopsy before definitive treatment of cervical metastatic carcinoma. Laryngoscope 1978; 88:594.

Mitsuyasu RT. Clinical variations and stages of Kaposi's sarcoma. Semin Oncol 1987; 14:13.

Osteen R, Wilson R. Lymph nodes and subcutaneous masses. In: Branch WT, ed. Office practice of medicine. Philadelphia: WB Saunders, 1987:1125.

Schroer K, Franssila K. Atypical hyperplasia of lymph nodes. Cancer 1979; 44:1155.

Sinclair S, Beckman E, Ellman L. Biopsy of enlarged superficial lymph nodes. JAMA 1972; 228:602.

Steinbergh AD. Angioimmunoblastic lymphadenopathy with dysproteinemia—NIH conference. Ann Intern Med 1988; 108:575.

Infectious Diseases

Isolation Techniques

Nelson M. Gantz, MD

79

Isolation techniques to prevent nosocomial transmission of infections from patient to patient, from patient to health care worker, and from health care worker to patient have been recommended by the Centers for Disease Control. In the past, the guidelines were based on the specific infection or were initiated by a category of infection such as blood, enteric, or wound precautions. Both of these systems depend on the patient's diagnosis. Recently, an alternative system has been recommended that utilizes universal precautions for all patients (Fig. 79-1). Masks are indicated in patients with varicella, herpes zoster, congenital rubella, staphylococcal pneumonia, Group A streptococcal pharyngitis, *Mycobacterium tuberculosis* infection, and respiratory syncytial virus (RSV) infection.

Reverse isolation or protective isolation refers to use of gowns, gloves, and masks for those who have contact with a patient with granulocytopenia. No benefit has been demonstrated using protective isolation versus standard hospital care in patients with profound neutropenia. Recently, however, use of protective isolation was effective in reducing the infection rate in a pediatric intensive care unit.

References

Klein BS, Perloff WH, Maki DG. Reduction of nosocomial infection during pediatric intensive care by protective isolation. N Engl J Med 1989; 320:1714.

Lynch P, et al. Rethinking the role of isolation practices in the prevention of nosocomial infections. Ann Intern Med 1987; 107:243.

Update: Universal precautions for prevention of transmission of human immunodeficiency virus, hepatitis B virus, and other bloodborne pathogens in health-care settings. MMWR 1988; 37:377.

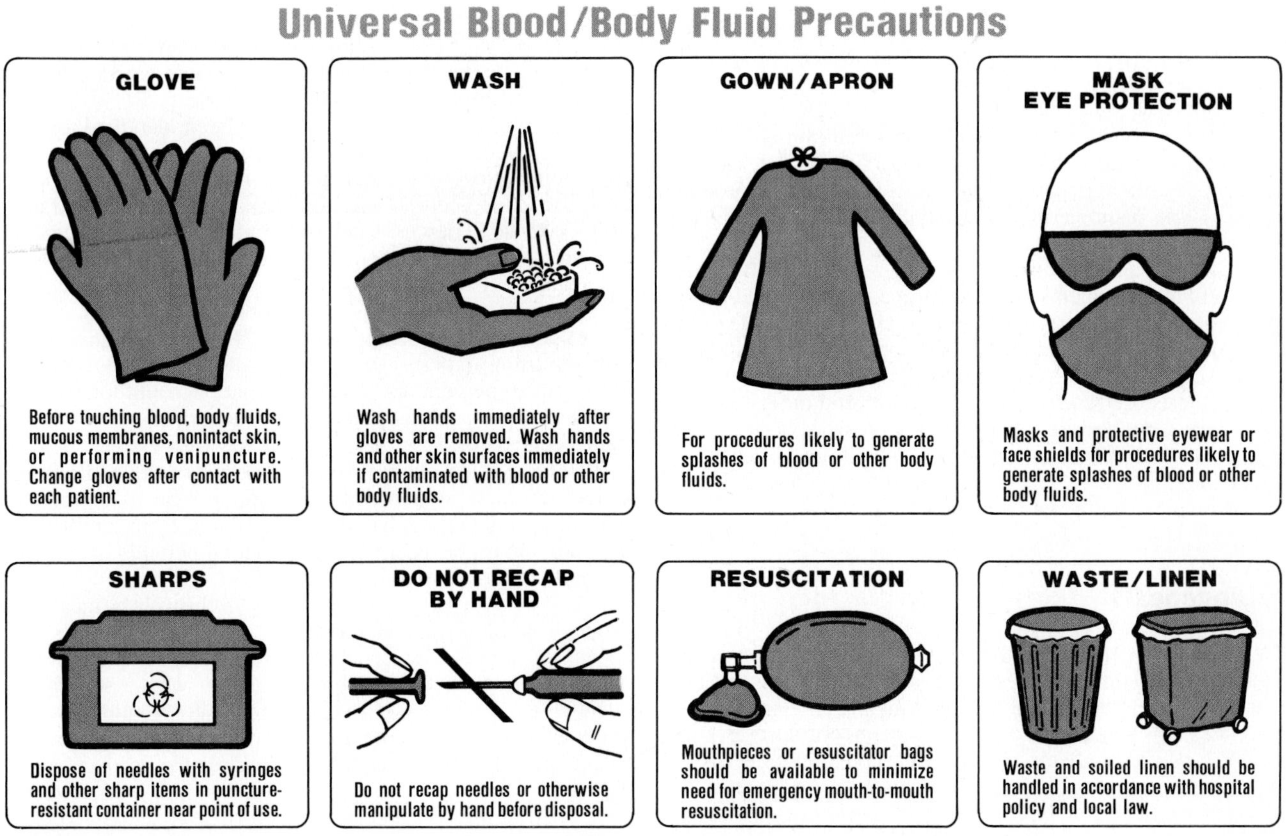

Universal Blood/Body Fluid Precautions
GLOVE
Before touching blood, body fluids, mucous membranes, nonintact skin, or performing venipuncture. Change gloves after contact with each patient.
WASH
Wash hands immediately after gloves are removed. Wash hands and other skin surfaces immediately if contaminated with blood or other body fluids.
GOWN/APRON
For procedures likely to generate splashes of blood or other body fluids.
MASK EYE PROTECTION
Masks and protective eyewear or face shields for procedures likely to generate splashes of blood or other body fluids.
SHARPS
Dispose of needles with syringes and other sharp items in puncture-resistant container near point of use.
DO NOT RECAP BY HAND
Do not recap needles or otherwise manipulate by hand before disposal.
RESUSCITATION
Mouthpieces or resuscitator bags should be available to minimize need for emergency mouth-to-mouth resuscitation.
WASTE/LINEN
Waste and soiled linen should be handled in accordance with hospital policy and local law.

Figure 79-1 Universal blood and body fluid precautions. (Used by permission of Brevis Corp., Salt Lake City, Utah.)

Acquired Immunodeficiency Syndrome

Patrick G. Fairchild, MD

Definition

Acquired immunodeficiency syndrome (AIDS) is a condition that represents the end stage of infection with the human immunodeficiency virus (HIV). First recognized in the early 1980s, it is a clinical state of immunosuppression with multisystem manifestations that usually results in death. Severe impairment of the immune system leads to the development of unusual and life-threatening opportunistic infections and malignancies. More than half the patients afflicted with this disease have died.

Etiology

In 1983, a human lentivirus, now referred to as the human immunodeficiency virus-1 (HIV-1), was identified by researchers in the United States and France as the infectious agent responsible for AIDS. Multiple other names have been used for this virus, including HTLV-III (human T-cell lymphotrophic virus-3), LAV (lymphadenopathy-associated virus), and ARV (AIDS-associated retrovirus).

HIV-1 is classified as a retrovirus because it utilizes reverse transcriptase, a DNA polymerase, which transcribes RNA into DNA. It also possesses important structural and regulatory proteins. These include GP-120 and GP-41, which are specific envelope glycoproteins on the outer surface of the virus. Another important component of the viral genome, P24, is located in the core region and is a marker of virus replication.

HIV isolates from different individuals demonstrate significant genetic variations, particularly in the envelope glycoprotein region. These dissimilarities have significantly hampered vaccine development.

Recently, another human retrovirus, designated HIV-2, has been identified in patients from West Africa and western Europe. HIV-2 appears to cause a syndrome that is indistinguishable from AIDS. Although HIV-1 and HIV-2 share many similarities, there are marked differences in the envelope regions. Consequently, serologic tests used to screen blood donors and other individuals for HIV-1 antibody may not detect the presence of HIV-2. No cases of HIV-2 infection acquired in the United States have been documented; however, HIV-2 infection has been found in patients who have immigrated into the United States.

Pathogenesis

HIV seems to have a special affinity for infecting a specific subset of lymphocytes commonly referred to as T4 helper cells or CD4 lymphocytes. The first step in infection involves the attachment of HIV to a CD4-specific antigen on the lymphocyte surface. This specific receptor-binding site is also found on monocytes, macrophages, neurons, and possibly gastrointestinal cells. Recent evidence suggests that HIV infection of gastrointestinal cells, monocytes, macrophages, and neurons may also occur independently of this specific CD4 receptor-binding site interaction. Macrophages can release high levels of virus for long periods of time and have been implicated as a persistent reservoir of infection as well as a major means of transporting HIV throughout the body. After binding to the CD4 receptor, the HIV uncoats and is ultimately incorporated into the host-cell genome. HIV subsequently replicates by using host cellular machinery. Infection appears to be lifelong.

After infection with HIV, CD4 lymphocytes become dysfunctional or die. How HIV kills CD4 cells is unknown, but the destruction of the helper T4 cell ultimately leads to significant defects in cell-mediated immunity. Impairment of the immune response interferes with the effective clearance of viruses, fungi, protozoa, mycobacteria, and selected bacteria, which may lead to the development of opportunistic infections. The increased incidence of malignancy in AIDS patients is also probably the result of impaired cell-mediated immunity, but the exact mechanisms have not been elucidated. It may involve abnormalities in tumor surveillance, cellular cytotoxic activity, cytokine production, and the activation of oncogenic viruses.

Epidemiology

By the middle of 1990, approximately 140,000 cases of AIDS in the United States had been reported to the Centers for Disease Control (CDC). At least 1 million individuals in the United States are thought to be infected with HIV, and approximately 360,000 cases of AIDS are expected to occur in the United States by 1991. AIDS has been reported in all 50 states, but major urban centers, like San Francisco and New York City, account for the majority of cases. AIDS has been reported in more than 100 countries throughout the world, and millions of people worldwide are known to be seropositive for HIV.

Several important risk factors have been identified for the acquisition of HIV infection. In the United States, these include male homosexual or bisexual activity (60 percent), intravenous drug use (21 percent), male homosexual activity plus intravenous drug use (7 percent), heterosexual contact with a member of a high-risk group (5 percent), hemophilia (1 percent), and receipt of blood or blood products (2 percent). Approximately 3 percent of AIDS patients have no identifiable risk factor.

Minorities are overrepresented in the AIDS epidemic. Current reporting indicates that 27 percent of those afflicted are black and 16 percent are Hispanic. Whites account for 56 percent, and the remaining 1 percent are of unknown or other racial backgrounds.

HIV has been isolated from multiple body fluids and tissues, including blood, semen, vaginal fluid, cervical tissue, breast milk, tears, and saliva. It has also been isolated from cerebrospinal fluid, the retina, central and peripheral nervous system tissue, and the gastric mucosa.

Transmission of HIV occurs almost exclusively by means of contact with blood, semen, or vaginal secretions. HIV does not appear to be spread by casual contact. The most efficient mode of transmission appears to be inoculation with a significant quantity of infected blood. In the United States, routine screening of all blood and plasma donors for HIV antibody has essentially eliminated HIV-infected blood and plasma products from the nation's blood supply. Intravenous drug use is an efficient means of transmission, and the majority of newly acquired cases of HIV infection appear to be occurring in this group. Intravenous drug users are thought to represent the most important route of HIV transmission into the heterosexual and pediatric populations.

Pediatric HIV infection is a tragic phenomenon. Approximately 2,400 cases of pediatric AIDS in the United States were reported to the CDC by mid-1990. Transmission of HIV from an infected mother to an infant may occur in utero, during parturition, or through breast milk after childbirth. The rate of transmission from mothers to infants is high, estimated at 30 to 35 percent. Failure to thrive, recurrent bacterial and fungal infections, and neurologic abnormalities are common manifestations. Because of the high rate of morbidity and mortality associated with AIDS in children, women at high risk for HIV infection (prostitutes, intravenous drug users, or the sexual partners of men at risk for HIV infection) should be counseled and screened for HIV infection before becoming pregnant.

In the United States, sexual transmission of HIV has occurred primarily among homosexual men. In central Africa, where heterosexual transmission is the primary mode of spread HIV infection is equally distributed between men and women. Heterosexual transmission occurs from men to women and from women to men. The risk of HIV infection following a single sexual contact with an infected person is unknown, but it is estimated to be 1 in 300.

There is a small but definite risk of HIV infection for individuals working in the laboratory or hospital setting. To date, approximately 20 health care workers have become infected with HIV after skin puncture with a needle contaminated by blood or body fluids from an HIV-infected patient. The risk of HIV infection by needle stick is quite low; it is estimated to be 0.4 percent. A small number of health care workers have become infected after cutaneous or mucous membrane exposure to blood from an HIV-infected individual.

Serotesting

The diagnosis of HIV infection is usually made by demonstrating the presence of antibody to the virus. The HIV antibody tests use inactivated HIV antigen in an enzyme-linked immunosorbent assay (ELISA). The ELISA is a very sensitive test, and it may yield false-positive results. Therefore, further confirmation is performed by means of another serologic assay, usually the western blot analysis, which is highly specific. The sensitivity and specificity of serotesting in a high-risk population is 99 percent under optimal laboratory conditions. Another new technique that employs gene amplification, the polymerase chain reaction, has been used to detect very small quantities of HIV DNA.

Persons who have recently experienced acute primary HIV infection may have a negative ELISA test because insufficient time may have elapsed to produce levels of HIV antibody high enough to permit detection. This may account for the rare cases of HIV transmission via blood products, even though the blood donor had been appropriately screened. Recently, rapid diagnostic assays have been developed that directly detect HIV antigens rather than HIV antibody, which, it is hoped, will obviate this problem.

HIV testing should be performed only for legitimate medical reasons, and then only with the permission of the patient or guardian. HIV test results should remain confidential.

Clinical Manifestations

Acute primary infection is characterized by a mononucleosis-like syndrome that develops after a 3- to 6-week incubation period. Clinical illness is often manifested by fever, rigors, arthralgias, myalgias, lymphadenopathy, sore throat, headache, diarrhea, and rash. A lymphocytic meningitis is occasionally present. In most patients, the acute signs and symptoms gradually subside over 2 to 3 weeks.

The time to seroconversion after a critical exposure appears to vary from individual to individual. Seroconversion to HIV usually occurs 8 to 12 weeks after exposure. Some cases have been reported with seroconversion occurring longer than 1 year after a known exposure.

Following resolution of acute primary infection, most patients appear to recover fully and remain asymptomatic. A period of latency subsequently ensues that may last from months to years in different individuals. During this time, subtle subclinical immunologic abnormalities may develop. These persons represent the vast majority of those individuals infected with HIV. They usually have serologic evidence of an antibody response to HIV without complaints or findings indicative of HIV-related disease.

Early in the course of HIV infection, some individuals develop the syndrome of persistent generalized lymphadenopathy (PGL), which is characterized by generalized enlargement (>1 cm) of lymph nodes, lasting at least 3 months and involving at least two extrainguinal sites, that cannot be explained by another illness or medication. A quantitative T-cell deficiency may not be present, and there are usually no defects in delayed hypersensitivity. Patients with this syndrome may not feel ill.

As the immune system becomes further impaired, some patients develop a clinical syndrome referred to as AIDS-related complex (ARC). This condition is characterized by a constellation of signs and symptoms that include intermittent fever, fatigue, weight loss, diarrhea, and generalized lymphadenopathy (Table 80-1).

As HIV continues to ravage the immune system and host defenses become further impaired, patients become susceptible to a variety of opportunistic infections, malignancies, and neurologic abnormalities. Some of these conditions establish the diagnosis of AIDS.

The case definition of AIDS was created by the CDC in 1982 for epidemiologic surveillance. It has also worked well for clinical purposes. The CDC modified and added several refinements to the case definition in 1985, when HIV antibody testing became available. The case definition was then revised again in 1987, when an expanded clinical spectrum of HIV-associated diseases became apparent.

The current criteria to meet the CDC definition for AIDS are organized into categories that depend upon the results of laboratory testing for HIV antibody. If the results of HIV antibody testing are unknown and the patient has no other reason for underlying immunodeficiency, the presence of any of the indicator diseases listed in Table 80-2 is considered presumptive evidence of AIDS. If HIV antibody test results are positive and the patient has evidence of any of the indicator diseases listed in Table 80-3, the patient is considered to have AIDS. This is independent of other factors that may cause the patient to be immunodeficient.

Many HIV-infected patients first seek medical attention for signs or symptoms of an opportunistic infection. For many, this is the initial manifestation of AIDS. Before the use of prophylactic agents, *Pneumocystis carinii* pneumonia was the first manifestation of AIDS in 65 percent of patients. As can be seen in

Table 80-1 AIDS-Related Complex

Clinical finding	Laboratory abnormality
Lymphadenopathy > 3 mo	Helper T4 cells < 400/mm^3
Fever over 100°F > 3 mo	T4 helper/T8 suppressor ratio < 1.0
Weight loss > 10%	Leukopenia
Fatigue	Thrombocytopenia
Persistent diarrhea	Anemia
Night sweats	Elevated serum globulins
	Reduced blastogenesis
	Anergy to skin tests
	Positive HIV antibody test

* This condition is defined by a combination of any two of the clinical findings and any two of the laboratory abnormalities listed in this table.

Table 80-2 Diseases That Indicate AIDS When HIV Antibody Testing Is Negative or Unknown*

Candidiasis of the esophagus, trachea, bronchi, or lungs
Cryptococcosis, extrapulmonary
Cryptosporidiosis with diarrhea persisting > 1 mo
Cytomegalovirus disease of an organ other than liver, spleen, or lymph nodes in a patient > 1 mo of age
Herpes simplex virus infection causing a mucocutaneous ulcer that persists longer than 1 mo; or bronchitis, pneumonitis, or esophagitis of any duration affecting a patient > 1 mo of age
Kaposi's sarcoma affecting a patient < 60 yr of age
Lymphoma of the brain (primary) affecting a patient < 60 yr of age
Lymphoid interstitial pneumonia or pulmonary lymphoid hyperplasia affecting a child < 13 yr of age
Mycobacterium avium complex or *Mycobacterium kansasii* disease, disseminated (at a site other than or in addition to lungs, skin, or cervical or hilar lymph nodes)
Pneumocystis carinii pneumonia
Progressive multifocal leukoencephalopathy
Toxoplasmosis of the brain affecting a patient > 1 mo of age

* Only if the patient has no other reasons for immunodeficiency.

Table 80-4 Opportunistic Infections Associated with AIDS

Clinical diseases	Etiologic agents
Pneumonia	*Pneumocystis carinii, Aspergillus fumigatus, Candida, Cryptococcus neoformans, Legionella, Nocardia, Mycobacterium avium-intracellulare, Mycobacterium tuberculosis,* cytomegalovirus
Persistent gastroenteritis	*Cryptosporidium, Isospora belli*
Mucous membrane disease	*Candida* (thrush), Epstein-Barr virus, herpes simplex virus, varicella zoster virus
Esophagitis	*Candida,* herpes simplex virus, cytomegalovirus
Meningitis, encephalitis, central nervous system abnormalities	*Toxoplasma gondii, C. neoformans,* papovavirus (progressive multifocal leukoencephalopathy), cytomegalovirus
Disseminated infections with multiple findings	*M. avium-intracellulare, M. tuberculosis, C. neoformans, Histoplasma capsulatum, A. fumigatus, Candida,* zygomycoses, *T. gondii, Strongyloides stercoralis,* herpes simplex virus, cytomegalovirus

Tables 80-2 and 80-3, many of the numerous opportunistic infections that have been identified are AIDS-defining conditions. Some of these are listed in Table 80-4.

Several types of malignancy may be diagnostic of AIDS. These include epidemic Kaposi's sarcoma, non-Hodgkin's lymphoma, and primary central nervous system lymphoma. Although not diagnostic of AIDS, Hodgkin's disease and squamous cell carcinoma have been reported to occur with increased frequency in HIV-infected individuals.

Neurologic disease also occurs as the direct result of HIV infection of nervous tissue and may have multiple presentations. Dementia, chronic meningitis, spinal cord myelopathy, and cranial and peripheral neuropathy have been described. These conditions are often clinically debilitating. Because HIV can directly infect brain cells, any effective therapeutic antiviral agent must be able to penetrate the blood-brain barrier.

The CDC has created a special clinical classification system for patients with HIV infection. Individuals are assigned to one of four mutually exclusive groups based on their cumulative illness (Table 80-5). The entire range of HIV-related diseases, from initial infection (group 1) and the asymptomatic state (group 2) to more advanced stages of illness (group 4 C–E), are represented. Patients in group 4 have profound immunodeficiency. Opportunistic infection, malignancy, and neurologic disease are common in this category. Group 4 C2 signs, such as oral candidiasis, oral hairy leukoplakia, and disseminated mucocutaneous zoster, are associated with an increased risk of development of AIDS in subsequent years. Although symptoms may resolve, the

Table 80-3 Diseases That Indicate AIDS When HIV Antibody Test Results Are Positive*

Bacterial infections, multiple or recurrent
Coccidioidomycosis, disseminated
HIV encephalopathy
Histoplasmosis, disseminated
Isosporiasis with diarrhea persisting > 1 mo
Kaposi's sarcoma at any age
Lymphoma of the brain (primary) at any age
Non-Hodgkin's lymphoma of B-cell type or unknown immunologic phenotype
Any mycobacterial disease caused by mycobacteria other than *Mycobacterium tuberculosis,* disseminated
Disease caused by *M. tuberculosis,* extrapulmonary
Salmonella septicemia, recurrent
HIV wasting syndrome

* Independent of other causes for immunodeficiency.

Table 80-5 Centers for Disease Control Classification System for HIV Infection*

Group 1	Acute infection
Group 2	Asymptomatic infection
Group 3	Persistent generalized lymphadenopathy with nodes 1 cm or larger at two or more extrainguinal sites for more than 3 mo
Group 4	Other diseases associated with HIV Constitutional disease: fever or diarrhea for more than 1 mo or 10% involuntary weight loss Neurologic disease: dementia, myelopathy, or peripheral neuropathy Secondary infectious diseases One or more symptomatic or invasive infectious diseases: *Pneumocystis carinii* pneumonia, chronic cryptosporidiosis, isosporiasis, toxoplasmosis, extraintestinal strongyloidiasis, candidasis (esophageal, bronchial, or pulmonary), cryptococcosis, histoplasmosis, mycobacterial infection with *Mycobacterium avium* complex or *Mycobacterium kansasii,* chronic herpes simplex virus infection, chronic cytomegalovirus infection, and progressive multifocal leukoencephalopathy Oral candidiasis, oral hairy leukoplakia, multidermatomal herpes zoster, recurrent *Salmonella* bacteremia, nocardiosis, tuberculosis Secondary cancers: Kaposi's sarcoma, non-Hodgkin's lymphoma, primary central nervous system lymphoma Other conditions, e.g., chronic lymphoid interstitial pneumonitis

* *Adapted from* MMWR 1986; 35:334.

patient's status within the classification schema remains unchanged.

The natural history of HIV infection is still unclear. Years of follow-up will be required before it can be fully understood. There appears to be remarkable variation among individuals with regard to clinical manifestations and the rate of disease progression. In some early published studies, as many as 35 percent of HIV-infected homosexual men developed AIDS within 3 to 5 years after initial infection. Although recent information suggests that the use of prophylactic agents against *Pneumocystis carinii* pneumonia and the early use of antiviral therapy directed against HIV have a favorable impact on the natural course of disease, once AIDS develops, it appears to be a universally fatal disease.

Some Specific Disease States Associated with AIDS

Pneumocystis carinii Pneumonia

Pneumocystis carinii pneumonia is the major cause of mortality in AIDS patients. Its onset tends to be insidious. Patients usually present with fever, dyspnea, and a nonproductive cough. The chest radiograph typically reveals bilateral interstitial infiltrates. Bronchoalveolar lavage via fiberoptic bronchoscopy is most commonly used to make the diagnosis. Occasionally, a transbronchial biopsy is required. At some centers, the organism has been detected in expectorated sputum samples.

Treatment usually consists of therapy with either trimethoprim-sulfamethoxazole or pentamidine. Therapy with either agent is typically continued for 21 days. Unfortunately, both of these medications have significant side effects. At least 40 percent of patients with HIV infection have adverse reactions to sulfa drugs that are manifested mainly as fever, rash, and leukopenia. Parenteral administration of pentamidine may cause hypotension, hypoglycemia, and renal insufficiency. The latter adverse reactions may be eliminated or minimized when delivered as an aerosol, and recent studies have demonstrated the efficacy of this route of administration in mild to moderate cases.

Although approximately 85 percent of patients recover from their initial episode of *Pneumocystis carinii* pneumonia, 50 percent will relapse within the first year without prophylaxis. The recovery rate from subsequent episodes of *Pneumocystis carinii* pneumonia is much lower than for initial episodes. As a result, prophylactic regimens have been developed to prevent recurrence. Currently used agents include trimethoprim-sulfamethoxazole, dapsone, and pentamidine.

Cryptococcal Meningitis

Cryptococcal meningitis typically presents subtly with headache and fever, but many patients have few central nervous system symptoms or physical findings. The classic signs of meningeal irritation are often absent. Lumbar puncture usually yields a normal cerebrospinal fluid formula or mild pleocytosis. Cryptococcal antigen testing is usually positive at high titer, and fungal cultures often grow *Cryptococcus neoformans*.

Intravenous amphotericin B (with or without flucytosine) has been the accepted standard therapy. Fluconazole, a new oral agent, has been shown to be as effective as amphotericin with fewer side effects in uncomplicated cases. Ketoconazole is not effective for central nervous system disease. Following acute treatment, patients require life-long suppressive therapy with either amphotericin or fluconazole.

Central Nervous System Toxoplasmosis

Toxoplasmosis is the most common cause of space-occupying lesions of the central nervous system in AIDS patients. Headache is common, and patients often exhibit fever, focal neurologic deficits, and seizures. Cerebrospinal fluid usually reveals a nonspecific lymphocytic pleocytosis. Computed tomography (CT) scanning of the head with contrast typically demonstrates ring-enhancing lesions. Brain biopsy is sometimes necessary to establish a definitive diagnosis and to exclude other causes of mass lesion, such as neoplasm, in patients who do not respond to empirical therapy for toxoplasmosis. Serologic testing of blood and cerebrospinal fluid may be useful. The mainstay of treatment is combination therapy with pyrimethamine and a sulfonamide. Folinic acid is given to counteract the folate antagonist effect on hematopoiesis. Because of the high incidence of adverse reactions to sulfa, alternative agents that are active against the *Toxoplasma gondii* organism are under investigation. Because the relapse rate after initial treatment is approximately 50 percent, long-term suppressive therapy is often required.

Kaposi's Sarcoma

Kaposi's sarcoma is a vascular malignancy characterized by violaceous nodules (Fig. 80-1). In AIDS patients, Kaposi's sarcoma often exhibits widespread cutaneous and visceral dissemination. Response to therapy is variable. Alpha-interferon may yield a favorable response in up to 40 percent of patients, but its use is limited by severe flulike symptoms. Vinblastine, vincristine, bleomycin, and adriamycin have been used for more aggressive cases with varying degrees of success. Radiation therapy may be useful for selected lesions.

Antiviral Therapy

At present, there is no cure for HIV infection. Azidothymidine (AZT), now called zidovudine (ZDV), is the only agent that has been shown to improve the clinical and laboratory status of patients with HIV infection. Zidovudine is a thymidine analog that inhibits reverse transcriptase activity and, hence, the replication of HIV. Patients with advanced HIV infection on ZDV appear to live longer and have an improved quality of life. They also experience fewer opportunistic infections. The major toxicity of ZDV is bone marrow suppression. Anemia and leukopenia are common and may necessitate an alteration in dosage. Approximately one-third of patients with severe ARC or AIDS who are on chronic ZDV therapy may require intermittent blood transfusions. The incidence of hematologic side effects is significantly reduced with the newly recommended lower dosage of ZDV (100 mg PO every 4 hours while awake).

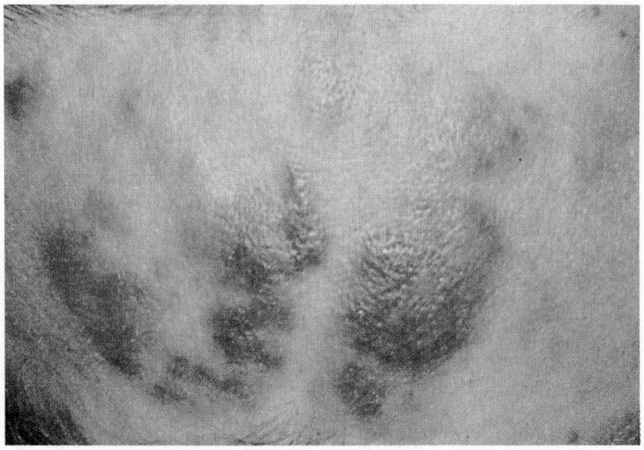

Figure 80-1 Violaceous color and nodularity of Kaposi's sarcoma.

Infectious Diseases

ZDV is well absorbed orally and is widely distributed throughout the body. It is metabolized by the liver via glucuronidation. Drugs that interfere with glucuronidation, such as acetaminophen, may lead to increased ZDV serum levels and increase the potential for toxic side effects. An important characteristic of ZDV is its ability to penetrate the blood-brain barrier. Concentrations in the central nervous system are approximately 30 to 50 percent of serum concentrations.

Initially, ZDV was approved by the Food and Drug Administration only for use in (1) patients with AIDS who have a history of *Pneumocystis* pneumonia, or (2) severe ARC patients with a CD4 count of less than 200. Recent studies have demonstrated definite benefit for patients with mild ARC or asymptomatic HIV infection who have fewer than 500 CD4 cells.

Multiple other antiviral agents as well as immune modulators are under investigation. Ultimately, the successful treatment of HIV infection may involve the combination of a potent antiviral agent with an immunopotentiating agent capable of reconstituting the immune system.

Advice for Health Care Workers

Because the majority of individuals infected with HIV do not display signs or symptoms, health care workers should treat all blood and body fluids from every patient as if they were potentially infectious. This concept has been referred to as "universal precautions" (see Chapter 79, "Isolation Techniques"). Always use gloves when drawing blood or handling any body fluid, and wear an impermeable gown and eye goggles or shields whenever blood or body-fluid splattering is anticipated. All mucocutaneous exposures or needle-stick punctures that involve HIV-contaminated blood or body fluids should be reported to the infection control department. A prophylactic trial with ZDV following massive exposure to HIV in health care and laboratory workers was discontinued because of low enrollment. Although routinely advocated at some centers, the use of ZDV after a critical exposure has not been recommended by the CDC because of the lack of supportive data. The role of ZDV for prophylaxis in various types of exposures remains to be determined. Surfaces contaminated with HIV-infected material can be disinfected with a 1-to-10 dilution of sodium hypochlorite (household bleach).

References

Centers for Disease Control. Recommendations for prevention of HIV transmission in health-care settings. MMWR 1987; 36:15.

Centers for Disease Control. Revision of the CDC surveillance case definition for acquired immunodeficiency syndrome. MMWR 1987; 36:42.

Centers for Disease Control. Public health service statement on management of occupational exposure to human immunodeficiency virus, including considerations regarding zidovudine postexposure use. MMWR 1990; 39:1.

Chuck SL, Sande MA. Infections with *Cryptococcus neoformans* in the acquired immunodeficiency syndrome. N Engl J Med 1989; 321:794.

Fischl MA, et al. The efficacy of azidothymidine (AZT) in the treatment of patients with AIDS and AIDS-related complex: A double-blind, placebo-controlled trial. N Engl J Med 1987; 317:185.

Fischl MA, et al. The safety and efficacy of zidovudine (AZT) in the treatment of subjects with mildly symptomatic human immunodeficiency virus type 1 (HIV) infection. Ann Intern Med 1990; 112:727.

Glatt A, Chirgwin K. *Pneumocystis carinii* pneumonia in human immunodeficiency virus–infected patients. Arch Intern Med 1990; 150:271.

Luft BJ, Remington JS. Toxoplasmosis encephalitis. J Infect Dis 1988; 157:1.

Richman DD, et al. The toxicity of azidothymidine (AZT) in the treatment of patients with AIDS and AIDS-related complex: A double-blind, placebo-controlled trial. N Engl J Med 1987; 317:192.

Volberding PA, et al. Zidovudine in asymptomatic human immunodeficiency virus infection. N Engl J Med 1990; 322:941.

81 Prophylaxis Against Rheumatic Fever and Endocarditis

Neil R. Blacklow, MD

The physician is frequently confronted with an otherwise healthy patient who has previously had rheumatic fever or has a heart murmur. Such a patient must stimulate the physician to think in terms of preventive medicine, i.e., to consider the need for prophylactic therapy directed against the development of rheumatic fever or bacterial endocarditis. These represent two different problems that are contrasted in Table 81-1. The problems need to be considered separately and must not be confused.

One problem is that of the healthy patient with a well-documented history of rheumatic fever. Compared with other persons, this individual clearly has an increased risk of another attack of illness. Such recurrent illness greatly increases the likelihood of subsequent development of rheumatic heart disease, if it is not already present. Because either symptomatic or asymptomatic infection of the pharynx with group A streptococci is necessary for the subsequent appearance of acute rheumatic fever, continuous antibiotic prophylaxis is essential in order to prevent the chain of events of streptococcal infection, rheumatic fever, and rheumatic valvular heart disease.

The second problem is that of the healthy patient who has a heart murmur. Certain of these patients seem to be at risk for the development of bacterial endocarditis when they undergo certain procedures that are commonly accompanied by a transient bacteremia. Although controlled studies have not been performed to establish the effectiveness of intermittent antibiotic prophylaxis in these patients at these times of transient bacteremia, such prophylactic measures are generally recommended.

This chapter discusses the indications for use of prophylactic antibiotic therapy directed against rheumatic fever and bacterial endocarditis, and points out the forms of therapy that should be used.

Table 81-1 Antibiotic Prophylaxis

	Rheumatic fever	Bacterial endocarditis
Timing	Continuous	Intermittent
Targeted problem	Group A streptococci	Anticipated bacteremia
Dose	Low dose	Higher dose
Indication	History of rheumatic fever or rheumatic heart disease	Valvular heart disease plus anticipated bacteremia

Distinction Between Prevention of Rheumatic Fever and Bacterial Endocarditis

It is very important not to confuse the antibiotic prophylactic measures directed against rheumatic fever with those directed against bacterial endocarditis. Antibiotic prophylaxis against rheumatic fever is *continuous,* because it is directed against acquisition of group A streptococcal infection, whereas antibiotic prophylaxis against bacterial endocarditis is *intermittent,* as it is used only at times of anticipated bacteremia. These two different preventive measures are often confused. Consider, for example, the patient with rheumatic valvular heart disease who may not receive antibiotic prophylaxis against potential endocarditis at the time of a dental extraction because he is already receiving penicillin prophylaxis against rheumatic fever. However, the continuous low doses of penicillin that are sufficient to prevent rheumatic fever are inadequate to prevent bacterial endocarditis. This is in part due to the frequent presence of partially penicillin-resistant viridans streptococci in the oropharynx of patients who are receiving continuous low-dose penicillin prophylaxis against rheumatic fever; therefore, these patients require an alternative prophylactic antibiotic regimen against bacterial endocarditis that avoids the use of oral penicillin.

Prophylaxis Against Rheumatic Fever

Indications

Continuous antibiotic prophylaxis should be given to all patients with a well-documented history of rheumatic heart disease. Such prophylaxis is a highly effective preventive measure. What is uncertain, however, is the duration of prophylaxis for a given patient. Some authorities recommend that prophylaxis be given indefinitely to all individuals, which implies lifelong prophylaxis. It is clear, however, that with advancing age, the risk of streptococcal infection and recurrent rheumatic fever becomes markedly reduced in older adults without heart disease or close exposure to school children. Thus, lifelong prophylaxis may be excessive for some patients. There are no absolute answers to the question of duration of prophylaxis, but one practical approach for low-risk individuals without recurrent rheumatic fever is to continue prophylaxis for at least 5 to 7 years in adults and until age 21 in children who have also had at least 5 to 7 years of prophylaxis. However, high-risk individuals should have lifelong prophylaxis; these individuals include those with established rheumatic heart disease, those who have had multiple attacks of rheumatic fever, those living in crowded conditions, and those often exposed to persons with group A streptococci, such as schoolteachers. If a prosthetic or biosynthetic heart valve has been inserted in a patient with rheumatic heart disease, prophylaxis should still be continued, probably for life.

Prophylactic Antibiotic Regimens

Benzathine penicillin G, given intramuscularly once a month, is the drug of choice. Oral agents, including penicillin, sulfadiazine, or erythromycin, may also be administered on a daily basis, but they are less effective than the monthly penicillin regimen, probably because of diminished patient compliance.

Prophylaxis Against Bacterial Endocarditis

Indications

The indications for prophylaxis against bacterial endocarditis are based on two main considerations: (1) patients with cardiac lesions that predispose to endocarditis, and (2) events that are likely to produce bacteremia.

The groups of patients with cardiac lesions predisposing to endocarditis are generally considered to be those with (1) rheumatic valvular heart disease; (2) aortic or mitral valves with calcific or atherosclerotic changes; (3) mitral valve prolapse/click murmur syndrome when associated with mitral insufficiency; (4) prior history of endocarditis; (5) various congenital lesions, including bicuspid aortic valve, patent ductus arteriosus, Fallot's tetralogy, ventricular septal defect, coarctation of aorta, and Marfan's syndrome; and (6) prosthetic or biosynthetic heart valves. These six groups of patients should receive prophylaxis against endocarditis. Unfortunately, only approximately one-half of patients with endocarditis have had known underlying heart disease, making antibiotic prophylaxis impossible for the other half.

Many medical events and procedures may be associated with transient bacteremia; however, certain procedures have a greater risk of high-grade transient bacteremia than others. The following procedures deserve prophylaxis in the six groups of patients with the aforementioned cardiac lesions:

1. Dental procedures with gingival bleeding: dental extraction, dental cleaning, periodontal surgery (e.g., gingivectomy)
2. Procedures involving the airways: tonsillectomy, bronchoscopy with a rigid bronchoscope
3. Genitourinary manipulations: cystoscopy, transurethral prostatic resection, urethral dilation, insertion or removal of urethral catheter*
4. Gastrointestinal tract surgery: cholecystectomy, intestinal surgery
5. Gynecologic and obstetric conditions: dilation and curettage of uterus, vaginal delivery (complicated)
6. Manipulation of septic foci: incision and drainage of abscesses

Patients with prosthetic or biosynthetic heart valves are at unusually high risk of endocarditis, and the following additional procedures deserve prophylaxis in these individuals:

1. Procedures involving the airways: nasotracheal intubation, fiberoptic bronchoscopy*
2. Gastrointestinal procedures: sigmoidoscopy, barium enema, colonoscopy, liver biopsy, upper gastrointestinal endoscopy
3. Hemodialysis*

It is generally thought that prophylaxis is *not* indicated for the following procedures in all patients with valvular heart disease: orotracheal intubation, nasotracheal suctioning, insertion or removal of intrauterine device, vaginal delivery (uncompli-

* Indications for prophylaxis are uncertain.

cated), cardiac catheterization and angiographic procedures, pacemaker insertion, peritoneal dialysis.

Patients with cardiac lesions that predispose to endocarditis must be informed of their need for antibiotic prophylaxis for indicated procedures so that they can notify or remind their dentist, physician, or surgeon accordingly.

Prophylactic Antibiotic Regimens

Note that antibiotic prophylaxis against bacterial endocarditis is intermittent and should be given only at the time of anticipated bacteremia. Generally, prophylaxis should be initiated by the parenteral or oral route, started about 1 hour before the procedure, and continued for one dose given 6 to 8 hours after the procedure, after which it should be stopped because anticipated bacteremia will no longer be present. Antibiotic prophylactic regimens are quite specific and narrow because they are directed only against the few organisms that commonly produce bacterial endocarditis following medical procedures: (1) *Streptococcus viridans* following dental procedures and upper respiratory tract surgical procedures; (2) *Enterococcus* following urinary, gynecologic, and gastrointestinal procedures; (3) coagulase-positive staphylococci following incision and drainage of skin abscesses.

Specific antibiotic prophylactic regimens, including dosages, are recommended by the Committee on Prevention of Bacterial Endocarditis of the American Heart Association. In general, these recommendations are as follows:

1. For dental procedures and upper respiratory tract surgical procedures, administer penicillin, ampicillin, or amoxicillin. If the patient is allergic to penicillin or is receiving continuous oral penicillin for prevention of rheumatic fever, administer vancomycin or erythromycin.
2. For urinary, gynecologic, and gastrointestinal procedures, administer penicillin or ampicillin, plus gentamicin. If the patient is allergic to penicillin, administer vancomycin and gentamicin.
3. For incision and drainage of skin abscesses caused by coagulase-positive staphylococci, administer penicillinase-resistant penicillin. If the patient is allergic to penicillin, administer a cephalosporin or vancomycin.

References

American Heart Association Committee Report. Prevention of bacterial endocarditis. Circulation 1984; 70:1123A.

American Heart Association Committee Report. Prevention of rheumatic fever. Circulation 1984; 70:118A.

Durack DT. Current issues in prevention of infective endocarditis. Am J Med 1985; 78(suppl 6B):149.

Durack DT. Current views on prevention. In: Sande MA, Kaye D, Root RK, eds. Endocarditis. New York: Churchill Livingstone, 1984: 213.

Jacoby I, Mandell LA, Weinstein L. The chemoprophylaxis of infection. A brief review of recent studies. Med Clin North Am 1978; 62:1083.

Kaye D. Prophylaxis for infective endocarditis: An update. Ann Intern Med 1986; 104:419.

Prevention of bacterial endocarditis. Med Lett 1989; 31:112.

82 Positive Purified Protein Derivative Skin Test for Tuberculosis

Sarah H. Cheeseman, MD

Definitions

The purified protein derivative tuberculin test, Mantoux test, and Tine test are all names for skin tests for tuberculosis. Infection is indicated by the presence of delayed cutaneous hypersensitivity to a protein antigen derived from *Mycobacterium tuberculosis.* The standard antigen is Tween-stabilized purified protein derivative (PPD), and it is injected intradermally for the PPD or Mantoux test. A less purified antigen, called old tuberculin (OT), which is administered by multiple puncture (Tine test) or patch techniques, is sometimes used in screening for tuberculosis. For diagnostic purposes, however, the Tine test must always be confirmed by performing a standard PPD test. Those who display a delayed hypersensitivity response to PPD (see the section on performance and interpretation) are called *reactors.* The clinical problem is the determination of the state of activity of a reactor's tuberculous infection. We consider the following concepts in this chapter:

1. Active disease—a syndrome or radiologic evidence of ongoing organ damage by replicating mycobacteria, such as progressive pulmonary tuberculosis.
2. Skin test conversion—an increase of at least 10 mm in the skin test reaction over a period of 2 years (at least 15 mm for persons over 35 years of age). A patient with skin test conversion has become infected with tuberculosis in the interval since the negative test.
3. "Old healed" or "quiescent" tuberculosis—radiologic or historical evidence of past active disease that is currently nonprogressive and not characterized by proliferation of mycobacteria.

Patients with a positive PPD test but none of the preceding features are designated as *merely reactors* in this chapter. This means that the only present sign of their tuberculous infection is the positive skin test.

Performance and Interpretation

The tuberculin test is used as a diagnostic or a screening test. As a diagnostic aid in identifying clinically suspected tuberculous *disease,* a positive PPD test is a "rapid diagnostic test," pending confirmation by culture. As a screen for asymptomatic tuberculous *infection,* the PPD test may be performed (1) as part of routine health care, (2) in response to an exposure to a case of infectious tuberculosis, (3) because of an occupation that makes exposure likely (health care worker) or poses special risks of transmission (such as the possibility of infecting young children), or (4) in anticipation of therapy that could reactivate tuberculosis, such as steroids. It is very important to screen persons found to have antibody to the human immunodeficiency virus (HIV).

To perform the standard PPD skin test, inject 0.1 ml containing 5 tuberculin units (TU) of PPD intradermally. A proper intradermal injection raises a wheal with a pigskin texture that is somewhat painful; the wheal and pain disappear within the first few hours. Failure to locate the injection correctly, as by inadvertent subcutaneous injection, may lead to false-negative results. The test is usually placed on the volar surface of the forearm. It should be on a relatively flat area, because placement too close to the antecubital fossa may make it difficult to distinguish the induration of a positive test from the natural rise of the brachioradialis muscle belly. Reading is best accomplished by feeling with the pad of a finger and marking the point at which a rise is felt on each side. Running a ballpoint pen along the skin until it meets the edge, where it will deviate, is another way to be sure the induration is measured correctly. Do not read erythema alone.

The test is read 48 to 72 hours after application. If 10 mm of induration is observed, it is a definite positive result. Five to 10 mm of induration is sometimes called intermediate; these results must be interpreted in the light of the circumstances for which the test was performed. In screenings of healthy populations, reactions of 5 to 10 mm in diameter are usually the result of previous infection with atypical mycobacteria, especially in the southern United States.

When true tuberculous infection is much more likely than infection with an atypical strain, such as in contacts of known cases of active tuberculosis or in patients with lesions on chest radiographs compatible with healed tuberculosis, reactions between 5 and 10 mm in diameter are considered significant and treated as positives. The 5-mm criterion is also applied to persons infected with HIV. For this reason, it is much more useful to record a numerical value rather than "positive" or "negative."

A special problem in interpretation of skin tests is the patient who has received bacille Calmette-Guérin (BCG), a strain of *Mycobacterium bovis* used for active immunization. BCG does not always produce skin test reactivity, although it often does, and it is not completely protective against tuberculosis. Those who have had BCG are generally not followed with skin tests on a regular basis, but reactivity is thought to wane with time. The American Thoracic Society recommends interpreting tuberculin tests in BCG recipients exactly as one does the reaction in patients who have not been vaccinated. Certainly, contacts of known cases and patients suspected of having active disease should be assumed to have real infection and not just a vaccine-induced cross reaction to the skin test. The same reasoning holds for immigrants from hyperendemic areas; even though use of BCG may be common, so is tuberculous infection. If a person with a history of BCG vaccination has a negative skin test reaction, it would be very important to repeat it in a week or two, looking for the booster phenomenon. If none occurs, the patient can be followed with PPD tests like any other tuberculin-negative individual, and conversion can be diagnosed as described previously.

Diagnostic Approach

The presence of a positive PPD test implies infection with tubercle bacilli. The primary infection replicated in the lungs, spread locally by way of lymphatics, and was disseminated throughout the body by the hematogenous route, as illustrated in Figures 82-1 and 82-2. The apices of the lungs, kidneys, liver, bones (especially vertebrae), and meninges are all sites of predilection for seeding and thus places to look for active disease. In evaluating the positive PPD test, one attempts to determine the status of the tuberculous infection.

In this regard, tuberculin convertors, those with active dis-

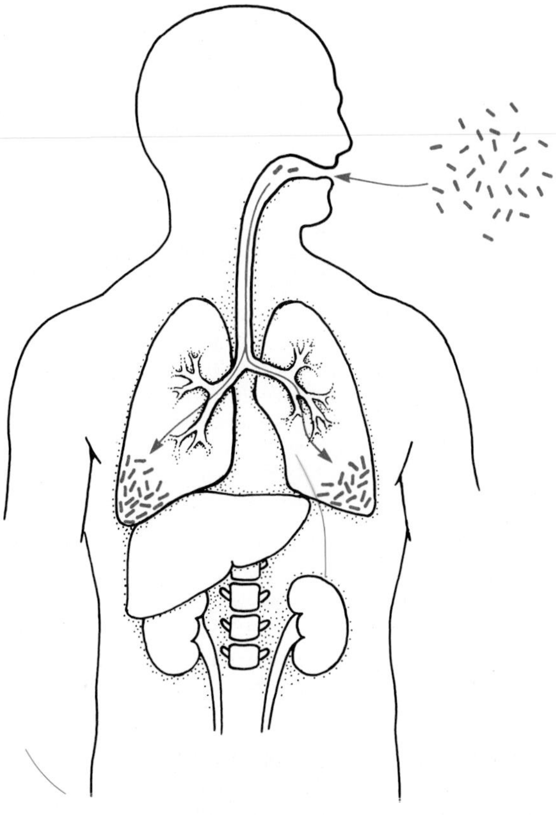

Figure 82-1 Aerosol infection by the tubercle bacillus. The organism is inhaled and multiplies in the lower lobes of the lungs. Spread to local lymphatics and the pulmonary vein results.

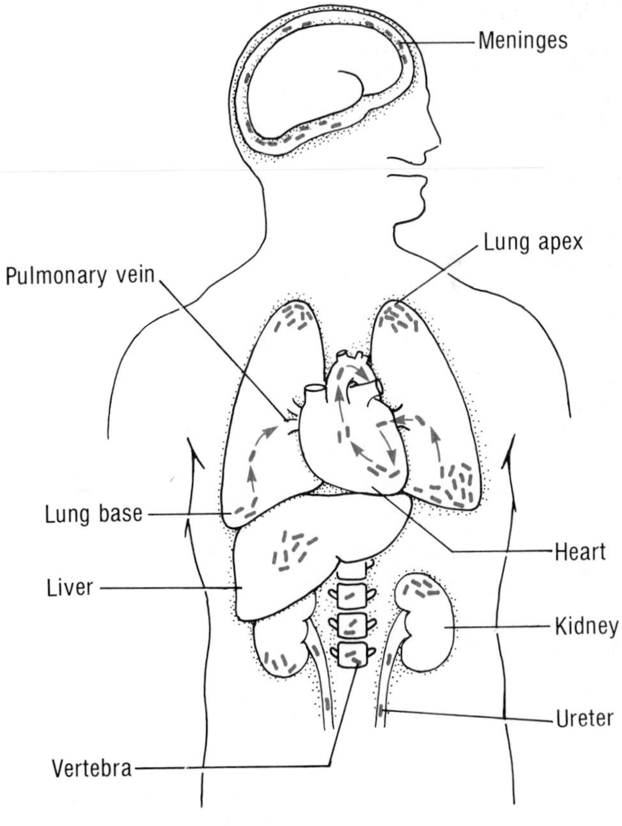

Figure 82-2 Hematogenous dissemination of tuberculous infection. Once the organism enters the pulmonary vein, it travels throughout the circulation and is deposited preferentially in areas of high P_{O_2} or high blood flow.

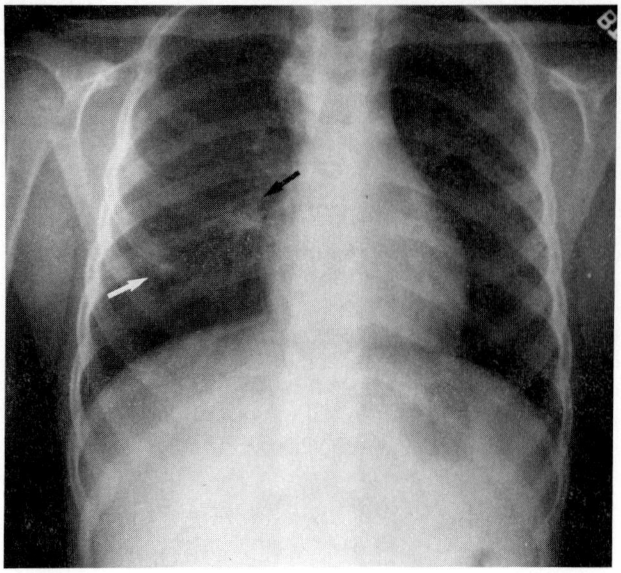

Figure 82-3 A calcified granuloma (*white arrow*) and enlarged lymph nodes (*black arrow*) constitute the Ghon complex in this patient with tuberculosis.

ease, and those with evidence of old healed tuberculosis are differentiated from those who are merely reactors. A convertor is a newly infected person. Because the risk of active tuberculosis is highest during the first 3 years after infection, emphasis is placed on identification and treatment of these individuals.

Review of the patient's history and records should answer two questions: Is the tuberculosis infection old or new? Is the tuberculosis infection active or inactive?

A search for the results of previous skin testing should include recollection of Tine tests, Mantoux tests, or patch tests performed at school, in the Armed Forces, upon discovery of a tuberculous contact, or as a routine for hospital and food service workers and teachers. A previous chest radiograph with calcified granulomas or a Ghon complex (peripheral calcification plus enlarged lymph node; Fig. 82-3) in a patient who does not come from an area highly endemic for histoplasmosis or coccidioidomycosis tells us that the patient probably had his or her infection, and thus a positive skin test, at the time those chest radiographs were taken. A history of prolonged pleurisy without known cause may well represent tuberculosis. Treatment in a sanatorium, therapeutic pneumothorax, and thoracoplasty strongly suggest that the patient had tuberculosis in the pre- or early chemotherapy era. Patients with these characteristics are unlikely to be convertors; it is more likely that they have old tuberculosis. It is important to determine what, if any, specific chemotherapeutic treatment they have received. The dates at which the important drugs were introduced are useful in this regard (streptomycin—1947; isoniazid—1956). Thus, patients treated before 1947 can be assumed to have received no chemotherapy, whereas patients who received drug treatments between 1947 and 1956 can be assumed to have had streptomycin alone. These patients are at particularly high risk for subsequent reactivation, as they have never received tuberculocidal therapy.

Certain groups of tuberculin-positive patients are regarded as being newly infected in the absence of prior known results of PPD tests. These include contacts of patients with active infectious tuberculosis and, because of the general low rate of tuberculosis in the United States, people under 21 years of age. Immigrants from areas where tuberculosis is much more common, such as Southeast Asia or Haiti, are of course more likely to have acquired their infection and skin test reactivity prior to arrival in the United States.

The possibility of active tuberculosis must also be considered in anyone with a positive skin test. Patients need not manifest the classic constitutional symptoms of fever, night sweats, and weight loss to have active tuberculous disease. Sizable cavities may be present in the lungs in patients who have a new cough as their only symptom. Genitourinary tuberculosis is usually afebrile, with a presentation simulating tumor, stones, or pyogenic infection. On the other hand, a patient who has had a positive PPD test for many years should not be subjected to repeated diagnostic procedures and alarms. The careful history should be the primary screening test, and one should look for (1) new coughs or change in an old one; (2) hemoptysis; (3) pleuritic chest pain; (4) hematuria; (5) flank pain; (6) scrotal swelling or history of recurrent "abscess"; (7) back pain, especially in the lower thoracic or upper lumbar regions; (8) neck mass; and (9) fever and weight loss.

An algorithm for the evaluation and management of the patient with a positive PPD test is presented in Figure 82-4.

Laboratory Studies

At the time a positive tuberculin test is first noted, a chest radiograph should be obtained. If this shows abnormalities compatible with tuberculosis, sputum should be obtained for smear and culture on at least three occasions. Morning gastric aspirates, representing the respiratory secretions swallowed during the night, may be cultured if sputum cannot be produced, but they should not be used for smears because false-positive results are possible owing to harmless saprophytes. Patients with positive sputum have active disease. Patients with abnormal chest films due to old healed tuberculosis who have not received tuberculocidal therapy should receive preventive isoniazid as described in the section Treatment Considerations.

If the chest radiograph is clear and the patient is asymptomatic, no further laboratory studies need be performed. If the patient has constitutional symptoms or any of the complaints listed previously, a search for extrapulmonary disease should be conducted. The most common form of extrapulmonary tuberculosis is cervical lymphadenitis, with a firm large node easily palpable on physical examination. Excisional biopsy with acid-fast bacillus smear and culture of the tissue provides the diagnosis. The second most common location is the genitourinary system, for which urinalysis provides an easy and inexpensive screening test. Hematuria and "sterile" pyuria are clues to follow-up with an intravenous pyelogram, in search of tuberculosis and the other significant diagnoses these findings suggest. Three specimens of first morning urine should be submitted for acid-fast bacillus culture to confirm the diagnosis. Fever of unknown origin or unexplained weight loss in the PPD-positive patient warrants a complete blood count with differential (almost any form of hematologic abnormality can be produced by tuberculosis involvement of the bone marrow), serum alkaline phosphatase levels, and acid-fast bacillus cultures of urine and any tissue obtained, in the search for miliary tuberculosis. Bone marrow biopsy is positive in 30 to 40 percent and liver biopsy in 60 to 70 percent of cases of miliary disease.

Yearly chest radiographs are no longer recommended for asymptomatic tuberculin reactors, but one should obtain a film when such a patient develops persistent respiratory symptoms, such as a cough that does not go away after a cold.

Management of the Hospitalized Patient

Patients with abnormal chest radiographs compatible with tuberculosis must be considered infectious until they are proved to be noninfectious by careful comparison with past radiographs or negative sputum smears for acid-fast bacilli. These radiographic abnormalities are most commonly apical cavities, fluf-

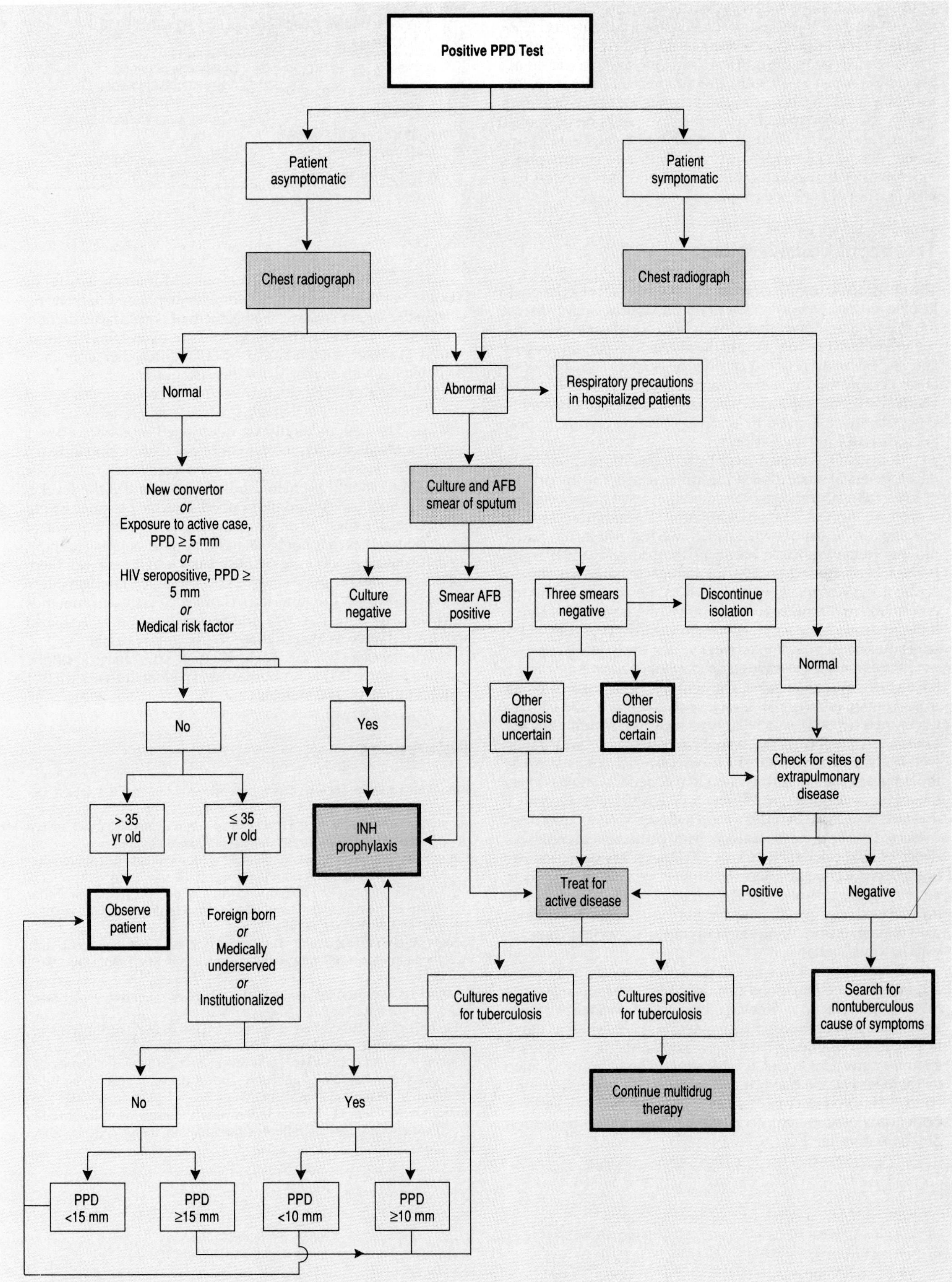

Figure 82-4 Algorithm for the evaluation of a patient with a positive PPD test. AFB = acid-fast bacillus, HIV = human immunodeficiency virus, INH = isoniazid.

finess around old granulomas, streaking from the hila to the apices, or actual retraction of the hila toward the apices. If the patient with a positive PPD test and an abnormal chest radiograph is admitted to the hospital, he or she must be placed in a private room on respiratory precautions until three or four sputum smears are negative. Patients may travel for diagnostic studies wearing a mask. Elective surgery should be postponed until the absence of infectivity is established. It is far better to err on the side of a few days of precautions than to embark on the mop-up campaign after roommates, visitors, and countless hospital personnel have been exposed.

Table 82-1 Medical Conditions Associated with High Risk of Tuberculosis

Silicosis	Conditions requiring prolonged high-dose corticosteroid therapy and other immunosuppressive therapy
Gastrectomy	
Jejunoileal bypass	
Weight 10% or more below ideal body weight	Malignancies, including leukemia and lymphoma
Diabetes mellitus	

Treatment Considerations

The decision to treat a patient with a positive PPD test is based on the diagnostic categories described previously. Active disease must be defined and treated with appropriate multiple drug regimens based on the site and the likelihood (pending culture and susceptibility reports) of drug resistance. Isoniazid resistance is common enough to warrant inclusion of at least two alternative agents in patients who have received prior treatment, especially those marked by poor compliance, and those from Southeast Asia and the Caribbean.

Conversion is treated "prophylactically," i.e., to prevent the development of active disease regardless of age. The importance of tuberculin conversion as an indication for therapy is underscored by the fact that serial cultures of sputum and gastric washings in 12 sailors who had converted within the past 6 months yielded tubercle bacilli in 10. Conversion represents real infection, not "exposure," as so many euphemistically describe it. Some patients treated early in the course of skin test conversion may actually revert to tuberculin negativity There is little point in repeating documented positive PPD tests in patients outside this category, except to demonstrate anergy.

Treatment of those designated *merely reactors* involves a balance of risks and benefits. The only drug with proven efficacy in preventing tuberculosis is isoniazid. The major side effect of isoniazid is hepatitis, which has been the cause of death in some cases. Susceptibility to this complication increases with age as well as the slowness with which one's liver enzymes acetylate the drug. Assessment of the expected risk-benefit ratio has led to the recommendation that reactors over age 35 be treated only if they are at special risk. This group includes recent convertors, contacts of active cases, patients with chest radiographic evidence of old healed tuberculosis, HIV-infected persons, intravenous drug users, and those with other conditions known to increase the risk of tuberculosis, as listed in Table 82-1. Tuberculin reactors over age 35 who have been in stable coexistence with their infection for a period of time are watched clinically without drug therapy.

Tuberculin reactors less than 35 years of age are treated according to the likelihood that their skin test represents true tuberculosis infection. Thus, members of high-incidence groups are treated if their reaction is 10 mm or greater, whereas members of low-incidence groups are treated only if their reaction is 15 mm or greater. Of course, all reactors at high risk (as defined in Table 82-1) are treated, and those with HIV infection, recent contact with an infectious case of tuberculosis, and radiographic evidence of old tuberculosis are treated for skin test induration of 5 mm or more.

The duration of preventive isoniazid therapy is 6 to 12 months, with HIV-infected and immunosuppressed persons receiving the longer course. The problem of prophylactic therapy for patients exposed to isoniazid-resistant tuberculosis is unresolved. Many recommend the use of rifampin, either alone or in combination with isoniazid, for this situation.

Patients should be taught to recognize and promptly report the clinical features of hepatitis, such as fever, anorexia, and malaise. The patient should be questioned monthly to detect such symptoms and remind him or her of their importance. If a patient develops fever or symptoms of hepatitis, SGOT (AST) or SGPT (ALT) should be measured promptly, and if the level is elevated, isoniazid should be stopped. Enzyme elevations without symptoms may occur in as many as 10 to 20 percent of patients, and they may not be an indication for stopping therapy, so that routine monitoring of these laboratory tests is not helpful. In patients who are over age 35 or who have underlying liver disease, however, the American Thoracic Society recommends periodic liver function tests and reconsideration of isoniazid therapy if the levels exceed three to five times normal.

Whenever a choice is made *not* to use prophylactic isoniazid for a positive PPD test, physician and patient must realize that regular follow-up is essential.

References

American Thoracic Society. The tuberculin skin test. Am Rev Respir Dis 1981; 124:356.

American Thoracic Society. Treatment of tuberculosis and other mycobacterial diseases. Am Rev Respir Dis 1983; 127:790.

Centers for Disease Control. Screening for tuberculosis and tuberculous infection in high-risk populations, and the use of preventive therapy for tuberculous infection in the United States: Recommendations of the Advisory Committee for the Elimination of Tuberculosis. MMWR 1990; 39(RR-8):1.

Comstock GW, Edwards PQ. The competing risks of tuberculosis and hepatitis for adult tuberculin reactors. Am Rev Respir Dis 1975; 111:573.

Howard TP, Solomon DA. Reading the tuberculin skin test. Arch Intern Med 1988; 148:2457.

Kent OC, et al. Tuberculin conversion: The iceberg of tuberculous pathogenesis. Arch Environ Health 1967; 14:580.

Koplan JP, Farer LS. Choice of preventive treatment for isoniazid-resistant tuberculous infection: Use of decision analysis and the Delphi technique. JAMA 1980; 244:2736.

Snider DE Jr, Caras GJ, Koplan JP. Preventive therapy with iosoniazid: Cost-effectiveness of different durations of therapy. JAMA 1986; 255:1579.

Hepatitis Exposure

Sarah H. Cheeseman, MD

83

Definition

The clinical problem of hepatitis exposure is the determination of what, if any, prophylactic measures are appropriate. These include precautions to prevent unnecessary infective exposures and the administration of biologic preparations that can diminish the risk of infection with hepatitis A, B, and perhaps non-A, non-B hepatitis, once exposure has occurred. This problem should be considered whenever one makes the diagnosis of viral hepatitis, and when needlesticks and other accidental exposures to hospital personnel occur.

Prevention of hepatitis is desirable for several reasons:

1. When clinical illness occurs, it may be prolonged and occasion much loss of time from work or school.
2. A small proportion of those who become ill develop severe acute liver dysfunction, called fulminant hepatitis or acute yellow atrophy, and this syndrome carries a 60 percent mortality rate.
3. Hepatitis B and non-A, non-B hepatitis (now termed hepatitis C) may progress to chronic liver disease, with resultant disability and early death.
4. Hepatitis B and C may also lead to a chronic carrier state, in which those infected serve as reservoirs of the virus and continued potential sources of infection for the population. It should be emphasized, however, that very rarely is a single individual shown to be responsible for multiple other infections, and the carrier state should not exclude one from any activities except donating blood.
5. There is an association between hepatitis B surface antigen (HBsAg) carriage and the development of hepatocellular carcinoma, at least in hyperendemic areas such as the Far East. Thus, it is desirable to prevent establishment of the carrier state whenever possible.

Management of hepatitis exposure depends upon defining the type of hepatitis and the type of exposure.

Etiology

Hepatitis A is now known to be the usual form of what used to be called "infectious hepatitis," which is spread by the fecal-oral route, water, and food. It is characterized by a rather abrupt onset, high levels of transaminases, and the absence of chronic liver disease or a carrier state as sequelae. In contrast, hepatitis B, the major component of what was once called "serum hepatitis," is transmitted by blood, needles, or intimate exposure to body secretions (which may be blood contact on a microscopic scale, with serum contaminating the secretions that reach the recipient's capillary beds through breaks in the skin or mucous membranes). Hepatitis B tends to have a more subacute onset and smoldering course than hepatitis A. Hepatitis with the clinical and epidemiologic characteristics of serum hepatitis in which markers of hepatitis B virus activity are not detected is called non-A, non-B hepatitis or hepatitis C. Hepatitis having the epidemiologic features of infectious hepatitis, but not diagnosed as being due to hepatitis A by laboratory tests, has also been called non-A, non-B hepatitis, but recently has been named hepatitis E. There are probably still more non-A, non-B agents to be defined. Delta hepatitis or hepatitis D occurs in individuals who are positive for HBsAg. Epstein-Barr virus and cytomegalovirus cause abnormal liver function tests as part of the infectious mononucleosis syndrome and occasionally present as full-blown viral hepatitis without other features of mononucleosis. Other forms of hepatitis, such as yellow fever, are found in the tropics and thus occasionally in travelers. In hospitalized Americans, "hepatitis" is frequently due to toxic or idiosyncratic reactions to drugs.

Exposure

Patients with hepatitis A excrete the virus in their feces for up to 2 weeks before the onset of illness; in the week after onset, only 50 percent have virus in stool, and this drops to 25 percent in the second week. Thus, relevant exposure is to feces or anything contaminated by stool, particularly in the 2 weeks prior to illness. This encompasses household contacts, close associates, and anyone who has eaten food prepared by the infected person, as hands are easily contaminated by stool. Spread is particularly likely when many children are kept together, as in day-care centers, especially if the children are still in diapers (increasing the stool-to-hand contact of their care providers). No spread by blood in a natural setting has been documented. Rarely, hepatitis A can be transmitted by a blood transfusion.

The blood of a patient with hepatitis B may contain detectable virus-specific antigen for as long as 1 month before onset of illness and for a variable period after resolution of the clinical syndrome. For hepatitis B, the exposures of interest include the following:

1. Direct exposure to blood, as in a laboratory or dialysis unit
2. Dental manipulations in which the patient bleeds and the dentist or hygienist is likely to have minute cuts from the teeth
3. Needle sharing, as by drug addicts or in clinics where nondisposable needles are used
4. Transfusion (donor blood units are screened to eliminate those with detectable HBsAg, but some may still be able to transmit hepatitis B)
5. Sexual intercourse of all varieties
6. Vertical transmission from mother to newborn, mostly during the birth process, but some transplacental infections may occur
7. Household contacts, presumably via close sharing of secretions apart from coitus
8. Human bites

Merely sharing a room (as in hospitals) or casual contact does not constitute a risk for hepatitis B exposure.

Diagnostic Approach

The history must establish the type and timing of exposure, and the review of systems and physical examination should seek evidence of active current hepatitis, such as fever, dark urine, light stools, anorexia, scleral icterus, hepatomegaly, or right upper quadrant tenderness. The reason for this lies in the fact that household contacts of patients with hepatitis A may have been exposed to the same source of infection at the same time as the index patient, and that those at risk for hepatitis B infection by the modes listed previously tend to have recurring exposures. Prophylaxis is of no benefit if the recipient already has disease.

Note that both hepatitis A and B often produce asymptomatic, "anicteric" infection. For this reason, laboratory studies, including transaminase levels and specific virus markers, are usually necessary. Fortunately, in both hepatitis A and B, it is possible to make a laboratory diagnosis from a single serum specimen obtained at the time of first presentation with symptoms, and it is also possible to screen for past infection. Thus, one can determine both the infectivity of the "donor" and the susceptibility of the "recipient."

IgM anti-HA is an antibody of the IgM class directed against the hepatitis A virus. It is present early in acute hepatitis A infection and becomes undetectable after 1 to 3 months. Its presence in serum is indicative of current or recent hepatitis A infection (Fig. 83-1).

HBsAg is excess viral surface coat material that is detectable in blood of the infected person as early as 1 week after exposure and is uniformly present at the onset of acute illness. In some patients, the HBsAg is cleared as symptoms subside (Fig. 83-2); in others, it may persist up to 6 months; and in those who go on to become chronic carriers (approximately 5 to 10 percent), it persists indefinitely (Fig. 83-3). HBsAg is not by itself an infectious particle, but it is the most widely available marker of hepatitis B virus (HBV) infection: all those who carry it are considered to be infectious.

Antibody to the hepatitis B surface antigen (anti-HBs) develops at the time of or after clearance of HBsAg following natural infection, and as a response to immunization with hepatitis B vaccine. Once present, it remains positive and indicates immunity to hepatitis B infection.

Antibody to hepatitis B core antigen (anti-HBc) appears at variable times in the course of acute hepatitis B, often while the patient is still symptomatic, and correlates with expression of viral core antigen in liver cells. In some patients, there is a period between disappearance of HBsAg and appearance of anti-HBs when anti-HBc is the only detectable marker of HBV infection; blood is infectious to recipients at this stage. Anti-HBc seems to persist for a lifetime, often in association with anti-HBs. Thus, a patient carrying either or both antibodies has already been infected by HBV and is not susceptible to reinfection from new exposures; the blood of a patient who has anti-HBc in the absence of anti-HBs should be considered infectious. The presence of IgM anti-HBc indicates an acute hepatitis B infection.

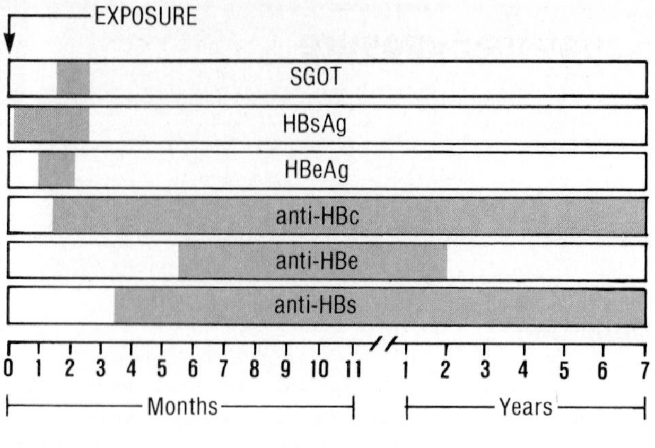

Figure 83-2 Typical laboratory features of acute hepatitis B with recovery. (*From* Krugman S. Viral hepatitis, type B: Studies on natural history and prevention reexamined. N Engl J Med 1979; 300:102; with permission.)

Hepatitis B e antigen (HBeAg) is also associated with the core of the virus and thus active viral replication. In virtually all patients positive for HBsAg, either e antigen or anti-e is detectable. The presence of HBeAg denotes high infectivity, but its absence (usually marked by the presence of anti-HBeAg) does not guarantee that blood is not infectious. Thus, the status of e antigen is not clinically helpful, although it is of great interest to researchers. HBeAg usually appears later than HBsAg and disappears earlier, although both may persist indefinitely.

All of these antigens and antibodies are detected by commercially available radioimmunoassay methods. Because of the need to screen donor blood units for HBsAg, blood banks usually perform these tests. Table 83-1 lists the charge to the patient for these examinations. A test for antibody to hepatitis C will become available for blood bank use in 1990, but the test usually does not produce positive-results during the acute symptomatic illness. In practice the diagnosis of non-A, non-B hepatitis is made when HBsAg, anti-HBc, and IgM anti-HA are not found in

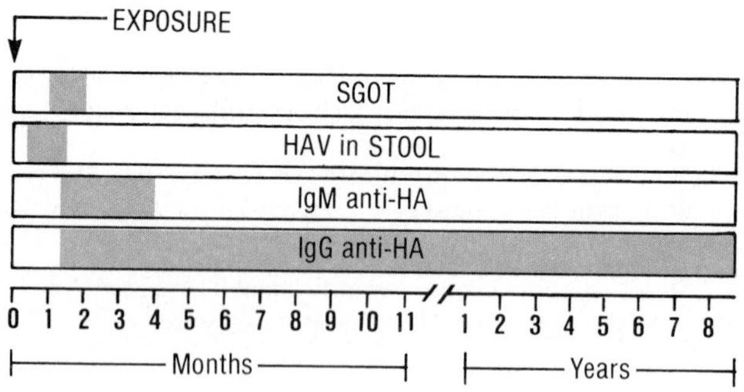

Figure 83-1 Typical laboratory features of acute hepatitis A. (*From* Krugman S. Viral hepatitis, type B: Studies on natural history and prevention reexamined. N Engl J Med 1979; 300:102; with permission.)

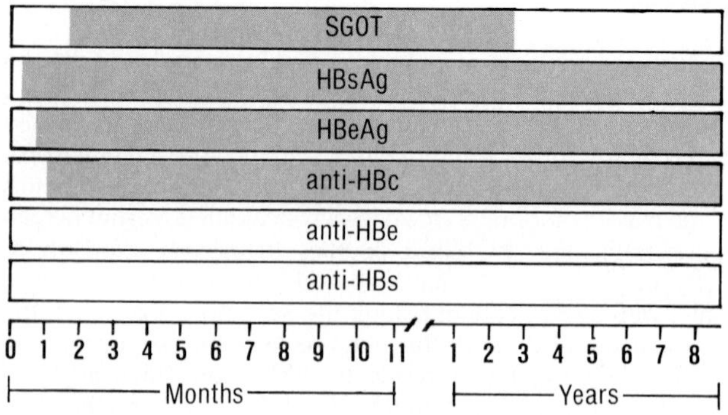

Figure 83-3 Typical laboratory features of acute hepatitis B followed by a carrier state. (*From* Krugman S. Viral hepatitis, type B: Studies on natural history and prevention reexamined. N Engl J Med 1979; 300:103; with permission.)

Table 83-1 Representative Costs of Serologic Tests for Hepatitis

Test	Cost
HBsAg	$25
Anti-HBs	$23
Anti-HBc	$23
HBeAg	$33.60
Anti-HBe	$33.60
IgG and IgM anti-HA	$23

Table 83-2 Representative Costs of Biologics for Prophylaxis Against Hepatitis

Biologic preparation	Cost
Immune globulin	$3.25/10 cc
Hepatitis B immune globulin	$141/5 ml
Hepatitis B vaccine	$139/dose (three-dose series)

the blood of a patient with hepatitis. Strictly speaking, active Epstein-Barr virus and cytomegalovirus infection must also be excluded for an episode of hepatitis to be classified as non-A, non-B, but management of the contact must usually take place before the results of studies for Epstein-Barr virus and cytomegalovirus are available.

Prophylactic Methods

Prevention by avoidance of exposure is obviously the first prophylactic method to be considered. Good hand washing and sanitary facilities are the basics of this approach for hepatitis A; care in the handling of needles and blood specimens to avoid accidental inoculation is necessary to avoid exposure to hepatitis B and C. Universal precautions are indicated for all patients admitted to the hospital. Biologic preparations used in hepatitis prophylaxis, along with their costs, are listed in Table 83-2.

Immune globulin (IG), made from the pooled sera of many donors, contains enough antibody to hepatitis A to be protective when given within 1 week of exposure. It is indicated for household and day-care contacts of cases. There is also one study suggesting that IG may protect against non-A, non-B hepatitis when given before transfusion to patients expected to receive multiple blood units, as in open-heart surgery, but this has not been confirmed. An IG preparation made from the serum of donors with high levels of anti-HBs, called hepatitis B immune globulin (HBIG), has been shown to be protective when given within 48 hours of needlestick exposure to hepatitis B or to infants of HBsAg-carrier women within 48 hours of birth. Hepatitis B vaccine is indicated for all hospital personnel. A combination of HBIG and vaccine is useful for hepatitis B exposure in both medical personnel and in newborns. At present, HBIG is recommended for sexual partners of patients with acute hepatitis B, newborn infants of carrier mothers, and hospital personnel who have not been immunized with hepatitis B vaccine but who have substantial exposure to hepatitis B, as by needlestick, accidental ingestion of blood, or a bite inflicted by a carrier.

Prophylaxis for Hospital Personnel After Exposure

Figure 83-4 is an algorithm for determining the need for and type of prophylaxis for personnel exposed to hepatitis. It is based on the need to give HBIG within 48 hours of exposure and the assumption that IG has some protective efficacy against post-transfusion non-A, non-B hepatitis. The uncertainty of this latter benefit makes the recommendation for IG use optional.

The history is used to determine whether the exposure fulfills the conditions for transmission outlined earlier. In the hospital setting, such "critical exposures" are needlesticks involving used needles, contamination of cuts and abrasions with blood or serum, and introduction of blood onto ocular or buccal surfaces, such as occurs if blood is splashed. Hospital exposure to hepatitis A occurs less commonly than parenterally transmitted hepatitis, but it may occur when a patient has fecal incontinence. Evaluation of the patient who is the potential source of infection involves review of the chart for liver function tests, the clinical impression as to the cause of any abnormalities (one would not wish to treat employees prophylactically for exposure to a case of cholecystititis or drug-induced liver disease), and past history that would place the patient at high risk of hepatitis B or non-A, non-B hepatitis. Serum from the patient is submitted for HBsAg testing as well as for SGOT (AST) and SGPT (ALT) levels, if they have not been determined recently.

The algorithm does not include determination of susceptibility of the exposed person, because only the HBsAg test is done frequently enough to fit within the time constraints for action. If serologic results on the exposed individual are available, the presence of either anti-HBs, anti-HBc, or HBsAg would negate the need for HBIG and hepatitis B vaccine. The presence of an adequate level of anti-HBs as a result of hepatitis B immunization would also eliminate the need for HBIG. Serum should be obtained from the exposed individual prior to administration of HBIG and one dose of vaccine. If no antibody is present, the employee should be urged to continue the hepatitis B vaccine series to obviate the problems of future exposure. The recognition of continuing risk, combined with the time, trouble, and possible discomfort of the management of this exposure, make this an excellent opportunity to discuss the usefulness of hepatitis B vaccine with the employee.

Similarly, individuals who are known to have anti-HA do not require prophylaxis for contact with hepatitis A, but note that the relative costs of IG and serologic testing will favor IG administration, unless the serologic information happens to have been obtained at some time in the past. Note that in hospital exposure situations, IG may be given for non-A, non-B hepatitis as well as hepatitis A; therefore, IG should not necessarily be omitted because an exposed staff member is positive for anti-HA.

Prophylaxis for Household (Nonhospital) Contacts, Including Sexual Contacts

Household contacts are treated prophylactically with IG for hepatitis A. There is a high risk of hepatitis B in sexual partners of patients with acute hepatitis B that has been shown to be reduced by giving these partners HBIG. There is a lower, but definable, risk for other household contacts, even those of carriers who are not acutely ill, which still probably derives from blood contact (it was correlated with sharing of razors and washcloths in one study). For these continuing exposures, the hepatitis B vaccine offers a more logical approach than passive immunization. It is probably wise to treat sexual partners and highly susceptible household contacts (e.g., an immunosuppressed person) with HBIG and begin vaccine simultaneously,

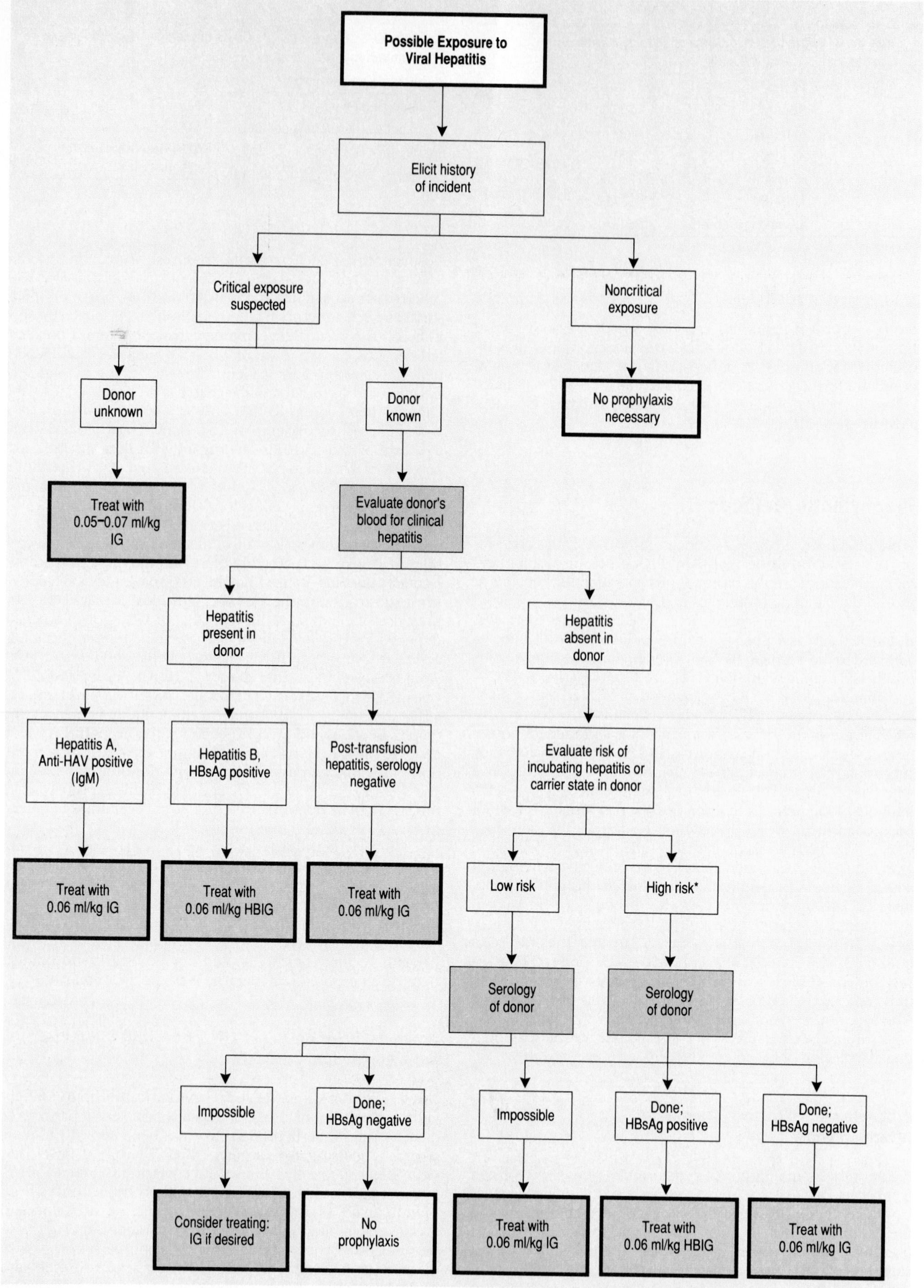

Figure 83-4 Algorithm for the management of individuals with possible exposure to viral hepatitis. Donors at high risk for incubating hepatitis or a carrier state include those with a history of undefined hepatitis or elevated liver function tests in association with a history of multiple blood transfusions, dialysis, or drug abuse and those who recently received multiple bloood products.

and to screen other members of the household for markers of past infection and give hepatitis B vaccine to those who are negative, if the index patient remains seropositive for more than 3 months.

References

Centers for Disease Control. Protection against viral hepatitis: Recommendations of the Immunization Practices Advisory Committee (ACIP). MMWR 1990; 39(RR-2):1.

Centers for Disease Control. Prevention of perinatal transmission of hepatitis B virus: Prenatal screening of all pregnant women for hepatitis B surface antigen. MMWR 1988; 37:341.

Goodman RA, et al. Nosocomial hepatitis A transmission by an adult patient with diarrhea. Am J Med 1982; 73:220.

Knodel RG, et al. Efficacy of prophylactic gamma-globulin in preventing non-A, non-B post-transfusion hepatitis. Lancet 1976; 1:557.

Szmuness W, et al. Hepatitis B vaccine. Demonstration of efficacy in a controlled clinical trial in a high-risk population in the United States. N Engl J Med 1980; 303:833.

Infection in the Compromised Host

Richard H. Glew, MD

84

During the past few decades, dramatic advances have been made in the therapy of various malignancies, with resultant improvement in the prognosis of patients with leukemia, lymphoma, and solid tumors. Similarly, progress in transplantation has resulted in increased numbers and survival of patients undergoing homotransplantation of kidney, heart, bone marrow, liver, and other organs and tissues. Unfortunately, these patients with neoplasia and transplants exhibit increased susceptibility to and mortality from infection. Thus, infections are responsible for approximately three-quarters of all deaths in patients with acute leukemia or following organ transplantation, and they are a major factor in the deaths of one-half to three-quarters of lymphoma patients.

Opportunistic, life-threatening infections also occur with increased frequency in patients who are receiving therapy with cytotoxic agents or adrenocorticosteroids for other conditions, such as connective tissue disorders. Over the last decade, severe and unusual infections have also been noted to occur with high frequency in patients with HIV-1–associated acquired immunodeficiency syndrome (AIDS), which is most commonly noted in homosexual and bisexual men, parenteral drug users, hemophiliacs and other recipients of blood products before mid-1985, Central Africans, and female sexual partners of patients with HIV-1 infection.

Etiology

In all such immunocompromised patients, increased susceptibility to infection results from the following factors: (1) immune defects inherent in the primary disease, (2) mechanical complications of the underlying disease, (3) immune defects related to systemic therapy (i.e., chemotherapy) of the disease, and (4) defects in mechanical barrier defenses due to radiotherapy and surgery (Table 84-1). By careful evaluation of the predisposing factors operative in the individual patient, one can better estimate which of the myriad of bacteria, fungi, viruses, or protozoa known to produce severe infections in the compromised host are likely to be operative in a particular patient.

Anatomic Barriers

In patients with solid tumors, infection commonly results from local complications of the malignancy, such as obstruction, perforation, or necrosis. Thus, one can expect to see recurrent pneumonia developing distal to an obstructing endobronchial tumor, multiple episodes of cholangitis in the patient with a biliary tract malignancy, and free peritonitis or pericolonic abscess in the patient with a colon carcinoma. In patients with acute leukemia, bacteremia and fungemia can arise through defects in skin and mucous membranes related to thrombocytopenia-induced integumentary hemorrhages or chemotherapy-induced mucositis. Finally, in any patient with malignancy, supportive measures involving intravenous access (for medications or nutrition), surgery, and irradiation can also contribute to breakdown of local defenses and lead to severe bacterial and fungal infections. Transfusion of blood products can result in transmission of cytomegalovirus infection or hepatitis (usually due to hepatitis C—formerly non-A, non-B—viruses).

Polymorphonuclear Leukocytic Defects

Polymorphonuclear leukocytes (PMNs) and macrophages defend against infection caused by bacteria and opportunistic fungi. Accordingly, patients with severe neutropenia (secondary to acute leukemia, cytotoxic chemotherapy, or bone marrow suppression due to metastatic tumor or adverse drug reaction) are especially likely to develop overwhelming, disseminated infections due to various bacteria, including common pathogens such as gram-negative bacilli (in particular, *Escherichia coli, Klebsiella pneumoniae,* and *Pseudomonas aeruginosa*) and staphylococci (including *Staphylococcus aureus* and the more resistant non-*aureus* species, such as *Staphylococcus epidermidis*), as well as several fungal organisms, including *Candida* species, *Aspergillus* species, and the phycomycetes (*Mucor*). Invasive and disseminated fungal infections become more common with increasing duration or repeated episodes of neutropenia and after repeated, prolonged courses of broad-spectrum antibiotic therapy.

Antibody-Mediated Immunity

B-lymphocyte function and antibody production often are impaired in untreated patients with chronic lymphocytic leukemia, non-Hodgkin's lymphomas, multiple myeloma, and hypogammaglobulinemia and dysgammaglobulinemia syndromes. To a certain degree, they are also impaired in patients who are receiving high-dose corticosteroid therapy. Impaired antibody response predisposes patients to infections due to encapsulated bacteria, such as *Streptococcus pneumoniae, Haemophilus in-*

Table 84-1 Altered Host Defenses in the Immunocompromised Patient

Mechanical factors		
Defective locus	*Disease or factor*	*Common infecting organism*
Skin/mucous membranes	Acute leukemia Cytotoxic chemotherapy Intravenous lines	Enterobacteriaceae *Pseudomonas aeruginosa* *Staphylococcus aureus* Fungi (*Candida, Mucor, Aspergillus*)
Organ/viscus perforation, obstruction	Solid tumor Lymphoma Surgery Irradiation	Lung: mouth anaerobes Bowel: Enterobacteriaceae, *Bacteroides*, other anaerobes
Immunologic factors		
Defective locus	*Disease or factor*	*Common infecting organism*
Phagocytes	Leukemia (acute, chronic) Lymphoma Cytotoxic chemotherapy Irradiation Corticosteroids	Enterobacteriaceae *Pseudomonas aeruginosa* *Staphylococcus aureus* Fungi (*Candida, Mucor, Aspergillus*)
Humoral immunity (B lymphocytes)	Chronic lymphocytic leukemia Multiple myeloma Splenectomy Hypogammaglobulinemia Corticosteroids AIDS (especially in children)	*Streptococcus pneumoniae* *Haemophilus influenzae* *Neisseria meningitidis* (Enterobacteriaceae)
Cell-mediated immunity (T lymphocytes)	Lymphoma Corticosteroids Irradiation AIDS	Viruses (CMV, HSV, VZV) Protozoa (*Pneumocystis carinii, Toxoplasma gondii*) Fungi (*Cryptococcus neoformans, Histoplasma capsulatum, Coccidioides immitis, Candida*) Helminths (*Strongyloides stercoralis*) Mycobacteria *Nocardia, Listeria monocytogenes*

Abbreviations: AIDS = acquired immunodeficiency syndrome, CMV = cytomegalovirus, HSV = herpes simplex virus, VZV = varicella zoster virus.

fluenzae, and infections with certain gram-negative bacilli (Enterobacteriaceae and *Pseudomonas aeruginosa*) occur with increased frequency as well.

Splenectomy, which is employed in the diagnosis and therapeutic staging of patients with Hodgkin's disease, also predisposes patients to fulminant and life-threatening infections due to encapsulated bacteria (Coker et al, 1983). Although most common in patients undergoing splenectomy for malignancy or reticuloendothelial disease, overwhelming postsplenectomy bacteremia can occur in any splenectomized patient, including patients whose spleen is removed for benign conditions (hemolytic anemia, thrombocytopenia) or following trauma.

Cell-Mediated Immunity

Delayed hypersensitivity, which is dependent on T lymphocytes, is impaired in patients with lymphoproliferative disorders, particularly Hodgkin's disease and other lymphomas, chronic lymphocytic leukemia, and malnutrition, and in transplant recipients or other patients receiving therapy with corticosteroids, antithymocyte globulin, or extensive irradiation. Patients with T-lymphocyte abnormalities are highly susceptible to frequent, severe infections due to viruses (varicella zoster virus, cytomegalovirus, herpes simplex virus), fungi (*Cryptococcus neoformans, Histoplasma capsulatum, Coccidioides immitis, Candida* species), intracellular bacteria (*Listeria monocytogenes*), mycobacteria (*Mycobacterium tuberculosis* as well as atypical mycobacteria, such as *Mycobacterium avium-intracellulare*), protozoa (*Pneumocystis carinii, Toxoplasma gondii*), and helminths (*Strongyloides stercoralis*).

Infections due to a similar wide spectrum of organisms have been observed to occur frequently in patients with AIDS. Although most opportunistic infections that occur in the HIV-1 infected, immunosuppressed patient reflect T-lymphocyte deficiency and are caused by viruses, mycobacteria, fungi, and protozoa, recurrent and severe bacterial infections due to encapsulated bacteria (*Streptococcus pneumoniae, Haemophilus influenzae*), *Salmonella* species, and *Listeria monocytogenes* are noted as well, especially in children (Table 84-2). Patients with AIDS may also suffer infection due to intestinal cryptosporidiosis and frequently develop severe and unusual malignancies such as rare cell types of non-Hodgkin's lymphoma and widespread Kaposi's sarcoma.

Diagnostic Approach

General

For several reasons, the appearance of fever in the immunocompromised host often is perplexing, and one should always be greatly concerned by its presence. First, one must attempt to distinguish between fever due to the underlying disease itself (or its therapies) and pyrogenic response to infections. Second, local symptoms or physical signs of infection may be less striking in the neutropenic host or the patient receiving anti-inflammatory agents, especially corticosteroids, than in the patient who is immunologically intact. Third, the sites of infection and possible infecting organisms in the compromised host are far more diverse than those encountered in most patients. Fi-

Table 84-2 Fever in Patients with Immunosuppression due to Human Immunodeficiency Virus-1

Neoplasia
Non-Hodgkin's lymphoma
Kaposi's sarcoma with liver involvement

Infections
Viral
- Cytomegalovirus: disseminated, enteritis, encephalitis
- Herpes simplex virus: extensive mucocutaneous lesions
- Varicella zoster virus: disseminated

Bacteria
- Pyogenic bacteria (*Haemophilus influenzae, Streptococcus pneumoniae*): pneumonia, sinusitis, bacteremia
- *Salmonella* species: recurrent bacteremia
- *Listeria monocytogenes:* bacteremia, meningitis
- *Mycobacterium avium-intracellulare:* disseminated
- *Mycobacterium tuberculosis:* disseminated

Fungi
- Mucosal infection: *Candida* species, *Aspergillus* species
- Dissemination: *Cryptococcus neoformans, Histoplasma capsulatum, Coccidioides immitis*

Protozoa
- *Pneumocystis carinii:* pneumonia
- *Toxoplasma gondii:* encephalitis, disseminated
- *Cryptosporidium* species: enteritis

nally, the alacrity of progression and mortality rates of many infections in the immunocompromised host are markedly exaggerated, leaving the clinician little margin for diagnostic and therapeutic error. Accordingly, in the compromised host, all episodes of fever or other complaints suggestive of infection (chills, sweats, dramatically increasing malaise or fatigue, cough, shortness of breath, abdominal pain, dysuria) must be evaluated promptly and thoroughly. Moreover, unless one concludes after thorough evaluation that the fever appears almost certainly noninfectious or an uncomplicated, localized source of infection can be found, and the patient appears relatively well, admission to hospital should be automatic, particularly in the febrile, neutropenic patient.

History and physical examination should be performed promptly initially, and be repeated frequently. Obtain background information on the nature and course of the primary disease, the types of therapy employed, and previous complications of each. For example, patients receiving cytotoxic agents (resulting in neutropenia) are particularly prone to the development of bacterial infections, especially with gram-negative bacteria, whereas patients with lymphoma or AIDS or those receiving corticosteroids are especially susceptible to infections with *Pneumocystis carinii, Listeria monocytogenes,* mycobacteria, and cytomegalovirus. Local symptoms should prompt special attention to the organ systems highlighted, but meticulous examination of high-risk areas, such as the oropharynx, the anorec-

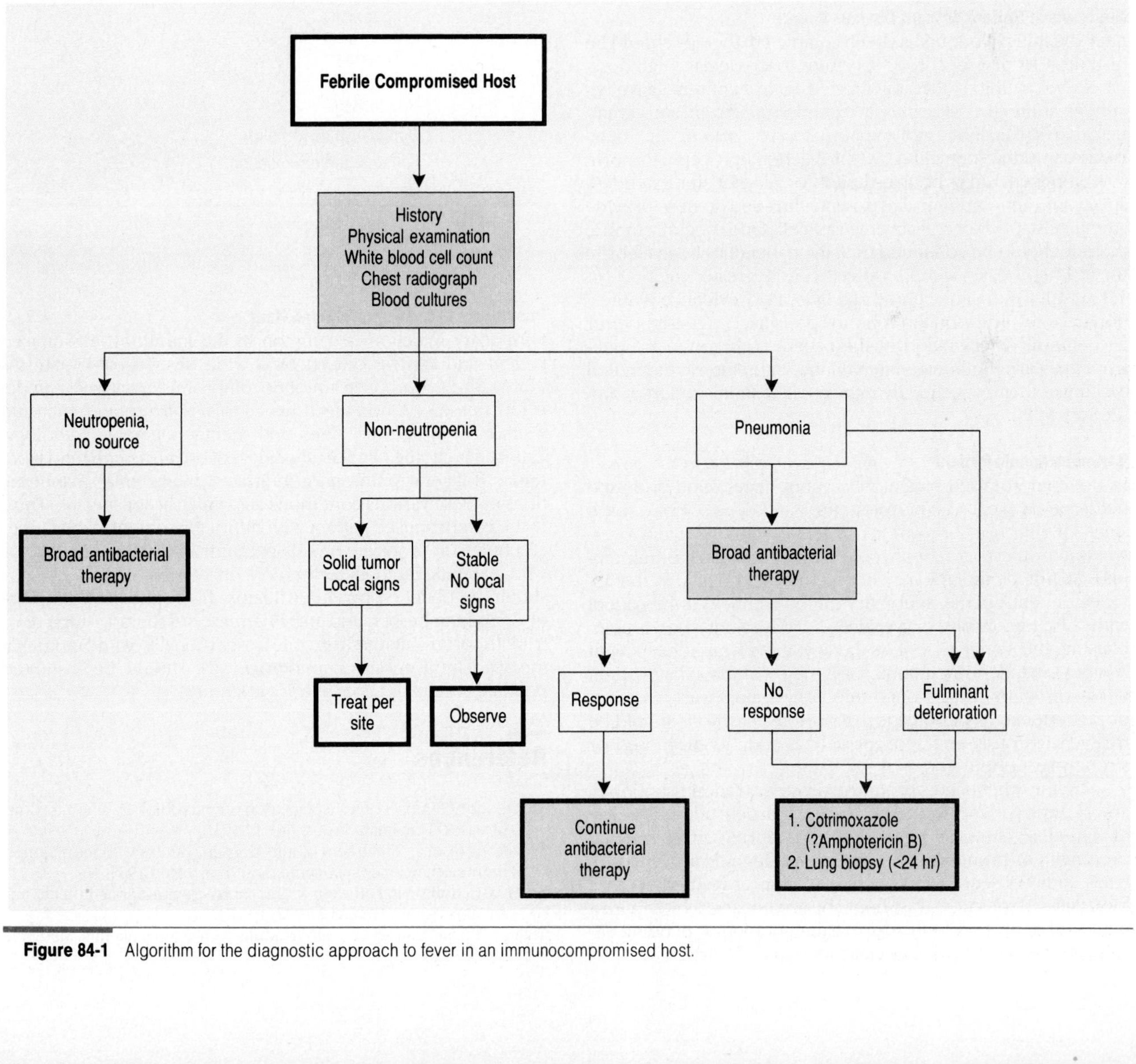

Figure 84-1 Algorithm for the diagnostic approach to fever in an immunocompromised host.

tal region, skin, lungs, abdomen, and optic fundi, is vital in all patients.

Routine laboratory studies in the febrile compromised host generally should include (1) cultures of blood and urine; (2) serum chemistries, in part to screen for possible hepatitis due to cytomegalovirus or one of the transfusion-related hepatitis viruses, and in part to provide baseline data (e.g., creatinine levels) to monitor for possible adverse reactions to subsequent antibiotic therapy; and (3) chest radiograph. The following additional studies should be dictated by local findings: (1) Gram stain and culture of sputum, if obtainable in patients with cough, tachypnea, or shortness of breath; (2) aspiration or biopsy (for smear, culture) of suspicious skin lesions; (3) lumbar puncture, in patients with altered mental status or stiff neck; and (4) arterial blood gases in the patient with AIDS, lymphoma, or other T-lymphocyte difficulties who presents with progressive cough, dyspnea, or bilateral pulmonary infiltrates.

Even when the aforementioned diagnostic approach is followed (Fig. 84-1), an infectious etiology will be documented in only one-half to two-thirds of febrile, neutropenic patients. Because routine cultures are unlikely to provide useful information for at least 1 to 2 days, one should begin broad-spectrum parenteral antibiotic therapy in most compromised patients with fever while awaiting the results of pending cultures and other studies.

Specific

Neutropenic Patient Without Obvious Source

After the initial work-up has been completed, therapy should be instituted to provide broad-spectrum, bactericidal, high-dose, parenteral antibiotic therapy directed against gram-negative bacilli (an aminoglycoside plus an extended-spectrum, anti–gram-negative penicillin) and *Staphylococcus aureus* (a beta-lactamase stable penicillin). A third-generation cephalosporin (or imipenem) may be substituted for at least the extended-spectrum, anti–gram-negative penicillin, and it may provide adequate staphylococcal coverage as well. Once begun, empiric therapy should be continued until the patient has been afebrile for at least 3 days, with blood cell counts greater than 500 to 1,000 PMNs/mm^3, and clinical and laboratory evidence of infection have resolved. On the contrary, prolonged, persistent fever and clinical deterioration of the patient with continued neutropenia warrant ultimate intervention with empiric parenteral antifungal therapy, generally intravenous administration of amphotericin B.

Non-neutropenic Patient

In the compromised patient who is not manifesting profound neutropenia (i.e., $\geq$1,000 PMNs/mm^3) and does not have local signs of infection or obvious systemic signs of acute overwhelming infection (e.g., hypotension, confusion), blind, empiric, antibiotic therapy may not be indicated. Thus, in the absence of neutropenia, antibiotics can be withheld if the patient with solid tumor shows no evidence that local infection is complicating the malignancy or its therapy; if the lymphoma patient does not manifest pneumonia; or if the renal transplant patient does not demonstrate wound infection, urinary tract infection, or pneumonia. It is axiomatic that obvious infections should be treated vigorously and appropriately as soon as diagnosed or strongly suspected.

On the other hand, chronic corticosteroid administration in any of these patients would necessitate transient administration of high-dose, stress-supportive steroids during an episode of prolonged or pronounced fever. Because high-dose corticosteroids could obscure subsequent evolution of fever as well as local signs of infection, this should be accompanied by administration of appropriate broad-spectrum antibiotics, pending results of laboratory tests, especially indicated cultures.

Table 84-3 Causes of Acute Pulmonary Disease in Immunocompromised Patients

Infectious
Bacteria
Streptococcus pneumoniae
Haemophilus influenzae
Pseudomonas aeruginosa
Enteric gram-negative bacilli
Staphylococcus aureus
Legionella pneumophila
Nocardia species
Mycobacteria
Protozoa
Pneumocystis carinii
Toxoplasma gondii
Viruses
Cytomegalovirus
Herpes simplex virus
Fungi
Aspergillus species
Candida species
Mucor species
Cryptococcus neoformans
Parasites (*Strongyloides stercoralis*)
Noninfectious
Primary disease
Malignancy (primary or metastatic)
Vasculitis
Drug toxicity
Bleomycin
Busulfan
Cytoxan
Hemorrhage
Congestive heart failure
Leukoagglutinin reaction
Radiation

Pneumonia in the Compromised Host

Pulmonary infection is common in the immunocompromised patient and can be caused by a wide diversity of organisms (Table 84-3). Moreover, immunocompromised patients can develop numerous noninfectious causes of acute and subacute pulmonary symptoms, signs, and roentgenographic pathology. Unfortunately, the clinical (shortness of breath, cough) and laboratory (bilateral pulmonary infiltrates, hypoxemia) manifestations of these various conditions are similarly nonspecific. Thus, in the compromised patient with diffuse pneumonia who fails to respond to appropriate broad-spectrum antibacterial therapy or who exhibits rapid deterioration on admission, lung biopsy should be obtained by either flexible fiberoptic bronchoscopy or open-lung biopsy, and anti-*Pneumocystis* therapy (high dose trimethoprim-sulfamethoxazole), occasionally with antifungal therapy (intravenous amphotericin B), should be instituted pending results of histopathologic studies.

References

Alexander JW. Impact of transplantation on microbiology and infectious diseases. Transplant Proc 1980; 12:593.

Armstrong D, et al. Treatment of infections in patients with the acquired immunodeficiency syndrome. Ann Intern Med 1985; 103:738.

Bodey GP, Bolivar R, Fainstein V. Infectious complications in leukemic patients. Semin Hematol 1982; 19:193.

Chang HY, et al. Causes of death in adults with acute leukemia. Medicine 1976; 55:259.

Coker DD, et al. Infection among 210 patients with surgically staged Hodgkin's disease. Am J Med 1983; 75:97.
Gill FA, et al. The relationship of fever, granulocytopenia and antimicrobial therapy to bacteremia in cancer patients. Cancer 1977; 39:1704.
Mattay RA, Greene WH. Pulmonary infections in the immunocompromised patient. Med Clin North Am 1980; 64:529.
Meunier-Carpentier F, Kiehn TE, Armstrong D. Fungemia in the immunocompromised host. Am J Med 1981; 71:363.
Notter DT, et al. Infections in patients with Hodgkin's disease: A clinical study of 300 consecutive adult patients. Rev Infect Dis 1980; 2:761.
O'Neal BJ, McDonald JC. The risk of sepsis in the asplenic adult. Ann Surg 1981; 194:775.
Pizzo PA, Young LS. Limitations of current antimicrobial therapy in the immunocompromised host: Looking at both sides of the coin. Am J Med 1984; 76:101.
Seligmann M, et al. Immunology of human immunodeficiency virus infection and the acquired immunodeficiency syndrome. Ann Intern Med 1987; 107:234.
Sickles EA, Greene WH, Wiernik PH. Clinical presentation of infection in granulocytopenic patients. Arch Intern Med 1975; 135:715.
Springmeyer SC, et al. The role of transbronchial biopsy for the diagnosis of diffuse pneumonias in immunocompromised marrow transplant recipients. Am Rev Respir Dis 1982; 126:763.
Winston DJ, et al. Infectious complications of human bone marrow transplantation. Medicine 1979; 58:1.

Human and Animal Bites

Irving Jacoby, MD

85

Definitions

Bites are lesions of the body caused by the mouths of humans or animals. They may be closed injuries, such as contusions or hematomas, which generally do not require intervention. The bites of large herbivores commonly fall into this group. Alternatively, the skin may be broken, with resultant abrasion, laceration, puncture wound, or large-scale avulsion injury. These open injuries may affect the airway or vital organs, resulting in life-threatening emergencies. Contamination by saliva of breaks in the skin acquired either previously or simultaneously may result in lesions that must be managed as true bites.

Epidemiology

In the United States, most animal bites are those by dogs, which account for about 90 percent of all bites. Cats account for an additional 5 percent; rodents and humans about 2 to 3 percent; and all other species, less than 1 percent. From 1979 through 1988, approximately 15 deaths per year resulted from the bites of domestic dogs. Working and sporting dogs, such as German Shepherds, are more likely to be biters, but an alarming increase in fatalities, particularly in infants, due to attacks by pit bulls has been identified in the last decade. In Africa, there are many more injuries and deaths from large mammals, including lions, tigers, and leopards.

Clinical Considerations

Bite wounds may cause local or systemic disease through any of the following mechanisms. Direct local trauma causes interruption of the skin and, frequently, an underlying structure. The result can be life threatening; e.g., interruption of the arterial blood supply by a bite may cause major hemorrhage. Damage to the airway may cause respiratory distress. Perforation of the thorax may result in either a simple or a tension pneumothorax. Local wound infections can cause serious illness in the form of cellulitis, abscess, necrotizing fasciitis, or localized wound tetanus. Osteomyelitis may develop from direct inoculation or contiguous or bacteremic spread Local wound inflammation may be due to an allergic reaction to some component of the animal (e.g., insect bites). Necrosis of skin may occur from the direct action of toxin from the brown recluse spider (*Loxosceles reclusa*) and, less commonly, from other spiders.

Systemic illness may result from the spread of bacterial or viral disease via the blood stream. For example, rat bite fever may develop from infection with *Streptobacillus moniliformis* or *Spirillum minus* organisms. Primate bites result in poorly characterized viral syndromes, whereas hepatitis B can be transmitted by human bites. Cat scratch disease bacillus has been identified as the causative agent of cat scratch disease, which can be transmitted by scratches or bites. Although human immunodeficiency virus type 1 (HIV-1) is secreted in the saliva of many HIV-positive patients, the concentration of virus is 1/1,000 to 1/10,000 that found in serum of infected patients. Transmission does not appear to occur readily; thus, bites are not yet considered to be a significant exposure by the Centers for Disease Control (CDC).

The elaboration of a toxin is another mechanism for development of systemic illness. The development of tetanus from the toxin of *Clostridium tetani* is the classic example. Toxic shock syndrome has recently been reported from an infected human bite. Envenomation, as from a poisonous snake, the black widow spider (*Lactrodectus mactans*), and other venomous creatures, is a third mechanism by which bites can cause systemic illness. The result may be neurologic, hematologic, cardiovascular, or necrotoxic pathology with poisonous snake envenomations, or hypertension and muscle cramps, especially of the chest and abdomen, with black widow spider bites.

Diagnostic Approach

In most cases the diagnosis of animal bite is obvious from the presenting complaint; with human bites, however, some social stigma may be attached to the injury. Patients may attempt to conceal the exact cause of the injury as a human bite. This most frequently occurs in the setting of an abrasion or laceration on the dorsum of the hand, at the level of one of the distal metacarpal heads or over a metacarpophalangeal joint. This common injury results from one person striking another in the mouth and hitting the victim's incisor tooth. In addition to the skin injury, the extensor tendon may be damaged in the stretched position that it assumes with the fist clenched. With relaxation of the hand, the site of the tendon injury may be concealed because it retracts proximal to the skin break; thus, the contaminated tendon becomes enclosed and may escape appropriate debridement or irrigation if not seen early. Hand injuries from dog and human bites have the highest incidence of infection of any part of the body.

When any patient presents with a bite wound, the first considerations must be first aid and wound management. Does the wound affect the airway? Is breathing compromised? What is the status of the circulation? Is there significant hemorrhage? If the answer to any of these questions is "yes," the specific problem must be dealt with from the viewpoint of Advanced Life Support. Otherwise, a more complete history may be obtained.

The timing of the bite and type of animal involved must be documented. Bites from carnivores like raccoons, foxes, wolves, skunks, and bats entail a high risk of rabies transmission. Squirrels, chipmunks, and other strict herbivores are not associated with rabies carriage. Rats, even when infected with rabies, generally do not carry the virus in the saliva and, hence, carry a low risk of rabies transmission. If there is a possibility that the animal may be rabid, it is important to document whether the patient was bitten or licked on an open wound or mucous membrane. Ideally, any animal that has bitten a human should be identified, captured, and observed to see if it is behaving normally. If the attack was unprovoked, the animal must be kept under observation for 10 days. If the animal becomes ill while under observation, laboratory examination by fluorescent antibody of the brain of the animal must be conducted to detect rabies. If positive, one dose of rabies immune globulin (RIG) for passive immunization, plus active immunization with five doses of human diploid cell vaccine, must be given to the nonimmune individual. These steps must be taken in addition to local wound management. The decision to institute rabies prophylaxis requires knowledge of the usual tendencies of the specific animal involved, as well as local factors, such as the presence of animal rabies in a given area of the country. If any question exists as to the presence of animal rabies in a given species, local health department officials should be contacted.

A tetanus vaccination history must be elicited from each patient with any open wound. Knowledge of whether the patient has received a primary series of at least three inoculations, negating the need for tetanus antitoxin (immune globulin) for dirty wounds, and whether there has been an additional booster of tetanus toxoid in the previous 10 years for a clean wound, or in the previous 5 years for a dirty wound or a puncture wound, will enable the physician to decide on appropriate intervention.

Management of Human, Dog, and Cat Bite Wounds

The infection rate of clean, nonbite lacerations is roughly 3 to 5 percent. The infection rate for dog bites is variously reported in the 6-to-12 percent range, whereas cat and human bite wounds become infected with an incidence ranging from 15 to 60 percent of cases. The prognosis for risk of infection in a dog or cat bite wound depends a great deal on what is done to the wound at the time it is seen, if infection is not already present, and on its location. Bites that come to the attention of a physician more than 24 hours after the event have higher infection rates. Risk is also higher if the patient is older than 50 years of age.

Irrigation of a bite wound reduces subsequent risk of infection dramatically. The infection rate in irrigated wounds is about one-fifth that of unirrigated wounds. Proper irrigation requires the use of a sterile liquid irrigant that, under continuous pressure, exerts a mechanical surface cleansing of the wound surface. Administration of 150 to 250 ml of either normal saline or povidone-iodine solution in a 20- or 35-cc syringe with a 19-gauge needle or catheter tip will be adequate to deliver necessary pressure. Larger volumes will of course be necessary for larger wounds. Puncture-type bite wounds, more common with cats than dogs, are almost impossible to irrigate properly because the track remains closed. Thus, the infection risk is four times greater for puncture wounds than for other wounds.

If rabies is suspected, some authorities advocate swabbing the wound surface with 1 percent benzalkonium chloride on cotton swabs, then rinsing with sterile saline solution. Other authorities have recommended debriding the entire surface of the open wound, when possible. This consists of cutting a thin layer of tissue off the entire wound surface, including the corners, to reduce the amount of contamination.

Debridement should be done regularly in all bite wounds, even when rabies is not suspected but particularly when suturing is to be done. Debridement in one series reduced the infection rate from 69 percent to only 12 percent with dog bites. Debridement of puncture wounds is difficult and time consuming, but it should be done when gross contamination is evident.

The question of suturing bite wounds has been controversial over the years. The pendulum has swung from the strict advocacy of never suturing bite wounds. The present consensus is to close dog bite wounds, with good surgical toilette, unless they occur on the hands, where the highest risk of infection occurs. According to most authorities, cat bite wounds and human bite wounds should be left open, unless an undesirable plastic result would remain, such as with bites of the face and ears.

Bites of the hand have an unusually high predilection for becoming infected, because of the multiplicity of poorly vascularized structures. Data for dog bites show an infection rate ranging from 30 percent to 36 percent or higher when they occur on the hand. Adequate irrigation and debridement are nearly impossible because of the complicated anatomy; thus, hand bites should always receive special consideration, and closed-fist injuries should be approached aggressively. Irrigation should be thorough, with 1 percent povidone-iodine solution. Although one study showed that complications and eventual outcome were the same whether the wounds were sutured or left unsutured, this has not been a uniform observation. Hence, wounds of the hand should be left open, and the hand should be immobilized and elevated. Radiographs should be obtained to search for gas in joint spaces, which signifies violation of the joint capsule; fractures; or foreign bodies, such as tooth fragments. Those patients with diffuse swelling suspicious for joint involvement, tenosynovitis, or abscess should be admitted to the hospital for intravenous antibiotic therapy and incision and drainage.

Antibiotic Selection

At least 42 species of aerobic and anaerobic bacteria and several species of fungi have been identified in human saliva, whereas more than 64 species of bacteria have been identified in gingival scrapings and the oral and nasal fluids of dogs.

Despite the large numbers and species of bacteria, routine antibiotic therapy is not indicated for simple bite lacerations. Exceptions to this rule occur in the following situations: high-risk wounds caused by human and cat bites that penetrate the skin; bites of the hand; and bites occurring in patients at high risk for serious infection (e.g., the elderly; patients with poor vascularity and difficulty in healing, such as diabetics; patients with peripheral vascular disease; and patients with radiation changes of the skin). Treatment of patients with indwelling hardware, such as artificial heart valves, joints, or other prosthetic material, is prudent, despite the lack of studies in these patients. Asplenic patients are also at risk of overwhelming infection, so they should be treated.

Routine culturing and Gram staining of fresh wounds is

neither cost-effective nor productive. These studies are helpful, however, in established purulent infections to select an appropriate antibiotic regimen.

When used for outpatients, antibiotics should be chosen to cover the organisms most frequently associated with infections, although it is clear that there is not one single choice that can cover every ultimate pathogen. The most frequent pathogens are *Staphylococcus aureus* and the mouth anaerobes *Peptococcus, Peptostreptococcus,* and *Bacteroides* species. Other mouth organisms, such as *Eikenella corrodens* and *Fusobacterium,* from human bites, and *Streptococcus viridans, Staphylococcus aureus, Pasteurella multocida,* and dysgonic fermenter 2 (DF-2), from dog and cat bites, are potential pathogens. Enteric gram-negative infections are much less common, but may still occur, and should be considered in patients whose bite wounds become infected despite coverage for gram-positive infection, or in patients admitted with sepsis or extensive local infection from a bite wound. Many infections are mixed, with cultures growing both aerobic and anaerobic organisms. Antibiotic coverage can be refined when the offending organisms have been identified. When more than one antibiotic regimen may have similar coverage, the least expensive one should be chosen.

References

Callaham M. Controversies in antibiotic choices for bite wounds. Ann Emerg Med 1988; 17:1321.

Centers for Disease Control. Diphtheria, tetanus and pertussis: Guidelines for vaccine prophylaxis and other preventive measures. MMWR 1985; 34:405.

Centers for Disease Control. Guidelines for prevention of transmission of human immunodeficiency virus and hepatitis B virus to health-care and public-safety workers. MMWR 1989; 38(suppl 6):14.

Centers for Disease Control. Rabies prevention. MMWR 1980; 29:265.

Rest JG, Goldstein EJC. Management of human and animal bite wounds. Emerg Med Clin North Am 1985; 3:117.

Sacks JJ, Sattin RW, Bonzo SE. Dog-bite related fatalities from 1979 through 1988. JAMA 1989; 262:1489.

Wasserman GS. Wound care of spider and snake envenomations. Ann Emerg Med 1988; 17:1331.

Musculoskeletal

Monarticular Arthritis

James L. McGuire, MD
David F. Giansiracusa, MD

Definition

Monarticular arthritis is the general term applied to the involvement of a single joint with swelling, pain, or limitation of motion. Although diagnostic emphasis is placed on the acute presentation, chronic arthritis involving one joint is also a common clinical problem.

Acute Monarticular Arthritis

Etiology

The common causes of acute monarticular disease include (1) septic (staphylococcal, gonococcal), (2) crystal-induced (gout, pseudogout, hydroxyapatite), and (3) traumatic arthritis. Together they constitute 90 percent of the etiologies of this presentation. A direct approach to diagnosis is necessitated by the potentially rapid joint destruction caused by a septic process in a closed space. In addition, many of the classic connective tissue diseases can manifest in one joint. Osteoarthritis may present acutely if superimposed trauma or crystal shedding occurs. Similarly, the chronic inflammatory arthritis group, including Reiter's syndrome and rheumatoid arthritis, may present in this fashion. These disorders are discussed in the section on chronic monarticular arthritis.

Diagnostic Approach

Examination of the joint fluid is critical to the correct diagnosis. This analysis, coupled with a history, permits determination of the most likely diagnosis and treatment (Fig. 86-1).

History

From a historical point of view, the joint involved and the abruptness of onset, with or without fever or chills, start the differentiating process. A history of a similar attack in the past with complete resolution, a family history of gout or uric acid kidney stones, and long-term diuretic therapy for hypertension in an adult man or postmenopausal woman make gout a strong possibility. Acute arthritis of the knee in an elderly individual, particularly in the setting of hyperparathyroidism, raises concern about acute calcium pyrophosphate arthritis, termed *pseudogout,* whereas a flare of osteoarthritis may be due to calcium hydroxyapatite crystal-induced inflammation. The sudden onset of knee pain, aggravated by weight bearing in an elderly individual, may indicate spontaneous osteonecrosis, also termed *avascular necrosis* or *ischemic necrosis* of bone. Obviously, a history of recent trauma to the joint needs to be elicited. Because gonococcal infection may disseminate from a genitourinary focus and cause migratory arthralgias, skin rash, and monarticular arthritis, the history should include questions about sexual activity, genitourinary symptoms (penile or vaginal discharge, pelvic pain), fever, and skin rash. Because septic arthritis caused by other bacteria tends to seed previously diseased joints by hematogenous spread, the history of a flare of a single joint in a patient with rheumatoid arthritis or osteoarthritis with an infectious site such as pneumonia, cellulitis, endocarditis, or urinary tract infection is an important historical point. Because joint sepsis may also occur as a result of a penetrating injury, inquiring about such an injury and about a previous joint injection is important.

Physical Examination

The pattern of joint involvement may be diagnostic. For example, arthritis of the first metatarsophalangeal joint is strongly suggestive of gout. The knee and the wrist are the most common joints for a pseudogout attack. However, the knee may be involved in a variety of joint diseases. Fortunately, knee joint fluid can be readily obtained. A careful examination of the knee for ligamentous or cartilage abnormalities is mandatory if a history of locking, buckling, giving way, or a sense of knee unsteadiness exists. The presence of erythema diffusely around the involved joint is characteristic of both crystal-induced arthritis and sepsis. History and physical examination should search for extra-articular manifestations such as pneumonia, cellulitis, abrasions that appear to be infected, pustules on the skin (staphylococcal or gonococcal disease), penile or vaginal discharge (gonococcal disease, Reiter's syndrome), subcutaneous nodules (rheumatoid arthritis, gouty tophi), and ecchymosis (trauma), which may be important clues to the diagnosis of arthritis.

Laboratory Studies

Plain radiographs are usually negative in cases of acute monarticular arthritis, regardless of the etiology, except for soft-tissue swelling, but they may reveal signs of osteomyelitis or unsuspected trauma. Look for the presence of calcification of the articular cartilage, termed *chondrocalcinosis* (calcium pyrophosphate), or so-called rat bite or punched-out erosions with sclerotic margins (gout).

The most important aspect of the laboratory evaluation is joint fluid analysis, which should include (1) crystal analysis, (2) Gram stain and culture, (3) glucose (low in septic joints), (4) cell count (white blood cell count elevated in inflammation, red blood cell count elevated in hemarthrosis). (Synovial fluid analysis is discussed in more detail in Chapter 96, "Laboratory and Radiographic Abnormalities in Rheumatic Diseases.")

Subsequent laboratory tests, including a complete blood count, serum urate and calcium levels, erythrocyte sedimentation rate, rheumatoid factors, and blood cultures, may be indicated on the basis of the clinical presentation and synovial fluid findings.

Crystal-induced arthritis can be diagnosed by the demonstration of offending crystals under polarizing light microscopy. Monosodium urate crystals (gout) are needle-shaped and negatively birefringent. The crystals are yellow when parallel to the plane of light coming through the microscope. The mnemonic PYG (*p*arallel *y*ellow *g*out) may be helpful in remembering this relationship. Calcium pyrophosphate dihydrate (CPPD) crystals are often short and rectangular and positively birefringent. The crystals are blue when parallel to the plane of light coming through the microscope. If CPPD crystals are observed within synovial fluid leukocytes, this establishes the diagnosis of pseudogout. Such fluid should always be cultured and examined

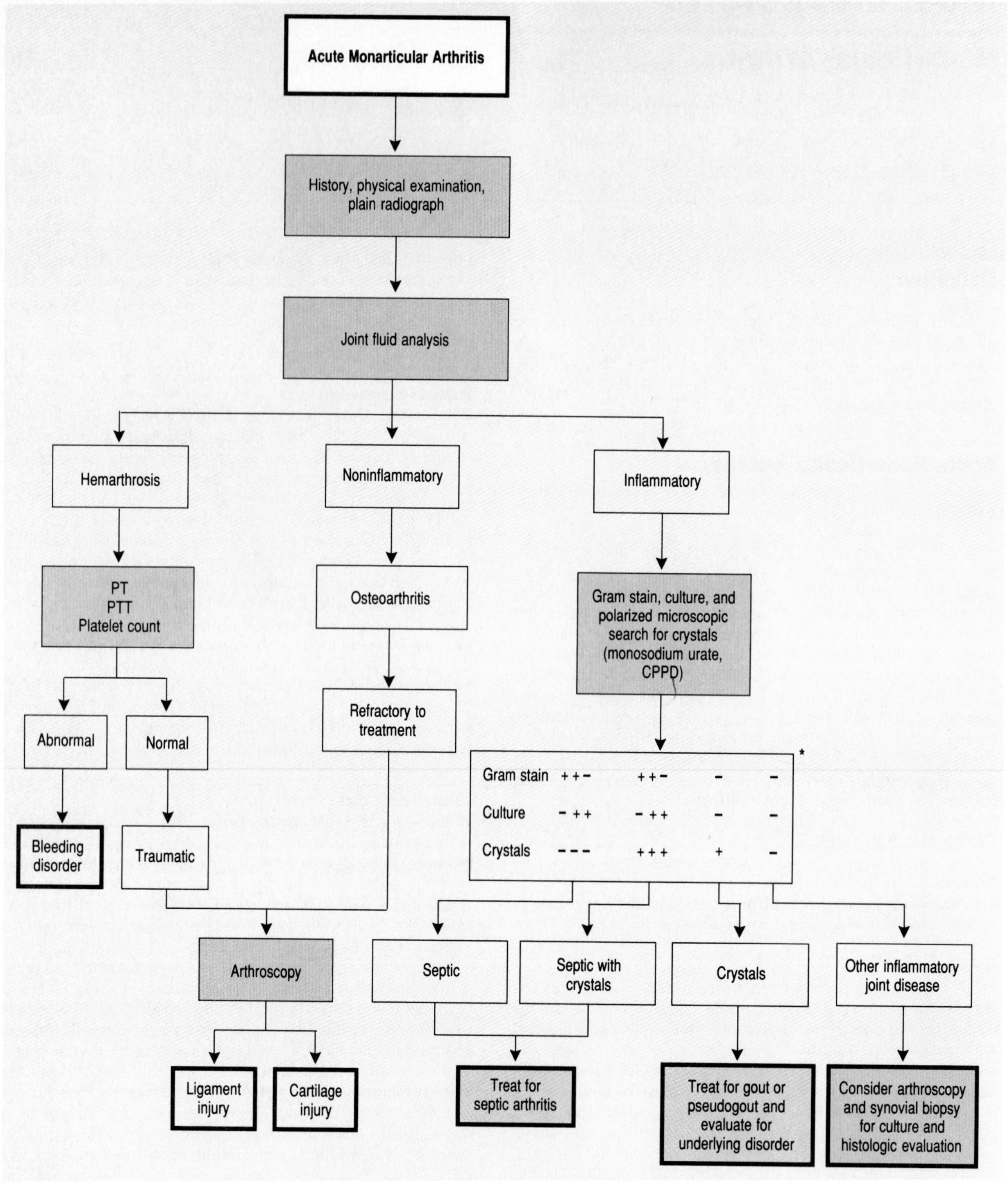

Figure 86-1 Algorithm for the diagnostic approach to the patient with acute monarticular arthritis. CPPD = calcium pyrophosphate dihydrate, PT = prothrombin time, PTT = partial thromboplastin time. *Possible combinations of Gram stain, culture, and crystal analysis.

by Gram stain, because septic arthritis may coexist with pseudogout and gout.

Risk factors for gout include age over 30 in men, postmenopausal age in women, history of uric acid stones, heavy alcohol ingestion, long-term diuretic therapy, low doses of aspirin, and obesity. Risk factors for pseudogout and chondrocalcinosis include aging, hyperparathyroidism, hypothyroidism, hypomagnesemia, diabetes mellitus, hemochromatosis, Charcot joints, and familial CPPD disease.

Because an adverse prognosis of septic arthritis is directly related to the length of time before recognition, infection within a joint must be diagnosed and treated as promptly as possible. Staphylococcal arthritis is identified on the Gram stain in approximately two-thirds of cases and is confirmed by the culture.

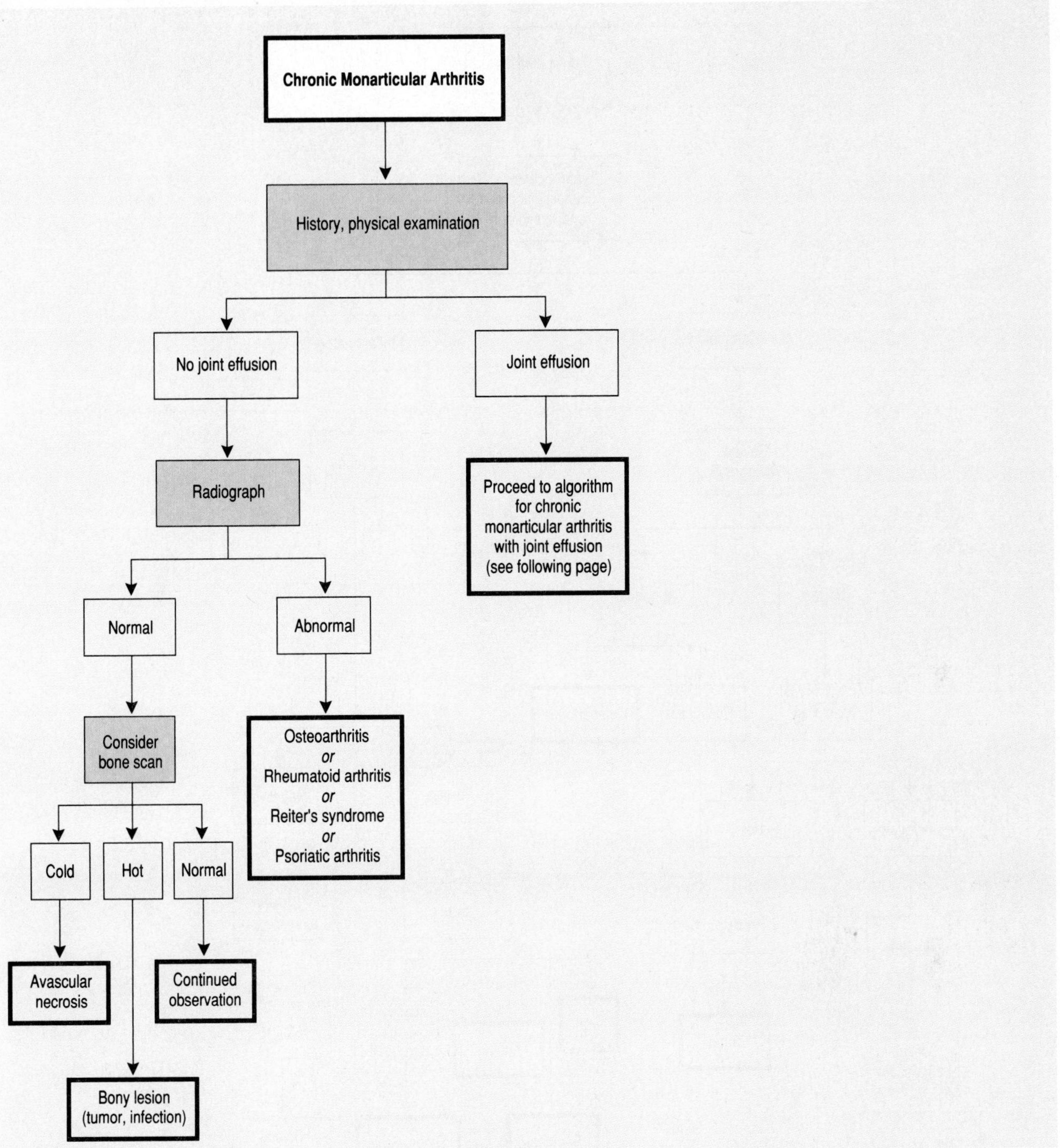

Figure 86-2 Algorithm for the diagnostic approach to the patient with chronic monarticular arthritis.

Figure continues on following page

Gonococcal arthritis is much less frequently seen on Gram stain and less frequently grows on culture. If a history of recent sexual contact exists, search carefully for extra-articular manifestations of disseminated gonococcal infection. In the presence of the skin lesions, the term *gonococcal arthritis-dermatitis syndrome* is used. Although previously rare, gram-negative bacteria are becoming a more common cause of septic arthritis, especially in the elderly and in immunosuppressed individuals. Treatment consists of antibiotics and adequate drainage.

Acute trauma to the joint with disruption of structural elements often causes a hemarthrosis. Sometimes hemarthrosis can occur spontaneously, especially in hemophiliacs and individuals who are anticoagulated. (See the discussion of synovial fluid in Chapter 96, "Laboratory and Radiographic Abnormalities in Rheumatic Diseases.")

The definition of traumatic arthritis as the result of "internal derangement," which includes ligamentous injury, chondromalacia patellae, meniscal tears, and loose bodies within the joint, has been greatly advanced by arthroscopy. This tool alone or in combination with an arthrogram allows accurate definition of the problem. Obviously, these invasive procedures are not done on all patients with a swollen knee, but they can be justified in those patients whose symptoms persist despite conservative measures (cold application, splints, non-weight bearing). Consultation with an orthopedist is an appropriate aspect of the evaluation and management of traumatic arthritis. Magnetic res-

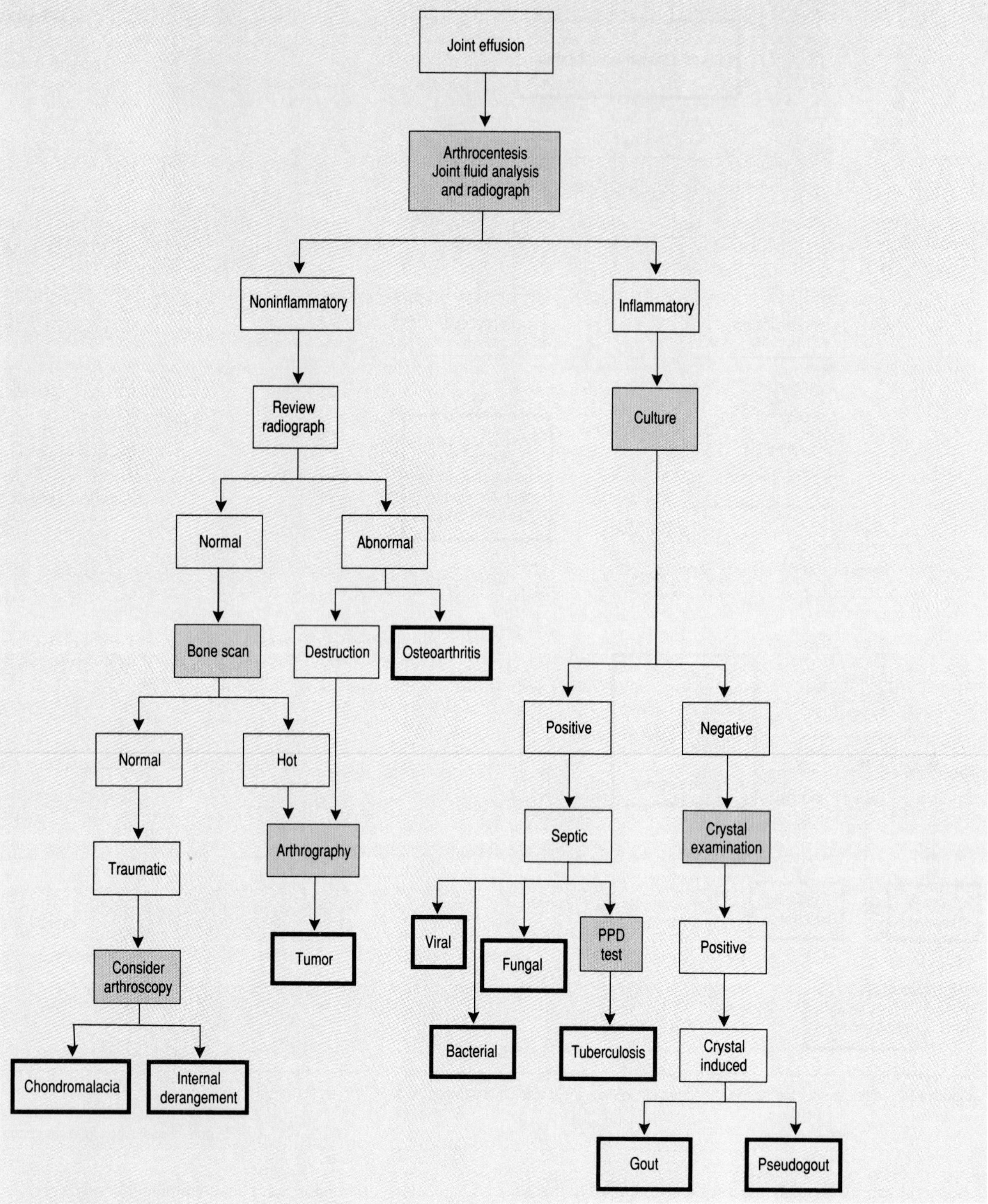

Figure 86-2 *Continued* PPD = purified protein derivative.

onance imaging (MRI) is a helpful, noninvasive technique to visualize ligamentous and meniscal injuries.

Chronic Monarticular Arthritis

Chronic monarticular arthritis (greater than 2 months' duration) is a common rheumatologic dilemma. Etiologies of chronic arthritis encompass all of the causes of acute inflammatory and noninflammatory monarticular and polyarticular arthritides. Any of the chronic disorders can present acutely if there is intercurrent trauma (hemarthrosis, internal derangement), crystal shedding (pseudogout in osteoarthritis), or infection. A systematic diagnostic approach must be applied (Fig. 86-2). Whereas in acute monarthritis the radiograph is usually normal, in chronic monarthritis, the plain radiologic evaluation and the joint fluid examination represent the diagnostic cornerstones. However, some chronic monarticular problems remain undiagnosed despite the most complete work-up, including synovial biopsy.

A noninflammatory monarticular presentation is classic for osteoarthritis. A large weight-bearing joint is often unilaterally involved. Occasionally, one of the smaller joints (distal interphalangeal, proximal interphalangeal, first carpometacarpal) in the hand is involved. Radiographic changes of a narrowed sclerotic (as opposed to demineralized) joint in a classic distribution should be considered diagnostic. When the radiograph is normal in a large joint, two important causes must be excluded.

First, structural joint problems such as cartilage and ligament tears, chondromalacia, and local bursitis may cause chronic pain and swelling. (These are discussed in Chapter 91, "Disorders of the Hip," Chapter 92, "Disorders of the Knee," and Chapter 94, "Foot and Ankle Pain.") The precipitating incident may have occurred many years before (a football injury) or may not be identified at all. The widespread use of arthroscopy has done much to clarify this differential diagnosis.

Second, avascular necrosis of bone, also termed *osteonecrosis* and *ischemic necrosis* of bone, is a common "x-ray negative" problem. The hip, shoulder, and knee are the most frequently involved joints. The diagnostic clues are a history of pain that is markedly worsened with weight bearing and use and the presence of risk factors, including steroid therapy, severe local trauma (hip fracture), hemoglobinopathies, hyperlipidemia, systemic lupus erythematosus, alcoholism, previous radiation therapy, and sickle cell disease. Underwater-tunnel workers exposed to high barometric pressures can develop avascular necrosis even if slow decompression is done. In elderly individuals, osteonecrosis may occur spontaneously (spontaneous osteonecrosis of the knee, or SONK).

The inflammatory causes, defined by joint fluid, of chronic monarticular arthritis can be grouped into septic, crystal-induced, and connective tissue diseases.

The causes of septic arthritis are similar to those of the acute presentation, but several deserve discussion. Tuberculous arthritis is usually manifested by pain and swelling over many months in a weight-bearing joint (hip, knee, ankle, spine). Active pulmonary disease is usually not apparent when the diagnosis of tuberculous arthritis is made. The final diagnosis rests on the demonstration of organisms by culture or special acid-fast stains performed on the synovial fluid or synovial biopsy specimens. A low glucose level is characteristic of this inflammatory joint fluid. The purified protein derivative (PPD) skin test is characteristically positive.

Lyme disease, a result of infection with the tick-borne spirochete *Borrelia burgdorferi,* may cause a chronic arthritis, generally of large joints, in approximately 10 percent of infected individuals. Histories of exposure to appropriate ticks, of tick bites, of the characteristic skin lesion of erythema chronicum migrans, and of neurologic or cardiac involvement consistent with Lyme disease help establish the diagnosis, which is confirmed by specific IgG antibodies against the Lyme spirochete.

Chronic bacterial monarthritis is uncommon unless inadequate therapy had been given for an acute septic process or unless a foreign body such as a hip prosthesis is present within the joint. Recently, cases of chronic sepsis of the sternoclavicular joints and sacroiliac joints with gram-negative bacteria in intravenous heroin users have been reported. Rarely do the common causes of acute septic joints (staphylococcal, gonococcal) recur chronically.

Occasionally, a "septic" arthritis may escape all diagnostic tests, especially when linked to a virus. Rubella is usually polyarticular but may remain confined to a single joint.

The incidence of the crystal-induced arthritides (gout, pseudogout) is reversed in the chronic monarticular disease. Gout is a rare cause of chronic monarthritis, although urate crystals can be demonstrated in some joints with only minimal signs of inflammation. On the other hand, pseudogout, demonstrated by the radiographic presence of articular chondrocalcinosis, is a common cause of smoldering or chronic monarthritis, which commonly affects the knees and wrists.

The connective tissue diseases may present with chronic single-joint involvement before their polyarticular involvement becomes manifest. Diagnostic techniques rely on the parameters discussed for polyarticular disorders. Rheumatoid factors, especially in high titers, HLA-B27 positivity, and synovial biopsy may help in making the diagnosis.

Neuropathic joints, also called Charcot joints, are found in a relatively classic pattern in some disease states. Tabes dorsalis results in a neuropathic arthritis of the lower extremity (knee). Joint fluid may reveal much cartilage debris and CPPD crystals. Diabetic neuropathy is a common cause of neuropathic joints in the feet, especially the tarsus. The upper limb (shoulder, elbow) may be involved in the cervical spinal cord condition of syringomyelia. In most cases, the radiographic findings include a destructive degenerative arthritis with an abundance of free bone fragments, osteophytes, and chondrocalcinosis.

References

Fletcher MR, Scott JT. Chronic monarticular synovitis. Ann Rheum Dis 1975; 34:171.

Goldenberg DL. Bacterial arthritis. In: Infections in the rheumatic diseases. In: Espinoza L, ed. New York: Grune & Stratton, 1988:3.

Goldenberg DL. Acute monarticular arthritis. In: Cohen AS, ed. Rheumatology and immunology. New York: Grune & Stratton, 1979:113.

Goldenberg DL, Reed JT. Bacterial arthritis. N Engl J Med 1985; 312:764.

McCarty DJ, ed. Crystalline deposition diseases. Rheum Dis Clin North Am 1988; 14:253.

McCune WJ. Monarticular arthritis. In: Kelley WN, et al, eds. Textbook of rheumatology. 3rd ed. Philadelphia: WB Saunders, 1989:442.

Persellin RH, Pope RM. Chronic monarticular arthritis. In: Cohen AS, ed. Rheumatology and immunology. New York: Grune & Stratton, 1979:117.

Richardson ML, ed. Magnetic resonance imaging of the musculoskeletal system. Radiol Clin North Am 1986; 24:135.

Schumacher H Jr, ed. Primer on the rheumatic diseases. 9th ed. Atlanta: The Arthritis Foundation, 1988.

Polyarthritis

David F. Giansiracusa, MD

William F. Winchell, MD

Definition

Polyarthritis refers to inflammation of a number of joints that is usually accompanied by pain and structural changes. The term *synovitis,* which literally means inflammation of the joint synovial membrane, is sometimes used as a synonym for arthritis.

Anatomy of Joints

Joints are composed of articular cartilage, which covers the ends of bones (so-called subchondral bone); synovial fluid, which is enclosed by the synovial membrane, which produces the fluid; the subsynovial connective tissues; the joint capsule, which envelops the synovial membrane and serves as a site of attachment for tendons (connective tissue structures connecting muscles to bones); and ligaments, which attach bones to bones. Nerves innervate and blood vessels perfuse the joint capsule, subsynovial connective tissue, synovial membrane, periosteum, subchondral bone, tendons, and ligaments. In contrast, the articular cartilage and synovial fluid do not contain nerves and blood vessels (see Fig. 87-1).

The components of a joint may be affected to varying degrees by different forms of arthritis. For example, osteoarthritis is characterized predominantly by damage of the articular cartilage and subchondral bone, whereas in inflammatory forms of arthritis such as rheumatoid arthritis, the synovial membrane and synovial fluid are the sites of initial involvement, and only later are the articular cartilage and subchondral bone affected.

Etiology

Polyarthritis may be the result of structural joint damage (traumatic and osteoarthritis), infection, neurologic disease (Charcot's arthropathy), crystal deposition (monosodium urate [gout], calcium pyrophosphate dihydrate [pseudogout], and hydroxyapatite), or an immunologic reaction to an infectious agent (as in rheumatic fever, polyarthritis during the prodrome of viral hepatitis B, and some cases of polyarthritis associated with Lyme disease and the arthritis of inflammatory bowel disease). A large number of inflammatory joint diseases, including the connective tissue diseases (such as rheumatoid arthritis, systemic lupus erythematosus, systemic sclerosis, polymyositis) and sarcoidosis, appear to be mediated by immunologic processes, but the actual etiologies of the disorders are *not* known.

Table 87-1 lists the most common causes of acute and chronic polyarthritis. (Chronic is arbitrarily defined as a process with a duration of more than 6 weeks.) As is evident from this table, many articular diseases may occur as acute or chronic processes. The exact order of frequency depends on demographic features.

Diagnostic Approach

The majority of rheumatic diagnoses are made on the basis of clinical information obtained by history and physical examination. Radiographic and laboratory evaluation generally help to confirm the clinical diagnosis or to establish the extent of joint disease.

In some forms of polyarthritis, specifically osteoarthritis, the joint disease is not accompanied by extra-articular manifestations. In some inflammatory forms of polyarthritis, such as rheumatoid arthritis and Reiter's syndrome, the joint disease and the extra-articular features may be manifest to an equal degree. In still other diseases, such as systemic lupus erythematosus, the joint disease may be rather minor compared with the involvement of other organ systems such as the skin, kidneys, lungs, heart, nervous system, gastrointestinal tract, and blood.

History

The most common symptom for which an individual with arthritis seeks medical attention is pain. Table 87-2 lists the essential historical features of joint pain.

Certain forms of polyarthritis have a predilection for a particular sex and age group. For example, the incidence of

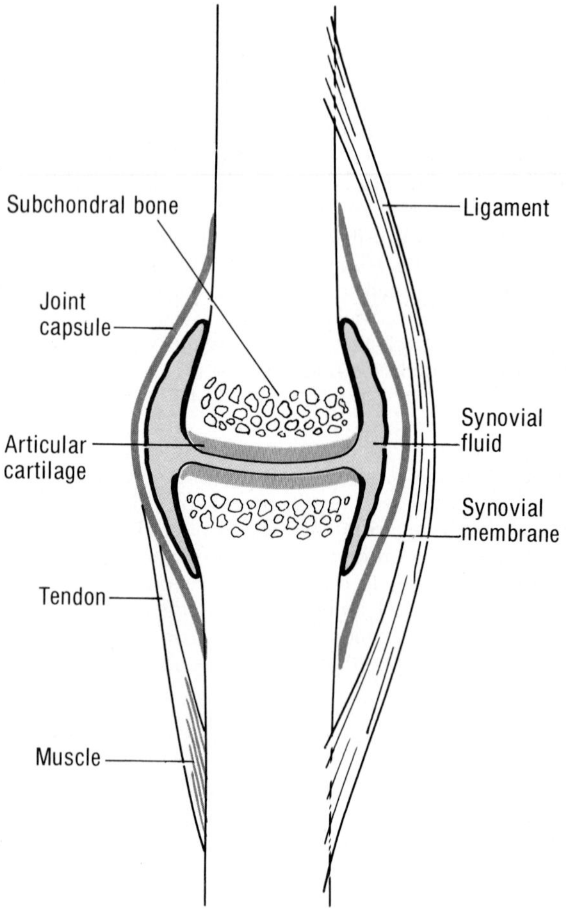

Figure 87-1 Diagram of the anatomy of a joint.

Table 87-1 Common Causes of Acute and Chronic Polyarthritis

Acute polyarthritis	Chronic polyarthritis
Rheumatoid arthritis	Osteoarthritis
Systemic lupus erythematosus	Rheumatoid arthritis
Acute rheumatic fever	Systemic lupus erythematosus
Gonococcal arthritis	Psoriatic arthritis
Reiter's syndrome	Reiter's syndrome
Ankylosing spondylitis	Arthritis of inflammatory bowel disease
Psoriatic arthritis	Lyme arthritis
Arthritis of inflammatory bowel disease	Sarcoid arthritis
Arthritis associated with viral hepatitis B	Hypertrophic osteoarthropathy
Rubella arthritis	Tophaceous gout
Arthritis of sarcoid and erythema nodosum	Calcium pyrophosphate dihydrate arthropathy
Arthritis associated with vasculitis	
Gout and pseudogout (these commonly present as monarticular arthritis)	

systemic lupus erythematosus, rheumatoid arthritis, and gonococcal arthritis is greatest among women of child-bearing age. Pseudogout and osteoarthritis are most common in elderly individuals. Gouty arthritis generally develops in men over 40 years old and in postmenopausal women.

The onset of polyarthritis of acute rheumatic fever, systemic lupus erythematosus, Lyme arthritis, and polyarticular gout tends to be migratory, in contrast with rheumatoid arthritis and osteoarthritis, in which previously affected joints remain inflamed as new joints become involved (so-called additive onset).

Involvement of a particular joint(s) may make specific diagnoses more likely, but rarely is the pattern of involvement diagnostic. For example, symmetric involvement of wrists and metacarpophalangeal (MCP) joints of the fingers is typical for rheumatoid arthritis, but this pattern may also be seen in systemic lupus erythematosus and in one form of psoriatic arthritis. However, the combination of symmetric synovitis of the wrists, proximal interphalangeal (PIP) joint, and MCP joints associated with ulnar deviation at the MCP joints, interosseous muscle atrophy, and subcutaneous nodules over pressure points is essentially diagnostic of rheumatoid arthritis. In some forms of polyarthritis, typically rheumatoid arthritis, the joint involvement is symmetric, meaning that the same joints on both sides of the body are involved. In contrast, the pattern of joint involvement in the most common form of psoriatic arthritis and gouty arthritis tends to be asymmetric.

Table 87-2 Essential Historical Features of Polyarthritis

Age and sex of affected individual
Nature of onset
Acute vs. insidious
Migratory vs. additive
Post-traumatic vs. nontraumatic
Distribution of joint involvement
Specific joints involved
Symmetry vs. asymmetry
Provoking and relieving factors: effect of particular motions, rest, previous treatment
Severity
Course of joint disease
Episodic
Constant with periods of improvement
Persistent
Progressive
Associated symptoms
Local: joint swelling, erythema, warmth, and stiffness
Systemic: detailed review of symptoms (see Table 87-3)
Socioeconomic status

Severity of the joint disease may be assessed by an evaluation of functional impairment or disabilities. Questions should attempt to assess what the individual *can* and *cannot* do with regard to occupational and household tasks, personal hygiene, recreational activities, and sexual relationships.

Consideration of the socioeconomic status of the arthritic individual is essential when assessing functional limitations and planning a treatment program. Personal support mechanisms, availability of community services, degree of immobility, and proximity to shopping and public transportation all need to be identified.

Rheumatic diseases in which family history is particularly important are osteoarthritis of the distal interphalangeal (DIP) and PIP joints, the spondyloarthropathies (Reiter's syndrome, psoriatic arthritis, and ankylosing spondylitis), hemoglobinopathies, gout, pseudogout, and rheumatoid arthritis.

In some instances, the extra-articular manifestations of the diseases may be even more helpful in making a diagnosis than is the pattern of joint involvement. As such, a detailed review of systems (Table 87-3) may suggest the presence of a multisystemic disease (such as systemic lupus erythematosus, rheumatoid arthritis, sarcoidosis, disseminated gonococcal infection, Reiter's syndrome) of which arthritis is a presenting complaint. A detailed drug history should be obtained to identify medications that may cause a drug-induced lupus-like syndrome (hydralazine, procainamide, antiepileptic drugs, and others) or a hypersensitivity reaction (penicillins, sulfonamides, thiazides, and others). A history of a bleeding disorder or use of anticoagulants is important in the evaluation of acutely swollen and painful joints.

Physical Examination

Because many forms of polyarthritis are a component of a multisystemic disease, the physical examination includes a thorough general examination with emphasis on the skin and nervous system as well as a detailed joint exam. During the general physical examination, the examiner should search specifically for the findings listed in Table 87-4. Physical examination of the joints is outlined in Table 87-5.

Radiographic Evaluation

Plain joint radiographs are an integral part of the evaluation of polyarthritis. The particular joints that are chosen for study depend on (1) the degree of involvement; (2) the likelihood of obtaining the greatest diagnostic yield, such as radiographs of the wrists and hands in a suspected rheumatoid patient versus radiographs of the sacroiliac joints and lumbosacral spine in a patient suspected of having ankylosing spondylitis; (3) the need to assess severity or progression of involvement of a specific joint; and (4) the need to evaluate for a cause of joint pain other than arthritis, such as a fracture or calcific tendonitis. The characteristic radiographic features of the common forms of arthritis are displayed in Table 96-1 in Chapter 96, "Laboratory and Radiographic Abnormalities in Rheumatic Diseases."

Laboratory Studies

Accessible synovial fluid should *always* be obtained and thoroughly analyzed. (See the section on synovial fluid analysis in Chapter 96.)

Table 87-3 Rheumatic Review of Systems

Symptoms	Disease(s) in which symptoms occur	Symptoms	Disease(s) in which symptoms occur
Constitutional		**Gastrointestinal**	
Unintentional weight loss, unexplained fevers, easy fatigability	RA, SLE, vasculitis, AS, Reiter's syndrome, sarcoidosis	Pain on swallowing (odynophagia)	SLE, Raynaud's disease, Sjögren's syndrome, RA (cricoarytenoid arthritis)
Mucocutaneous		Difficulty swallowing (dysphagia)	Scleroderma, SLE, Raynaud's disease, Sjögren's syndrome, RA, myositis
Malar erythema	SLE, dermatomyositis, MCTD	Nausea, vomiting, diarrhea, abdominal pain	SLE, vasculitis
Rashes	SLE, dermatomyositis, MCTD, psoriasis, Reiter's syndrome, juvenile RA, acute rheumatic fever, cryoglobulinemia, vasculitis, Sjögren's syndrome, scleroderma, gonococcal arthritis	Chronic diarrhea	Inflammatory bowel disease
		Genitourinary	
		Penile discharge, pain on urination (dysuria), vaginitis	Reiter's syndrome, gonococcal infection
Finger- and toenail pitting, ridging, elevation	Psoriasis, Reiter's syndrome	Pain with intercourse	Sjögren's syndrome, Behçet's syndrome
Dry eyes and/or mouth	Sjögren's syndrome	**Musculoskeletal**	
Oral ulcers	SLE, Reiter's syndrome	Joint pain, swelling, erythema, tenderness, stiffness	Inflammatory arthritis
Digital ulcers	Vasculitis (RA, SLE, scleroderma), Raynaud's phenomenon, cryoglobulinemia	Muscle aching and stiffness	SLE, RA, polymyalgia rheumatica, hypothyroidism
Subcutaneous nodules	RA, SLE, acute rheumatic fever, gout, sarcoid	Weakness (see Chapter 93, "Limb Pain and Weakness")	Polymyositis, dermatomyositis, SLE, RA, sarcoid
Annular lesion	Erythema chronicum migrans (Lyme disease)	Muscle tenderness	Polymyalgia rheumatica, severe polymyositis, SLE, RA
Eyes		**Neurologic**	
Dryness, excessive tearing, feeling of sand in eyes	Sjögren's syndrome	Headaches and visual problems	GCA, SLE, Lyme disease
Pain on exposure to light	Reiter's syndrome, AS	Scalp tenderness	GCA
Eye pain with or without redness	RA, SLE, AS, Reiter's syndrome, GCA, Behçet's syndrome, sarcoidosis	Depression	GCA, polymyalgia rheumatica, SLE, RA
Cardiovascular		Tingling, burning, numbness of hands or feet	Osteoarthritis with nerve impingement, RA, SLE, hypothyroidism, vasculitis, Lyme disease
Pleuritic chest pain	SLE, familial Mediterranean fever, RA, vasculitis, Reiter's syndrome, scleroderma		
Shortness of breath	SLE, RA, vasculitis		
Hemoptysis, epistaxis	Vasculitis, Wegener's granulomatosis, SLE		
Pallor (blanching cyanosis)	SLE, scleroderma, Raynaud's disease		
Redness of hands, feet	Vasculitis		

Abbreviations: AS = ankylosing spondylitis, GCA = giant cell arteritis, MCTD = mixed connective tissue disease, RA = rheumatoid arthritis, SLE = systemic lupus erythematosus.

Routine laboratory work, specifically complete blood counts with differential and platelet counts, blood urea nitrogen (BUN), creatinine, urinalysis, electrocardiogram, and chest radiographs should be scrutinized for evidence to suggest a possible cause of the polyarthritis. For example, leukopenia, anemia, thrombocytopenia, hematuria, proteinuria, red cell casts, an elevated BUN, and pleural effusion in a patient with polyarthritis suggest the diagnosis of systemic lupus erythematosus.

Measurement of at least one of the acute-phase proteins (see Chapter 96), usually the Westergren erythrocyte sedimentation rate (ESR), should be done to evaluate for laboratory evidence of inflammation.

Additional routine laboratory studies that may help to establish a diagnosis are liver function studies (elevated in the prodromal phase of hepatitis B) and serologic tests for syphilis (a false-positive result occurs in about 25 percent of patients with

Table 87-4 Physical Findings That May Provide Clues to Diagnosis of Polyarthritis

Physical findings	Disease(s) in which findings occur
Loss of hair (alopecia)	SLE
Oral ulcers	SLE, Reiter's syndrome, Behçet's syndrome
Conjunctivitis (iritis), uveitis	Sjögren's syndrome (often present in RA and SLE), ankylosing spondylitis, Reiter's syndrome, sarcoidosis, JRA, Behçet's syndrome, SLE
Cytoid bodies	SLE
Butterfly rash	SLE
Violaceous (lilac) or heliotrope discoloration of upper eyelids	Dermatomyositis
Sweaty palms, thenar and hypothenar erythema	Rheumatoid arthritis, SLE
Psoriatic rash, nail pitting	Psoriatic arthritis
Digital infarcts, ulcers	Digital vasospasms or vasculitis (RA, SLE, bacterial endocarditis)
Subcutaneous tender nodules	RA, SLE, gout (tophi), acute rheumatic fever
Erythematous, tender nodules over pretibial regions	Erythema nodosum (sarcoidosis)
Edematous or atrophic thickening of skin	Scleroderma
Erythematous plaques with scales over extensor surfaces of knuckles, elbows, knees	Dermatomyositis, SLE, psoriasis
Red macules and papules and annular lesions	Erythema chronicum migrans of Lyme disease
Palpable purpura	Vasculitis
Pleural effusion	SLE, RA
Pericarditis	Any connective tissue disease
Aortic insufficiency	Acute rheumatic fever, SLE, RA, ankylosing spondylitis, Reiter's syndrome
Restricted chest expansion	Spondylitis
Lymphadenopathy	SLE, RA, JRA, sarcoidosis, lymphoma
Hepatomegaly and splenomegaly	SLE, RA, JRA, sarcoidosis, infections (viral, bacterial endocarditis)
Penile rash or discharge, vaginitis	Reiter's syndrome, gonococcal arthritis
Polyneuritis, mononeuritis	Vasculitis (polyarteritis, SLE, RA)
Long-tract signs and weakness	Compressive myelopathy (RA, osteoarthritis, spondylitis)
Peripheral nerve entrapment (carpal tunnel syndrome, tarsal tunnel syndrome)	RA, gout, hypothyroidism, amyloidosis

Abbreviations: JRA = juvenile rheumatoid arthritis, RA = rheumatoid arthritis, SLE = systemic lupus erythematosus.

Table 87-5 Examination of Joints in Polyarthritis

Inspection: swelling, erythema, alignment, deformity, active range of motion of joints; overall distribution and symmetry of joint involvement

Palpation (of joints, tendons, bursal regions, and muscles): soft tissues vs. bony swelling; joint effusion; nodules; tenderness; warmth; crepitus on motion; muscle mass, tone, and strength

Passive range of motion

Provocative maneuvers: stress joints for instability; stress tendons

Posture and gait

lupus). Serologic testing for Lyme disease, specifically measurements of IgG and IgM titers to the infectious Lyme spirochete *Borrelia burgdorferi,* is now widely available.

Other, more elaborate (and usually more expensive) tests should be ordered on the basis of clinical diagnostic considerations and knowledge of the specificity, sensitivity, and implications of such tests. These tests include the antinuclear antibodies (ANA), antibodies to double-stranded deoxyribonucleic acid (DNA), rheumatoid factor, uric acid, complement levels, immunoprotein electrophoresis, serum protein electrophoresis (SPEP), quantitative immunoglobulin levels, and cryoglobulin and circulating immune complex determinations. (See Chapter 96 for more information about these tests.)

Establishing a Diagnosis of Polyarthritis

Establishing a specific diagnosis of polyarthritis depends on the collection and interpretation of historical, physical, radiographic, and laboratory evidence in the presence of extra-articular manifestations of rheumatic diseases. Because the etiology of many forms of polyarthritis is unknown, many rheumatic diagnoses are defined on the basis of a constellation of clinical and laboratory features. As such, making the diagnosis of a specific rheumatic disease almost always depends on the total picture rather than on one particular historical fact, physical finding, radiographic finding, or laboratory result. The notable exceptions are the identification of monosodium urate or calcium pyrophosphate crystals within synovial fluid leukocytes, which establishes the diagnosis of gouty arthritis or pseudogout (calcium pyrophosphate dihydrate deposition disease), respectively, and positive synovial fluid Gram stains and cultures, which establish the diagnosis of septic arthritis. It is especially important to establish the diagnosis of septic arthritis, for which specific therapy exists and which, if left untreated, may rapidly result in joint damage and functional impairment.

Table 87-6 lists clinical aspects of polyarthritis and associated features that may help in establishing a specific diagnosis. In some instances, even after thorough examination, information is inadequate to establish a diagnosis. In such cases, continued observation may allow formulation of a specific diagnosis at a later time.

Table 87-6 Clinical and Laboratory Features of Common Forms of Polyarthritis

Diagnosis	Historical features	Joints involved	Physical findings
Osteoarthritis	Middle-aged onset Gradual additive onset F > M Progressive pain, loss of motion, deformity Initially, pain only with weight bearing or motion of affected joint With progression, pain at rest and at night Morning stiffness minimal (usually 10–15 min)	Weight-bearing joints Cervical and lumbar spine Hips Knees DIP, PIP joints of fingers IP and CMC joints of thumbs MTP joint of great toe Bilateral but not symmetric (wrists, shoulders, elbows, ankles *not* involved)	Bony enlargement Joint deformity Joint-line tenderness Crepitus and pain with motion Loss of motion ± erythema, effusion, instability
Rheumatoid arthritis	Insidious, additive onset associated with prolonged (>1 hr) morning stiffness F > M Peak onset 15–50 yr of age	Symmetric involvement of large and small joints (PIP, MCP, wrist, elbow, shoulder, spine, hip, knee, ankle, tarsal, MTP joints) and cervical spine (thoracic and lumbar spine and DIP joints *not* involved)	Slight erythema Fusiform soft-tissue swelling Warmth and tenderness Restricted range of motion Muscle atrophy Flexion contractures Ulnar deviation of fingers Subcutaneous nodules
Acute rheumatic fever	Peak onset 5–15 yr of age Migratory polyarthritis	Migratory involvement of large extremity joints lasting days to weeks	Erythema, swelling, tenderness of affected joints
Systemic lupus erythematosus	Women much more frequently affected during child-bearing years (15–45) than men Joint disease may be a major or very minor aspect of this systemic illness	Symmetric involvement of finger, wrist, elbow, knee, and ankle joints	Joint and often tendon swelling, tenderness, and mild erythema
Reiter's syndrome	Peak onset late teens through 40s	Asymmetric involvement of foot and toe joints, often with tendonitis Joints of low back (sacroiliac, intervertebral, and apophyseal spinal joints)	Marked erythema, swelling, tenderness "Sausage appearance" of involved toe or finger Loss of back motion
Ankylosing spondylitis	Peak onset late teens through 40s Men more severely affected than women Profound morning low-back pain and stiffness	Joints of low back with progressive ascent up spine Hips, shoulders, knees less frequently affected	Loss of back motion and of normal spinal curvature Tender sacroiliac joints
Psoriatic arthritis	Insidious onset, almost always in individual with psoriatic skin disease of one of four types of joints (see next column)	1. Asymmetric involvement of a few peripheral joints (MTP of feet and IP of fingers and toes) 2. Symmetric pattern indistinguishable from rheumatoid arthritis 3. Involvement of spine that is similar to ankylosing spondylitis 4. Extremely destructive form of peripheral arthritis (arthritis mutilans)	Diffuse erythema and swelling of entire finger or toe; associated with psoriatic rash Fingernail pitting Loss of back motion when spine is involved

Laboratory features	Radiographic features	Course of joint disease	Extra-articular manifestations
Acute-phase proteins not elevated Noninflammatory joint fluid	Localized loss of cartilage Bony sclerosis Bone cysts Osteophytes	Progressive May have acute exacerbations	None
Elevated ESR, CRP, and other acute-phase proteins Rheumatoid factor 70–80% ANA < 50% Inflammatory joint fluid	Soft-tissue swelling Diffuse loss of joint space Small erosions at joint margins Bone cysts (bony sclerosis and osteophytes *not* present) Periarticular demineralization	10% remitted 80% smoldering with remissions and relapses 10% relentlessly progressive	Fatigue, depression Systemic involvement (eye, muscle, lung, heart, blood vessels, lymphatic system)
Antibodies to streptococcal antigens (antistreptolysin O) Elevated ESR and other acute-phase proteins	Soft-tissue swelling	90% subside in ≤ 3 mo	Fever Carditis Chorea Subcutaneous nodules Erythema marginatum
Elevated ESR antibodies to nuclear antigen in almost 100% Antibodies to DNA and to Smith antigen are specific Rheumatoid factor and elevated gamma globulins frequent Mildly inflammatory joint fluid	Soft-tissue swelling Absence of joint damage	Joint disease is usually transient, responsive to treatment, and *nondestructive*	Multisystemic involvement; fever, weight loss, fatigue, skin rash, mouth sores, hair loss; renal (glomerulonephritis); lung (pleuritis, pneumonitis); heart (pericarditis, myocarditis); nervous system (seizures, psychosis, organic brain syndrome, neuropathy); hematologic (hemolytic anemia, leukopenia, thrombocytopenia)
Elevated acute-phase proteins Inflammatory joint fluid HLA-B27 usually positive	Soft-tissue swelling Fluffy appearance of lining of bone (periosteum) Sacroiliac joint sclerosis, erosions, and fusion	Variable: self-limited, persistent	Conjunctivitis Urethritis Balanitis Keratoderma blennorrhagica Mucosal ulcers
Elevated acute-phase proteins HLA-B27 usually positive	Sacroiliac joint changes Bony bridges between vertebral bodies (syndesmophytes)	Progressive May burn out, leaving deformities	Aortic root involvement Conjunctivitis, uveitis Upper-lobe interstitial fibrosis
Elevated acute-phase proteins Inflammatory joint fluid	Destructive changes of small finger and toe joints Sacroiliac and spinal changes similar to Reiter's syndrome and ankylosing spondylitis	Usually persistent	Psoriatic rash Nail pitting

Table continues on the following page

Table 87-6 (*Continued*)

Diagnosis	Historical features	Joints involved	Physical findings
Gonococcal arthritis (see discussion of septic arthritis in Chapter 86, "Monarticular Arthritis")	Acute migratory onset Polyarthritis Sexually active F > M Dissemination during pregnancy and menses	Small and large extremity joints	Fever Pustules on erythematous hemorrhagic base Tendonitis Later, monoarthritis
Polyarticular gout (see discussion of gout in Chapter 86, "Monarticular Arthritis")	Acute, excruciating pain Men > 40 yr or postmenopausal women	Monarticular or asymmetric polyarticular MTP, great toe, ankle, knee, wrist, MCP, IP joints, and elbows	Swelling Erythema Fever ± tophi
Polyarticular calcium pyrophosphate dihydrate deposition disease (pseudogout)	F > M Incidence increased in elderly Either acute or chronic arthritis	Knees, wrists, and less commonly the MCP joints in a mon- or polyarticular fashion	Erythema Swelling Tenderness Loss of motion of affected joint(s)

Diagnosis	Laboratory features	Radiographic features	Course of joint disease	Extra-articular manifestations
Gonococcal arthritis	Elevated acute phase proteins Positive blood, joint, or urethral, vaginal, pharyngeal, rectal cultures Very inflammatory joint fluid	Soft-tissue swelling Joint effusions	Responsive to antibiotic therapy	(As per history and physical examination)
Polyarticular gout	Visualization of monosodium urate crystals within synovial fluid leukocyte is diagnostic	Punched-out erosions, joint-space loss, bone cysts, and localized soft-tissue swellings with stippled calcification in chronic gout	Episodic, progressing to chronic, destructive arthritis	Fever Peripheral leukocytosis
Polyarticular calcium pyrophosphate deposition disease (pseudogout)	Visualization of rhomboid-shaped positively birefringent crystals within synovial fluid leukocytes and negative Gram stain and cultures of synovial fluid	Linear or punctate calcification of articular cartilage (articular chondrocalcinosis)	Chronic with exacerbations and remissions	CPPD may be associated with hypothyroidism, hyperparathyroidism, hypomagnesemia, hemochromatosis, and diabetes mellitus

Abbreviations: ANA = antinuclear antibodies, CMC = carpometacarpal, CPPD = calcium pyrophosphate dihydrate deposition disease, CRP = C-reactive protein, DIP = distal interphalangeal, ESR = erythrocyte sedimentation rate, F > M = more women than men are affected, HLA = human leukocyte antigen, IP = interphalangeal, MCP = metacarpophalangeal, MTP = metatarsophalangeal, PIP = proximal interphalangeal.

References

Cohen AS, Bennett JC, eds. Rheumatology and immunology. 2nd ed. Orlando: Grune & Stratton, 1986.

Espinoza L, et al, eds. Infections in the rheumatic diseases. Orlando: Grune & Stratton, 1988.

Katz WA. The diagnosis of monarticular and polyarticular rheumatic disorders. In: Katz WA, ed. Rheumatic diseases: Diagnosis and management. 2nd ed. Philadelphia: JB Lippincott, 1988:751.

McCarty DJ, ed. Arthritis and allied conditions. 11th ed. Philadelphia: Lea & Febiger, 1989.

Moskowitz RW. Acute polyarthritis (Chap. 6). Subacute and chronic polyarthritis (Chap. 7). In: Moskowitz RW. Clinical rheumatology. 2nd ed. Philadelphia: Lea & Febiger, 1982:101, 118.

Polly HF, Hunder GG. Rheumatologic interviewing and physical examination of the joints. 2nd ed. Philadelphia: WB Saunders, 1978.

Schumacher HR, ed. Primer on the rheumatic diseases. 9th ed. Atlanta: The Arthritis Foundation, 1988.

Sergent JS. Polyarticular arthritis. In: Kelley WN, et al, eds. Textbook of rheumatology. 3rd ed. Philadelphia: WB Saunders, 1989:455.

Back Pain

88

David F. Giansiracusa, MD
Harold A. Wilkinson, MD
James L. McGuire, MD

The causes of low-back pain are numerous (Table 88-1). Back pain may be the result of disorders within the back itself or pathology elsewhere that results in radiation or referral of pain to the back. The specific etiology of back pain can often be established if the examiner performs a thorough history and physical examination and correctly interprets appropriate laboratory and radiographic studies.

History

The interviewer should elicit a thorough description of the back pain, noting the following: quality (tingling, aching, dull, sharp, burning), location, radiation, intensity, duration, nature of onset, course (intermittent, persistent, progressive), pattern of discomfort over the course of each day, and aggravating as well as relieving factors. The interviewer should also determine any associated symptoms, weakness or numbness, bowel or bladder dysfunction, and the degree of the resultant functional impairment (disability).

Most cases of back pain may be described as (1) radicular, (2) deep or poorly localized, or (3) well localized. Radicular pain is usually unilateral and is characterized by radiation into the lower leg. It is often felt in the lower back, buttock, or posterior thigh as well, but pain in these areas that does not radiate distally into the leg is usually *not* radicular but related to bones or joints. Radicular discomfort in the leg indicates pressure on or injury to a lumbar nerve root(s). The specific pattern of pain radiation or neurologic loss may help to identify the specific nerve root(s) that is (are) affected. When the nerve roots that contribute to the sciatic nerve are involved, the process is termed *sciatica*. Although sciatica often is due to nerve root impingement by a ruptured or herniated disk, other processes that cause nerve root damage (such as nerve infarct secondary to diabetes mellitus or vasculitis) or bony impingement (such as by a facet joint osteophyte in the case of lateral recess lumbar spinal stenosis, and forward subluxation of the lower lumbar vertebrae, so-called spondylolisthesis) may be responsible for the radicular pain, as may be a mass lesion within the spinal canal.

Poorly localized pain may suggest a diffuse back disorder, any process accompanied by generalized paraspinous muscle spasm, or an intra-abdominal, intraperitoneal, or intrapelvic process with a wide distribution of referred pain.

In contrast, localized pain may allow the patient to direct the examiner to the specific site of pathology, such as a discrete tender point in the soft tissues, or at the level of an infected intervertebral disk or vertebral body compression fracture.

The nature of the onset and course of the presenting complaint can often provide valuable diagnostic clues. For example, pain from a dissecting aneurysm, back strain, or osteoporotic vertebral compression fracture may develop acutely. In contrast, pain due to osteoarthritis of the spine or spondylitis tends to have an insidious onset and chronic course.

The pattern of pain during the course of the day may help limit the differential diagnoses. The pain associated with mechanical problems such as back strains, osteoporotic compression fractures, and herniated disks tends to be minimal on waking in the morning and worsens with the course of the day's activities. In contrast, the pain of inflammatory back disease (spondylitis) such as ankylosing spondylitis, psoriatic spondylitis, spondylitis associated with inflammatory bowel disease, and Reiter's syndrome tends to be most severe (and associated with stiffness) on awakening in the morning.

The relationship of pain to activity is extremely important diagnostically. Many causes of back pain are aggravated by bending or lifting, but ambulation specifically aggravates the discomfort caused by spinal stenosis, and recumbency may aggravate the pain of intraspinal neoplasms. Osteoarthritis of lumbar facet joints tends to cause pain that is aggravated with back extension.

Identification of associated symptoms is of paramount importance. For example, the history of back pain associated with weight loss, night sweats, chills, feverishness, and tender nodules on the fingertips (Osler's nodes) raises a strong concern of bacterial endocarditis. Low-back pain in an individual with a history of pain on urination, conjunctivitis, and heel pain may be due to spondylitis associated with Reiter's syndrome, whereas back pain associated with nausea, vomiting, and abdominal pain in an alcohol abuser may be due to pancreatitis.

Physical Examination

Examination of the spine should concentrate on four areas. First, a careful general examination should be performed, with special attention given to the pelvis, abdomen, and rectum. This is critical for diagnosing problems that originate in locations other than the back, such as from aortic aneurysms, in the gallbladder or pelvic organs, and from malignant diseases.

Second, the back itself is examined for palpable, tender local trigger points, muscle tenderness and spasm, spinal deformity (scoliosis), kyphosis, cutaneous lesions (pilonidal sinus, midline nevi), and range of motion. The latter is best described in terms of degree of motion in forward, backward, and lateral bending. Straight-leg raising suggests nerve root entrapment if distal sciatic leg pain is produced, or problems with hip or lower back bones and joints if pain in the lower back and buttocks is elicited. Tenderness over areas of vertebral osteomyelitis or metastatic cancer may be more apparent on percussion than on palpation.

The third aspect of the physical assessment of the back is a thorough examination of the hip, because arthritis of this joint can manifest as back pain.

Finally, the neurologic examination must be done carefully. Early in the disease course, findings can be very subtle. Close attention must be paid to deep tendon reflexes, muscle-group strength testing, and the sensory examination in order to localize a radiculopathy. Sacral and perianal sensory testing and testing of rectal sphincter tone are important to document cauda equina dysfunction. In general, the level of nerve impingement can be predicted from the physical findings (Table 88-2); however, computed tomography (CT), magnetic resonance imaging (MRI), myelography, and surgery may still demonstrate nerve root compression at a different level from that suspected clinically. Algorithms for the diagnostic approach to back pain after a complete history and physical examination are shown in Figure 88-1.

Table 88-1 Common Causes of Back Pain

Mechanical:
- Trauma: fracture, ligmentous tears, muscle strain, disk rupture, retroperitoneal hematoma
- Acute or chronic muscle strain or spasm
- "Flabby back syndrome"
- Degenerative disk disease
- Intervertebral disk herniation or rupture
- Arachnoiditis
- Spinal stenosis or lateral recess stenosis
- Spondylolisthesis
- Pseudarthrosis of spinal fusion
- Acquired pseudomeningocele (after trauma or surgery)

Arthritis:
- Ankylosing spondylitis
- Spondylitis associated with psoriasis, Reiter's syndrome, inflammatory bowel disease, or *Yersinia histolytica* infection
- Osteoarthritis of facet joints and intervertebral joints
- Aseptic (inflammatory) diskitis
- Gout
- Rheumatoid arthritis

Infectious:
- Retroperitoneal abscess
- Epidural abscess
- Intervertebral septic diskitis
- Osteomyelitis
- Myalgias of back muscles associated with bacterial endocarditis

Bony disease affecting the spine:
- Osteoporosis with compression fractures
- Osteomalacia
- Paget's disease of bone
- Malignancy metastatic to spine
- Multiple myeloma

Primary spinal tumors:
- Lipoma
- Teratoma
- Epidermoid
- Chordomas
- Hemangioblastomas
- Gliomas: ependymomas, astrocytomas
- Meningiomas
- Schwannomas (neurofibroma)

Pain referred to low back (particularly from retroperitoneal structures):
- Dissecting aortic aneurysm
- Pancreatitis, pancreatic carcinoma
- Cholecystitis
- Penetrating peptic ulcer
- Lymphoma
- Pyelonephritis
- Nephrolithiasis
- Disease of pelvic organs
- Rectal or prostatic cancer

Psychogenic

Radiographic Evaluation

Routine radiographic evaluation of the lumbar spine includes the standard anteroposterior (AP), lateral, and oblique views. Special AP pelvic radiographs in which the beam is directed 30 to 40 degrees above the horizontal may help to evaluate the sacroiliac joints. Oblique views may be valuable in evaluating facet joints and sacroiliac joints. Polytomography or CT should be used if one area is suspect or obscured by other structures. The presence of osteopenia (demineralization) or osteoarthritic changes on radiographs are a common finding in the elderly. Although these conditions may cause pain, their presence radiographically does not prove that osteopenia or osteoarthritis is the cause of the patient's discomfort. Alternative explanations must also be considered.

The intervertebral disk spaces are radiolucent. Therefore, degenerative disk disease can only be appreciated on plain radiographs as narrowing of the space(s) between the vertebral bodies or localized degenerative changes, neither of which is diagnostic of disk rupture.

Myelography is extremely helpful in diagnosing lumbar disk rupture, but it may be normal despite disk rupture or may be abnormal because of degenerative spurs. Myelography usually provides definitive evidence of intraspinal tumors or arachnoiditis.

The radioisotope bone scan using technetium-99 is a sensitive but nonspecific test for evaluating early inflammatory, neoplastic, and metabolic bone disorders before findings can be detected by plain-film radiographs. Unfortunately, a normal bone scan may be observed in a variety of diseases, including mechanical back problems, traumatic injuries, and even multiple myeloma.

CT scans have become an excellent noninvasive adjunct to the myelogram for defining the volume and shape of the spinal canal and the presence of disk herniation. Moreover, the CT scan may identify mass lesions in the spine, pelvis, or retroperitoneal region that previously could be visualized only by more invasive studies such as arteriography and lymphangiography.

High-resolution images, particularly of soft tissues, that are obtained without the use of ionizing radiation are characteristics of MRI that have made this a valuable noninvasive procedure in evaluating for disk herniations, intramedullary mass lesions, arachnoiditis, and even infiltrative marrow processes.

Pelvic and abdominal ultrasonography may be helpful in evaluating causes of pain referred to the back. Discography and epidural venography or epidurography may help to define pathology in the intervertebral disks and spinal canal, respectively.

Text continues on page 376

Table 88-2 Physical Findings of Lumbar Nerve Root Compression Due to Disk Rupture

Level of disk	Nerve root	Deep tendon reflex	Muscle weakness	Sensory loss
L2-L3	L3	—	Hip flexion and knee extension	Anterior thigh
L3-L4	L4	Patellar	Knee extension and foot inversion	Medial aspect of the foot
L4-L5	L5	Tibialis anterior*	Dorsiflexion of foot and first toe	Dorsum of the foot and anterior shin
L5-S1	S1	Achilles	Plantar flexion and eversion of the foot	Lateral aspect of the foot and calf

* This reflex is usually difficult to elicit even in normal individuals.

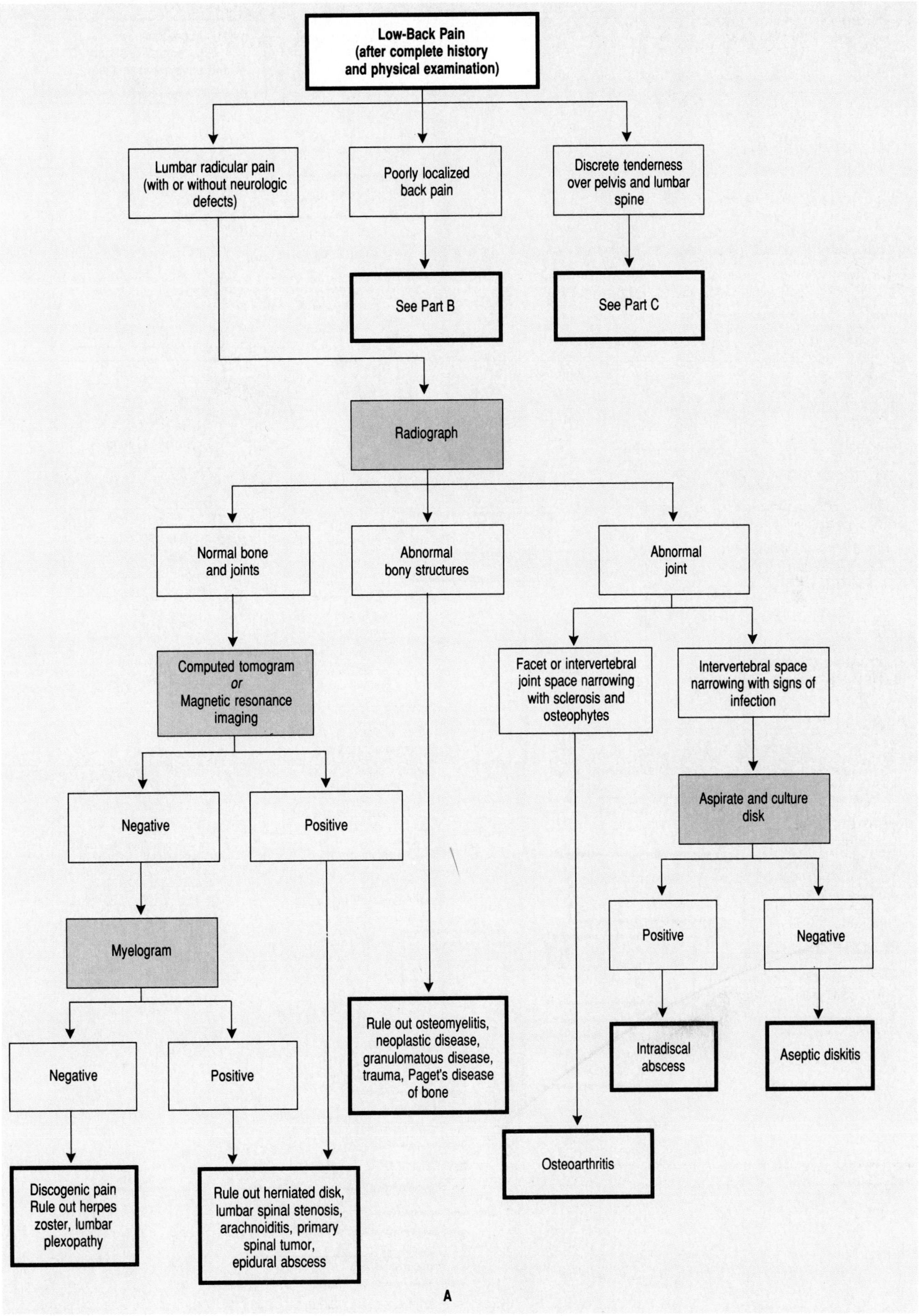

Figure 88-1 Algorithm for the diagnostic approach to back pain. (**A**) Lumbar radicular pain.

Figure continues on following page

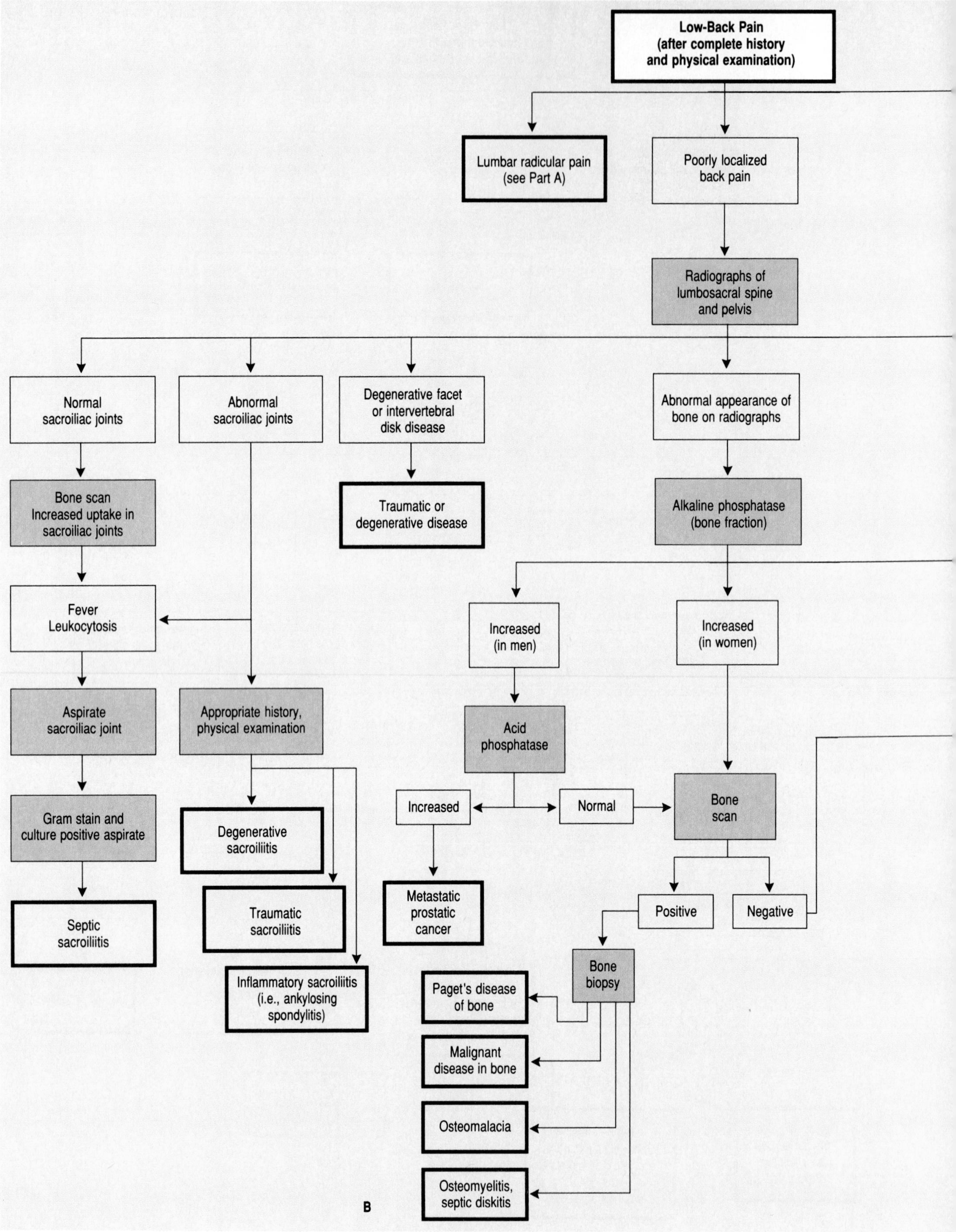

Figure 88-1 (**B**) Poorly localized back pain.

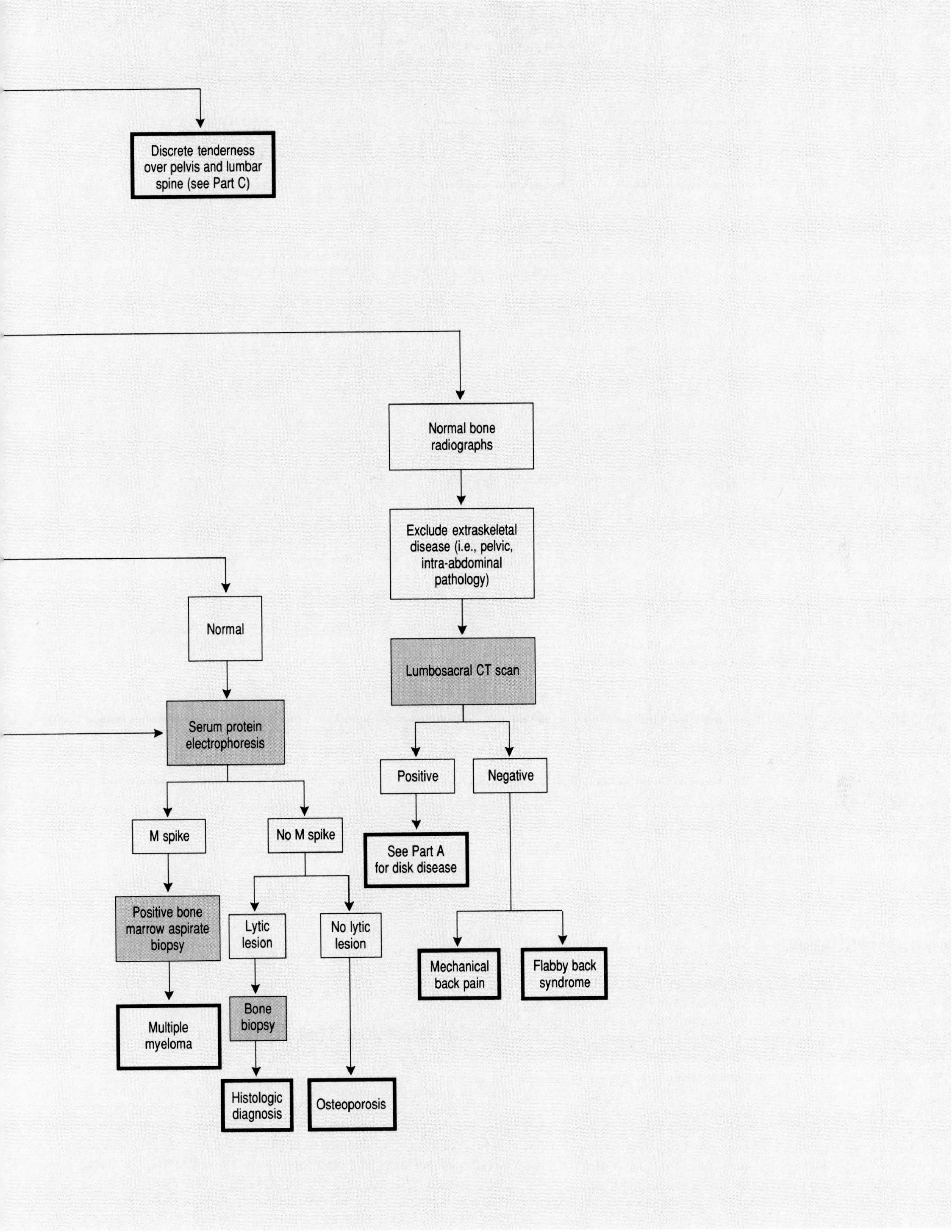

Figure continues on following page.

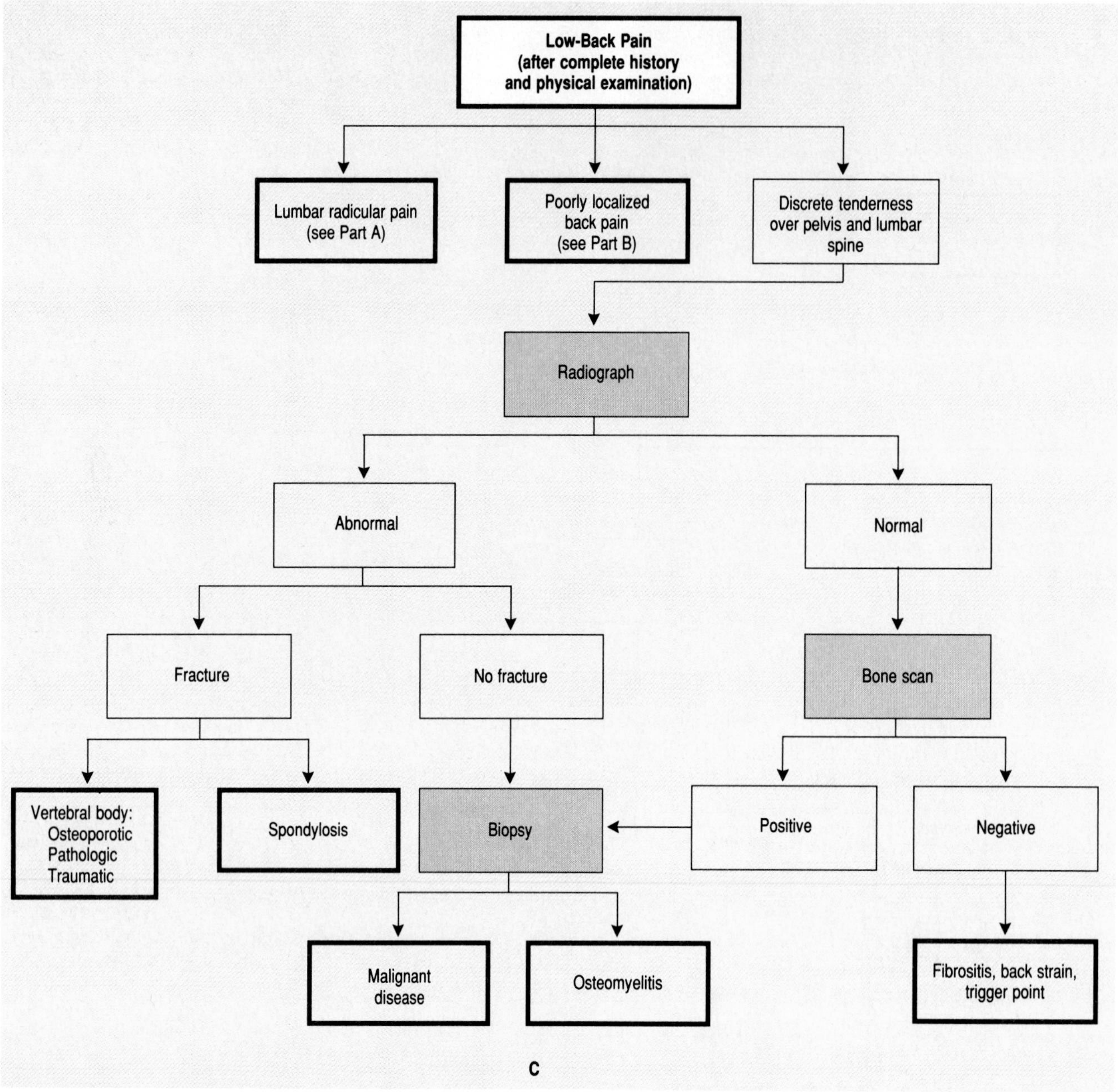

Figure 88-1 (**C**) Discrete tenderness over pelvis and lumbar spine.

Laboratory Studies

The laboratory can give valuable clues to the cause of back pain. Alkaline phosphatase is elevated in a variety of bone disorders (Paget's disease of bone, osteomalacia, multiple myeloma, neoplastic disease metastatic to bone), whereas it is normal in osteoporosis. The acid phosphatase and prostate specific antigen (PSA) levels are elevated in metastatic prostate cancer but normal in all other common bone diseases. An elevated erythrocyte sedimentation rate (ESR) is nonspecific but helpful in differentiating mechanical disorders from inflammatory, infectious, and neoplastic disorders, which elevate the ESR. The presence of leukocytosis, especially when associated with a left shift, suggests a septic process or marrow involvement. The urinalysis and stool guaiac should be examined for evidence of renal and bowel disease. Recently, the availability of HLA-B27 testing has become widespread in the evaluation of chronic back disorders and, when coupled with the appropriate history and physical findings of sacroiliitis, even in the absence of radiographic changes, suggests the presence of a spondyloarthropathy.

Specific Disorders That Cause Back Pain

The most common cause of back pain, the so-called flabby back syndrome, is characterized by pain in the soft tissues as a result of poor muscle tone (caused by inactivity, obesity, or neuromuscular disease) and poor posture, which leads to muscle fatigue and discomfort. Often there is no history of antecedent trauma. Some back stiffness and pain on motion are common. The back pain may be chronic and punctuated by acute exacerbations. Physical examination may reveal limited back motion, tenderness to palpation and percussion, and pain referred in a dermatomal distribution. Abnormal neurologic findings are characteristically absent.

Localized myofascial trigger points and generalized fibrositis are soft-tissue disorders that cause back pain. Fibrositis is a chronic, painful disorder in which tender points occur in a stereotypic distribution over the bony pelvis and in the lumbar paraspinous and gluteal muscles. Isolated trigger points are discrete for pain and tenderness at muscle-insertion sites onto bone, most commonly at the posterior iliac spinous processes. Little relief is afforded either condition by therapeutic doses of aspirin or other anti-inflammatory drugs. Muscle relaxants may be nearly curative of fibrositis but rarely relieve muscle-insertion trigger-point pain. Heat almost always helps, whereas changes in weather may aggravate the symptoms. The patient with fibrositis often complains of "good days and bad days" with intermittent morning stiffness. Patients may be emotionally labile and cry spontaneously during the interview. A history of trauma is more often obtained with myofascial trigger points than fibrositis and may cause confusion with mechanical low-back problems. All laboratory test results are normal in both groups of patients. The dramatic, instantaneous response to local anesthetic injections into myofascial and fibrositic tender points may be both diagnostic and therapeutic, especially if these are coupled with injection of steroids. Biopsies of soft tissues have not identified any evidence of inflammation. Fibrositis may be a pain syndrome that results from excessive muscle tension and a nonrestorative sleep disorder, and myofascial trigger points seem to result from excessive muscle tension, which is often perpetuated by an underlying painful process in the back.

Pain due to a herniated disk may be preceded by a snapping or popping sensation in the back, often in association with trauma. The back pain tends to be severe and incapacitating and later radiates in the distribution of the affected nerve. The patient often lists to the unaffected side and has difficulty standing, walking, and sitting. Lumbar muscle spasm and tenderness are usually present. Maneuvers that increase intra-abdominal pressure, such as coughing, sneezing, and straining, and straight-leg raising and extension of the knee while the patient is sitting typically increase the back and radicular pain. The specific neurologic findings depend on the level of the disk protrusion(s) (see Table 88-2).

The presence of daily, prolonged morning stiffness, limited back flexion, sacroiliitis on pelvic radiographs, syndesmophytes on lumbosacral spinal films, and frequently a positive HLA-B27 define a group of disorders labeled spondyloarthropathies. The HLA-B27 antigen is present in approximately 50 to 90 percent of individuals with inflammatory sacroiliitis or spondylitis; it also occurs in approximately 10 percent of the normal Caucasian population. As such, the presence of the HLA-B27 antigen is consistent with a spondyloarthropathy, but it is not diagnostic in and of itself. The diagnosis is also dependent on the *history* of morning low-back pain and stiffness, the *physical findings* of restricted back motion and sacroiliac joint tenderness, and *radiographic evidence* of sacroiliitis, often associated with radiographic changes of spondylitis. (A discussion of ankylosing spondylitis, the spondylitis of inflammatory bowel disease, Reiter's disease, and psoriatic arthritis is also included in Chapter 87, "Polyarticular Arthritis.") It should be noted that Reiter's disease, especially when predated by an infection such as *Shigella, Salmonella, Yersinia,* or *Campylobacter,* is also called reactive arthritis.

Diseases of bone may cause diffuse, dull back pain. Osteomalacia characteristically causes poorly localized back pain. The presence of an elevated alkaline phosphatase level and a low serum phosphate level combined with pseudofractures seen on radiographs makes the diagnosis. In contrast, osteoporosis is not usually a painful disorder until either an acute vertebral body compression fracture occurs or altered alignment of the spine results in mechanical low-back strain. Paget's disease of bone commonly involves the vertebrae and pelvis. Pain can result from the involved bone itself, pathologic fractures, or the resultant premature osteoarthritis caused by the bone's nonyielding character. Laboratory and radiographic features of Paget's disease of bone are elevated levels of alkaline phosphatase, cortical and trabecular thickening and bone enlargement on radiographic studies, and increased activity on bone scans. (See Chapter 138, "Musculoskeletal Pain in the Elderly," for more discussion of these bone diseases.)

Other causes of back pain due to bony involvement are metastatic, malignant, and infectious disease. Prostate cancer frequently metastasizes to the lumbar spine and pelvis and is associated with elevated acid phosphatase and PSA levels. Other types of metastatic malignancies, most commonly carcinoma of the breast, kidney, lung, thyroid, and ovary, cause combinations of back pain, radicular pain, and neurologic deficits. Percussion tenderness is characteristic over the level of spinal involvement. Multiple myeloma can manifest as back pain. Radiographs show either discrete osteolytic "punched-out" lesions or diffuse demineralization. Osteomyelitis of a vertebral body typically causes back pain and chills. The physical examination usually reveals fever, paraspinal muscle tenderness and spasm, spine tenderness on percussion, and limited back motion. Although radiographs are often negative, particularly in early disease, technetium bone scans, as well as gallium or white blood cell scans, are usually positive. Epidural abscess usually causes back pain before radiculopathy develops; radiculopathy may be secondary to local septic vasculitis and, therefore, may be abrupt in onset and permanent.

Back pain may be referred from a number of pathologic processes within the thorax, abdomen, retroperitoneum, or pelvis, rather than emanate from structures in the back itself (see Table 88-1). Such referred pain tends to be poorly localized. CT, MRI, ultrasonic scans of the abdomen, intravenous pyelograms, and pelvic and rectal examinations have improved the diagnostic accuracy in the previously "hidden" retroperitoneal area.

References

Arnett FC. Seronegative spondylarthropathies. Bull Rheum Dis 1987; 37(1):1.

Borenstein DG, Wiesel SW. Low back pain. Philadelphia: WB Saunders, 1988.

Calin A, ed. Spondylarthropathies. New York: Grune & Stratton, 1984.

Finneson BE, Katz WA. The lower back and pelvis. In: Katz WA, ed. Diagnosis and management of rheumatic diseases. 2nd ed. Philadelphia: JB Lippincott, 1988:104.

Hall H. Examination of the patient with low back pain. Bull Rheum Dis 1983; 33(4):1.

Macnab I. Backache. Baltimore: Williams & Wilkins, 1977.

Moskowitz RW. Low back pain. In: Clinical rheumatology. 2nd ed. Philadelphia: Lea & Febiger, 1982:283.

Sheon RP, Moskowitz RW, Goldberg VM. The low back. In: Soft tissue rheumatic pain. 2nd ed. Philadelphia: Lea & Febiger, 1987:159.

Spengler DM. Low back pain. New York: Grune & Stratton, 1982.

Stanton-Hicks M, Boas R. Chronic low back pain. New York: Raven Press, 1982.

Hand Complaints

89

David F. Giansiracusa, MD

Steven L. Strongwater, MD

The hand performs a multitude of important functions. Pain, weakness, numbness, and deformity often prompt medical attention and may be due to trauma, skin or soft-tissue infection, muscle cramps, arthritis, tendonitis, vascular or neurologic disorders, or the shoulder-hand syndrome (reflex sympathetic dystrophy) (Table 89-1). Diagnosis of a specific problem is paramount, not only in guiding appropriate treatment but also in providing clues to the presence of a systemic disease.

Diagnostic Approach

A thorough history should include the nature and onset of symptoms; the duration, frequency, constancy, severity, location, and radiation of pain; aggravating and alleviating factors; the presence or absence of color changes, swelling, stiffness, parethesias, and functional impairment; and the effects of rest and exercise. Attempts should be made to localize the discomfort to the skin, tendons, joints, bones, muscles, nerves, or blood vessels by history and physical examination.

A patient may have a sense of swelling even though the hand may not appear swollen on inspection. A more objective and reliable indication is a history of inability to remove a ring or wear gloves that previously fit.

The complaint of stiffness following inactivity, usually most profound on awakening, may also be difficult to elicit by history. Morning stiffness is suggested by difficulty opening jars and turning knobs on doors until "loosening up," after which it is no longer difficult to perform these routine tasks. Prolonged and profound morning stiffness is a common feature of rheumatoid arthritis, and its duration actually reflects the activity of the disease.

Numbness, burning, tingling, heaviness, clumsiness, and weakness suggest that the primary cause of hand pain is neurologic. Determining the exact location of the symptoms and pattern of radiation will permit localization of the lesion (see Table 89-1). The complaint of weakness must be distinguished from functional loss due to pain as opposed to true motor weakness due to direct nerve injury (e.g., carpal tunnel syndrome).

Table 89-1 Common Causes of Hand Pain and Dysfunction

Trauma:
  Thermal trauma (cold, heat)
  Sprain
  Dislocation
  Fracture
  Contusion
	Arthritis

Skin and soft-tissue infections:
  Paronychia
  Furuncle
  Dermatitis
  Cellulitis
  Felon
	Vascular disorders:
	  Obstructive peripheral vascular disease
	  Thrombophlebitis
	  Digital vasospastic disorders (Raynaud's phenomenon)
	  Vasculitis

Muscle cramps	Neurologic disorders:
	  Neuritis
	  Neuropathies
	  Nerve compression or entrapment

Tendonitis	

Swelling, erythema, tenderness, and pain on motion of a joint suggest an inflammatory joint process, known as arthritis or synovitis. In contrast, the inability to move a finger with initial effort until it suddenly gives way, termed "triggering," indicates involvement of the tendon apparatus. Other symptoms suggestive of tendonitis include snapping, clicking, and a rubbing sensation as well as swelling and tenderness when stressing the tendon.

A final and very important aspect of the history regarding hand complaints is the evaluation of the presence and severity of functional impairment. Questions such as "Can you open jars, button clothing, cut your meat, lift objects with your hands, and write with a pen or pencil?" address these issues. A distinction should be made between fine and gross motor functional impairment. Does the severity of the functional impairment(s) vary throughout the course of the day or with a particular activity? Patients with rheumatoid arthritis tend to have the greatest dysfunction on awakening, in contrast to those with osteoarthritis, who have the greatest difficulty with repetitive activity.

Physical Examination

The physical examination of the hand begins with the introductory handshake, when the muscle and soft tissue mass, strength, temperature, moisture, presence of gross deformities, and degree of tenderness can be assessed. Casual inspection of the hands during the interview, when hand posture, ease of holding an object, and pointing can be observed, provides additional information.

As is the case with physical examination of other areas of the body, the general examination of the hand should proceed in an orderly fashion, beginning with inspection and palpation.

Inspection of the hands (Fig. 89-1) should include examination of the overall configuration of the hands, muscle mass, color, skin creases, ulcers, hair pattern, swelling, and deformities. Fingernails should be examined for pitting, ridging, splinter hemorrhages, and clubbing. Areas of erythema and swelling should be evaluated to determine whether they represent a joint, a tendon, or a more generalized process such as cellulitis. Although swelling of the metacarpophalangeal joints may not be apparent in the extended position, loss of the normally present "valleys" between the knuckles when a closed fist is made may reveal swelling. Inspection should also encompass assessment of active joint motion, including hand grasp. When evaluating range of motion, remember that loss of motion may be a result of disease in the bone, joint, muscle, tendon, nerve, or soft tissues.

Palpation is performed to evaluate muscle mass (particularly the interosseous muscles and muscles of the thenar and hypothenar eminences), to assess joint swelling, to distinguish bony from soft-tissue proliferation, to localize nonarticular tenderness, and to evaluate vascular integrity (checking the radial pulse and capillary filling). Stress maneuvers of a particular tendon may be performed to localize the presence of tendonitis or a tear.

Because neurologic symptoms that are appreciated in the hands may be the result of nerve impingement proximal to the

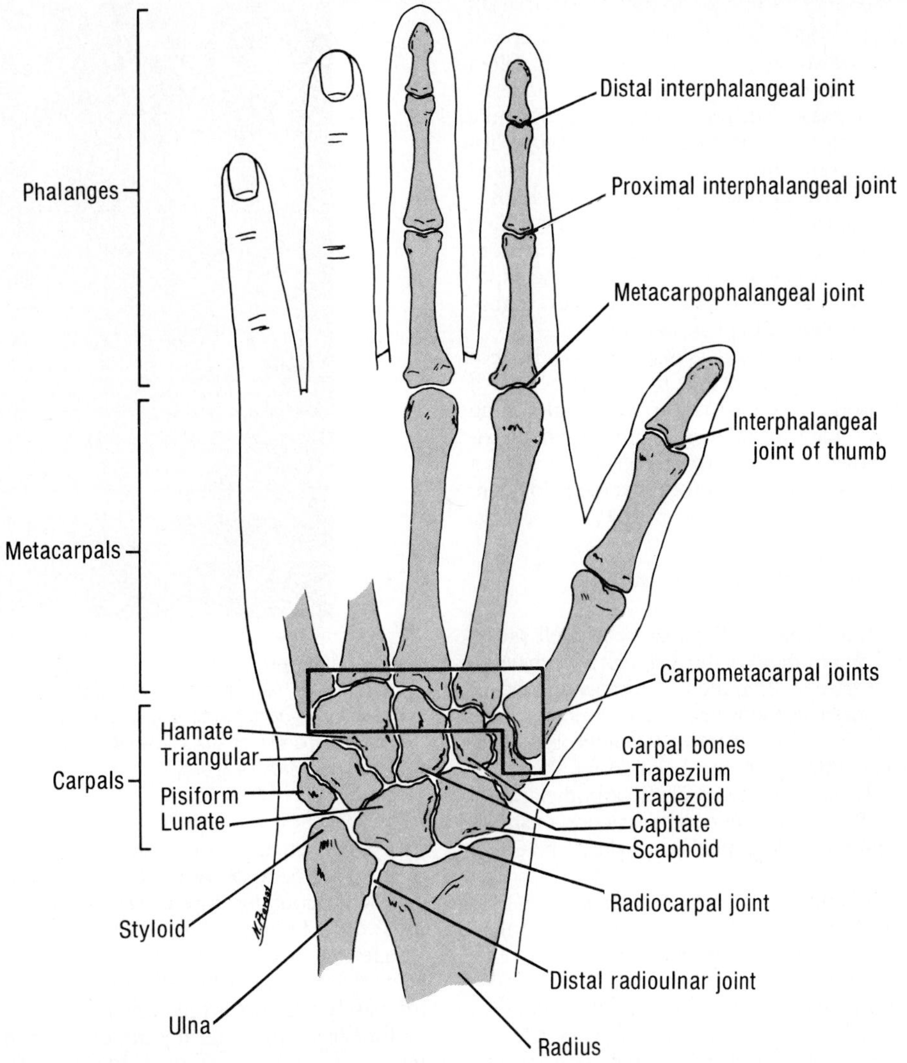

Figure 89-1 Diagram of the anatomy of the hand.

hand, neurologic examination of the hand should include an examination of the neck, shoulder, and arm. The hand should be evaluated for sensory and motor functions, which include testing of grip and pinch strength.

Approach to Specific Hand Complaints

The following discussion of hand disorders is organized in terms of the region of involvement (i.e., finger problems) and the structural nature of the disorder (i.e., tendonitis, arthritis).

Disorders of the Fingernails and Soft Tissues of the Fingers

Common problems of the nails and soft tissues of the fingers include fingernail pitting, ridging, lifting of the fingernail off its bed (called onycholysis), subungual (below the fingernail) hemorrhages, inflammation of the sides of the fingernails (paronychia), clubbing, ulcers around the fingernails and around the distal tips of the fingers, loss of distal finger-pad pulp, thickening of the skin of the fingers, and skin discoloration.

A variety of diseases may express themselves in abnormalities of the fingernails (see references for further discussion of the diagnostic significance of fingernail abnormalities). Fingernail ridging and pitting commonly occur after trauma to the nail's growth plate but also as manifestations of psoriasis. Onycholysis may be seen in individuals with psoriasis, hyperthyroidism, and fungal infections. Subungual splinter hemorrhages may be a sign of embolization or vasculitis. The latter may occur as a feature of a connective tissue disease or of bacterial endocarditis. Tender, erythematous nodules on the distal finger pads (called Osler's nodes), fever, and constitutional symptoms suggest the latter. Subungual splinter hemorrhages, ulcers on the distal fingertips, and frank gangrene of the distal fingers are suggestive of connective tissue disease–associated vasculitis. A common and benign cause of subungual hemorrhages is minor trauma. Subungual discoloration in the absence of trauma should raise concern for melanoma.

Ulcers on the distal ends of the fingers, particularly when associated with loss of tissue of the distal finger pulp and thickening of the skin of the fingers, is suggestive of digital vasospasm, or Raynaud's phenomenon. The classic presentation of Raynaud's phenomenon is a triphasic color change. Initial pallor or blanching of the fingers is followed by a dark-bluish, cyanotic discoloration, which then resolves after a painful erythematous phase. This phenomenon is often precipitated by exposure to cold or emotional stress. Although this history, in combination with physical findings, is adequate to establish a diagnosis clinically, in less clear situations a "cold pressor test" may be needed to confirm the presence of digital vasospasm. Digital vasospasm may occur as an isolated disorder, in which case it is called Raynaud's disease, or it may exist as a component of an underlying connective tissue disease (such as scleroderma, systemic lupus erythematosus), cryoglobulinemia, or hematologic disease (such as Waldenström's macroglobulinemia with blood hyperviscosity), or occlusive vascular disease (atherosclerosis, Buerger's disease). In the latter cases, digital vasospasm is called Raynaud's phenomenon. Cold injury such as frostbite, vibratory trauma (prolonged use of rivet gun or jack hammer), and exposure to chemicals such as polyvinyl chloride are also pathogenically associated with Raynaud's phenomenon.

Thickening of the skin of the fingers that is taut or "bound-down," perhaps with loss of motion of the fingers, may occur as a result of repeated episodes of digital vasospasm. If thickening and the "bound-down" character of the skin are present proximal to the knuckles, however, one must be concerned about a more generalized process, such as scleroderma (see Hoffman, 1980, for further discussion of digital vasospasm).

Joint Diseases of the Fingers and Wrists

Nearly all forms of joint disease, inflammatory as well as degenerative, may affect one or more of the 33 joints in each hand. Inflammatory joint disease is extremely common and has a variety of manifestations. The following is a discussion of the differential diagnosis of arthritis of the distal interphalangeal (DIP) joint, the proximal interphalangeal (PIP) joint, the metacarpophalangeal (MCP) joint, the wrist, and the carpometacarpal (CMC) joint (see Fig. 89-1). A more general discussion of arthritis is included in Chapter 86, "Monarticular Arthritis," and Chapter 87, "Polyarthritis."

Common causes of arthritis of the DIP joints of the fingers and the IP joints of the thumbs are osteoarthritis, psoriatic arthritis, and gouty arthritis. The gradual development of "knobby" enlargement of the DIP joints, often associated with angular deviation of the distal phalanges, which is seen most often in middle-aged women with a positive history of other affected female family members, is characteristic of nodal osteoarthritis. This arthropathy frequently affects the PIP joints and the CMC joint at the base of the thumb. Nodal osteoarthritis is generally associated with painless deformities, although erythema, local tenderness, and pain may be pronounced at the affected joint early in the course of this disorder. Palpation reveals bony nodules at the DIP joints, which are called Heberden's nodes. Bony nodules at the PIP joints are called Bouchard's nodes. Radiographs reveal narrowing, bony sclerosis, cysts, and bony spurs (osteophytes), which are typical features of osteoarthritis (Fig. 89-2). Osteoarthritis manifested by prominent erythema, pain and swelling of the DIP or PIP joints of the hands and rarely the metacarpal joints, associated central erosions, joint space narrowing, subchondral sclerosis, and osteophytes is referred to as inflammatory erosive osteoarthritis. This form of osteoarthritis of the finger joints is most common in postmenopausal women.

One or more red, tender, painful DIP joints, a true synovitis, is characteristic of psoriatic arthritis, particularly when accompanied by fingernail pitting and ridging or redness, swelling, and tenderness of the PIP and MCP joints and phalanges of the same finger (the so-called sausage digit). There may be a personal or family history of psoriasis. Physical examination might reveal evidence of nail pitting, ridging, and onycholysis, as well as psoriatic skin lesions about the umbilicus, gluteal cleft, scalp and hairlines, extensor surfaces of the knees, elbows, and axillary and submammary skin folds. Radiographs of joints affected by psoriatic arthritis may reveal only soft-tissue swelling. However, severe bone and joint erosions that result in resorption of periarticular bone may be seen in arthritis mutilans, the most severe form of psoriatic arthritis (Fig. 89-3).

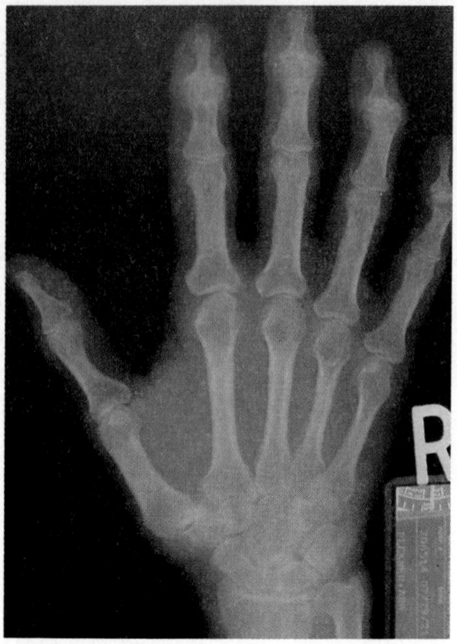

Figure 89-2 Radiograph of the hand of a patient with osteoarthritis, demonstrating joint space narrowing, bony sclerosis, and bony spurs of the distal interphalangeal joints of the fingers creating Heberden's nodes.

When gout develops in a DIP joint, typically only one joint is involved, although less frequently PIP, MCP, and wrist joints may be affected concurrently. Commonly, a history can be elicited of acute episodes of arthritis that last for 5 to 10 days and involve the base of the great toe (classical podagra, gout affecting the first metatarsophalangeal joint, or the ankle or knee). Podagra most commonly occurs in middle-aged men and presents with the rapid onset of excruciating pain. The diagnosis is suspected on the basis of the history and is confirmed by visualization of needle-shaped, negatively birefringent monosodium urate crystals within synovial fluid leukocytes aspirated from the affected joint(s).

Septic arthritis must be considered when one is faced with an acutely inflamed, painful, tender DIP joint. As discussed in Chapter 86, "Monarticular Arthritis," appropriate evaluation includes aspiration of the inflamed joint, Gram stain and culture of synovial fluid, synovial fluid analysis (synovial fluid glucose, mucin clot, white blood cell counts, and differential), blood cultures, and radiographs of the affected joint. Radiographs are obtained for two reasons: to exclude the presence of osteomyelitis in the adjacent bone, and to establish a "baseline" for future comparison.

As discussed previously, the PIP joints may be affected by gout, osteoarthritis, and psoriatic arthritis. However, the most common cause of arthritis of the PIP joints is rheumatoid arthritis.

Rheumatoid arthritis should be suspected in patients who present with the insidious onset of fusiform swelling, pain, and tenderness of all of the PIP joints in a symmetric pattern. This presentation, when associated with symmetric polyarthritis of the MCP joints and wrists, ulnar deviation of the fingers at the MCP joints, interosseous muscle atrophy, extensor tenosynovitis manifested by swelling and tenderness over the dorsum of the hands and wrists, and subcutaneous nodules (most commonly over the extensor surfaces of the elbows), is characteristic of

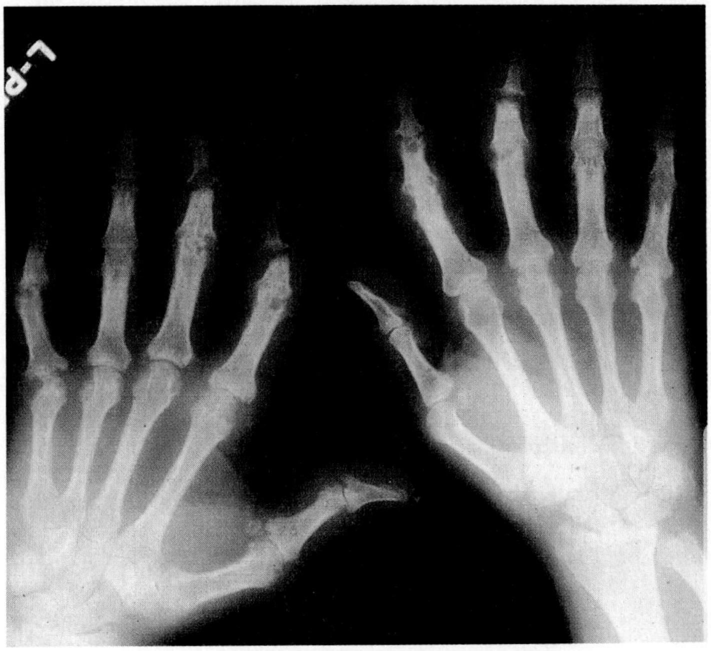

Figure 89-3 Radiograph of the hands of a patient with destructive psoriatic arthritis, demonstrating severe erosions of multiple distal interphalangeal (DIP) joints of the fingers with less severe disease of the proximal interphalangeal and metacarpophalangeal joints. The DIP involvement helps to distinguish psoriatic arthritis from rheumatoid arthritis, because DIP disease tends not to occur in rheumatoid arthritis.

rheumatoid arthritis (Fig. 89-4). Arthritis of the DIP joints almost never occurs as a major component in rheumatoid arthritis. In early disease, radiographs may reveal only soft-tissue swelling. As the disease progresses, demineralization of the bone adjacent to the joint, so-called periarticular demineralization, as well as loss of joint space, erosion of the margins of the joints, and malalignment at the affected joint may be seen (Fig. 89-5). A rheumatoid factor (IgM-anti-IgG) is present in the sera of 70 to 80 percent of patients with rheumatoid arthritis (see Chapter 96, "Laboratory and Radiographic Abnormalities in Rheumatic Diseases," for further discussion of rheumatoid factors).

Rheumatoid arthritis, gout, and psoriatic arthritis may all affect the MCP joints. By contrast, osteoarthritis rarely affects the MCP joints unless there has been prior injury such as trauma or infection. Hemochromatosis and calcium pyrophosphate dihydrate deposition (CPPD) disease may cause an arthritis of the MCP joints that resembles osteoarthritis radiographically. The latter may be manifested clinically as pseudogout. Elevation of the serum ferritin level or elevation of the iron–to–total iron binding capacity, as well as other stigmata, including liver disease and diabetes mellitus, support the diagnosis of hemochromatosis. The diagnosis of CPPD disease causing arthritis of the MCP joints is supported by the presence of linear calcifications of the articular cartilage of the joints as well as calcification in the triangular cartilage just distal to the ulnar styloid. CPPD disease is confirmed by visualization of rhomboid-shaped, positively birefringent crystals within the synovial fluid leukocytes aspirated from the affected joint when synovial fluid is examined under the polarizing microscope (see the section on synovial fluid analysis in Chapter 96, "Laboratory and Radiographic Abnormalities in Rheumatic Diseases").

Common causes of arthritis that affects the wrists are rheumatoid arthritis, gouty arthritis, psoriatic arthritis, and CPPD disease. Although osteoarthritis may cause pain along the radial aspect of the wrist owing to arthritis at the joint at the base of the thumb (the CMC joint), primary osteoarthritis does not affect the true wrist joint unless a pre-existing anatomic abnormality is present (ulnar plus deformity) or trauma has injured the joint. The presence of an acute arthritis of the wrist, particularly when seen in a sexually active individual in association with tendonitis, should raise suspicion of gonococcal arthritis. Evaluation should include a pelvic examination; urethral, rectal, vaginal, throat, and blood cultures; and aspiration, Gram stain, and cultures of the affected joint.

In addition to osteoarthritis of the CMC joint of the thumb, another common musculoskeletal problem that may cause pain along the radial aspect of the wrist, and may be confused with wrist arthritis, is tendonitis of the thumb abductor and extensor tendons, the abductor pollicis longus (APL), and the extensor pollicis brevis (EPB). Tendonitis at this site is called DeQuervain's stenosing tenosynovitis. Pain along the radial aspect of the wrist that is aggravated by thumb motion, particularly abduction and extension, is common. Physical examination demonstrates tenderness along the affected tendons in the region of the radial styloid. Pain with abduction of the thumb against resistance as well as ulnar deviation of the wrist while the thumb is held within a closed fist (the so-called Finklestein sign) support the diagnosis of DeQuervain's tenosynovitis.

The following disorders affect either specific joints in the hand or multiple hand and wrist joints simultaneously: systemic lupus erythematosus, dermatomyositis, mixed connective tissue disease, arthritis associated with inflammatory bowel diseases, multiple myeloma, sickle cell anemia, hyperthyroid arthropathy, hypertrophic osteoarthropathy, the hyperextensible joint syn-

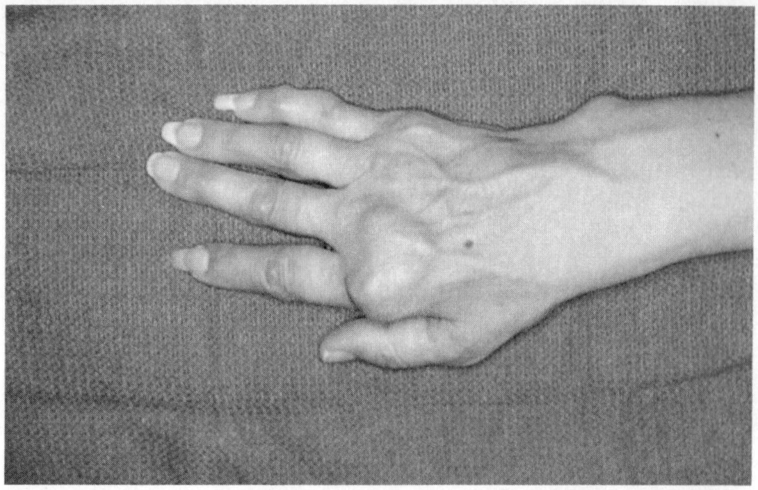

A

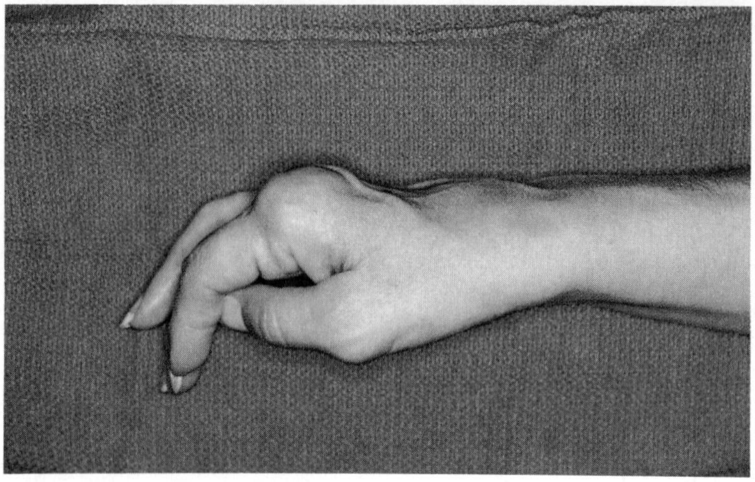

B

Figure 89-4 (**A**) Rheumatoid arthritis of the hand demonstrating synovitis with subcutaneous nodules of the proximal interphalangeal joints, metacarpophalangeal joints, and wrist with ulnar deviation of the fingers. (**B**) Lateral view of the same rheumatoid hand demonstrating synovial proliferation of the thumb and index finger metacarpophalangeal (MCP) joints and of the wrist and palmar subluxation of the index finger at the MCP joint.

drome, sarcoid arthropathy, and, as stated previously, rheumatoid arthritis, osteoarthritis, psoriatic arthritis, gout, and septic arthritis. The diagnosis of many of these conditions depends as much or more on the extra-articular features of the diseases as on the specific nature of the arthritis. The more common disorders are discussed in Chapter 87, "Polyarthritis."

Inflammation of the Tendon (Tendonitis, Tenosynovitis)

Pain and swelling in a linear fashion, aggravated by activity corresponding to the anatomy of a tendon, should suggest the diagnosis of tendonitis. The flexor and extensor tendons of the fingers, the abductor and extensor tendons of the thumb (DeQuervain's tenosynovitis), and the tendons of the wrist may become inflamed as a result of trauma (including overuse), infection (particularly gonococcal infection and rarely mycobacterial infection), gout, rheumatoid arthritis, the spondyloarthropathies (ankylosing spondylitis, Reiter's syndrome, and psoriatic arthritis), and other connective tissue diseases such as systemic lupus erythematosus, mixed connective tissue disease, and scleroderma. Hyperlipidemias, tumors of tendon sheaths, including pigmented villonodular synovitis, and infiltrating processes such as amyloidosis may also cause tendonitis. Amorphous calcium hydroxyapatite deposits in tendon sheaths may incite an inflammatory reaction that is pathophysiologically similar to gout and that presents as acute tendonitis. This entity is known as calcific tendonitis or calcific periarthritis and can be readily diagnosed radiographically.

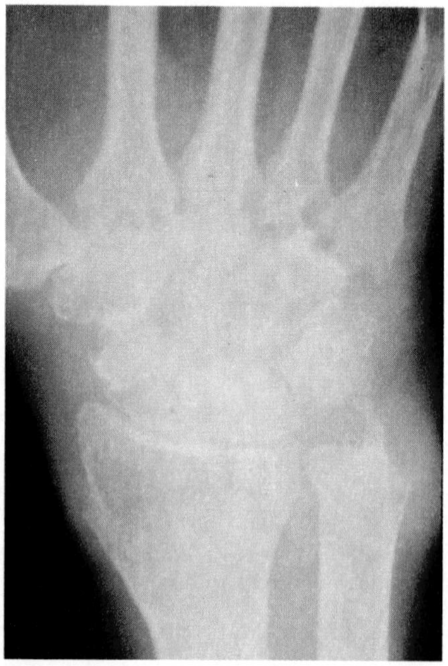

Figure 89-5 Radiograph of the hand of a patient with erosive rheumatoid arthritis of the wrist, demonstrating soft-tissue swelling over the ulnar styloid, narrowing of the joint spaces of the wrist, and erosions of the ulnar styloid and of the proximal heads of the metacarpal bones.

With subacute and chronic tendon inflammation, patients may complain of inability to move a joint with initial effort until the joint suddenly gives way (so-called triggering), which is associated with a snapping or rubbing sensation along the course of the tendon. This is due to nodular enlargement of the tendon, particularly at sites where retinacula hold tendons in place, or stenosis of the tendon sheaths. Thickening and even nodularity may be palpated along the tendon, most commonly along the finger flexor tendons overlying the MCP joints. The most common cause of tendon nodules is rheumatoid arthritis. Tophaceous deposits in chronic intercritical gout and cholesterol deposits in type 4 hyperlipoproteinemia may also cause tendon nodules.

Although not intrinsically involving flexor tendons, a condition called Dupuytren's contracture may cause progressive flexion deformities of the fourth and fifth fingers due to thickening of the palmar fascia. This occurs predominantly in middle-aged and older men. Dupuytren's contracture typically leads to difficulty in using the fingers owing to the progressive flexion deformities. Physical examination reveals thickening and often a palpable nodule along the palmar aponeurosis, most frequently of the fourth and fifth fingers.

Other conditions that may cause flexion contractures of the fingers are diabetic cheiroarthropathy, scleroderma, traumatic scars, ischemic contractures, congenital flexor deformities, chronic reflex sympathetic dystrophy (shoulder-hand syndrome), and arthritis.

Burning, Tingling, and Numbness in the Hand

"Pins and needles" tingling, numbness, a heavy sensation, and clumsiness of the hand are complaints suggestive of nerve impingement. The most common etiologies of these complaints in the hand include pressure on a cervical nerve root due to osteoarthritis in the spine (so-called cervical spondylosis with cervical radiculopathy), cervical disk herniation, compression of the median nerve in the carpal tunnel (so-called carpal tunnel syndrome), and ulnar nerve entrapment at the elbow or in the ulnar (Guyon's) canal at the wrist.

The distribution of symptoms helps in determining the site of nerve root injury. Radiation of pain down the radial aspect of the forearm and into the thumb and index finger associated with sensory loss in this distribution, weakness of wrist extensors and flexors, and diminished or absent biceps and brachial radialis deep tendon reflexes are findings consistent with impingement of the *sixth cervical nerve root.* Pain on the dorsum of the forearm; sensory loss in the index, middle, and fourth fingers associated with decreased or absent triceps deep tendon reflexes; and weakness of triceps and wrist flexors and extensors are indicative of compression of the *seventh cervical nerve root.* Pain in the ulnar aspect of the forearm associated with sensory loss in the fourth and fifth fingers, diminished triceps reflex, and weakness of the finger extensors and interossei muscle may reflect impingement of the *eighth cervical nerve root.* An oblique-view radiograph of the cervical spine may reveal bony impingement of the affected cervical neuroforamen from cervical spondylosis, but magnetic resonance imaging (MRI) or myelography may be required to diagnose cervical disk herniation.

Median nerve compression, also known as the *carpal tunnel syndrome,* presents with burning paresthesias on the thenar aspect of the thumb radiating into the thumb, index, and middle fingers (the distribution of the median nerve in the hand). Occasionally this discomfort awakens patients from sleep, is aggravated by flexion or extension of the wrists, and is relieved with rubbing, dangling, or shaking of the hands. Physical examination early in the course of the condition may be normal. However, lancinating pain that radiates into the first three fingers by tapping on the volar aspect of the wrist (Tinel's sign) or reproduction of the symptoms during 60 seconds of forced wrist flexion (Phalen's maneuver) support the diagnosis of median nerve entrapment at the wrist. As the nerve compression progresses, numbness in the median nerve distribution associated with impaired sensation on examination, loss of pinch strength between thumb and index finger, and thenar muscle atrophy may develop. Occasionally, the individual may have pain radiating in a retrograde fashion up the arm, as proximally as the shoulder. Nerve conduction studies and electromyograms (EMGs) are helpful in documenting and assessing the severity of compression.

The causes of carpal tunnel syndrome include repetitive wrist motion (as in the case of carpenters); conditions causing vulnerability of peripheral nerves, such as diabetes mellitus and renal failure; disorders associated with increased tissue mass, such as synovitis of the wrist (particularly rheumatoid arthritis); pregnancy; hypothyroidism; acromegaly; and amyloidosis. In some cases, carpal tunnel syndrome is familial and presumably develops as a result of a genetically determined small carpal tunnel. Frequently, no underlying disorder can be found. In addition to a thorough history and physical examination, evaluation should include testing for diabetes mellitus, hypothyroidism, and renal impairment.

Much less common sites of nerve compression in the upper extremity are compression of the ulnar nerve in the elbow (cubital tunnel) or in the wrist (Guyon's canal), which presents with tingling of the fourth and fifth fingers. This is usually the consequence of rheumatoid arthritis of the elbow and wrist joints or repetitive minor trauma. Thoracic outlet obstruction may also cause tingling or numbness of the hand. (See Chapter 90, "The Shoulder.")

In the evaluation of an individual with tingling or numbness in a hand, it is important to distinguish localized symptoms from symptoms presenting in a symmetric manner in the hands and feet, the so-called stocking-and-glove pattern, which suggests a peripheral neuropathy.

Puffy Hands

Puffy hands may occur as a result of trauma, arthritis, allergic reaction, infection, excessive heat, venous or lymphatic obstruction, other causes of increased soft tissue or bone mass, such as idiopathic cyclic edema and acromegaly, and a condition called the shoulder-hand syndrome, or reflex sympathetic dystrophy. (See Chapter 90, "The Shoulder," and Chapter 94, "Foot and Ankle Pain.") Bilateral puffy hands may also be the initial manifestation of a connective tissue disease (scleroderma, mixed connective tissue disease, systemic lupus erythematosus, rheumatoid arthritis), hypothyroidism, anasarca, or superior vena cava obstruction.

References

Canoso JJ. Hands, wrists and elbows. In: Cohen AS, ed. Rheumatology and immunology. New York: Grune & Stratton, 1979:1.

Hoffman G. Raynaud's disease and phenomenon. Am Fam Physician 1980; 21(1):91.

Katz WA. Hands and wrists. In: Katz WA, ed. Rheumatic diseases: Diagnosis and management. 2nd ed. Philadelphia: JB Lippincott, 1988:27.

Kozin F. Painful shoulder and the reflex sympathetic dystrophy syndrome. In: McCarty DJ, ed. Arthritis and allied conditions. 11th ed. Philadelphia: Lea & Febiger, 1989:1509.

Nakano KK. Neurology of musculoskeletal and rheumatic disorders. Boston: Houghton Mifflin, 1979.

Schumacher HR Jr, ed. Primer on the rheumatic diseases. 9th ed. Atlanta: The Arthritis Foundation, 1988.

Sheon RP, Moskowitz RW, Goldberg VM. The wrist and hand. In: Soft tissue rheumatic pain. Philadelphia: Lea & Febiger, 1987:112.

The Shoulder

Katherine S. Upchurch, MD

David F. Giansiracusa, MD

90

Definition

The shoulder is one of the most complex structures in the human musculoskeletal system. It is composed of three large bones (the humerus, scapula, and clavicle), four joints (the sternoclavicular, acromioclavicular, scapulothoracic, and glenohumeral), and three muscle groups (the scapulohumeral, the axiohumeral, and the scapulothoracic). Because of this complexity and because a variety of somatic and visceral lesions are characterized by referred pain to the shoulder, the diagnosis of the cause of shoulder pain may be difficult.

Anatomy

The joints of the shoulder in anterior view are shown in Figure 90-1A. Musculature of clinical importance includes the rotator cuff muscles (supraspinatus, infraspinatus, teres minor, and subscapularis), which are incorporated into the capsule of the shoulder at the tuberosities of the humerus; the deltoid muscle, which covers most of the glenohumeral joint and rotator cuff; the trapezius, which runs from the cervical spine to the clavicle, acromion, and crest of the scapula; and the long head of the biceps, which passes through the glenohumeral joint space, attaching to the posterior aspect. Also important are the structures for the neural and vascular supply of the upper extremity, which, if compromised, may produce shoulder pain in association with certain other symptoms. The location of the subacromial bursa, the most important of the several bursae from a clinical point of view, is shown in Figure 90-1B.

Etiology

Common etiologies of shoulder pain are shown in Table 90-1 and discussed more fully in the section "Specific Diagnoses."

Diagnostic Approach

As with other joints in the body, correct diagnosis of complaints referable to the shoulder requires careful history taking, physical examination, and the use of appropriate diagnostic studies.

History

Patients complaining of shoulder pain should be carefully questioned concerning the location of the pain, the nature of the pain (e.g., type of onset, precipitating or alleviating factors, presence of systemic symptoms, or involvement of other joints). With the exception of the acromioclavicular joint (derived from the C4 dermatome), all parts of the shoulder are innervated by the C5 dermatome; shoulder pain from any structure may thus be perceived as pain that may extend from the deltoid area down the outside of the arm to the level of the wrist. The most common site of shoulder pain is in the lower part of the deltoid area, where the supraspinatus tendon inserts. Pain in this location is almost never referred from visceral disease. Pain directly over the acromioclavicular joint implies intra-articular or periarticular pathology in that joint. Pain in any other part of the arm, shoulder, or neck may be due to virtually any extrinsic or intrinsic shoulder lesion. Bilateral shoulder pain suggests an underlying systemic disorder rather than localized pathology.

The type of onset of shoulder pain as well as its pattern of occurrence may provide clues to diagnosis. Sudden onset of pain following trauma or heavy lifting suggests fracture, dislocation, or muscular or tendon tear (rotator cuff, biceps tendon). Subacute pain in the setting of repeated movement of the shoulder may be due to tendonitis or bursitis, an impingement syndrome secondary to rotator cuff disease, adhesive capsulitis, or an arthritic process.

Pain in either shoulder with exertion should be considered of cardiac origin until proven otherwise. Typically, this pain will be relieved by rest or by sublingual nitroglycerin, and it will be recurrent. Furthermore, the patient will not describe concomitant stiffness in the area of pain.

The pain of tendonitis and bursitis is aggravated by initial motion of the affected extremity and by lying on the involved side. When severe, it may be unremitting and worse at night.

Shoulder pain associated with fever, chills, or a warm, erythematous shoulder with restricted motion should always raise concern about septic arthritis. Joint aspiration for stains and cultures is required. Predisposing factors for joint sepsis include an infectious site such as pneumonia, endocarditis, cellulitis, urinary tract infection, a history of a penetrating injury, underlying malignancy, alcoholism, diabetes mellitus, renal failure, and intravenous drug abuse.

The presence of associated symptoms may suggest an underlying systemic disorder. In rheumatoid arthritis, for example, polyarticular arthritis as well as generalized fatigue and malaise are prominent. The presence of vague weakness and stiffness in the hip and shoulder girdle in an elderly individual suggests polymyalgia rheumatica as the underlying disorder. Pain in the shoulder may be due to intra-abdominal pathology. Shoulder pain that is related to respiration suggests pulmonary infarction, pleuritis, or pericarditis. Subjective shoulder-girdle weakness, if bilateral, is suggestive of a myopathic process such as polymyositis, and it should prompt the examiner to focus carefully on the neurologic examination. Unilateral weakness may indicate cervical nerve root diseases or disorders of the brachial plexus. Pain only in certain positions of the shoulder, particularly when accompanied by paresthesias, weakness, swelling, and coldness, suggests thoracic outlet syndrome.

Physical Examination

Examination of the shoulder should include all aspects of the composite shoulder, as discussed previously. Each of the joints, bones, bursae, tendons, ligaments, and musculature should be examined for deformities, muscle atrophy, erythema and warmth, swelling and effusions, tenderness, and range of motion. In addition, a full neurologic examination should be performed, checking carefully for abnormal muscle strength, sensation, and reflexes. Particular aspects of inspection, palpation, and range of motion examination are mentioned in the following section.

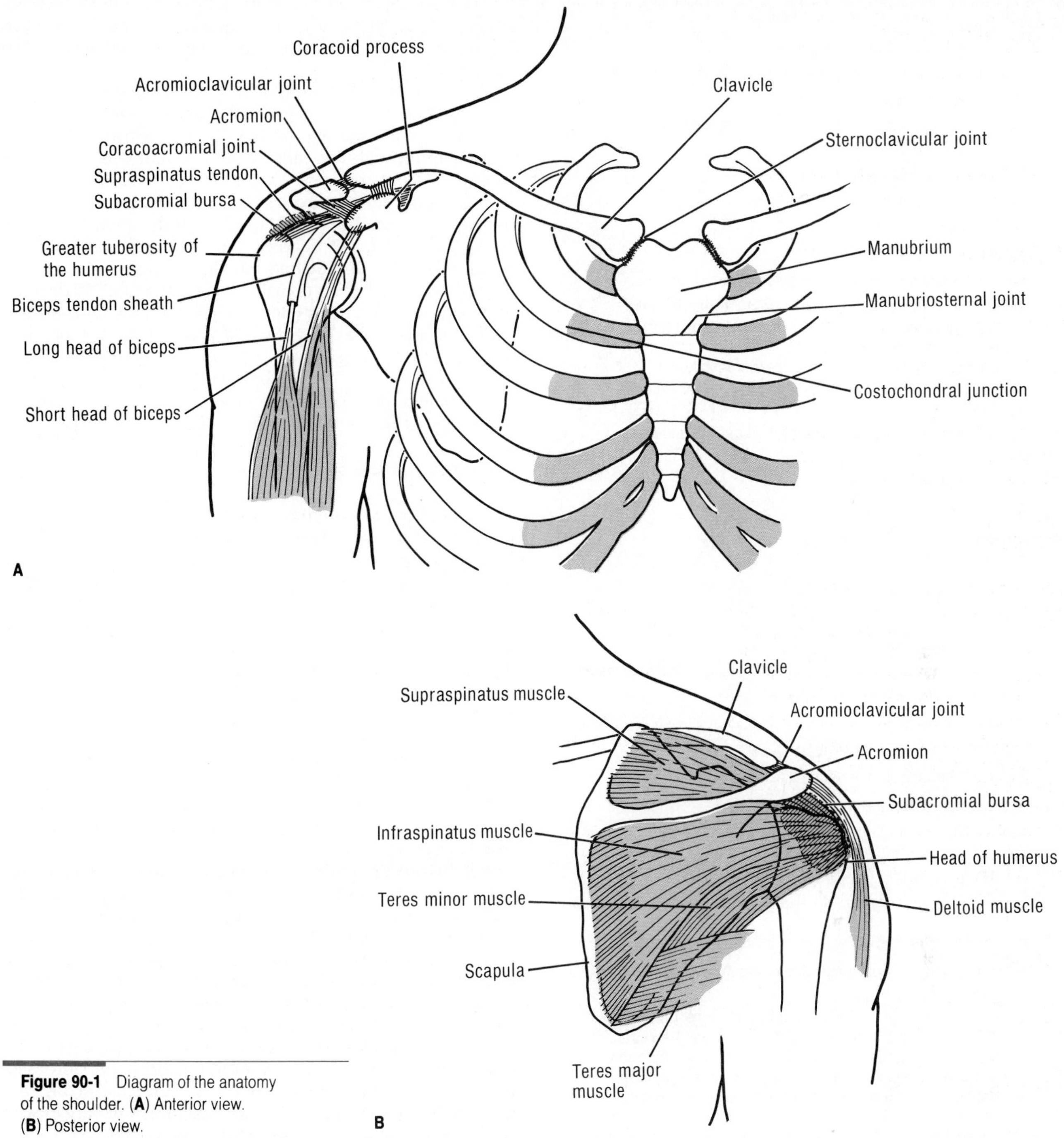

Figure 90-1 Diagram of the anatomy of the shoulder. (**A**) Anterior view. (**B**) Posterior view.

Inspection

Swelling of the shoulder or neck is uncommon, although occasionally glenohumeral effusions may be seen just beneath the coracoid process. When this joint communicates with the subdeltoid bursa, the effusion may be prominent. Arthritis, bursitis, or tendonitis may produce localized erythema or warmth. Asymmetry of the shoulders due to swelling, muscle atrophy, or deformity is often readily apparent on inspection. Squaring of a normally rounded deltoid muscle may be caused by a ruptured supraspinatus tendon or deltoid muscle atrophy. Anterior subluxation of the shoulder may produce a hollow beneath the acromioclavicular joint. Paget's disease may produce bowing of the clavicle or humerus. Congenital abnormalities of neurologic or vascular supply, such as neurofibromatosis, may cause atrophy or hypertrophy of the affected part.

Palpation

Localized areas of tenderness should be sought by carefully palpating possible sites of intrinsic disease. In the setting of bicipital tendonitis, the biceps tendon is exquisitely painful to palpation, accentuated by forcibly externally rotating the shoulder or by having the patient flex his or her elbow and supinate his or her forearm against resistance. The subdeltoid bursa and subacromial bursa may be sites of point tenderness if these structures are inflamed. In addition, pain produced by subacromial bursitis may be provoked when the shoulder is abducted against resistance. Diffuse tenderness, especially directly over the glenohumeral joint, suggests true synovitis of the joint. In cases of acute cervical strain or nerve root compression, the trapezius muscle may be tender to palpation, and pain may be aggravated by neck motion.

Table 90-1 Common Causes of Shoulder Pain

Diseases confined to the shoulder:
Tendonitis (noncalcific), supraspinatus; rotator cuff, biceps
Tendonitis (calcific), supraspinatus; rotator cuff, biceps
Rupture syndromes (rotator cuff rupture, partial and complete), bicipital rupture
Adhesive capsulitis ("frozen shoulder")
Bursitis (subacromial, subdeltoid)
Acromioclavicular syndromes
Milwaukee shoulder syndrome
Diseases of systemic origin with shoulder involvement:
Inflammatory arthropathies (rheumatoid arthritis, juvenile rheumatoid arthritis, ankylosing spondylitis, psoriatic arthritis, acute rheumatic fever, pseudogout, infectious arthritis, enteropathic arthropathy, systemic lupus erythematosus, polymyalgia rheumatica, sickle cell anemia, hemophilia)
Noninflammatory osteoarthropathy (osteoarthritis, usually secondary)
Traumatic injuries to the shoulder:
Acromioclavicular separation
Dislocations (anterior, posterior)
Direct capsular injury
Fractures
Nerve injuries
Bony lesions of the shoulder:
Malignancy metastatic to bones or soft tissues of the shoulder
Bony tumors (primary)
Paget's disease of bone
Metabolic bone diseases (osteomalacia)
Avascular necrosis of the humeral head
Infectious diseases of the shoulder:
Septic arthritis
Osteomyelitis
Septic tenosynovitis
Septic bursitis
Reflex sympathetic dystrophy (shoulder-hand syndrome)
Visceral and somatic syndromes producing pain referred to the shoulder:
Visceral diseases (pulmonary infarction, pleuritis, pericarditis, perforated viscus, ectopic pregnancy, subdiaphragmatic abscess, gallbladder disease, Pancoast's tumor, coronary insufficiency and myocardial infarction, dissecting aortic aneurysm, hiatal hernia, esophageal spasm, esophageal cancer)
Cervical lesions (cord tumor, herniated disk [C5-6], cervical spondylitis with nerve root compression, brachial plexitis, herpes zoster, thoracic outlet syndromes, ankylosing spondylitis)
Distal musculoskeletal lesions (carpal tunnel syndrome, synovitis of the elbow with nerve entrapment, "tennis elbow")

Range of Motion

Normal shoulder motion involves normal functioning of all shoulder structures described previously. Most shoulder motion, however, takes place in the glenohumeral joint. Clinically important ranges of motion that should be examined both actively and passively include extension (35 degrees from neutral), flexion (95 degrees to 100 degrees from neutral), adduction (25 degrees to 30 degrees), abduction (90 degrees before scapular movement), and external and internal rotation (90 degrees). Full passive range of motion in the setting of shoulder disease is common, even with marked limitation of active motion. For this reason, all ranges of motion should be observed actively and passively.

In the setting of rotator cuff disease, as the arm is abducted from 60 degrees to 120 degrees, the acromion impinges upon the rotator cuff (see Fig. 90-1B). Because active and passive movement through this range causes pain, this is termed the painful arc. In a complete rotator cuff tear, the individual has pain and only several degrees of motion when attempting to initiate shoulder abduction. However, if the shoulder is passively abducted to 90 degrees, the individual may hold this position by using the deltoid muscle. In contrast, in a partial rotator cuff tear, there is no pain on abduction until 60 degrees. The pain continues to 120 degrees, and then the remainder of abduction is painless. Most other disorders of the shoulder limit motion to some degree, although the findings are generally more diffuse and less specific than in the rotator cuff syndromes.

Shoulder pain of cardiac origin is not accompanied by tenderness or limitation of motion in the shoulder itself.

Laboratory Studies

Few laboratory studies have specific diagnostic value in the evaluation of a patient with shoulder pain. The erythrocyte sedimentation rate (ESR), a complete blood count, and rheumatoid factor may suggest underlying rheumatoid arthritis or other arthropathies. An elevated alkaline phosphatase level suggests osteomalacia, Paget's disease, a healing fracture, or an infectious or neoplastic bony lesion. Culture of joint fluid may reveal an infectious etiology for shoulder pain, and other synovial fluid studies may help distinguish between inflammatory and noninflammatory processes.

Radiographic Evaluation

Radiographic examination of the shoulder should be performed in all cases in which intrinsic (as opposed to referred) shoulder pain is suspected. The standard view is an anteroposterior view with both internal and external rotation views of the humerus. The axillary view is particularly helpful in assessment of the glenohumeral joint space as well as shoulder dislocation. A chest radiograph with apical lordotic views is also often useful to evaluate for cervical rib or intrathoracic pathology with referred pain to the shoulder. Calcific deposits in the rotator cuff or bursae may be seen in the setting of calcific bursitis, tendonitis, and a subacromial spur in patients with shoulder impingement syndrome. Juxta-articular erosions, joint-space narrowing, and osteopenia may be seen in rheumatoid arthritis. Chondrocalcinosis may be visualized in the hyaline cartilage of the glenohumeral joint. Narrowing of the acromiohumeral gap with abduction is suggestive of a full-thickness rotator cuff tear. In addition, shoulder radiographs may reveal primary or metastatic bony lesions, Paget's disease of bone, fractures, or bone infection (osteomyelitis).

Other Diagnostic Studies

Fluoroscopy of the shoulder is helpful in evaluating for shoulder subluxations and impingements as well as in guiding arthrocentesis of the glenohumeral joint and biopsy of osseus lesions. Arthrography also helps to confirm intra-articular needle positioning for joint aspiration.

Arthrography is the most useful study for evaluation of suspected rotator cuff tears and is an excellent way to distinguish between complete and incomplete tears. The presence of dye in both the bursa and joint space is diagnostic of a complete rupture. Arthrography may also be helpful in evaluation of suspected adhesive capsulitis or recurrent shoulder dislocations.

Arthrographic findings of adhesive capsulitis are excessive resistance to intra-articular injection of contrast and a small joint space.

Tomography and bone scanning may be useful in evaluating bony abnormalities seen on plain-film radiographs or if underlying metastatic malignant lesions or Paget's disease is suspected in the setting of normal plain-film radiographs. Computed tomography (CT) is helpful in evaluating shoulder dislocations and abnormal anatomic relationships of the glenohumeral joint and acromioclavicular joint. It may also be used to evaluate the patient with osteomyelitis and to detect periosteal bone formation and the extent of marrow involvement. CT can demonstrate foreign bodies, soft-tissue abscesses, lytic and blastic lesions, and lesions of the brachial plexus. Magnetic resonance imaging (MRI), because of its ability to demonstrate noninvasively the anatomic structures of the shoulder, is used to evaluate the rotator cuff.

Specific Diagnoses

Although a complete review of all possible etiologies of shoulder pain is beyond the scope of this chapter, several points referable to each category of disorders described in Table 90-1 are discussed in this section.

Disorders Confined to the Shoulder

The following comments referable to the diagnosis of pain syndromes arising from structures in and about the shoulder joint are amplified in the monograph on the shoulder by Bland et al (1977).

Although several distinct periarthritic syndromes can be identified as etiologies of shoulder pain, the following syndromes refer to the same basic pathologic process: supraspinatus tendonitis, rotator cuff tendonitis, subacromial bursitis, subdeltoid bursitis, and calcific tendonitis. More general terms that also refer to similar processes include periarthritis, adhesive capsulitis, frozen shoulder, and adhesive bursitis. It is likely that the common mechanism of these disorders is an initial lesion in the supraspinatus tendon with subsequent spread to contiguous structures, the specific structure determining the clinical syndrome.

The rotator cuff syndromes most commonly involve the supraspinatus tendon and are most frequently secondary to degenerative changes in the setting of minor recurrent rotator cuff tears (partial or complete). They rarely occur in young individuals, even in the setting of severe trauma. This diagnosis implies underlying pathology such as chronic tendonitis or rheumatoid arthritis. The specific clinical syndromes of intrinsic shoulder disease are differentiated in Table 90-2. Severe rotator

Table 90-2 Common Disorders Confined to the Shoulder

Disorder	Presentation	Physical findings	Laboratory studies
Rotator cuff syndromes:			
Tendonitis (noncalcific)	Middle-aged patient; history of shoulder stress; dull ache in deltoid area that is increased with abduction and worse at night	Diffuse tenderness of shoulder; pain on forced abduction; relief of symptoms with lidocaine infiltration	Negative
Tendonitis (calcific)	Abrupt onset of severe aching pain; all motion uncomfortable; pain worse at night	No movement of shoulder allowed by patient; marked muscle spasm	Calcium deposits between acromion and humeral head
Rupture syndromes	Abrupt shoulder pain in deltoid area in middle-aged (>50 yr) patient, usually following exertion	Arm can be passively but not actively abducted to 90 degrees; supraspinatus, infraspinatus atrophy after 3 wk; severe muscle spasm	Humeral head high on the glenoid with abduction arthrography to differentiate partial from complete tears
Bicipital syndromes:			
Tendonitis	Chronic pain in anterior aspect of the shoulder with muscle spasm and trapezius pain; no history of trauma	Extreme tenderness, bicipital groove produced by flexion of shoulder against resistance	Occasional osteopenia of greater tuberosity of humerus
Rupture	History of stiffness, shoulder pain, and a "snap," an abrupt, sharp pain with acute strain	Lump at site of contracted muscle; inability to flex elbow	
Frozen shoulder	Painful shoulder with progressive immobility; pain is severe, worse at night; precipitating event (see text)	Passive range of motion is impossible	Patchy osteopenia of humeral head; cystic changes; joint-space narrowing
Bursitis	Pain that may be localized or diffuse	Point tenderness in location of involved bursa	Negative comment: Bursitis is rarely an isolated condition, but it is usually associated with tendonitis
Acromioclavicular syndromes	Pain located in superior aspect of the shoulder	Localized tenderness over acromioclavicular joint exaggerated by horizontal abduction	Negative

cuff disease with secondary degenerative disease of the glenohumeral joint may occur in elderly individuals in association with basic calcium phosphate (hydroxyapatite) crystals. This process, occasionally referred to as "Milwaukee shoulder," can cause shoulder pain with restricted motion, joint crepitus, and glenohumeral joint effusions.

Diseases of Systemic Origin with Shoulder Involvement

For a more complete discussion of this group of disorders, see Chapter 87, "Polyarticular Arthritis." Of the inflammatory arthropathies, rheumatoid arthritis and juvenile rheumatoid arthritis are the most likely to involve the shoulder. Despite the fact that gout occurs in most joints of the body, it rarely affects the shoulder, unlike pseudogout, which not uncommonly involves the shoulder.

Primary osteoarthritis of the shoulder is uncommon; when symptoms, clinical examination, and radiographic findings suggest advanced osteoarthritis, an underlying primary etiology (such as ochronosis, hemochromatosis, avascular necrosis) or particular occupational or recreational stresses should be suspected.

Traumatic Injuries

The traumatic lesions listed in Table 90-1 are those seen most frequently in an orthopedic practice; rarely is a rheumatologist consulted for diagnosis and management of these injuries. In most instances, the onset is abrupt, following a readily identifiable traumatic episode.

Bony Lesions

Bony lesions of the clavicle, scapula, humeral head, and acromion may produce shoulder pain. Of these, malignancy metastatic to bone is the most common. Malignancies that are likely to metastasize to bone include those of the breast, kidney, thyroid, ovary, lung, and prostate, and melanoma. An underlying malignancy should be suspected if shoulder radiographs reveal a lytic or blastic lesion, particularly if the patient has known malignant disease or has systemic symptoms suggestive of this (see Chapter 108, "Bone Pain and Bone Metastasis"). Paget's disease is diagnosed by the classic roentgenographic findings of coarsened trabecular bone with thickened cortices and increased bone dimension. Avascular necrosis should be suspected when radiographs reveal the characteristic subcortical lucencies or "crescents" and "step-down" lesions, especially if the patient has a history of corticosteroid use, renal transplantation, systemic lupus erythematosus, diabetes mellitus, alcoholism, or sickle cell anemia, which are the most prominent among many factors that predispose to this lesion.

Reflex Sympathetic Dystrophy

This disorder, which is of uncertain etiology, has been called by many names in the past, including Sudeck's atrophy, shoulder-hand syndrome, and causalgia. Clinically, it is characterized by a painful stiff shoulder and then dystrophic changes of the ipsilateral hand (pain, swelling, hyperhidrosis, pigmentary changes). This may follow certain precipitating events, including myocardial infarction, cerebral thrombosis, cervical spondylitis, calcific tendonitis, or trauma to the shoulder, arm, or hand. At any time in the course of this disorder, the contralateral side may become similarly involved. Immobilization and an underlying central nervous system mechanism mediated in the sympathetic limb are the likely mechanisms. Rapidly developing patchy osteoporosis of the shoulder girdle is the characteristic radiographic finding. Perfusion radionuclide bone scans reveal increased uptake in the affected bone and soft tissues even before radiographic changes may be apparent.

Table 90-3 Common Thoracic Outlet Syndromes

	Presentations	Physical findings	Tests
Scalenus anticus syndrome	Intermittent or constant pain, paresthesias, ulnar distribution	Tenderness over scalenus anticus muscle; positive Adson's maneuver	Shoulder and neck radiographs should be done on all patients suspected of these syndromes. If arterial compression is suspected, angiography may be indicated. If venous compression is suspected, venography is indicated.
Cervical rib			
Neural compression	Pain, paresthesias, atrophy, ulnar or medial distribution, left affected more often than right	Occasional palpation of rib in supraclavicular fossa, positive Adson's maneuver	
Arterial compression	Pain, pallor, coldness, intermittent claudication of affected extremity	Occasional palpation of rib in supraclavicular fossa, positive Adson's maneuver	
Venous compression	Swelling of affected extremity	Occasional palpation of rib in supraclavicular fossa; positive Adson's maneuver; also, edema and venous distention of affected extremity	
Hyperabduction syndrome	Severe pain, paresthesias in upper extremity on awakening	Positive hyperabduction test	
Costoclavicular syndrome	Pain, paresthesias in shoulders with "military positioning"	Positive costoclavicular maneuver	

Visceral and Somatic Syndromes That Produce Symptoms Referable to the Shoulder

For diagnostic points concerning visceral syndromes that produce shoulder pain, consult a general medicine text. Compression of the spinal cord at the cervical level or of the brachial plexus may produce segmental and radicular signs in the upper limbs. In compression at the cervical level, these signs are combined with long-tract signs in the lower extremities. The specific findings in the upper extremity depend on the nerve roots that are involved. Underlying causes of cervical radiculopathies include cervical spondylosis, herniated disks, and intra- or extramedullary tumors. The mid and lower cervical spine are most likely to be involved. Generally, there may be loss of power and bulk in muscles of the shoulder girdle and arms. These and sensory deficits should suggest intraspinal compression. Absent biceps, brachioradialis, or triceps reflexes suggest C5, C6, or C7 involvement, respectively. Sensory deficits in the radial border of the forearm and thumb suggest C6 cord segment or nerve root involvement; in the index and middle finger, C7 involvement; and in the ring and little fingers, C8 involvement. The tendency of tumors of the superior sulcus of the lung, so-called Pancoast's tumors, to invade the stellate ganglion, which may cause a Horner's syndrome and invade cervical nerve roots, emphasizes the importance of ordering apical lordotic chest radiographs in the evaluation of such a patient.

Thoracic outlet syndromes are those disorders in which clinical symptoms result from compression of the brachial plexus or the subclavian artery or vein, the structures for the neural and vascular supply to the upper extremity that exit to the arm at the root of the neck. Symptoms include paresthesias, pain, loss of strength in any part of the shoulder or arm, and swelling and coolness of the affected extremity. Clinical findings depend upon the precise site of compression, but they include cyanosis, decreased skin temperature, diminished sensation (all modalities), muscle atrophy, edema, reduction of peripheral pulses during certain maneuvers, a blood pressure decrement in the involved extremity, and reflex changes. Adson's maneuver is a useful test that is positive in many thoracic outlet syndromes. The patient is seated, with chin raised and head turned to the symptomatic side. During deep inspiration, the patient holds his or her breath. A positive test is one in which clinical symptoms are reproduced, because diminution in the radial pulse in this setting may be normal. The costoclavicular maneuver, positive in the costoclavicular syndrome, is performed by forcing the patient's shoulders downward and posteriorly, and the hyperabduction test (often positive in the hyperabduction syndrome) is performed by having the patient hyperabduct his or her arms. As in the case of Adson's maneuver, these tests are positive only if symptoms are reproduced. Some common thoracic outlet syndromes are differentiated in Table 90-3.

References

Bland JH, Merrit JA, Boushey DR. The painful shoulder. Semin Arthritis Rheum 1977; 7:21.

Eversmann WW Jr. Compression and entrapment neuropathies of the upper extremity. J Hand Surg 1983; 8:759.

Katz WA, Bland JH. Shoulders, neck and thorax. In: Katz WA. Rheumatic diseases: Diagnosis and management. 2nd ed. Philadelphia: JB Lippincott, 1988:76.

McCarty DJ, ed. Crystalline deposition diseases. Rheum Dis Clin North Am 1988; Volume 14, Number 2.

Matsen FP, Kirby RM. Office evaluation and management of shoulder pain. Orthop Clin North Am 1982; 13:453.

Neer CS: Impingement lesions. Clin Orthop 1983; 173:70.

Rizk TE, Pinals RS. Frozen shoulder. Semin Arthritis Rheum 1982; 11:440.

Sarforis DJ, Resnick D. Imaging the painful shoulder. What studies to order. J Musculoskeletal Med 1988; 5(7):21.

Thornhill TS. Painful shoulder. In: Kelley WN, Harris ED, Ruddy S, et al. Textbook of rheumatology. 3rd ed. Philadelphia: WB Saunders, 1989:491.

Warren RF. Shoulder pain. In: Beary JF III, Christian CL, Johanson NA, eds. Manual of rheumatology and outpatient orthopedic disorders. 2nd ed. Boston: Little, Brown, 1987:81.

Disorders of the Hip

91

Katherine S. Upchurch, MD

David F. Giansiracusa, MD

Definition

The hip is a major weight-bearing joint that is centrally involved in ambulation in man. The ability to assess correctly the etiology of complaints referable to the hip and nearby pelvic structures requires an understanding of the anatomy of both the articular and periarticular structures, which is represented in Figure 91-1. As can be seen, disorders affecting the true synovium-lined joint, any of several nearby bursae or bony structures, and the vascular supply to the region may cause symptoms referable to the hip.

Etiology

Common etiologies of hip disease are shown in Table 91-1. Although a detailed discussion of each disorder listed in Table 91-1 is beyond the scope of this chapter, Table 91-2 differentiates the most common causes of hip pain.

Diagnostic Approach

History

Although some serious disorders of the hip are painless, hip pain is the most frequent complaint. Generally, history taking from a patient with hip pain should be designed to (1) define the precise anatomic site of the pain and, if possible, distinguish between periarticular and articular disease; (2) delineate the clinical characteristics of the complaint; and (3) investigate the possibility of underlying causes of the complaint (e.g., systemic illness). Because the hip joint is innervated by the obturator, sciatic, and femoral nerves, arthropathies of the hip may produce pain in the anterior or posterior aspects of the hip as well as the groin. In contrast, the pain of bursitis is typically more discretely localized. Pain directly overlying the greater trochanter of the femur, for example, is often secondary to trochanteric bursitis, a diagnosis that eliminates the need for further diagnos-

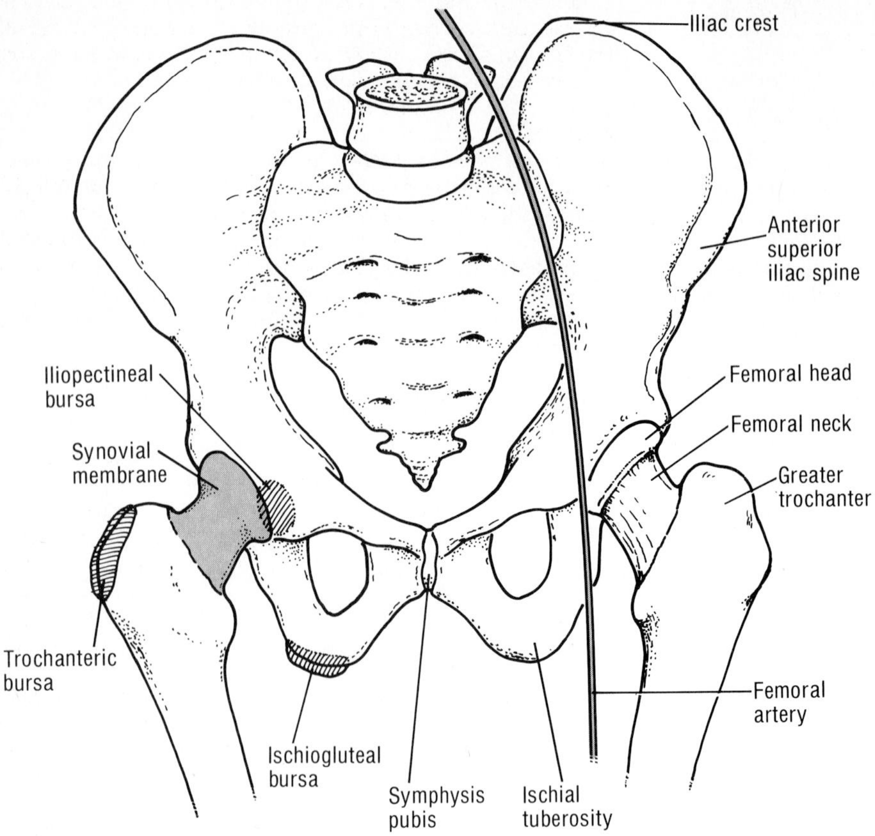

Figure 91-1 The articular and periarticular structures of the hip.

tic tests. Pain that is "lightning-like in character" and begins in the back or buttocks but travels down the leg is most likely secondary to nerve root compression from a number of possible causes, the most common of which is a herniated disk.

In addition to anatomic localization of the complaint, precise clinical characteristics should be defined. Information should be obtained about the patient's age at onset of the complaint, its subsequent time course (e.g., acute, subacute, chronic), the quality of the pain, and factors that exacerbate or alleviate the symptoms. Patients with pain referable to the hip joint dating from childhood or adolescence may have had unrecognized dislocation of the hip with subsequent early-onset osteoarthritis. Patients who are adolescents at the time of presentation should be suspected to have a slipped femoral epiphysis, which most commonly occurs in obese male adolescents. Patients with acute or subacute complaints should be carefully questioned about the possibility of any underlying traumatic event, bearing in mind that many such events may not be appropriately interpreted by the patient.

Identification of exacerbating or relieving factors may also aid in diagnosis. Hip pain secondary to osteoarthritis is typically exacerbated by weight bearing and relieved by rest, whereas hip pain secondary to rheumatoid arthritis may actually improve with activity and be worse in the early morning after a night of bed rest. The pain of trochanteric bursitis may be aggravated by hip abduction, going up and down stairs, or lying on the involved side. Pain due to trochanteric bursitis frequently radiates down the anterolateral aspect of the thigh to the knee, and as such may be misconstrued as a knee problem. The pain of iliopectineal bursitis, in contrast, is exacerbated by walking with normal strides or by extension and flexion of the hip. Pain in the area of the ischial tuberosity that is worsened by sitting could be due to ischiogluteal bursitis.

Patients with hip pain should be questioned carefully about other musculoskeletal and systemic complaints to assess the possibility of a related underlying illness. Symmetric polyarticular pain and swelling of chronic duration is suggestive, for example, of rheumatoid arthritis, which rarely involves the hip alone but often produces significant hip synovitis in association with synovitis of other joints. Sacroiliac or back pain suggests the possibility of underlying ankylosing spondylitis. A history of fevers, recent pelvic surgery, or the presence of a prosthetic hip joint mitigates for infection as the underlying cause of hip pain. Systemic symptoms such as weight loss, fatigue, and malaise may raise the question of an underlying malignancy. Diffuse bone pain may be secondary to Paget's disease or to metastatic bone lesions. Hip pain in an individual who has been treated with a course of corticosteroids or who has a history of renal transplant, diabetes mellitus, or alcoholism may be due to avascular necrosis of the femoral head. The pain due to avascular necrosis is characteristically aggravated by weight bearing. Exercise-induced hip and thigh pain may be due to atherosclerotic compromise to the iliac arteries rather than an underlying musculoskeletal disease.

Physical Examination

Examination of the hip should include an evaluation of stance and gait, inspection for overt swelling or muscle atrophy, evaluation for localized tenderness or pain on motion, assessment of range of motion, and evaluation for hip deformities and discrepancies in leg length. In addition, the lumbar spine, knees, legs, feet, and abdomen should be examined carefully.

Stance and Gait

An assessment of stance may reveal pelvic tilt or inequality in leg lengths. Measurements of anatomic leg length are made from the anterior-superior iliac crest to the medial malleolus with the legs directly in line below the trunk. Anatomic leg length is generally equal in persons with joint diseases, although defor-

Table 91-1 Common Causes of Hip Pain

Articular Disorders Producing Hip Pain
Noninflammatory arthropathies
Primary osteoarthritis*
Secondary osteoarthritis (ochronosis, hemochromatosis)
Inflammatory arthropathies
Rheumatoid arthritis*
Juvenile rheumatoid arthritis
Infectious arthritis (rare)
Other (ankylosing spondylitis, psoriatic arthritis, pseudogout, enteropathic arthropathy, polymyalgia rheumatica, systemic lupus erythematosus, hemophilia, sickle cell disease, gout)
Pigmented villonodular synovitis
Synovial tumors
Periarticular Disorders Producing Hip Pain
Bursitis
Trochanteric bursitis*
Iliopectineal bursitis
Ischiogluteal bursitis
Myositis (dermatomyositis, polymyositis)
Skeletal Disorders Producing Hip Pain
Malignancy metastatic to the bones or soft tissues of the pelvis*
Avascular necrosis of the femoral head*
Paget's disease of bone*
Fracture of the femoral neck, of the pubic rami
Metabolic bone diseases
Osteomalacia
Transient painful osteoporosis
Bone tumors (primary)
Slipped femoral epiphysis
Osteitis pubis
Extrinsic Disorders with Pain Referred to the Hip
Herniated disk syndromes and lumbar plexopathies*
Vascular disorders (Leriche's syndrome [iliac artery compromise])
Obturator or psoas abscess
Renal colic
Pelvic inflammatory disease
Hernia syndromes

* Indicates most common entities.

mity may produce relative discrepancy in leg lengths, an example being the adduction deformity of the hip that is often seen in degenerative joint disease. Pelvic obliquity may compensate for relative inequality in leg length and can be identified by placing both hands on the patient's anterior-superior iliac crest and observing whether the line between them is horizontal.

Assessment of gait may reveal several abnormalities in patients with hip disease. An *antalgic gait* is one in which the weight of the body is shifted to the *involved* side in order to avoid pain secondary to abductor muscle spasm. A *Trendelenburg* gait is one in which the weight is shifted to the normal limb because of weakness in affected abductor musles; this eliminates support for the pelvis when weight is borne on the involved hip.

Inspection and Palpation

Inspection and/or palpation of the hip and thigh should be performed to identify localized areas of tenderness and swelling, although overt effusions of the synovium or bursae are rarely identified in the hip because of the overlying musculature. The groin also should be checked for hernias and lymphadenopathy.

Range of Motion

Normal range of motion of the hip joint is discussed in detail in Polly and Hunder (1978). The normal ranges of motion of the hip include flexion (neutral to 120 degrees with knee flexed), extension (neutral to minus 30 degrees), internal rotation (neutral to 45 degrees), and external rotation (neutral to 45 degrees).

Internal rotation while the hip is flexed to 90 degrees is the first range of motion to be impaired with intrinsic hip disease, but this is also frequently impaired in elderly patients without hip disease.

Deformity

Deformities such as flexion contractures may not be noticed when the patient is lying supine in bed but should be sought while the patient is in the prone position. Adduction contractures of the hip may also occur, most commonly after prolonged inflammation of the hip joint. Other common deformities include the external rotation and abduction deformity seen in femoral neck fractures and the internal rotation deformity seen in posterior dislocations.

Radiographic Evaluation

Radiographs should include an anteroposterior view of the pelvis, to allow for comparison between hips, and a lateral view of the affected hip. If disease is suspected to be present in the lower back with referred pain to the hip, lumbosacral spine films, including oblique views, should be obtained. Radiographs of the hips may reveal characteristic and diagnostic changes. In osteoarthritis, for example, the typical findings include narrowing of the superior (weight-bearing) region of the joint space, which reflects loss of articular cartilage, subchondral sclerosis, osteophytes, and discrete subchondral cysts. In rheumatoid arthritis, uniform narrowing of the joint space is seen secondary to diffuse destruction of articular cartilage. Periarticular erosions may be present in the rheumatoid hip, but osteophytes are absent unless there is secondary osteoarthritis. Infectious arthritis may produce rapid loss of joint space secondary to cartilage destruction as well as signs of bone destruction. Rarely, calcification in soft tissues may be seen in the periarthritic syndromes, such as in the region of the abductor tendon insertion or in the greater femoral trochanter in some cases of trochanter bursitis. The radiograph may be diagnostic in congenital hip displasia, Legg-Calvé-Perthes disease, and the slipped femoral epiphysis syndrome. Computed tomography (CT) may provide clarification of the bony or soft-tissue abnormalities identified on plain-film radiographs. Computed tomograms are more sensitive in detecting changes of osteonecrosis (avascular or ischemic necrosis) than are plain-film radiographs. Over the past several years, magnetic resonance imaging (MRI) has been demonstrated to be a very sensitive and noninvasive technique to document the presence of osteonecrosis.

Laboratory Studies

Results of blood studies in patients with hip pain may be nonspecific. These should include complete blood count with differential, erythrocyte sedimentation rate (ESR), and rheumatoid factor if rheumatoid arthritis is considered possible on clinical grounds. An elevated leukocyte count with a left shift is suggestive of infection, whereas an elevated ESR suggests an underlying inflammatory, infectious, or malignant process. Blood cultures should always be obtained when fever is present.

Other Diagnostic Studies

Aspiration of the hip, preferably under fluoroscopy, should be performed if infection is a consideration. Synovial fluid should be examined in the manner described in Chapter 96, "Laboratory and Radiographic Abnormalities in Rheumatic Diseases." Arthrography may be useful to demonstrate localized disorders such as synovial tumors. Bone scanning identifies the presence of bony lesions such as avascular necrosis of the femoral head, metastatic bony lesions, or early Paget's disease. CT and MRI recently have been useful in the identification of both extrinsic

Table 91-2 Differentiation of Selected Causes of Hip Pain

Diagnosis	History	Physical findings	Laboratory findings	Radiographic findings
Disorders That Produce Generalized Hip Pain				
Primary and secondary osteoarthritis	Chronic groin pain, worse with weight bearing, relieved by rest, nocturnal in advanced disease	Pain on motion; decreased range of motion progressing with advanced disease	Normal except in case of underlying disease (e.g., hemochromatosis)	Superior joint-space narrowing; osteophytes; subchondral cysts
Rheumatoid arthritis	Subacute to chronic, episodic pain that is worse in the morning; possible improvement of pain with ambulation; systemic symptoms (fatigue, malaise) are common; other joint involvement plus bilateral hip involvement common; female predominance	Pain on motion; tenderness to palpation; decreased range of motion progressing with advanced disease; rarely, effusions are felt; flexion contractures; asymmetric leg length	Anemia; elevated ESR; positive rheumatoid factor common	Diffuse joint-space narrowing; periarticular erosions; osteopenia protrusio acetabulae
Ankylosing spondylitis	Subacute to chronic diffuse pain; back pain common; male predominance	See osteoarthritis; also, flexion contractures and decreased mobility of spine	Positive HLA-B27 ~90%	Often normal; sacroiliitis on pelvic films
Disorders That Produce Generalized Hip Pain				
Pseudogout	Subacute diffuse pain	See osteoarthritis	Calcium pyrophosphate crystals in synovial fluid	Chondrocalcinosis common
Infectious arthritis	Acute, subacute, or chronic pain; fever; malaise; more common in children	See osteoarthritis; flexion contractures in infants; effusions occasionally palpable	Elevated WBC and ESR; occasionally, positive blood cultures; positive synovial Gram stains and cultures	Early radiographs may be normal, progressing to severe destructive changes
Pigmented villonodular synovitis	Chronic diffuse pain without trauma; most common in young adults	See osteoarthritis	Synovial fluid dark, bloody	Soft-tissue density without calcification; bony lesions on one side of joint
Synovial and soft-tissue tumors	Chronic diffuse pain	Depends on exact location and nature of tumor	MRI or CT helpful to demonstrate mass lesion	Tissue diagnosis by biopsy
Disorders That Produce Localized Hip Pain				
Trochanteric bursitis	Lateral hip pain with or without radiation to knee; worse at night and with pressure, flexion, rotation, and abduction	Exquisite point tenderness over trochanteric bursa (*Note:* lidocaine infiltrate diminishes pain—diagnostic maneuver.)	Normal	Occasionally, trochanteric bursal calcium deposits
Iliopectineal bursitis	Pain at lateral border of triangle bounded by inguinal ligament, sartorius, adductor longus; pain increased with forced flexion, with or without anterior thigh radiation	Tenderness over iliopectineal bursa	Normal	Negative
Ischiogluteal bursitis	Buttock pain worse with sitting (weaver's bottom), with or without radiation down posterior leg; pain worse at night and on bending forward	Tenderness over ischial tuberosity (with hip flexed to expose this)	Normal	Negative
Osteitis pubis	Groin discomfort after exercise in athletes, exacerbated by sprinting, long strides; also occurs after pregnancy	Tenderness over symphysis pubis, pelvic bone on full flexion of legs or passive abduction of hips	Normal	Fraying at corner of symphysis; periosteal elevation; osteopenia

Table 91-2 (*Continued*)

Diagnosis	History	Physical findings	Laboratory findings	Radiographic findings
Hernia syndromes (inguinal, femoral)	Groin pain with anterior mass on lifting and Valsalva maneuver (inguinal)	There may or may not be limitation of hip motion	Normal	Barium enema may show incarceration
Skeletal Disorders That Produce Hip Pain				
Metastatic malignant pelvic or femoral lesions	Generalized or localized pain	Preserved joint motion; tenderness over involved bone	Depends on primary lesion (breast, prostatic, thyroid, renal, lung, gastrointestinal most common)	Lytic or blastic lesion; pathologic fractures. (*Note:* Bone scan is useful.)
Bone tumors (primary)	Generalized or localized pain	Variable depending on size, type of tumor		Often diagnostic, with pattern depending on type of tumor. (*Note:* Bone scan is useful.)
Paget's disease	Generalized or localized pain	Polyostotic bony deformities common; limitation of motion when joint involved	Elevated alkaline phosphatase level common	Coarsened trabecular pattern of bone. (*Note:* Bone scan is positive before radiographs.)
Osteomalacia	Diffuse bone pain; proximal muscle weakness	Children: bow-legged deformities. Adults: pain on motion, but preserved range of motion	Depends on underlying disorder	Osteopenia; pseudofractures. (*Note:* Bone biopsy is useful.)
Transient painful osteoporosis	Migratory lower extremity pain (ankle, knee, hip)	Muscle atrophy; pain on motion of affected joint	Normal	Patchy osteopenia of involved joint. (*Note:* Bone scan is positive.)
Avascular necrosis of femoral head	Pain at rest or on motion; renal transplant, steroid use, diabetes mellitus, alcoholism, and trauma are common underlying conditions	Normal, or pain on motion of the hip	Normal	Step-down lesions; diffuse spotty increase in radiodensity. (*Note:* Bone scan, biopsy, MRI positive before radiograph.)
Femoral neck fractures	Acute pain following trauma, often in elderly women	Extremity held in external rotation, abduction	Normal	Fracture; osteopenia often present
Slipped femoral epiphysis	Diffuse hip pain in a growing adolescent, with or without knee or anterior thigh radiation	Pain on forceful internal rotation	Normal	Hip radiographs show slipped epiphysis
Disorders with Referred Hip Pain				
Obturator or psoas muscle abscess	Diffuse, subacute, or chronic pelvic or hip pain; history of genitourinary tract infection or surgery common; fever; malaise	Preserved range of motion of joint; fluctuant mass may be palpable	Peripheral leukocytosis; elevated ESR	Negative unless bony involvement. (*Note:* CT or MRI may be diagnostic.)
Renal colic	Crampy costovertebral angle pain radiating to groin; fever	Lower quadrant costovertebral angle tenderness	Hematuria	Intravenous pyelogram demonstrates renal calculus (may be seen on plain film on occasion)
Herniated disk syndrome	See Chapter 88			
Vascular disorders (Leriche's syndrome)	Buttocks, leg pain brought on by walking; impotence	Decreased femoral and distal pulses common	Normal	Negative. (*Note:* Arteriogram shows vascular occlusive disease.)
Pelvic inflammatory disease	Diffuse pelvic pain and tenderness	Positive pelvic exam	Peripheral leukocytosis	Negative

Abbreviations: CT = computed tomography, ESR = erythrocyte sedimentation rate, MRI = magnetic resonance imaging, WBC = white blood cell count.

lesions causing hip pain (psoas or obturator, abscess, tumor) and intrinsic lesions (synovioma, bone tumors).

References

Katz WA. Hips and thighs. In: Katz WA, ed. Rheumatic diseases: Diagnosis and management. 2nd ed. Philadelphia: JB Lippincott, 1988:123.

Partridge REH. Low back and hip pain. In: Cohen AS, ed. Rheumatology and immunology. New York: Grune & Stratton, 1979:136.

Polly HF, Hunder GG. Rheumatologic interviewing and physical examination of the joints. 2nd ed. Philadelphia: WB Saunders, 1978.

Schumacher HR Jr, ed. Primer on the rheumatic diseases. 9th ed. Atlanta: The Arthritis Foundation, 1988.

Sculco TP. Hip pain. In: Beary JF, Christian CL, Johanson NA, eds. Manual of rheumatology and outpatient orthopedic disorders. 2nd ed. Boston: Little, Brown, 1987:104.

Sheon RP, Moskowitz RW, Goldberg VM. The hip and thigh region. In: Soft tissue rheumatic pain. Philadelphia: Lea & Febiger, 1987:207.

Disorders of the Knee

David F. Giansiracusa, MD

Katherine S. Upchurch, MD

92

The knee is composed of (1) articular cartilage overlying the femoral condyles, tibial plateaus, and undersurface of the patella; (2) the patella, distal femur, and proximal tibia; (3) the medial and lateral menisci; (4) the knee synovial membrane and joint capsule; (5) the patellar apparatus, which is composed of the quadriceps tendon, patella, and infrapatellar ligament; and (6) the four principal stabilizing ligaments of the knee—the medial (tibial) collateral, the lateral (fibular) collateral, and the anterior and posterior cruciate ligaments. The following six bursae are located in close proximity to the knee: the suprapatellar (quadriceps) bursa, which is proximal (cephalad) to and almost always continuous with the knee joint; the prepatellar bursa (overlying the patella); the anserine bursa (located along the inferomedial aspect of the knee joint); the deep infrapatellar bursa (located under the patellar ligament); the superficial infrapatellar bursa (located over the patellar ligament); and the bursa under the semimembranous tendon (Fig. 92-1).

Etiology

The structures of the knee may be affected by a variety of traumatic, infectious, inflammatory, and neoplastic processes. Table 92-1 lists the common disorders of the knee. Differentiation of selected disorders that produce knee pain is presented in Table 92-2.

Common forms of arthritis that may affect the knee are osteoarthritis, traumatic arthritis, crystal-induced arthritis (gout, pseudogout), infectious arthritis (including Lyme arthritis), and rheumatoid arthritis, as well as arthritis associated with psoriasis, Reiter's syndrome, ankylosing spondylitis, rheumatic fever, systemic lupus erythematosus, and sarcoidosis. For further discussion of arthritis, see Chapter 86, "Monarticular Arthritis," and Chapter 87, "Polyarthritis."

Diagnostic Approach

History

Always obtain a thorough general history when evaluating knee pain. Specific attention should be given to the age of the patient; history of trauma; the location, distribution, and nature of the pain; factors that aggravate and relieve the pain; and the occurrence of swelling and a limp. Certain conditions that are the result of vigorous physical activity and traumatic sports injuries, such as chondromalacia patellae (degeneration of the undersurface of the patellae) and meniscal and ligamentous tears, as well as pain and tenderness of the tibial tubercle at the insertion of the patellar ligament (Osgood-Schlatter disease) tend to occur in adolescents and young adults, whereas disorders such as osteoarthritis, gouty arthritis, spontaneous osteonecrosis of the knee (SONK), and anserine bursitis usually occur in middle-aged and elderly individuals.

Trauma may result in dysfunction of the patellar apparatus; ligamentous injury, which may manifest as joint instability; meniscal injury, which may result in locking of the knee (the inability to extend the knee fully); and pain localized to the medial or lateral joint lines. Knee trauma may also cause a traumatic arthritis characterized by an often bloody knee effusion or fracture. In an individual who has deposition of monosodium urate or calcium pyrophosphate dihydrate crystals in the articular structures of the knee, trauma may induce an acute attack of gouty arthritis or pseudogout, respectively.

Knee pain due to arthritis may be diffuse. It may be felt in the hip, thigh, or lower leg as well as the knee. Disorders may cause pain that can be localized to the anatomic site (e.g., bursa, tendon, ligament, or meniscus). Identification of particular activities and positions of the knee joint that aggravate the pain may be helpful in making the diagnosis.

Always look for associated symptoms because the knee problem may be only one component of a systemic disease. (See review of systems in Table 87-3 in Chapter 87, "Polyarthritis.")

Aggravation of knee pain during weight bearing with the knee in flexion (such as standing from a sitting position, climbing stairs, riding a bicycle) suggests patellar disease (chondromalacia patellae, osteoarthritis of the patellofemoral joint). Pain on twisting the knee or squatting is consistent with meniscal disease. Pain that is relieved with rest and aggravated by weight bearing is typical for osteoarthritis of the femorotibial aspect of the knee joint and for osteonecrosis and osteochondritis dissecans of the femoral condyle(s) or tibial plateau(s).

Physical Examination

Inspect the knees with the individual standing to assess genu valgus (knock-knees), genu varus (bow-legs), and hyperextension (genu recurvatum) deformities. Observe the gait for a limp and gross discrepancy in leg length. While the individual lies supine with legs extended, inspect the knees for flexion contractures (inability to extend the knees fully), erythema, and swelling. Swelling that is located predominantly, if not exclu-

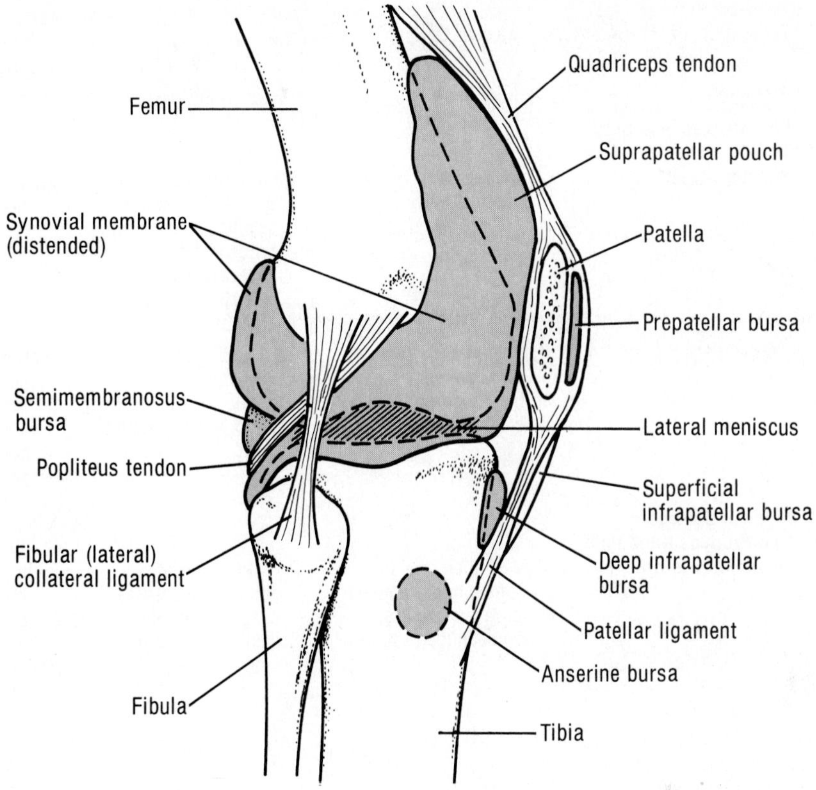

Figure 92-1 Lateral view of the knee.

sively, on the top of the patella suggests inflammation of the prepatellar bursa, whereas swelling on the medial, lateral, and cephalad (superior) aspects of the patella suggests synovial swelling or knee effusion. Active and passive range of motion should also be observed.

Palpate the prepatellar, infrapatellar, lateral, medial, and inferomedial aspects of the knee for local tenderness, which may indicate prepatellar bursitis, infrapatellar bursitis, patellar ligamentous injury, lateral and medial ligamentous or meniscal pathology, and anserine bursitis, respectively. Palpate the posterior aspect of the knee for swelling and tenderness indicative of a popliteal cyst, aneurysm of the popliteal artery, or a mass lesion.

Table 92-1 Common Causes of Knee Pain

Periarticular Disorders
Bursitis (prepatellar, infrapatellar, anserine)*
Tendonitis*

Articular Disorders
Rheumatoid arthritis,* osteoarthritis,* gout, pseudogout,* and other arthropathies, including spondyloarthropathies and Lyme arthritis
Chondromalacia patellae*
Popliteal (Baker's) cyst
Osteochondritis dissecans
Synovial osteochondromatosis

Traumatic Causes of Knee Pain
Ligamentous injuries (sprains)*
Meniscal tears
Fractures

Bone Disorders
Metastatic malignant lesions
Paget's disease of bone
Avascular (aseptic) necrosis
Osteomyelitis

* Most common disorders.

Swelling and pain in the calf and lower leg may be the consequence of dissection or rupture of a popliteal cyst. Because this condition may appear similar to the presentation of deep vein thrombophlebitis, the term *pseudothrombophlebitis* has been used to describe lower leg pain and swelling secondary to the ruptured cyst. (The crucial management point is that patients with calf swelling and pain *must be evaluated with impedance plethysmography or venography to evaluate for deep vein thrombophlebitis,* because this condition is potentially fatal as a result of pulmonary embolism. *Only when deep vein thrombophlebitis has been excluded* may one proceed with the evaluation and management of the ruptured popliteal cyst.) Palpate the hamstring tendons for tenderness.

Both legs should be measured from the anterior-superior-iliac spine (ASIS) to the superior aspect of the medial malleoli to evaluate for discrepancy in leg length. The circumference of both thighs should be measured 10 cm above the patellae as part of the evaluation of atrophy of the hamstring and quadriceps muscles.

Specific maneuvers may then be performed to elicit local pathology. A small knee effusion may be detected by gently massaging the medial aspect of the knee toward the suprapatellar pouch, then stroking the lateral aspect of the suprapatellar pouch and knee in a distal direction. The appearance of a bulge or fluid wave that fills the medial knee depression documents the presence of an effusion ("bulge sign"). Appreciation of a ballotable patella is a less reliable sign of a knee effusion, because the patella may be ballotable in an obese knee, even in the absence of excessive synovial fluid.

McMurray's test is a maneuver to detect a diseased meniscus. A positive test consists of a palpable click over the joint line while the knee is simultaneously extended (from a flexed position) as medial and then lateral stress is applied.

Examination for stability of the knee consists of stressing the collateral and cruciate ligaments while inspecting and palpating for deviation or slippage of the joint. With the leg extended, the integrity of the medial collateral ligament is tested by attempting to abduct the lower leg at the knee. The lateral

Table 92-2 Differentiation of Selected Causes of Knee Pain

Diagnosis	History	Physical findings	Laboratory and radiographic findings	Other
Periarticular Disorders That Produce Knee Pain				
Bursitis*	Localized pain; history of repeated stress	Point tenderness; erythema, warmth, swelling over involved bursa (inferomedial aspect of knee—anserine; overlying patella—prepatellar)	Laboratory: usually negative	Septic bursitis associated with peripheral leukocytosis, and inflammatory bursal fluid with positive Gram stain or cultures
Tendonitis	Localized pain over involved tendon; history of repeated or acute trauma	Pain on palpation of involved tendon; pain on motion (depending upon involved tendon)	Laboratory: usually negative; elevated peripheral WBC if tendonitis is due to gout or disseminated gonococcal infection	
Articular Disorders That Produce Knee Pain				
Rheumatoid arthritis*	Painful knee swelling, often bilateral; other joint involvement; worse in the morning	Erythema; warmth; effusion; decreased range of motion; flexion contracture (late)	Laboratory: positive rheumatoid factor (80%); elevated ESR; inflammatory effusion Radiographic: juxta-articular demineralization; marginal erosions; diffuse joint-space narrowing	
Osteoarthritis*	Painful or painless swelling aggravated by weight bearing; often history of past trauma, surgery, or repeated stress; may be unilateral or bilateral	Effusion (noninflammatory); palpable spurs; crepitus and pain on motion; decreased range of motion (late)	Laboratory: negative Radiographic: joint-space narrowing (lateral or medial); subchondral cysts and sclerosis; hypertrophic spurs	
Other arthropathies	See Chapters 86 and 87			
Chondromalacia patellae*	Intermittent anterior knee pain and swelling that is worse on rising from squat and climbing stairs; often in young person	Crepitus anteriorly; effusion; full range of motion	Laboratory: negative Radiographic: negative or (late) posterior patellar sclerosis; irregularity; spurring; decreased joint space	Air arthrography may show cartilage indentation; arthroscopy may show irregularity of underside of patella
Baker's cyst	Painful or painless swelling of medial aspect of popliteal fossa; often associated with underlying disease (osteoarthritis, rheumatoid arthritis, etc.) but may be isolated; calf swelling if ruptured	Medial bulge, popliteal fossa; edema of calf if ruptured, with pain on dorsiflexion of ankle (so-called Homan's sign)	Laboratory: negative unless there is underlying disorder	CT or echography if rupture not suspected; arthrography if rupture suspected
Osteochondritis dissecans	Insidious diffuse pain; momentary locking; often in a young person	Tenderness of femoral condyles on deep palpation with knee flexed	Laboratory: negative Radiographic: loose body seen on tunnel views of intercondylar notch	
Synovial osteochondromatosis	Diffuse pain; swelling	Effusion; limitation of knee motion	Laboratory: noninflammatory effusions with loose bodies Radiographic: calcifications within joint cavity	Loose bodies detected at arthroscopy
Synovial and soft-tissue tumor	Generalized or localized knee pain (depends on specific lesion)	Effusion; soft-tissue mass may be palpable	Laboratory: negative Radiographic: soft-tissue mass may be seen; bony involvement by intrasynovial or soft-tissue tumor may be seen	Arthrography or CT may demonstrate synovial or soft-tissue tumor, respectively

Table 92-2 (*Continued*)

Diagnosis	History	Physical findings	Laboratory and radiographic findings	Other
Pigmented villonodular synovitis	Persistent monarticular swelling and pain	Effusion; occasionally, palpable focal mass	Laboratory: hemarthrosis with orange-red hue Radiographic: joint-space narrowing; erosions; multiloculated cysts	Air arthrogram shows tissue-like masses; biopsy for diagnosis
Traumatic Causes of Knee Pain*				
Meniscal injuries (lateral or medial)	Lateral or medial knee pain; history of "knee twisting" (may not be prominent); patient often over 30 yr old	Tenderness of lateral or medial aspect of knee; McMurray's sign often present; pain on hyperabduction (medial meniscus)	Laboratory: negative	Arthrography, arthroscopy, or MRI may show torn meniscus
Ligamentous injuries	Severe knee pain; limitation of motion following acute trauma	Effusion; severe pain on motion; instability (type and degree depend on specific ligamentous tear)	Laboratory: hemarthrosis Radiographic: stress radiographs in children may show epiphyseal plate separation	Surgical confirmation
Other: see standard orthopedic text.				
Bone Lesions That Produce Knee Pain				
Metastatic malignant lesions	Bone pain (diffuse or localized)	Tenderness over involved bone	Laboratory: consistent with underlying disease Radiographic: lytic or blastic lesions	Bone scan and MRI positive before plain films
Paget's disease of bone	Bone pain (diffuse or localized)	Tenderness to palpation; generalized bony deformities if polyostotic	Laboratory: alkaline phosphatase increased Radiographic: sclerotic bone with coarsened trabeculation	
Avascular necrosis	Progressive knee pain (associated with diabetes mellitus, systemic lupus erythematosus, alcoholism, steroid therapy, sickle cell anemia)	Negative	Laboratory: negative Radiographic: evolution of medial condylar flattening; subchondral cysts	Bone scan, MRI, biopsy positive before plain films
Osteomyelitis	Acute or chronic pain and warmth	No effusion; tenderness over involved bone; fever	Laboratory: elevated WBC and ESR Radiographic: periosteal elevation, sequestrated bone	Bone scan positive before plain radiographs
Primary bone tumors	Bone pain (diffuse or localized)	Tenderness over involved bone	Laboratory: usually negative Radiographic: depends on type of tumor	CT useful in evaluation of extent of lesion

Abbreviations: CT = computed tomography, ESR = erythrocyte sedimentation rate, MRI = magnetic resonance imaging, WBC = white blood cell count.
*(*Note:* If suspected, orthopedic consultation should be obtained.)

collateral ligament is tested by attempting to adduct the lower leg in relation to the knee. Instability of the knee due to disease of the cruciate ligaments is assessed by pulling and pushing on the lower leg just below the knee joint while the patient is supine and the knee is flexed to 90 degrees. Anteroposterior instability (the so-called drawer sign) during this maneuver suggests torn cruciate ligaments.

Laboratory Studies

Routine laboratory studies include complete blood count with differential and measurement of acute-phase proteins such as the Westergren erythrocyte sedimentation rate (ESR). A diagnostic arthrocentesis and thorough synovial fluid analysis should always be performed when an undiagnosed knee effusion is identified (see synovial fluid analysis in Chapter 96, "Laboratory and Radiographic Abnormalities in Rheumatic Diseases"). A swollen, erythematous, prepatellar bursa should be aspirated and the bursa fluid analyzed and cultured.

Radiographic Evaluation

Routine plain films include anteroposterior and lateral views. Because these studies are often performed while the patient is supine, the radiographs may not provide a true assessment of joint space. Thus, if one wishes to assess joint-space narrowing (loss of cartilage as occurs in osteoarthritis, rheumatoid arthritis, and other forms of inflammatory arthritis), an anteroposterior view while the patient is standing, so-called weight-bearing films, should be ordered. Special views using plain films include tunnel, patellar, and stress views.

The tunnel view is the best plain-film radiograph for evaluating the appearance of intercondylar spines as well as for demonstrating a loose body within the knee joint or osteochondritis dissecans. Patellar (sunrise) views (taken with knee held in flexion so that the patella appears as a rising sun between the femoral condyles; hence the name *sunrise views*) are helpful in evaluating for patellar disorders. These views may demonstrate (1) narrowing of the joint space between the patella and the distal femur, (2) malalignment of the patella relative to the medial and lateral femoral condyles, (3) lateral and medial patellar osteophytes, (4) irregularities of the undersurface of the patella, and (5) fracture.

Other Diagnostic Studies

Special radiographic studies and imaging techniques are the arthrogram, bone scan, and arthroscopy. The arthrogram is particularly useful to define disease of the menisci and dissection or rupture of a popliteal cyst. Computed tomography (CT) and ultrasonography are two noninvasive techniques that may demonstrate the presence of popliteal cysts. However, the arthrogram demonstrates dissection or rupture much better than either of these tests. Bone scans are helpful in evaluating for osteonecrosis, infection in bone (osteomyelitis), and inflammatory joint disease, in which case the scan reveals increased uptake in the inflamed regions. In contrast, bone scans are generally normal in cases of structural knee problems such as meniscal disease.

Arthroscopy is being used (1) to evaluate for chondromalacia patellae; (2) to visualize and resect meniscal tears; (3) to inspect the cartilage surfaces and synovium; (4) to perform directed synovial biopsies for culture and histologic exam, as well as synovectomy; (5) to evaluate the integrity of the cruciate ligament; and (6) to remove small loose bodies from the joint.

Magnetic resonance imaging (MRI) has been documented to demonstrate the anatomy of the knee and to be particularly helpful in noninvasively demonstrating soft-tissue knee pathology such as meniscal and ligamentous tears and joint effusions, abnormalities of articular cartilage, osteonecrosis of the knee, and tumor in and about the knee joint.

References

Johanson NA. Knee pain. In: Beary JF III, Christian CL, Johanson NA, eds. Manual of rheumatology and outpatient orthopedic disorders. Boston: Little, Brown, 1987:108.

Johnson RP. Mechanical disorders of the knee. In: McCarty DJ, ed. Arthritis and allied conditions. 11th ed. Philadelphia: Lea & Febiger, 1989:1390.

Katz WA. Knees and legs. In: Katz WA, ed. Rheumatic diseases: Diagnosis and management. 2nd ed. Philadelphia: JB Lippincott, 1988:134.

Katz RS, et al. The pseudothrombophlebitis syndrome. Medicine 1977; 56:151.

Mink JH, Reicher MA, Crues JV III. Magnetic resonance imaging of the knee. New York: Raven Press, 1987.

Polley HF, Hunder GG. Rheumatologic interviewing and physical examination of the joints. 2nd ed. Philadelphia: WB Saunders, 1978.

Schumacher HR Jr, ed. Primer on the rheumatic diseases. 9th ed. Atlanta: The Arthritis Foundation, 1988.

Sheon RP, Moskowitz RW, Goldberg VM. The knee. In: Soft tissue rheumatic pain. 2nd ed. Philadelphia: Lea & Febiger, 1987:217.

Limb Pain and Weakness

93

David F. Giansiracusa, MD

James L. McGuire, MD

Ann Gateley, MD

Definition

Pain and weakness are common complaints of both the hospitalized and the ambulatory patient. The clinician must decide whether weakness is a consequence of muscle (myopathy), nerve (neuropathy), or articular (arthropathy) disorders or, alternatively, of a functional or psychogenic basis.

Etiology

The causes of limb pain and weakness are listed in Table 93-1. The conditions that may cause weakness of the respiratory muscles are amyotrophic lateral sclerosis, myasthenia gravis, Guillain-Barré syndrome, Duchenne's muscular dystrophy, and inflammatory and noninflammatory myopathies (rarely).

History

A patient with weakness may complain of feeling fatigued or tired, or may describe limb heaviness rather than limb weakness. The clinician must ask specific questions about functional capacity in order to localize the affected muscle and quantify the weakness. Temporal relationships are important (morning versus later in the day), as is the relationship of strength to exercise (cramping after exertion, improvement, or exacerbation). Pose questions that help distinguish proximal weakness (difficulty standing up from a sitting position or lifting arms above the head) from symptoms indicative of distal muscle weakness (difficulty grasping objects or standing on one's toes). Double vision, drooping of the eyelids, and difficulty swallowing, chewing, and breathing are bulbar signs, and they may indicate a primary neurogenic rather than myopathic disorder.

Many neuromuscular disorders are familial; therefore, a family history of weakness in other relatives should be obtained.

Questions directed at identifying evidence of underlying endocrine, metabolic, dietary, or inflammatory disorders as well as a careful drug history are important because they may have a profound effect on strength. Potassium-depleting diuretics, steroids, thyroid medications, and alcohol can all cause a myopathy. Other medications can cause fatigue without weakness through central sedation. Ingestion of undercooked or raw pork or, more rarely, beef might suggest trichinosis.

Sleep disturbances and loss of appetite may reflect endogenous depression, a psychogenic cause of weakness. Numerous medical consultations or invasive procedures may raise the possibility of a psychogenic component of the weakness.

Pain is often a difficult symptom to separate from weakness. Some types of limb pain may be exacerbated by exercise, whereas others are relieved by exercise (vascular insufficiency versus restless leg syndrome). Questions regarding the onset of pain (acute versus insidious) are important. Complaints of pain

Table 93-1 Classification of Pain and Weakness

Condition	Degree of weakness*	Degree of pain*†
Inflammatory muscle disease (dermato- and polymyositis)	+ to ++++	0 to ++
Noninflammatory myopathies		
Metabolic		
Hypothyroidism	+ to ++++	0 to +++
Hypokalemia	+ to ++++	0 to +
Hypophosphatemia	+ to ++++	0 to ++
Hypomagnesemia	+ to ++++	0
Hypercortisolism (Cushing's syndrome, exogenous steroid administration)	+ to ++++	0
Inherited		
Dystrophic	+ to ++++	0
Nondystrophic (metabolic)	+ to ++++	0 to ++++
Drug	+ to ++++	0 to ++
Infectious myopathies		
Viral	+ to ++++	0 to ++++
Trichinella	+ to ++++	0 to +++
Neurogenic		
Amyotrophic lateral sclerosis	+ to ++++	0
Peripheral neuropathies	+ to ++++	0 to ++++
Poliomyelitis	+ to ++++	0
Myasthenia gravis	+ to ++++	0
Guillain-Barré syndrome	+ to ++++	0 to +++
Central nervous disease		
Cerebrovascular accidents	0 to ++++	0
Tumor	0 to ++++	0
Demyelinating disease (multiple sclerosis)	0 to ++++	0 to +
Psychogenic weakness		
Depression	0	0 to ++
Hysteria	0 to ++++	0 to ++++
Malingering	0 to ++++	0 to ++++
Inflammatory joint disease (arthritis‡/tendonitis)	0 to +++	+ to ++++
Polymyalgia rheumatica	0	+ to ++++
Nocturnal leg cramps	0	0
Thrombophlebitis	0	0 to ++++
Ruptured Baker's cyst	0 to +	+ to ++++
Bone disorders		
Fractures	0	++ to ++++
Paget's disease	0	0 to ++
Osteomalacia§	0 to ++	+ to ++++
Osteonecrosis	0	+ to ++++
Cellulitis	0	+ to ++++

*0 to ++++; 0 = none, ++++ = severe.
† Pain may interfere with strength testing.
‡ Some inflammatory diseases such as rheumatoid arthritis and systemic lupus erythematosus may have myositis as a component.
§ Phosphate depletion may cause myopathy in patients with osteomalacia.

involving more than one limb suggest a generalized (myopathy, polymyalgia rheumatica) rather than a regional problem (overuse syndrome). Occasionally, pain may be associated with limb weakness, but any painful process may interfere with effort; therefore, subjective "weakness" may be described.

Physical Examination

Physical evaluation of patients with pain or weakness includes inspection of muscle mass as well as posture and gait, palpation of muscle mass and tone, assessment of strength, examination for joint or muscle tenderness, and neurologic testing to include, at a minimum, testing of deep tendon reflexes and sensation.

Various scales of muscle weakness have been devised. The Medical Research Council 1 to 5 gradation (Table 93-2) is commonly used, but most myopathic problems range between 4 and 5, so clear-cut delineation and comparison may be difficult. The strength of the neck and hip flexors, the abductors of the shoulders, and the distal musculature should be assessed. Weak muscles generally fail to withstand progressive resistance. Unexpected giving way of a muscle to applied force may point to a *painful* musculoskeletal process or factitious weakness.

Look for cutaneous manifestations associated with inflammatory muscle or systemic disorders (polymyositis). A dusky violaceous (heliotrope) rash of the eyelids and scaly, erythematous papules over the knuckles (Gottron's papules) are classic signs of dermatomyositis. A malar rash that affects the face is suggestive of systemic lupus erythematosus; splinter hemorrhages suggest vasculitis; and dry, thickened skin suggests hypothyroidism.

Laboratory Studies

Weakness can be assessed by studying serologic or electrical abnormalities. Regarding the former, the hallmark of muscle disease is increased blood levels of the enzyme creatine phosphokinase (CPK). Other enzymes that may be elevated in the serum are aldolase, aspartate aminotransferase (AST, also referred to as serum glutamic-oxaloacetic transaminase [SGOT]), alanine aminotransferase (ALT, also referred to as serum glutamic-pyruvic transaminase [SGPT]), and lactate dehydrogenase (LDH). Serum phosphate, calcium, magnesium, thyrotropin, and thyroxine levels should also be checked. Antinuclear antibodies (ANAs) are present in approximately one-third of patients with dermatomyositis or polymyositis, usually in low titer. The Westergren erythrocyte sedimentation rate (ESR) may be normal or high. Because inflammatory myositis may accompany other collagen vascular disorders, these studies must be interpreted with caution.

Other important tests include nerve conduction studies (NCS) and electromyography (EMG), which help in distinguishing myopathic from neuropathic disease. Within the spectrum of myopathic patterns, polymyositis is usually diagnosed if a characteristic triad of increased insertional activity, decreased

Table 93-2 Medical Research Council Grading of Strength

5	Normal
4	Muscle force able to overcome gravity and moderate resistance
3	Muscle force able to overcome gravity only
2	Able to move body part with gravity eliminated
1	Examiner able to observe only flickers of muscle contraction
0	No movement or identifiable muscle contraction

amplitude, and an interference pattern with mild effort is present. EMG may help identify affected muscles. The contralateral muscles may then be chosen as the optimal sites for biopsies. The actual muscles studied with EMG needles should not be biopsied, because the needle trauma may cause artifact that resembles the histologic changes seen in myositis.

The definitive study for evaluation of muscle weakness is a muscle biopsy. The quadriceps or deltoid muscle, depending on clinical weakness and EMG findings, is an appropriate site. The inflammation of polymyositis may be dramatic. The demonstration of *Trichinella* on muscle biopsy is diagnostic. Patients with metabolic myopathies, polymyalgia rheumatica, and myasthenia gravis characteristically have normal muscle biopsy findings.

Special Problems

Polymyositis is an inflammatory myopathy. The diagnosis relies on (1) weakness, (2) CPK elevation, (3) an abnormal EMG, and (4) characteristic findings on muscle biopsy. Dermatomyositis is present when polymyositis is accompanied by a characteristic rash. Weakness without significant pain is usual. Polymyositis is grouped with the other connective tissues and may be associated with a low incidence of both ANA and rheumatoid factor positivity. In the elderly population, the diagnosis of polymyositis or dermatomyositis should prompt a thorough history, physical examination, and routine health maintenance studies to search for an underlying neoplasm. Muscle weakness in patients with cancer may also be due to processes independent of myositis.

Disorders with a negative muscle biopsy constitute most of the causes of muscle weakness and fall under the categories of toxic (e.g., drug-related) metabolic- or endocrine-related myopathy. Hypokalemia, most commonly as a result of diuretic therapy, may cause diffuse muscle weakness. CPK elevations have been reported. The classic endocrine myopathy that causes CPK elevations is hypothyroidism, which may also present with muscle weakness and normal CPK values. Primary hyperparathyroidism may cause a proximal myopathy due to phosphate wasting.

Muscle pain without weakness occurs in two common clinical settings: some forms of infectious myopathies and polymyalgia rheumatica. Viruses, including human immunodeficiency virus (HIV), which may also cause an inflammatory myopathy, and toxoplasmosis infections are associated with prominent myalgias, especially in the early phase. These should be distinguished from the severe infectious myopathies associated with *Trichinella*. Prominent systemic complaints of the latter include fever, muscle tenderness, and edema. Laboratory studies may reveal an eosinophilia, low ESR, and a marked increase in CPK activity. Polymyalgia rheumatica presents in the elderly as proximal muscle aching. It may start acutely in one or all of the limb girdle muscles and posterior neck. Morning stiffness may be severe and several hours in duration, with symptoms improving as the day proceeds. There is usually a history of fatigue and often depression. CPK levels, electromyograms, and muscle biopsies are normal. Elevation of the ESR to above 50 mm per hour is characteristic, and a normochromic, normocytic anemia is common. The rapid improvement of clinical symptoms within several days with low doses of steroids is so dramatic as to be diagnostic of polymyalgia rheumatica.

Restless leg syndrome and nocturnal leg cramps are additional examples of painful processes without associated weakness. These are less serious in nature than those entities described previously and are very common. In each, the diagnosis is made on the basis of a characteristic history, as the physical examination is usually normal.

Nocturnal leg cramps, occurring in all age groups, are described as an intermittent, usually unilateral, spasm that occurs during sleep, and are characterized by a hard, drawing feeling in the calf, foot, or rarely the thigh. The cramps are relieved by moving, rubbing, or applying heat to the affected muscle. Try to determine whether an underlying electrolyte disorder is contributing to the problem, although potassium, calcium, and magnesium levels are usually normal. Nocturnal leg cramps usually improve when the patient gets up and walks, in marked contrast to cramps due to claudication, which occur with and worsen during activity.

Restless leg syndrome is usually found in middle-aged and elderly patients. The problem can occur when the patient is awake or asleep, but it seems to be most troublesome at night. The features are characteristic and include bilateral diffuse discomfort that is variably described as a burning, gnawing, jumping, or crawling sensation. The cause of the discomfort is unknown, although some feel that it is a manifestation of chronic anxiety or tension.

Muscle dystrophy is a family of degenerative myopathies that can be present in adulthood as weakness of selected muscle groups. The CPK elevation, the muscle biopsy, and even the EMG results may be confused with polymyositis. Myasthenia gravis is a neuromuscular disorder that results from antibodies directed against acetylcholine receptors in the motor end-plate. The clinical presentation of muscle weakness, which often affects the ocular muscles as well, that gets worse with exercise or as the day progresses suggests myasthenia gravis, in contrast to the muscle weakness in polymyositis, which is constant and is minimally affected by rest. In myasthenia gravis, the CPK level and muscle biopsy are normal, whereas the EMG demonstrates decremental potentials with rapid repetitive stimulation.

No discussion of limb weakness and pain would be complete without a caution that cervical spine osteoarthritis is capable of presenting as both upper limb weakness and pain (cervical radiculopathy) and leg weakness (long-tract involvement). This emphasizes the importance of performing a careful neurologic examination of the patient who presents with the complaint of weakness.

References

Bradley WB, Tandan R. Inflammatory diseases of muscle. In: Kelley et al, eds. Textbook of rheumatology. 3rd ed. Philadelphia: WB Saunders, 1989:1263.

Calabrese LH. The rheumatic manifestations of infection with the human immunodeficiency virus. Semin Arthritis Rheum 1989; 18:225.

Fontneau NM, Chad DA. Differential diagnosis of myositis. IM—Intern Med Specialist 1988; 1:85.

Kagen LJ. Polymyositis/dermatomyositis. In: McCarty DJ, ed. Arthritis and allied conditions. 11th ed. Philadelphia: Lea & Febiger, 1989:1092.

Mastalgia FL. Inflammatory diseases of muscle. Boston: Blackwell Scientific, 1988.

Miller ML, Phelps P. Weakness. In: Kelley WN, et al, eds. Textbook of rheumatology. 3rd ed. Philadelphia: WB Saunders, 1989:462.

Moskowitz RW. Clinical rheumatology. Philadelphia: Lea & Febiger, 1982.

Nakano KK. Neurology of musculoskeletal and rheumatic disorders. Boston: Houghton Mifflin, 1979.

Sheon RP, Moskowitz RW, Goldberg VM. Soft tissue rheumatic pain. 2nd ed. Philadelphia: Lea & Febiger, 1987.

Strongwater SL. Clinical overview: Polymyositis and dermatomyositis. Mt Sinai J Med 1988; 55:435.

Foot and Ankle Pain

94

David F. Giansiracusa, MD

Steven L. Strongwater, MD

Complaints referable to the foot and ankle are extremely common. The foot plays an integral role in both dynamic (locomotion) and static functions (support). It may be affected by a multitude of mechanical (static disorders), inflammatory, vascular, or neurologic disorders. Most often, pain is the presenting complaint. Table 94-1 lists common causes of foot and ankle pain.

Diagnostic Approach

A discussion of problems affecting the foot may be organized into disorders affecting the (1) forefoot, which is composed of the toe metatarsophalangeal joints (balls of the feet); (2) midfoot (arch of the foot); (3) heel (hindfoot); and (4) ankle (Fig. 94-1).

History

The location, character, duration, nature of onset, radiation, and aggravating and attenuating factors as well as associated symptoms are important in determining the cause of foot pain. Localizing complaints to one of four regions of the foot (the forefoot, midfoot, hindfoot, and ankle) helps to focus on a particular diagnosis.

Individuals should be specifically questioned regarding trauma; previous episodes of joint pain, swelling, and redness; and activities that precipitate or aggravate the particular problem. Because many of the causes of foot pain may be manifestations of systemic disease (rheumatic, vascular, neurologic), a complete medical history and a detailed review of systems relating to these areas are of crucial importance.

The presence of swelling, erythema, or heat in association with pain suggests an inflammatory process. Alternatively, pain with walking could indicate vascular or neurogenic claudication as well as any number of other static, bone, or miscellaneous processes (Table 94-1).

Tingling (paresthesias), dysesthesia, burning, numbness, or weakness suggests pain resulting from nerve irritation or compression. Common sites of nerve compression that may manifest as foot pain include lumbosacral spine disease (lumbar disk herniation, lumbar spinal stenosis, radiculitis), posterior tibial or peroneal nerve disorders at the level of the knee (compression from a Baker's cyst, direct pressure, or compartment syndrome), or compression of the posterior tibial nerve at the medial aspect of the ankle in the tarsal tunnel.

Physical Examination

Physical examination of the foot, in addition to a thorough general examination, should include observation of gait for a limp; of stance; of deformities (Fig. 94-2) such as flat feet, talipes irregularities, or malalignment; of the joints for swelling, tenderness, erythema, and range of motion; of the skin for calluses, warts, corns, atrophy, color, temperature, hair distribution, and other rashes; of toenails for ridging and pitting (onycholysis, pitting, and ridging occur in psoriatic arthritis and Reiter's syndrome); of peripheral pulses; and of shoes for abnormal wear.

Laboratory Studies

If an osseus (bony) lesion or inflammatory process is suspected, obtain plain-film radiographs of the foot. Additional studies such as arthrocentesis, synovial fluid analysis, bone and joint scans, and serologic determinations (rheumatoid factor, antinuclear antibody, tissue typing for HLA-B27) may also be helpful and are discussed in Chapter 87, "Polyarticular Arthritis," and Chapter 96, "Laboratory and Radiographic Abnormalities in Rheumatic Diseases."

Forefoot Pain

Common causes of forefoot pain include arthritis affecting the interphalangeal joints of the toes, hammer and cock-up toes, corns, ischemic peripheral vascular disease, Raynaud's phenomenon, and cellulitis.

Table 94-1 Common Causes of Foot and Ankle Pain

Static Disorders
Foot strain
Flat feet (pes planus)
High arches (pes or talipes cavus)
Ankle deformities
Toe deformities (hallux valgus, rigidus, hammer toe, cock-up toe)
Corns, bunions, calluses, plantar warts
Inflammatory Disorders
Acute arthritis (gout, pseudogout, gonococcal arthritis-dermatitis syndrome)
Chronic arthritis (rheumatoid arthritis, psoriatic arthritis, Reiter's syndrome)
Tendonitis, bursitis, tenosynovitis, plantar fasciitis
Vascular Disorders
Ischemia (atherosclerosis, diabetes mellitus), arterial embolism
Vasospastic disease (Raynaud's phenomenon), cryoglobulinemia
Venous insufficiency, dependent edema (multiple etiologies)
Neurologic Disease
Peripheral neuritis
Entrapment syndromes (posterior tibial nerve entrapment, termed tarsal tunnel syndrome)
Compartmental syndromes in the lower leg
Peripheral neuropathy (e.g., alcoholic, diabetic)
Bone Disease and Disorders
Traumatic and pathologic fractures
March or stress fractures
Osteomyelitis
Osteochondritis
Calcaneal spurs
Miscellaneous
Soft-tissue trauma (muscles/ligaments)
Cellulitis
Sudeck's atrophy (reflex sympathetic dystrophy)
Morton's neuroma
Tumors
Osteoarthritis

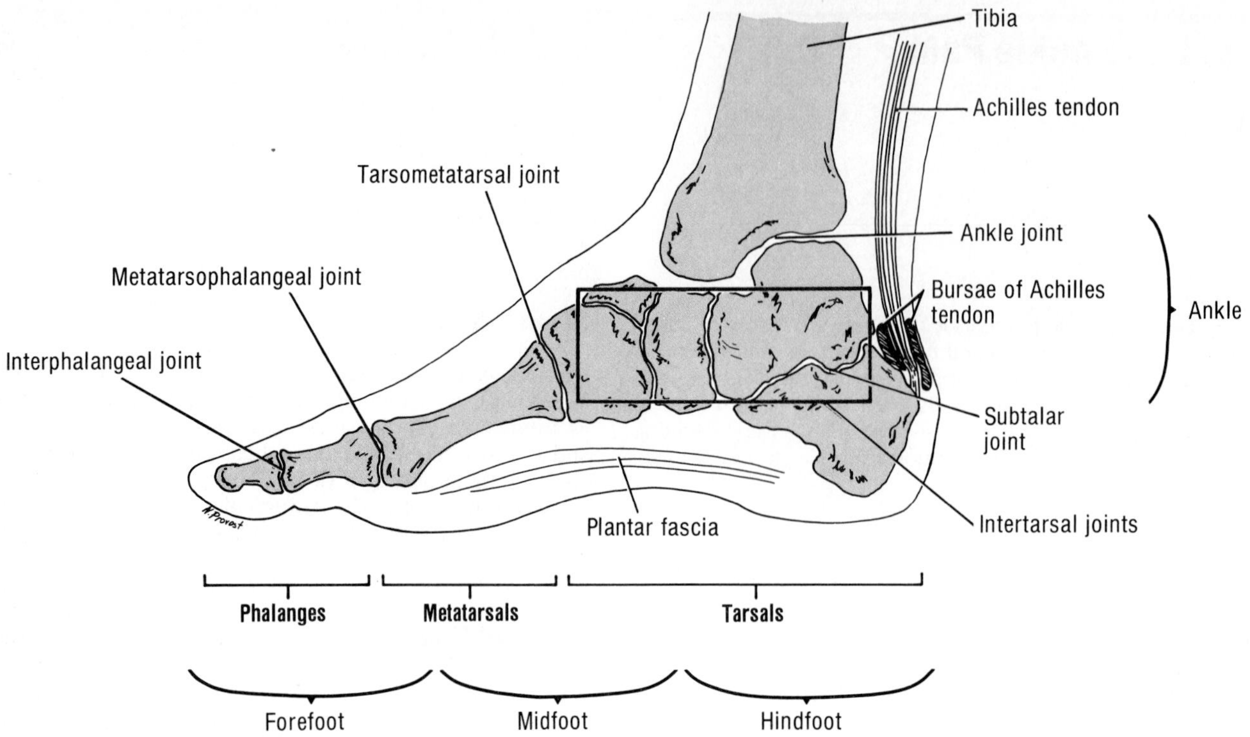

Figure 94-1 Anatomy of the foot.

Toe Pain

The painful red swollen toe suggests an inflammatory process that is either rheumatic or infectious in nature. A history of skin abrasion or identification of a fissure between digits in the setting of a tender streak up the foot or leg, tender inguinal lymphadenopathy, fever, and a peripheral blood leukocytosis strongly suggest an infectious process such as cellulitis. Evaluation should include blood cultures in the toxic patient and radiographs, the latter to evaluate for the possibility of osteomyelitis.

When severe peripheral vascular disease is the cause of the toe pain, a history of foot or calf pain with walking that is relieved with rest (so-called claudication) may be elicited. Examination may reveal skin atrophy, including loss of hair, thinning and coolness of the skin, pallor when the foot is raised, and diminished dorsalis pedis and posterior tibialis arterial pulses. Ulcers may occur in ischemic vascular disease, particularly at pressure points.

The individual who has vasospastic disease (Raynaud's phenomenon) as well as complaints related to the feet often complains of symptoms affecting the fingers. A typical history for Raynaud's phenomenon includes a history of episodic coolness and blanching (white discoloration) that is followed by dusky cyanosis (blue discoloration) and then, upon rewarming, by hyperemia and pain. In severe cases of Raynaud's phenomenon, periungual and finger-pad ulcerations may complicate the disease. An evaluation for a systemic connective tissue disease should be undertaken (see Chapter 87, "Polyarthritis").

Arthritis of the toe interphalangeal joints, particularly when accompanied by tenosynovitis or periostitis of the phalanges, may result in a painful, diffusely red, swollen, tender toe(s). Such a presentation is characteristic of Reiter's disease or psoriatic arthritis (see Chapter 87, "Polyarthritis").

Metatarsal Pain

Common causes of pain at the base of the toes (balls of the feet) are arthritis of the metatarsophalangeal (MTP) joints, bursitis over the medial aspect of the base of the great toe, metatarsalgia, Morton's neuroma, and plantar fasciitis at its distal insertion.

A variety of rheumatic diseases may affect the MTP joints, including rheumatoid arthritis, psoriatic arthritis, and Reiter's syndrome (see Chapter 87, "Polyarthritis"). Gouty arthritis and osteoarthritis commonly involve the first MTP joint (i.e., the joint at the base of the great toe). Gout tends to be an episodic, excruciatingly painful inflammatory form of joint disease that most commonly affects middle-aged men. Concurrent signs of inflammation in the dorsum (arch or instep) of the foot or involvement of multiple ipsilateral joints, such as the ankle, suggests a diagnosis of polyarticular gout. Arthrocentesis with crystalline analysis reveals needle-shaped (negatively birefringent) crystals within synovial fluid leukocytes (see Chapter 96, "Laboratory and Radiographic Abnormalities in Rheumatic Diseases") to confirm this diagnostic impression. Radiographs may reveal a characteristic nonmarginal erosion in advanced disease. Painful, warm, erythematous swelling of the bursa on the medial aspect of this great toe can mimic gouty arthritis, but it can be differentiated by bursal fluid analysis.

In contrast to the sudden episodic, intensely painful attacks of gouty arthritis, osteoarthritis of the first MTP joint is characterized by the insidious onset of pain, deformity (bunion formation), and loss of range of motion. Characteristic findings of MTP osteoarthritis on radiographs include joint-space narrowing, subchondral bony sclerosis, cyst formation, and osteophytes or spurs. Painful restricted motion of the great toe due to osteoarthritic spurs is termed hallux rigidus.

Pain in the MTP joints (balls of the feet) that is aggravated by weight bearing and sometimes associated with thick, tender

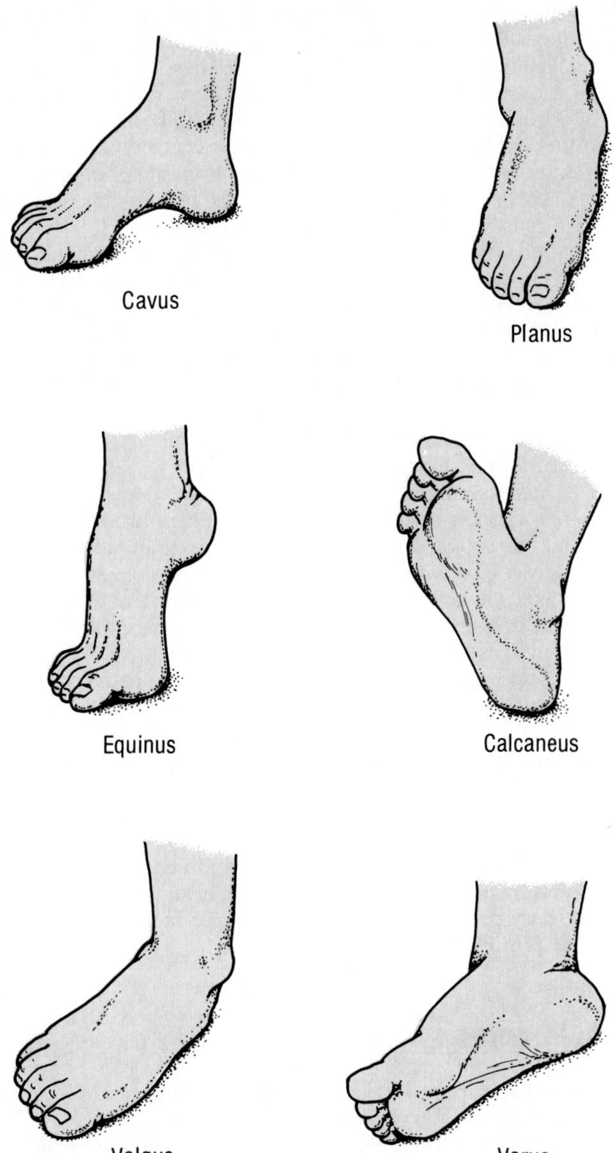

Figure 94-2 Types of talipes.

calluses on the undersurface of the foot is called metatarsalgia. This problem may be due to a structural problem (i.e., shoes that do not fit correctly) or rheumatic disease, most frequently rheumatoid arthritis. When a distinct point of tenderness (sometimes a nodule) can be localized between, rather than over, the third and fourth toes, Morton's neuroma is a likely diagnosis. Another cause of metatarsalgia is inflammation of the plantar fascia where it inserts on the metatarsal heads.

Midfoot Pain

Because the midfoot is composed of the longitudinal arch, the metatarsal and tarsal bones and joints, the middle portion of the plantar fascia, extensor and flexor tendons of the toes, and associated soft tissues, inflammation in any of these structures may result in pain affecting the midfoot.

Pain in the region of the metatarsal bones associated with localized tenderness and swelling after excessive walking, hiking, or marching is consistent with a stress or march fracture. Radiography may not reveal the fracture until a bony callus has formed; however, the diagnosis can readily be made by bone scan. Gouty arthritis may affect the instep. The presence of low-grade discomfort and bony overgrowth and swelling in the joints of the arch (the tarsal joints) suggests neuropathic (Charcot's) arthropathy. Pain in the arch of the foot associated with an excessively high arch (pes cavus) or flat feet (pes planus) is consistent with mechanic or static foot problems (see Fig. 94-2).

Hindfoot Pain

The heel is probably the most common site of hindfoot pain. Hindfoot pain is less often due to arthritis of the subtalar joint, which results in pain during active and passive inversion (adduction, supination, internal rotation) and eversion (abduction, pronation, external rotation) and occurs as a result of gout, rheumatoid arthritis, or trauma (ligamentous sprains, strains).

Pain along the plantar (weight-bearing) aspect of the heel may be due to inflammation of the plantar fascia at its site of origin on the calcaneus. A spur may ultimately form that is tender on direct palpation and identifiable on a lateral-view radiograph of the foot. Periostitis of the calcaneus at the insertion of the plantar fascia is a frequent component of the spondyloarthropathies (psoriatic arthritis, Reiter's syndrome, ankylosing spondylitis). Mechanical foot problems, such as flat feet (pes planus), may also inflame the plantar fascia at its attachment to the periosteum owing to excessive stress.

Pain affecting the posterior superior aspect of the heel, often associated with tenderness to palpation and discomfort on dorsiflexion of the foot (which stresses the Achilles tendon), may be due to inflammation of the Achilles tendon or of the bursa(e), which are superficial to or beneath the Achilles tendon (see Fig. 94-1). Because inflammation of these structures as well as of the plantar fascia is a common component of the spondyloarthropathies (Reiter's syndrome, the arthritis associated with psoriasis, inflammatory bowel disease, and ankylosing spondylitis), patients with these forms of heel pain should be evaluated for a more generalized systemic disorder (see Chapter 87, "Polyarthritis").

The presence of a painless or painful discrete area of swelling along the Achilles tendon (nodules) raises the possibility of a tendinous xanthoma (seen in hyperlipoproteinemia), "pump bumps" due to local trauma from shoes, rheumatoid nodules (seen in patients with rheumatoid arthritis), or gouty tophi.

Pain in the heel that is aggravated by weight bearing and localized by examination to the calcaneus may be due to a bony process such as calcaneal fracture (in which case a history of trauma is likely), osteomyelitis, and, if occurring in a child or adolescent, calcaneal epiphysitis. Radiographic studies are the first step in evaluating these disorders.

Disorders That Cause Diffuse Foot Pain

Disorders that cause diffuse foot pain are often associated with swelling. These include cellulitis, edema from any cause (see Chapter 22, "Edema"), generalized arthritis or tendonitis in the foot, and trauma.

Sudeck's atrophy or reflex sympathetic dystrophy (RSD) is an unusual, painful condition that results in generalized foot swelling. This condition generally affects one foot to a greater degree than the other, and most commonly occurs after trauma and a period of immobilization (a classic example is a tibial fracture treated with casting). RSD may evolve through several stages. The initial stage is characterized by a swollen, clammy, cool foot that has a diffusely cyanotic discoloration and is painful to move and tender to touch. Perfusion bone scans characteristically reveal markedly increased uptake in the affected area during this phase. As the process evolves, cutaneous atrophy, which is manifested by tightening of the skin and soft tissues in association with loss of motion, develops. The characteristic radiographic appearance of the foot bones is patchy demineralization. Ultimately, if not treated appropriately, the foot may become nonfunctional.

Burning, Tingling, and Numbness in the Foot

Burning, tingling, and numbness generally indicate either pressure on or disease of the nerves that innervate the foot. Impingement of lumbar nerve roots (so-called lumbar radiculopathy) by osteoarthritic spurs arising from the lumbar facet joints is a common cause of such symptoms. Specific sensory and motor symptoms of lumbar nerve root compression(s) are discussed in Chapter 88, "Back Pain." Compression of the peroneal or posterior tibial nerves in the region of the knee and entrapment of the posterior tibial nerve along the medial malleolus of the ankle (so-called tarsal tunnel syndrome) are other causes of sensory loss and weakness in the foot.

Burning paresthesias and numbness, when present in both feet (and often in both hands) in a symmetric pattern, are suggestive of peripheral neuropathy. Diabetes mellitus is the most common cause of peripheral neuropathy; however, the list of causes is numerous and includes other metabolic disorders, deficiency states, infectious processes, vascular disease, genetically determined disorders, drug toxicity, and organic and metal poisons.

The Ankle

The ankle actually consists of two joints, the true ankle joint (articulation of the tibia and fibula with the tarsus, the tibiotalar joint), at which flexion and extension of the ankle occur, and the subtalar (talocalcaneal) joint, which allows inversion and eversion of the ankle. Historical evaluation and physical examination should attempt to localize the pain to either or both of these joints.

The ankle may be affected by trauma or a number of arthritic disorders; alternatively, it may appear swollen but painless because of local edema. The latter may result from local venous insufficiency, thrombophlebitis, or systemic diseases such as nephrosis, congestive heart failure, and portal hypertension (see Chapter 22, "Edema"). Historically, swelling that worsens with standing is characteristic of dependent edema. In contrast, painful swelling that is more severe in the morning, even before getting out of bed, suggests ankle arthritis.

Common causes of arthritis of the true ankle joint are rheumatoid arthritis, gouty arthritis, systemic lupus erythematosus, psoriatic arthritis, and Reiter's syndrome. Other less common causes include sarcoid and the periarthritis of erythema nodosum. Osteoarthritis does not generally affect the ankle. (Osteoarthritis of the ankle should raise concern of neuropathic [Charcot's] arthropathy, the most common cause being diabetic neuropathy.) Gouty and rheumatoid arthritis are the most common causes of inflammation of the subtalar joint.

Inflammation of the structures around or near the ankle (such as the capsule of the joint), Achilles tendonitis, and cellulitis may be confused with ankle arthritis. The presence of a tender, erythematous streak up the leg (indicative of lymphangitis) or tender, swollen inguinal lymph nodes (lymphadenopathy) suggests a cellulitis. Marked swelling around the ankle with retention of good ankle motion may occur in periarthritis secondary to sarcoidosis and Reiter's syndrome. (See Chapter 87, "Polyarthritis," for further discussion.)

Ankle sprains (muscle and connective tissue tears) are a common cause of ankle pain. An antecedent history of trauma should be sought. The ankle should be examined for swelling, tenderness, ecchymosis, altered range of motion, and ligamentous laxity. Obtain routine radiographs to rule out fractures. If no fractures are radiographically apparent, stress views may be helpful to assess the extent of ligamentous injury.

Ankle pain and swelling may also be the result of a stress fracture, particularly of the distal fibula or tibia, which may develop secondary to trauma or even normal weight-bearing stresses, particularly in an elderly individual with osteoporosis, in patients with rheumatoid arthritis with osteopenia, or even in a person with fairly normal bone mass who is subjected to unusual stress such as excessive jogging on hard surfaces (stress fractures, shin splints). Plain-film radiographs may not reveal any abnormalities until callus forms during healing, whereas a bone scan may reveal increased uptake before radiographs demonstrate positive findings.

References

Calabro JJ. Foot pain. In: Cohen AS, ed. Rheumatology and immunology. New York: Grune & Stratton, 1979:144.

Calabro JJ. Knees, ankles and feet. In: Cohen AS, ed. Rheumatology and immunology. New York: Grune & Stratton, 1979:27.

Katz WA, Sbarbaro JL. Feet and ankles. In: Katz WA, ed. Rheumatic diseases: Diagnosis and management. 2nd ed. Philadelphia: JB Lippincott, 1988:156.

Moskowitz RW. The painful foot. In: Clinical rheumatology. 2nd ed. Philadelphia: Lea & Febiger, 1982:307.

Sheon RP, Moskowitz RW, Goldberg VM. The ankle and foot. In: Soft tissue rheumatic pain. Philadelphia: Lea & Febiger, 1987.

Wood BT. Foot pain. In: Kelley WN, et al, eds. Textbook of rheumatology. 3rd ed. Philadelphia: WB Saunders, 1989:526.

Osteopenia

John L. Stock, MD

95

Definition

There is a relentless physiologic decline in the mass of bone tissue after peak levels are achieved in early adulthood. *Osteopenia* is defined as a reduction of bone mass below "normal." If "normal" is defined as peak bone mass at maturity, then osteopenia becomes a physiologic process common to all persons. Osteopenia is suspected clinically when increased lucency of bone is noted on standard radiographs. This will be the working definition for the following discussion. Given that a loss of almost 50 percent of the bone mass is necessary before any changes are seen on plain-film radiographs, many persons with significant amounts of bone loss will not be discovered until they sustain fractures.

The finding of osteopenia suggests an underlying *metabolic bone disease,* which is defined as a generalized disorder of bone related to a disturbance in body metabolism. Most of the metabolic bone diseases are caused by an imbalance between bone formation and bone resorption. The differential diagnosis of osteopenia involves determination of the individual type or types of metabolic bone disease contributing to the bone loss in order to direct therapy. Strict distinctions of the metabolic bone diseases are made on a pathologic basis. *Osteoporosis* is characterized as a decrease in bone mass per unit volume of bone with a normal ratio of mineral to extracellular organic matrix (osteoid). Various pathologic subtypes of osteoporosis have been described that depend on whether the bone-resorbing cell (osteoclast) activity or the matrix-forming cell (osteoblast) activity is affected. *Osteomalacia* is defined by a decrease in the rate of osteoid mineralization. Osteomalacic bone has wide osteoid seams with an increased number of osteoid seams per unit area of bone. The bone mass in osteomalacia may be decreased, normal, or even increased. *Osteitis fibrosa cystica* (OFC) is characterized as an increase in bone resorption that is mediated by parathyroid hormone–stimulated osteoclast activity and leads to a decrease in bone mass.

Because bone biopsies are rarely performed on the many patients who have osteopenia, more practical working definitions of these metabolic bone diseases are often used. Osteoporosis is clinically suggested when a bone mass below the fracture threshold is reached. The clinical diagnosis of osteoporosis is usually made when a patient sustains a fracture and is found by radiographic examination to have osteopenia. Osteomalacia is practically defined in this discussion as the bone disease resulting most commonly in the adult population from significant vitamin D deficiency, usually due to inadequate intake, malabsorption, or lack of sunlight exposure. OFC is the bone disorder resulting from hyperparathyroidism and is less common than it was in the past because primary hyperparathyroidism is usually diagnosed at an early and relatively asymptomatic stage by routine chemistry screening.

These working definitions are complicated by the fact that any person with osteopenia may simultaneously have more than one type of histologic metabolic bone disease contributing to the decrease in bone mass. A common example is the patient with chronic renal failure whose bones often display components of all the various processes just described. Another example is the postmenopausal woman who has significant osteoporosis as well as vitamin D deficiency–mediated osteomalacia. Because the therapy for the patient found to have osteopenia by radiographic studies depends on the various pathologic component metabolic bone diseases, the differential diagnosis of osteopenia becomes important. The magnitude of the problem is staggering given the more than 100,000 wrist fractures, 200,000 hip fractures (with approximately 15 percent mortality), and 500,000 vertebral crush fractures that occur in United States every year. Billions of dollars are spent for acute care alone.

Etiology

The majority of patients with osteopenia identified on radiographs are postmenopausal women with histologic osteoporosis. Less than 10 percent of these women have another histologic metabolic bone disease, such as osteomalacia or OFC, significantly contributing to their reduced bone mass. Men and premenopausal women with osteopenia have these other metabolic bone diseases more frequently. In adults, the most common cause of osteomalacia is vitamin D deficiency, usually due to poor nutrition or gastrointestinal disease such as malabsorption. Less frequently, drugs such as anticonvulsants or antacids are implicated. OFC is caused by hyperparathyroidism.

There are two distinct clinical syndromes of osteoporosis. The incidence of distal forearm (Colles') fractures and vertebral crush fractures in women increases soon after menopause. These bones consist mainly of trabecular or spongy bone. The incidence of hip, proximal humerus, proximal tibia, and pelvic fractures increases slowly with aging and then exponentially in later life in both men and women. These bones contain more cortical or solid bone. The pathogenesis of fractures in these syndromes may be different, and for any patient with osteoporosis there are probably multiple risk factors for the development of bone loss (Table 95-1).

A genetically determined small frame may result in less than optimal bone mass prior to the physiologic decline that begins to occur shortly after maturity. Many of these patients have a strong family history of osteoporosis. Local factors such as mechanical stresses may affect coupling between bone resorption

Table 95-1 Risk Factors for Osteoporosis

Small frame or family history of osteoporosis
Immobilization or sedentary lifestyle
Nutritional factors
Poor calcium intake
Smoking
Alcohol
Endocrine abnormalities
Hypogonadism
Hyperthyroidism
Hypercortisolism
Diabetes mellitus
Other
Drugs (heparin)
Malignancy (multiple myeloma)
Renal failure

and formation, and immobilization or sedentary lifestyle may predispose to bone loss. General nutrition and overall calcium balance play important roles in determining and maintaining bone mass. Inadequate dietary calcium, decreased calcium absorption with age, or increased renal loss of calcium may be important. Use of alcohol and tobacco may predispose to osteoporosis. Bone formation and resorption are exquisitely sensitive to hormones. Loss of estrogen at menopause accelerates the physiologic decline in bone mass; hypogonadism in men causes similar problems. Other hormonal disorders such as hyperthyroidism, hypercortisolism, and diabetes mellitus may affect bone mass. Other factors, including drugs such as heparin, malignant conditions such as multiple myeloma, and metabolic disturbances such as chronic renal failure, may also contribute to osteoporosis.

Diagnostic Approach

Osteopenia is usually discovered incidentally when patients undergo radiographic evaluation for other medical indications. The majority of these patients are older women with postmenopausal osteoporosis. The aim of diagnosis is to select those patients with histologic components of the other and more reversible metabolic bone disease as well as to uncover potentially reversible risk factors for osteoporosis.

History

The age, sex, and menstrual status of the patient are the most important historical details in determining the level of suspicion for potentially reversible processes. A postmenopausal woman at any age will most likely have osteoporosis, whereas in a menstruating woman or in any man, other diagnoses must be more fully entertained. Osteoporosis is usually asymptomatic unless there have been recent fractures, which present as a sudden sharp pain, most commonly in the vertebrae, wrist, or femoral neck. Less often, patients complain of diffuse and chronic pain, especially in the lower back. In contrast, patients with a significant component of osteomalacia have fewer fractures but complain of vague diffuse pain and tenderness that may be increased by muscle strain. They may also have pronounced muscle weakness. Unusually, osteomalacia may be associated with symptomatic hypocalcemia, so that a history of tingling, cramping, seizures, and tetany should be sought. Because the most common cause of osteomalacia in adults is nutritional vitamin D deficiency, a careful history of the patient's diet and sun exposure should be obtained.

Inquire about weight loss, diarrhea, bulky stools, and previous gastrointestinal surgery in order to rule out malabsorption of vitamin D. Long-term therapy with antacids or anticonvulsant medications can also cause osteomalacia and thus should be included in the drug history. The rare patient with severe OFC will complain of diffuse bone pain and may sustain fractures at sites of advanced bone resorption or "brown tumors." More commonly, patients with mild hyperparathyroidism complain of fleeting arthralgias or may have no skeletal symptoms at all, despite radiographic osteopenia. In some of these patients, constitutional symptoms such as anorexia, constipation, and fatigue or muscle weakness, and history of renal stones, hypertension, and peptic ulcer disease may suggest the diagnosis of hyperparathyroidism. In summary, historical assessment of menstrual status in women, review of symptoms of hypocalcemia and hypercalcemia, and evaluation of the skeletal and gastrointestinal tracts may suggest a particular metabolic bone disease.

Look for reversible risk factors for osteoporosis in the history, especially in any man or premenopausal woman with osteopenia. Changes in weight and body build, appetite, temperature tolerance, sexual function, and so forth may suggest endocrine disorders. A careful drug history and review of constitutional symptoms may uncover other reversible processes (see Table 95-1).

Physical Examination

This is probably the least sensitive means of diagnosis in patients with osteopenia. Careful palpation of the spine may reveal areas of tenderness corresponding to compression fractures in osteoporosis. The usual signs associated with the endocrine disorders in Table 95-1 may be helpful. More diffuse tenderness elicited by pressure on the ribs, tibiae, or iliac crest suggests underlying osteomalacia, as may unexplained proximal muscle weakness or signs of hypocalcemia, such as a positive Chvostek's sign. Skeletal deformities, including leg bowing, sclerosis, or pigeon chest, may be found in patients with severe, longstanding osteomalacia. There are few reliable physical signs of hyperparathyroidism and OFC.

Laboratory Studies (Table 95-2)

The presence of osteopenia may be confirmed and quantitated by more specific measures of bone mass or density. This is most commonly done using dual-photon absorptiometry or computed tomography (CT) scanning. The role of bone-density determinations in the evaluation of patients with osteopenia or suspected osteoporosis is controversial. This test should not be used for mass screening, but it is valuable in quantitating bone loss in patients with osteopenia or clinical osteoporosis, as well as for other selected indications. Serum measurements of parameters of mineral metabolism may be useful in suggesting the presence of a particular metabolic bone disease. As shown in Table 95-3, the serum calcium, phosphorus, alkaline phosphatase, parathyroid hormone, and 25-hydroxyvitamin D levels are usually normal in patients with predominant histologic osteoporosis, and abnormalities in these values may suggest the presence of osteomalacia or OFC.

Plain-film radiographs are generally not sensitive or specific enough to help diagnose early disease. Radiographic studies may suggest the predominance of a particular metabolic bone disease, but the process is usually far advanced and obvious by other criteria when this occurs. In severe osteoporosis, there may be collapse or biconcavity of the vertebrae, the so-called codfish appearance. Pseudofractures (Looser's zones) or lucent bands perpendicular to the periosteum that correspond to actual small stress fractures may suggest advanced osteomalacia. Subperiosteal resorption, especially in the hand bones, is pathognomonic for OFC. Other radiographic signs of hyperparathyroidism include resorption of the distal ends of the clavicles, thinning of the lamina dura of the teeth, and widening of

Table 95-2 Laboratory Studies That May Be Used in the Evaluation of Patients with Osteopenia and Their Costs

Study	Cost
Calcium, phosphorus, alkaline phosphatase, creatinine, liver enzymes	$90
25-hydroxyvitamin D	$75
Serum and urinary immunoelectrophoreses	$75
24-hour urinary calcium and creatinine	$30
Free thyroxine index	$45
Testosterone	$65
Luteinizing hormone and follicle-stimulating hormone	$85
Bone density (by dual-photon absorptiometry)	$95
Bone biopsy	$500–$1,000

Table 95-3 Laboratory Studies for Evaluation of Patients with Metabolic Bone Diseases*

	Osteoporosis	Osteomalacia (nutritional)	Osteitis fibrosa cystica
Serum calcium	Normal	Decreased	Increased
Phosphorus	Normal	Decreased	Decreased
Alkaline phosphatase	Normal†	Increased	Increased
Parathyroid hormone	Normal	Increased	Increased
25-hydroxyvitamin D	Normal	Decreased	—

* Assuming normal renal function.
† May be increased in presence of recent fracture.

the symphysis pubis. In more advanced and severe hyperparathyroidism, lytic lesions or "brown tumors" corresponding to areas of intense osteoclastic bone resorption may be seen.

Laboratory studies are also useful in confirming clinically suspected reversible risk factors for osteoporosis. Such tests include the serum free thyroxine index in suspected hyperthyroidism; serum cortisol after a midnight dose of dexamethasone to rule out Cushing's syndrome; luteinizing and follicle-stimulating hormone (LH and FSH) in women with questionable menopausal status; testosterone, LH, and FSH in men with possible hypogonadism; and a postprandial blood sugar level in patients with questionable glucose tolerance. Serum and urine immunoelectrophoreses followed by bone marrow biopsy, if indicated, will usually confirm the diagnosis of multiple myeloma. Finally, a subgroup of patients with osteoporosis may have a significant renal leak of calcium contributing to their negative calcium balance. Because there is potential therapeutic intervention for this problem, a 24-hour measurement of urinary calcium and creatinine may be useful in any patient with osteoporosis.

In men, premenopausal women, or selected postmenopausal women, the diagnosis may still be unclear after all of the aforementioned indirect studies are performed. In these patients, a bone biopsy after a regimen of tetracycline can often lead to a definitive diagnosis. Undecalcified bone is studied for osteoid, relative osteoclastic activity, and mineral apposition rate. This procedure is uncomfortable and usually requires day hospitalization for anesthesia. The total expense of a bone biopsy ($500 to $1,000) as well as the special expertise necessary to process and interpret the samples dictate its use only in selected patients.

References

Aurbach GD, Marx SJ, Spiegel AM. Metabolic bone disease. In: Williams RH, ed. Textbook of endocrinology. 7th ed. Philadelphia: WB Saunders, 1985:1218.

Frame B, Parfitt AM. Osteomalacia: Current concepts. Ann Intern Med 1978; 89:966.

Health and Public Policy Committee, American College of Physicians. Bone mineral densitometry. Ann Intern Med 1987; 107:932.

Riggs BL, Melton LJ III. Involutional osteoporosis. N Engl J Med 1986; 314:1676.

Riggs BL, Wahner HW. Bone densitometry and clinical decision-making in osteoporosis. Ann Intern Med 1988; 108:293.

Laboratory and Radiographic Abnormalities in Rheumatic Diseases

Robert A. Yood, MD

96

This chapter discusses laboratory studies that are frequently used to evaluate rheumatic complaints. However, abnormalities often are not limited to rheumatic diseases. Test results must be interpreted in the context of the clinical situation; conversely, the clinical situation must be taken into account when determining which tests to order. The reflex reaction that leads one to order a battery of tests when presented with a case of "arthritis" cannot be tolerated; rather, specific tests should be obtained depending on the clinical presentation. For example, an elderly man with inflammation of the first metatarsophalangeal joint probably has gout, so it makes little sense to order a rheumatoid factor and an antinuclear antibody test in the initial evaluation of this patient. The following are the most commonly ordered laboratory tests that may have abnormal results in the patient who presents with rheumatic complaints.

Erythrocyte Sedimentation Rate and C-Reactive Protein

The acute-phase response is the name given to a characteristic increase in the concentration of certain plasma proteins, including C-reactive protein (CRP), in response to most forms of tissue injury. This response is most often measured by the erythrocyte sedimentation rate (ESR) or occasionally CRP levels. Erythrocytes usually sediment slowly, but elevated plasma proteins (especially fibrinogen) enhance rouleaux formation, allowing more rapid erythrocyte sedimentation. Although both CRP and fibrinogen are synthesized by the liver and both tend to be elevated in inflammatory processes, the synthesis of each is independent. As such, the magnitudes of CRP and ESR elevations may be discordant.

The two most common techniques for measurement of the ESR are the Wintrobe and Westergren methods. In the Wintrobe method, undiluted blood is allowed to sediment for 1 hour in a 100-mm tube, and the distance from the top of the plasma to the top of the sedimenting red cells is recorded as the ESR. Because the maximum Wintrobe ESR is 100 mm minus the hematocrit, the degree of elevation of the Wintrobe ESR is limited. In the Westergren method, diluted blood sediments for 1 hour in a 200-mm tube. The Westergren sedimentation rate is more sensitive for patients with moderately or severely elevated ESRs; therefore, it is preferred for monitoring activity in chronic inflammatory diseases. The normal value of the Westergren ESR is usually given as 0 to 10 mm per hour for men and 0 to 15 mm per hour for women. However, the upper limit of normal increases with age, and an ESR of 30 to 40 mm per hour may be normal for an elderly patient.

Most forms of tissue injury, including infection, infarction, and other types of inflammation, result in an acute-phase response. Thus, the ESR and CRP are nonspecific, but they are often used as screening tests for organic disease and for monitoring activity of chronic inflammatory disease, such as rheumatoid arthritis. In patients with musculoskeletal pains, the sedimentation rate is often used to help classify the problem as an inflammatory disease, in which there is usually an elevated ESR (e.g., rheumatoid arthritis, psoriatic arthritis, polymyalgia rheumatica), or a noninflammatory disease (e.g., osteoarthritis, fibrositis), in which the ESR is normal. This distinction is not absolute, as patients with early or mild inflammatory arthritis may have a normal sedimentation rate and patients with noninflammatory arthritis may have an elevated ESR due to other causes. A Westergren ESR of 100 mm per hour or more in patients in a general hospital is associated with bacterial infections in about one-half, connective tissue diseases in about one-third, and malignancy in about one-sixth of patients. In referral centers, the frequency of malignancy among patients with grossly elevated ESRs is much higher.

Serum Protein Electrophoresis and Immunoelectrophoresis

Serum protein electrophoresis divides serum proteins into albumin and alpha-1, alpha-2, beta-, and gamma-globulin fractions. Elevations of alpha-2 and, to a lesser extent, alpha-1 proteins are found in acute inflammation, whereas a polyclonal increase in gamma globulin is often seen in chronic inflammatory disorders such as chronic infection, connective tissue diseases, or chronic liver disease. The findings of a homogeneous monoclonal protein (M-component) on protein electrophoresis should lead one to perform an immunoelectrophoresis to confirm the presence of the monoclonal protein and to determine its immunoglobulin class and light-chain type. The immunoelectrophoresis is more sensitive than the protein electrophoresis for detecting monoclonal proteins and should be performed when multiple myeloma, Waldenström's macroglobulinemia, heavy-chain disease, or primary amyloidosis is suspected. Monoclonal proteins may be found in these disorders as well as in lymphoma. The terms *benign monoclonal gammopathy* and *monoclonal gammopathy of undetermined significance* have been used to denote the presence of a monoclonal protein in patients without evidence of these disorders. An undetermined number of these patients with benign monoclonal gammopathy will later develop myeloma, macroglobulinemia, or amyloidosis. No good criteria are available for determining which cases will progress to these illnesses, and periodic re-examination of these patients is essential.

Rheumatoid Factor

A rheumatoid factor is a circulating immunoglobulin that reacts with an Fc portion of IgG; thus, a rheumatoid factor is an antibody directed against an antibody. These anti-antibodies have been termed *rheumatoid factors* because they are frequently associated with rheumatoid arthritis. They are also found in a large number of diseases as well as in many healthy individuals. Although there is evidence that rheumatoid factors modify the immune response, the pathogenic significance (if any) of rheumatoid factors remains unknown.

Various techniques exist for detecting rheumatoid factor. The most commonly used method involves mixing test serum with latex particles (latex fixation test) that have been previously coated with IgG. The IgM rheumatoid factor in the test serum binds with the IgG, resulting in agglutination of the latex particles.

Because rheumatoid factor is found so frequently in patients with rheumatoid arthritis, its presence is helpful in supporting that diagnosis; however, a positive rheumatoid factor is not diagnostic of rheumatoid arthritis. Rheumatoid factor is present in about 80 percent of cases of rheumatoid arthritis, 90 percent of cases of Sjögren's syndrome, 30 percent of cases of systemic lupus erythematosus, and about 10 percent of cases of juvenile rheumatoid arthritis, as well as in some cases of scleroderma and other connective tissue diseases. Rheumatoid factor is frequently found in certain chronic diseases, such as leprosy, subacute bacterial endocarditis, tuberculosis, and chronic liver disease, as well as some malignant diseases, such as multiple myeloma, Waldenström's macroglobulinemia, and lymphoma. In addition, rheumatoid factor is present in approximately 5 percent of normal people, especially the elderly. A titer should be obtained in all cases in which a rheumatoid factor is found. The concentration of rheumatoid factor is helpful in determining the significance of a positive test. Patients with a positive rheumatoid factor but without rheumatoid arthritis usually have a relatively low titer (1:320 or less). Thus, one must use all available clinical information and be wary of misdiagnosing rheumatoid arthritis in, for example, an elderly patient with osteoarthritis and a positive rheumatoid factor.

Just as the presence of rheumatoid factor does not establish a diagnosis of rheumatoid arthritis, a negative or low-titer rheumatoid factor does not exclude this diagnosis. Patients with rheumatoid arthritis who do not have the rheumatoid factor (seronegative rheumatoid arthritis) usually have a less severe disease than those with a positive rheumatoid factor, who are more likely to have rheumatoid nodules, bony erosions, pulmonary involvement, or vasculitis. When rheumatoid factor is present early in cases of rheumatoid arthritis, it usually remains present indefinitely. Titers usually do not correlate with disease activity, although the titer may decrease with sustained remission or as a result of treatment with gold, penicillamine, or immunosuppressive agents. It is rarely helpful to obtain serial rheumatoid factor tests in patients with known seropositive rheumatoid arthritis.

LE Cell and Antinuclear Antibody

The LE cell phenomenon, first reported by Hargraves in 1948, was a major breakthrough that led to a clearer understanding of systemic lupus erythematosus (SLE). The LE cell is a neutrophil that has phagocytized nuclear material from a second leukocyte following incubation in serum containing antibody reactive with deoxyribonucleoprotein. The LE cell is found in approximately 70 percent of patients with SLE, but it is not specific for this disease.

Testing for LE cells has largely been supplanted by the more sensitive antinuclear antibody (ANA) test, which is positive in at least 95 percent of cases of SLE. Thus, the ANA is an excellent screening test for SLE. The ANA is usually detected by an indirect immunofluorescent technique. The test serum is placed on a microscope slide containing a thin section of tissue such as mouse liver. If ANA is present in the serum, it binds with nuclear material in the tissue section. After the slide is washed, anti-immunoglobulin antiserum conjugated to a fluorescein dye is placed on the slide, and the slide is again washed. The antiserum binds to any ANA that has previously bound to the cell nuclei. Under a fluorescent microscope, the nuclei show bright green fluorescence if the test is positive. Although the concept underlying the testing for ANA is straightforward, the test is difficult to perform, and many laboratories have problems with false-positive results. As with rheumatoid factor, the titer of ANA should be determined. Higher titers are most often associated with SLE. The ANA test may be positive in other diseases, including about 20 percent of cases of rheumatoid arthritis and about 40 percent of cases of scleroderma. The ANA test is positive in

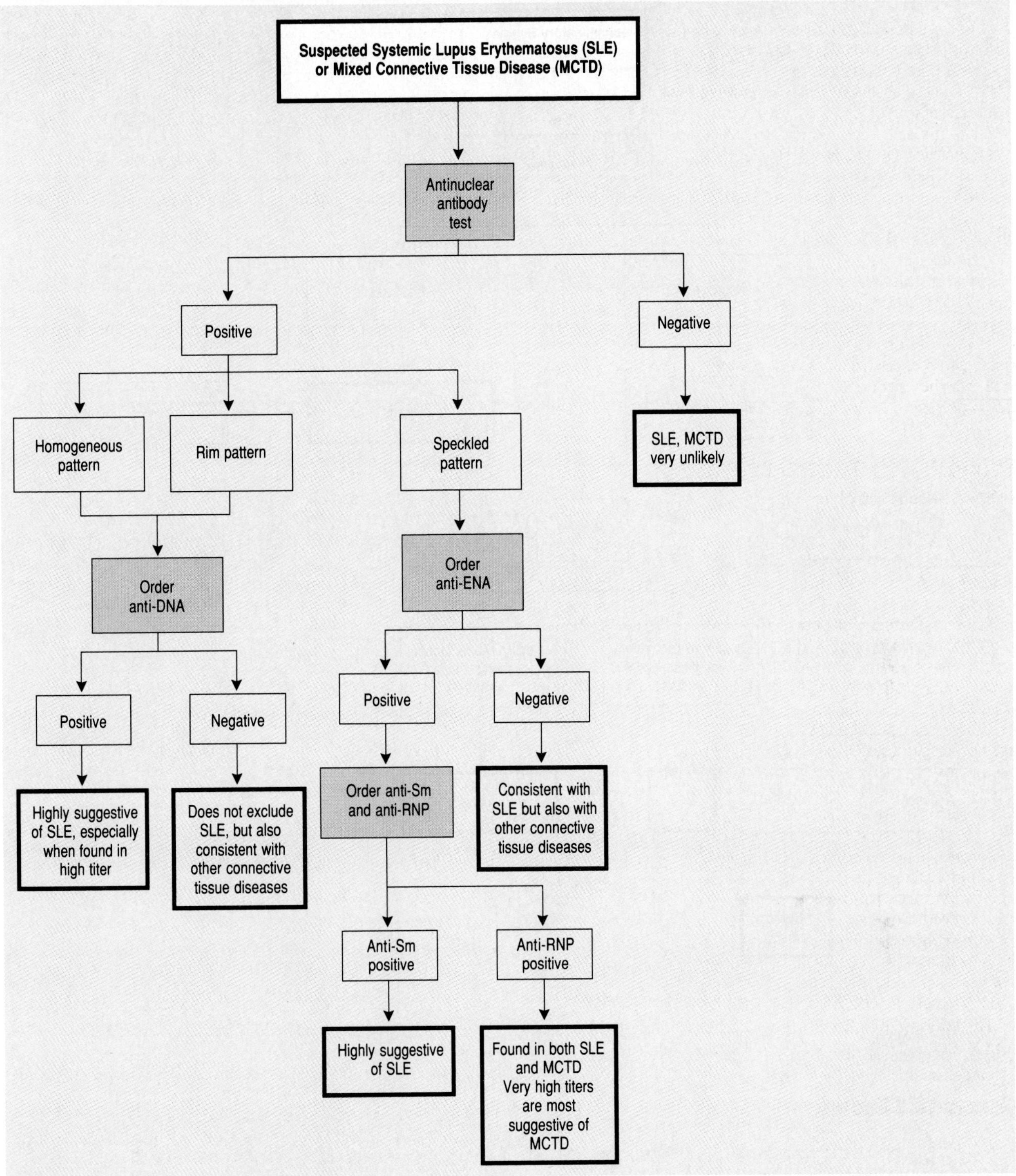

Figure 96-1 Algorithm for the evaluation of suspected systemic lupus erythematosus and mixed connective tissue disease. Anti-DNA = antibody to DNA, anti-ENA = antibody to extractable nuclear antigen, anti-RNP = antibody to ribonucleoprotein, anti-Sm = antibody to Smith antigen.

virtually all patients with mixed connective tissue disease (MCTD) and drug-induced lupus. It is also present in some patients with discoid lupus erythematosus, juvenile rheumatoid arthritis, Sjögren's syndrome, and other autoimmune diseases such as chronic active hepatitis, Hashimoto's thyroiditis, and myasthenia gravis. Like rheumatoid factor, the ANA test may be positive in some normal persons, especially the elderly.

The four most common patterns of ANA fluorescent staining are homogeneous, speckled, peripheral, and nucleolar. In the homogeneous (or diffuse) pattern, the entire nucleus is stained, indicating antibodies of nucleoprotein. This is the most common type and is nonspecific; it is present in some patients with SLE as well as in many other conditions. However, ANA with a homogeneous pattern may also represent antibodies to double-stranded DNA. The speckled pattern appears as speckles of fluorescence within the nucleus. This pattern may reflect antibodies to extractable nuclear antigen (ENA), which is composed in part of the Smith (Sm) antigen and ribonucleoprotein. This is the most common pattern in scleroderma, but it may be seen in SLE, rheumatoid arthritis, Sjögren's syndrome, MCTD,

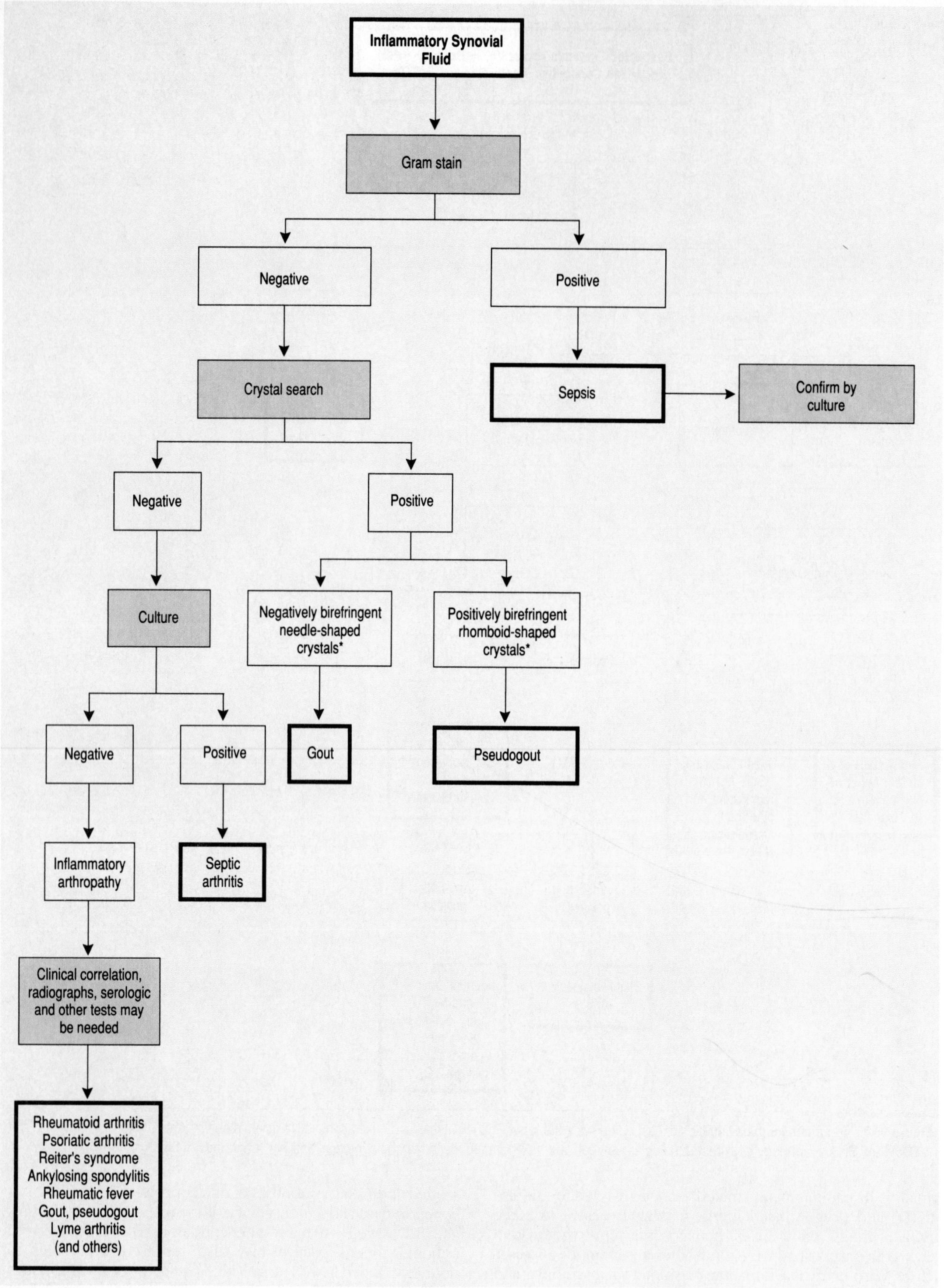

Figure 96-2 Analysis of synovial fluid. *Synovial fluid containing birefringent crystals should also be cultured to evaluate for concurrent joint sepsis.

Table 96-1 Differential Diagnosis by Joint Fluid Groups

Group 1 (noninflammatory)	Group 2 (inflammatory)	Group 3 (septic)	Hemorrhagic
Degenerative joint disease	Rheumatoid arthritis	Bacterial infections	Hemophilia or other hemorrhagic diathesis
Trauma	Acute crystal-induced synovitis (gout and pseudogout)		Trauma with or without fracture
Osteochondritis dissecans	Reiter's syndrome		Neuropathic arthropathy
Osteochondromatosis	Ankylosing spondylitis		Pigmented villonodular synovitis
Neuropathic arthropathy	Psoriatic arthritis		Synovioma
Subsiding or early inflammation	Arthritis accompanying ulcerative colitis and regional enteritis		Hemangioma and other benign neoplasm
Hypertrophic osteoarthropathy	Rheumatic fever		
Pigmented villonodular synovitis	Systemic lupus erythematosus		
	Progressive systemic sclerosis (scleroderma)		

and other conditions. The peripheral (or rim) pattern is characterized by staining of the periphery of the nucleus. Because this pattern may indicate antibodies to DNA, it is the most specific (but not sensitive) for SLE. The nucleolar pattern is the one found least frequently and occurs when only the nucleoli stain; this pattern is most specific for scleroderma.

Because a positive ANA test may be due to autoantibodies reactive with one or more nuclear components, further definition of these antibodies may increase the diagnostic information (Fig. 96-1). These autoantibodies are found almost exclusively in patients who are ANA-positive, so that the most economical and rational diagnostic approach entails use of the ANA as a screening test for SLE or MCTD. Although ANAs are often sought in the evaluation of other autoimmune disorders, their presence may not have specific diagnostic significance. If the ANA test is positive in a homogeneous or rim pattern, a test for antibodies to double-stranded DNA should be ordered. If the ANA pattern is speckled, an antibody to ENA test can be ordered, and this can be further tested for the presence of antibodies to Sm antigen and ribonucleoprotein. Some laboratories perform specific tests for antibodies to Sm antigen and ribonucleoprotein without doing a determination for antibodies to ENA. Because the ANA pattern may be technically difficult to determine or may even vary in a single patient depending on the concentration of serum used, some laboratories and clinicians test for antibodies to double-stranded DNA, Sm antigen, and ribonucleoprotein as well as other antigens in all patients with a positive ANA test. This process of evaluating a positive ANA test is important, because antibodies against double-stranded DNA and the Sm antigen are found primarily in SLE, whereas high titers of antibodies to ribonucleoprotein are characteristic of MCTD.

In addition to antibodies to DNA, Sm antigen, and ribonucleoprotein, other clinically important autoantibodies are being described in the current medical literature. Among them are anticentromere antibody (associated with Raynaud's phenomenon and the CREST variant [*c*alcinosis, *R*aynaud's *e*sophageal dysfunction, *s*clerodactyly, *t*elangiectasias] of scleroderma), anticardiolipin antibody (associated with arterial and venous thrombosis and fetal loss in SLE), and antineutrophil cytoplasm antibody (associated with Wegener's granulomatosis).

Complement

The complement system consists of 18 plasma proteins that interact sequentially to affect systems of inflammation. Complement levels are most often measured either by total hemolytic complement (CH_{50}), which measures the ability of test serum to lyse 50 percent of a suspension of sheep red blood cells coated with antibody, or by immunodiffusion measurement of specific complement components. Because C3 is common to both the classical and alternate complement pathways, the C3 level is often used as a guide to the activity of the entire complement system.

Low complement levels may be due to genetic deficiencies of complement components, severe liver disease, malnutrition, or, much more commonly, in vivo utilization of complement. This occurs commonly in SLE and other immune complex diseases, including certain cases of vasculitis. The determination of complement levels is not useful as a screening test; it should be reserved for patients with known SLE or for those in whom immune complex disease or vasculitis is suspected. In these patients, low complement levels often reflect disease activity, and serial measurements may be helpful in assessing therapeutic response and prognosis.

Table 96-2 Examination of Joint Fluid

Measure	Normal	Group 1 (noninflammatory)	Group 2 (inflammatory)	Group 3 (septic)
Clarity	Transparent	Transparent	Translucent-opaque	Opaque
Color	Clear	Yellow	Yellow to opalescent	Yellow to green
Viscosity	↑	↑	↓	Variable
WBC (per mm^3)	<200	200–2,000	2,000–100,000	>100,000
Polymorphonuclear leukocytes	<25%	<25%	50% or more	75% or more
Culture	Negative	Negative	Negative	Often positive
Mucin clot	Firm	Firm	Friable	Friable
Glucose (mg/dl)	Nearly equal to blood	Nearly equal to blood	>25, lower than blood	<25, much lower than blood

Synovial Fluid Analysis

Synovial fluid analysis is the one test in rheumatology that may be absolutely diagnostic. Even when not diagnostic, synovial fluid analysis may categorize effusions into noninflammatory, inflammatory, or severely inflammatory categories, thereby aiding diagnosis (Fig. 96-2 and Table 96-1). The key tests on synovial fluid include cell count and differential, Gram stain and culture, and search for crystals using the polarizing microscope. Other tests, including mucin clot test, viscosity, glucose, and complement levels, may occasionally be helpful (Table 96-2). Noninflammatory effusions usually have a white blood cell (WBC) count less than 3,000/mm^3 (predominantly mononuclear) and are due to such illnesses as osteoarthritis and SLE. Inflammatory effusions have a WBC count between 3,000 and 50,000/mm^3 (often predominantly polymorphonuclear) and are due to such illnesses as rheumatoid arthritis, Reiter's syndrome, psoriatic arthritis, rheumatic fever, gout or pseudogout, and occasionally bacterial infections. The demonstration under the polarizing microscope of the needle-shaped, strongly negatively birefringent monosodium urate crystals establishes the diagnosis of gout, whereas the finding of square or rhomboid-shaped, weakly positively birefringent calcium pyrophosphate dihydrate crystals is diagnostic of pseudogout. Very inflammatory fluid with WBC counts greater than 100,000/mm^3 is usually due to bacterial infection but may occasionally be due to gout or rheumatoid arthritis. The Gram stain is positive in about one-half to two-thirds of cases of septic arthritis (see Fig. 96-2). Hemorrhagic effusions may be due to trauma, hemorrhagic diathesis such as hemophilia or anticoagulation, sickle cell disease, pseudogout, pigmented villonodular synovitis, osteoarthritis, or neuropathic (Charcot's) joints. If fat or marrow elements are seen in hemorrhagic synovial fluid, intra-articular fracture is likely.

HLA-B27

The human leukocyte antigens (HLA) are controlled by genes located on the sixth human chromosome. A number of specific HLA markers occur more frequently in certain diseases. The HLA-B27 antigen is present in approximately 80 to 90 percent of individuals who have ankylosing spondylitis and Reiter's syndrome, and about 50 percent of patients with spondylitis associated with inflammatory bowel disease and psoriasis. However, *caution* must be exercised in interpreting the presence of the HLA-B27 antigen, because its presence in a patient with back pain does *not* establish the diagnosis of spondylitis, as 8 percent of healthy caucasian individuals possess the HLA-B27 antigen. Therefore, HLA-B27 should not be used as a screening test in the evaluation of a patient with back pain, but it should be obtained when there is a clinical suspicion of ankylosing spondylitis or Reiter's syndrome. In the individual with clear-cut ankylosing spondylitis as determined by history, physical examination, and radiographic findings, the HLA-B27 is not needed for diagnosis and need not be obtained.

Lyme Disease Testing

Lyme disease, a multisystemic disorder, is caused by the ixodid tick-borne spirochete *Borrelia burgdorferi*. Clinical features of the disease include a rash characterized as an expanding erythematous macule or papule with red, somewhat raised borders and partial central clearing that is often accompanied by a flu-like illness with severe headache, stiff neck, chills, fevers, myalgias, arthralgias, and severe malaise approximately 1 to 4 weeks after the tick bite. Within several weeks, approximately 10 percent of patients develop carditis with atrioventricular block and, less commonly, myopericarditis and, rarely, cardiomegaly. Several weeks to months later, approximately 15 percent of affected individuals may develop neurologic manifestations, including meningitis, mild encephalitis, cranial neuritis, and radiculitis. Musculoskeletal manifestations consist of migratory joint pain, tendonitis, bursitis, and myalgias early in the illness. Weeks to months later, approximately 50 percent of patients develop a true arthritis, generally involving one or a few joints, most commonly the knees, but small- and large-joint polyarthritis may occur. Approximately 10 percent of patients will develop a large-joint chronic erosive arthritis.

Specific IgM and IgG antibodies against the Lyme spirochete may now be measured. The IgM antibody levels rise during the first several weeks and reach maximum titers at 3 to 6 weeks, whereas IgG antibodies rise more gradually and reach maximum titer months after the initial infection, generally when arthritis is present. Positive antibody titers in the context of the appropriate clinical setting help make the diagnosis of Lyme disease and distinguish this from other rheumatic diseases. Some asymptomatic individuals, however, particularly in endemic areas (Atlantic seaboard, Wisconsin, parts of the Pacific coast), have elevated antibodies without having disease.

Table 96-3 Radiographic Features of Common Forms of Arthritis

Rheumatoid Arthritis
- Soft-tissue swelling
- Joint effusion
- Periarticular demineralization
- Diffuse joint-space narrowing
- Erosions at margins of joints
- Joint malalignment
- *Lack* of bony proliferation (osteophytes)

Osteoarthritis
- Localized (nonuniform) joint-space narrowing
- Sclerosis of subchondral bone (bone under articular cartilage)
- Marginal osteophytes
- Subchondral bone cysts

Gout
- Joint effusions
- Nodules or lobulated soft-tissue masses near joints, often with irregular opaque deposits (tophi)
- Bony erosions with sclerotic margins and overhanging edges

Calcium Pyrophosphate Dihydrate Deposition Arthropathy (Pseudogout, Articular Chondrocalcinosis)
- Punctate calcification of menisci of knees and triangular cartilage of wrists
- Linear-appearing calcification in hyaline articular cartilage

Ankylosing Spondylitis and Spondylitis Associated with Psoriasis, Reiter's Syndrome, and Inflammatory Bowel Disease
- Sacroiliac joints
  - Blurring
  - Reactive sclerosis
  - Narrowing and obliteration
  - Ankylosis
- Vertebral joints
  - Superficial erosions of anterosuperior and inferior vertebral bodies
  - Squared appearance of vertebral bodies
  - Vertical ossifications from vertebral body margins (so-called syndesmophytes)
  - Ossification of spinal ligaments

Peripheral Arthritis of Psoriasis and Reiter's Syndrome
- Resorption of distal phalangeal tufts
- Soft-tissue swelling
- Extensive articular bone destruction ("whittled down" or "pencil-in-cup" deformity)
- Large, asymmetric syndesmophytes (paraspinal ossifications)
- "Fluffy" periostitis

Radiographic Features

Radiographic features of common forms of arthritis are listed by diagnosis in Table 96-3. For discussion of the distribution of joint involvement and other clinical features, see Chapter 87, "Polyarthritis."

References

Bedell SL, Bush BT. Erythrocyte sedimentation rate: From folklore to facts. Am J Med 1985; 78:1001.

Cohen AS, ed. Laboratory diagnostic procedures in the rheumatic diseases. 3rd ed. Orlando: Grune & Stratton, 1985.

Craft JE, Grodzicki RL, Steere AC. Antibody response in Lyme disease: Evaluation of diagnostic tests. J Infect Dis 1984; 149:789.

Falk R, Jennette JC. Anti-neutrophil cytoplasmic autoantibody with specificity for myeloperoxidase in patients with systemic vasculitis and idiopathic necrotizing and crescentic glomerulonephritis. N Engl J Med 1988; 318:1651.

Fritzler MJ. Antinuclear antibodies in the investigation of rheumatic diseases. Bull Rheum Dis 1985; 35:1.

Kyle RA. Monoclonal gammopathy of undetermined significance. Am J Med 1978; 64:814.

Lockshin MD, et al. Antibody to cardiolipin as a predictor of fetal distress or death in pregnant patients with systemic lupus erythematosus. N Engl J Med 1985; 313:152.

McCarty DJ. Synovial fluid. In: McCarty DJ, ed. Arthritis and allied conditions. 11th ed. Philadelphia: Lea & Febiger, 1989:69.

Resnick D, Niwayama G. Diagnosis of bone and joint disorders. 2nd ed. Philadelphia: WB Saunders, 1988.

Sarkozi J, et al. Significance of anti-centromere antibody in idiopathic Raynaud's syndrome. Am J Med 1987; 83:893.

Schumacher HR Jr, ed. Primer on the rheumatic diseases. 9th ed. Atlanta: The Arthritis Foundation, 1988.

Sox MC Jr, Liang MH. The erythrocyte sedimentation rate: Guideline for rational use. Ann Intern Med 1986; 104:515.

Neurology

Headache

Cynthia B. Passarelli, MD

Although everyone has experienced a headache at some time, few individuals seek medical attention. The patient who does present complaining of headache usually does so because of a change in the pattern or quality of the headache. Although the patient may not state it directly, often the underlying fear of a brain tumor precipitates the visit.

Etiology

Pain-Sensitive Cranial Structures

An understanding of the causes of headache begins with an appreciation of the pain sensitivity of various extracranial and intracranial structures. Pain-sensitive extracranial structures include skin, subcutaneous tissues, muscles, arteries, and periosteum. Intracranially, the dura at the base of the brain, the dural arteries, the venous sinuses and their tributaries, the intracranial arteries at the base of the brain, and the fifth, seventh, ninth, and tenth cranial nerves are sensitive to pain. The brain parenchyma is not sensitive to pain; nor are the skull, most of the dura, most of the pia arachnoid and choroid plexuses, and the ependymal linings of the ventricles. Stimulation of the upper cervical nerves can also result in pain at the back of the head or the neck, which would be perceived as a headache. Wolff and others have determined that the basic mechanisms that result in pain from intracranial processes include (1) displacement of the venous sinuses or traction on the veins that feed them; (2) traction on the middle meningeal arteries; (3) traction of the large arteries at the base of the brain or their main branches; (4) inflammation, distention, or compression of intracranial arteries; and (5) compression or inflammation of any of the other intracranial pain-sensitive structures.

Stimulation of the pain-sensitive structures in the anterior and middle cranial fossae causes pain to be conveyed along the fifth cranial nerve and usually results in a frontal headache. The posterior fossa and infratentorial structures are supplied by the ninth and tenth cranial nerves as well as the upper three cervical nerves, and pain in this region is perceived as pain in the occipital and neck regions.

Neurologic Headache Syndromes

There are classic headache syndromes for which the pathogenesis as well as the treatments are known; therefore, it is worthwhile to try to classify the type of headache that the patient is experiencing.

Migraine

Migraine is frequently a familial, recurrent category of headache. It is found in approximately 3 to 5 percent of the general population and occurs twice as often in women as in men. Onset is usually during childhood or adolescence, but migraine can occur during any time of life.

The word *migraine* is derived from the Greek *hemikrania,* meaning pain on one side of the head. The headaches are usually unilateral at onset, but they may spread and become generalized. The headaches are throbbing in quality and often are accompanied by nausea and vomiting. The frequency of the headaches is variable, but they usually do not occur more often than every few weeks. The duration also varies, with each attack lasting from a few hours to 1 to 2 days. Migraines often begin soon after awakening, but can also begin at any time of day. The headache usually reaches its peak intensity after a half hour, and during a severe attack, the patient may appear acutely ill, looking pale and experiencing photophobia, nausea, and vomiting. These patients often seek a dark, quiet room, and sleep usually relieves the headache.

The migraine event may be precipitated by chocolate, nuts, monosodium glutamate, foods containing nitrites, red wines or any type of alcohol, and other substances. Hormonal changes such as pregnancy or menses can also bring on attacks. The etiology of migraine has long been thought to be vascular in nature. An initial phase of intracranial vasospasm, either asymptomatic or, if sufficient to lead to localized ischemia, symptomatic, precedes a secondary phase of vascular dilatation with associated "throbbing" headache. Recent data and theories have suggested an entirely different pathogenesis related to disturbances of serotonin metabolism within brain-stem pathways that modulate pain transmission.

The three major subtypes of migraine are classical, complicated, and common. Classical migraine is a headache that is preceded by a prodromal disturbance in neurologic function. Most often this is a visual disturbance such as a scintillating scotoma, zigzag lines, fortification spectra (so called because of their resemblance to a fort's battlements), or a homonymous field defect, but the deficit may also be numbness and tingling of the lips or one hand, mild aphasia, hemiparesis, loss of consciousness, vertigo, ataxia, or other focal neurologic disturbance. If the neurologic deficit spreads, it is characteristically a slow progression over minutes, rather than seconds, as would occur during a seizure or transient ischemic attack. The neurologic deficits typically last 15 to 30 minutes and resolve before the headache begins. In some patients, the neurologic deficit may persist during the headache and may last as long as several days after the headache has ended. This type of headache is known as a complicated migraine. Common migraine is a throbbing, "sick" headache occurring without a neurologic prodrome. The headache phase follows a similar pattern as in the other types.

During a patient's lifetime, attacks may occur with or without the prodrome, or the prodrome may occur alone, without a headache following (known as migraine equivalent). The headache, if unilateral, may occur on different sides during separate attacks, although there may be a predominance of one side.

Migraines have a tendency to begin in childhood or adolescence and to decrease in frequency with age, but there may be an increase in attacks during menopause. New onset of migraines may occur during later life, but if they are accompanied by neurologic deficits in this older population, it is especially important to rule out transient ischemic attacks as a cause of transient neurologic deficits.

Cluster Headaches

Also known as Horton's headache, or histaminic cephalalgia, this syndrome is also a recurrent type of vascular headache. It is typically seen in middle-aged men, many of whom smoke. Inheritance plays only a minor role in this type of headache. The attacks may occur 1 to 3 hours after falling asleep, and the patient is awakened from a sound sleep with the full-blown headache syndrome. The attacks tend to recur, sometimes with more than one attack during a single 24-hour period. These headaches may occur frequently for several days or weeks; hence the name *cluster*. During this time, alcohol may precipitate an attack, whereas during the headache-free intervals of months to years, alcohol does not cause a headache.

The pain of the headache is strictly unilateral. It is located in and behind the eye and may radiate to the forehead and temple. The pain is much more severe than that of migraine and is deep and nonthrobbing. The characteristic accompanying features of the headache are injection of the conjunctiva and tearing of the affected eye, ipsilateral nasal congestion and rhinorrhea, increased perspiration, and occasional flushing and edema of the cheek. Ipsilateral ptosis and miosis may be present during and shortly after a headache episode. Nausea and vomiting are usually absent. During an attack, the patient is in great distress because of the excruciating pain and often holds the affected side of his face while pacing the floor. The individual attacks are stereotypic in nature and consistently occur on the same side of the head.

Because cluster headaches can be reproduced by intravenous injection of histamine, it was originally believed that the syndrome was caused by spontaneous release of histamine. This notion has not been borne out by further experimentation, and cluster headaches are now believed to reflect a cyclic neurochemical disturbance.

Muscle-Contraction Headache

Often called tension headache, this entity is the type of headache seen most commonly in clinical practice. It occurs more often in women than in men. Muscle-contraction headaches usually have

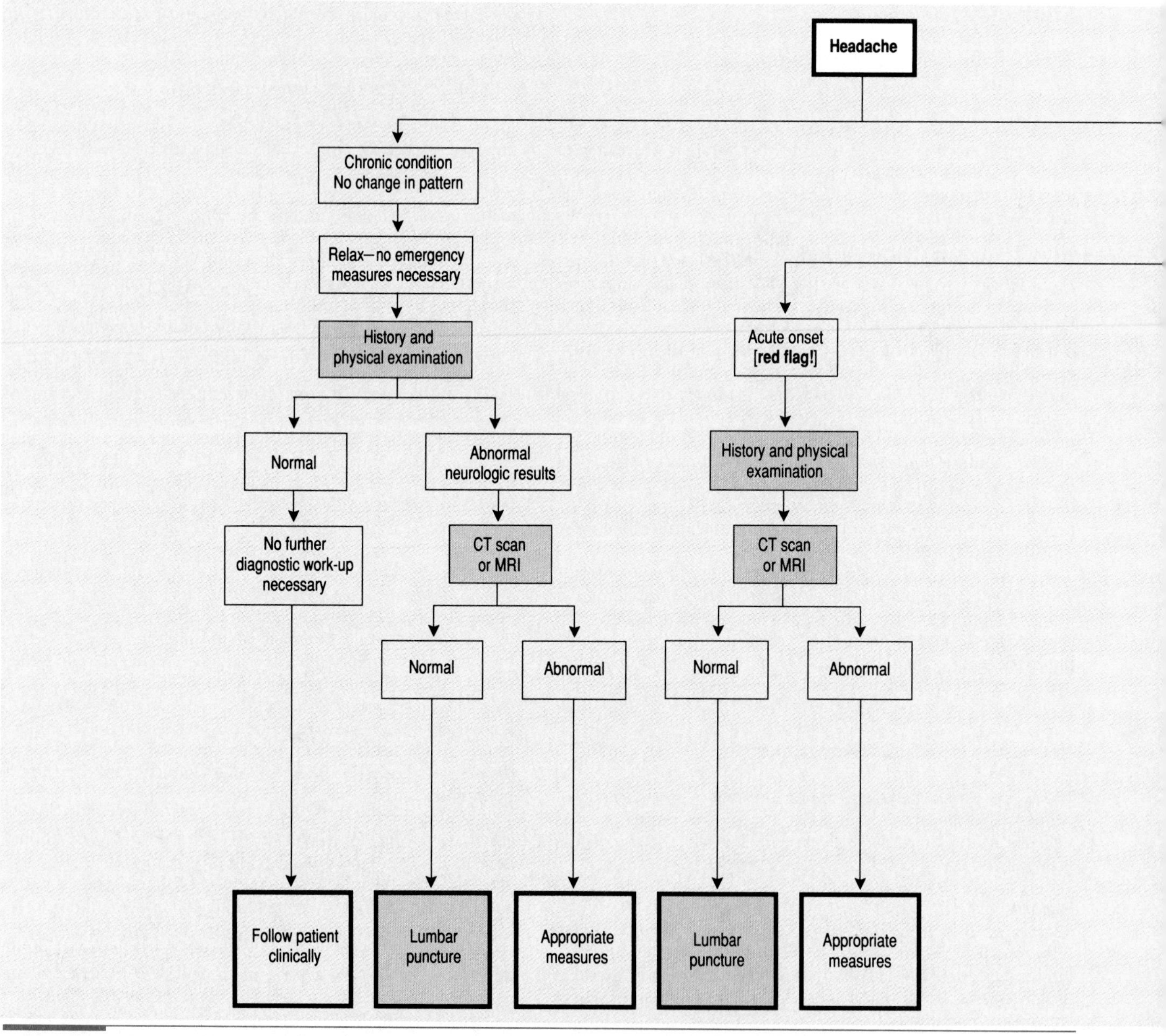

Figure 97-1 Algorithm for the diagnostic evaluation of patients with headache. CT = computed tomography, MRI = magnetic resonance imaging.

their onset in adult life but are occasionally seen in children and adolescents. The headache is usually bilateral, often beginning suboccipitally or bitemporally and then spreading to involve any area of the head. The pain is characteristically a steady, nonpulsatile tightness or pressure sensation ("bandlike" or "viselike") at both temples or at the occiput and neck. The onset of the headache may be gradual, and the headache may last for days, weeks, or even months and years. The headache is often present on awakening, although it rarely awakens the patient from sleep as does migraine or cluster. The headaches occur frequently in depressed or anxious individuals and are increased in frequency and intensity during times of stress. Other constitutional signs of depression, such as feelings of hopelessness and helplessness, insomnia, and early morning awakening, should be pursued by the physician. Chronic analgesic abuse is a common cause of chronic daily headache that can be clinically similar to a muscle contraction headache.

The pain is caused by sustained contraction of cranial and cervical muscles. A vicious cycle may develop in which the headache increases the patient's anxiety, which then leads to further muscle spasm and pain. A sustained muscle-contraction headache may also be a complication of an event that began as a vascular, post-traumatic, or sinus headache. These mixed headache syndromes are often difficult diagnostic dilemmas and require the examining physician to take a careful, detailed history.

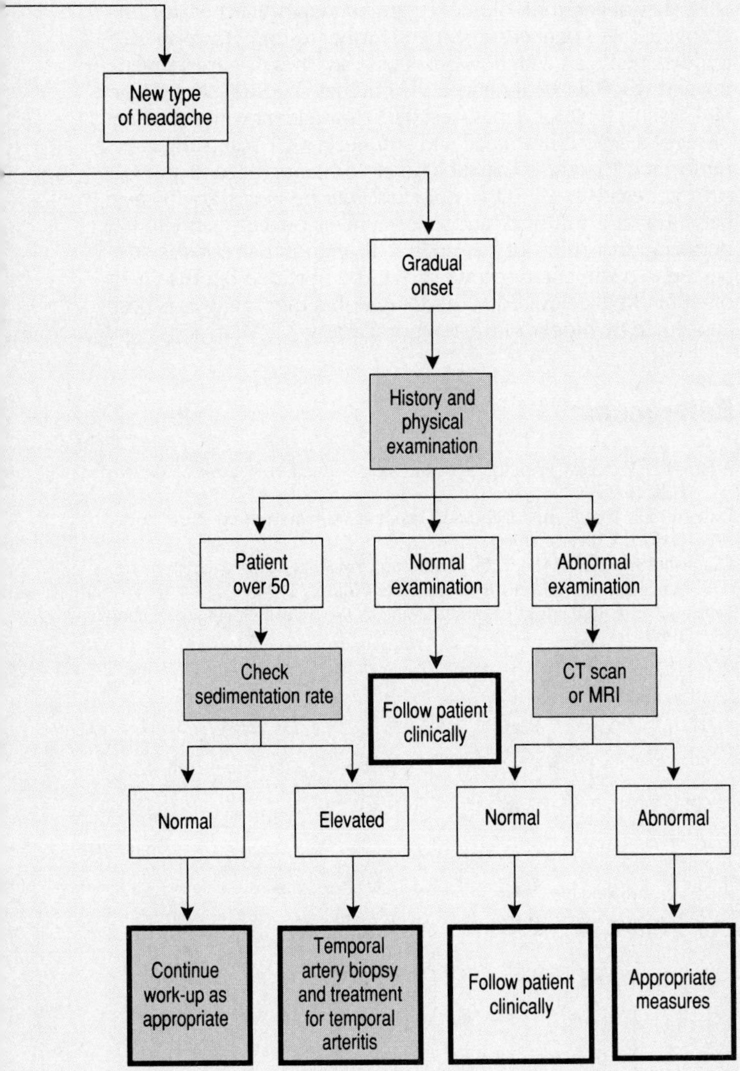

Figure 97-1 *Continued*

Post-traumatic Headache

Head or neck trauma may result in either chronic or recurrent headaches of variable intensity. Although a subdural hematoma should be a diagnostic consideration, most often the headache is related to extracranial structures and may be secondary to muscle contraction or local tissue damage. Head trauma can precipitate migraine attacks in predisposed individuals.

Headache is a common feature of the "post-traumatic syndrome," other symptoms of which include anxiety, insomnia, decreased ability to concentrate, light-headedness, easy fatigability, and emotional lability. This self-limited entity is often misdiagnosed as depression. The headache associated with a chronic subdural hematoma may be unilateral or generalized, constant and aching, and may be accompanied by focal neurologic signs and a changing mental status (varying from mild confusion to coma).

Mass Lesions (Abscesses, Tumors, and Hematomas)

The headache caused by a mass lesion is usually a dull, deep, aching pain. The headache may be intermittent, varying with activity and changes in position. It is often worse in the morning and may awaken the patient during the night. As the mass enlarges, the headache tends to increase in frequency and severity. Supratentorial masses tend to refer pain frontally, whereas masses in the posterior fossa may cause suboccipital or neck pain. If the headache is unilateral, it is usually ipsilateral to the mass. Depending on the location of the mass, there may be focal neurologic findings. Nausea and vomiting may occur if increased intracranial pressure develops.

The mechanism for the headache in space-occupying lesions is traction or displacement of the large arteries, veins, venous sinuses, or pain-sensitive cranial nerves.

Meningeal Irritation

A subarachnoid hemorrhage (bleeding from an aneurysm or arteriovenous malformation) usually results in abrupt onset of an excruciating headache that the patient classically describes as the worst in his life. Accompanying signs may include changed mental status, focal neurologic signs (which vary depending on the site of the underlying lesion and hemorrhage), and nuchal rigidity.

In some cases of aneurysmal rupture, the patient may have had a prodrome of a headache or a focal neurologic event that may have been caused by leaking of the aneurysm in the days or weeks prior to its rupture.

Meningitis and Meningoencephalitis

In cases of inflammation of the meninges, the patient usually complains of severe generalized throbbing pain that may be associated with nuchal rigidity. If the irritation involves the entire extent of the meninges, the patient may also complain of back pain. Accompanying signs and symptoms will depend on the causative organism.

Cranial Arteritis

Also known as temporal arteritis or giant cell arteritis, this syndrome must be considered in any patient with the onset of a headache after the age of 50. The patient typically complains of increasing headache that may be throbbing or constant and usually involves the temporal areas either unilaterally or bilaterally. The disease is caused by granulomatous inflammatory lesions of medium-sized cranial arteries, most often involving the temporal arteries. On examination, the affected temporal artery may be thickened, tender, and nonpulsatile, but it can also appear normal. Systemic signs and symptoms of malaise, anorexia, and a low-grade fever are common. Fifteen to 20 percent of patients may have accompanying proximal muscle pain, a syndrome known as polymyalgia rheumatica. It is important to diagnose and treat this disease early, because blindness may result if the arteritis spreads to involve the ophthalmic artery. These patients typically have a markedly elevated erythrocyte sedimentation rate. If the diagnosis is suspected, corticosteroid therapy should be started immediately. The diagnosis can be confirmed with temporal artery biopsy.

Headaches Related to Medical Illnesses

Many medical diseases can cause headache. A partial list includes hypertension, fever, chronic lung disease with hypercapnia, acute anemia, carbon monoxide exposure, hypothyroidism, corticosteroid withdrawal, hypoglycemia, Cushing's syndrome, and carcinoid tumors.

Diagnostic Approach

An algorithm for the diagnostic evaluation of patients with headache is shown in Figure 97-1.

History

Evaluation of any headache begins with a thorough history and physical examination. The historical characteristics of the headache often make the diagnosis apparent. Among the most important parameters are the qualities of the headache. Is it throbbing? Pressure or viselike? Dull or aching? What are the location? Does the headache occur exclusively on one side of the head? Does it begin in one area and then radiate? What are the pattern and duration? Does the pain increase gradually, or is it of full intensity at the onset? Are there any foods or activities that seem to precipitate a headache? Is it related to the menstrual cycle? Ask the patient what he usually does when he has a headache. A patient suffering from a migraine is usually unable to carry on a normal day's activities and seeks out a dark, quiet room to lie down. In contrast, a patient with a cluster headache usually holds the affected side of the face and paces the floor. Determine whether the patient has any warning aura before the headache starts and whether there is any accompanying nausea or vomiting.

If the patient is experiencing the headache during the interview, observation of his behavior can often be informative. Does the patient appear ill or uncomfortable? Or, at the other extreme, is the patient sitting and smiling while describing, in a detached manner, the excruciating headache he is experiencing? The answers to questions like these often implicate one of the classical headache syndromes.

Physical Examination

The physical examination should begin with vital signs. During the general physical exam, one should pay special attention to the eye, performing a funduscopic examination to look for entities such as papilledema or hemorrhage; to the sinuses, using transillumination and palpation to look for evidence of sinusitis; and to the neck, looking for nuchal rigidity and signs of cervical arthritis. Palpation of the temporalis muscles and posterior cervical muscles may determine whether muscular contraction and tenderness are present.

Each patient presenting with a headache should have a complete neurologic exam. Look for a change in mental status or a focal neurologic deficit.

Laboratory Studies

The diagnostic evaluation depends on the patient's physical findings and the physician's diagnostic suspicions. Obviously, not every patient with a headache needs a computed tomographic (CT) or magnetic resonance imaging (MRI) scan. The patient who has had a 20-year history of classical migraine attacks that began in adolescence and whose headaches are unchanged does not necessarily need further testing. However, the middle-aged man with new onset of headaches that are worsening and who has focal neurologic findings should have a CT or MRI scan to look for a mass lesion. In any patient with the acute onset of a severe headache and stiff neck, a CT scan should be performed to rule out a subarachnoid hemorrhage. If the CT scan is negative, a lumbar puncture will be necessary. In any patient with a stiff neck and fever, lumbar puncture should be performed to rule out meningitis. If temporal arteritis is suspected, a sedimentation rate should be obtained because it is often markedly elevated in this disease, but the diagnosis is best confirmed by biopsy of the temporal artery.

References

Adams RD, Victor M. Principles of neurology. 4th ed. New York: McGraw-Hill, 1989.

Dalessio DJ. Wolff's headache and other head pain. 5th ed. New York: Oxford University Press, 1987.

Diamond S, Dalessio DJ. The practicing physician's approach to headache. 4th ed. Baltimore: Williams & Wilkins, 1986.

Patten J. Neurological differential diagnosis. New York: Springer-Verlag, 1987.

Coma

Justin A. Zivin, MD, PhD

98

Definition

Coma has been defined in numerous ways. In ancient Greece, the term referred to sleep, but in the usual modern medical context, coma indicates that a patient is alive but unresponsive to verbal or noxious stimuli. The word can no longer be used with precision because of the multiple definitions that have accumulated in the medical literature and the difficulties of distinguishing coma from stupor, confusional states, and other entities. It is not helpful to record that a patient is comatose; what is useful is to note carefully the maximal state of arousal of which the patient is capable at the time of examination. In that way, improvement or deterioration at later evaluations can be adequately judged.

Etiology

Coma, of course, is merely a symptom of profound dysfunction within the central nervous system. Any medical problem that causes severe dysfunction of *both* cerebral hemispheres or the reticular activating system of the brain stem will produce coma. Traditionally, these medical problems have been segregated into two broad categories, surgical and medical causes. Surgical problems include head trauma and other structural lesions that cause increased intracranial pressure. This chapter is primarily confined to the medical causes of coma, although diagnosis and initial management of inapparent head trauma are included. The general categories of medical problems that produce coma are structural damage, metabolic disorders, and epilepsy.

The types of structural lesions that can cause coma include strokes and tumors. Any lesion that produces severe damage to both hemispheres (one damaged hemisphere will not cause coma) or the brain stem can cause coma. The list of such structural lesions is lengthy and includes brain-stem hemorrhages or infarctions, strokes of the hemispheres, cerebellar hemorrhages or infarction, primary or secondary tumors, and extracerebral blood collection such as subdural or epidural hematomas. Any lesion that does not directly damage the brain stem usually causes coma by producing increased intracranial pressure (because the cranial cavity is essentially a closed space with little room for an expanding mass), which squeezes both hemispheres or the brain stem. No tumor within the brain can be considered truly benign. Even if it is growing slowly and does not invade surrounding tissue, it can eventually become large enough to cause increased pressure and secondary damage to the brain.

Almost any metabolic disorder can cause coma. If the metabolic disturbance becomes sufficiently severe, neuronal function in the critical brain areas will eventually be disturbed and the patient will become comatose. The most common metabolic causes of coma include drug intoxication, hypoxia, hyper- or hypoglycemia, infections, electrolyte or pH disturbances, or dysfunction of other organs such as liver, kidney, or various endocrine glands.

Epileptic patients may appear to be comatose both during the seizure and during the postictal phase. During the seizure, the patient may not show any grossly apparent signs of tonic or clonic motions and is usually unarousable. This may occur in any type of epilepsy, but it is particularly common during psychomotor or petit mal status epilepticus. If a grand mal seizure has not been observed, the patient may appear to be comatose while in the postictal state.

Of course, combinations of problems may cause coma. Diabetics frequently have vascular disease and may become comatose after a stroke with superimposed hyperglycemia. Patients who are drug intoxicated may develop respiratory insufficiency, which may produce anoxic brain damage. Many other combinations also are common causes of coma.

Diagnostic Approach

Because coma is an emergency, a relatively standardized routine must be used for the initial care and evaluation of such patients (Table 98-1). If the cause of coma is immediately apparent, such as obvious head trauma or cardiac arrest, appropriate specific therapy should be instituted. Frequently, the cause of unresponsiveness is not immediately clear. In such circumstances, whether the patient is found unarousable on the floor at home or whether a hospitalized patient is discovered to be comatose by a member of the medical team, the initial response is to secure a patent airway, determine whether the patient is breathing, and establish whether the heart is beating (the ABCs). If not, resuscitation should be initiated.

After recording vital signs, the next step is to examine the patient briefly. The patient should be disrobed, and a cursory inspection should be conducted in which the examiner looks for obvious signs of trauma or any signs of movement, such as a repetitive twitching of a part of the body, which may be the only indication of seizure. Four signs should be recorded immediately and assessed repeatedly: (1) size and symmetry of pupils, (2) presence and type of spontaneous eye movements, (3) best motor response to noxious stimuli, and (4) respiratory pattern. Many patterns of pupil size and reactivity may be present. Three particularly important patterns are small reactive pupils, which usually indicate intoxication; large unreactive pupils, which frequently indicate hypoxia; and unequal pupils, which may indicate structural lesions. Observation of extraocular movements may be helpful. If roving eye movements are present, coma is usually not deep, and asymmetric movements suggest structural lesions. Other patterns may also be present. For testing best motor responses, a noxious stimulus should be applied. This testing should not in itself cause an injury (sticking a pin into a comatose patient is frequently a poor stimulus and may cause damage). Good methods are to squeeze the side of a pen into a nail bed or carefully squeeze the supraorbital ridge. In this way, sensation in each extremity and the face can be checked. Look especially for asymmetric movements or signs of decorticate or decerebrate posturing. Finally, the pattern of respiration should be recorded. This is especially important because comatose patients frequently are intubated, and later examiners may not be able to assess the respiratory pattern.

Table 98-1 Initial Evaluation of a Comatose Patient

1. Establish that coma is present (patient unresponsive to verbal and noxious stimuli).
2. Ensure that vital signs are stable (airway, breathing, circulation). If vital signs are unstable, begin (a) basic life support, (b) advanced life support.
3. Perform brief examination to assess
   a. Pupil size and symmetry
   b. Spontaneous eye movements
   c. Best motor response
   d. Respiratory pattern
4. At initial blood collection, obtain
   a. Glucose
   b. Electrolytes
   c. SMA 12
   d. Complete blood count
   e. Arterial blood gas
   f. Toxicology screen
5. Begin initial therapy with
   a. Thiamine
   b. Glucose
   c. Naloxone
6. Perform more thorough physical examination and obtain any history possible.
7. Order more detailed tests, such as
   a. Electrocardiogram
   b. Oculovestibular testing
   c. Lumbar puncture (if necessary and not contraindicated by high intracranial pressure, or focal findings on exam)
   d. Radiographs (skull, neck, chest)
8. Decide whether coma is attributable to a structural, metabolic, or epileptic cause, then obtain
   a. Computed tomography or magnetic resonance imaging scan
   b. Arteriogram, if necessary (after consultation)
   c. Electroencephalogram

After this quick evaluation, blood samples should be drawn immediately for glucose, electrolytes, SMA 12, complete blood count, arterial blood gases, and toxicology screen. It is most important that blood glucose be drawn before any glucose is given to the patient. Intravenous lines should be placed, and unless there is some known contraindication, all patients should receive a rapid intravenous infusion of 50 g of glucose, 100 mg of thiamine, and 0.4 mg of naloxone. If there is a rapid response to glucose, it may be necessary to give more. Naloxone may cause the pupils of a patient with miosis to dilate, but this alone is not proof of narcotic intoxication, and a repeat dose may be required.

The next step is to complete a more thorough physical examination. The physical examination of a comatose patient should proceed according to the same sequence used in alert patients, but some of the responses will be simplified. A detailed physical exam is required. First, the general examination is conducted, with special attention paid to skin lesions. Look through the hair for signs of trauma. Breath odor may be particularly important (e.g., hepatic coma, diabetic ketoacidosis). The cardiovascular examination should be complete. Care should be taken to prevent neck movement unless trauma can be unequivocally excluded.

The neurologic examination is also conducted in a simplified, but normal, fashion. Testing of mental status is not possible except as noted. Fundi should be examined, without dilatation if at all possible. Neck flexion should be checked if there is real concern about meningitis, but one should avoid this if neck injury is a major concern. Noxious stimuli give information about the status of both motor and sensory systems. Coordination or gait cannot be tested, but one should look carefully for muscle movements such as fasciculations or shivering. Deep tendon reflexes in comatose patients are notoriously unreliable, but they should be recorded while special attention is paid to possible asymmetries; the same is true of plantar stimulation.

One should then perform a rapid series of tests, including measurement of temperature with a thermometer that is capable of recording hypothermic temperature. An electrocardiogram should be obtained. Oculocephalic testing in patients who have not sustained neck trauma is important; oculovestibular tests should be performed in all others unless bilaterally perforated tympanic membranes are present.

This concludes the initial emergency evaluation, which usually takes less than 5 to 10 minutes. Several other tests, such as skull, neck, and chest films, are highly desirable. By the time the radiographs are obtained, some of the results of the initial laboratory studies should be available, along with the results of the physical examination. At this point, one can consider the next level of decisions.

Starting at the time of initial admission or recognition that a patient is comatose, it is essential to have at least one member of the medical team try to obtain the history. If family or friends are available, they usually provide helpful information. Indigents frequently have no wallet, but they may have scraps of paper in their pockets listing phone numbers; call these numbers. Find out where the patient was found (ambulance drivers usually know; don't let the drivers leave without giving details). The phone company usually keeps a "reverse directory" that will allow you to call phones in the immediate vicinity of the spot where the patient was found. There are many more tricks to this particularly urgent form of detective work, but obtaining information about a patient's history and condition before he or she became comatose is usually worth the effort. If a hospitalized patient becomes comatose, a detailed evaluation of medication sheets is frequently helpful.

Once this stage in the evaluation is reached, it is usually possible to make some preliminary assessments if the diagnosis is not already obvious. For example, the detailed physical examination may disclose traumatic lesions, or the patient may begin to have a tonic-clonic seizure, indicating that epilepsy is present. If the etiology of coma is still obscure, it is important to attempt to distinguish between metabolic and structural lesions. If there are focal neurologic signs, structural lesions are likely. A history of relatively rapid loss of consciousness or abrupt onset of focal symptoms suggests structural lesions. If the patient shows signs of rapid progression of deficits, papilledema, decerebrate or decorticate posturing, and the like, immediate neurologic or neurosurgical consultation should be obtained. Computed tomography (CT) or magnetic resonance imaging (if available), arteriography, or possibly even immediate decompressive surgery is indicated.

If there is a history of loss of consciousness after a period of generalized malaise, and the patient is febrile and has a stiff neck, a lumbar puncture is indicated, but only if disks are flat and there are no focal neurologic signs. If cerebral abscess is a consideration, the lumbar puncture should be deferred until after a CT scan, if the scan can be obtained quickly.

Thereafter, if the problem seems metabolic, the next most useful tests are evaluation of the blood studies that were obtained, especially the arterial blood gas reading, and if the studies to this point are normal, an electroencephalogram may be of benefit. Subsequent to these rapid evaluations, the pace of the work-up usually slows somewhat. Leads indicated by the initial studies should be investigated in more detail. It is impossible to indicate all the therapeutic maneuvers that could then be pursued because they will depend on the cause of the coma.

Summary

Coma is a medical emergency, and the main objectives are to keep the patient alive, to make a diagnosis as quickly as possible, and to perform the procedures in a calm and organized manner so that the patient is not subjected to any unnecessary risk. Some early treatment may be necessary to stabilize the patient and prevent irreversible damage; however, until a diagnosis is made, it is wise not to be too aggressive in initiating therapy, because incorrect treatment in the absence of a diagnosis may complicate an already confusing picture. With the exceptions of maintaining adequate vital signs and oxygenation, administering glucose and thiamine, starting antibiotics in an infected patient, stopping status epilepticus, and performing appropriate surgical procedures in those who will benefit from emergency surgery, there is usually time to evaluate the patient more carefully and to gain help from consultants. Specific therapy can then be initiated.

References

Caronna JJ. The comatose patient: Diagnosis, treatment, and prognosis. In: Henning RJ, Jackson DL, eds. Handbook of acute critical care neurology. New York: Praeger, 1985.

Fisher CM. The neurological examination of the comatose patient. Acta Neurol Scand 1969; 45(36):1.

Plum F, Posner JB. The diagnosis of stupor and coma. 3rd ed. Philadelphia: FA Davis, 1980.

Sabin TD. Coma and acute confusional state in the emergency room. Med Clin North Am 1981; 65:15.

Gait Disturbances

Paul T. Gross, MD

99

The ability to stand, balance, and walk depends on an intact nervous system functioning in a coordinated manner. After the first year of life, walking is generally performed without conscious effort, but walking is a deceptively complex act, requiring proper function of upper motor neurons, basal ganglia, cerebellum, motor and sensory nerves, neuromuscular junction, muscle, and skeleton. When walking is disturbed, there are two possible presentations. The patient may come to the physician because of difficulty with walking, or, alternatively, an unsuspected neurologic abnormality may be discovered by the physician's observation of a gait disturbance. Thus, not only is it useful to be able to diagnose and treat an impaired gait but observation of gait is one way to screen a patient for a neurologic disorder.

Etiology

The commonest causes of gait disturbance are pain and orthopedic injury or deformity. Among neurologic illnesses, central nervous system dysfunction resulting from cerebral palsy, stroke, head injuries, drugs, or cranial mass is the most common cause of gait disturbance. In the elderly, the combination of multiple sensory deficits, such as impaired vision, hearing, and peripheral sensation, leads to impaired ambulation. Other neurologic causes of gait disturbance, such as disorders of the spinal cord, nerve, muscle, and neuromuscular junction, are less common.

Muscle and Neuromuscular Junction

Most patients with muscle disease have proximal muscle weakness. Impaired ambulation is manifested at first by difficulty climbing stairs or by difficulty rising from the ground or a chair. With more advanced weakness, a "waddling" gait is seen. Weakness of the hip joint and trunk results in a lordotic posture, and the patient is seen to twist the pelvis from side to side, at times almost throwing the leg forward with each step.

Congenital myopathies and muscular dystrophies are common causes of muscle weakness in children and young adults. Polymyositis and endocrine and metabolic myopathies are more common in adults. In myasthenia gravis, there is usually, but not always, weakness of the neck, eye and lid muscles, and increased muscle fatigue with prolonged use. This is best tested by a repetitive, forceful attempt to displace the abducted arm or flexed head. Important findings in most patients with muscle and neuromuscular junction illnesses include fairly symmetric abnormalities; intact mentation, sensation, and stretch reflexes; and absent Babinski's sign. Because part of cerebellar testing depends on good proximal muscle strength, this portion of the examination should be interpreted with caution.

Motor Nerve

Patients with disorders of the peripheral motor nerve generally have weakness of the most distal muscles. The "steppage" or "foot slapping" gait is characteristic of this type of illness. There is a tendency to trip over one's feet and, because of foot drop (weak dorsiflexion) or flail foot (weak dorsiflexion and plantar flexion), the patient must, with each step, lift the knee sufficiently to elevate the dangling toes off the ground. At bedside examination, the muscles of the distal arms and legs may show weakness and atrophy, and in anterior horn cell disease, fasciculations (visible twitching of muscles at rest) are common. Diffuse, symmetric neuropathies may be found in patients with diabetes, uremia, alcoholism, and nutritional deficiency, or as part of a Guillain-Barré syndrome. Familial and idiopathic neuropathies are among the most common types, however. Some diseases of the motor nerve, such as amyotrophic lateral sclerosis and polio, are often asymmetric and may present with proximal or bulbar weakness. Childhood anterior horn cell disease (Kugelberg-Welander disease) often presents as a proximal weakness. Diseases of the peripheral motor nerve usually result in loss of reflexes, loss of sensation if mixed motor and sensory nerves are also involved, and Babinski's sign if concomitant upper motor neuron involvement is present, as in many cases of amyotrophic lateral sclerosis.

Sensory Loss

This category includes loss of proprioceptive, visual, and vestibular input. Proprioceptive loss, resulting in sensory ataxia, may occur with peripheral neuropathy or in disease of the posterior column of the spinal cord. The patient's walking is improved by watching the feet, and when this is prevented by darkness or visual difficulty, walking becomes impaired. A positive Romberg's test and proprioceptive loss in the toes are the relevant positive physical findings. If the proprioceptive loss is part of a peripheral neuropathy, findings of impaired motor nerve function may be present as well. Causes of neuropathy and symptoms of coexisting motor nerve dysfunction were described earlier. If the proprioceptive loss is from spinal cord disease, there may be associated upper motor neuron findings, such as spasticity and Babinski's sign, or a sensory level over the trunk may be demonstrated. Relevant illnesses include multiple sclerosis, spinal cord tumor, vitamin B_{12} deficiency, and Friedreich's ataxia.

It is common, especially in the elderly, to see gait impairment secondary to multiple sensory defects, such as impaired vision, hearing, vestibular function, and proprioception. Lack of self-confidence compounded by fear of falling as well as diminished strength and cerebellar function and joint disease may make the underlying sensory deficit less tolerable. Correction of vision and hearing loss and use of a cane to increase proprioceptive input are often helpful measures for these patients.

Central Nervous System

The supraspinal control systems are of three principal types: cerebellar, basal ganglia, and upper motor neuron. Loss of each results in a characteristic gait disturbance.

Cerebellar Disorders

Patients with cerebellar dysfunction walk with a broad-based gait and have special difficulty with tasks in which balance is essential, such as tandem gait or heel and toe walking. The patient may not be able to assume Romberg's position and, because vision may substitute somewhat for impaired cerebellar function, Romberg's test may appear "positive." Some patients with cerebellar disease hold their elbows as well as their knees away from the trunk as they walk and stand, creating a characteristic appearance. Additional helpful findings include impaired heel-to-shin or finger-to-nose testing, impaired speech, rebound phenomenon, and nystagmus. Body tone and stretch reflexes may be diminished. Important negative findings are the absence of proximal muscle weakness and sensory loss. Important causes of cerebellar ataxia include drug toxicity (anticonvulsants, sedatives, 5-fluorouracil), tumors, and cerebellar degeneration, which may be idiopathic or familial or associated with alcohol or malignancy.

Basal Ganglia Disorders

Basal ganglia disorders result in impaired motor control without marked weakness, cerebellar disturbance, or sensory loss. Typically, natural spontaneity of movement is lost. It becomes difficult to initiate body movements, and the patient appears somewhat stiff while walking. There is a loss of associated movements, such as the ability to swing the arms and to change facial expression. The inertia encountered when an attempt is made to initiate walking is complemented by an inability to stop suddenly. There is a tendency to fall backward (retropulsion). Much is often made of the "marche a petit pas," or short-stepped walk, of patients with Parkinson's disease. In most cases, the diagnosis can be made before this stage is reached. The two commonest basal ganglia disorders, by far, are Parkinson's disease and the extrapyramidal (basal ganglia) disorder induced by the major tranquilizers.

Upper Motor Neuron Disorders

The third major central nervous system gait disorder is that which results from impairment of the upper motor neuron (spasticity). This may be unilateral or bilateral. With unilateral illness, a characteristic form of weakness and gait disturbance involves the opposite (if the lesion is above the medulla) side of the body. With severe weakness the patient is unable to walk, but with milder involvement there is selective weakness of foot dorsiflexion, knee extension, and hip flexion. The patient learns to lock the knee, keeping the lower leg in extension, and the thigh and leg are circumducted in a semicircle from back to front as the patient walks. In very mild cases, there is impaired heel walking on one side. The sound of the plantar-flexed foot rubbing along the floor may be heard, and when the shoe is examined, it is found to be worn under the ball of the foot rather than at the heel. Weakness of upper extremity extensors is an additional helpful observation. On examination, there may be increased stretch reflexes and muscle tone and Babinski's sign on the involved side. Common causes of unilateral upper motor neuron dysfunction include stroke, subdural hematoma, and brain tumor. Bilateral lesions may be found with cerebral palsy ("cerebral diplegia"), spinal cord disease, and multiple sclerosis, in which there may be associated cerebellar and sensory lesions.

In normal pressure hydrocephalus, a gait apraxia is present. The patient has great difficulty initiating gait or may be unable to walk despite intact strength, sensation, and cerebellar function, and only mild spasticity. Although the individual movements necessary for walking can be carried out, the ability of the brain to "put it all together" may be lacking. The patient stands with feet apart, and may appear to have the feet glued to the floor. With great effort, halting steps may be made. Other diagnostic features include incontinence, dementia, and large lateral ventricles.

Non-neurologic Causes

Any patient with unexplained gait impairment should be questioned about pain in the feet, knees, hips, abdomen, or elsewhere, and this information should be incorporated into the diagnostic impression. Orthopedic conditions not always associated with pain, such as shortened leg, dislocated hip, or scoliosis, may lead to impairment of gait and should be considered. Prolonged bed rest, especially in the elderly, usually results in gait impairment, possibly secondary to weakness, fear, and impaired central nervous system control. In this situation, gait disturbance should only be diagnosed after the patient has been gradually mobilized for days to weeks, depending on the length of bed rest. Orthostatic hypotension, at times associated with prolonged bed rest, should also be considered in hospitalized patients who have difficulty walking.

Malingering and conversion reactions are possible causes of gait disturbance. Malingering may range from a well-intended effort to convince the physician that something is wrong to an effort to deceive for secondary gain. In conversion reaction a conscious effort to deceive is not present. One relatively common observation in malingering or conversion is that, in an effort to alter the gait, the patient may perform feats of great skill. For example, while attempting tandem gait, the patient may lean to one side and move one foot and two arms briskly through the air but not fall. In another presentation, the leg is dragged limply behind the patient—a gait disturbance that conforms to no known "organic" illness.

As personal experience is gained in the observation of the various gait disorders, gaits that do conform to known patterns become more obvious.

Diagnostic Approach

The approach to gait disturbances is summarized in Figure 99-1.

History

Helpful clues that lead to the cause of a gait disturbance may be obtained from the history. Difficulty climbing steps, getting up from a chair, and washing one's hair suggest a proximal muscle disorder. Poor balance and falls may be early symptoms of disease of the cerebellum or basal ganglia. Tripping over one's feet and a frequently sprained or broken ankle are found in motor neuropathies, and the inability to walk in a dark room suggests sensory nerve or posterior column spinal cord (proprioceptive) loss. Most patients with neurologic or orthopedic disability find walking more difficult after prolonged exertion or at the end of the day. If this is a particularly prominent part of the history, myasthenia gravis should be suspected.

Physical Examination

The examination of gait includes observation of the patient's best relaxed walking and performance of specialized tasks that stress various parts of the nervous system. These observations often direct attention to the part of the nervous system that is impaired. Subsequent testing of strength, sensation, and coordination during the formal neurologic examination may help to confirm the original observations.

For the initial portion of the gait examination, the patient is asked to walk naturally for 20 or more feet at a fairly brisk pace or is observed while walking from the waiting room. A normal person is able to get up briskly from a chair and start to walk without hesitation. The heels strike the floor first, and the foot is kept partially dorsiflexed so that it is not necessary to lift the foot far off the floor to prevent tripping over the toes. Most persons can walk with the feet only 2 to 4 inches apart and still avoid kicking themselves or falling. The movements should be fluid and symmetric when the sides are compared. The arms are close to the body and swing gently with slow walking and more vigorously with a brisk gait.

Observation of abrupt turning, starting, and stopping may demonstrate abnormalities of balance and inertia, as seen in basal ganglia disorders. Tandem walking (walking on a line) may bring out the balance problems seen with cerebellar defects. Heel and toe walking is an excellent measure of tibialis anterior and gastrocnemius/soleus strength, respectively, because these muscles are quite strong and may be difficult to test at the bedside. Romberg's test is primarily a measure of proprioceptive function. First, the patient is asked to stand with the feet together and the eyes open. This position ("Romberg's position") requires good cerebellar and vestibular function and good leg strength. A patient with poor proprioception can maintain this posture as long as the eyes are open, because any sway is perceived visually and corrected. At this point, instructions are given to close the eyes so that a fall ("positive Romberg") can be avoided only if sway is detected by intact proprioception. If the patient is unable to maintain Romberg's position even with the

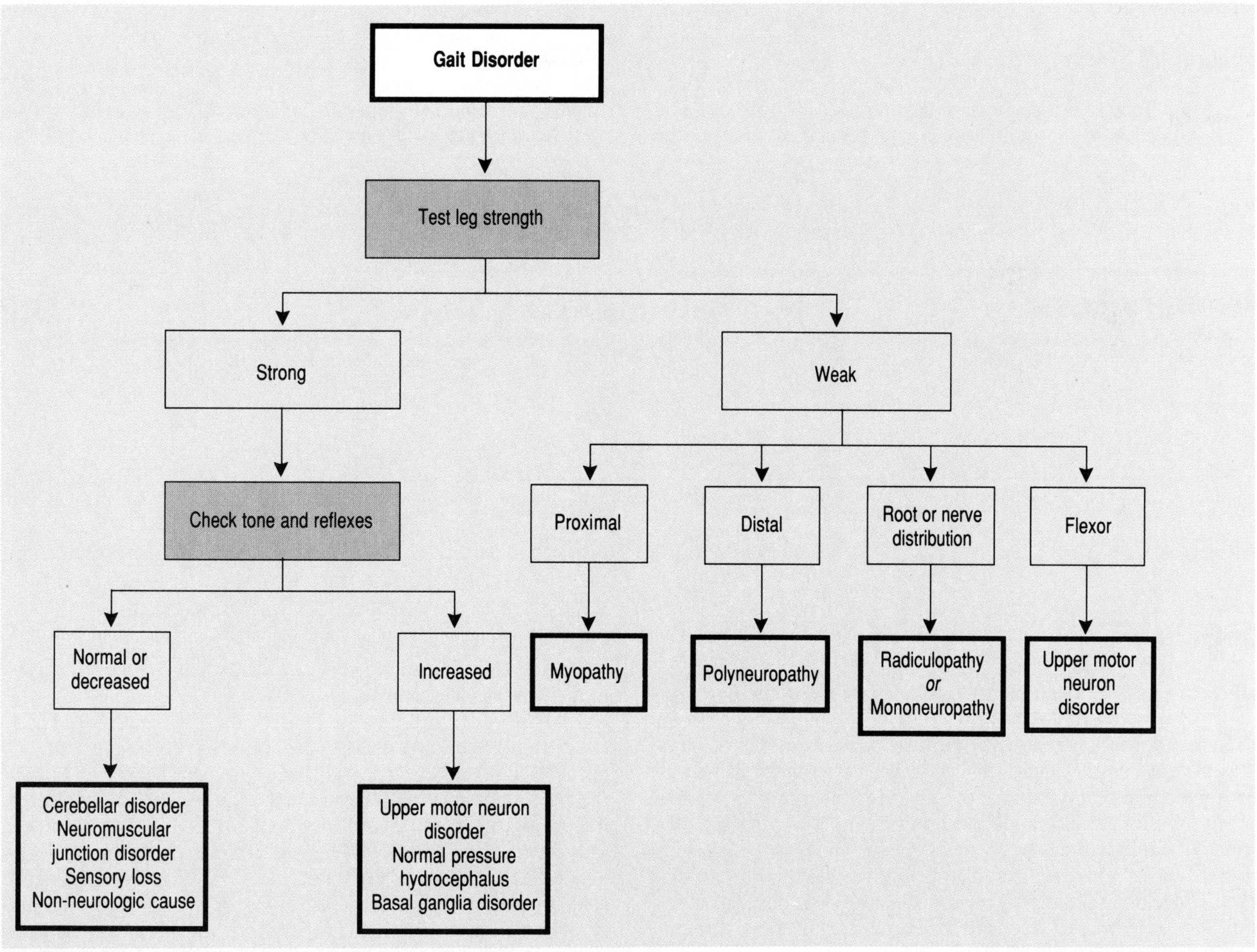

Figure 99-1 Algorithm for the evaluation of gait disturbance.

Table 99-1 Suggested Diagnostic Tests for Gait Disorders

Suspected problem	Blood/lab	Radiographic	Other
Myopathy	CPK, aldolase, electrolytes, thyroid function	None	EMG/NCS, muscle biopsy
Polyneuropathy	Glucose	None	EMG/NCS
Mononeuropathy or sensory (neuropathy)	Creatinine, protein immunoelectrophoresis, sedimentation rate, thyroid function, vitamin B_{12}, glucose	None	None
Radiculopathy	None	Spine x-ray (EMG/NCS), CT or MRI of spine, myelogram	None
Upper motor neuron	None		
Cerebellar	Thyroid function, vitamin B_{12}	MRI scan	
Neuromuscular junction	Acetylcholine, receptor antibody	CT of chest	EMG/NCS
Sensory (spinal cord)	Vitamin B_{12}	MRI of spine	None
Basal ganglia	None	MRI of brain	None
Normal pressure hydrocephalus	None	CT or MRI of brain	None

Abbreviations: CPK = creatine phosphokinase, CT = computed tomography, EMG = electromyogram, MRI = magnetic resonance imaging, NCS = nerve conduction study.

eyes open, the test can be modified, e.g., by separating the feet.

Most people can perform tandem walking until the fifth or sixth decade and heel and toe walking through the seventh and eighth decades. As experience with examinations is gained, an observer is able to appreciate acceptable limits of performance for each age group.

Laboratory Studies

Once one arrives at a suspected anatomic localization of a gait disturbance based on the history and physical examination, the laboratory can be used selectively to arrive at a specific etiologic diagnosis. The selective use of laboratory studies is illustrated in Table 99-1.

Reference

Adams RD. Aging and human locomotion. In: Albert M, ed. Clinical neurology of aging. New York: Oxford University Press, 1984.

Memory Loss

Sandra L. Horowitz, MD

100

Definition

Much of our understanding about memory has come from patients who have lost the ability to remember. Memory has been used in different contexts over the years, and most of us think of it as reminiscences of earlier life. To Freud, memory was a key with which he could explore the unconscious mind and its use of suppression, sublimation, and repression. The physical substrate of memory has been investigated, and DNA, RNA, and protein have been implicated in primitive species, but experiments have been difficult to reproduce in independent laboratories. We know more about the structural organization of memory in the brain from studies of patients who have lost memory, who are called amnesics. Amnesia means the loss of the ability to form memories despite an alert state of mind. Thus, patients in acute confusional states who are not attending to their surroundings, or aphasics who have decreased comprehension, should not be classified as amnesic. A clear sensorium is a prerequisite to an accurate diagnosis of amnesia.

Memory is traditionally divided into (1) immediate recall, (2) the ability to learn, and (3) the ability to reproduce with total accuracy information that has been received. There is a limit to the amount of information that can be immediately recalled, and this is not true memory. It is not consolidated or stored and can only be recalled for a short period of time. The ability to learn, which neurologists call recent memory, refers to the presence of selection and registration of information to be stored. Retrieval of information is the third step, where the memory has been incorporated into an individual's fund of information to be accessed as needed. This is remote memory, and it is usually the most resilient to disease.

Pathology of Amnesia

The following anatomic areas have been implicated in the genesis of amnesia:

1. Mammillary bodies are involved in Korsakoff's psychosis. They are at the base of the hypothalamus and are part of the limbic system.
2. The destruction of the dorsal medial nucleus of the thalamus, in isolation and with other structures, has been reported to result in amnesia.
3. Damage to the hippocampus and parahippocampal structures in the medial temporal region as a result of trauma, vascular and infectious disease, and epilepsy can result in amnesia.
4. The fornix connects the mammillary bodies to the hippocampus, forming part of the limbic system.

History and Physical Examination

Memory can be tested easily at the bedside, although standardized formal psychological tests can complement this testing with quantitative data. Usually, the clinician can assess memory adequately if certain principles are used.

Immediate recall should be examined because it confirms both the attention level of the patient and his or her ability to deal with new material. Repetition of a series of random digits slowly and clearly stated by the examiner is an adequate test.

Most people can remember a string of seven digits (± 2), and this is somewhat related to IQ and anxiety. If the patient fails to repeat four digits, there is no evidence that he or she is following or comprehending the commands; more complex operations can be tested, but interpretation should be guarded.

The ability to learn new material is tested by giving the patient three or four words that are unrelated and not relevant to the hospital setting, such as "baseball, cabbage, red, freedom." Have the patient repeat them to be sure he or she has attended the command, and remind the patient that you will return to ask for the words. Then, after 3 to 5 minutes of other examination, ask for the newly learned words. Most people remember this easily, but if there are difficulties, categorizing clues may be given, although it should be noted as a failed test. Three objects in the patient's room can then be given in the same fashion, as this is an easier task with visual as well as verbal clues. Patients with verbal comprehension difficulties can be presented with three simple designs that they are asked to reproduce after 3 to 5 minutes. Patients with minor difficulties may remember the four words, but if the patient is given a supraspan list of 10 words, which usually takes two to four trials, he or she will fail to learn this. All of these tests are designed to show that information can be learned and stored.

History taking can also contribute to your assessment of memory. Orientation to date, place, physician, hospital room number, and means and circumstances of arrival to the hospital are all memory-laden questions. Retrieval of old information is often tested by asking the patient to recite a list of presidents' names. One should also include more detailed questioning, e.g., about recent current events and more remote historic events. School and armed-service records are well-learned pieces of information. Questions should be structured so that the examiner can develop a sense for a temporal progression in memory loss.

An amnesic patient may have preserved immediate recall but a severe reduction in the ability to learn new material (anterograde amnesia). Remote memory testing assesses preservation of the more remote information, with increasing decay as most recent facts are covered (retrograde amnesia). Confabulation is a dramatic manifestation of acute amnesia in which the patient offers bizarre responses that go beyond merely incorrect and may have a fantastic quality. Confabulation occurs when the patient does not remember that he or she does not remember. The patient has lost the ability to monitor responses and be self-corrective. Bilateral frontal lobe dysfunction has been implicated in confabulation.

Forgetting is a different type of memory dysfunction in which the patient is unable to retrieve information that may remain in storage. The problem is in activation of the retrieval process. Everyone experiences forgetting to various degrees.

Etiology

Korsakoff's Psychosis

This is the classic example of amnesia. It occurs most often in people with chronic severe alcoholism, and it relates most probably to dietary deficiency of thiamine (vitamin B_1). Many cases of Korsakoff's psychosis begin with Wernicke's encephalopathy, usually after prolonged drinking of alcohol with little or no nutrient intake. Ataxia, oculomotor problems, and confusion occur with the encephalopathy. If the patient is not treated with thiamine, the amnesic syndrome becomes apparent within 3 to 5 days as the confusion clears. Most patients with Korsakoff's psychosis confabulate and have retrograde amnesia that may span several years prior to the onset of illness. Older information tends to be retained, and patients can manipulate old knowledge with surprising competence. New learning is markedly deficient. Most patients eventually improve, and in a study by Victor et al (1989), 25 percent were able to return to previous employment, 25 percent could work at a reduced level, 25 percent got along at home, and 25 percent needed custodial care.

Post-traumatic Amnesia

After major brain trauma the patient is often confused and may be agitated. The amnesia that follows consists of an inability to learn new material, which usually lasts for a few hours from the time of injury but may continue for weeks or months.

The accompanying retrograde amnesia may involve more than the post-traumatic period and include days to years prior to the event. This retrograde amnesia shrinks over days to weeks and eventually involves just the period during which the actual trauma and post-traumatic amnesia occurred, which may remain as a permanent gap or lacuna in memory.

Amnesic Stroke

Infarction in the territory of the posterior cerebral arteries involving the medial temporal region can cause amnesia. Branches of the posterior cerebral artery that supply the hippocampus in the medial temporal lobe are thought to be involved. This is usually bilateral, but unilateral left hemisphere disease has been reported. Visual symptoms of cortical blindness or hemianopsia often coexist. Transient global amnesia most likely represents transient vascular insufficiency in branches of the posterior cerebral circulation. Episodes have an abrupt onset and last up to 24 hours; they usually do not recur, but there may be a lacuna for the episode.

Postoperative Amnesia

Amnesia follows unilateral temporal lobectomy only if the remaining temporal lobe is functioning abnormally. Lobectomy is done in patients who have intractable epilepsy with seizures arising from one temporal lobe.

Hypoxic Amnesia

After a patient survives cardiac arrest and the subsequent coma, a confusional state usually ensues. An amnesic syndrome often follows that can last for months to years. Permanent disability in learning new material may result, but often some improvement occurs, usually in the first year.

Postinfectious Amnesia

Encephalitis, particularly when due to herpes simplex virus, which has predilection for the temporal lobes and limbic structures, can cause amnesia. Other neurologic syndromes of aphasia, dementia, or personality change can also be present. After recovery, amnesia may remain as a residual deficit.

Psychogenic Amnesia

In times of high stress a person may dissociate from his or her environment by creating a state of amnesia. The striking feature of this amnesia is that memory of personal information tends to be preferentially affected. Concomitant psychological disease should be sought.

Memory Disturbances in Dementia

Dementia is an increasingly common and complex source of memory dysfunction. It was previously defined as an irreversible loss of mental ability, but now an increasing number of diseases associated with dementia are treatable. Thyroid dysfunction, vitamin B_{12} deficiency, meningoencephalitis, Parkinson's disease, normal pressure hydrocephalus, side effects of medication, and cerebrovascular disease are some of the causes of dementia that are potentially reversible. These conditions have signs or symptoms other than changes in mental status that aid in diagnosis. The associated memory loss may reflect confusion and inattention in the toxic metabolic conditions. Immediate recall and continuous performance tests are impaired. The memory disturbance of Parkinson's disease is associated with forgetfulness, inattention, and slowness of retrieval functions.

Alzheimer's disease refers to the primary dementing process that runs a progresssive deteriorating course and affects several mental capacities simultaneously. Amnesia figures prominently, but aphasia, agnosia, apraxia, and decreased ability to abstract and perform constructions also are usually present to varying degrees. The amnesia of Alzheimer's disease affects both recent and remote memory and usually extends further back than in Korsakoff's psychosis.

References

Adams RD, Victor M. Principles of neurology. 4th ed. New York: McGraw-Hill, 1989.
Albert ML. Subcortical dementia. In: Katzman R, Terry RD, Bick KL, eds. Alzheimer's disease: Senile dementia and related conditions. New York: Raven Press, 1978:173.
Albert ML, Feldman RG, Willis AL. The "subcortical dementia" of progressive supranuclear palsy. J Neurol Neurosurg Psychiatry 1974; 37:121.
Benson DF. Amnesia. South Med J 1978; 71:1221.
Caine ED, Ebert MH, Weingartner H. An outline for the analysis of dementia: The memory disorder of Huntington's disease. Neurology 1977; 27:1087.
Cummings J, Benson DF, LoVerme S Jr. Reversible dementia. JAMA 1980; 243:2434.
Fisher CM, Adams RD. Transient global amnesia. Acta Neurol Scand 1964; 40(suppl 9):7.
Mercer B, Wepner W, Gardner H, et al. A study of confabulation. Arch Neurol 1977; 34:429.
Victor M, Adams RD, Collins GH. The Wernicke-Korsakoff syndrome. 2nd ed. Philadelphia: FA Davis, 1989.
Victor MJ, et al. Memory loss with lesions of hippocampal formation. Arch Neurol 1961; 5:543.

Numbness and Tingling

Lawrence M. Kulla, MD

101

Definition

The initial step in the evaluation of numbness and tingling is to have the patient clarify exactly what is meant by "numbness." Does he or she mean weakness, decreased sensation, abnormal sensation, or some combination of the above? A number of more precise terms are used by clinicians to refer to the symptoms and signs of sensory disturbance. *Paresthesia* is a symptom of abnormal sensation, such as tingling, pins and needles, or crawling sensations. *Dysesthesia* implies painful abnormal sensations. *Hypesthesia* and *anesthesia* refer to decreased and complete loss of sensation, respectively. *Hypalgesia, analgesia,* and *hyperalgesia* refer to decreased, absent, and heightened sensitivity to pain, respectively.

History

The clinician needs to direct attention to the exact location of the sensory disturbance. If the patient states that his or her hand is numb, it is useful to ask if only certain fingers are affected, or if both the front and back of the hand are affected. A general knowledge of the anatomy of the peripheral nervous system is essential in interpreting this information. The age, sex, and occupation of the patient, as well as the mode of onset, duration of symptoms, aggravating and alleviating factors, associated symptoms, and medical or surgical illnesses are also important aspects of the patient's history.

Physical Examination

The physical examination should include a careful neurologic examination, with particular attention paid to the symptomatic area. Primary sensory modalities such as touch, pain, temperature, position, and vibration, as well as stereognosis, graphesthesia, and double-simultaneous stimulation should be tested. Often it is instructive to "map out" on the patient's skin the area of sensory disturbance. After the history and physical examination have been performed, the physician attempts to localize the disturbance to either the central or peripheral nervous system or occasionally to a non-neurologic cause.

Peripheral Nervous System

Peripheral nervous system diseases may be grouped conveniently into generalized neuropathies, mononeuropathies, multiple mononeuropathies, radiculopathies, and plexopathies.

Generalized Neuropathies

In generalized neuropathies (polyneuropathies), all nerves of the body are affected, those with the longest axons being most vulnerable. The axons thus degenerate in a distal-to-proximal fashion. Sensory symptoms are often prominent and consist of symmetric distal hypesthesia, pins-and-needles paresthesias, or burning dysesthesias. These symptoms first affect the feet, then the hands, producing the characteristic "stocking and glove" distribution. Physical examination reveals distal weakness, atrophy, sensory loss, and hypoactive or absent distal reflexes. Symptoms may develop acutely, but more commonly develop subacutely or chronically. A wide variety of causes have been identified (Table 101-1); thus, a careful occupational, medical, and family history is essential. In patients whose diagnosis is not apparent from the history and physical examination, the laboratory evaluation should include a chest film, complete blood count, SMA-12, serum glucose, B_{12}, folate, thyroid functions, sedimentation rate, serum protein electrophoresis, and electromyelogram (EMG). Additional studies such as lumbar puncture, malignancy search, and nerve biopsy are performed when appropriate.

Mononeuropathies

Mononeuropathies are injuries to one peripheral nerve; they are usually the result of nerves being stretched, compressed in a tight compartment, or traumatized where they lie superficially or adjacent to bone. Mononeuropathies may result from vascular infarction of a nerve, as in vasculitis or diabetes; multiple mononeuropathies (mononeuritis multiplex) may occur in these settings. Mononeuropathies are an important cause of sensory and motor complaints in one extremity and are diagnosed by history, physical examination, and EMG. Only those specific mononeuropathies that have prominent sensory components are discussed here.

Median neuropathies are the most common mononeuropathy of the arm, typically occurring at the wrist. At this level, the nerve travels in a tight compartment with the flexor tendons, roofed by the transverse carpal ligament. Entrapment at this level is referred to as the carpal tunnel syndrome. Patients complain of tingling paresthesias or painful dysesthesias of the hand that often awaken them at night. Although the median nerve supplies the palmar aspect of the first 3½ digits, patients frequently complain that the whole hand feels numb. Occasionally, the discomfort shoots up the forearm and arm. Vasospastic symptoms in the fingers resembling Raynaud's phenomenon may also occur. Physical examination reveals hypesthesia in a median sensory distribution, often with sparing of the thenar eminence. The extent of the sensory loss is variable, but the tips of the fingers are usually maximally affected. Symptoms may be reproduced by the percussion of the median nerves at the wrist (Tinel's sign) or by forced flexion of the wrist for 30 to 60 seconds (Phalen's maneuver). If the entrapment is longstanding, there may be weakness and atrophy of thenar muscles. The syndrome is more common in women (3 : 1) and, although often idiopathic or occupationally related, may be associated with pregnancy, diabetes, hypothyroidism, amyloidosis, rheumatoid arthritis, gout, and acromegaly.

Numbness along the medial aspect of the hand should suggest the possibility of an *ulnar neuropathy*. Ulnar neuropathies are common, but they are less frequent than median neuropathies. They typically occur at the elbow (cubital tunnel syndrome) or less commonly at the wrist (Guyon's canal). The neuropathy may develop years after trauma to the elbow (tardy ulnar palsy). With lesions at the wrist, the sensory disturbance affects only the palmar aspect of the last 1½ digits, whereas both the palmar and dorsal aspects of the hand are affected with lesions at the elbow. Weakness, if present, will affect intrinsic hand muscles supplied by the ulnar nerve but will spare the thenar muscles supplied by the median nerve. With lesions at the elbow, the flexor carpi ulnaris and the flexor digitorum profundus to the fourth and fifth digits also may be affected. Ulnar neuropathies must be distinguished from C8 radiculopathies as well as from lesions of the medial cord of the brachial plexus (see Chapter 89, "Hand Complaints").

Mononeuropathies of the leg with prominent sensory complaints are much less common than either mononeuropathies of the arm or radiculopathies of the leg. Probably the most common sensory mononeuropathy of the leg is due to a lesion of the lateral femoral cutaneous nerve (meralgia paresthetica). Patients complain of tingling paresthesias along the lateral aspect of the thigh. This nerve, which arises from the L2 and L3 roots within the lumbar plexus, is a purely sensory nerve. Meralgia paresthetica is believed to result from low-grade continuous trauma at the level of the inguinal ligament or tensor fascia lata. It has been anecdotally reported to be more common in both obese patients and obese patients who have recently lost weight. The syndrome is usually self-limited and resolves within a few weeks or months.

Femoral neuropathies typically are manifested by prominent weakness of the iliopsoas and quadriceps muscles. Numbness along the medial aspect of the knee and calf, however, may be due to an injury to a sensory branch of the femoral nerve, the saphenous nerve. Isolated saphenous neuropathies are rare, but they are occasionally secondary to degenerative disease of the knee or injury during surgical procedures such as vein stripping.

The terminal segment of the tibial nerve, like the median nerve, travels in a tight compartment at the level of the medial malleolus in company with a group of tendons and is roofed by a flexor retinaculum. Entrapment at this level produces the tarsal tunnel syndrome, which is characterized by burning of the soles of the feet and, later, weakness of the intrinsic foot muscles. This syndrome is much rarer than carpal tunnel syndrome.

Table 101-1 Major Causes of Peripheral Neuropathy

Inherited
- Autosomal dominant, e.g., Charcot-Marie-Tooth*
- Autosomal recessive, e.g., Dejerine-Sottas disease, Refsum's disease, Tangier disease, abetalipoproteinemia, porphyria, leukodystrophy
- X linked, e.g., Fabry's disease

Nutritional, e.g., folate, thiamine, B_6, B_{12} deficiency*

Metabolic, e.g., diabetes, hypothyroidism, uremia, amyloidosis*

Toxic*
- Industrial, e.g., acrylamide, carbon disulfide, organophosphates, volatile solvents, thallium, arsenic, lead
- Drugs, e.g., ethanol, gold, isoniazid, disulfiram, nitrofurantoin, vincristine

Infectious
- Diphtheria, leprosy†
- Immune mediated, e.g., Guillain-Barré,* chronic inflammatory demyelinating polyneuropathy (CIDP),* neuropathy associated with paraproteinemia*

Vasculitis, e.g., rheumatoid arthritis, Wegener's granulomatosis, polyarteritis nodosa, mixed cryoglobulinemia

Neoplastic*
- Metabolic product of cancer, e.g., amyloid, macroglobulin, cryoglobulin
- Paraneoplastic "remote" effect of cancer (cause unknown)

* Common.
† Uncommon in United States, but common worldwide.

Radiculopathies

Radiculopathy, or damage to a nerve root, is another important cause of extremity numbness. It can be difficult to distinguish between a mononeuropathy and a radiculopathy on sensory testing alone, because each discrete region of skin is supplied by a peripheral nerve that, in turn, is derived from a nerve root. For example, the index finger is supplied by fibers of the C6 root that travel in the median nerve. Additional information is provided by the motor and reflex changes. If weakness is present in the distribution of several peripheral nerves, but primarily one nerve root, the symptoms are probably due to a radiculopathy. Conversely, if the weakness and sensory disturbance can all be explained by a lesion of one peripheral nerve, a mononeuropathy is the likely cause. A similar argument holds for the reflex changes.

Radiculopathies most commonly result from either acute or chronic degenerative disk disease and occur most frequently at cervical and lumbosacral levels. Patients often complain of neck or low back pain that radiates into an extremity, or of an electric-shock–like discomfort precipitated by coughing, sneezing, or Valsalva maneuver. Radiculopathies that occur at unusual levels (thoracic or high lumbar) should suggest the possibility of a diabetic radiculopathy, meningioma, or metastatic tumor. The clinical features of the common radiculopathies are listed in Table 101-2.

Diagnostic studies include spine films, computed tomographic (CT) scan, magnetic resonance imaging (MRI) scan, EMG, and myelography. In patients with typical histories for radiculopathy with purely sensory symptoms, the initial therapy is conservative and spine films alone are often sufficient. They will not demonstrate an acutely herniated disk, but they will show chronic degenerative changes and will screen for neoplasms. In patients with suspected motor radiculopathies, CT and, more recently, MRI scanning are extremely sensitive anatomic tests. EMG will demonstrate motor radiculopathies at any level and can detect lesions such as plexopathies or mononeuropathies, which might mimic radiculopathies. Myelography is usually reserved for patients with myelopathy or severe or refractory motor symptoms who are considered candidates for surgery.

Plexopathies

Plexopathies do not commonly result in isolated extremity numbness. Trauma, radiation, and cancer are the most commonly recognized causes of brachial plexus lesions, but cases are often idiopathic. In many cases, pain and weakness predominate. The thoracic outlet syndrome refers to compression of the brachial plexus or subclavian artery as it approaches the axilla. Although commonly discussed, this syndrome is quite rare. The two distinct aspects of the syndrome are the neural and vascular components. Vascular compression may result in positional arm numbness and pallor or repeated episodes of arm pain associated with blanching and swelling of the hand. Adson's maneuver (Table 101-3) may obliterate the radial pulse and reproduce the symptoms, although the pulse may be obliterated in many asymptomatic individuals. The neurologic symptoms consist of paresthesias in the axilla and medial forearm, i.e., lower plexus, often associated with weakness in median and ulnar innervated muscles. Patients with primarily positional arm symptoms may respond to simple exercises designed to widen the thoracic outlet. In patients with suspected lower plexus involvement, EMG, search for cervical rib, and occasionally arteriography are indicated.

Central Nervous System

In central nervous system diseases, the distribution of the sensory disturbance does not suggest a root or peripheral nerve dysfunction. In addition, the associated symptoms and signs often point to central nervous system pathology.

Multiple sclerosis, a demyelinating disease of the central nervous system, may produce a variety of sensory symptoms. The patient may complain of a tight, bandlike sensation about

Table 101-2 Clinical Features of Common Radiculopathies

	Distribution of pain or paresthesias	Sensory loss (if present)	Motor deficit	Reflex changes	Other clinical features
C5	Shoulder and lateral border upper arm	In distribution of pain	Deltoid, supraspinatus, rhomboid	Biceps, brachioradialis	C5 and C6 are the most frequently affected roots in chronic cervical spondylosis
C6	Lateral forearm, thumb, and index finger	In distribution of pain	Biceps, brachioradialis, supinator	Biceps, brachioradialis	
C7	Posterior arm, mid-forearm, middle finger (often diffuse)	Often maximal in middle finger	Triceps, pronator teres, wrist and finger	Triceps	Most frequently affected root in acute cervical disk herniation (70% of cases)
C8	Medial forearm, medial hand	In distribution of pain	Extensor indices proprius, intrinsic hand muscles	Finger flexors (variable)	
L5	Hip, groin, posterolateral thigh, lateral calf, dorsum of foot	Often maximal over great toe	Extensor hallucis longus, tibialis anterior, tibialis posterior, peroneus longus	Tibialis posterior (variable)	L5 and S1 lesions account for 90–95% of all lumbosacral radiculopathies caused by disk herniation
S1	Midgluteal region, posterior thigh and calf to the heel, and lateral aspect of foot	Maximal in lower leg and lateral foot	Gluteus maximus, hamstrings, plantar flexors of foot	Achilles tendon	

Table 101-3 Adson's Maneuvers

1. The chin is rotated toward the symptomatic extremity and elevated to hyperextend the neck. Upon deep inspiration, the patient's symptoms may be reproduced.
2. In a second maneuver, with the chin rotated and hyperextended as described above, the examiner applies downward traction on the affected extremity.
3. In the third maneuver, the patient rotates the chin to the opposite side and abducts the affected shoulder to 90 degrees. The examiner attempts to hyperextend the shoulder. A positive test reproduces the patient's symptoms.

the trunk or of paresthesias affecting virtually any part of the body. He or she may also note an electric-shock–like sensation running down the spine associated with flexion of the neck (Lhermitte's sign). This is not specific for multiple sclerosis, but it is thought to reflect posterior column dysfunction. Occasionally, patients experience paroxysms of facial pain, similar to trigeminal neuralgia. In order to establish a diagnosis of multiple sclerosis, the physician must demonstrate by history, physical examination, and laboratory tests that there are lesions disseminated in space (multiple levels of the neuraxis) and time (previous exacerbations).

Cerebrovascular disease may present with prominent sensory complaints. Symptoms may either be transient, as in transient ischemic attack, or permanent, as in completed stroke. Sensory symptoms may be associated with hemiparesis, aphasia, hemianopsia, or other neurologic deficits, or may occur in isolation. The sensory symptoms may affect half the body, the face and arm, the hand alone, or half the face and the opposite side of the body. The distribution of the sensory symptoms and the associated signs should fit into a vascular territory. In addition, a history of hypertension, previous stroke, or valvular or ischemic heart disease, as well as the presence of craniocervical bruits, is extremely useful in supporting a vascular basis for the sensory disturbance.

Although paraplegia or quadriplegia is often the most obvious sign of *myelopathy,* it may not be present initially when sensory symptoms may predominate. Patients may complain initially only of numbness or paresthesias affecting the feet. Associated signs include leg spasticity, hyperactive reflexes with extensor plantar signs, loss of position and vibration sense in the toes, and bowel and bladder dysfunction. A discrete sensory level may not be present initially, but one should search for it carefully.

Migraine may also produce transient hemisensory symptoms. The neurologic symptoms generally last between 5 and 15 minutes, are often followed by headache, and characteristically spread slowly from one area of the body to another, over minutes. The history is critical in migraine, and the slow march of symptoms, as well as a history of stereotyped episodes, associated headaches, and a positive family history are important in establishing a diagnosis (see Chapter 97, "Headache").

Episodic sensory disturbances may also be a manifestation of a *seizure* disorder. The disturbance may generalize secondarily to produce a tonic-clonic seizure, or it may remain isolated. Sensory symptoms often begin at the lips, fingers, or toes and spread to adjacent areas. In contrast to migraine, however, the symptoms advance over seconds, rather than minutes. Electroencephalography is the diagnostic test for seizures, and in cases of focal epilepsy, a careful search for underlying focal pathology such as arteriovenous malformation or tumor should be undertaken (see Chapter 103, "Seizures").

Non-neurologic Causes

Hyperventilation is a common cause of episodic numbness. The symptoms occur in a characteristic distribution, affecting the perioral regions and fingertips bilaterally. Patients occasionally complain of associated light-headedness or, paradoxically, shortness of breath, which induces further hyperventilation. It may not be apparent to the patient or initially even to the observing physician that the patient is overbreathing. The symptoms may be induced by anxiety or may have no obvious precipitant. The diagnosis is established by the history, distribution of numbness, and reproduction of the patient's symptoms by volitional hyperventilation. In this event, the patient should be reassured that the symptoms are benign. Not all sensory symptoms precipitated by hyperventilation are benign, however. Paresthesias or dysesthesias due to either peripheral or central nervous system disease may be accentuated by the change in pH that accompanies hyperventilation.

Psychiatric disorders such as conversion symptoms and malingering are also important causes of numbness. Excellent discussions of these topics can be found elsewhere. One should be cautioned, however, that an inability to make a neurologic diagnosis or an inability to demonstrate an abnormality on sensory testing should not, on that basis alone, lead to a diagnosis of psychiatric illness.

References

Adams RD, Victor M. Principles of neurology. 4th ed. New York: McGraw-Hill, 1989.

DeJong RN. Neurologic examination. 4th ed. Hagerstown, MD: Harper & Row, 1979:721.

Dyck PJ. Definition and basis of classification of hereditary neuropathy with neuronal atrophy and degeneration. In: Dyck PJ, et al, eds. Peripheral neuropathy. 2nd ed. Philadelphia: WB Saunders, 1984.

Kopell HP, Thompson WAL. Peripheral entrapment neuropathies. Huntington, NY: Robert L. Krieger, 1976.

Nakano KN. Neurology of musculoskeletal and rheumatic disorders. Boston: Houghton Mifflin, 1979.

Patten J. Neurological differential diagnosis. New York: Springer-Verlag, 1987.

Spence AM. Pain and sensory disturbance in the extremities. In: Swanson PD, ed. Signs and symptoms in neurology. Philadelphia: JB Lippincott, 1984.

Sunderland S. Nerves and nerve injuries. 2nd ed. Edinburgh: Churchill Livingstone, 1978.

Dizziness

James A. Russell, DO

102

Dizziness is a nonspecific symptom that may be the result of disease at many levels of the nervous or cardiovascular systems. The subjective complaint is often accompanied by a paucity of signs. Therapy is usually symptomatic and often unrewarding. In addition, despite its frequently benign etiology, dizziness may be the initial or cardinal symptom of an underlying sinister and at times potentially treatable disease.

Despite this pessimistic prelude, a physician who possesses some knowledge of vestibular anatomy and employs a rational approach to the dizzy patient will be able, in many cases, to identify the underlying problem. Patients with self-limited disease can then be reassured and treated symptomatically. Those with more serious problems can be identified, and appropriate investigations and therapy can be initiated.

Functional Neuroanatomy

The vestibular system, along with the visual and proprioceptive systems, serves to orient the body in space. The anatomic substrate of this system is the vestibular end organ (three semicircular canals, a utricle, and a saccule), the vestibular division of the eighth cranial nerve, the four vestibular nuclei in the caudal pons, and the multitude of their central connections. The vestibular labyrinth acts as a transducer to convert the mechanical forces of rotation, linear acceleration, and gravity to electrical impulses that tonically bombard the vestibular nuclei. From here afferent signals travel to the cerebral cortex, cerebellum, spinal cord (via the vestibulospinal tracts), extraocular muscles (via the medial longitudinal fasciculus), and reticular formation. In this manner, consciousness of movements (cortex) and coordinated reflex movements of postural and extraocular muscles occur, maintaining our bodies in appropriate relationship to gravity and our eyes fixed on objects of interest. Disorders of this system result in the illusion of movement (vertigo) as well as imbalance and disordered eye movements (nystagmus).

Understanding the nystagmus produced by unilateral peripheral vestibular dysfunction is facilitated by understanding the normal relationship between the semicircular canals and extraocular movements. There are two pairs of three semicircular canals: horizontal, anterior, and posterior. These lie within the bony labyrinth such that the horizontal canal is tilted 30 degrees cephalad to the horizontal plane, with each of the other canals oriented 90 degrees away from the other in the x-, y-, and z-axes. Ipsilateral stimulation of any of these canals results in contraction of a yoked pair of extraocular muscles (Table 102-1), with concomitant relaxation of the antagonistic pair. For example, rotational movement perceived by the right posterior canal will result in contraction of the right superior oblique and the left inferior rectus muscles; consequently, the eyes will be conjugately depressed and rotated to the left. Conversely, destruction or inhibition of the entire labyrinth on one side will result in an imbalance of the normally equal tonic input to extraocular muscles. As the vertical vectors cancel in the normal ear, there will be a resultant horizontal and rotational movement toward the affected ear.

Nystagmus of peripheral vestibular origin can be induced by either pathologic or physiologic influences. Instillation of cold or warm water in the external ear canal represents a form of the latter. As stated previously, vestibular end-organ damage tends to encompass all ipsilateral semicircular canals, resulting in a slow conjugate horizontal-rotary eye movement toward the affected ear. Despite the tradition of naming nystagmus by its fast phase, it is the slow phase that is the initial and abnormal component. The compensatory fast phase is then unconsciously mediated by the frontal cortex. Teleologically speaking, this fast phase serves to reposition the eyes to the midline, where the object of interest can be clearly focused upon the fovea.

Disordered postural movements mediated by vestibulospinal tracts are also common in vestibular disorders. In peripheral vestibular disorders, the illusion of vertigo results in the sensation of the environment moving toward the fast phase of nystagmus or toward the good ear. If visual fixation is abolished, past pointing will occur in the opposite direction (toward the affected labyrinth or slow phase of nystagmus) in an attempt to compensate for the illusion of movement.

History

The history obtained from the dizzy patient is critically important. If the diagnosis is not strongly suspected by the end of the history, the odds of identifying the etiology are greatly reduced. Four critical pieces of information must be obtained: a description of the patient's dizziness, its temporal course, the factors that provoke it, and the identity of associated symptoms. The patient must be allowed to describe the symptoms in his or her own words, preferably without using the word *dizzy.*

Baloh (1988) has divided dizziness into five separate categories. In some patients the abnormal sensation is one of movement, usually rotatory, although occasionally linear, which is termed *vertigo* and implies dysfunction of the vestibular system. Often the actual rotatory sensation occurs only at the peak of the illness and is preceded or followed by a light-headed sensation. The physician should be aware that patients may use a variety of descriptive terms to describe their vertigo. A sense of giddiness, drunkenness, swimming, or floating is commonly reported. A second category of dizzy patients is those who describe presyncopal light-headedness. This may occur with chronic anxiety or hyperventilation, diffuse atherosclerotic cerebrovascular disease, or global central nervous system hypoperfusion on the basis of arrhythmia, orthostatic hypotension, valvular heart disease, or carotid sinus hypersensitivity. A third group

Table 102-1 Extraocular Muscles Stimulated by Individual Canal Stimulation

Canal stimulated	Ipsilateral	
Horizontal	Medial rectus	Lateral rectus
Posterior	Superior oblique	Inferior oblique
Anterior	Superior rectus	Inferior oblique

Adapted from Baloh RW, Honrubia V. Clinical neurophysiology of the vestibular system. 2nd ed. Philadelphia: FA Davis, 1989.

of patients describe disordered balance or disequilibrium. The sensation is peripheral, not cephalic, and occurs only when standing or walking. Various disorders of the cerebellar or proprioceptive systems are often at fault in addition to bilateral vestibular disease. The fourth category consists of those with visual distortion. This may be the result of anything that interferes with visual acuity, including a new refractive prescription, cataract surgery, or disordered eye movements. The last category—individuals with multiple sensory impairments in whom no one cause is responsible—may be the most difficult to define. Typically, these patients suffer from reduced visual acuity and hearing and have decreased proprioception, usually on the basis of a mild peripheral neuropathy.

Attention is then directed to the timing of the symptoms. Vertigo measured in seconds is typical of benign positional vertigo. Vertebrobasilar transient ischemic events typically last 5 to 10 minutes. As a general rule, hours are required for an attack of Meniere's disease to subside. The symptoms of vestibular neuronitis or infarction of the labyrinth are characteristically measured in days to weeks, as would an attack of multiple sclerosis. Persisting vertigo that lasts for months is not typical of vestibular disease.

Because the vestibular labyrinth serves to detect movement, it stands to reason that movement frequently precipitates or exacerbates vestibular symptoms. Benign positional vertigo is precipitated by sudden head turning, frequently with turning in bed in the early morning. With far less frequency, dizziness with head turning may be caused by compression of the vertebral arteries in the neck or by carotid sinus hypersensitivity. Vertigo with extreme head extension probably represents a normal physiologic variant in most individuals. Dizziness precipitated by standing is invariably secondary to orthostatic hypotension. Dizziness precipitated by loud noises (Tulio's phenomenon) may occur in Meniere's syndrome. Cough-initiated vertigo suggests a perilymphatic fistula.

Acute vestibular disorders are commonly associated with nausea and vomiting, visual distortion (illusion of movement), and disordered equilibrium. A pressure or fullness in the ear suggests that the lesion is at the level of the labyrinth. Hearing loss and tinnitus can occur with lesions at the level of the labyrinth, the internal auditory canal, or cerebellopontine angle. The presence of ipsilateral facial weakness in association with hearing loss favors the internal auditory canal, whereas facial numbness and ipsilateral extremity incoordination imply a lesion of the cerebellopontine angle. Vertigo that arises from a lesion within the brain-stem parenchyma would, in most instances, occur in association with diplopia, binocular visual disturbance, dysarthria, ataxia, or motor and sensory symptoms of the extremities. As the vestibular labyrinth is represented on the cortex of the temporal lobe, complex partial seizures may express their aura at least in part as vertigo. Altered awareness noted by an observer would be an expected associated finding.

Physical Examination

One of the most important aspects of the physical examination of the dizzy patient is an attempt to reproduce the patient's symptoms if the localization of the lesion is not clear from the history alone. The dizziness simulation battery outlined by Drachman and Hart (1972) was designed for this purpose and is presented in an abbreviated form in Table 102-2. Orthostatic blood pressure measurements, carotid sinus massage, and the potentiated Valsalva maneuver are all designed to reproduce and identify three common causes of syncope. In the latter, the patient arises from a squatting position with the breath forcibly exhaled against a closed glottis. The Barany chair will produce vertigo in any normal individual. The Nylen-Barany maneuver will allow documentation of positional vertigo by quickly bringing the patient from the sitting position to the supine position with head rotated and hyperextended. The hyperventilation maneuver will reproduce the light-headed sensation produced by hyperventilation. Turning rapidly on command while walking will be poorly accomplished by those with disequilibrium.

Table 102-2 Dizziness Stimulation Battery

1. Supine and standing blood pressure at 1 and 3 min
2. Potentiated Valsalva maneuver
3. Carotid sinus massage with electrocardiographic monitoring
4. Nylen-Barany maneuver
5. Barany chair rotation
6. Hyperventilation for 2 min
7. Rapid turn on walking

A careful examination of the external ear canal and tympanic membrane is, of course, important. Evidence of infection, hemorrhage, glomus tumor, herpetic vesicles, and cholesteatoma is sought. A fistula test should also be performed. If there is pathologic communication between the middle and inner ear chambers, an increase in pressure in the external canal created by a pneumatic bulb attached to an otoscope will produce a burst of vertigo and nystagmus.

The neurologic examination should be complete but focused particularly on gait and cranial nerve function. During an acute vestibular attack, the patient will be unsteady but will retain the ability to walk independently. With eyes closed, the patient will veer or fall toward the affected ear. The sensitivity of this test may be increased by maintaining the feet in a tandem posture. This can be maintained for approximately 30 seconds in a healthy individual under the age of 50 years. If the patient is asked to bring his or her arms overhead while keeping the eyes closed and then to return the arms to their original position, the patient will deviate (past point) toward the bad ear as well. Poor coordination of the extremities in the presence of visual cues is not consistent with a vestibular disorder. The manifestations of vestibulospinal tract dysfunction will be rapidly compensated for and will be subtle or inapparent within a few days in the case of vestibular neuronitis.

Cranial nerve examination should include assessment of visual acuity, facial movement, facial sensation, extraocular movements, and hearing, but one should also search for the presence or absence of nystagmus. Nystagmus may be roughly divided into three categories: nystagmus that is present in the primary position of gaze, nystagmus that is apparent only with eccentric gaze, and nystagmus that is brought out only with change in head position (Baloh, 1983). During acute vestibular symptoms of peripheral etiology, horizontal-rotary nystagmus will be present in primary position and will increase in intensity with gaze toward the affected ear. The nystagmus will always be unidirectional, with the slow phase always directed toward the affected ear. This nystagmus will resolve quickly. It is distinguished from other forms of primary position nystagmus by its suppression with visual fixation, a property that can be tested with the use of +20 lens (Frenzel glasses). Nystagmus that is present in the primary position that is not suppressed with visual fixation is either congenital, if longstanding, or indicative of brain-stem or cerebellar disease, if acquired.

Positional nystagmus is characteristically brought about with the use of the Nylen-Barany maneuver. In benign positional vertigo, a torsional nystagmus beating upward and away from the dependent ear is observed. It begins a few seconds after the assumption of the provocative position, fatigues within 30 seconds or so, and habituates with repetitive trials. Positional nystagmus without these characteristics is usually of central origin (Baloh, Honrubia, Jacobsen, 1978).

Nystagmus that is present only with eccentric gaze, with the exception of transient physiologic nystagmus at the extremes of gaze, is usually of central origin. The most common form is gaze paretic nystagmus, in which the fast phase of nystagmus is always in the direction of gaze. This is frequently the result of vestibulotrophic drugs such as phenytoin or barbiturates.

In summary, peripheral vestibulopathy is characterized by unidirectional horizontal-rotary nystagmus, with the fast phase directed toward the good ear and with amplitude increasing as gaze is directed toward the fast phase. The slow phase of nystagmus, past pointing tests, and Romberg's sign are directed toward the affected ear. During the acute phase, nystagmus may be present in the primary position, but it is suppressed in all stages by visual fixation. After the acute phase, nystagmus may not be overt but can be brought about by the use of Frenzel lenses, which suppress visual fixation but allow physician's observations. Any deviation from these characteristics should lead the clinician to suspect a central vestibular disorder.

Etiology

Most of the definable causes of vertigo are listed in Table 102-3. They can be classified into etiologies of peripheral, central, or systemic origin. Only a summary of the more common or significant types is presented here.

Vestibular neuronitis is thought to be a condition analogous to Bell's palsy. It tends to occur in clusters in the spring and early summer, frequently following a viral illness. This pattern suggests a viral etiology. Vertigo, emesis, and disequilibrium develop over hours and gradually resolve over a few weeks.

Benign positional vertigo may occur in all ages, but it is more common in the elderly. It may develop idiopathically or in response to a variety of insults, including head trauma. Characteristically, brief episodes of vertigo (30 seconds) are precipitated by head turning. Ninety percent resolve spontaneously in 6 months.

Meniere's syndrome has been historically overdiagnosed. It is characterized by fluctuating episodes of ear fullness, tinnitus, hearing loss, and at times incapacitating vertigo that typically persists for 3 to 6 hours. Fifty percent of cases become bilateral. There is often excessive concern that an acoustic neuroma may be the underlying cause of vertigo. In actuality, slowly progressive, usually unilateral hearing loss is the most common symptom of an acoustic neuroma. Vertigo is relatively rare, because the gradual compression of the vestibular division of the eighth cranial nerve and the vestibular mismatch it creates are readily overcome by central compensation.

Vertigo may occur as a symptom of vertebrobasilar insufficiency but rarely does so in isolation, producing for the most part coexistent symptoms such as binocular visual loss or distortion, diplopia, dysarthria, ataxia of the trunk and limbs, or motor and sensory symptoms of the face and extremities.

Vertigo may occur with multiple sclerosis, but it is a rare presenting symptom.

A variety of systemic diseases may result in vertigo, including a number of the vasculitides, dysproteinemias, polycythemia, syphilis, diabetes, and hypothyroidism.

Table 102-3 Causes of Dizziness and Vertigo

Peripheral
Peripheral vestibulopathy—acute, recurrent, vestibular neuronitis, labyrinthitis
Benign positional vertigo
Post-traumatic vertigo
Vestibulotoxic drugs—aminoglycosides
Meniere's syndrome
Other—otosclerosis, perilymphatic fistula, focal ischemia
Central
Brain-stem ischemia
Demyelinating disease—multiple sclerosis, remote effects of carcinoma
Cerebellopontine angle tumor
Intrinsic brain-stem lesions—tumor, arteriovenous malformations
Seizure disorders (rare)
Spinocerebellar degeneration
Systemic
Drugs—alcohol, anticonvulsants, sedative-hypnotics, antihypertensives
Infections—syphilis, meningitis
Hypotension
Endocrine—diabetes, hypothyroidism
Vasculitis—collagen vascular disease, temporal arteritis, drug-induced
Other—polycythemia, dysproteinemia, sarcoid and other granulomatous disease

Ancillary Testing

Ancillary testing procedures should be utilized to pursue a specific diagnostic consideration, not as screening tools. If a diagnosis is not suspected clinically, further testing will have a low yield in identifying the correct diagnosis and may provide false-positive information. No one test is indicated in every patient.

The primary value of standard audiometric testing is to identify the presence or absence of hearing loss and to further distinguish between a conductive and a sensorineural hearing loss. In Meniere's disease it may identify variable sensorineural hearing loss, a pattern suggestive of this disorder. If sensorineural hearing loss is present, further audiologic testing and brain-stem auditory evoked responses will usually allow distinction between a cochlear and retrocochlear lesion. Electronystagmography may prove helpful if done properly. It allows the objective recording of eye movements under a number of provocative conditions. Its major role is to allow separation of peripheral from central disorders of eye movement control.

Brain-stem auditory evoked potentials may be useful in the detection and the intraoperative monitoring of the patient with a cerebellopontine angle mass. They are relatively sensitive although nonspecific in the detection of acoustic neuromas.

Neuroimaging procedures are rarely indicated in a patient with uncomplicated dizziness. If there is clinical suspicion of a parenchymal lesion of the brain stem or cerebellum, magnetic resonance imaging (MRI) is the imaging procedure of choice. In the case of cerebellopontine angle tumors, particularly small intracanalicular acoustic neuromas, MRI with gadolinium has become the gold standard. If pathology of the bony labyrinth is suspected, computed tomographic (CT) scanning at 2- to 3-mm intervals through the petrous temporal bones with bone windows is the procedure of choice.

Therapy

Fortunately, vertigo is more often than not a self-limited symptom, and reassurance that this is so is a key first step in therapy. Whenever possible, identification and treatment of the underlying disease are indicated.

A variety of antihistamines, anticholinergic drugs, phenothiazines, and other tranquilizers have been employed in the symptomatic management of acute vertigo. Although there have been some suggestions that these drugs may delay central compensatory responses to peripheral vestibular imbalance, they are often helpful in suppressing what is otherwise a frightening and disabling symptom. Most vestibular suppressant agents have sedative effects. This may actually be desirable when treating acute vertigo. It can be a limiting side effect in the management of recurrent or chronic vertigo, however. One can counter sedative side effects with stimulants such as methylphenidate, although side effects must be closely monitored.

Vestibular desensitization exercises also have a role in the management of benign positional vertigo (Brandt and Daroff, 1980). An explanation is required to enlist the patient's cooperation, inasmuch as the exercises initially increase vertigo. Meniere's syndrome may respond to sodium restriction and diuretic therapy. Destructive procedures such as labyrinthectomy or vestibular neurectomy have been used in intractable cases.

References

Baloh RW. History and bedside examination of the dizzy patient. Vail, CO: Syllabus for the 9th Annual Clinical Brain Conference, 1988:1.
Baloh RW. The clinical neurosciences. Vol 2. New York: Churchill Livingstone, 1983:841.
Baloh RW, Honrubia V. Clinical neurophysiology of the vestibular system. 2nd ed. Philadelphia: FA Davis, 1989.
Baloh RW, Honrubia V, Jacobsen K. Benign positional vertigo: Clinical and oculographic features in 240 cases. Neurology 1978; 37:371.
Brandt TH, Daroff RB. Physical therapy for benign paroxysmal positional vertigo. Arch Otolaryngol 1980; 106:484.
Brandt T, Daroff RB. The multisensory physiological and pathological vertigo symptoms. Ann Neurol 1980; 7:195.
Drachman DA, Hart CW. An approach to the dizzy patient. Neurology 1972; 22:323.
Leigh RJ, Zee DS. The neurology of eye movements. Philadelphia: FA Davis, 1983.
Troost BT. Dizziness and vertigo. American Academy of Neurology Meetings. Minneapolis: American Academy of Neurology, 1981.

Seizures

Bruce S. Zaret, MD

103

Definition

The word *epilepsy* is derived from the Greek word *epilepsia,* meaning "to be seized by forces from without." A seizure is the clinical manifestation of an abnormal, sudden, excessive, and disorderly discharge of cortical neurons. Epilepsy is defined as the repeated occurrence of seizures in the absence of an acute precipitating systemic cause of brain insult. By definition, a diagnosis of epilepsy is not appropriate if only one seizure is documented, when recurrent seizures occur secondary to processes such as hypoglycemia and hypocalcemia, or when they occur in children in association with fever. Only one-third of individuals with a generalized motor seizure have an additional seizure within 3 years after the first episode.

Epilepsy historically has been divided into symptomatic, sympathetic, and idiopathic varieties. *Symptomatic epilepsy* refers to a recurrent seizure disorder secondary to an identifiable and usually acquired structural nervous system process. *Sympathetic epilepsy* refers to a recurrent seizure disorder reflecting central nervous system irritability that results from systemic dysfunction of other organs or metabolic systems (i.e., uremia, hypoglycemia). When no etiology is identifiable, recurrent seizures have been termed *idiopathic.*

Epilepsy may also be divided into primary and secondary generalized forms. *Primary generalized epilepsy* connotes generalized seizures, usually of absence and tonic-clonic varieties, which are idiopathic in origin and often are associated with an increased genetic risk for such seizures. These individuals usually have normal neurologic and mental status examinations. *Secondary generalized epilepsy* refers to seizures, often of mixed clinical types, that occur in the setting of organic brain dysfunction, often manifesting as mental retardation and focal neurologic deficits.

Centrencephalic epilepsy is similar in concept to primary generalized epilepsy. Centrencephalic epilepsy suggests a pathophysiologic origin for seizures in which synchronous bihemispheric cortical discharges occur secondary to activation from a midline pacemaker, which historically has been postulated to be the thalamus.

Clinically, generalized seizures may be classified by their electroencephalographic (EEG) patterns into those that begin simultaneously in both hemispheres (*primary bilateral synchrony*) and those that begin focally and spread to involve the other hemisphere secondarily (*secondary bilateral synchrony*).

International League Against Epilepsy Classification of Seizures

Seizures are currently classified according to the revised International League Against Epilepsy (ILAE) classification, which was adopted in 1981. Under this system, seizures are categorized as either partial or generalized, depending upon whether a clear focal onset to the event can be determined using both clinical and EEG data.

Partial Seizures

Partial seizures are simple if not associated with an alteration in consciousness, and complex if consciousness is impaired. An *aura* is a symptom of a partial simple seizure that corresponds to its anatomic site of origin. Partial simple seizures may be manifested by focal motor activity that may spread according to somatotopic cortical organization (jacksonian march), somatosensory or special sensory symptoms (visual, auditory, olfactory, gustatory, vertiginous), autonomic signs or symptoms (including epigastric sensation, pallor, sweating, flushing, piloerection, and pupillary dilation), or psychic symptoms (dysphasia, dysmnesia, illusions, structured hallucinations, cognitive impairment, or affective symptoms).

Complex Partial Seizures

Complex partial seizures (CPS) are often preceded by simple symptoms manifested as the aura during which consciousness is not impaired. CPS may be divided into three types on the basis of clinical observations derived from simultaneous closed-circuit televised EEG recordings of the seizures.

Type 1 CPS consist of three phases: phase 1, motionless

stare; phase 2, stereotypic automations, including lip smacking and pursing, chewing, blinking, and nonpurposeful fumbling with clothes; phase 3, quasipurposeful reactive automatisms with response to verbal and painful stimulation and amnesia for the event. Type 1 CPS originate from within the temporal lobe.

Type 2 has only two phases, being devoid of the initial phase of motionless staring. Type 2 CPS are of extratemporal origin from frontal and occipital lobes as well as from the somatosensory cortex. Phase 1 components vary depending upon the site of origin. Frontal lobe origin is often associated with adverse head and eye movements, the assumption of a fencing posture, and clonic jerks of the contralateral face, trunk, or limbs mixed with stereotypic automatisms. Occipital lobe origin may be associated with contraversive eye movement or clonic jerks of the eyes and eyelids mixed with stereotypic automatisms. With either frontal or occipital onset, phase 2 consists of quasipurposeful complex automatisms, amnestic confusion, and gradual recomposure, with response to verbal and painful stimulation.

Type 3 CPS, the rarest of the three types, consist of sudden loss of consciousness lasting 2 to 3 minutes and resembling syncope (temporal lobe syncope), followed by partial responsiveness, formed speech, and reactive automatisms that last for about 2 minutes before full recovery is achieved.

The term *temporal lobe seizure* has been replaced by the term *complex partial seizures,* because these seizures can derive from extratemporal origins in the frontal, occipital, and parietal lobes.

Generalized Seizures

Generalized seizures are those that reflect bilateral symmetric cortical discharge and may be either primary or due to secondary electrical synchrony (partial onset with secondary spread). Generalized seizures are of the following varieties: tonic-clonic, clonic-tonic-clonic, absence, tonic, clonic, atonic (astatic), and myotonic. These varieties have been grossly divided into major motor or grand mal (tonic-clonic and clonic-tonic-clonic), minor motor (tonic, clonic, atonic, myoclonic), and petit mal (absence) types.

Absence Seizures

Absence seizures are characterized by brief (usually less than 60 seconds' duration) staring episodes during which the individual demonstrates impairment of consciousness. Absence seizures may be associated with clonic, atonic, tonic, or myoclonic components and may also be associated with autonomic changes and with stereotypic automatisms identical to those seen in partial complex seizures. Note that automatisms are not specific for CPS. Absence seizures may be clinically distinguished from CPS by their duration (shorter than CPS), their EEG pattern, and, most important, by the immediate return of normal mental status after the termination of an absence seizure. The EEG in absence seizures reveals a generalized paroxysm of 3-Hz spike and slow wave activity. The onset of absence is rare before age 3, most common between ages 4 and 11, and uncommon after age 20. Up to 50 percent of these patients may have one or more generalized tonic-clonic seizures.

Atypical absence seizures are clinically similar to typical absence seizures but have a more heterogeneous EEG picture that consists of features other than the typical 3-Hz spike and slow-wave complex.

Major Motor Seizures

Tonic-clonic seizures (grand mal) may be preceded by a succession of generalized muscular jerks that usually last several seconds and are frequently accompanied by a "jerky" state. This initial clonic state is accompanied by immediate loss of consciousness and the development of tachycardia, mydriasis, and hypertension. These jerks tend to be in flexion, causing sudden loss of postural tone and sometimes resulting in serious injury.

This initial clonic phase is followed in succession by a tonic and then a clonic phase, the *clonic-tonic-clonic seizure.* The tonic phase usually lasts 10 to 20 seconds and consists of tonic contraction of facial, axial, and appendicular muscles. This results in opening of the mouth and eyes and initial flexion posturing of the limbs, with a "hands-up" configuration of the arms. Tonic contraction in flexion yields to a phase in extension during which the mouth snaps shut, often resulting in tongue biting, and forced prolonged expiration against a spasmodic glottis, resulting in a tonic cry. The body assumes an opisthotonic attitude, with spontaneous extensor posture of the large toes.

The second clonic phase lasts about 30 seconds and consists of an initial generalized muscle "trembling," followed by a succession of brief violent flexor spasms of the entire body. Tongue biting may also occur during the clonic phase. Apnea during the tonic phase and ineffective respiration in the clonic phase often result in hypoxemia and cyanosis.

After cessation of the clonic activity, there is a brief period marked by muscular flaccidity, which also affects the bladder and its sphincters, resulting in passive emission of urine. This is then followed in about 5 seconds by the return of intense tonic muscular contraction, lasting seconds to minutes, during which forced jaw closure may again cause tongue biting. Pupillary and superficial reflexes are absent in the postictal state, during which the patient may appear comatose. The postictal state is usually marked by gradual recovery of full consciousness and is often associated with complaints of fatigue, muscle aches, and headache. The patient is amnesic for all components of the generalized seizure.

Physical examination after the seizure may reveal focal neurologic deficits such as a hemiparesis (Todd's paralysis), which usually lasts less than 24 hours. The finding of a postictal focal deficit may suggest that the seizure had a partial onset, which is an important clinical distinction because generalized seizures of partial onset have a much higher association with focal organic cerebral pathology than those without focal onset.

Minor Motor Seizures

Tonic seizures are usually seen in children with a history of mental retardation and slow (less than 3 Hz) spike and slow wave complexes on the EEG. Tonic seizures may produce muscle contraction involving the trunk or the extremities. A brief "cry" may occur at the onset of the event. The patient assumes a posture similar to the flexion phase of the tonic component of a tonic-clonic seizure, which has already been described. These seizures may begin slowly or abruptly and last from a few seconds to a minute.

Clonic seizures are seen almost exclusively in early childhood. They consist of initial muscle hypotonia or a brief generalized tonic spasm that results in loss of postural tone. The child then manifests a series of generalized symmetric or asymmetric clonic jerks of the extremities that last from 1 to several minutes. The degree of postictal alteration in consciousness is often related to the duration and severity of the seizure. Clonic seizures may be seen in the setting of both primary and secondary generalized epilepsies.

Myoclonic seizures consist of single or multiple brief jerks that may be generalized or partial in distribution. They must be distinguished from myoclonic activity secondary to dysfunction within the brain stem or spinal cord and from physiologic myoclonus, such as that seen in light sleep. The EEG in myoclonic seizures often reveals a generalized poly spike and slow wave complex pattern that precedes or coincides temporally with the clinical myoclonic jerk. Myoclonic seizures may be seen in association with uremia, hepatic failure, and cerebral anoxia in adults. In children it is often associated with other minor motor seizures as part of a picture of mental retardation. Myoclonic seizures may occur as part of myoclonic epilepsy syndromes secondary to degenerative central nervous system diseases. Owing to the brief duration of the myoclonic seizure, consciousness is not usually impaired.

Atonic seizures consist of sudden diminution in muscle tone that may be fragmentary, resulting in head drop and jaw opening, or total, resulting in a sudden loss of postural tone with loss of consciousness (the epileptic drop attack). In the akinetic form of this entity, there is less severe impairment of consciousness, maintenance of posture, and the patient appears motionless. The EEG in atonic (and akinetic) seizures reveals a generalized complex of synchronous 10-Hz multiple spike activity admixed with slow waves.

Other Seizure Disorders

No discussion of the classification of epilepsy and seizures would be complete without consideration of important clinical syndromes and terminology not encompassed within the ILAE classification.

The Lennox-Gustaut syndrome consists of a variety of generalized seizures, predominantly tonic, tonic-clonic, atonic, akinetic, and myoclonic, which begin between the ages of 1 and 5 years. It is associated with an EEG picture of slow (less than 3 Hz) spike and slow wave activity. Mental retardation is often present (up to 90 percent by age 5), and refractoriness to anticonvulsants is common. A variety of etiologies, including inherited metabolic abnormalities, perinatal and postnatal disorders, and congenital dysplastic or dysgenetic conditions, have been suggested.

Infantile spasms (salaam seizures) consist of a brief initial rapid contraction of neck, trunk, and bilateral limb musculature, followed by a tonic phase of sustained contraction that usually lasts 2 to 10 seconds. These contractions may be flexor, extensor, or of mixed variety. The onset of infantile spasms is before 1 year of age in 86 percent of patients. These patients may also have other generalized seizures. The triad of infantile spasms, arrest of psychomotor development, and the EEG pattern of hypsarrhythmia has been called the *West syndrome.* The term *hypsarrhythmia* denotes an extremely disorganized EEG picture of slowing and multifocal spike and slow wave activity. West syndrome occurs in the clinical setting of a large number of presumed causes, only the minority of which are amenable to treatment (phenylketonuria, pyridoxine deficiency, hypoglycemia, and central nervous system infections). West syndrome can be treated with adrenocorticotropic hormone (ACTH), which decreases the seizures and EEG abnormalities, although a beneficial effect on the associated mental and motor disabilities is less clearly defined.

Benign focal epilepsy of childhood (sylvian seizures and mid-temporal spike foci) is an important electroclinical syndrome. It consists of sensorimotor symptoms involving one side of the tongue, mouth, and face and is accompanied by the inability to speak or swallow without the loss of consciousness. Nocturnal seizures may be adversive or generalized. The symptoms are due to epileptiform activity emanating from the inferior rolandic cortex near the sylvian fissure. It usually occurs between ages 4 and 10 years and is associated with a genetic predisposition to seizures in first-degree relatives. It is a "benign" syndrome because it demonstrates a clear trend toward spontaneous remission of seizures, allowing discontinuation of anticonvulsant therapy.

Generalized seizures of tonic-clonic and partial complex varieties are often preceded by nonspecific complaints that have been termed the *prodrome.* Unlike an aura, the prodrome is not an ictal equivalent. Prodromal symptoms include depression, headache, insomnia, fatigue, and irritability. Patients may experience prodromal myoclonic jerks days or hours before a generalized tonic-clonic seizure, suggesting that a seizure will soon ensue.

Reflex epilepsy consists of generalized or partial seizures, often of myoclonic or tonic-clonic variety, that can be associated with a clear precipitant. Varieties of reflex epilepsy include reading, startle, eating, musicogenic, and photosensitive epilepsy. Identification of a clear precipitant is important because, as in the case of photosensitive epilepsy, the environment may be manipulated to reduce the offending stimulus.

The last term that will be considered is *febrile seizure.* Febrile seizures occur between the ages of 6 months and 5 years in the clinical setting of an acute febrile illness. The seizure usually consists of a generalized tonic-clonic event, although pure tonic and clonic forms have been reported. Focal aspects, or febrile seizures longer than 15 minutes in duration or occurring more than once in a 24-hour period, have been termed *complex febrile seizures.* Children with recurrent or complex febrile seizures are at increased risk of developing subsequent nonfebrile seizures.

Etiology and Incidence

The incidence of epilepsy is greatest in the first 6 months of life. The incidence of nonfebrile convulsions declines from 912 new cases per 100,000 per year after the first month of life to 240 per 100,000 per year at 6 months of age. By age 4 or 5 years, the rate further declines to 60 to 80 per 100,000 per year. In the Rochester study of epilepsy from 1935 to 1964, the incidence of epilepsy was greatest between ages 0 and 15 years, plateaued between 15 and 50 years, and subsequently rose after the age of 50. The cumulative incidence of recurrent seizures in the population is 0.7 percent at age 10, 1.1 percent at age 20, 1.7 percent at age 40, and 3.2 percent by age 80.

The etiology of recurrent seizures varies significantly in each age group. In newborns and infants, genetic metabolic defects, hypoglycemia, hypocalcemia, pyridoxine deficiency, congenital brain defects, and perinatal injuries are the most common etiologies. Central nervous system infections, perinatal or subsequent brain injury, perinatal anoxia, tumors, and toxins contribute to seizure development in the 2- to 10-year-old group. Idiopathic etiology, trauma, and congenital defects are the common causes in the 10- to 18-year-old age group. Similarly, these disorders, plus alcohol and drug addiction, are important in the early adult years (ages 18 to 25 years). The incidence of seizure disorders secondary to tumor and vascular disease increases significantly after the age of 50. Central nervous system degenerative disorders are also an important etiology in the elderly population.

Differential Diagnosis

Clues that help to delineate epileptic seizures from other types of episodes include abrupt onset, brief duration, rapid recovery, and stereotypic genuine loss of awareness. Despite these clues, it may be difficult at times to distinguish focal and generalized seizures from symptoms associated with other clinical conditions.

Nonepileptic focal transient neurologic sensorimotor deficits can occur as a result of other forms of central nervous system (CNS) dysfunction. Demyelinating disease (multiple sclerosis), CNS tumor, subdural hematoma, and CNS ischemia (complicated migraine or hemispheric transient ischemic attack) can produce transitory neurologic deficits. Hypoglycemia can also cause focal neurologic weakness or induce loss of consciousness.

Loss of muscle tone with or without associated loss of consciousness may present the clinician with a difficult differential diagnosis. Cataplectic attacks are characterized by generalized loss of muscle tone and are often induced by an emotional stimulus. During cataplectic episodes, deep tendon reflexes are lost and consciousness is not impaired. This diagnosis may be made by eliciting a history of other companion symptoms of narcolepsy, sleep paralysis, and hypnagogic hallucinations. Episodes of loss of consciousness without motor activity are usually secondary to syncope. Orthostatic hypotension, cardiac arrhythmias, illnesses associated with reduced cardiac output, or situations associated with reduction in cardiac venous return (Valsalva maneuver, cough, micturition) may contribute to the development of syncope. Syncope is often characterized by an initial ill feeling that is followed by nausea or vomiting and associated with pallor and perspiration. Vision may seem to dim, and tinnitus can occur. If unconsciousness persists for 15 to 20 seconds, brief mild clonic jerks of the extremities or, rarely, a generalized tonic-clonic convulsion can occur. Confusion, headache, and drowsiness, common sequelae of a generalized convulsive seizure, do not follow an uncomplicated syncopal episode. Recurrent tonic extensor spasms without loss of consciousness may occur secondary to multiple sclerosis and are not associated with loss of consciousness. These spasms may be abolished by treatment with the anticonvulsant carbamazepine.

Breath-holding spells are a common cause of loss of consciousness in children. Hysteria must be considered in the differential diagnosis of both partial and generalized seizures in adults and children. Failure of hysterical seizures to follow known physiologic patterns greatly contributes to their recognition. Patients with hysterical grand mal events may talk during an event or purposefully react to painful stimuli; often these "seizures" can be precipitated and terminated at the suggestion of the examiner. Preservation of pupillary reaction and deep tendon reflexes militates against the diagnosis of a true grand mal seizure in these patients. Absence of epileptiform activity on the "ictal" EEG is the surest way of establishing the diagnosis of pseudoseizures. Documentation of pseudoseizures is important for therapeutic reasons because they often occur in individuals with a documented seizure disorder.

Psychogenic fugue states and rage attacks with or without psychosis must be distinguished from partial complex seizures. Alcoholic "blackouts," hypoglycemia, and transient global amnesia may produce episodes of alteration in sensorium without loss of consciousness.

Myoclonic activity of focal or generalized varieties may be secondary to subcortical central nervous system dysfunction within the brain stem or spinal cord secondary to anoxic-metabolic or structural etiologies. Nocturnal myoclonus in light sleep is a common occurrence in normal individuals.

Diagnostic Approach

History

A thorough history outlining the events occurring before, during, and after a seizure is important. The correct classification of the seizure type often determines successful treatment, because different seizure types respond better to specific classes of anticonvulsant therapy. History of an aura, type of motor activity and its duration, presence of automatisms and postictal confusion or lethargy should be sought. A history of Todd's paralysis suggests a partial onset for a seizure. Symptoms of tongue biting and urinary incontinence associated with loss of consciousness are suggestive of a generalized convulsive seizure. Clues to the presence of nocturnal generalized convulsive seizures include diffuse morning muscle aches and enuresis.

A complete pre- and postnatal history should be obtained in any child or young adult with seizures. A history of bleeding, infection, or medication use during the pregnancy may suggest an intrauterine insult responsible for the epilepsy. The remote development of mesial temporal (horn of Ammon) sclerosis may be associated with birth trauma; a history of low birth weight, abnormal presentation, prolonged labor, or use of forceps should be sought. Patients or their parents should be questioned about immediate neonatal difficulties, and a profile of developmental language and motor milestones should be constructed. A history of febrile seizures in the patient or siblings is relevant because there is an increased risk of febrile and idiopathic single or recurrent seizures in such individuals compared with controls. Complex febrile seizures also suggest a greater risk of subsequent nonfebrile seizures.

A family history of epilepsy suggests an increased risk in the patient and often the diagnosis of a primary generalized epilepsy.

Precipitants that may be associated with a seizure include sleep deprivation, drug ingestion, noncompliance with anticonvulsants, pregnancy, or stimuli associated with the reflex epilepsies. Alcohol or barbiturate withdrawal may be associated with absence seizures.

A history of remote head trauma or loss of consciousness often provides evidence suggesting previous organic cerebral damage that may be responsible for the seizure. A history of systemic illnesses is crucial; uremia, hepatic failure, hypoglycemia, hypocalcemia, hypomagnesemia, and acute porphyric attacks all may be associated with seizures. Prior neurologic impairment secondary to stroke, tumor, abscess, and encephalitis may produce delayed onset of seizures several years after acute resolution.

Physical Examination

Every patient with a seizure should undergo a complete neurologic examination. It is beyond the scope of this discussion to outline all of the elements of the standard neurologic examination, so the reader is referred to standard texts. Certain aspects of the examination are relevant and are mentioned here. The presence of dysmorphic head and eye features such as hypertelorism or optic dysplasia may suggest developmental abnormalities within the brain that are often associated with seizures. Children or individuals with a family history of seizures should be examined in a darkened room with a Wood's lamp for the presence of neurocutaneous stigmata, i.e., ash leaf and café au lait spots associated with the phacomatoses, one of the most important of which is tuberous sclerosis.

If a clear precipitant appears to be associated with the clinical events in question, an attempt should be made to reproduce the circumstances, so that the clinician can observe the process first hand. Hyperventilation for 3 to 5 minutes is an extremely potent stimulus in producing absence seizures. The diagnosis can often be readily confirmed during the initial patient encounter with this activation technique. Reproduction of symptoms such as dizziness, light-headedness, and perioral and extremity tingling during hyperventilation suggests the diagnosis of hyperventilation syndrome. Photosensitive or other reflex epilepsies can often be documented by reproducing the precipitant during the examination.

Hysterical seizures can often be suggested to begin and end on cue from the clinician; patients with pseudoseizures may have a seizure after an injection of saline that they have been told could promote such an event.

Lastly, if the diagnosis of carotid sinus hypersensitivity is suggested by the history, carotid sinus massage under electrocardiographic (EKG) monitoring may confirm the diagnosis.

Laboratory Studies

The EEG is extremely important in the diagnosis of epilepsy because it provides data on physiologic brain activity, in contrast to the computed tomographic (CT) scan, which provides data on brain structure. The EEG records cerebral activity from the surface of the skull with an array of electrodes placed according to a system that divides the head circumference and anteroposterior and transverse distances into 10- and 20-percent intervals (the 10-20 classification system). This information is usually displayed on 16 channels of recording that are derived by hooking up the electrodes in different patterns, or montages. A large body of information is available regarding the amplitude and frequency of activity in the awake and asleep states of normal adults and children. The EEG is examined for evidence of abnormal slow or paroxysmal activity; the latter includes spikes and sharp waves. Because focal or generalized epileptiform activity (spikes, sharp waves, spikes and slow wave complexes) may occur in individuals without a history of seizures, the EEG is *not* diagnostic of epilepsy unless an actual seizure is recorded. Many individuals with epileptiform activity on the EEG without a history of seizures have a positive family history of epilepsy.

Because the EEG rarely records an actual ictal episode, the interictal EEG must be relied upon to reflect expressions of different seizure types. Partial seizures are characterized by focal spikes or sharp waves; the area of focal discharge often corresponds to the clinical characteristics of the seizure. The finding of an area of consistent cortical irritability in the setting of clinically generalized convulsive seizures suggests a partial onset of these events with secondary electrical generalization.

Generalized synchronous 3-Hz spike and slow wave complexes are very characteristic of absence seizures. Slow spike and slow wave complexes (under 2.5 Hz) are usually seen as part of the Lennox-Gustaut syndrome. Fast spike and slow wave complexes, greater than 3 Hz, are often associated with inherited and secondary metabolic disturbances. Multiple spikes (poly spikes) and slow wave complexes are often associated with myoclonic seizures. The pattern of hypsarrhythmia, which consists of diffusely distributed polymorphic slow waves admixed with multifocal spike activity, is characteristic of infantile spasms.

The percentage of interictal records in patients showing epileptiform activity varies with the different seizure types: absence, 80 to 90 percent; tonic-clonic, 30 to 40 percent; and myoclonic, 50 to 60 percent.

Electroencephalography is routinely performed with hyperventilation for 3 to 5 minutes and photic stimulation using a bright light at a frequency of 1 to 25 flashes per second. Besides accentuating the 3-Hz spike and slow wave complexes of absence seizures, hyperventilation may also promote focal and other forms of generalized epileptiform activity. Patients may develop spike activity in a generalized distribution, or it may be limited to the occipital regions in response to photic stimulation. The epileptiform activity may be limited to the duration of the photic stimulation (photoparoxysmal response), or it may outlast the photic stimulus (photoconvulsive response). The photoconvulsive response carries a high association with clinical epilepsy, especially primary generalized epilepsies. The photoparoxysmal response is less specific because it may also be seen in association with central nervous system irritability from conditions such as alcohol or drug withdrawal.

Sleep is a potent activator of epileptiform activity. Epileptiform activity may not be seen in a routine awake recording, whereas it may be quite prominent in the sleep portion of the recording. In addition, the yield of interictal abnormalities may be further increased by depriving the patient of sleep.

New advancements in EEG include ambulatory EEG, which offers the advantage of recording the patient for 24 hours while in his usual routine and surroundings. The ambulatory recording is similar in concept to the ambulatory Holter EKG monitor.

Specific clinical data regarding seizures may also be obtained by performing split-screen closed-circuit televised monitoring with the EEG (CCTV/EEG), the latter obtained via a cable attached to the electrodes (*cable telemetry*) or broadcast via FM frequencies (*radio telemetry*). Revisions in the 1981 ILAE seizure classification are largely based on data derived from CCTV/EEG monitoring.

Skull radiographs are of limited usefulness in the evaluation of epilepsy. They may provide information when abnormal calcifications, such as those secondary to cytomegalic inclusion virus or toxoplasmosis infection or associated with tuberous sclerosis or Sturge-Weber disease, are seen. The CT scan has largely replaced the need for skull radiographs. Any patient with a newly diagnosed seizure of partial clinical or electrical onset should undergo CT scanning of the head to rule out tumor or other structural dosage. The yield on CT scanning is lower in patients with generalized seizures, especially among the primary generalized epilepsies.

Patients with acute onset of seizures should also have serum electrolytes, calcium, magnesium, and glucose levels evaluated. A toxicology screen may also be helpful. Because poor compliance with anticonvulsant regimens is the most common cause of poorly controlled epilepsy, serum anticonvulsant levels are useful in documenting the noncompliance. Anticonvulsants in toxic ranges may themselves at times produce a deterioration in seizure control.

Therapy

Only general principles of anticonvulsant therapy are considered at this time. First, choose the appropriate anticonvulsant for the seizure type being treated. For example, ethosuximide is effective against absence seizures but ineffective in the treatment of other seizure types. Second, use the maximal dosage of one drug before instituting a second; polypharmacy rarely proves superior to monotherapy. Third, use only the amount of drug necessary to control the seizures. Too often clinicians treat the serum drug level and not the patient. "Therapeutic" normative values for anticonvulsants represent the range at which most patients achieve an anticonvulsant effect without developing toxic side effects. Patients may have anticonvulsant protection from subtherapeutic levels of an anticonvulsant. Dosage increases to provide higher serum anticonvulsant levels should be entertained only when the patient's seizures are not well controlled. Finally, match the dosaging of the anticonvulsant to the serum half-life of the drug. Anticonvulsants such as phenobarbital and dilantin, which have long half-lives, may be administered once daily, whereas agents with shorter half-lives, such as carbamazepine, valproic acid, and ethosuximide, require multiple daily doses.

Reference

Lechtenberg R. Seizure recognition and treatment. New York: Churchill Livingstone, 1990.

Porter RJ. Management of convulsive seizures. In: Asbury AK, McKhann GM, McDonald WI, eds. Diseases of the nervous system. Philadelphia: WB Saunders, 1986.

Weakness

David A. Chad, MD

104

Weakness is a prominent symptom of most general medical illnesses. Patients with heart disease, renal insufficiency, anemia, malignancy, and gastrointestinal disorders, for example, complain of weakness at some time during the course of their illness. However, direct examination of the strength of different muscle groups may not reveal loss of power. In many cases, pain, reduction in cardiopulmonary reserve, and depression contribute to an overall lack of energy—a sensation described by the patient as fatigue or "weakness." (Fatigue is discussed in Chapter 30.) However, some diseases produce decreased muscle strength per se by interfering with the function of either the central or peripheral nervous system.

Definition

Weakness is the quality we detect in a muscle when it is incapable of resisting a force we think it should resist. This is obviously a highly subjective definition, but in practice it seems to work. The physician generally begins by testing muscle strength against gravity alone. For example, if the patient can hold his or her arm out at the side (abduction), then the muscle (deltoid) resists gravity and is graded as at least 3 on a scale of 0 to 5. (This scale has been worked out by the Medical Research Council [MRC]). MRC 5 corresponds to full, or normal, strength; MRC 4, to strength that is obviously less than normal yet enough to overcome mild to moderate force in excess of gravity alone; MRC 2 indicates that the subject can exert force but only with gravity eliminated; and MRC 1 indicates only a flicker of movement.

For clinical purposes, and to simplify discussion, weakness can be divided into two broad categories based on the presence or absence of associated neurologic findings: the first is weakness caused by a lesion of the upper motor neuron (UMN), and the second, weakness caused by a lesion of the lower motor neuron (LMN). Table 104-1 summarizes the characteristics associated with these two types of weakness.

This chapter considers the central and peripheral nervous system locations affected by diseases that produce muscle weakness. These locations include the cerebral hemispheres, cerebellum, brain stem, spinal cord, nerve roots, peripheral nerves, neuromuscular junction, and muscle. Disturbances at each of these levels produce a characteristic distribution and temporal evolution of weakness.

Table 104-1 Categories of Weakness

	Upper motor neuron	Lower motor neuron
Site of lesion	Corticobulbar or corticospinal fibers or their cell bodies	Anterior horn cell or its axon (peripheral nerve)
Tone	Increased	Normal or decreased
Reflexes	Increased	Decreased to absent
Pathologic reflex	Present (Babinski's sign)	Absent
Atrophy	No*	Yes
Fasciculations	No	Yes

* Disuse atrophy may occur.

Localization Overview

In approaching weakness, the physician's first task is to localize the causative lesion. The physician must discover where in the nervous system the disease process acts to produce a given constellation of symptoms and signs.

Cerebral hemisphere disturbances produce contralateral hemiparesis. Weakness is of the UMN type. Because neural centers controlling movement are adjacent to those involved in higher integrative somatosensory and visual functions, weakness is often associated with a disorder of language or body and space orientation, sensation, or visual fields.

Cerebellar disorders produce ataxia rather than weakness per se. However, an ataxic clumsy limb caused by a lesion of a cerebellar hemisphere can sometimes be difficult to distinguish from weakness caused by a lesion of a cerebral hemisphere. Some clues to the presence of a cerebellar lesion are normal or somewhat reduced reflexes on the affected side (pendular reflexes), disturbances of ocular muscle control (nystagmus), and dysarthria. In addition, the gait of cerebellar disease is usually strikingly abnormal; it is an ataxic staggering gait that is not seen in cerebral hemispheric disorders.

In *brain-stem* disorders, weakness is accompanied by cranial nerve, sensory, and cerebellar abnormalities. This constellation of findings is a result of the anatomic organization of the brain stem: pyramidal fibers coursing through the anterior portions of the brain stem are adjacent to brain-stem nuclei, sensory fibers, and fibers connecting brain-stem nuclei with the cerebellum. As in disturbances of the cerebral hemisphere, the weakness is of the UMN type.

Disorders of the *spinal cord* produce weakness of the UMN type. Most lesions disrupting motor pathways also disturb sensory pathways because ascending sensory systems run close by the descending corticospinal tracts. Important clues to a spinal cord localization are incontinence (bladder and bowel) and a sensory "level" (sensation abnormal below the level of spinal cord pathology).

Peripheral nerve disorders (peripheral neuropathy) produce weakness of the LMN type. In some peripheral neuropathies, cranial nerves are involved. Peripheral neuropathies often also produce sensory signs.

Disorders of the *neuromuscular junction* produce pure motor syndromes that affect predominantly cranial nerve–supplied muscles. Fatigability and fluctuation in strength are important clues to a nerve-muscle junction localization.

Diseases of *muscle* tend to produce weakness of the neck flexors and extensors, the shoulder and pelvic girdle muscles, and the proximal muscles of the limbs. Cranial nerve–supplied and distal limb muscles are usually spared. There are a few exceptions to this pattern; distal muscles may be involved early in the course of myotonic dystrophy, and ocular muscles are usually the first to be involved in certain inherited ophthalmoplegias and some metabolic myopathies (usually those with mitochondrial involvement).

Diagnostic Approach

History

A detailed history will provide enough information for the physician to identify the level in the nervous system at which the disease process acts to produce weakness, and may even allow the nature of the disease process to be discerned. What is the pattern of weakness? Is there involvement of the face, the arm, and the leg, which would suggest a hemisphere location? Are both legs affected, suggesting a spinal cord location? Is weakness generalized and present in the limbs and cranial nerve–supplied muscles, suggesting a peripheral neuropathy? Or are limb girdle and proximal muscles alone affected and other muscles relatively spared, indicating muscle as the locus of involvement?

The rate of onset of weakness needs to be considered. Does weakness in a hemiparetic distribution come on acutely, as in stroke? Has generalized weakness of the limbs and cranial nerve–supplied muscles come on gradually, over a course of months, as in a slowly progressive peripheral neuropathy? Or have symptoms of cranial nerve–supplied muscles appeared over a period of days in association with respiratory dysfunction, suggesting a disorder at the nerve-muscle junction?

The presence of abnormalities other than weakness is also important in helping to reach a diagnosis. Is weakness associated with disturbance of higher intellectual function, as in hemisphere lesions? Is weakness joined by sensory disturbances (numbness and tingling), suggesting peripheral neuropathy? Lack of associated features is also important in allowing a diagnosis to be made. For example, a pure motor syndrome affecting cranial nerve–supplied muscles that tends to fluctuate in severity and produces little in the way of limb muscle symptoms strongly suggests myasthenia gravis, a disorder of the neuromuscular junction. If historical features indicate that either nerve or muscle is affected, family history, which is always helpful, becomes vitally important, because a number of neuropathies and myopathies are inherited.

Noting the presence of associated illnesses such as neoplasms, infections, and collagen vascular disorders is helpful in deciding upon the cause of weakness. For example, if a patient with a collagen vascular disorder, such as rheumatoid arthritis, developed rapidly progressive weakness associated with numbness and tingling, a neuropathy caused by vasculitis would be seriously considered. If a patient with breast cancer developed proximal muscle weakness, inflammatory myopathy would be likely.

Physical Examination

A major goal of the physical examination of the weak patient is to establish whether the weakness is of the UMN or the LMN type. Table 104-1 reviews the characteristics of both types of weakness.

Laboratory Studies

History and physical examination almost always allow precise localization of the lesion producing the weakness. Laboratory studies are helpful primarily in identifying the nature of the weakness-producing pathologic process. (Rarely, even after history and physical examination, some doubt about localization lingers; in these instances, laboratory studies contribute to lesion localization.) If the site of the lesion is thought to be the hemispheres, cerebellum, or brain stem, computed tomography (CT) and magnetic resonance imaging (MRI) will identify most structural lesions and suggest their underlying nature (i.e., stroke or tumor). If a structural lesion is not seen, metabolic, infectious, and inflammatory conditions need to be considered, and examination of the cerebrospinal fluid (CSF) is often helpful. If the lesion is localized to the spinal cord, CT, MRI, or myelography is often needed to exclude a structural, surgically treatable lesion. If none is identified, CSF studies will help to identify demyelinating illnesses (multiple sclerosis) and inflammatory disorders.

Neurodiagnostic testing will often help to define the nature of a neuropathy (whether axons or myelin is primarily affected) and its distribution (mononeuropathy multiplex versus polyneuropathy). Electrodiagnostic testing is also helpful in reaching a diagnosis of myasthenia gravis or botulism. Needle electrode examination may help to define the nature of an underlying myopathy (e.g., polymyositis versus corticosteroid-induced myopathy). Muscle diseases generally produce increases in the enzymes creatine kinase and aldolase; thus, their measurement will help to recognize weakness caused by myopathy. (Diseases of nerve and neuromuscular junction are not generally associated with large increases in muscle enzymes.)

Specific Disease Entities Affecting the Nervous System

Cerebral Hemispheres

Let us consider three different common disease processes (stroke, brain tumor, generalized cerebral hypoperfusion) that affect the cerebral hemispheres.

A common cause of *stroke* is cerebral embolism originating from a thrombus lodged in either the left atrium (a consequence of mitral stenosis) or the left ventricle (a result of a large anterior wall myocardial infarction). The usual presentation is the sudden onset of a hemiparesis on the side opposite the affected hemisphere. If the left hemisphere is affected, weakness is associated with aphasia.

In a patient with a *brain tumor* situated, for example, in the right frontal lobe, there may be a history of slowly progressive change in personality and behavior as well as gradually increasing hemiparesis. In these cases, weakness is an important clue to the localization of the tumor, but it is a relatively unimportant manifestation of the lesion.

Several days following resuscitation after a *cardiac arrest,* there may be bilateral weakness involving the proximal portions of the arms and legs. These patients are able to flex their fingers but unable to elevate their arms to shoulder level. Similarly, they may be able to flex and extend at the toes and ankles but are unable to lift their legs up off the bed. In addition, there are subtle disturbances of higher integrative function. The pathology in these patients is bilateral, involving areas of cortex in the watershed zones of the middle, anterior, and posterior cerebral arteries.

Brain Stem

Common causes of brain-stem pathology are brain-stem stroke, hemorrhage, and demyelination. Typically, in a brain-stem stroke, arm and leg weakness come on suddenly. Superficially, the pattern of weakness may resemble that seen when the locus of pathology is in the cerebral hemisphere. Upon careful inspection, however, the clinician may detect involvement of one or more cranial nerves. For example, in a brain-stem infarct involving the ventral portion of the mid-brain, in addition to face, arm, and leg weakness of the UMN type, there is contralateral paresis of the third cranial nerve. Such a combination of long-tract and cranial nerve findings is virtually pathognomonic for brain-stem pathology. Brain-stem hemorrhage usually produces quadriplegia, hypotension, respiratory abnormalities, and coma. Brain-stem demyelination (commonly multiple sclerosis) may be manifested by an episode of face, arm, or leg weakness that lasts for a couple of days and then resolves. Episodes of weakness may be joined by bouts of sensory loss, dysarthria, diplopia, and vertigo.

Spinal Cord

Common spinal cord problems include tumors, metabolic abnormalities, and demyelinating and degenerative conditions. A mid-thoracic spinal cord tumor may, for example, produce the gradual onset of leg weakness and urinary incontinence. Examination discloses bilateral leg weakness of the UMN type and a mid-thoracic sensory level.

A metabolic disturbance, e.g., vitamin B_{12} deficiency, produces the gradual onset of leg weakness and difficulty in walking. Physical examination reveals weakness of the UMN type in both legs and grossly abnormal joint position sense in the feet. Such a combination of weakness and sensory loss reflects involvement of the corticospinal tracts and the posterior columns, respectively.

In multiple sclerosis, episodes of arm or leg weakness come abruptly and resolve over a short period of time. Other features include episodes of numbness, sphincter disturbance, and radicular pain in thoracoabdominal areas.

An example of a degenerative condition is amyotrophic lateral sclerosis, which causes weakness in the trunk, limbs, respiratory, and cranial nerve–supplied muscles. Weakness of the LMN type is caused by degeneration of anterior horn cells. In addition to anterior horn cell involvement, there is degeneration of descending corticobulbar and corticospinal tract, which leads to superimposed weakness of the UMN type. Most patients note that weakness develops in subacute fashion over weeks to months. After the disease has been present for a number of years (generally about 3 years), the patient suffers from generalized weakness and usually succumbs to respiratory failure caused by respiratory muscle involvement.

Peripheral Nerve

There are four main clinical types of peripheral neuropathy. The first is a distal, symmetric subacute polyneuropathy. The clinical features include distal, mixed motor-sensory loss, with the legs more involved than the arms, and possible recovery upon treatment or avoidance of a toxin. The causes of such a neuropathy are legion, including vitamin deficiency, remote effect of carcinoma, uremia, diabetes, immune-mediated disturbances, and toxins.

The second is an acute, fulminant polyneuropathy. Its clinical features include ascending paralysis that is usually mainly motor. Cranial nerves are often affected. Patients with these conditions may require ventilatory assistance. The patient usually recovers. The most common cause of such a neuropathy is the Guillain-Barré syndrome.

The third is a proximal, asymmetric, primarily motor mononeuropathy multiplex. In this condition there is the sudden onset of numbness and pain in the territory of a peripheral nerve. Hours to days later such symptoms occur in the territory of another peripheral nerve. There is a variable temporal evolution, and the process is often painful. There is a tendency for the patient to recover. The usual causes of such a pattern are vasculitis and diabetes.

Last is a chronic, recurrent peripheral neuropathy. The clinical features include enlarged nerves and a chronic course. There is distal, motor-sensory involvement. The CSF protein is often elevated. Chronic, immunologically mediated demyelinating neuropathies may respond to corticosteroid therapy. Some of these neuropathies are inherited.

Neuromuscular Junction

Two major categories of disorder affect the neuromuscular junction. The most common abnormality of the postsynaptic region is myasthenia gravis. Disorders of the presynaptic region include botulism and a syndrome associated with neoplasia (usually small cell carcinoma of the lung), called Lambert-Eaton myasthenic syndrome.

In myasthenia gravis, findings are restricted to the motor system. Patients present with weakness referable to cranial nerve–supplied muscles. Ocular muscles are usually the first involved, leading to ptosis and diplopia. In the course of the illness, limb girdle and proximal limb muscle weakness often develop. A hallmark of myasthenic weakness is easy fatigability.

Patients with botulism, caused by the toxin produced by *Clostridium botulinum,* present with the acute onset of severe and rapidly spreading weakness that begins hours to several days after ingestion of contaminated food. The weakness first affects bulbar musculature and later respiratory and limb muscles. Autonomic nervous system involvement leads to dry mouth and loss of potency.

In Lambert-Eaton myasthenic syndrome, a paraneoplastic autoimmune disorder, ocular muscle weakness is not prominent, but there is weakness of limb girdle and proximal muscles of the arms and legs. Paradoxically, weak muscles become stronger with exercise.

Muscle

Diseases of muscle (myopathic conditions) can be confused with those of nerve, anterior horn cell (neurogenic conditions), and neuromuscular junction. However, careful clinical examination and wise interpretation of laboratory studies can usually help to distinguish among these categories of disease. As we have seen, muscle diseases have a predilection for proximal muscle involvement, whereas peripheral neuropathies tend to produce weakness first in distal muscles. In muscle diseases, stretch reflexes are usually normal; in peripheral neuropathy, reflexes are depressed or absent. In both peripheral neuropathies and anterior horn cell diseases, muscle atrophy is often quite prominent; in the latter, fasciculations are usually seen. Fasciculations are never seen in myopathies, and atrophy of the disuse type is a late occurrence. As noted, myasthenia gravis produces ocular involvement early on, whereas most muscle diseases do not. In addition, easy fatigability is a hallmark of myasthenia and not generally a major factor in the myopathies or neuropathies. In myopathies, there should be no involvement of the sensory system, whereas in neuropathies, sensory loss and paresthesias are common.

Muscle diseases can be divided into two categories: the inherited and the acquired. Muscular dystrophies are inherited, slowly progressive disorders. They generally begin in childhood or adolescence and, as time passes, cause progressive loss of strength. Some, such as Duchenne-type dystrophy, lead to profound weakness and a wheelchair-bound existence; others, such as myotonic and facioscapuloperoneal dystrophy, cause relatively mild weakness that does not require a wheelchair. Congenital myopathies are generally recognized at birth; in most patients, weakness is slowly progressive and does not result in inability to walk.

In contrast to the slow progression and long natural history of the inherited conditions, the acquired diseases of muscle have a much quicker tempo. Polymyositis and dermatomyositis usually produce weakness over weeks to months; most of the endocrine myopathies have a similar time course. Metabolic myopathies may even occur abruptly: myoglobinuric and hypokalemic myopathies may produce profound generalized weakness within hours. The infectious myopathies are generally associated with muscle pain and elevated body temperature.

References

Adams RD, Victor M. Principles of neurology. New York: McGraw-Hill, 1986.

Brooke MH. A clinician's view of neuromuscular diseases. 2nd ed. Baltimore: Williams & Wilkins, 1986.

Garcia CA. Patient with muscle weakness. In: Weisberg LA, Strub RL, Garcia CA. Decision making in adult neurology. Toronto: BC Decker, 1987:193.

Walton JA, ed. Disorders of voluntary muscle. 5th ed. New York: Churchill Livingstone, 1988.

Acute Toxicity of Cancer Chemotherapy

Thomas W. Griffin, MD

Chemotherapy has become an extremely important therapeutic modality in the treatment of neoplastic disease because it is the only readily available systemic therapy for cancer at the present time. Because 50 to 60 percent of adult patients with malignancy present with either macroscopic or microscopic metastases at the time of cancer diagnosis, the major local and regional forms of therapy, surgery and radiation, are effective in inducing cure in only 40 to 50 percent of patients with malignancy. Therefore, in lieu of major breakthroughs in the earlier diagnosis of cancer, a systemic form of treatment that is capable of eradicating malignant cells distant from the primary cancer is extremely important. Although the therapeutic index in cancer chemotherapy remains relatively narrow compared with other commonly used therapeutic modalities in medicine, significant recent advances have been made in the chemotherapy of malignant disease. Curative chemotherapy is now available for Hodgkin's disease, some forms of non-Hodgkin's lymphoma, childhood acute lymphocytic leukemia, choriocarcinoma of the uterus, testicular cancer, and several others. In addition, palliation of symptoms and, in some cases, increase in useful life span can be achieved with appropriate chemotherapy for many other tumor types.

Present chemotherapy has two major limitations: (1) the development or emergence of malignant cells that are resistant to the chemotherapeutic agents employed, and (2) the lack of selectivity of chemotherapeutic agents. This lack of selectivity results in the narrow therapeutic index found with most chemotherapeutic agents, which is due to the many basic biochemical similarities between normal and neoplastic tissues. Because of this lack of selectivity, the physician and patient must balance the expected benefits of treatment against the anticipated or possible side effects when assessing a therapeutic program.

The decision to use chemotherapy in any given patient involves several concerns (Table 105-1). First, the natural history of the tumor must be considered, including its histologic type and its known responsiveness (or lack thereof) to chemotherapy, e.g., lymphoma (responsive) versus pancreatic carcinoma (nonresponsive). The doubling time of the tumor has a broad but imprecise role in determining tumor responsiveness in that rapidly growing tumors generally are more sensitive to chemotherapy. Far-advanced tumors are less responsive to chemotherapy, and these debilitated patients are much more susceptible to the toxicities of the drugs. The patient's performance status, nutritional status, presence of active infection, history of previous treatment with chemotherapy or radiation therapy, and psychological and social status all enter into the decision whether or not to use chemotherapy. Thus, the commitment to start a course of chemotherapy should be made only after careful consideration. Extensive preclinical and clinical studies indicate that the dose and dose rate of chemotherapy are extremely important in producing meaningful antitumor responses. Chemotherapy given at reduced doses or on haphazard or half-hearted schedules usually produces toxicity without meaningful benefit. The use of low-dose chemotherapy for "psychological" reasons can rarely be justified in clinical practice.

As noted previously, most chemotherapeutic agents and regimens have narrow therapeutic ratios, and mild to moderate degrees of toxicity are seen in most patients who receive chemotherapy. Any physician involved in the use of chemotherapy should be extremely well versed in the incidence, prevention, and treatment of the side effects associated with chemotherapeutic agents. In addition, physicians not directly involved with the administration of these agents need to have an understanding of the various toxicities because they are commonly called upon to support patients through periods of toxicity. Also, an understanding of the toxicities helps primary physicians to be more realistic counselors for their patients who are considering entering a chemotherapeutic protocol. This chapter reviews the commonly seen acute complications of cancer chemotherapy, which are defined as those toxicities seen typically within 1 year of the administration of the chemotherapeutic agent. Chronic toxicities of cancer chemotherapy (those occurring after several years) are reviewed in Chapter 106.

General Principles

There are two general categories of acute toxicity from chemotherapy. The first is common to a large number of chemotherapeutic agents of different chemical structure and class. Most of the currently available chemotherapeutic agents are directed against the DNA synthetic mechanism within cells. Therefore, it is not surprising that the majority of acute side effects of chemotherapy are expressed in those areas of the body with rapid cell turnover: the gastrointestinal mucosa, the hair follicle, and the replicating blood elements in the bone marrow (Table 105-2). The second category includes a number of poorly understood side effects that chemotherapeutic agents have on parenchymal organs such as lung, liver, and heart.

Table 105-1 Factors to Be Considered When Making Decisions About Cancer Chemotherapy

Patient	Tumor
Age	Histology and tissue of origin
Physiologic status	Tumor bulk and extent
Nutritional status	Tumor growth rate
Psychological status	
Concomitant illnesses	

Table 105-2 Acute Toxicities Common to a Number of Chemotherapeutic Agents

Depression of the bone marrow resulting in Leukopenia Thrombocytopenia Anemia
Nausea and vomiting
Loss of hair (alopecia)
Ulceration of the mucous membranes (mucositis)

Therefore, the doses and schedules of administration of chemotherapeutic agents must be based on the mechanism of action of the individual drugs, clinical pharmacology, and the time required for normal tissues to recover from the acute toxicities.

Chemotherapeutic toxicities are often exacerbated by concomitant medical problems or the administration of interacting drugs (Table 105-3). The myelosuppression seen with a great variety of chemotherapeutic agents is much more severe in patients who have received previous bone marrow irradiation. Similarly, the onset of a congestive cardiomyopathy may be seen with lower doses of doxorubicin in patients who have received previous radiation to the mediastinum and myocardium. Medical conditions that interfere with the metabolism or excretion of therapeutic agents may increase the toxicity of these drugs. Several chemotherapeutic drugs are metabolized by the biliary system, and a patient with liver or biliary dysfunction can experience increased toxicity with such a drug. Methotrexate is excreted by the kidneys and can produce greatly increased toxicity in the presence of renal dysfunction. Drug interactions are also important. Salicylates displace methotrexate from its binding sites on albumin and can increase methotrexate toxicity. Also, the antileukemic drug 6-mercaptopurine is ordinarily metabolized by the enzyme xanthine oxidase. The concurrent administration of allopurinol, a potent xanthine oxidase inhibitor, can alter the metabolism of this drug and increase its toxicity. Chemotherapeutic agents may also interact synergistically with ionizing radiation such as therapeutic x-rays and ultraviolet light. For instance, a "recall reaction" consisting of markedly increased skin erythema and inflammation can be seen in patients who receive doxorubicin or actinomycin D shortly after a course of radiation therapy. This inflammation is characteristically limited to the area of the body that had previously been irradiated. A number of chemotherapeutic agents, notably 5-fluorouracil, methotrexate, and others, may act as photosensitizers and produce increased susceptibility to inflammation and damage induced by sunlight. Finally, as noted previously, idiosyncratic or allergic reactions may occur with a variety of chemotherapeutic agents. Anaphylaxis has been known to occur with administration of the antitumor antibiotic bleomycin, cisplatin, and others.

Hepatotoxicity

Several chemotherapeutic agents are known to cause hepatic toxicity to various degrees. One can see such mild effects as a transient elevation of liver enzymes, or the damage may be severe enough to result in permanent cirrhosis of the liver. The nitrosourea compounds bischloroethylnitrosourea (BCNU), lomustine (CCNU), and streptozotocin can cause mild elevations of serum transaminases, alkaline phosphatase, and bilirubin, but these liver function values generally return to normal upon withdrawal of the offending agent from the chemotherapeutic regimen. The antimetabolite methotrexate, a dihydrofolate reductase inhibitor, is known to be associated with liver dysfunction. Methotrexate therapy often causes elevations of serum glutamic-oxaloacetic transaminase (SGOT) and lactate dehydrogenase (LDH), and patients treated orally with this agent are twice as likely to become afflicted with fibrosis or cirrhosis of the liver than are patients on an intermittent intravenous regimen. There is also some evidence that methotrexate may act as a carcinogen to the liver. Azathioprine and 6-mercaptopurine are antimetabolites that are also frequently used in renal transplant patients and cancer chemotherapy. These agents not only cause an increase in liver enzymes, but their use can also result in the development of intrahepatic cholestasis as well as parenchymal cell necrosis. Elevated liver enzymes can also be seen with administration of cytosine arabinoside. The antibiotic mithramycin, which was used in the past to treat testicular carcinoma and is now used to treat refractory tumor hypercalcemia, is considered the most hepatotoxic of the chemotherapeutic agents. The many effects that this drug has on the liver include large elevations of SGOT and LDH, milder elevations of alkaline phosphatase, acute hepatic necrosis, and decreased synthesis of the coagulation factors II, V, VIII, and X. Finally, L-asparaginase, a drug used frequently in children with acute lymphoblastic leukemia, causes hepatotoxic effects such as fatty changes, decreased serum proteins and coagulation factors, and liver enzyme elevations.

Myelosuppression

Bone marrow toxicity is the most important and typically the dose-limiting toxicity of the majority of chemotherapeutic agents. If treatment deaths occur following chemotherapy, they are usually due to infection related to chemotherapy-induced leukopenia or to bleeding due to thrombocytopenia related to chemotherapy. The onset of myelosuppression following use of a given therapeutic agent varies from drug to drug, although general guidelines are available. Typical cell-cycle–specific chemotherapeutic agents affect the rapidly proliferating pool of blood precursors in the bone marrow (from the myeloblasts to the promyelocytes). Destruction of this cohort of myeloid precursors leads to a predictable decrease in the peripheral white blood cell (WBC) count approximately 10 to 14 days after drug administration. This is generally followed by the rapid recovery of a normal WBC count. Other chemotherapeutic agents affect stem cells, leading to myelosuppression, which occurs later, as well as a delayed recovery of normal blood cell counts. In the majority of instances, myelosuppression secondary to chemotherapy is relatively brief (3 to 5 days) and self-limited. The incidence of severe infection rises dramatically when the granulocyte count is less than 1,000 cells per cubic millimeter (total granulocyte count = total WBC count × % granulocytes).

The management of the leukopenic patient is a special clinical problem. The profoundly immunosuppressed and leukopenic patient may not mount an inflammatory response in the presence of infection. For example, the patient may have soft-tissue infections without clinical evidence of cellulitis, or pneumonitis without infiltrates on chest radiograph. Often, the only evidence of infection in these patients is fever. The most common infecting organisms are bacterial, especially gram-negative rods, including *Pseudomonas*. Without proper treatment, these patients may succumb rapidly to overwhelming sepsis. Therefore, after appropriate examinations and cultures,

Table 105-3 Drugs and Treatments That Increase the Toxicity of Chemotherapy

Chemotherapeutic agent	Interacting drug or treatment	Clinical result	Mechanism and comments
Doxorubicin	Radiation	Skin and soft-tissue inflammation	Radiation recall
Methotrexate	Salicylates	Mucositis	Displacement of methotrexate from albumin binding sites
Mercaptopurine	Allopurinol	Myelosuppression	Inhibition of xanthine oxidase

these patients require coverage with broad-spectrum antibiotics. (See Chapter 73, "Leukocytosis and Leukopenia").

Mucocutaneous Toxicity

Complete or partial hair loss in both male and female patients is a psychologically devastating event. Hair loss due to chemotherapy is caused by damage to rapidly dividing cells within the germinal portion of the hair bulb. This is not a universal side effect of chemotherapy, but it occurs much more commonly with certain agents (such as doxorubicin, actinomycin D, and others). Other chemotherapeutic agents such as methotrexate, 5-fluorouracil, and cisplatin may cause mild hair thinning to partial hair loss but rarely produce generalized alopecia. Hair loss with chemotherapy is usually reversible after the completion of chemotherapy. Patients should be informed of the temporary nature of the hair loss. Furthermore, they should be warned prior to the onset of any significant alopecia, and provision should be made for the "prophylactic" acquisition of a suitable hairpiece or wig. If this hairpiece is obtained before the hair is lost, a very close match to the patient's natural hair color and texture usually can be obtained. Patients should also be forewarned that, upon regrowth, the hair is often of a slightly different texture and color. Normal hair grows only approximately 2 mm per week, so reversal of alopecia, even with cessation of chemotherapy, is usually a slow process. On occasion, for unexplained reasons, some patients show little or no alopecia in situations in which it is expected. Also, occasionally, scalp hair will regrow despite continued chemotherapy.

Preventive measures such as the scalp tourniquet have been introduced in the clinic. Some success with this technique, either alone or in combination with scalp cooling, has been described with several relatively low dose chemotherapeutic regimens. However, with higher doses, this technique seems to have at best delayed the onset of alopecia or perhaps to have slightly lessened its severity. Scalp tourniquets should not be used in diseases with wide systemic dissemination such as leukemia or oat cell lung cancer.

The alopecia associated with chemotherapeutic agents is perhaps most devastating in regard to its effect on the patient's self-esteem. Although the availability of wigs of excellent quality has made social interactions more accessible to these patients, their personal and especially sexual relations may be profoundly affected. Patients facing this chemotherapeutic toxicity require the support of their physicians, family, and friends.

A disastrous but avoidable cutaneous complication of chemotherapy is the local infiltration of a vesicant drug. A vesicant chemotherapeutic agent is a drug that is ordinarily used intravenously but that can cause severe tissue inflammation and necrosis if extravasation from the vein occurs. The major drugs associated with such reactions include doxorubicin, actinomycin D, mitomycin C, mithramycin, BCNU, dacarbazine (DTIC), nitrogen mustard, vincristine, vinblastine, and several others. The skin ulceration and inflammation that result from extravasation of such drugs can be an extremely difficult problem to manage. The necrotic process may be continued over several months, and skin grafting on a poorly vascularized base may be necessary. The only successful management of this problem is its complete avoidance in the first place. Any person responsible for the intravenous administration of these drugs should be aware of the correct procedures. This includes injection through the side arm of a freely running intravenous infusion under continuous observation. If there is even suspicion of minimal tissue infiltration, the infusion should be discontinued.

Chronic skin changes, specifically hyperkeratosis and hyperpigmentation, are commonly seen with the antitumor antibiotic bleomycin. Bleomycin is a polypeptide antibiotic used in treatment of lymphoma, squamous cell carcinoma, testicular cancer, and several other malignancies. This drug is concentrated in squamous tissues and seems to have a unique predilection for affecting the skin. Toxicity is related to both total dose level and duration of administration. Skin changes occur especially on the dorsum of the hands and feet as well as in areas of local trauma. The skin changes are typically slowly reversible after the drug is discontinued. This toxicity may be highly symptomatic, disfiguring, and incapacitating. Hyperpigmentation of the skin has also been described in association with a number of other chemotherapeutic agents.

Chemotherapy-Induced Mucositis

Ulceration of the mucous membranes can be one of the most painful toxicities induced by antitumor chemotherapy. In addition, mucosal ulceration in a patient with concomitant leukopenia and immunosuppression can lead to sepsis and death. Chemotherapy-induced mucositis is typically seen with antimetabolite drugs such as 5-fluorouracil, methotrexate, and antibiotics such as doxorubicin, actinomycin D, and bleomycin. This toxicity occurs earlier than myelosuppression, commonly 4 to 6 days after the start of treatment. Attempts at symptomatic control include using a mixture of an antibiotic (tetracycline) and an antifungal (mycostatin) medication in a mouthwash and paying attention to good oral hygiene. Local anesthetics applied topically can give brief, partial relief. Severe oropharyngeal mucositis that occurs in a patient whose nutritional status is marginal can induce significant nutritional compromise because of interference with oral intake. Mucositis is typically self-limiting and reversible, but it can be severely symptomatic to the individual patient. Again, the best management of this condition is to attempt to avoid doses of chemotherapeutic agents that are capable of producing mucositis.

Pulmonary Toxicity

Pulmonary toxicity has been associated with a variety of chemotherapeutic agents. Generally, it is infrequent and sporadic, but in two clinical settings it may be dose-limiting and catastrophic. The first is the total dose-related pulmonary toxicity of bleomycin, and the second is the cumulative dose-related pulmonary toxicity of nitrosoureas. The final common pathway of lung injury appears to be pulmonary fibrosis. Histologically, it is difficult, if not impossible, to differentiate bleomycin pulmonary toxicity from idiopathic diffuse interstitial pulmonary fibrosis. Early preclinical studies on bleomycin indicate that the drug was preferentially concentrated in squamous tissues, particularly the lung and skin. Electron microscopic studies in man have shown a decrease in type 1 pneumocytes and changes in type 2 pneumocytes following bleomycin administration.

Bleomycin pulmonary toxicity is often heralded by the development of a dry, hacking cough followed by exertional dyspnea. Symptoms may develop during the course of drug treatment or 1 to 3 months after stopping the drug. The earliest physical findings are fine, crackling bibasal rales, although rhonchi and occasionally a pleural friction rub may also be audible. The earliest radiographic manifestations of bleomycin lung toxicity are fine, reticular bibasilar infiltrates that may progress to bibasilar alveolar and interstitial infiltrates, progressive lower lobe involvement, and consolidation. Blood gas analyses commonly show low oxygen and bicarbonate concentration. Serial determinations of carbon monoxide diffusing capacity (D_{CO}) may be of value in monitoring the subclinical pulmonary effects of bleomycin. It is generally believed that serial pulmonary function tests should be performed in all patients receiving bleomycin.

Bleomycin lung toxicity is strongly dose-related. The incidence significantly increases at doses greater than 500 units. In doses of bleomycin lower than 400 to 500 units, there is still a constant but low incidence of definite bleomycin lung toxicity. The incidence significantly increases with cumulative doses greater than 500 units. Risk factors for bleomycin lung toxicity include advanced age, pre-existing lung disease, and previous radiation therapy. High-dose oxygen support during anesthesia may also be a significant risk factor. It has also been suggested that concurrent cyclophosphamide treatment may increase susceptibility to bleomycin lung toxicity. Patients with lymphoma may also be at an advanced risk. However, there is some suggestive evidence that bleomycin given as a continuous infusion may be associated with decreased risk.

A number of other chemotherapeutic agents have been associated with pulmonary toxicities. There is suggestive, but not definitive, evidence that cyclophosphamide, procarbazine, melphalan, mitomycin C, and BCNU are also pulmonary toxins. Methotrexate pulmonary toxicity appears to be related to hypersensitivity to the drug. The pulmonary toxicity associated with the alkylating agents appears most commonly to be progressive pulmonary fibrosis associated with prolonged drug therapy.

Cardiac Toxicity

Doxorubicin and its related congener, daunorubicin, are the only chemotherapeutic agents that are frequently associated with cardiac damage. The cardiac toxicity of doxorubicin can be divided into two broad categories. Acute effects on the heart are manifested by electrocardiographic abnormalities. The incidence of electrocardiographic abnormalities associated with the administration of doxorubicin ranges from 0 to 41 percent of patients receiving the drug. These changes include primarily nonspecific ST-T wave changes, sinus tachycardia, premature ventricular and atrial contractions, and low-voltage QRS complexes. These changes appear to be more common if the patient has previously had an abnormal baseline cardiogram. They do not seem to be predictive of the development of doxorubicin-induced cardiomyopathy. On the other hand, sudden death possibly due to an arrhythmia during doxorubicin administration has been reported.

The most serious cardiac toxicity associated with doxorubicin therapy is drug-induced cardiomyopathy. This toxicity, when it occurs, has a mortality as high as 61 percent. There is no doubt that the total dose (greater than 450 mg/m^2) of doxorubicin administered to a patient is the most significant risk factor for the development of drug-induced cardiomyopathy; single dosages of 50 mg/m^2 or higher place the patient at higher risk. Other risk factors include the schedule, age over 70 years, pre-existing cardiac disease, prior mediastinal radiotherapy, and coadministration of other cytotoxic drugs such as cyclophosphamide or mitomycin C.

The clinical presentation of doxorubicin cardiotoxicity is nonspecific. Tachycardia may be the first sign. The patient usually presents with symptoms of congestive heart failure (CHF) with shortness of breath, or a nonproductive cough. The usual signs of CHF, including distended neck veins, gallop rhythm, ankle edema, hepatomegaly, and cardiomegaly, are present. Pathologic findings are nonspecific and can be seen with other cardiomyopathies. Electron microscopic changes reveal vacuolization of myocytes as well as dilated mitochondria.

Recent attention has focused on methods of predicting which patients will develop doxorubicin cardiomyopathy. A number of tests, including QRS voltage, serial systolic time intervals, and echocardiography, have been suggested. Probably the most promising noninvasive technique to predict doxorubicin-induced cardiomyopathy is radionuclide cineangiography. The use of percutaneous biopsy of the myocardium to assess damage has also been attempted at several centers. Overall, despite a wide variety of tests, no one has been completely accepted as being predictive for development of doxorubicin-induced CHF. A summary of possible methods of monitoring for cardiomyopathy is shown in Table 105-4.

Table 105-4 Techniques to Predict Development of Doxorubicin-Induced Cardiomyopathy

Systolic time intervals

Echocardiography: an ejection fraction < 30% may indicate cardiomyopathy

Electrocardiogram: decreased QRS voltage

Cardiac catheterization: comprehensive assessment of cardiac function

Radionuclide cineangiocardiography: indications of cardiomyopathy include the following:
- Decrease in ejection fraction > 15% from pretreatment
- Ejection fraction < 45%
- Failure to increase ejection fraction by more than 5% with exercise

In conclusion, doxorubicin cardiomyopathy can be prevented in the majority of patients by dose limitation. Better methods of identifying those patients who have developed subclinical myocardial damage from doxorubicin and are therefore at risk for clinical toxicity are greatly needed. In addition, further attempts to develop less cardiomyopathic dose schedules as well as investigations of the use of alternative anthracyclines are underway.

Genitourinary Toxicity

A number of chemotherapeutic agents have major toxicity directed at the kidney. These drugs include cisplatin, streptozotocin, and methotrexate. These drugs cause renal dysfunction by

Table 105-5 Neurotoxicity of Chemotherapeutic Agents

Drug	Mechanism	Frequency	Clinical manifestations
Vinca alkaloids	Axonal damage	Common and dose-limiting	Decreased deep tendon reflexes,
Vincristine	—		paresthesias (numbness and tingling of fingertips)
Vinblastine	—	Uncommon	Abdominal pain, constipation, ileus
L-Asparaginase	Drug-induced metabolic disorders	Common	Lethargy, somnolence, confusion
Fluorouracil	Cerebellar dysfunction (? fluorocitrate)	Rare (1–3%)	Ataxia, dysmetria, nystagmus
Procarbazine	Monoamine oxidase inhibition	Uncommon	Sedation, confusion, peripheral neuropathy
Cisplatin	Segmental demyelination	Common	Paresthesias, "stocking-glove" peripheral neuropathy, high-frequency hearing loss

Table 105-6 Some Common Chemotherapeutic Agents and Their Side Effects

	MTX	CTX	ADR	Cisplatin	5-FU	VCR	Ara-C	Bleo	VP16
Bone marrow toxicity	X	X	X		X		X		X
Alopecia	X	X	X		X	X			X
Skin toxicity								X	
Vesicant effects			X			X			X
Mucositis	X		X		X			X	
Nausea and vomiting	X	X	X	X	X	X	X		X
Malabsorption	X								
Neurotoxicity				X	X	X			
Fever								X	
Nephrotoxicity	X			X					
Cystitis		X							
Arrhythmias			X						
Immunosuppression	X	X							
Interstitial pneumonitis	X	X						X	

Abbreviations: MTX = methotrexate, CTX = cyclophosphamide, ADR = adriamycin (doxorubicin), 5-FU = 5-fluorouracil, VCR = vincristine, Ara-C = cytosine arabinoside, Bleo = bleomycin, VP16 = etoposide.

Table 105-7 Costs of Commonly Used Chemotherapeutic Regimens

Protocol	Drugs	Dose*	Days		Price†
FAM	Fluorouracil	900 mg	1, 8, 29, 36		$ 48.00
	Doxorubicin	45 mg	1, 36		246.88
	Mitomycin	15 mg	1		315.78
				Total	$ 610.66
Advanced ovarian cancer	Doxorubicin	105 mg			$ 342.72
Protocol induction	Cisplatin	105 mg	1		709.02
				Total	$1,051.74
Consolidation	Cyclophosphamide	150 mg	1–14		$ 23.25
	Hexamethylmelamine	225 mg	1–14		3.50
	Fluorouracil	900 mg	1, 8		25.00
				Total	$ 51.75
Advanced colorectal cancer	Methotrexate	150 mg	1, 8		$ 114.02
	Fluorouracil	900 mg	1,8		24.00
	Leucovorin	15 mg	2 (10 doses)		3.50
				Total	$ 141.52
MOPP	Mechlorethamine	9 mg	1, 8		$ 105.30
	Vincristine	2 mg	1, 8		137.92
	Procarbazine	150 mg	1–14		10.65
	Prednisone	60 mg	1–14		5.20
				Total	$ 259.07
CMF	Cyclophosphamide	150 mg	1–14		$ 23.30
	Methotrexate	60 mg	1, 8		75.60
	Fluorouracil	900 mg	1, 8		24.00
				Total	$ 122.90
ABVD	Doxorubicin	37.5 mg	1, 14		$ 111.20
	Bleomycin	15 mg	1, 14		114.84
	Vinblastine	9 mg	1, 14		47.91
	Dacarbazine (DTIC)	225 mg	1–5		17.30
				Total	$ 291.25
High-dose cisplatin	Cisplatin	225 mg	2		$1,181.70
	Etoposide	150 mg	1–5		10.00
				Total	$1,191.70
Leukemia protocol induction	Cytosine arabinoside	150 mg	1–7		$ 118.93
	Daunorubicin	6.75 mg	1, 2, 3		45.00
				Total	$ 163.93

damaging the tubules rather than the glomerulus. Toxicity is dependent on the dose of the agent used as well as on the schedule of administration.

Cisplatin is a heavy metal compound that has major activity against a number of solid tumors. Nephrotoxicity is a major factor that limits the use of this agent. This drug can cause an acute tubular necrosis that is similar to heavy metal nephropathy. This toxicity may be avoided by aggressive hydration with normal saline, with or without the use of mannitol. The toxicity of cisplatin may be potentiated by pre-existing renal disease or by the concurrent use of other nephrotoxic agents such as aminoglycoside antibiotics.

Methotrexate in high dose has also been associated with acute renal failure. These renal effects can be successfully avoided through the use of aggressive hydration and alkalinization schemes.

Streptozotocin, an agent that is useful in the treatment of islet cell tumors, is associated with acquired Fanconi's syndrome, consisting of acute tubular necrosis and renal tubular acidosis. This renal toxicity is related to the dose and rate of streptozotocin administration, as well as the urine output of the patient.

Finally, cyclophosphamide has been associated with bladder toxicity in the form of hemorrhagic cystitis. This is related to the excretion of toxic metabolites of cyclophosphamide in the urine and may be avoided with adequate hydration. Symptoms of cystitis include urgency, frequency, and dysuria. Almost universally, a mild microscopic hematuria is also present. The cystitis is usually self-limiting, resolving within 2 to 6 weeks after cessation of the drug. However, severe hemorrhagic cystitis may be a medical emergency. Control of severe bleeding may require cystoscopy with clot removal, fulguration of discrete bleeding sites, and instillation of sclerosing agents such as formalin. Because the cystitis appears to be related to the concentration of cyclophosphamide metabolites that appear in the urine, hydration prior to administration of the drug may prevent its occurrence. Liberal use of fluids is recommended both on the day prior to treatment and for 24 hours thereafter, and the patient should be encouraged to void frequently.

Neurotoxicity

Chemotherapeutic agents have been associated with neurologic toxicities of various sorts. The best described toxicity is related to the vinca alkaloids, particularly vincristine. Vincristine is unique among the antineoplastic agents in that its neurologic toxicity is its dose-limiting factor. Early manifestations of the neurologic effects of this drug are the loss of deep tendon reflexes and the onset of distal paresthesias. Cranial nerve palsy, autonomic neuropathy, and syndrome of inappropriate antidiuretic hormone secretion (SIADH) are seen with high cumulative doses of vincristine. Toxicity is typically symmetric, dose-related, and reversible. The peak dose levels obtained following administration appear to have a better correlation with toxicity than does the overall cumulative dose. Other drugs reported to cause neurotoxicity are listed in Table 105-5. The first indications of neurologic toxicity are usually tinnitus and hearing loss, especially in the high-frequency ranges. 5-Fluorouracil has been reported to induce cerebellar ataxia, especially with long-term treatment schedules. L-Asparaginase has been associated with the syndrome of lethargy, confusion, and disorientation. Hexamethylmelamine has been described as causing a symmetric peripheral neuropathy. The use of high-dose or intrathecal methotrexate, especially when combined with cranial radiation, has been known to cause a progressive encephalopathy.

Summary

In summary, a wide number of acute complications can result from cancer chemotherapy. Many of these are predictable, some are reversible, and others are preventable. The complications associated with specific agents are summarized in Table 105-6.

Finally, Table 105-7 lists the financial cost of chemotherapy to the patient. This also is a "complication" and may prove to be a source of severe stress to the patient with cancer who in many cases is either unable to work because of the disease and the therapy, or is elderly and already retired and living on a fixed income.

Late Complications of Chemotherapy

Thomas W. Griffin, MD

106

Definition

Recent improvement in cancer treatment has led to increased numbers of long-term, disease-free survivors. Because patients with cancer live longer, greater concern has been focused on the late toxic effects that chemotherapeutic drugs have on the health and quality of life of these survivors. Two major problems that have emerged are gonadal injury from chemotherapy and the development of second malignancies.

Pathophysiology

Effects of Chemotherapeutic Drugs on Gonadal Function

Gonadal dysfunction is commonly seen as a late complication of chemotherapy. Important determinants of the degree of gonadal injury are the age and sex of the patient and the total dose of the chemotherapeutic drug received. Age is important in that extreme vulnerability to chemotherapy-related gonadal damage may occur during puberty. Men and women differ in their sensitivity to gonadal dysfunction induced by drugs. Men commonly develop gonadal dysfunction with infertility but retain normal Leydig cell function. Women, on the other hand, may suffer impaired fertility and early ovarian failure. Different classes of drugs vary in their potential for inducing gonadal toxicity. The alkylating agents (nitrogen mustard, cyclophosphamide, melphalan, and many others) have the most severe effects. These factors are considered in more detail in the following paragraphs.

Age of Patient at Time of Treatment. The gonads of prepubertal children are relatively insensitive to chemotherapeutic drugs because of the low levels of circulating gonadotropins prior to puberty. Doses of chemotherapeutic drugs that produce gonadal damage in adolescents and adults produce limited effects in the prepubertal child. This reduced vulnerability is relative, and high cumulative doses of drugs, especially if associated with radiation to the gonadal area, may produce permanent damage to the ovaries.

Gonadal Dysfunction in Men. Gonadal dysfunction in men consists of infertility and low sperm counts, with retained male hormonal function and libido. This is because the cytotoxic drugs exert more damage on the germinal epithelium, which is necessary for sperm production, than on the Leydig cells, which are responsible for male hormone production. Qualitative sperm abnormalities (reduced motility, morphologic changes) may also be seen. Prepubertal boys sustain less gonadal injury from cytotoxic drugs than do adolescents or adults. As many as 90 percent of postpubertal males treated with combination chemotherapy (MOPP) for Hodgkin's disease may develop irreversible sterility. The incidence may be somewhat less with the drugs used to treat acute leukemia. Male patients at high risk for development of irreversible sterility should be informed of this possibility prior to the initiation of therapy.

Gonadal Dysfunction in Women. Alkylating agents are known to cause ovarian damage similar to that caused by radiation therapy. Abnormal ovarian function during chemotherapy is frequently manifested by irregular menstrual cycles or amenorrhea. Young women commonly recover normal ovarian function and fertility. However, women who are within several years of natural menopause may develop irreversible ovarian failure. Gonadal damage may be decreased by the use of oral contraceptives during chemotherapy. Biopsy of the ovary after long-term treatment with an alkylating agent frequently shows absence of ova and no evidence of follicular maturation. The reversibility of this gonadal failure is related to the total dose and duration of the drug received.

Effect on Pregnancy Outcome and Progeny. Despite the frequent adverse effects of chemotherapeutic agents on gonadal function and their documented mutagenicity and teratogenicity in animal models, present evidence suggests that women who received chemotherapy give birth to normal infants in the majority of cases. Moreover, no apparent increase in the incidence of chromosomal or congenital abnormalities has been reported in the offspring of patients who have received chemotherapy. These facts are of value in counseling patients who have received chemotherapy regarding the potential risks to their offspring.

Second Malignancies Associated with Chemotherapeutic Agents

The development of acute leukemia caused by prior chemotherapy that was administered for the treatment of hematologic malignancy, solid tumors, or non-neoplastic disease has become a significant problem. Increased risk of leukemia has been described to follow chemotherapy treatment for such cancers as multiple myeloma, Hodgkin's disease, non-Hodgkin's lymphoma, and chronic lymphocytic leukemia. Time to onset of the leukemia from the start of chemotherapy has been observed to be relatively short, approximately 3.5 to 4.5 years. Pancytopenia and increased myeloblasts in the bone marrow often precede overt acute leukemia. The usual course of the acute leukemia is rapid progression to death in 1 to 2 months. Antileukemic therapy only infrequently produces a complete remission. In Hodgkin's disease, combined-modality treatment schemes with both radiation and chemotherapy seem to be synergistic in increasing the leukemia risk. In patients who have received both combined intensive radiotherapy and chemotherapy, the risk of developing an acute leukemia has been estimated to be more than 100 times that predicted.

Blayney and colleagues (1987) studied a group of 192 patients who had been treated for Hodgkin's disease with the highly successful MOPP (mechlorethamine, vincristine, procarbazine, and prednisone) chemotherapy regimen. A known complication of MOPP therapy plus radiation is the development of acute nonlymphocytic leukemia and its precursor, a pancytopenic myelodysplastic syndrome. They found that when patients survived for 11 or more years after MOPP therapy, they were no longer at increased risk of developing acute leukemia. Sixty-three patients underwent bone marrow aspiration, and all were found to have normal marrow morphology. The authors go on to suggest that the risk of leukemia, which is significant during the first 11 years following treatment, can be minimized by reserving the use of combined modality approaches for patients in whom it is evident that radiation alone or chemotherapy alone will not be curative.

Cases of acute nonlymphocytic leukemia have been known to occur after treatment for such solid tumors as cancer of the breast, cancer of the ovary, lung cancer of both the small and non-small cell types, as well as other tumor types. Of great concern has been the description of over 60 cases of acute leukemia in patients with non-neoplastic disease that were treated with chemotherapeutic agents. The majority of these patients had rheumatoid arthritis, advanced renal disease, or renal transplants.

In contrast to acute leukemia, in which the incidence for patients receiving chemotherapy can be 100 times that of normal people, fewer solid tumors have been described in patients who had been treated with chemotherapy. The best-documented solid tumor is the bladder cancer that can occur following chronic bladder fibrosis induced by cyclophosphamide. However, it is now being recognized that the risk of developing solid tumors is higher than was initially predicted.

Tucker and associates (1988) evaluated 1,507 patients who had been treated at Stanford University Medical Center for Hodgkin's disease since 1968. Eighty-three of these patients developed second primary malignancies more than a year after the diagnosis of Hodgkin's disease, excluding nonmelanoma skin cancer. The patients were studied on the basis of what type of therapy they had undergone, what type of second cancer developed, and when the second cancer was discovered. Of the 83 patients studied, 28 developed leukemia, 9 developed non-Hodgkin's lymphoma, and the remaining 46 developed various types of solid tumors. At 15 years after initial diagnosis of Hodgkin's disease, the mean cumulative risk of any second cancer was 17.6 percent, whereas the general population would have only a 2.6 percent risk of developing cancer during the same time period. Although the risk of leukemia seemed to plateau at 3.3 percent after approximately 9 years, the risk of developing a solid tumor continued to rise dramatically after 10 years, with a 13.2 percent risk at 15 years. Variations in the risk of second cancer in patients from different treatment groups were also noted. One treatment group that had received radiotherapy and gold had a very high risk of lung cancer as compared with other treatment groups. The risk of leukemia was somewhat higher, as compared with the general population, in those patients who had received radiotherapy alone. However, when adjuvant chemotherapy had been added, the risk of leukemia was substantially increased. This study reveals that the risk of developing second malignancies, especially solid tumors, continues to rise for at least 15 years after diagnosis and treatment of Hodgkin's disease.

In a study of the occurrence of cutaneous malignant melanoma after treatment for Hodgkin's disease, Tucker and coworkers (1985) found that 6 patients in a group of 1,405 with Hodgkin's disease had developed melanoma. This represents a significant increase over the expected incidence rate of 0.77 in this population (a relative risk of 8). The majority of these melanomas were large invasive lesions, despite the fact that the patients had been followed quite closely. Two of these six patients eventually developed a second primary melanoma. Five of the six patients had evidence of dysplastic nevus syndrome. The authors go on to say that the increased risk of malignant melanoma after treatment for Hodgkin's disease is not unlike that observed in other immunocompromised patients. In fact, histologic examination of the lesions in these patients revealed only a sparse inflammatory response to the tumor, in contrast to the intense lymphocyte-macrophage infiltration usually found in association with melanoma. The authors conclude that those Hodgkin's patients with the dysplastic nevus syndrome are at highest risk for developing cutaneous malignant melanoma and should be carefully monitored with frequent skin examinations.

Investigators in the field of obstetrics and gynecology have also been looking at the incidence of second neoplasms as a result of cancer therapy. Tucker and Fraumeni (1987), in reviewing several studies on the risk of second cancer after treatment for gynecologic malignancies, concluded that the risk is small. However, women receiving pelvic radiation are at some increased risk for the development of second tumors in the pelvic area from 5 to 20 or 30 years after radiation. Additionally, women who are treated with radiotherapy for cervical and endometrial cancers have a somewhat increased risk of leukemia. The chemotherapeutic agents that are frequently used for the treatment of ovarian cancer, especially the alkylating agents, also increase the risk of developing leukemia in a dose-dependent manner.

Rustin and colleagues (1983) looked at 457 long-term survivors after chemotherapy for gestational trophoblastic tumors. The women had received a variety of cytotoxic drugs and various schedules. However, all but two had received methotrexate during treatment. Of the entire patient group, one woman developed intraductal carcinoma of the breast, and another woman succumbed to acute myelomonocytic leukemia. These two cases of secondary neoplasms were, in fact, less than would be expected. The authors concluded that the use of methotrexate for treatment of choriocarcinoma and invasive moles does not place the patient at increased risk for developing second neoplasms.

Although tremendous advances have been made in the field of pediatric oncology, with survival rates for acute lymphocytic leukemia approaching 80 to 90 percent, there are concerns about the long-term effects of the chemotherapy regimens being used.

In a study of the development of leukemia after therapy for childhood cancer, Tucker and her group (1987) noted that the increased risk is due almost entirely to alkylating agents. Of a cohort of 9,170 children who had been diagnosed with cancer at least 2 years previously, 22 developed secondary leukemia. Upon further study, a strong dose-response relationship was discovered between leukemia risk and the total dose of alkylating agents received. Those patients who had initially been diagnosed and treated for Hodgkin's disease or Ewing's sarcoma had a much greater risk of developing leukemia, especially acute nonlymphocytic leukemia, than the remainder of the cohort. This appears to be due to the fact that the therapeutic regimens developed to treat these cancers included large cumulative doses of alkylating agents. There also appears to be a somewhat increased risk of leukemia in those patients who had received doxorubicin, even after controlling for the cumulative dose of the alkylating agent. The authors conclude by reminding the reader that tremendous successes have been achieved in pediatric oncology owing to the development of combination chemotherapy protocols that include the use of alkylating agents. Therefore, the physician must weight the potential benefit of using these drugs against the risks when determining treatment plans for patients.

The etiology of second cancers induced by chemotherapeutic agents is not well understood. A number of mechanisms have been suggested, including immunosuppression by these agents. However, most of the evidence points toward the mutagenic property of these drugs as having the major contribution. Most of the patients who have developed second malignancies have been treated with alkylating agents. Alkylating agents damage the genetic material by cross-linking DNA during the resting phase of the cell cycle. This effect is similar to that of radiation, and the acute leukemias seen in these patients appear similar to the acute leukemia that has been described to occur following radiation exposure. Chromosomal abnormalities are frequently detected in bone marrow cells prior to the development of the leukemia, suggesting that direct damage to DNA by the cytotoxic drugs is responsible for the onset of malignancy.

References

Blatt J, et al. Pregnancy outcome following cancer chemotherapy. Am J Med 1980; 69:8218.

Blatt J, Poplack DG, Shjerins RJP. Testicular function in boys after chemotherapy for acute lymphoblastic leukemia. N Engl J Med 1981; 304:1121.

Blayney DW, et al. Decreasing risk of leukemia with prolonged follow-up after chemotherapy and radiotherapy for Hodgkin's disease. N Engl J Med 1987; 316:710.

Chapman RM. Gonadal injury resulting from chemotherapy. Am J Industr Med 1983; 4:149.

Chapman RM. Effect of cytotoxic therapy on sexuality and gonadal function. Semin Oncol 1982; 9:84.

Chapman RM, Sutcliff SP. Protection of ovarian function by oral contraceptives in women receiving chemotherapy for Hodgkin's disease. Blood 1981; 58:849.

Kyle RA. Second malignancies associated with chemotherapeutic agents. Semin Oncol 1982; 9:131.

Rustin GJS, et al. No increase in second tumors after cytotoxic chemotherapy for gestational trophoblastic tumors. N Engl J Med 1983; 308:473.

Simone J. Late complications of treatment of children with leukemia and lymphoma. In: Rosenberg S, Kaplan H, eds. Malignant lymphomas. New York: Academic Press, 1982:663.

Tucker MA, et al. Cutaneous malignant melanoma after Hodgkin's disease. Ann Intern Med 1985; 102:37.

Tucker MA, et al. Leukemia after therapy with alkylating agents for childhood cancer. J Natl Cancer Inst 1987; 78:459.

Tucker MA, et al. Risk of second cancers after treatment for Hodgkin's disease. N Engl J Med 1988; 318:76.

Tucker MA, Fraumeni JF. Treatment-related cancers after gynecologic malignancy. Cancer 1987; 60:2117.

Breast Mass

Joel H. Schwartz, MD

107

Definition

It is estimated that in 1991 breast cancer will account for 29 percent of all cancers in women and 18 percent of all deaths from cancer in women. As such, it represents the most common cancer in women and the second most common cause of death from cancer. It is estimated that there will be 150,000 new cases in 1991 and 44,000 deaths. Currently, 1 in 10 women develops breast cancer over the course of a lifetime. Many studies have been conducted assessing the roles of various screening methods in detecting preclinical lesions, i.e., *before* the lesions become palpable. It is not the purpose of this chapter to review these screening studies but rather to outline the approach to the evaluation of an already palpable mass in the breast, either discovered by the patient herself or discovered by the physician during routine physical examination.

History

The clinician should try to elicit the following information from the patient about the lump in her breast:

1. Ask whether this patient has any risk factors associated with an increased incidence of breast cancer (see section below).
2. Ask how and when the lump was discovered.
3. Ask how the lump felt when originally discovered and whether there has been a perceptible change over the period of observation.
4. What is the location of the lump in the breast? What is its size? What is its texture? Is it moveable? Have there been any overlying skin changes (redness or dimpling)? Have there been any changes in the nipple?
5. Is the lump tender?
6. Has there been any nipple discharge? If so, what was the nature of this discharge (e.g., bloody, cloudy, clear)?
7. Has the patient had a history of any prior breast problems?
8. Is the patient taking any medications currently?
9. On what day of the menstrual cycle (if the patient is premenopausal) is the patient being examined?

Assessment of Who Is at High Risk for the Development of Breast Cancer

The clinician should obtain the following information in order to assess a patient's relative risk of breast cancer:

1. Age of the patient. Both the incidence and death rate from breast cancer increase with age. Only 1 percent of breast cancer occurs in women less than 30 years of age; 75 percent of all breast cancer occurs in women over the age of 40.
2. Family history of breast cancer. Mothers, sisters, and daughters (i.e., first-degree relatives) of patients with unilateral breast cancer have about a 1.2- to 1.8-fold higher risk of developing breast cancer than the general population. The risk in relatives increases to about ninefold if the patient was both premenopausal and had bilateral disease. Susceptibility to breast cancer is thought to be transmitted through both the paternal and maternal lines.
3. Previous breast cancer. This increases the risk of breast cancer by about five- to tenfold. These first three risk factors are the most important.
4. Age at first birth. The earlier a woman has her first birth, the lower the incidence of breast cancer. Women who have a child in their thirties actually have a higher risk than women who have never given birth at all.
5. Menstrual activity. Early menarche increases the risk of breast cancer, but, more important, early menopause (under age 45), either natural or surgically induced, protects against the development of breast cancer.
6. History of other cancers, specifically, ovarian cancer, endometrial cancer, cancer of the colon or rectum, and cancer of the salivary glands. There seems to be an increased risk of breast cancer in patients who have been previously diagnosed as having these other cancers.

Note that answers to these questions can help determine whether a particular patient is in a high-risk group for the development of breast cancer. If a lesion is clinically suspicious, however, it needs to be investigated regardless of whether the patient is thought to be at high risk for the development of breast cancer.

Physical Examination

The patient should be studied in both the sitting and supine positions. The following descriptive information about the breast, mass, and related anatomic areas should be provided:

1. Size, preferably measured with a ruler or other device rather than estimated.
2. Location in the breast.
3. Consistency of the mass.
4. Fixation of the mass.
5. Any skin changes such as reddening, thickening, or an orange peel–like appearance (peau d'orange). Any scaling or erythema of the nipple, which might indicate a particular type of condition known as Paget's disease of the nipple, should be noted.
6. Inversion of the nipple.
7. Any discharge from the nipple and its color and consistency (serous, serosanguinous, watery, and bloody discharges are significant, being associated with cancer 14 percent of the time).
8. Any swelling or reddening of the arm.
9. Any palpable axillary, supra-, or infraclavicular nodes.
10. Is the lump in question the only palpable abnormality in the breast, or are there other nodules, cysts, or lumps palpable in that breast or both breasts?

It should be noted that features of "lumps" usually associated with benignity are not totally reliable: 60 percent of breast cancers are moveable, 40 percent have regular borders, and 40 percent feel soft or cystic.

Differential Diagnosis

It is worthwhile, at this point, to consider the differential diagnosis of a solitary lump and of multiple lumps in the breast. In the premenopausal population, approximately one of every six breast lumps biopsied proves malignant, whereas in the postmenopausal population, five of every six such lumps are malignant. Of operations on breast masses, about 80 percent are for benign lesions and about 20 to 30 percent are for malignant lesions. Fibrocystic disease accounts for about 36 percent of the lesions, cancer for about 27 percent, fibroadenomas for about 20 percent, and other less frequent diagnoses for the remaining percentages. In fibrocystic disease the lesions are commonly bilateral and multiple, causing fullness and tenderness, particularly premenstrually; these occur with a median age of about 30 years and a range of 20 to 49 years. Fibroadenomas are usually more solid and rubbery, as well as painless, but are also frequently multiple and bilateral; these occur with a median age of about 20 years and a range of 15 to 39 years. Cancers are usually solitary, unilateral, hard, irregular, and painless.

Diagnostic Approach

First, let us consider a premenopausal patient who tells you that she has bilaterally tender breasts but is particularly concerned about a "lump" that she discovered in the upper outer quadrant of the left breast. From the history, you note that the patient is premenstrual. Examination reveals bilaterally nodular breasts, and the lump that the patient has felt is very similar to, but perhaps somewhat larger than, the other "nodules" that are felt in both breasts. A possible course of action would be to have the patient return approximately 3 days after cessation of her menses, i.e., on day 8 of her menstrual cycle. At this time, the influences of estrogen and progesterone on breast tissue are minimal. Upon re-examination of the breast, you find that there is much less tenderness and that all of the nodules, including the one that the patient discovered, are smaller. Cyclic physiologic changes are very common, and observation of the patient may be the best course.

Next consider the same premenopausal patient who complains of a "lump" in her breast. Examination may reveal the same lump as in the preceding situation, but re-examination on day 8 of the menstrual cycle reveals no diminution in the size of this lump. In this instance, the presence of malignancy would have to be ruled out with further diagnostic studies, which are elucidated in the following sections.

Aspiration of a Breast Mass

To further investigate the lump, a needle aspiration should be performed in the office. The skin overlying the area is swabbed with an alcohol swab. The "lump" is immobilized between the second and third fingers of one hand, and a syringe with a #20 needle is thrust into the center of the mass. After the needle has entered the mass, any fluid present in the mass is collected by suction. If the mass completely disappears and the fluid is clear, one may be certain that a cyst has been aspirated and the fluid may be discarded. If, on the other hand, the fluid is bloody, it should be sent for cytologic analysis. If a solid mass is encountered, the needle should be moved back and forth multiple times during suctioning in order to obtain a specimen for analysis. The material obtained is then applied to a slide, which is then sprayed with fixative.

If the mass completely disappears after removal of nonbloody fluid, mammography (see subsequent section) should be performed. If the mammogram is negative, a repeat physical examination every few months should be conducted to detect any recurrence of the cyst.

If the mass does not completely disappear after fluid is aspirated, or if the fluid is bloody, excision is indicated. Any residual mass that cannot be aspirated also needs to be excised. There is a false-negative rate of between 5 and 20 percent with aspiration (i.e., aspiration diagnosis is negative for malignancy when a malignancy is present). The false-positive rate (i.e., the aspiration diagnosis is recorded as cancer, when actually a benign lesion is present) is about 1 to 2 percent.

Figure 107-1 is an algorithm for the diagnostic evaluation of a breast mass by fine-needle aspiration biopsy.

Needle Biopsy in the Surgeon's Office

In instances in which an aspiration is unsuccessful or in which uncertainties still exist about the nature of the "lump," the patient may be referred to a surgeon. The surgeon may wish to perform a needle biopsy under local anesthesia. There is a false-negative rate of up to 19 percent but a very low false-positive rate. A report of "unsatisfactory for examination" or a report of "benign tissue" is usually followed by excision of the lump. Some surgeons excise the lump straightaway without doing a needle biopsy first.

Mammography

Mammography is important for a number of reasons in the assessment of patients with palpable breast lesions. Mammography may show more than one area of malignancy within a breast with obvious malignancy and may show carcinoma of the contralateral breast. It may show conclusively that a lesion is malignant. In the frequently encountered "lumpy" or "nodular" breast, mammography may show that one of the lesions is malignant. This is particularly useful in a breast that is too lumpy overall for one to be certain that a more suspicious, discrete lump is or is not present.

In the premenopausal patient described previously, mammography is utilized both in the patient whose mass disappears after aspiration, to detect recurrent lesions, and in the patient whose mass persists and will be biopsied anyway, to detect other suspicious areas.

One of the most important points that can be made about mammography is that it is a better technique in older patients in whom there is a better contrast between the carcinoma and the underlying breast stroma (decreased glandular tissue and more fat). In the postmenopausal patient with a mass, aspiration may be attempted or mammography may be done first. If either procedure fails to reveal malignancy, however, and findings persist, biopsy is indicated.

If one is clinically suspicious about a breast mass, a negative mammogram, or one that indicates that the lesion is benign, should not be accepted as definitive evidence of benignity. In this instance, the definitive procedures elucidated previously still need to be carried out regardless of the benign-appearing nature of the lump on mammography. Generally, an 8 to 15 percent false-negative rate for mammography is quoted. As expected, younger patients, because of the greater density of the breast, have a somewhat higher false-negative rate. Again, it cannot be overemphasized that a normal mammogram would not necessarily imply the absence of cancer; clinically suspicious lumps still need to be evaluated with aspiration or biopsy procedures.

Ultrasonography

Ultrasound is useful in distinguishing cystic from solid lesions when the lesions are 6 to 7 mm in size or greater. It can then direct the examiner to a further procedure—aspiration cy-

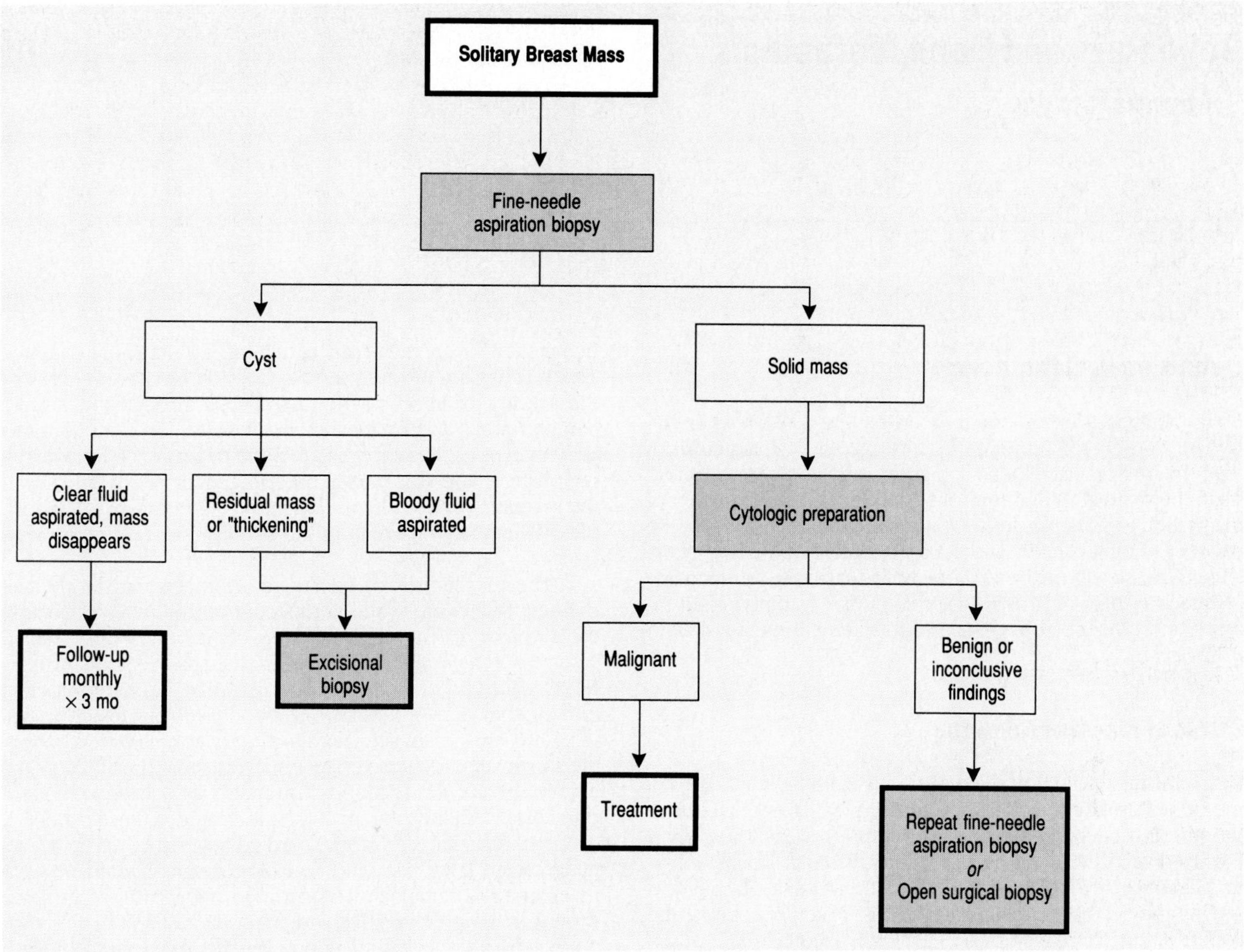

Figure 107-1 Algorithm for the diagnostic evaluation of breast mass by fine-needle aspiration biopsy. (Algorithm designed by Michael D. Wertheimer, MD.)

tology, often under ultrasound control, or biopsy. Note that mammography is superior to ultrasonography in distinguishing benign from malignant disease.

References

Blamey RW, Elston CW. The diagnosis of breast cancer. Clin Oncol 1982; 1:821.

D'Orsi CJ, Wilson RE, eds. Carcinoma of the breast: Diagnosis and treatment. Boston: Little, Brown, 1983.

Frable WJ. Thin needle aspiration biopsy: A personal experience with 469 cases. Am J Clin Pathol 1976; 65:168.

Gravelle IH. Diagnostic imaging in breast cancer. Clin Oncol 1982; 1:795.

Harris JR, et al, eds. Breast diseases. Philadelphia: JB Lippincott, 1987.

Leis HP Jr. The diagnosis of breast cancer. CA 1977; 27:209.

Love S, Gelman RS II, Silen W. Fibrocystic "disease" of the breast—a non-disease? N Engl J Med 1982; 307:1010.

Mushlin AI. Diagnostic tests in breast cancer. Ann Intern Med 1985; 103:79.

Stoll BA, ed. Risk factors in breast cancer. Chicago: Year Book Medical Publishers, 1976.

Bone Pain and Bone Metastasis

Thomas W. Griffin, MD

108

Definition and Incidence

Bone metastases are secondary growths that develop when detached, transported tumor fragments that have separated from the primary neoplasm lodge and grow in bone. Cancer metastasis to the bone is a common event during the natural history of many solid tumors in adults. Of the common malignancies, the majority of lung cancers and over 40 percent of breast cancers will metastasize to the bone. Bone is also the most common site of dissemination of prostate cancer. Of the common solid tumors, only cancer of the colorectum infrequently metastasizes to the bone.

Clinical Manifestations

Pain is the most common symptom associated with metastases to the bone. Usually this pain develops gradually over weeks or months and becomes progressively more severe. The pain is localized and characteristically is severe at night, often awakening the patient from sleep. It is often lessened by physical activity and decreases in intensity during the day. In contrast, the pain from degenerative diseases generally increases with physical activity, is relieved by rest, and is noticed least at night. Patients often characterize the pain associated with bone erosion by tumor as deep, constant, dull, and boring. On physical examination, percussion tenderness is a highly reliable clinical sign of a discrete area of bone destruction by tumor. If bone pain associated with malignant disease is intensified by activity and associated with radiographic evidence of bone destruction, it may indicate the presence of a pathologic fracture or impending fracture. On occasion, this pattern of pain may reflect multiple small microfractures that are not apparent on plain radiographs. Pathologic fractures may occur in the pelvis, femur, humerus, and vertebral bodies. A pathologic fracture may also present as a sudden exacerbation of pain.

Pain in bone and associated musculoskeletal structures is a frequent complaint in clinical practice. It is important that the clinician be aware of features of the history and physical examination that help to differentiate benign from malignant etiologies of bone pain. Bone pain associated with benign causes is characteristically acute or subacute in onset, and it is commonly related to injury or unaccustomed physical activity. Typically, the pain is described by the patient as dull and aching in nature, in contrast to the boring pain of bone metastases. Benign pain is worse with movement and is relieved by rest. Frequently, pain from benign causes is episodic and related to recurrent minor trauma or physical exertion. However, the persistence of bone pain of any nature in an immobilized patient dictates consideration of a malignant etiology.

Mechanism of Pain in Bone Metastasis

The spread of cancer to bone may be by direct extension, as occurs frequently in cancer of the nasopharynx. However, the hematogenous spread of cancer to bone is much more common. This mechanism involves venous invasion by cancer cells, then the passage of intact, viable tumor cells through the vascular compartment, and establishment of secondary foci of tumor growth in bone. Direct spread to bone by cancer cells traversing lymphatic channels is rare. In prostate cancer, retrograde flow in the prostatic venous plexus and in the vertebral veins (Batson's plexus) may be important in the establishment of bone metastases.

The mechanism of pain in bone metastases is not well defined. Stretching of the periosteum of the involved bone by direct tumor pressure or weakening of the bone from mechanical stress at the tumor site may precipitate pain in some patients. Bone involvement may also cause pain by nerve entrapment, tumor expansion, or destruction of bone with collapse. This type of pain is most often seen with metastasis to a vertebral body or the sacrum and is characterized by its radicular quality. Note that vertebral body destruction is commonly associated with extradural disease; a myelogram may be indicated in these patients in order to rule out early spinal cord compression. Certainly, any patient with back pain and neurologic signs should undergo myelography or magnetic resonance imaging (MRI) of the spine. It must be emphasized that early treatment of a partial or complete spinal cord block may prevent the long-term sequela of paraplegia.

The mechanism of osteolysis by metastatic cancer deposits is complex. It may involve osteoclastic activity, release of enzymes from cancer cells, ischemia induced by the pressure of tumor growth, and other factors. Osteoclasts may be activated by the release of the lymphokine osteoclast activating factor (OAF), which is produced in hematologic malignancies, or other substances that are directly produced by tumor cells. A balance between osteoblastic and osteoclastic activity maintains the normal architecture of cortical bone. Metastases may shift this equilibrium toward excessive osteoclastic activity, resulting in bone destruction. The late stages of osteolysis appear to be related to the direct action of cancer cells. Finally, metastatic tumor in bone is associated with both active bone destruction and new bone formation. It is the latter reparative reaction by normal bone to the growing metastasis that gives rise to the metabolic abnormalities detected on bone scan.

Bone metastases are most commonly found in those bones associated with active marrow in the adult: spine, pelvis, ribs, skull, proximal femur, and humerus. The pattern of metastases is often related to the specific vascular areas that have been invaded. For example, neuroblastoma frequently involves the skull, shoulder girdle, and pelvis. Cancer of the prostate commonly involves the pelvis and lower spine. Arteries are very resistant to neoplastic invasion; therefore, the hands, feet, forearm, and distal tibia and fibula are rarely afflicted with bone metastases.

Diagnostic Approach

An algorithm for the diagnostic approach to bone pain in the cancer patient is presented in Figure 108-1.

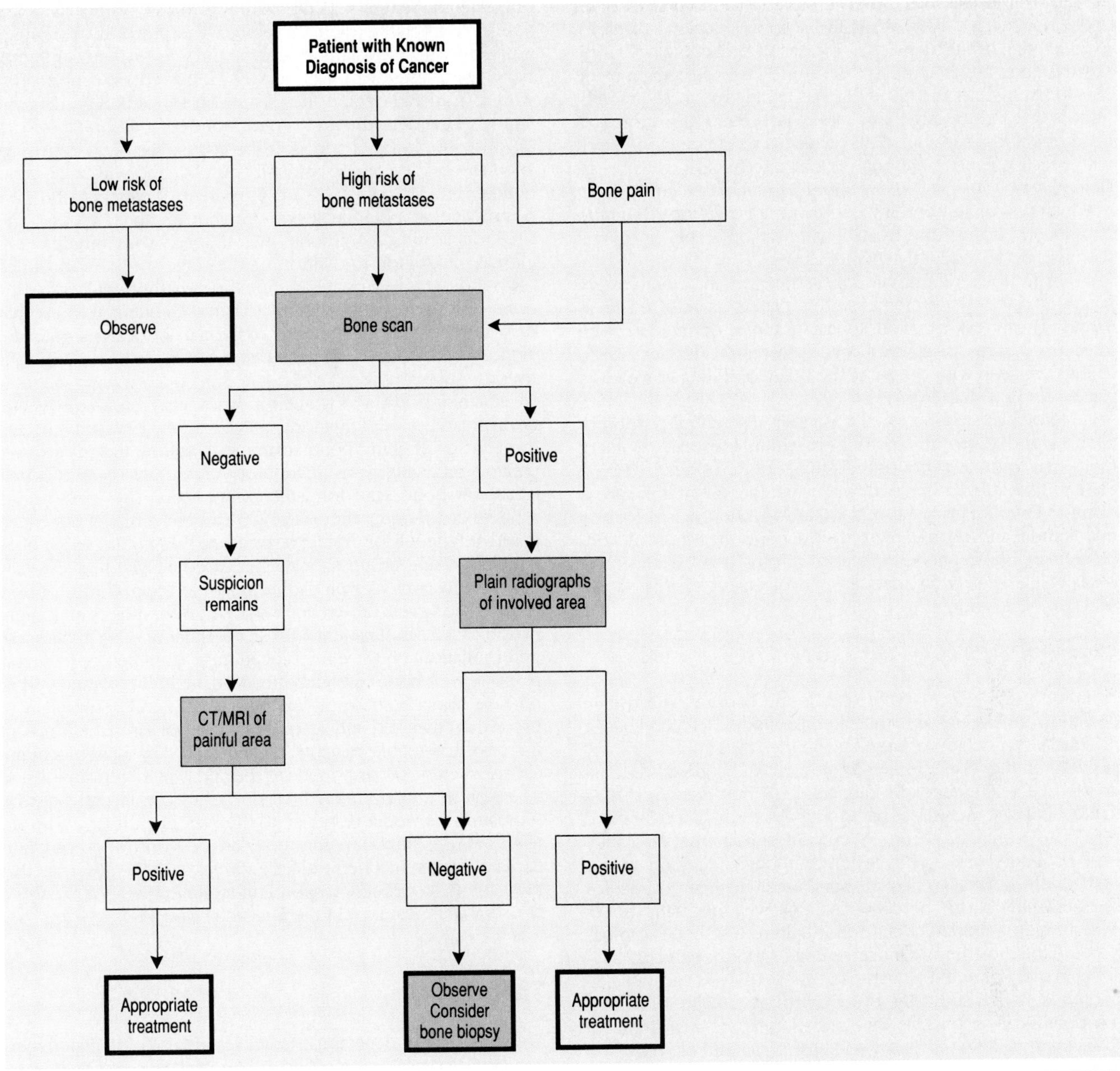

Figure 108-1 Algorithm for diagnostic approach to bone pain in the patient with cancer. CT = computed tomography, MRI = magnetic resonance imaging.

The diagnostic evaluation of bone metastases involves two major complementary diagnostic modalities: the bone radiograph ("plain films") and the radionuclide bone scan. The skeletal survey of bone metastases (metastatic bone series) is based on the predilection of metastases to involve the central skeleton, and consists of an anteroposterior and lateral view of the cervical, dorsal, and lumbosacral spine; a lateral view of the skull; and anteroposterior views of the pelvis and rib cage. However, plain radiographs are relatively insensitive for use as a screening test for bone metastases, and the skeletal survey has been supplanted by the radionuclide bone scan. The bone scan, which costs approximately $240, is more sensitive in the detection of bone metastases and has become an important technique in the staging and management of malignant disease.

Radiographs

Bone metastases are often characterized by their radiographic appearance. This appearance can be osteolytic (decreased bone density), osteoblastic (increased bone density), or mixed. Bone metastases may also appear as discrete morphologic alterations such as cortical lesions or vertebral pedicle loss.

Osteolytic lesions are associated with bone loss and erosion. The radiographic visibility of osteolytic lesions depends on their size and location and their effect on bone trabeculae and cortex. Lytic lesions from a malignancy usually have a ragged, uneven margin, whereas the margins of benign processes causing bone loss are typically sharp and smooth.

In the spine, the vertebral bodies as well as the pedicles may be involved. A loss of the outline of one or more of the pedicles may be the earliest sign of tumor involvement. Osteolytic bone lesions usually occur with the most aggressive cancers and are frequently seen with malignancies of the breast, kidney, and thyroid. Also, multiple myeloma may present with multiple osteolytic bone lesions involving the skull, spine, and long bones.

Osteoblastic bone lesions result from increased bone production in response to tumor involvement and produce a radiographic appearance of sclerotic areas with increased bone density. Osteoblastic changes may occur as isolated rounded foci in

Oncology

a bone or may produce a diffuse increase in the density of an entire bone (e.g., "ivory vertebra," seen in Hodgkin's disease). Even though bone density is increased on radiographs, the normal bony architecture is lost in the involved area and the tensile strength of the bone may be greatly reduced. Indolent tumors that induce large amounts of new bone formation produce osteoblastic lesions. This pattern is most commonly seen with prostate cancer, although it may also be seen with breast cancer, lymphoma, and other tumors. Osteoblastic changes occasionally occur in bone invaded by tumor that was thought to have been successfully treated with radiotherapy, hormonal therapy, and infrequently chemotherapy.

Finally, the radiographic appearance may show both osteolytic and osteoblastic elements; this pattern is referred to as *mixed.* These lesions often appear granular or mottled, with intermixed areas of increased and decreased density. Mixed lesions are seen with cancer of the breast and lung as well as a variety of other malignancies.

Metastases to bone usually lodge in the central portion of the bone and destroy the cortex from within. An isolated, solitary metastasis to bone is unusual. If such a lesion is detected on a plain radiograph, a bone scan will usually reveal multiple areas of involvement. Periosteal new bone formation or sclerosis is uncommon around the margin of a bone metastasis. A soft-tissue mass is also uncommon, although soft-tissue extension is occasionally seen with metastatic involvement of a vertebral body or the sternum.

Bone Scans

As noted previously, a bone scan is much more sensitive in detecting bone metastases than are plain films. Before a change in density can be appreciated on routine radiographs, 30 to 50 percent of the bone mineralization must be destroyed. Increased skeletal uptake of radionuclide (a "hot" lesion) is seen in areas of bone metastases because of increased blood flow and new bone formation. Up to 99 percent of bone metastases appear on bone scan as hot lesions, although approximately 1 percent are normal or "cold." Bone scans may be positive for metastases in up to 30 percent of patients with metastatic cancer without radiographic skeletal abnormalities. The bone scan has become the most important screening test for bone metastases at the present time. Previously used chemical tests such as alkaline phosphatase and urine hydroxyproline are less reliable. If the bone scan is positive and radiographs are negative in a patient with a known primary malignancy, an MRI or computed tomographic (CT) scan of the arch may demonstrate a lesion not yet visualized on plain films.

Although the bone scan is sensitive, it is relatively nonspecific (Table 108-1). Areas of increased uptake on bone scan may not represent metastatic disease. These areas may indicate previous trauma, radiation osteitis, surgery, osteomyelitis, osteonecrosis, osteoporosis, Paget's disease, osteoarthritis, spondylitis, or benign bone tumors. Trauma may give rise to a positive bone scan even when the trauma is remote. Therefore, the work-up of a patient with metastatic disease should involve screening for bone metastases with a bone scan, followed by confirmation with a plain radiograph. If a suspicion remains regarding the nature of the abnormality seen on bone scan, a bone biopsy or CT/MRI should be obtained. If the cortex has been destroyed, adequate biopsy can occasionally be obtained with a 22-gauge needle. In approximately 1 to 5 percent of patients who have destructive radiographic lesions, the bone scan is negative. This situation is most commonly encountered with multiple myeloma. In addition to confirming the bone scan abnormalities, plain radiographs can help define the structural integrity of the bone and evaluate the risk of fracture. Sequential scans may demonstrate the appearance of additional new lesions, but scans are not useful in following the disease progression of a specific lesion.

In their study of 53 women with advanced breast cancer and bone metastases, Coleman and collaborators (1988) investigated the efficacy of using bone scanning to follow the progress of patients receiving systemic therapy. All patients received a pretreatment bone scan for later comparison. The investigators found that 3 months after starting treatment, a repeat bone scan could not identify or predict response to therapy. In fact, 12 of 16 patients in one group showed increased activity in previously observed lesions as well as the presumed appearance of new lesions. However, repeat bone scans at 6 months revealed improvement in most patients. These investigators also made serial determinations of several biochemical parameters that correspond with bone osteoblast function, including alkaline phosphatase bone isoenzyme (ALP-BI) activity and osteocalcin (a protein synthesized and secreted by osteoblasts). The transient increase in osteoblast activity, as determined by these biochemical parameters, corresponded to the apparent deterioration and subsequent improvement seen on bone scan in patients who ultimately showed a response to the systemic therapy. The authors call this phenomenon the "flare response" and go on to explain that the biochemical flare should alert the physician that the patient is probably responding to systemic therapy despite worsening appearance of the 3-month bone scan.

Table 108-1 Diagnostic Pitfalls of the Bone Scan

False-Positive Scan
Osteoblastic response to tumor cell kill, representing healing
Tumor-induced structural defect with secondary osteoblastic effect
Incidental unrelated disease (e.g., osteoarthritis, trauma, Paget's disease, surgery)
Paraneoplastic bone changes (hypertrophic pulmonary osteoarthropathy)
False-Negative Scan
Symmetric distribution of disseminated tumor
Purely osteolytic lesions, e.g., multiple myeloma
Rapidly destructive lesions

Therapy

Treatment of bone metastases involves the use of radiation therapy both to relieve pain and to prevent fracture of weight-bearing bones. The presence of pathologic fractures may make pain relief with radiation therapy difficult and increase the need for orthopedic management. Bone metastases almost always imply incurable metastatic disease, and the aims of management should be patient comfort and quality of life. Localized radiation therapy is highly effective in relieving bone pain related to metastases. Lytic lesions in weight-bearing bones require special attention. Pathologic fractures should be anticipated. Internal fixation following radiotherapy should be considered in patients who have lytic lesions of weight-bearing bones in order to reduce the risk of pathologic fractures.

Lancaster and colleagues (1988) studied 57 actual or impending fractures of the humerus in patients who were terminally ill with cancer. Impending fracture was considered present when 50 percent or more of the cortex was involved and the patient reported pain in the area. The majority of the patients had either breast carcinoma or multiple myeloma, two neoplastic lesions that not infrequently metastasize to the appendicular skeleton. The authors compared various methods of treating pathologic fractures or impending fractures and found that those patients treated surgically had the best restoration of function and relief of pain. The best results were obtained with intramedullary fixation with a Küntscher rod. In the majority of the patients treated surgically, the tumor was curetted out and the defect was filled in with methyl methacrylate. Patients were also treated postoperatively with radiation, if necessary. On the other hand, another group of patients was managed nonsurgically with either a Velpeau's shoulder immobilizer or a plaster Velpeau's dressing and radiation therapy. This form of treatment was found to be less successful. The authors conclude that terminally ill cancer patients with fractures or impending fractures of the humerus due to metastatic lesions can benefit from the surgical intervention described.

References

Blair RJ, McAfee JG. Radiological detection of skeletal metastases: Radiographs versus scans. Int J Radiat Oncol Biol Phys 1976; 1:1201.

Brooker AF. Orthopedic approach to osseous metastases. In: Abeloff MD, ed. Complications of cancer. Baltimore: Johns Hopkins University Press, 1979:243.

Coleman RE, et al. Bone scan flare predicts successful systemic therapy for bone metastases. J Nucl Med 1988; 29:1354.

Galasko CSB. The pathological basis for skeletal scintigraphy. J Bone Joint Surg 1975; 57:353.

Lancaster JM, et al. Pathologic fractures of the humerus. South Med J 1988; 81(1).

Lokich J. Osseous metastases: Radiographic monitoring of therapeutic response. Oncology 1978; 35:274.

Malawer MM, Delaney TF. Treatment of metastatic cancer to bone. In: De Vita VT, Hellman S, Rosenberg SA, eds. Cancer: Principles and practice of oncology. 3rd ed. Philadelphia: JB Lippincott, 1989:2298.

Parker BR, Marglin S, Castellino RA. Skeletal manifestations of leukemia, Hodgkin's disease and non-Hodgkin's lymphoma. Semin Roentgenol 1980; 15:302.

Weiss L, Gilbert HA, eds. Bone metastasis. Boston: GK Hall, 1981.

109 Skin Signs of Internal Malignancy

Rita S. Berman, MD, MPH

A wide variety of skin signs have been associated with internal malignancies. Sometimes these cutaneous manifestations occur before an internal malignancy is recognized, and the skin findings can aid in making an early diagnosis.

Etiology

Cutaneous manifestations of internal cancers can be grouped into those that have malignant cells present in the skin and those in which no malignant cells are present in the skin. Cutaneous manifestations of internal neoplasms have many etiologies and can be conveniently classified as shown in Table 109-1. Some of the more common or well-known markers of cutaneous malignancies are discussed.

Table 109-1 Etiologies of Cutaneous Manifestations of Internal Neoplasms

Malignant Cells Present in the Skin
Infiltration of the skin by the malignancy, e.g., metastatic carcinoma
Skin changes induced by exposure to a carcinogen that also causes internal malignancy, e.g., arseniasis
Neoplasms of the skin associated with an increased risk of another primary internal malignancy, e.g., Kaposi's sarcoma associated with lymphoma
No Malignant Cells Present in the Skin
Skin changes due to metabolic products of malignancies, e.g., carcinoid syndrome
Skin changes due to abnormalities of other systems, e.g., jaundice
Idiopathic skin changes, e.g., acanthosis nigricans
Genetic diseases with skin manifestations and the tendency to develop internal malignancies, e.g., neurofibromatosis

Malignant Cells Present in the Skin

Infiltration of the Skin by Malignancy

Carcinoma

Up to 5 percent of patients with cancer develop skin metastasis. These metastases may be the presenting sign of the malignancy, but more commonly they occur later in the course of illness in a previously diagnosed patient. Malignancies spread to the skin via blood vessels, lymphatics, direct extension, and surgical implantation. Metastases that spread via the blood stream to skin usually occur early in the course of the disease, as seen in lung, kidney, and ovarian carcinoma. Those that spread via lymphatics appear in the skin later in the disease course, as in breast and oral cavity carcinoma (hence, metastases are usually associated with disseminated disease).

In men, the primary tumors that most commonly metastasize to skin, in order of frequency, are lung, colon, melanoma, and squamous cell carcinoma of the oral cavity. In women, the most common tumors are breast, colon, melanoma, and ovary.

The location of the skin lesion can give a clue to the originating site of the malignancy. The abdominal wall is the most common site for skin metastasis in men. In this instance, the primary tumor is often the colon. In women, the most common site is the chest wall, from breast carcinoma.

Skin metastases are commonly cutaneous or subcutaneous nodules that vary from flesh-colored, to erythematous, to purple. They may be single or multiple and may feel firm or hard to the touch. They may resemble benign skin lesions such as epidermal inclusion cysts, lipomas, neurofibromas, pyogenic granulomas, hemangiomas, or other malignancies, such as Kaposi's sarcoma (see later), lymphoma (see later), or even primary skin neoplasms. Skin lesions resembling erysipelas can be seen with breast carcinoma. Areas of scalp hair loss, known as alopecia neoplastica, result most commonly from breast carcinoma. Alopecia neoplastica must be distinguished from other scarring alopecias, especially those resulting from discoid lupus. Also, metastasis to skin can show areas of "hide-bound" skin, resembling changes seen in scleroderma.

A skin biopsy is necessary for the diagnosis. Histologic findings usually correlate with those of the primary tumor but may show a lesser degree of differentiation. Often it is only possible to classify skin metastasis into carcinoma or sarcoma, and identification of the primary tumor must be sought from clinical information, i.e., location of metastasis and age and sex of patient. Some histologic pictures are distinctive enough to permit identification of the primary site, as with "signet-ring cells," which are seen in metastasis from gastric carcinoma.

Leukemia

Infiltration of leukemia cells in the skin is not uncommon; it is most frequently seen in monocytic leukemias. Occasionally, the skin lesions appear before the diagnosis of leukemia. Lesions are usually macules, papules, nodules, and plaques. Colors range from pink, to red-brown, to "plum-colored," and lesions often feel indurated or firm.

Because the most frequent skin lesions in patients with leukemia are nonspecific and relate to drugs, infection, bleeding, and anemia, other causes for skin lesions must be taken into account. Purpuric lesions in patients with leukemia may not only represent leukemia cutis, but must be differentiated from leukocytoclastic vasculitis or a leukemid (autosensitization) reaction. Leukocytoclastic vasculitis has many causes, but of particular concern in patients with leukemia are sepsis and drug eruptions. Blood cultures should be obtained, and a skin biopsy should be evaluated for histopathology and cultured for bacteria, *Candida,* and fungi. A touch prep should be performed. This consists of gently touching the tissue specimen to a glass slide and then staining for leukemic cells (Wright-Giemsa stain), bacteria (Gram stain), and *Candida* and fungi (potassium hydroxide stain). Sometimes, it is clinically advisable to initiate therapy for sepsis before results of the preceding tests are back.

Paget's Disease of the Breast

Paget's disease of the breast consists of erythema, scaling, oozing, and crusting. It begins on one nipple and extends to the areola and surrounding skin. Itching and irritation may be an early symptom. Differential diagnosis includes eczema, psoriasis, and skin tumors such as Bowen's disease, squamous cell carcinoma, and basal cell carcinoma. If topical therapy fails to clear the lesion, a skin biopsy is necessary to make the diagnosis. In Paget's disease, the epidermis contains large, round cells with clear cytoplasm, which arise in almost every case from an underlying ductal adenocarcinoma of the breast.

Extramammary Paget's Disease

Extramammary Paget's disease affects areas where apocrine glands are found, especially on the genitalia, but also the inguinal region, upper thighs, and rarely the axilla. The lesions may consist of white, thickened plaques, or they may be eczematous, weeping with crusts or ulcerations. Itching and pain may be prominent. Lesions must be differentiated from eczema, fungal infections, candidiasis, leukoplakia, Bowen's disease, and squamous cell carcinoma. If, after appropriate topical therapy, the lesion does not respond, a skin biopsy must be performed. Histopathology is similar to that of Paget's disease of the nipple. In contrast to Paget's disease of the nipple, however, only about 50 percent of the cases in extramammary Paget's disease are associated with an underlying malignancy. These occur mainly regionally in the genitourinary tract, gastrointestinal tract, apocrine and eccrine glands, and, rarely, in the breast.

Lymphoma

Various skin manifestations occur in 50 percent of patients with lymphoma and can be the presenting feature of the disease. Cutaneous lesions with malignant cells are seen most frequently with histiocytic or lymphocytic lymphoma and only rarely with Hodgkin's disease. Lesions consist of papules, plaques, nodules, and tumors and range in size from a few millimeters to centimeters. Colors are characteristically pink, plum, or red to reddish brown, and the lesions have a firm, but not rock-hard, feel to them. Ulcerations rarely occur. Differential diagnoses include leukemia cutis, benign lymphocytic infiltrates, sarcoidosis, lupus erythematosus, and reaction to insect bite.

Nonspecific eruptions and symptoms occur much more frequently in Hodgkin's disease than in other lymphomas, and include generalized pruritus, exfoliative dermatitis, and acquired ichthyosis (discussed elsewhere in this chapter).

Mycosis fungoides is a T-cell lymphoma that has a predilection for the skin, but it can have visceral involvement as well. Patients may go through all three phases of the disease—eczematous stage to plaque stage to tumor stage. However, some patients present only in the later stages. The eczematous or erythematous stage may last years and consists of a nonspecific, unremitting dermatosis that can resemble eczema, psoriasis, or seborrhea. The histology may be nonspecific. In the plaque stage, the lesions are infiltrated and take on bizarre shapes with a haphazard distribution, as if paint had been splattered on the skin. The entire skin may be indurated and red, with scaling (exfoliative dermatitis) or without scaling (erythroderm). When an erythroderm is associated with lymphadenopathy and circulating abnormal T cells, this is known as Sezary syndrome. Tumors may develop from prior skin lesions or occur de novo.

Skin Changes Due to Exposure to a Carcinogen That Also Induces Internal Malignancy

Arsenical Keratosis

Prolonged ingestion of inorganic arsenic leads to arseniasis. Arsenic is found in insecticides, in well water, in old medications called Fowler's solution and Asiatic pills, and in other industrial and environmental sources. After a latent period of many years, punctate areas of hyperkeratotic papules called keratoses may arise on the palms and soles. These lesions must be distinguished from warts. Rarely, keratoses may develop skin cancers in them. Ingestion of arsenic may also lead to increased formation of other skin cancers as well as internal malignancies. A patient with these keratoses or a history of arsenic ingestion should be carefully evaluated for internal and cutaneous carcinoma.

Neoplasms of the Skin Associated with an Increased Risk of Another Primary Internal Malignancy

Bowen's Disease

Bowen's disease is squamous cell carcinoma in situ of the skin. When it is located on the glans penis, it is termed erythroplasia of Queyrat. Clinically the lesions may be well circumscribed, raised, or flat and may be erythematous with scale and crust.

Ulceration is a late change and usually signifies invasion into the dermis. Differential diagnoses include psoriasis, eczema, actinic keratosis, Paget's disease, and squamous cell and basal cell carcinoma. Histopathologic study is necessary to establish a diagnosis.

In about 5 percent of patients, Bowen's disease of the skin develops into invasive squamous cell carcinoma. Approximately one-third of these metastasize to internal organs. Patients with Bowen's disease, especially in non-sun-exposed areas, are at risk for development of internal cancers, and they should be evaluated for this. Arseniasis also can give rise to Bowen's disease.

Kaposi's Sarcoma

Kaposi's sarcoma may be a reactive process or a neoplastic process, which occurs most often in the skin but also can be extracutaneous. Skin lesions have a characteristic purple color, but they may vary from bluish to red to brown.

Single or multiple macules, papules, nodules, and plaques may be formed anywhere, but most commonly are limited to the lower legs. Although lesions of Kaposi's sarcoma are usually quite characteristic, sometimes they can be confused with vascular anomalies, such as pyogenic granulomas, hemangiomas, or vascular tumors. Biopsy should be performed.

In Western countries, 10 percent of cases of Kaposi's sarcoma are associated with lymphoma or leukemia. In Africa, the disease takes a more aggressive form but is not associated with a second malignancy. Kaposi's sarcoma is frequently seen in patients with acquired immunodeficiency syndrome (see Fig. 80-1, page 337).

No Malignant Cells in the Skin

Skin Changes Due to Metabolic Products of Malignancy

Carcinoid syndrome, usually associated with an underlying carcinoid tumor of the appendix and, less commonly, with the small intestine, or with a bronchial adenoma, can cause flushing. Addisonian hyperpigmentation is seen when certain carcinomas (especially oat cell carcinoma of the lung) produce a melanocyte-stimulating hormone and an ACTH-like peptide.

Pancreatic carcinomas can produce nodular fat necrosis, which consists of red, painful, subcutaneous nodules on the legs in association with fever, malaise, and arthralgias. Pathologic evaluations must be performed to differentiate this from other panniculitis (inflammation of the fat). Glucagon-secreting pancreatic tumors can produce a periorificial erythematous, annular eruption known as necrolytic migratory erythema. Circulating cryoproteins formed in multiple myeloma can cause Raynaud's phenomenon, in which fingers and toes develop pallor, cyanosis, and then hyperemia in response to cold. Amyloidosis can also be seen in multiple myeloma, and this appears clinically as small, yellowish, and sometimes hemorrhagic papules around the face (especially eyes and ears), scalp, and body folds.

Skin Changes Due to Abnormalities in Other Systems

Obstructive jaundice from metastatic or primary malignancy of the liver can give the skin and mucous membranes a generalized yellow hue, cause by deposition of the bile pigment bilirubin. Bleeding from thrombocytopenia can cause nonblanchable purpuric lesions, whereas anemic patients have a pallor. Herpes simplex and zoster both occur more frequently and more severely in patients with malignancies, especially those with Hodgkin's disease. Herpes zoster usually occurs after the malignancy has been diagnosed.

Idiopathic Skin Changes

Dermatomyositis

Dermatomyositis is a systemic disease that affects the skin and muscles. In adults, dermatomyositis has been associated with malignancies in 6 to 50 percent of cases. The four criteria used in diagnosis of dermatomyositis are as follows: (1) progressive symmetric proximal muscle weakness; (2) characteristic muscle biopsy with myositis; (3) elevated levels of muscle enzymes, including creatine phosphokinase (CPK), aldolase, serum glutamic-oxaloacetic transaminase (SGOT), or lactate dehydrogenase (LDH); (4) characteristically abnormal electromyogram; and (5) typical skin findings. All of these criteria do not have to be met to make the diagnosis of dermatomyositis. The dermatologic manifestations of dermatomyositis may be mild or severe, and all of the skin findings need not always be present.

Cutaneous lesions include a raised or flat red to red-purple fine scaly eruption found on the trunk, extremities, and face, especially in the malar areas. The rash may have a photodistribution. An edematous violaceous eruption on the upper lids is known as a heliotrope rash. Gottron's papules, also characteristic, are flat-topped lesions over the knuckles. There may be periungual erythema, cuticular telangiectasia, and cuticular overgrowth.

The differential diagnoses of dermatomyositis include lupus, scleroderma, mixed connective tissue disease, rheumatoid arthritis, trichinosis, toxoplasmosis, muscular dystrophy, thyroid disease, and other neurologic diseases. The work-up to differentiate among these conditions may include (1) a good history and physical examination, (2) muscle enzymes (CPK, SGOT, LDH, aldolase), (3) electromyogram, (4) nerve conduction studies, (5) muscle biopsy, (6) skin biopsy with immunofluorescence, if necessary, to try to distinguish it from systemic lupus erythematosus, and (7) thyroid function tests (see Chapter 110, "Paraneoplastic Syndromes").

Dermatomyositis is associated with malignancies in adults, but not in children. These patients should have a work-up for malignancy and close follow-up. The neoplasm may precede, coincide, or follow (by even years) the myositis. A relapse of dermatomyositis may herald recurrence of tumor or metastasis. All types of neoplasms are involved, with breast and lung the most common.

Malignant Acanthosis Nigricans

Malignant acanthosis nigricans is a distinctive dermatologic entity, with velvety, confluent hyperpigmented and hyperkeratotic plaques found in body folds, e.g., knuckles, axilla, neck, umbilicus, and nipples. Thickened skin of palms and soles may also occur. Although there are benign causes of acanthosis nigricans, some of these lesions indicate an underlying adenocarcinoma, most commonly of the stomach. The dermatoses may precede, occur with, or follow the diagnosis of the tumor, and the skin lesions follow a course similar to that of the tumor.

Migratory Thrombophlebitis

Migratory superficial thrombophlebitis occurring in the neck, trunk, or extremities should alert one to the possibility of an underlying cancer, most commonly of the pancreas. One or more veins can be palpated with tender cords, and the veins may be involved simultaneously or sequentially. This may be seen most often with virtually any adenocarcinoma. Pancreatic carcinoma is frequently found in patients at postmortem examination.

Adult-Onset Ichthyosis

Ichthyosis, which is a dermatosis of rhomboid scales, especially on the lower legs, usually is inherited. When it occurs de novo in an adult, it has been associated with an underlying malignancy, most frequently lymphoma. Scaling can also be seen in hypothyroidism and asteatosic eczema.

Pruritus

Pruritus, without any primary skin lesions, can be seen in Hodgkin's disease and less frequently in other lymphomas and carcinomas. The pruritus may precede Hodgkin's disease by several years. Other causes of pruritus must be ruled out, including dry skin, infestations, chronic renal failure, obstructive biliary disease, hyperthyroidism, and prebullous pemphigoid.

Erythema Multiforme

In erythema multiforme, a hypersensitivity syndrome, many types of lesions are present—macules, papules, urticarial lesions, and blisters. A characteristic lesion, the target lesion, may have a dusky center or a papule or vesicle at its center with concentric rings around it. Rarely, erythema multiforme is associated with underlying malignancy and also with radiation therapy for cancer.

Chronic Urticaria

Hives that last longer than 6 weeks are called chronic urticaria. Occasionally, chronic urticaria develops with underlying malignancies. Multiple other causes of chronic urticaria must be ruled out, including infections, collagen vascular diseases, drugs, foods, and food additives.

Genetic Diseases with Skin Manifestations and the Tendency to Develop Internal Malignancies

Gardner's Syndrome

Gardner's syndrome is a dominantly inherited disease with multiple epidermal cysts, dermoid tumors, lipomas, and fibromas. Also associated are osteomas and polyps of the colon, with a high incidence of adenocarcinoma of the colon.

Peutz-Jeghers Syndrome

Peutz-Jeghers syndrome, which is dominantly inherited, includes pigmented macules on lips, oral mucosa, and digits, and intestinal polyposis (especially of the small intestine). There is a low incidence of gastrointestinal adenocarcinomas.

The Complex of Myxomas, Spotty Pigmentation, and Endocrine Overactivity

Carney and associates (1985) described a new complex of findings that includes spotty pigmentation (lentigines and blue nevi), myxomatous masses (cardiac, cutaneous, and mammary), and endocrine overactivity of the adrenal and pituitary glands, with various testicular tumors. Other internal malignancies are rarely associated with this complex.

Neurofibromatosis

Neurofibromatosis is a dominantly inherited disorder that affects primarily the skin, bone, endocrine, and neurologic systems. Skin lesions include neurofibromas, café au lait spots, and axillary "freckles." Rarely, tumors of the central nervous system, pheochromocytomas, and sarcomas are seen.

Tuberous Sclerosis

Tuberous sclerosis, a dominantly inherited neurocutaneous syndrome, has several cutaneous manifestations, including hypopigmented macules; seizures; mental retardation; hamartomas in brain, kidney, and heart; and a low incidence of brain tumors.

Cowden's Disease

Cowden's disease, a newly described disease with autosomal dominant inheritance, consists of multiple mucocutaneous hamartomas and high incidence of later development of carcinomas. Lesions include flat-topped papules over the head and neck; wart-like papules over the wrists and dorsa of the hands; keratotic lesions on palms and soles; and multiple lipomas, cavernous hemangiomas, and other benign skin tumors, including trichilemmomas. This syndrome has a high association with fibrocystic breast changes, carcinoma of the breast, thyroid disease, including carcinomas, and gastrointestinal polyposis.

References

Braverman IM. Skin signs of systemic disease. 2nd ed. Philadelphia: WB Saunders, 1981.

Callen J. Cutaneous aspects of internal disease. Chicago: Year Book Medical Publishers, 1981.

Carney JA, et al. The complex of myxomas, spotty pigmentation and endocrine overactivity. Medicine 1985; 64:270.

Helm F, Helm J. Cutaneous markers of internal malignancies. In: Cancer dermatology. Philadelphia: Lea & Febiger, 1979:245.

McLean D, Haynes H. Cutaneous aspects of internal malignant disease. In: Fitzpatrick TB, Freedberg IM, eds. Dermatology in general medicine. 3rd ed. New York: McGraw-Hill, 1987:1917.

Rook A, Wilkinson DS, Ebling FJD. Cutaneous markers of internal malignancy. In: Rook A. Textbook of dermatology. 4th ed. Boston: Blackwell Scientific Publications, 1986:2348.

Sauer GC. Manual of skin disease. 5th ed. Philadelphia: JB Lippincott, 1986.

Shuster S. Dermatology in internal medicine. New York: Oxford University Press, 1978.

Paraneoplastic Syndromes

Thomas W. Griffin, MD

110

Paraneoplastic syndromes are effects that tumor has on a host that are not related to direct invasion, compression, or destruction by the primary tumor or its metastasis. Paraneoplastic syndromes are often related to production by the tumor of biologically active substances that circulate in the blood stream and alter the functions of distant organs.

As many as 50 percent of patients with malignancy may develop a paraneoplastic syndrome. The incidence of paraneoplastic phenomena varies with the tumor histology. For example, small cell carcinoma of the lung is commonly associated with a large variety of paraneoplastic syndromes, whereas carcinoma of the colon produces these effects infrequently.

Multiple mechanisms have been proposed for paraneoplastic syndromes. One of the best-documented mechanisms is the production of biologically active substances by the tumor tissue. These substances may be similar or identical to such naturally occurring hormones as antidiuretic hormone (ADH). Presumed but as yet unidentified biologically active substances also have been suggested as etiologic factors in cancer cachexia, hypertrophic pulmonary osteoarthropathy, and the diverse neurologic syndromes that can be seen with various types of malignancies. The tumor may also directly affect the immune function of the host, resulting in paraneoplastic phenomena. These effects may include autoimmunity, immune complex formation, and acquired immunodeficiency. Autoimmunity and immune complexes may lead directly to tissue damage, while acquired immunodeficiency may allow the development of atypical infections that may mirror a paraneoplastic event. In this regard, the syndrome of progressive multifocal leukoencephalopathy is of interest. This syndrome, long considered to be a manifestation of neurologic paraneoplasia, is now known to represent a viral infection of the central nervous system in an immunocompromised host.

Paraneoplastic syndromes offer specific clinical challenges to the physician caring for the patient with cancer, and they often present difficult diagnostic problems. The prompt recognition that a given symptom complex indicates the presence of a remote cancer may lead to the discovery of an occult, curable malignancy. Furthermore, successful treatment of these syndromes may be possible even when the underlying malignancy itself cannot be cured. Therefore, symptomatic management of these syndromes may add appreciably to the patient's comfort.

Features that suggest a paraneoplastic etiology of a clinical syndrome include the sudden onset and rapid progression of a symptom complex, the occurrence of a clinical syndrome in an atypical host (e.g., dermatomyositis in an elderly man), and the atypical clinical manifestations of a well-defined endocrine syndrome (e.g., Cushing's syndrome in a patient with lung cancer).

Hypercalcemia

Hypercalcemia is a relatively common finding in cancer patients; it can be defined as a serum calcium level greater than 10.5 mg/dl. The physiologic consequences of hypercalcemia are related to the level of ionized calcium in the serum. Ionized calcium constitutes about one-half of the serum calcium and is in equilibrium with calcium bound to serum proteins, especially albumin. Roughly, 0.8 mg of calcium is bound by 1 g of serum protein. Therefore, in severe hypoproteinemia, elevations of ionized calcium may exist even with normal levels of total serum calcium.

Approximately 7 percent of patients with cancer will have hypercalcemia at some point in their illness, and malignancy is the most common cause of hypercalcemia occurring in the hospitalized patient. The most common forms of cancer associated with hypercalcemia are multiple myeloma (70 percent) and breast cancer (50 percent). Other tumors commonly associated with hypercalcemia include squamous cell carcinoma of the lung (but not small cell carcinoma of the lung), carcinoma of the kidney, carcinoma of the pancreas, and many others.

There are many plausible mechanisms for the development of hypercalcemia in the patient with malignancy. Bone metastases with osteolytic changes probably cause hypercalcemia in a significant proportion of the patients. The simultaneous occurrence of primary hyperparathyroidism may also cause elevations in serum calcium. Tumors are sometimes able to produce biologically active compounds such as parathormone-related polypeptide, prostaglandins, or osteoclast activating factor (OAF), any of which could cause hypercalcemia by various mechanisms. OAF may be produced by such hematologic malignancies as multiple myeloma.

The symptoms and signs of hypercalcemia are manifested in four major physiologic systems. The neuromuscular signs and symptoms can include fatigue, severe muscle weakness, behavioral changes, stupor, and coma. Cardiovascular manifestations of hypercalcemia include electrocardiographic changes, hypertension, and a potentiation of the effects of the cardiac glycoside digitalis. Polydipsia, polyuria, dehydration (nephrogenic diabetes insipidus), hyperuricemia, renal tubular acidosis, and other manifestations of renal tubular dysfunction are among the renal effects often seen. The gastrointestinal signs and symptoms include anorexia, constipation, ulcers, and pancreatitis.

The differential diagnosis of hypercalcemia in the cancer patient must take into consideration the three major categories of this condition. The first is hypercalcemia related to the presence of metastatic cancer in bone, which is most likely to be associated with breast cancer and adenocarcinoma of the lung. Hypercalcemia can also be caused by the secretion of a humoral factor by the tumor without direct involvement of the bone by metastatic cancer. This is commonly seen in squamous cell carcinoma of the upper digestive tract and lung; carcinoma of the kidney, ovary, and pancreas; and hepatoma. Third, such benign conditions as primary hyperparathyroidism, thiazide diuretic therapy, hyperthyroidism, and immobilization can cause hypercalcemia in the cancer patient.

Syndrome of Inappropriate Antidiuretic Hormone Secretion

Syndrome of inappropriate antidiuretic hormone secretion (SIADH) results from the unregulated tumor production of antidiuretic hormone (ADH), which results in increased water retention by the kidney and leads to increased total body water and hyponatremia. This syndrome is common in clinical medicine and has been described with a variety of malignancies, including lung cancer, thymoma, pancreatic cancer, lymphoma, and several others. However, SIADH is most frequently encountered in lung cancer of the small cell (oat cell) type. As many as 10 percent of patients will have evidence of this syndrome during the clinical course of this tumor.

ADH is normally released from the posterior pituitary gland in response to increased plasma osmolarity or decreased plasma volume. The release of ADH is normally inhibited by decreased plasma osmolarity and increased plasma volume. The hormone acts by increasing water reabsorption in the renal collecting tubules. In SIADH, the tumor directly synthesizes and releases ADH. The increased plasma volume leads to an increased glomerular filtration rate and to a decrease in aldosterone secretion, which in turn causes the increased renal excretion of sodium. Therefore, the hyponatremia seems to result from both increased total body water and decreased body sodium.

Clinical manifestations are related to the rate of development of the hyponatremia; more severe symptoms occur in those patients who develop the syndrome more rapidly. Lethargy, nausea, anorexia, and weakness are common symptoms in patients with gradual development of hyponatremia. A more rapid course may be associated with convulsions, coma, and death.

The diagnostic criteria for SIADH include hypo-osmolality and hyponatremia of extracellular fluids, urine that is less than maximally dilute, absence of volume depletion, appreciable renal excretion of sodium, and normal renal and adrenal function.

Ectopic Adrenal Corticotrophic Hormone Syndrome

The ectopic adrenal corticotrophic hormone syndrome refers to the production by tumor tissue of adrenal corticotrophic hormone (ACTH) and related polypeptides. Excess amounts of this hormone can give rise to diverse metabolic consequences.

Ectopic production of ACTH has been known to be associated with a variety of malignancies, including small cell carcinoma of the lung, bronchial carcinoid, islet cell tumors of the pancreas, medullary carcinoma of the thyroid, pheochromocytoma, and a renal blastoma of the ovary.

The clinical syndrome results from the excess production of ACTH by the adrenal glands as a result of excess and sustained stimulation by the ectopic polypeptide. Biologically active ACTH is secreted by tumor tissue with varying proportions of biologically inactive prohormone and pre-prohormone.

Although slow-growing tumors that produce ACTH may produce the classic stigmata of Cushing's syndrome with truncal obesity, striae, buffalo hump, and moon facies, the syndrome commonly associated with small cell carcinoma of the lung does not fit this classic description. Instead the syndrome is characterized by severe muscle weakness, fatigue, weight loss, and pronounced metabolic abnormalities, specifically hypokalemia and metabolic alkalosis. Glucose intolerance and mild hypertension may also be present. These tumors are usually autonomous and are rarely suppressible with dexamethasone.

Cancer patients who complain of weakness should have their serum electrolytes measured. Hypokalemia and metabolic alkalosis (serum bicarbonate greater than 30 mEq/L) suggest the presence of ectopic ACTH syndrome. Further laboratory evaluation commonly reveals a plasma cortisol level greater than 40 μg/ml and an ACTH level greater than 200 pg/ml. The elevated cortisol and ACTH levels fail to suppress with both low-dose and high-dose dexamethasone.

Selected Other Paraneoplastic Syndromes

Hypertrophic Pulmonary Osteoarthropathy

Hypertrophic pulmonary osteoarthropathy (HPO) is a syndrome that may range from asymptomatic clubbing to a severe periostitis and polyarticular arthritis. When clubbing of the fingers is accompanied by subperiosteal new bone formation, the condition is referred to as hypertrophic osteoarthropathy.

Clubbing, with or without HPO, occurs in 5 to 12 percent of patients with intrathoracic tumors. However, it is only rarely seen in patients with tumors metastatic to the lung. Note that clubbing may be associated with a variety of benign etiologies, including cystic fibrosis, biliary cirrhosis, cyanotic congenital heart disease, and bacterial endocarditis.

The mechanisms for the development of HPO are unknown, but several etiologies have been proposed, including arteriovenous shunts, humoral factors produced by the tumor, and neurogenic factors.

Clubbing may occur slowly or abruptly and be either painless or painful. Periosteal new bone formation is usually seen initially along the shafts of the tibia, radius, and phalanges. A full-blown syndrome may involve the iliac crest, clavicles, and vertebral column.

The articular symptoms may precede both periosteal changes and clubbing. The joints most frequently involved are the knees, ankles, elbows, wrists, and metacarpophalangeal joints. Joint involvement is usually symmetric. The diagnosis of HPO may be made on the basis of radiologic evidence together with clinical signs and symptoms.

Periosteal thickening can be demonstrated radiographically, especially in the long bones of the forearms and legs and the tarsal and carpal bones. The bone scan may also be positive in areas of new bone formation. However, the serum alkaline phosphatase level is generally within normal limits.

Dermatomyositis

Dermatomyositis is a condition that is characterized by muscle weakness with inflammation and is accompanied by distinctive skin changes, which may be more or less accentuated in a given patient. This syndrome is only rarely associated with malignancy, and its clinical features are similar to those of idiopathic dermatopolymyositis. Although the exact relationship of dermatomyositis to malignancy has been questioned in recent years, occurrence of the syndrome in patients over age 40 (especially men) does have a clear-cut relationship to the presence of occult malignancy. The malignancies involved are the common visceral adenocarcinomas, including gastric, breast, lung, and prostate. Although the etiology of this syndrome is unknown, proposed mechanisms include humoral factors and autoimmunity.

The clinical manifestations of dermatomyositis include a polymyositis and characteristic skin rash. The rash typically consists of a violaceous erythema on exposed parts of the body, especially the malar areas and the eyelids. However, widespread areas of the body may show erythema and telangiectasias, especially the hands. Muscle disease (polymyositis) may occur with or without the skin rash and is characterized by proximal muscle weakness that progresses over weeks to months, with spontaneous remissions and exacerbations. Muscle pain, swelling, and tenderness may also be seen. Dysphagia is common, and weakness of the respiratory muscles may occur.

Laboratory studies may demonstrate elevated levels of serum muscle enzymes (creatine phosphokinase, aldolase, and transaminases). The urinary creatinine level is also often increased.

Electromyography can be used to demonstrate evidence of primary muscle degeneration (spontaneous fibrillations). A muscle biopsy can be used to document focal or diffuse necrosis of muscle fibers, regenerative activity, and an inflammatory reaction consisting of interstitial and perivascular infiltration of lymphocytes and plasma cells.

Acanthosis Nigricans

Acanthosis nigricans is a symmetric, verrucous, velvety hyperplasia of the skin with hyperpigmentation that ranges from brown to black. There are at least two different types of acanthosis nigricans. The more common type occurs in young women who have a form of insulin-resistant diabetes and loss of adipose tissue. In addition, forms of acanthosis nigricans similar to that which occurs with internal malignancy have been described in obesity. Acanthosis nigricans has been described in association with adenocarcinoma (especially of the stomach), lymphoma, and squamous cell carcinoma.

Proposed mechanisms include abnormal skin response to injury, hormonal substances produced by tumors, and viruses. The verrucous and papillary pigmented lesions tend to occur in skin flexures, particularly in the axilla and perineal areas. They may also occur in areas of repeated skin trauma. These lesions are usually symmetric, and pruritus is common. Malignant acanthosis nigricans usually runs a parallel course with the tumor. Its appearance most commonly precedes the diagnosis of a malignancy and therefore may be a clue to the presence of occult cancer (see Chapter 109, "Skin Signs of Internal Malignancy").

Eaton-Lambert Syndrome

Eaton-Lambert syndrome is an unusual condition that resembles myasthenia gravis with respect to muscle fatigability but differs in electromyographic and pharmacologic aspects. Eaton-Lambert syndrome is rare, but when it occurs, it is usually associated with an intrathoracic tumor that is typically, but not invariably, oat cell carcinoma of the lung.

The site of dysfunction is the neuromuscular junction, where acetylcholine released from axonal terminals by the nerve impulse is decreased. How this abnormality is induced by the tumor is unknown, although autoantibodies directed against the neuromuscular junction have been detected in some patients.

The syndrome is manifested by weakness and easy fatigability of the proximal muscles. Symptoms referable to the ocular and bulbar muscles (common in myasthenia gravis) are infrequent and mild. Aching in the thighs, paresthesias, and impotence may also be seen. Anticholinesterases, which are effective in relieving some of the symptoms of myasthenia gravis, are without effect in patients with Eaton-Lambert syndrome.

The classic diagnostic finding is seen on electromyogram. Patients with myasthenia gravis exhibit fatigue on repeated stimulation, whereas patients with Eaton-Lambert syndrome show facilitation (increase in amplitude of muscle action potentials).

References

Brown J, Winkelman RK. Acanthosis nigricans. Medicine 1968; 47:33.

Bunn PA, Ridgway EC. Paraneoplastic syndromes. In: DeVita VT, Hellman S, Rosenberg SA, eds. Cancer: Principles and practice of oncology. 3rd ed. Philadelphia: JB Lippincott, 1989:1896.

Griffin TW, Rosenthal PE, Costanza ME. Paraneoplastic and endocrine syndromes. In: Cancer manual. 7th ed. Boston: American Cancer Society, 1986:373.

Ruddon RW. Cancer biology. 2nd ed. New York: Oxford University Press, 1987.

Tagnon HJ, Hildebrand J. Paraneoplastic syndromes. Eur J Cancer Clin Oncol 1981; 17:969.

Red Eye

Edward L. Kazarian, MD

Most cases of red eye(s) will need to be treated by an ophthalmologist, but all physicans should be familiar with a working differential diagnosis. It is in this manner that the urgency of the situation can be assessed and proper treatment or referral given. Associated complaints such as loss of vision and pain indicate referable situations.

Definition

When patients complain of a red eye, they generally imply that the area over the sclera is red. This may vary from the mild, diffuse erythema associated with environmental irritants to the bright, diffuse, intense redness of subconjunctival hemorrhage. Because a wide variety of disorders can lead to a red eye, each is discussed individually. When evaluating patients with red eyes, one might use the following mnemonic (RED I's) as a reminder for differential diagnosis:

Red blood (subconjunctival hemorrhage)
Elevated intraocular pressure
Debris
Infection
Inflammation
Iritis
Injury

Red Blood (Subconjunctival Hemorrhage)

The red eye of subconjunctival hemorrhage is rather spectacular in appearance; fortunately, it is generally benign. Often the patient states during the history that the occurrence was spontaneous and that it was noted when he or she looked in the mirror in the morning. Associated symptoms are rare. Sometimes, the history of coughing, sneezing, or anticoagulant usage is given. If the hemorrhages are recurrent, the possibility of blood dyscrasia or hypertension should be considered.

On physical examination, the blood is usually very bright red and appears to be dissecting in the plane between the conjunctiva and sclera. Usually, the hemorrhage is unilateral and may involve the entire subconjunctival space or be loculated in a segmental fashion. The vision is normal, as are the cornea, pupils, motility, and pressures. After several days, the blood may turn to a reddish-purple hue before absorbing in several weeks. No specific treatment is indicated.

Elevated Intraocular Pressure

Elevated intraocular pressure is discussed in Chapter 137, "Vision Problems in the Elderly."

Debris

During the history, the patient often states that the eye is red and that some foreign particle apparently landed on the eye. Seek a history of any situation in which particles might have entered the eye, dating back at least several days. Occasionally, a foreign body may be asymptomatically dormant for several days on the surface of the eye. Foreign-body sensation will be a prominent feature, and if the debris is corneal, complaints of reduced vision, photophobia, and lacrimation might also be mentioned.

On physical examination, the visual acuity may be normal to moderately reduced because of photophobia and lacrimation. Occasionally, a drop of topical anesthetic is necessary in order to examine the eye properly. Look for debris on the lashes, cul-de-sacs, and conjunctival and corneal surfaces. The conjunctiva is mild to moderately red, and there is usually an increased erythema in the area or quadrant of the foreign body. Fluorescein dye instillation in the eye is very helpful in localizing corneal foreign bodies and abrasions. Areas where the foreign body is or has been usually stain bright green. If vertically stained scratches are noted on the cornea, a foreign body under the upper lid should be suspected. Always consider the possibility that the staining area may represent a herpetic dendrite. Because of this possibility and that of corneal infection, most corneal foreign bodies or abrasions should be seen and followed up by an ophthalmologist. Also, nonophthalmologists should not use topical steroids or steroid-antibiotic combinations for treatment of red eyes.

Infection

Conjunctivitis is the most common cause of red eye. The patient usually complains of diffuse redness that may vary from mild to severe in different cases. The onset is usually over a period of several days, but frequently it may be quite acute. Just prior to or beginning with the acute phase, the patient's eye(s) is crusted closed upon awakening in the morning. This morning crusting of an eye is a fairly reliable symptom to help differentiate conjunctivitis from other causes of red eye. The infection may be unilateral or bilateral, and the onset of the infection in each eye may be different. In many cases someone in the household has had similar symptoms in the recent past. Pain, foreign-body sensation, and decreased visual acuity are not major complaints; the infection may be viral, bacterial, or chlamydial.

On physical examination, the vision may be mildly or variably decreased, depending on how much inflammatory debris is present. The cornea is generally clear; corneal involvement should raise the suspicion of herpes simplex or possibly severe viral or bacterial keratoconjunctivitis. Corneal involvement is an indication for referral to an ophthalmologist. The pupils are normal, as are the pressures and motility. The bulbar and tarsal conjunctivae are red. Inflammatory debris is usually noted on the lashes and lid margins. Preauricular and submandibular nodes may be palpable and usually indicate viral or acute, severe bacterial conjunctivitis.

Treatment usually consists of antibiotic drops. Cultures may be obtained, but they are usually not necessary in routine cases of conjunctivitis. In fulminant cases with suspected bacterial involvement, cultures, Gram stains, and Giemsa stains are helpful. The patient, his or her relatives, and involved physicians should be aware that many cases of conjunctivitis are highly contagious.

Iritis

Iritis is an intraocular inflammation that frequently is of unknown etiology. Patients may be asymptomatic, but they often complain of decreased vision, deep ocular pain unlike foreign-body pain, photophobia, and lacrimation. Other symptoms are generally absent.

On physical examination, the visual acuity may be normal to significantly decreased. The involved eye(s) is usually mildly to moderately red. The erythema is frequently in an arcuate fashion following the corneal curvature. The erythema is more intense near the corneae limbus (ciliary flush) than nasally and temporally. Crusting and discharge are conspicuously absent. The pupil of the involved eye is usually slightly, but noticeably, smaller than the pupil of the contralateral eye. The pupils generally react normally unless the involved pupil is scarred down and irregular because of the intraocular inflammation. The intraocular pressure is usually normal to slightly decreased. When this diagnosis is suspected, the patient should be referred to an ophthalmologist.

Inflammation

Miscellaneous inflammatory conditions involving the eye can cause a red eye. Allergic conjunctivitis or toxic conjunctivitis from pollutants, contact lens solutions, and so forth is usually easily diagnosed with careful history. On examination, the conjunctiva is mildly erythematous. There may be a stringy mucoid discharge, but all else is generally normal. Corneal ulcer is a serious, generally acute infection of the cornea by bacteria or fungi. Pain and decreased vision are the usual complaints. Poor vision, severe red eye, and a localized gray, opaque haze in the affected part of the cornea is generally noticed. This is a severe emergency that requires immediate referral. Episcleritis and scleritis are inflammations of the episclera (the tissue between the sclera and the conjunctiva) and sclera, respectively. Pain and redness are the presenting symptoms; they are much more severe in scleritis. The inflammation is usually localized to one segment or quadrant of the globe; it appears to be much deeper in scleritis.

Injury

Most blunt and sharp injuries to the eye cause varying degrees of conjunctival erythema. A history of trauma or foreign body is usually readily obtainable. Examination or referral should be appropriate for each given ocular and periocular injury.

References

Allansmith MR. Vernal conjunctivitis. In: Duane T, ed. Clinical ophthalmology. Vol 4. Ch 9. Philadelphia: Harper & Row, 1986.

Dawson C. Follicular conjunctivitis. In: Duane T, ed. Clinical ophthalmology. Vol 4. Ch 7. Philadelphia: Harper & Row, 1979.

Gittinger JW Jr. Angle closure glaucoma. In: Gittinger JW Jr, Asdourian GK. Manual of clinical problems in ophthalmology. Boston: Little, Brown, 1988:55.

Gittinger JW Jr. Herpes simplex keratitis. In: Gittinger JW Jr, Asdourian GK. Manual of clinical problems in ophthalmology. Boston: Little, Brown, 1988:46.

O'Day DM, Jones BR. Herpes simplex keratitis. In: Duane T, ed. Clinical ophthalmology. Vol 4. Ch 19. Philadelphia: Harper & Row, 1987.

Simmons RJ, Belcher CD III, Dallow RL. Primary angle closure glaucoma. In: Duane T, ed. Clinical ophthalmology. Vol 3. Ch 3. Philadelphia: Harper & Row, 1985.

Tessler HH. Classification and symptoms and signs of uveitis. In: Duane T, ed. Clinical ophthalmology. Vol 4. Ch 32. Philadelphia: Harper & Row, 1987.

Vaughan D, Asbury T, Cook R. General ophthalmology. 11th ed. Los Altos, CA: Appleton & Lange, 1986:55, 78, 109, 129.

Wilson L. Bacterial conjunctivitis. In: Duane T, ed. Clinical ophthalmology. Vol 4. Ch 5. Philadelphia: Harper & Row, 1979.

Abnormalities of Tearing

Edward L. Kazarian, MD

112

Complaints related to lacrimal dysfunction are common in the adult population. Tears are composed of secretions from the major and minor lacrimal glands (water component), meibomian glands (lipid component), and goblet cells (mucin component). Most complaints are attributable to either decreased production of one component of the tear film or decreased ability to drain tears away from the eyes.

Dry Eyes

History

The symptoms of dry eye can be caused by a deficiency of any of the major components of the tear film. Complaints are frequently registered as dryness, itching, gritty or sandy feeling, burning, frequent need to blink or rub the eyes, and mild chronic redness. Dry eye symptoms usually increase as the day proceeds, being worse in the afternoon and evening. Dry conditions such as the winter air, air conditioning, and homes with wood or coal stoves tend to exacerbate the symptoms. Patients may complain of an unusual sensitivity to smoke-filled rooms or dusty areas. The symptoms generally vary, with patients having good and bad days.

Although most people with dry eyes have no associated systemic disease, the patient should be questioned for symptoms related to rheumatoid arthritis and other connective tissue diseases. Dry eyes, dry mouth, and connective tissue disorder form the classical triad of Sjögren's syndrome. A history of severe conjunctivitis in the past is relevant because conjunctivitis may have destroyed some of the secretory glands or ducts. Bell's palsy or eyelid abnormalities that affect the blinking mechanism and the manufacturing of tears are common causes of dry eyes. A medication history (including nonophthalmologic drugs) is important because diuretics and anticholinergics may cause dry eyes. A history of relief of the symptoms with over-the-counter eye drops suggests a benign cause.

Physical Examination

On superficial inspection, the eyes generally appear normal. The visual acuity is good, but many patients blink frequently to reach the best visual potential while reading the chart. It is important to check lid closure, because normal lid function is needed to spread tears over the eyes. The cornea and conjunctiva may appear to be less lustrous or moist than normal. The bulbar conjunctiva often is slightly and superficially erythematous in the palpebral fissure. There should be no discharge or drainage, but occasionally thick, stringy mucus is found in the lower cul-de-sac.

Although the diagnosis is frequently made on the basis of the history, Schirmer's test is often helpful for confirmation and to demonstrate to the patient the cause of the symptoms. A useful way to do Schirmer's test is to put one drop of topical anesthetic in each eye and then wait several minutes. After this interval, place a Schirmer paper strip into both cul-de-sacs with the strip overhanging the lower lids. If less than 10 mm of the filter strip is wet after 5 minutes, the test is positive for decreased tear function. Frequently, the first strip gives a negative result. In this case a repeat test (performed without adding more anesthetic) will eliminate some false-negative results. A negative Schirmer's test result does not necessarily rule out dry eye syndrome. One component of the tear film, such as mucin, may be deficient, yet enough of the hydrous component is manufactured to give a negative result. Generally, clinical judgement should prevail.

When Schirmer's test is performed as instructed, the false-positive and false-negative rates are about 20 percent. The main purpose of performing Schirmer's test is to document that dryness is the cause of the symptoms. When dry eyes are diagnosed, the patient should be treated symptomatically with artificial tears. If symptoms persist despite this therapy, or if Schirmer's test does not confirm dry eyes, ophthalmologic consultation is usually helpful.

Watering Eyes

History

If more tears are produced than can be drained away, the patient may complain of excessive tearing. The symptoms may range from a sensation of increased moisture over the eye to frank overflow of tears down the cheek. Patients may complain of recurrent infections in either eye. The symptoms are usually fairly constant, occurring essentially daily, and increase in windy or irritating environments when lacrimal secretion is increased by smoke, pollutants, and the like.

Physical Examination

The usual cause of the preceding symptoms is a decreased ability of the nasolacrimal system to drain away the tears. One should check the lid position to ensure that the lacrimal puncta are in proper position to absorb tears. Ectropion or entropion (outward turning or turning under of the eye lid) frequently causes malposition of the puncta. The patency of the puncta should also be assured by general inspection. Pressure over the nasolacrimal sac will cause purulent regurgitation from the puncta if the sac is obstructed and infection exists. If all the aforementioned checkpoints are normal, a relative decrease in drainage ability probably exists, and probing or irrigation by an ophthalmologist may be curative.

References

Gittinger JW Jr, Asdourian GK. Manual of clinical problems in ophthalmology. Boston: Little, Brown, 1988.

Lemp MA. Diagnosis and treatment of tear deficiencies. In: Duane T, ed. Clinical ophthalmology. Vol 4. Ch 14. Philadelphia: Harper & Row, 1980.

McCord CD Jr. The lacrimal drainage system. In: Duane T, ed. Clinical ophthalmology. Philadelphia: Harper & Row, 1980.

Tabbara KF. Tears. In: Vaughan D, Asbury T, Cook R. General ophthalmology. 11th ed. Los Altos, CA: Appleton & Lange, 1986:72.

Flashing Lights (Photopsia)

Edward L. Kazarian, MD

113

Complaints of the sensation of flashing lights, or photopsia, are fairly common after the age of 40. The two most common underlying causes are migraine phenomenon and vitreoretinal traction. Epileptic aura is a remote possibility. Each of these diagnostic possibilities must be positively identified and differentiated from the other causes, because each has a specific treatment.

History

The cause of photopsia can often be determined by careful questioning. A personal and family history of migraine should be sought. The prodromal scintillating scotoma of migraine may be described by the patient as a flashing light. With careful questioning, the patient may recall that there was a blind spot (scotoma) associated with this light effect. Frequently, the light effect appears in a somewhat jagged fashion around the edge of the scotoma. With migraines, the patient may be able to draw the scotoma and the flashing lights. The symptoms last about 20 to 30 minutes and may be associated with nausea, vomiting, and somnolence and followed by unilateral headache. The ocular signs may be the only symptoms, especially if the migraine begins later in life.

If epilepsy or migraine does not seem likely, one should have a high suspicion of vitreoretinal traction. As patients get older, the vitreous gel gradually becomes more liquid and sepa-

Table 113-1 Evaluation of Flashing Lights

Type	Timing	Associated symptoms	Diagnosis	Ophthalmologic referral
Jagged lines	Lasts >20 min	Scotoma Headaches	Migraine	Not necessary
Spark-like	Lasts several sec or more	Change of vision	Vitreoretinal traction	Urgent if new floaters exist, semiurgent if no floaters or only old floaters

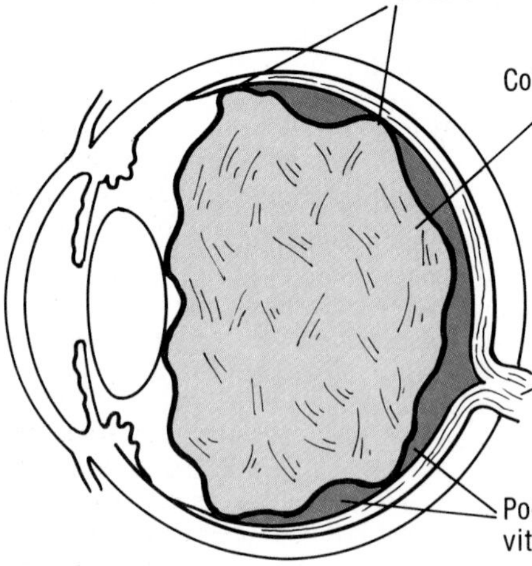

Figure 113-1 Abnormal areas of adhesion.

rates from the retina. With the normal separation of the vitreous from the retina, there are no areas of vitreoretinal traction (Fig. 113-1). The cleavage is generally clean, with the shrinking vitreous separating without areas of retinal traction. The risk of retinal traction is greatest after cataract surgery and in myopic patients. Because early treatment might prevent blindness, careful questioning should be done to ascertain the exact description of the light flashes. Frequently, they are described as periodic and recurring, minute, bright, momentary spots of light, as if a light flash from a camera took place. The symptoms may be more prominent in the dark (greater contrast) or with head movement (increased movement of the vitreous within the eye). The symptoms may be unilateral or bilateral. New-onset light flashes, followed by persistent "floaters" or, more ominously, by a sudden shower of new "floaters," or loss of part of the visual field strongly suggests vitreoretinal traction. The patient should be referred urgently for ophthalmologic evaluation. Chronic light flashes and old, unchanging floaters need no specific evaluation.

Physical Examination

Generally, the examination of the eye is unremarkable. The vision should be normal. External examination, pupils, motility, and confrontation fields should be unremarkable. If the visual acuity is decreased, a pupillary abnormality is noted, or a loss of part of the visual field is detected, immediate ophthalmologic referral is indicated. In general, all patients with new light flashes in this vitreoretinal traction category should have ophthalmologic evaluation (Table 113-1).

References

Asdourian GK. Retina and vitreous. In: Gittinger JW Jr, Asdourian GK. Manual of clinical problems in ophthalmology. Boston: Little, Brown, 1988:106.

Gittinger JW Jr. Fundus abnormalities. In: Ophthalmology: A clinical introduction. Boston: Little, Brown, 1984:220.

Gittinger JW Jr. Neuro-ophthalmology. In: Ophthalmology: A clinical introduction. Boston: Little, Brown, 1984:154.

Straatsma BR, Foos RY, Kreiger AE. Rhegmatogenous retinal detachment. In: Duane T, ed. Clinical ophthalmology. Vol 3. Ch 27. Philadelphia: Harper & Row, 1980.

Tasman W. The vitreous. In: Duane T, ed. Clinical ophthalmology. Philadelphia: Harper & Row, 1984:12.

Troost BT. Migraine. In: Duane T, ed. Clinical ophthalmology. Vol 2. Ch 19. Philadelphia: Harper & Row, 1987.

Vaughan D, Asbury T, Cook R. General ophthalmology. 11th ed. Los Altos, CA: Appleton & Lange, 1986:154.

Diplopia

Edward L. Kazarian, MD

114

Definition

Diplopia can be defined as seeing one object in two different places at the same time. Patients occasionally confuse other symptoms, such as blurred vision or dizziness, with double vision, but careful questioning should delineate the true nature of the complaint. If the examiner feels that the complaints represent true diplopia, an evaluation is usually indicated. This often requires the combined efforts of the patient's primary physician, neurologist, and ophthalmologist.

History

Careful questioning of patients with double vision is very important. One must differentiate first between monocular and binocular diplopia. The former is a double image perceived by one eye alone. This perception persists when the other eye is covered and, of course, disappears when the involved eye is covered. This type of diplopia represents an ophthalmologic problem rather than a neurologic or medical one. The double image is usually caused by cataracts, refractive error, or a postoperative state in which an extra iris opening has been made.

Binocular diplopia, on the other hand, may represent a more urgent problem that requires investigation. This type of diplopia persists only when both eyes are open and disappears when either eye is covered. In this circumstance, there is a misalignment of the two eyes because of either mechanical displacement in the orbit or an abnormality of one of the cranial nerves innervating an extraocular muscle.

Careful questioning should be directed toward the possibility of systemic disease such as diabetes, hypertension, thyroid disease, myasthenia gravis, or temporal arteritis. Also, the exact nature of the diplopia should be elicited. It is important to determine whether the symptoms are of sudden or gradual onset, or persistent or intermittent; whether the patient has a previous history of similar episodes or if this is a first-time occurrence; whether the diplopia is in a horizontal direction versus a vertical or oblique direction; or whether the symptoms worsen with any particular activity or time of day. This information is important in determining the possible etiologic factor. For instance, suddenness might suggest a vascular etiology, as occurs in hypertension, diabetes, or temporal arteritis. Gradual onset argues in favor of a breakdown in normal control of the eyes, such as occurs in a -phoria (misalignment of the visual axes), slow-growing intracranial mass, thyroid eye disease, or myasthenia gravis. Diplopia that is worse toward the end of the day, especially if it is associated with a history of a variable ptosis (a drooping of the upper eyelid) and increasing fatigue, is highly suggestive of myasthenia gravis. Ptosis may also be noted with third nerve palsy. If the symptoms are worse in the morning upon awakening, this may represent the increased orbital edema noted in thyroid disease. Strictly horizontal diplopia suggests a sixth nerve palsy. Vertical diplopia or combined vertical and oblique diplopia most likely represents a third or fourth cranial nerve palsy.

Physical Examination

Careful examination will often yield clues to the etiology of the binocular diplopia. The problem will be in the orbit, intracranial, or a local manifestation of a systemic disease. The visual acuity is usually normal. If the vision is decreased, and this decrease is a new complaint, the optic nerve is likely involved and diagnostic studies should be directed toward a vascular etiology or a lesion in the orbit or orbital apex. A dilated or sluggish pupil may represent ipsilateral third nerve palsy. Motility should be carefully observed. In complete third nerve palsy, there is usually ptosis, mydriasis, and a deviation of the involved eye down and out. (An easy way to remember this position of deviation is to recall that the third nerve innervates four of the six extraocular muscles. If you lost four of your six friends, you would likely also be down and out.) Esotropia associated with decreased abduction and a head turn to the involved side suggests sixth nerve palsy. A head tilt toward the opposite shoulder and torsional or oblique diplopia suggests fourth nerve palsy. Ptosis is consistent with both third nerve palsy and myasthenia gravis. Variability in the ptosis or a positive lid twitch or lid fatigue test is suggestive of myasthenia. Proptosis (protrusion of the eyeball) and orbital congestion suggest thyroid disease or orbital mass lesions. The fundus is usually normal, but diabetic or hypertensive retinopathy, optic atrophy, and papilledema may all be helpful clues for determining the correct diagnosis.

References

Gittinger JW Jr. Neuro-ophthalmology. In: Ophthalmology: A clinical introduction. Boston: Little, Brown, 1984:151.

Glaser JS. History taking. In: Duane T, ed. Clinical ophthalmology. Vol 2. Ch 1. Philadelphia: Harper & Row, 1978:1.

Glaser JS. Neuro-ophthalmologic examination: General considerations and special techniques. In: Duane T, ed. Clinical ophthalmology. Philadelphia: Harper & Row, 1981:1.

Parks MM, Mitchell PR. Cranial nerve palsies. In: Duane T, ed. Clinical ophthalmology. Vol 1. Ch 19. Philadelphia: Harper & Row, 1986.

Vaughan D, Asbury T, Cook R. General ophthalmology. 11th ed. Los Altos, CA: Appleton & Lange, 1986:14, 232.

Arterial Blood Gases

Rolf D. Hubmayr, MD

Richard S. Irwin, MD

Arterial blood gas analysis is the single most important laboratory test in the evaluation of respiratory and metabolic disorders. It includes the measurement of arterial blood gas tensions for oxygen (PaO_2) and carbon dioxide ($PaCO_2$), the arterial concentration of hydrogen ion (H^+), usually expressed as the negative logarithm (pH_a), and bicarbonate ion concentration (HCO_3^-). These values help in assessing the accuracy of gas exchange and acid-base homeostasis. Proper interpretation of these values requires a working knowledge of (1) the alveolar air equation, (2) the alveolar-arterial (A-a) oxygen tension gradient concept, (3) the Henderson-Hasselbalch equation, (4) the calculation of the H^+/PCO_2 ratio and its application in making therapeutic decisions, and (5) the differential diagnostic possibilities to consider for various acid-base disorders.

Normal Gas Exchange

Respiration is the interchange of gases between an organism and the medium in which it lives. In man, this process involves the uptake of oxygen (O_2) and the elimination of carbon dioxide (CO_2). The gas exchange between blood and atmosphere is a process that can be divided into two basic components: (1) the bulk flow of gas between the atmosphere and the terminal airways (alveolar ventilation), and (2) the transfer of gas between terminal lung regions and the pulmonary capillary blood.

Alveolar ventilation ($\dot{V}_A$) is the main determinant of CO_2 elimination and thus $PaCO_2$; normally, $PaCO_2$ remains fairly constant between 37 and 43 mm Hg. The following equation demonstrates what determines $PaCO_2$:

$$PaCO_2 = K \times \frac{\dot{V}CO_2}{\dot{V}_A}$$

K is a constant of proportionality, $\dot{V}_A$ is alveolar ventilation in liters per minute, and $\dot{V}CO_2$ is CO_2 produced in liters per minute. $\dot{V}CO_2$ reflects the metabolic rate and energy consumption of the organism. Unless a drastic change in the metabolic rate is observed, any change in the $PaCO_2$ reflects a change in alveolar ventilation.

The transfer of O_2 between the terminal lung regions and the pulmonary capillary blood depends on the partial pressure of O_2 in alveolar gas (P_AO_2) and determinants of the (A-a) PO_2 gradient (see below). The alveolar PO_2 can be calculated with the simplified form of the alveolar air equation:

$$P_AO_2 = P_IO_2 - \frac{PaCO_2}{R}$$

P_IO_2 represents partial pressure of O_2 in inspired gas; it is obtained by multiplying the atmospheric pressure of dry inspired gas by the fraction of inspired O_2 being breathed (F_IO_2). At sea level and breathing 21 percent O_2, this value can be assumed to be 150 mm Hg. R is the respiratory exchange ratio, which is assumed to be 0.8. Therefore, substituting into the alveolar air equation and assuming a normal $PaCO_2$ of 40 mm Hg,

$$P_AO_2 = 150 - \frac{40}{0.8} = 100$$

The alveolar air equation numerically expresses the reduction in the O_2 concentration of inspired air as it is taken up by pulmonary capillary blood and mixed with CO_2-rich gas in terminal lung units.

The (A-a) PO_2 Gradient Concept

In the absence of a diffusion impairment and ventilation ($\dot{V}$)/perfusion ($\dot{Q}$) mismatch, the P_AO_2 and the PaO_2 would be identical. The difference, therefore, between P_AO_2 and PaO_2 is the (A-a) PO_2 gradient; it is a measure of efficiency of gas exchange. Because diffusion impairment by itself is seldom a major cause of hypoxemia, the (A-a) PO_2 gradient is a sensitive index of $\dot{V}/\dot{Q}$ mismatch. In clinical practice, it is an extremely important test for detection of intrinsic pulmonary disease.

The normal (A-a) PO_2 gradient and therefore PaO_2 are affected by age and body position. Predicted normal values are as follows:

In the upright position, $PaO_2 = 104.2 - 0.27 \times \text{age (yr)}$
$(A\text{-}a)\ PO_2 = 2.5 + 0.21 \times \text{age (yr)}$

In the supine position, $PaO_2 = 103.5 - 0.42 \times \text{age (yr)}$

It is important to remember that there are disorders in which $\dot{V}/\dot{Q}$ mismatch, hypoxemia, and an elevated (A-a) PO_2 gradient occur only in a specific body position (see Chapter 28, "Dyspnea").

Abnormal Gas Exchange

An abnormality in gas exchange is identified by the presence of arterial hypoxemia or hypercapnia. Blood gas analysis helps to distinguish pulmonary from extrapulmonary disorders. Lung diseases are often associated with $\dot{V}/\dot{Q}$ mismatch as identified by an increase in the (A-a) PO_2 gradient. On the other hand, disorders of the respiratory pump (central drive, neuromuscular breathing apparatus, chest wall) lead to a decrease in the bulk flow of gas to and from the lungs, hypoxemia, and hypercapnia, but the (A-a) PO_2 gradient remains normal unless a pulmonary complication such as atelectasis arises.

In the following section, the differential diagnosis between $\dot{V}/\dot{Q}$ mismatch and right-to-left shunt as well as their impact on gas exchange are discussed.

Ventilation/Perfusion Mismatch

The nonlinear relation between arterial oxygen content and PaO_2 (oxyhemoglobin dissociation curve) explains why $\dot{V}/\dot{Q}$ mismatch leads to hypoxemia. Blood draining from a region of the lung that is underventilated relative to its perfusion (low $\dot{V}/\dot{Q}$) will have both a low PO_2 and a low O_2 content. Blood arising from lung units with excessive ventilation for the amount of perfusion (high $\dot{V}/\dot{Q}$) will have a higher than normal PO_2 but only a minimal improvement, if any, in O_2 content. This is due to the sigmoid shape of the oxyhemoglobin dissociation curve, which illustrates that there is relatively little increase in O_2 content above Po_2 values of 70 mm Hg. Consequently, areas of low $\dot{V}/\dot{Q}$ decrease the oxygen transfer into the blood far more than areas of high $\dot{V}/\dot{Q}$ mismatch increase it. The overall net result is that the PaO_2 is decreased and the (A-a) Po_2 gradient is increased.

CO_2 elimination is also affected by low $\dot{V}/\dot{Q}$ mismatch. In contrast to oxygen transfer, however, increasing bulk flow to units with normal or high $\dot{V}/\dot{Q}$ mismatch will augment CO_2 elimination further, because the CO_2 hemoglobin dissociation curve is nearly linear. This explains why patients with lung disease and $\dot{V}/\dot{Q}$ mismatch have normal or even lower than normal arterial CO_2 tensions until late in the course of their disease.

Right-to-Left Shunting

Right-to-left shunting refers to mixed venous (deoxygenated) blood going directly into the systemic arterial circulation without first being exposed to alveolar gas. This represents the most severe degree of $\dot{V}/\dot{Q}$ mismatch ($\dot{V}/\dot{Q} = 0$); therefore, it must also lead to hypoxemia and an increase in the (A-a) Po_2 gradient. There are three basic types of right-to-left shunts: (1) cardiac or great vessel, (2) pulmonary vascular, and (3) pulmonary parenchymal. A right-to-left shunt with abnormal communication between systemic and pulmonary circulation requires, in most instances, the presence of pulmonary hypertension. If shunting occurs on a pulmonary vascular level, it is usually related to an arteriovenous malformation. Finally, pulmonary parenchymal shunts will occur whenever blood goes through the normal pulmonary circulation channels, but the surrounding alveoli are either collapsed or filled with something other than gas (i.e., edema in the adult respiratory distress syndrome).

Hypoxemia from right-to-left shunts ($\dot{V}/\dot{Q} = 0$) can be differentiated from that due to $\dot{V}/\dot{Q}$ mismatch ($\dot{V}/\dot{Q}$ is low but greater than 0) by the administration of 100 percent O_2. In patients with lung disease and $\dot{V}/\dot{Q}$ mismatch, supplemental O_2 will increase the P_AO_2 of low $\dot{V}/\dot{Q}$ areas; therefore, an increase in PaO_2 is to be expected. In cardiac and great vessel as well as pulmonary vascular right-to-left shunts, where blood totally bypasses alveolar gas, an improvement in P_AO_2 cannot result in an increase in PaO_2. Finally, if part of the lung parenchyma is totally excluded from ventilation (i.e., lobar collapse, pulmonary edema, and so forth), supplemental oxygen cannot reach these zero $\dot{V}/\dot{Q}$ regions and PaO_2 remains relatively unchanged. Therefore, if 100 percent O_2 alleviates hypoxemia, $\dot{V}/\dot{Q}$ mismatch and lung disease are present. If it has no impact on the arterial oxygenation, a right-to-left shunt must be sought.

Alveolar Hypoventilation

Alveolar hypoventilation is defined as a decrease in alveolar ventilation for a given level of CO_2 production ($\dot{V}co_2$). A decrease in alveolar ventilation leads to a proportional increase in the $PaCO_2$ and therefore hypercapnia. Thus, alveolar hypoventilation implies hypercapnia and vice versa. Patients with lung disease and $\dot{V}/\dot{Q}$ mismatch often are able to maintain a normal $PaCO_2$ at the expense of increasing bulk flow (minute ventilation) and work of breathing. As the illness progresses, the increasing ventilatory demand cannot be met and alveolar hypoventilation is present despite large increases in minute ventilation. The diagnosis of alveolar hypoventilation and lung disease is readily established when an increase in the (A-a) Po_2 gradient is associated with hypercapnia.

Alveolar hypoventilation in the absence of $\dot{V}/\dot{Q}$ mismatch is indicative of disease of the respiratory pump (i.e., the central drive, the neuromuscular breathing apparatus, or the chest wall), but not the lung. In contrast to lung disease, the volume of gas entering the alveoli is less than normal and the diagnosis can be readily suspected by the presence of a normal (A-a) Po_2 gradient.

Hypoxemia

Five basic conditions can cause hypoxemia: (1) a low P_IO_2, (2) alveolar hypoventilation, (3) $\dot{V}/\dot{Q}$ mismatch, (4) right-to-left shunts, and (5) diffusion impairment. A low P_IO_2 and diffusion impairment are uncommon clinical problems. From the alveolar air equation it is clear that at constant P_IO_2 and R values, any increase in the $PaCO_2$ (alveolar hypoventilation) must lead to a fall in the P_AO_2. This in turn results in a lowered arterial oxygen tension.

In the evaluation of a patient with hypoxemia, the presence of alveolar hypoventilation can be assessed by the mere inspection of the $PaCO_2$. If it is normal, an increase in the (A-a) Po_2 gradient is present and $\dot{V}/\dot{Q}$ mismatch or right-to-left shunt must be suspected. When the $PaCO_2$ is increased but the (A-a) Po_2 gradient is normal, a disorder of the respiratory pump is present. If the (A-a) Po_2 gradient is also increased, $\dot{V}/\dot{Q}$ mismatch or right-to-left shunts must be contributing to the hypoxemia.

Respiratory Acid-Base Balance

Acid-base balance is clinically assessed from the arterial hydrogen ion (H^+) concentration. It can be expressed in nanoequivalents per liter (nEq/L) or as a negative logarithm thereof (pH_a). Table 115-1 shows how to estimate values of H^+ from pH over the physiologic range. Fortuitously, an H^+ concentration of 40 nEq/L corresponds to a pH of 7.40; moreover, for each 0.01 change in the pH, there is approximately a 1 nEq/L change in the H^+ concentration in the opposite direction.

The H^+ concentration is uniquely determined by the ratio between bicarbonate (HCO_3^-) and carbonic acid (H_2CO_3); i.e., $H^+ = H_2CO_3/HCO_3^-$ or $H^+ = K\,H_2CO_3/HCO_3^-$, where K is the dissociation constant for the reaction $H_2CO_3/H^+ + HCO_3^-$. Because $H_2CO_3 = 0.03 \times PaCO_2$, we can substitute for H_2CO_3 and write the Henderson version of the Henderson-Hasselbalch equation:

$$H^+ = 24 \times \frac{PaCO_2}{HCO_3}$$

It reflects the net availability of acid versus base and the resulting H^+ concentration in the body. $PaCO_2$ represents the acid level, whereas HCO_3^- is an index of the availability of base. Clinically, all acid-base disorders can be evaluated in terms of this basic equation.

In the description of an acid-base disturbance, it should be determined whether it is (1) a respiratory or metabolic disturbance, (2) a simple or a complicated disturbance, and (3) an acute or chronic process. A respiratory disturbance primarily affects the $PaCO_2$, whereas a metabolic disturbance alters the bicarbonate concentration. The simple disorder is characterized by a primary change in only one parameter, whereas a complicated or mixed disorder is characterized by a primary change in

Table 115-1 Relationship Between H^+ and pH

pH	True [H^+]	Estimated [H^+]*
7.1	79	70
7.2	63	60
7.3	50	50
7.35	45	45
7.4	40	40
7.5	32	30

* The H^+ concentration can be estimated by assuming a 1 nEq/L change in H^+ for each 0.01 change in pH.

Table 115-2 Respiratory Acid-Base Disorders

	Normal	Respiratory acidosis		Respiratory alkalosis	
		Acute	*Chronic*	*Acute*	*Chronic*
pH	7.40	7.24	7.34	7.48	7.42
H^+	40	56	46	32	38
$PaCO_2$	40	60	60	30	30
HCO_3^-	24	26	30	22	19
$\Delta H^+/\Delta PaCO_2$	—	16/20 = 0.8	6/20 = 0.3	8/10 = 0.8	2/10 = 0.2

both. An acute process is measured in minutes to hours, whereas a chronic process is measured in days to weeks or longer. The rest of this discussion is concerned only with primary respiratory disorders.

Respiratory Acidosis

Respiratory acidosis is the result of a disturbance of CO_2 elimination by the respiratory system. As the $PaCO_2$ increases, CO_2 enters red blood cells, where it combines with water under the influence of carbonic anhydrase to form carbonic acid. As carbonic acid dissociates, bicarbonate ions diffuse out of the cells into the plasma. Therefore, each 10 mm Hg increase in $PaCO_2$ is accompanied by a 2 mEq/L increase in the serum bicarbonate concentration. The H^+ concentration, which is uniquely determined by $PaCO_2$ and bicarbonate through the Henderson-Hasselbalch equation, concomitantly increases by 8 nEq/L. An acute respiratory acidosis is therefore present when the ratio of the change in H^+ concentration (ΔH^+) per change in $PaCO_2$ ($\Delta PaCO_2$) approximates 0.8 (see Table 115-2 for a specific example).

If the primary disturbance (i.e., CO_2 retention) persists, a metabolic compensation in the form of bicarbonate retention by the kidneys follows. This compensation becomes clinically apparent after 12 hours and is usually complete by 48 hours. Its net effect is to restore the ratio between $PaCO_2$ and bicarbonate and thus the pH toward normal. Therefore, in chronic respiratory disorders with CO_2 retention, the ratio of the $\Delta H^+/\Delta PaCO_2$ approaches 0.3 (see Table 115-2).

The clinical implication of the simple differentiation between acute and chronic respiratory acidosis is profound. Whereas the former implies an acute, potentially life-threatening process and therefore demands immediate therapeutic intervention, the latter indicates that the disturbance has been present for days, that a new steady state between $PaCO_2$ and the overall CO_2 excretion has been achieved, and that immediate therapeutic intervention will not be necessary. The importance of this differentiation cannot be overemphasized.

Table 115-3 Causes of Respiratory Acidosis*

Normal (A-a) Po_2 gradient	Elevated (A-a) Po_2 gradient
Central Nervous System Disorders	**Intrinsic Lung Diseases**
Drug overdose	Chronic obstructive pulmonary disease
Primary hypoventilation	Asthma
Myxedema	Cystic fibrosis
Spinal cord disease	Interstitial fibrosis
Peripheral Nervous System Disorders	**Chest Wall and Combined Lung Diseases**
Guillain-Barré syndrome	Scoliosis
Amyotrophic lateral sclerosis	
Post-poliomyelitis	
Multiple sclerosis	
Myasthenia gravis	
Botulism	
Chest Wall Disorders	
Thoracoplasty	
Ankylosing spondylitis	
Respiratory Muscle Disorders	
Polymyositis	
Muscular dystrophy	
Upper Airway Obstruction	
Epiglottitis	
Laryngeal disorders	
Tracheal stenosis	

* This is not an all-inclusive list, but it demonstrates the concept of dividing the causes of respiratory acidosis into those with a normal and those with an elevated (A-a) Po_2 gradient.

Differential Diagnosis of Respiratory Acidosis

As discussed in the chapter on respiratory failure and again summarized in Table 115-3, disorders of the respiratory system can be divided into those of the lung and those of the respiratory pump. As discussed previously, the (A-a) Po_2 gradient will usually differentiate those two broad categories. For further discussion of this topic, refer to Chapter 120, "Respiratory Failure."

Respiratory Alkalosis

In primary respiratory alkalosis, the $PaCO_2$ is decreased with an accompanying compensatory decrease in the bicarbonate level. Acute respiratory alkalosis decreases the arterial bicarbonate concentration by approximately 2 mEq/L for every 10 mm Hg

Table 115-4 Causes of Respiratory Alkalosis

Normal (A-a) Po_2 gradient	Elevated (A-a) Po_2 gradient
Central nervous system disorders	Gram-negative sepsis
Hormones and drugs	Endotoxemia
Salicylates	Hepatic failure
Catecholamines	Interstitial lung diseases
Progesterone	Pulmonary edema
Analeptic overdose	Pulmonary emboli
Thyroid hormone excess	Pneumonia
Pregnancy	Asthma
High altitude	Mechanical overventilation of abnormal lungs
Severe anemia	
Psychogenic hyperventilation	
Endotoxemia	
Mechanical overventilation of normal lungs	

decline in the $PaCO_2$. At the same time, the H^+ concentration falls by 8 nEq/L, such that the ratio of $\Delta H^+/\Delta PaCO_2$ approximates 0.8 (see Table 115-2).

The metabolic response, which may take up to 2 weeks to complete, is one of renal bicarbonate wasting. Chronic respiratory alkalosis is the only primary acid-base disorder in which the H^+ concentration and therefore pH_A is returned to normal by the compensatory metabolic action. In all other primary disorders, compensation tends to have a corrective action on the pH but is unable to normalize the H^+ concentration totally. In the case of chronic respiratory alkalosis, the $\Delta H^+/\Delta PaCO_2$ approximates 0.17 to 0.2 (see Table 115-2).

The causes of acute and chronic respiratory alkalosis are shown in Table 115-4. They can be divided primarily into those associated with lung disease and those not associated with lung disease, a categorization that can be made with the help of the (A-a) Po_2 gradient.

References

Narins RG, Emmett M. Simple and mixed acid-base disorders: A practical approach. Medicine 1980; 59:161.

Sorkin B, Goldring RM. Arterial blood gases: Hypoxemia and acid-base balance. In: Miller A, ed. Pulmonary function tests in clinical and occupational lung disease. New York: Grune & Stratton, 1986.

Stewart PA. Modern quantitative acid-base chemistry. Can J Physiol Pharmacol 1983; 61:1444.

Taylor AE, et al. Regulation of acid-base balance. In: Clinical respiratory physiology. Philadelphia: WB Saunders, 1989:239.

Clubbing

Earle B. Weiss, MD

116

Definition

Acquired or hereditary distal clubbing (Hippocratic fingers) is a physical sign characterized by a usually painless, bulbous enlargement of the distal digit of the fingers and at times the toes, accompanied by a softening of the nail bed. Pathologically, the major components of simple clubbing are a fibrous tissue hyperplasia in the segment between the nail and phalanx with lymphocytic extravasation, increased vascularity, and edema. The result is a decrease in the normal obtuse angle between the proximal soft tissue and the nail itself. This phenomenon, although relatively innocuous in itself, is important because its presence may signify a serious underlying disease, and its regression or progression may have important prognostic implications.

History

Typically, the early symptoms and signs of acquired clubbing are overlooked because of their subtle, insidious onset. Hence, digital deformation is generally observed by the physician and not the patient. In rare instances of acute clubbing, as seen with lung cancer or suppurative diseases, unusual tenderness or frank bulbous digital deformity may alert the patient to seek medical advice. Concurrent disease may exist even in severe form without clubbing or hypertrophic pulmonary osteoarthropathy (see later in this chapter); occasionally, acropachy (clubbing) may precede the disorder.

Examination and Measurement

The usual clinical method of diagnosing clubbing, aside from a softening and sponginess of the nail bed, is to measure the angle,

Supported by The Foundation for Research in Bronchial Asthma.

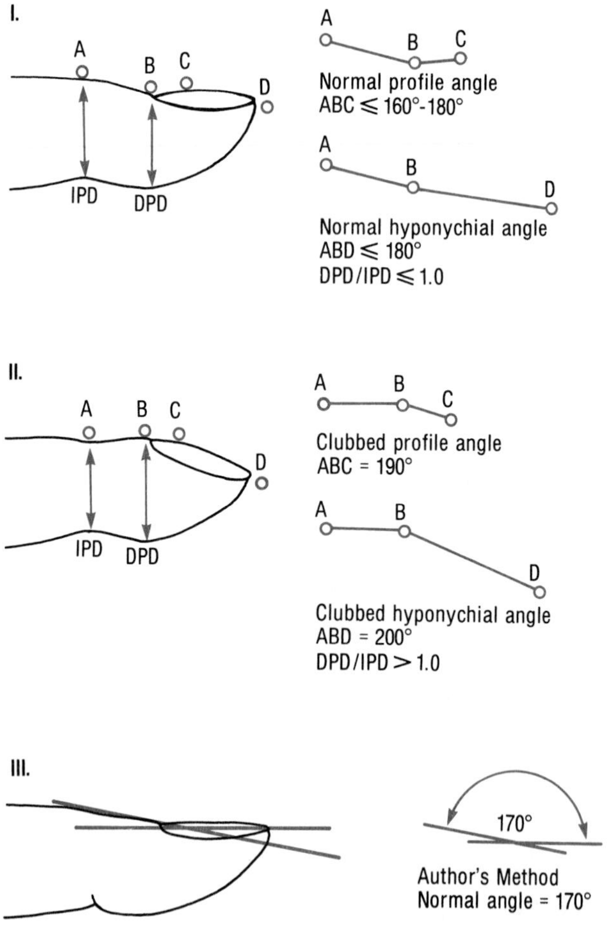

Figure 116-1 Measurement of clubbing. DPD = distal phalangeal depth, IPD = interphalangeal depth.

viewed laterally, described by the base of the nail and the adjacent dorsal surface of the terminal phalanx, the so-called base or profile angle (Fig. 116-1). Coexistent contiguous erythema, warmth, bulk of the terminal tuft, or increased nail curvature is not a sufficient criterion in itself. Normally, this angle is cited to be approximately 160 degrees, although no study has ever validated normal variations by this usual method of visual inspection. Angles greater than 180 degrees are generally considered abnormal. Nonetheless, visual estimates of this angle are largely subjective and therefore unreliable.

Using the following simple bedside method, however, it is possible to obtain accurate and reproducible measurements of the base angle. An affected digit is positioned firmly with its side on a piece of paper. A sharp-tipped pencil is then placed at the base of the finger and, while continuous pressure is applied along the finger tissue, the entire digit is outlined and the nail-proximal digit tissue edge noted. The resulting outline is then easily transcribed into two planes of nail and distal tissue base, from which the base angle can be directly measured. Normal profile angle values observed are similar to those obtained with other techniques: 172.7 degrees ± 4.1 degrees.

Several other features of the clubbing process may be noteworthy. Whereas advanced clubbing generally involves all fingers and toes, the early evolution begins in the thumb and index finger. Other associated physical examination findings include an increase in the nail curvature in coronal and longitudinal

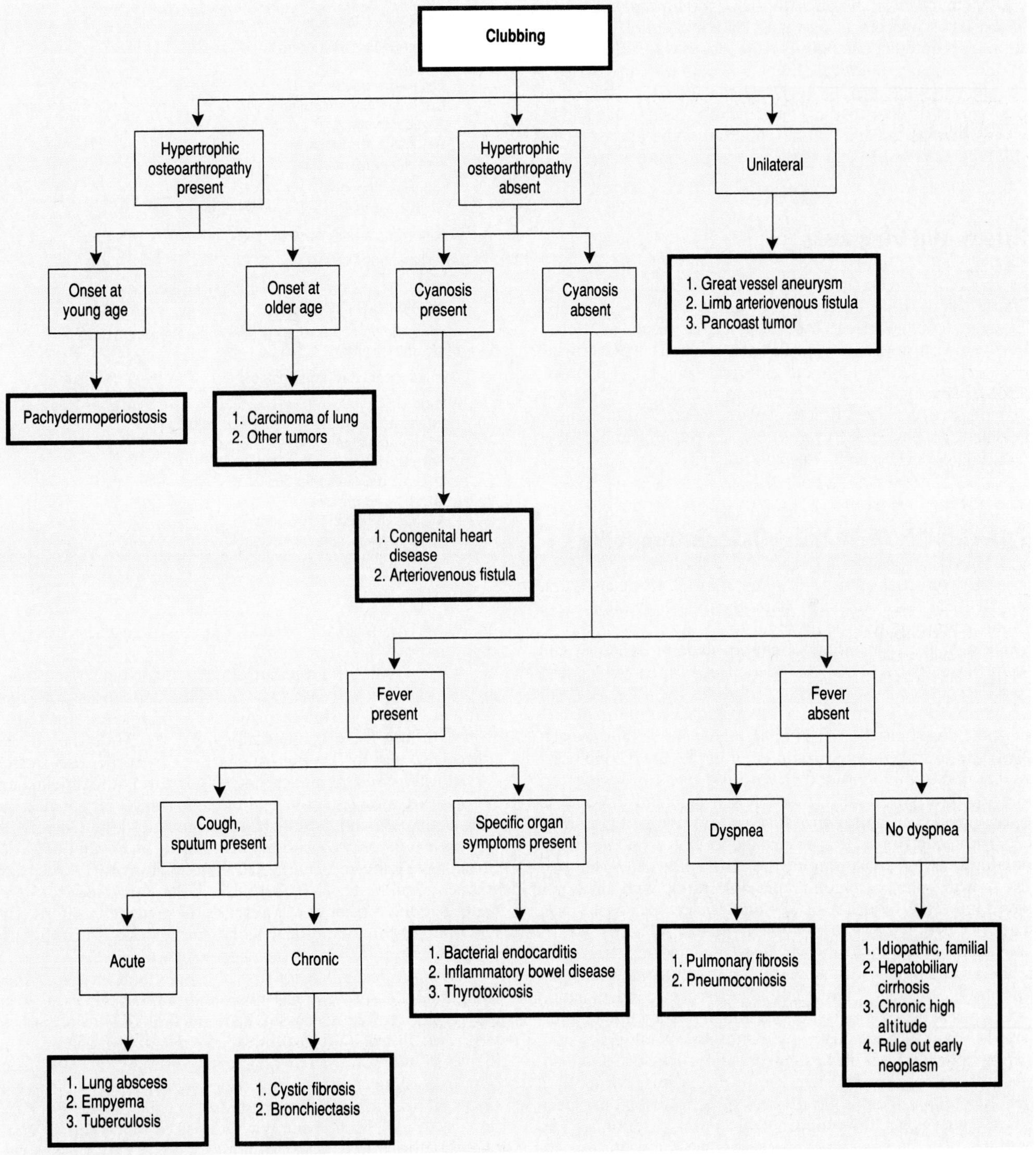

Figure 116-2 Algorithm for the diagnostic evaluation of clubbing.

planes. Also distinctive is an increased mobility of the nail on its bed such that the affected nail can be easily rocked by applying alternating pressure to the base and tip. (A degree of experience is required to distinguish pathologic from normal "rocking" motions.)

Etiology

The etiology of clubbing is always determined by precisely defining the causative clinical disorder (Fig. 116-2). In general, the degree of clubbing parallels the severity of the pulmonary disease; it may abate if the underlying disorder regresses. It is usually symmetric in distribution, but in certain congenital heart diseases the process is asymmetric. For example, only toe clubbing is noted in patent ductus arteriosus with a shunt reversal. Interestingly, unilateral clubbing occurs with aneurysms of the great thoracic vessels (e.g., subclavian artery, aorta), arteriovenous fistulae in the affected limb, ipsilateral Pancoast tumors, hemiplegia, and trauma. Tuberculosis, unless associated with empyema or bronchiectasis, is not a common cause.

Differential Diagnosis

Because of its diagnostic implications, this condition should be differentiated from other finger abnormalities: (1) simple "breaking" or curvature of the nail, a normal variant; (2) Heberden's osteoarthritic nodes; (3) chronic infectious digital arthritis with periarticular swelling and a normal nail bed; (4) chronic paronychia and felons; (5) epidermoid cysts of the osseous phalanges; (6) acromegalic bony enlargement; (7) posthemiplegic digital atrophy; and (8) acrosteolysis, a pseudoclubbing seen in people who work with vinyl chloride.

Table 116-1 Diseases Associated with Digital Clubbing

Idiopathic, familial
Acquired diseases
Heart disease
Cyanotic (congenital)
Bacterial endocarditis
Lung disease
Carcinoma of lung or pleura
Bronchiectasis
Lung abscess
Empyema
Tuberculosis (typically with apical bronchiectasis)
Pulmonary fibrosis, pneumoconiosis
Cystic fibrosis
Alveolar proteinosis
Gastrointestinal disorders
Regional enteritis
Ulcerative colitis
Cirrhosis (hepatic, biliary)
Amebic dysentery
Achalasia, peptic ulcer
Hepatic amyloidosis
Endocrine disorders
Thyrotoxicosis (thyroid acropachy)
Any chronic suppurative process
Arteriovenous fistulae
Rarer: repeated pregnancies, purgative abuse, syphilis, hemiplegic limbs
Hypertrophic osteoarthropathy (Marie-Bamberger syndrome)
Idiopathic
Familial pachydermoperiostosis
Acquired
Lung cancer (primary or metastatic to)
Pleural, especially mesothelioma
Thymus, thyroid carcinoma
Leiomyoma of esophagus
Thoracic lymphoma
Nasopharyngeal carcinoma
Chronic myelogenous leukemia

Hypertrophic Pulmonary Osteoarthropathy

Secondary or acquired hypertrophic pulmonary osteoarthropathy (HPO), also known as the Marie-Bamberger syndrome, is a distinct entity and must be distinguished from simple clubbing, with which it is commonly confused. Acquired HPO usually occurs in certain visceral disorders, but bronchogenic carcinoma accounts for 90 percent of all cases (Table 116-1). Pulmonary metastases rarely cause HPO. Digital clubbing may or may not be associated with HPO, although it is generally present. Digital perfusion patterns are different in these two conditions; in acquired clubbing, blood flow to the digits is augmented, whereas in acquired HPO, blood flow is shunted through arteriovenous communications to the sites of osteoarthropathy.

The syndrome of HPO occurs in 4 to 12 percent of patients with lung carcinoma, commonly with the epidermoid cell type, less so with adenocarcinoma, and only rarely with small cell carcinoma. HPO consists of a symmetric neoperiostitis with subperiosteal new bone formation in the distal diaphysis of the long bones of the forearms and legs (ulna and radius, 80 percent; tibia and fibula, 70 to 80 percent) and occasionally metacarpals and metatarsals. There is also a periarticular inflammation with synovial hypertrophy and joint effusion. The periosteum is raised by a new bone matrix and subsequent mineralization. Radiographically, this new subperiosteal bone formation appears as a thin layer separated from the normal cortex by a radiolucent line. Coexisting features of neurovasomotor instability include episodic swelling and blanching, diaphoresis, and paresthesia of the hands and feet. Pain is the chief clinical complaint as a result of these pathologic changes in the affected ankles, wrists, or tibiae. If digital clubbing coexists, it too is quite painful.

Occasionally, the osteoarthropathy involving wrists, knees, ankles, or elbows presents with swelling, tenderness, morning stiffness, and ankylosing deformities that mimic rheumatoid arthritis. In fact, these manifestations may resemble rheumatoid arthritis so closely that the patient may be erroneously treated for arthritis while the underlying osteoarthropathy remains unrecognized. However, the typical radiographic appearance of long bone periostitis is sufficiently diagnostic, if not essential, to distinguish these two entities. Furthermore, synovial fluid from the affected joints in HPO reveals a noninflammatory fluid that is sparse in leukocytes ($<2{,}000/mm^3$) and neutrophils (<15 percent), serving further to differentiate these two conditions. The tendency of this noninflammatory fluid to clot is also a fairly distinctive feature of pulmonary osteoarthropathy.

In some patients, exquisite periosteal tenderness elicited by manual pressure over the involved distal bones is a clue to an underlying remote neoplasm. Radionuclide Tc-99m phosphate bone scans reveal a typical linear isotopic accumulation along the periosteum of distal diaphyses that distinguishes HPO from bony metastases (with central or focal radiotracer density) in cases of carcinoma. Scans may also permit diagnosis of the process in patients presenting with early or vague clinical complaints before the characteristic conventional radiologic changes develop.

Primary or Familial Disorders

Secondary (acquired) clubbing and HPO are unrelated to two other rarer, but distinguishable, conditions: pachydermoperiostosis and primary or familial clubbing. Neither disorder is currently known to be associated with any underlying systemic disease.

Pachydermoperiostosis is a familial process (autosomal dominant) characterized by painless clubbing and HPO and particularly coarse facial features with deep furrowing of nasolabial and forehead folds. Hyperhidrosis in these sites is typical. The disorder usually appears at puberty and progresses insidiously for about a decade before becoming stationary. Often, a grotesque deformity of the fingers and toes accompanies the clubbing process. Early osseous changes identical with HPO are limited to the distal portions of long tubular bones, metacarpals, and metatarsals; later, all bones except the skull become affected.

Primary or hereditofamilial clubbing, which may occur in the absence of HPO, appears simply in the first or second decade of life, having been transmitted as an autosomal dominant process with low expression. It is not associated with an increased capillary circulation.

References

Coury C. Hippocratic fingers and hypertrophic osteoarthropathy. Br J Dis Chest 1960; 54:202.

Epstein O, Adjukiewicz AB, Dick R. Hypertrophic hepatic osteoarthropathy. Am J Med 1979; 67:88.

Fisher DS, Singer DH, Feldman SM. Clubbing: A review with emphasis on hereditary acropachy. Medicine (Baltimore) 1964; 43:459.

Hansen-Flaschen J, Nordberg J. Clubbing and hypertrophic osteoarthropathy. Clin Chest Med 1987; 8:287.

Lemen RJ, et al. Relationship among digital clubbing, disease severity, and serum prostaglandins F_2 and E concentrations in cystic fibrosis patients. Am Rev Respir Dis 1978; 117:639.

Lovibond JL. Diagnosis of clubbed fingers. Lancet 1983; 1:363.

Schumacher HR Jr. Articular manifestations of hypertrophic pulmonary osteoarthropathy in bronchogenic carcinoma: A clinical and pathological study. Arthritis Rheum 1976; 19:629.

Cough

117

Rolf D. Hubmayr, MD

Richard S. Irwin, MD

Pulmonary

Definition

To cough is to expel air from the lungs suddenly, usually in a series of efforts, with an explosive noise made by the opening of the glottis. Chronic persistent cough, one that is troublesome and present for more than 3 weeks, is never seen in healthy subjects; therefore, it is an important sign of disease. Cough may be initiated voluntarily or through reflexes triggered by irritation of receptors located in the nose, paranasal sinuses, pharynx, ear canals and drums, pleura, stomach, pericardium and diaphragm, and the tracheobronchial tree. Its physiologic significance is to protect the respiratory tract from foreign bodies and aid in lung clearance when the normal mucociliary defense mechanisms are overwhelmed.

On the other hand, cough may be harmful by causing adverse effects. For instance, syncope may be caused by cough. Although it is seen most commonly in men with obstructive lung disease, who generate intrathoracic pressures in excess of 300 cm H_2O, syncope has also been reported in children with asthma. The mechanical and neurally mediated consequences of cough, a modified Valsalva maneuver, are arterial hypotension and an increase in the cerebrospinal fluid pressure that, in its extreme form, may lead to cerebral hypoperfusion and loss of consciousness, e.g., cough syncope. Pneumothorax and mediastinal emphysema are other well-known complications of cough. Lastly, musculoskeletal pain and fractures of ribs may be consequences of coughing spells, particularly in the elderly.

Causes of Chronic Persistent Cough

Chronic persistent cough can be produced by a multiplicity of diseases affecting a variety of anatomic locations. Although virtually any process that stimulates cough receptors or afferent nervous pathways is capable of producing cough, common causes of chronic persistent cough, which account for over 90 percent of all patients seen, can be discussed under four general headings. Moreover, it is not unusual to identify more than one cause of chronic persistent cough in a given patient.

It is useful when confronted with the individual patient to answer four general questions:

1. Is the patient a cigarette smoker?
2. Does the patient have a postnasal drip?
3. Is there evidence of bronchial hyperreactivity?
4. Does the patient suffer from gastroesophageal reflux or aspiration?

Cigarette smoking is probably the most common cause of chronic persistent cough. Although the true incidence of the association between cough and smoking is unknown, direct counting of coughs has shown that individuals who smoke during a period of observation cough twice as often as those who do not smoke. In most large series, however, less than 50 percent of patients were smokers or ex-smokers. The selection bias and the tolerance of the smoker to the symptom cough are likely responsible for the underestimation of the true incidence in the literature.

Smoke may lead to cough by a variety of mechanisms. It can act as a nonspecific irritant to stimulate cough receptors and afferent nervous pathways or induce inflammatory changes in the mucosa of the respiratory tract. This in turn may cause mucous hypersecretion and its clinical correlates in lower and upper airways, chronic bronchitis and postnasal drip.

The majority of nonsmokers presenting with chronic persistent cough show evidence of a postnasal drip. It can be diagnosed when a patient describes a sensation of having something drip down into the throat or the need to clear the throat frequently, and when the physical examination of the nasopharynx and oropharynx reveals mucoid or mucopurulent secretions or a cobblestone appearance of the mucosa. In one large series, postnasal drip or asthma accounted for 72 percent of causes of persistent cough in adults. Postnasal drip can be found in persons with seasonal or perennial rhinitis, chronic sinusitis, and obstruction of the nasopharynx by enlarged adenoids. It is probably the common pathophysiologic mechanism of cough in a variety of diseases involving the nasopharynx.

Cough may be the only presenting symptom of diseases associated with hyperreactive airways. Bronchial hyperreactivity, as defined by an abnormal response to inhalation of bronchodilators or cholinergic agents, is typically seen in symptomatic asthmatics. However, a variety of insults may also render the airways hyperreactive. For instance, bronchial hyperreactivity has been described for as long as 2 months following viral infections of the respiratory tract and after inhalation of ozone.

Gastroesophageal reflux was responsible for persistent cough in 10 percent of all patients in one large series. In such cases, cough may be due to three mechanisms: (1) reflux of acid stomach contents may damage the esophageal mucosa and initiate cough by reflex activation of vagal pathways within the esophagus; (2) gastric contents may be inhaled and irritate receptors within the tracheobronchial tree; and (3) chronic aspiration may lead to chemical lung injury with fibrosis and concomitant increase in elastic recoil. This may initiate the cough reflex by activation of receptors within the lung parenchyma.

Having accounted for more than 90 percent of all causes, the remaining list of disorders associated with cough includes virtually all diseases of the cardiovascular and respiratory systems. A few deserve to be mentioned specifically. In rare cases bronchogenic carcinoma has chronic cough as its sole manifestation. This probably also holds true for respiratory tract infections with fungi and *Mycobacterium tuberculosis.* On the other hand, it is important to recognize that congestive heart failure can lead to troublesome cough in the absence of lung disease. Some rather unusual causes of cough have been described in the literature. They include osteophytes of the cervical spine, aneurysm of the ascending palatine artery, neurilemmoma of the vagus nerve, lobar sequestration, and hairs touching the tympanic membrane. It is important to note that psychogenic or habit cough is a rare condition.

Diagnostic Approach

If one systematically evaluates location of receptors and afferent nervous pathways that initiate the cough reflex, one should almost always be able to come to a specific diagnosis. Specific treatment will almost always be successful. Therefore, disappearance of cough with specific treatment is required to confirm one's initial diagnostic impression. In 80 percent of cases, the history alone will strongly suggest the diagnosis and also determine the appropriate use of laboratory tests.

Obviously, the smoker should be asked to discontinue his or her habit. Cessation of smoking is in a sense a diagnostic test as well as a form of specific therapy. In one study, 77 percent of smokers with a bronchial cough were free of symptoms when they stopped smoking—54 percent within 4 weeks. If cough persists or has been of recent onset, the presence of an endobronchial lesion, particularly carcinoma, should be strongly considered. Chest radiograph, sputum cytology, and flexible fiberoptic bronchoscopy are useful in this setting. A careful examination of ears, nose, and throat is also imperative. Remember that malignant cells found in sputum may indicate a carcinoma arising from the epiglottis or larynx in addition to the bronchi. Finally, it is important to screen for and quantitate any degree of pulmonary function impairment with spirometry and look for associated hyperreactive airways disease. Table 117-1 lists tests that are useful in the evaluation of the patient with cough.

It is extremely helpful to ask the patient to demonstrate what he or she means by cough. Frequently, the presence of throat clearing may point to postnasal drip. The physical examination might demonstrate phlegm in the back of the oropharynx. Inspection of the nose, transillumination of paranasal sinuses, and indirect laryngoscopy should rule out structural lesions such as polyps, enlarged adenoids, and tumors of the epiglottis and larynx. If sinusitis is suspected, radiographs of the paranasal sinuses may show mucosal thickening or air-fluid levels.

Another important piece of information concerns the timing of coughing spells. If the cough awakens the patient at night, it not only underscores the severity of the patient's complaint but may also point to nocturnal asthma, bronchiectasis, congestion of the lungs due to heart failure, or gastroesophageal reflux with aspiration. Asthma in a classic setting with episodic cough, wheezing, and dyspnea associated with a family history of asthma, hay fever, eczema, and exacerbation of symptoms in winter and during exercise should be easy to diagnose from history alone. The presence of blood and sputum eosinophilia may further support the diagnosis of asthma.

As pointed out previously, the common denominator of all diseases associated with hyperreactive airways, including asthma, is a reversible increase in expiratory flow demonstrated by spirometry. The patient is asked to perform a maximal, forced expiratory effort, and the volumes of air exhaled over the first second (FEV_1) and the entire vital capacity (FVC) are measured. A reduction in FEV_1/FVC ratio indicates airway obstruction, and the test is repeated after inhalation of a bronchodilator such as isoproterenol. An increase of more than 20 percent in the FEV_1 indicates reversibility of airway obstruction. A number of patients with hyperreactive airways disease, however, have normal or near-normal flows on baseline spirometry. Further improvement in expiratory flows following use of bronchodilators can therefore not be expected. In this population, the demonstration of hyperreactive airways rests on the provocation of airflow obstruction by inhalation of agents such as methacholine, a cholinergic agonist. After each incremental dose given as an

Table 117-1 Tests Useful in the Evaluation of the Patient with Cough

Complete blood count with differential blood count
Sputum examination for cytology
Acid-fast organisms
Fungi
Eosinophils, parasites
Radiograph of the chest
Radiograph of the paranasal sinuses
Gastrointestinal contrast studies
Esophagoscopy
Flexible fiberoptic bronchoscopy
Spirometry
With bronchodilators
With methacholine challenge

aerosol, spirometry is repeated. The test is terminated and regarded as positive if a reduction of more than 20 percent in the FEV_1 has occurred. Otherwise, it is carried out until a maximum dose of 195 dose units has been given. If a 20 percent reduction does not occur after 195 dose units, hyperreactive airways and asthma are not present.

Gastroesophageal reflux is probably the most difficult diagnosis to establish among the disorders commonly causing cough. This relates to the frequency of heartburn, the fact that gastroesophageal reflux is a common finding in healthy individuals, and the low sensitivity and specificity of laboratory tests at hand. Nevertheless, it is useful to examine a barium swallow for functional and anatomic disturbances of the upper gastrointestinal tract and to screen specifically for reflux of barium from stomach to esophagus. It is also possible to perform endoscopy with manometry and to pass a pH electrode into the lower third of the esophagus to look for acidity indicative of reflux.

There are patients in whom neither history, physical examination, nor chest radiograph provides a strong clue concerning the diagnosis. The most useful diagnostic tests in this setting are pulmonary function studies. The literature indicates that in as many as 40 percent of these patients, previously undiagnosed hyperreactive airways disease is found. It is much less clear how one should proceed if pulmonary function test results are normal. Aside from a general medical evaluation, these patients should have a detailed examination of ears, nose, and throat and probably should undergo fiberoptic bronchoscopy. Despite its low yield, bronchoscopy may reveal the presence of an endobronchial adenoma, a type of tumor that may grow rather slowly and not be apparent on radiographs. If the diagnosis is still in question, consider a detailed cardiac evaluation as well as an extensive gastrointestinal work-up before diagnosing psychogenic or habit cough.

References

Irwin RS, Rosen MJ, Braman SS. Cough: A comprehensive review. Arch Intern Med 1977; 137:1186.

Leith DE. Cough. In: Brain JD, et al, eds. Lung biology in health and disease. Vol 5. Respiratory defense mechanisms. Part 2. New York: Marcel Dekker, 1977:545.

SantAmbrogio G. Afferent pathways for the cough reflex. Bull Eur Physiopathol Respir 1987; 23(Suppl 10):19s.

The Breathless Patient

118

Rolf D. Hubmayr, MD

Richard S. Irwin, MD

Pulmonary

Definition

Shortness of breath (dyspnea) is a subjective complaint; therefore, different patients may describe it differently. To one, it may mean not being able to take a deep breath; to another, it feels like having to breathe too much; to a third, it simply means being uncomfortable during breathing. Some patients are breathless all the time, whereas others may experience shortness of breath only at rest, during exertion, or when lying down. Although there is no known specific peripheral receptor, neural pathway, or cortical location for the sensation of dyspnea, it is useful to consider the control of ventilation in understanding the neuropathophysiology of dyspnea.

Respiration can be thought of as being governed by a respiratory center (controller) that receives inputs from chemo- and mechanoreceptors of the cardiovascular and external respiratory systems (Table 118-1). Anatomically consisting of neuronal complexes within the upper brain stem, the controller is also connected to higher cortical centers and thus is under voluntary control. The respiratory center's output is transmitted via efferent nervous pathways to the respiratory muscles and to a higher integrated level, where input and output are compared; if input and output signals do not match, an alarm is triggered. This alarm is the sensation of dyspnea. Some of the chemo- and mechanoreceptors, which constitute the input to the respiratory system, are listed in Table 118-1. Not only do they inform the respiratory center whether the end products of respiration (i.e., oxygen uptake and carbon dioxide elimination) are normal but also, once compared with the output (i.e., neural drive), they provide a measure of efficiency.

Two examples should help to illustrate these points. A patient with myasthenia gravis, for instance, may have a relatively normal minute ventilation and normal arterial blood gases but be short of breath. Because there is a defect in the impulse transmission from nerve to muscle in myasthenia gravis, an increase in neural drive (output) is required to achieve an adequate tidal volume (input). This discrepancy between input and output may be perceived as dyspnea. Some patients with chronic obstructive pulmonary disease (COPD) complain of severe dyspnea despite relatively normal arterial blood gases. In

Table 118-1 Source of Input to the Respiratory Center

Mechanoreceptors
Cardiovascular system
Baroreceptors
Aortic arch
Left atrium
Respiratory system
Lung
Stretch receptors
Irritant receptors
J receptors
Respiratory muscles
Muscle spindles
Chest wall
Proprioceptors of the costovertebral joints
Chemoreceptors
Medulla
Carotid body

these "pink puffers," a variety of abnormal input signals are perceived. Irritant receptors and their afferent pathways provide information about bronchomotor tone and therefore airway resistance, which is increased in these patients. Muscle spindles and tendon organs of the diaphragm and intercostal and accessory muscle groups register the increase in tension generated as a result of high airway resistance and high lung volume breathing. Proprioceptors of the costovertebral joints register the increase in expansion of rib cage and, indirectly, lung volume. Neural drive has to increase appropriately in order to overcome the mechanical impairments, which are noted by the controller-alarm system and perceived as abnormal. (Note that in this latter example, supplemental oxygen would not be expected to alter any of the pathophysiologic determinants of dyspnea.)

If an imbalance between input and output persists, dyspnea is perceived unless the controller-alarm system adapts. This adaptation may explain why all patients with similar degrees of impairments do not complain of dyspnea. For instance, patients with chronic hypercapnic respiratory failure may not be short of breath. These "blue bloaters" accept a higher steady-state arterial carbon dioxide tension ($PaCO_2$) despite their transient ability to hyperventilate voluntarily and normalize their $PaCO_2$. They have adapted their controller-alarm system to accept hypercapnia instead of dyspnea.

Table 118-2 Causes of Dyspnea on Exertion

Ventilatory exercise limitation
Disorders associated with neuromuscular dysfunction (i.e., amyotrophic lateral sclerosis, myasthenia gravis)
Diseases affecting the mechanical properties of the chest wall (i.e., kyphoscoliosis, ankylosing spondylitis, obesity)
Disorders primarily affecting pulmonary gas exchange
Airways—chronic obstructive pulmonary disease, upper airway obstruction
Parenchyma—restrictive interstitial (sarcoid, idiopathic fibrosis, pneumoconioses)
Vasculature—pulmonary arteriolar hypertension, chronic pulmonary emboli
Pleura—effusions, fibrothorax
Cardiovascular limitations
Primary cardiac limitation
Heart muscle disease
Valvular heart disease
Pericardial disease
Abnormal arteriovenous connections
Pulmonary arteriovenous malformations
Patent ductus arteriosus
Intracardiac shunts
Anemia
Deconditioning

Etiology

In clinical practice, the majority of patients with dyspnea suffer from disorders of the respiratory or cardiovascular systems or they are deconditioned. Because it is possible to call upon a variety of compensatory mechanisms when stressed by disease or exercise, most patients with shortness of breath initially complain only during exertion. Therefore, a normal exercise capacity and the absence of exertional dyspnea in a patient who complains about shortness of breath at rest strongly suggest a psychogenic cause. The rest of this discussion is limited to relatively common diseases in which dyspnea is either the only or the leading symptom and in which dyspnea is exertional.

The most common lung diseases presenting with exertional dyspnea are those associated with airway obstruction. The obstruction can be either extrathoracic (i.e., vocal cord paralysis) or intrathoracic. In asthma, airway cooling caused by exercise-related increases in ventilation may aggravate bronchospasm and lead to exertional symptoms. Patients with chronic bronchitis and emphysema may accept a gradual decline in their exercise tolerance without symptoms and are often severely limited by the time they seek medical attention for dyspnea. Although less common from a purely statistical standpoint, pulmonary interstitial and chronic pleural diseases, pulmonary hypertension, and disorders of the respiratory pump may also have dyspnea as their sole manifestation. Diseases of the respiratory pump include disorders of the neuromuscular apparatus as well as abnormalities of the chest wall that affect its mechanical properties (Table 118-2).

Cardiovascular disorders manifesting as dyspnea on exercise can be divided into diseases of the heart muscle (i.e., cardiomyopathies), the valvular apparatus, or the pericardium, and conditions with abnormal arteriovenous connections. In young, otherwise asymptomatic patients, congenital heart disease with either valvular dysfunction or shunts is of prime concern. Later in life, emphasis shifts to coronary artery disease and ischemic cardiomyopathy, as well as occult valvular dysfunction. Two mechanisms are responsible for the exercise limitation and associated shortness of breath in patients with cardiac disorders: (1) cardiac output may be inadequate to satisfy the demand of the periphery, and (2) impaired left ventricular function will lead to pulmonary venous hypertension and edema.

Patients who are not physically fit also may complain of dyspnea. Their deconditioning, due to prolonged bed rest or a sedentary lifestyle, can be characterized as an "atrophy" of the cardiovascular response to exercise. It usually can be suspected from history; the diagnosis should be one of exclusion.

In patients with malignancies who present with exercise limitation, a number of factors may be operating. They are often malnourished and deconditioned, or anemic and suffering from cardiopulmonary toxicity due to chemotherapy and radiation therapy.

Dyspnea does not always mean pulmonary or cardiovascular dysfunction. In diabetic ketoacidosis and after ingestion of large doses of aspirin, it may be a leading symptom because of the compensatory increase in minute ventilation in response to metabolic acidosis. Finally, there are a number of patients in whom no organic cause can be found, even after thorough investigation. This so-called psychogenic dyspnea is a diagnosis of exclusion.

Diagnostic Approach

Baseline, Routine Considerations

In many cases the history and physical examination will help to categorize a disturbance as primary cardiovascular or respiratory. Exertional cough and wheezing may point to asthma, whereas chest pain suggests ischemic cardiomyopathy. Paroxysmal nocturnal dyspnea is present when the patient wakes from sleep, is short of breath, and has to sit on the edge of the bed. Although it is classically seen in patients with heart disease and pulmonary edema, it may be confused with nocturnal aspiration, nocturnal asthma, and bronchiectases, when pooled secretions empty into the central airways. Orthopnea or breathlessness on recumbency is a classic symptom of cardiac disease associated with pulmonary venous hypertension; however, it may also be seen in patients with bilateral phrenic nerve paralysis. Orthodeoxia, hypoxemia, and shortness of breath on standing may provide clues to the presence of liver disease with portopulmonary shunts or pulmonary arteriovenous malformations.

When patients complain of dyspnea even at rest, their organic functional impairment must be severe unless the symptom is psychogenic in cause.

If the history suggests a cardiac problem, chest radiography, electrocardiography (EKG), echocardiography, isotope scanning, and exercise tolerance testing may be indicated to describe structure and function of the cardiovascular system. If pulmonary disease is suspected, a chest radiograph, pulmonary function tests, and arterial blood gas analyses are indicated.

Special Considerations

Many times, the cause of dyspnea is not immediately apparent or there may be more than one potential cause of dyspnea. In these instances, the physician has to assess the relative contribution of every potential diagnostic possibility (see Table 118-2).

A few screening tests of respiratory, cardiovascular, and hematologic systems are essential at this initial stage of the work-up (Table 118-3). For instance, a complete blood count allows one to estimate red blood cell mass, a major determinant of the arterial oxygen content. The presence of anemia may indicate an underlying malignancy or blood loss, whereas polycythemia may point to chronic hypoxemia. Arterial blood gas analysis helps in the assessment of resting gas exchange; its interpretation is discussed in Chapter 115, "Arterial Blood Gases." A chest radiograph should be examined for the presence of cardiomegaly, evidence of pulmonary hypertension, air trapping, parenchymal infiltrates, and skeletal and pleural abnormalities. If the retrosternal space is encroached upon by the silhouette of the heart and if the hilar vascular shadows are prominent, an enlarged right ventricle and pulmonary hypertension may be present. Although all of these studies provide clues that the patient is not normal, further testing will be necessary in order to link them to the patient's complaint.

Pulmonary function tests document and characterize respiratory function impairment. The measurement of lung volumes and their subdivisions may reveal evidence of air trapping or restriction. Expiratory flow is reduced in patients with COPD. The degree of reversibility of airway obstruction can be assessed after inhalation of bronchodilators. In the absence of airway obstruction, a reduction in the maximum voluntary ventilation (the maximum amount of gas an individual can move in and out of the lungs) may be a sign of neuromuscular disease or a concomitant upper airway lesion. The neuromuscular output and therefore muscle strength can be further tested by observing the pressures an individual can generate during maximal inspiratory and expiratory efforts against an occluded airway. Finally, because the carbon monoxide diffusion capacity test correlates well with the amount of functional alveolar-capillary units, it is expected to be abnormal in disorders primarily involving the pulmonary capillary bed. It also may be the only abnormal test result in patients with interstitial lung diseases.

The resting EKG may indicate chamber hypertrophy, conduction abnormalities, arrhythmias, or ischemia and thus direct further attention to the cardiovascular system.

Because exertional dyspnea may be the only symptom suggesting asthma, bronchoprovocation testing (i.e., methacholine inhalational challenge; see Chapter 117, "Cough") may be required to establish the diagnosis. This test should be considered whenever the diagnosis is unknown and before invasive studies are ordered, even if baseline spirometry is normal.

The tests discussed so far reflect structure and resting function but not the output of the stressed respiratory and cardiovascular systems. Exercise testing will not only quantitate the degree of impairment but also characterize it as ventilatory or cardiovascular. A noninvasive exercise test is absolutely indicated in patients whose exertional dyspnea remains of unknown cause after initial screening studies and bronchoprovocation challenge. Historically, exercise testing developed as a diagnostic test for ischemic heart disease; thus, in its early days, most of the attention focused on exercise-induced changes in the electrocardiogram. It has since become apparent that much more information about the heart, lungs, and circulation can be derived from an exercise test. It is often possible to separate noninvasively whether exercise is ventilation- or cardiac-limited by observing the basic parameters of tidal volume, breathing frequency, heart rate, blood pressure, and attainable work rate. This information can be expanded by noninvasively measuring parameters of gas exchange such as oxygen uptake, carbon dioxide output, and arterial oxygen saturation. In selected patients, it may be indicated to further broaden the database by invasively determining the arterial blood gas tensions, blood lactate, cardiac output, and pulmonary artery and capillary wedge pressures.

Ventilatory limitation of exercise is suggested whenever there is an increase in minute ventilation out of proportion to oxygen uptake and work performed. Abnormalities of pulmonary gas exchange in response to exercise include a fall in the arterial oxygen saturation, and one often associated with a widening of the alveolar-arterial oxygen tension gradient and an increase in breathing frequency rather than tidal volume. Ventilatory exercise limitation may be caused primarily by diseases of the chest wall and neuromuscular output or by failure of the lungs to provide adequate gas exchange. Pulmonary vascular disorders such as primary pulmonary hypertension and interstitial lung diseases early in their course may escape detection on simple screening pulmonary function tests, resting blood gas analysis, and even chest radiographs. Therefore, if the exercise test indicates an unexpected abnormality of gas exchange, right-heart catheterization with measurements of pulmonary artery pressure and pulmonary vascular resistance should be considered. Furthermore, a transbronchoscopic or open thoracotomy lung biopsy may reveal radiologically occult interstitial lung disease.

Exercise is said to be cardiovascular-limited if ventilation parameters are normal and the attainable work rate (oxygen uptake) is reduced in spite of a normal or increased heart rate response. Although it may be difficult at times to separate poor cardiovascular performance due to heart disease from that due

Table 118-3 Tests Useful in the Work-Up of Patients with Dyspnea

Initial Screening

Complete blood count, arterial blood gases, chest radiograph, electrocardiogram, pulmonary function tests (lung volumes, spirometry before and after bronchodilators, carbon monoxide diffusion capacity)

Special Tests

- Bronchoprovocation test
- Flow-volume loops, forced inspiratory and expiratory pressures
- Exercise test (noninvasive or invasive)
  - If ventilatory impairment
    - Right-heart catheterization
    - Bronchoscope with transbronchoscopic lung biopsy
    - Thoracotomy
  - If cardiovascular impairment
    - Echocardiography, isotope scanning
    - Right- and left-heart catheterization
    - Coronary angiography
  - If deconditioned
    - Repeat exercise test after training period

to deconditioning, the latter is reversible with exercise training, and this can be objectively assessed. In the case of cardiovascular exercise limitation, echocardiography may not only demonstrate valvular lesions but also provide data about chamber size and myocardial function. Isotope scans may be useful in the evaluation of cardiac performance and function and allow estimates of the magnitude of shunts. However, if valvular or ischemic heart diseases are suspected, right- and left-heart catheterization with coronary angiography may ultimately be required.

References

Bates DV, Macklem PT, Christie RV. Pulmonary function and dyspnea. In: Bates DV. Respiratory function in disease. 3rd ed. Philadelphia: WB Saunders, 1989.

Killian KJ, Campbell EJM. Dyspnea. In: Roussos C, Macklem PT, eds. The thorax. Vol 29. Part B. New York: Marcel Dekker, 1985:787.

Wasserman K, et al. Pathophysiology of disorders limiting exercise. In: Principles of exercise testing and interpretation. Philadelphia: Lea & Febiger, 1987.

Hemoptysis

Rolf D. Hubmayr, MD

Richard S. Irwin, MD

119

Definitions

Hemoptysis, literally translated from the Greek, means "blood coughing." However, the medical literature has arbitrarily restricted the term to conditions in which blood arises from the lower respiratory tract, i.e., below the vocal cords. Its incidence has been reported to be as high as 6 percent in a random adult population and 30 percent in patients with pulmonary diseases. It usually leads to immediate consultation with a physician because of fears of death, tuberculosis, and bronchogenic carcinoma.

When blood arises from sites other than the lower respiratory tract, the condition is called *pseudohemoptysis.* It may be caused when blood from the oral cavity, nares, pharynx, and tongue drains to the back of the throat and initiates a cough. Patients with bleeding from the upper gastrointestinal tract may vomit (*hematemesis*) and subsequently aspirate blood. Although an occasional patient cannot distinguish the source of his or her bleeding, hematemesis may be differentiated from true hemoptysis because of the coffee-ground character of the expectorate and the absence of the bubbly appearance of bloody sputum. *Serratia marcescens,* a facultative gram-negative bacillus, may colonize or infect the respiratory tract of debilitated patients and produce a red pigment that may be confused with blood. However, sputum culture and the lack of red blood cells on a microscopic examination of the sputum usually point to the correct diagnosis. Finally, self-inflicted injuries or other bizarre tactics in the malingering patient seeking hospitalization present a challenging diagnostic problem when the source of bleeding is not obvious.

It is of considerable therapeutic importance to further qualify and quantitate the observation of hemoptysis. It may be scant, producing the appearance of streaks of bright red blood in the sputum, or profuse, with the expectoration of a large volume of blood. Massive hemoptysis, defined as the expectoration of 600 ml of blood in 48 hours, is associated with excessive mortality and requires immediate, usually surgical, intervention. Gross or frank hemoptysis is defined as expectoration of a quantity of blood that is less than massive, but more than scant blood streaking.

Common Causes of Hemoptysis

It is useful to divide the common causes of hemoptysis into several categories, as shown in Table 119-1. They include disorders of the tracheobronchial tree, cardiovascular system, hemostasis, and the pulmonary parenchyma itself.

When considering disorders of the tracheobronchial tree, one is usually dealing with infectious, inflammatory, or neoplastic disorders. These most commonly include acute tracheobronchitis, chronic bronchitis, and bronchiectasis, on the one hand, and pulmonary carcinoma and bronchial adenoma, on the other hand.

Pulmonary infarction, mitral stenosis, and congestive heart failure account for the majority of cardiovascular disorders associated with hemoptysis. Even though tuberculosis is a frequent diagnostic consideration, virtually any pulmonary parenchymal disorder, including pneumonia from any cause, may lead to the expectoration of blood. Although hematologic disorders are comparatively rare causes of hemoptysis, anticoagulation therapy, thrombocytopenia, and disseminated intravascular coagulation (DIC) may contribute to the development of hemoptysis as a result of coexisting pulmonary parenchymal disorders. Finally, hemoptysis can be seen following thoracic invasive procedures. However, they should not pose a differential diagnostic problem.

Diagnostic Approach

Table 119-2 outlines a systematic diagnostic approach to the problem of hemoptysis. Utilizing this approach, one can find the cause of hemoptysis in the majority of patients. However, in up to 18 percent of patients, a specific cause will not be determined. This is called idiopathic or essential hemoptysis; it is seen most commonly in men between the ages of 30 and 50 years. Prolonged follow-up of these patients almost always fails to reveal the source of bleeding, even though 10 percent will continue to have occasional episodes.

History, physical examination, chest radiograph, and routine laboratory tests usually narrow the differential diagnostic

Table 119-1 Most Common Causes of Hemoptysis

Tracheobronchial Disorders
Acute tracheobronchitis*
Chronic bronchitis*
Bronchogenic carcinoma*
Bronchiectasis*
Cystic fibrosis*
Bronchial adenoma
Tracheobronchial trauma
Foreign body aspiration
Invasive mediastinal tumor
Endobronchial metastases
Tracheoesophageal fistula
Bronchial telangiectasia
Bronchopleural fistula

Cardiovascular Disorders
Pulmonary infarction*
Mitral stenosis*
Congestive heart failure*
Aortic aneurysm
Pulmonary artery aneurysm
Pulmonary arteriovenous fistula
Congenital heart disease
Pulmonary hypertension
Pulmonary venous varix
Superior vena cava syndrome
Fat embolization

Hematologic Disorders
Anticoagulant therapy
Hemophilia
Leukemia
Thrombocytopenia
Lymphoproliferative disease
Disseminated intravascular coagulation

Localized Parenchymal Disease
Acute and chronic nontuberculous pneumonia*
Paragonimiasis*
Pulmonary tuberculosis*
Lung abscess
Lung contusion
Aspergilloma
Metastatic carcinoma
Bronchopulmonary sequestration
Wegener's granulomatosis
Lipoid pneumonia

Diffuse Parenchymal Disease
Systemic lupus erythematosus
Idiopathic pulmonary hemosiderosis
Goodpasture's syndrome
Uremic lung
Wegener's granulomatosis
Legionnaire's disease

Other
Idiopathic*
Iatrogenic (lung biopsy, bronchoscopy, cardiac catheterization)

* This listing is not meant to be all-inclusive; however, the asterisk (*) does identify all the common causes in each category.

Table 119-2 A Systematic Diagnostic Approach to Hemoptysis

Initial and Routine
History
Physical examination
Complete blood count, chest radiograph
Coagulation studies (prothrombin time, partial thromboplastin time, and platelets)
Quantitate hemoptysis
Consider fiberoptic bronchoscopy

Tracheobronchial Disorders
Expectorated sputa for tubercle bacilli, fungi, cytology, parasites
Bronchoscopy
Bronchography

Cardiovascular Disorders
Arterial blood gases
Electrocardiogram
Echocardiogram
Ventilation/perfusion lung scans
Pulmonary angiogram and aortogram
Cardiac catheterization

Hematologic Disorders
Coagulation studies (sophisticated or special)
Bone marrow

Localized Parenchymal Diseases
Expectorated sputa for parasites, tubercle bacilli, fungi, cytology
Tomograms
Aspergillus serum precipitins
Lung biopsy with special stains

Diffuse Parenchymal Diseases
Expectorated sputa for parasites, tubercle bacilli, fungi, cytology
Blood urea nitrogen, creatinine, antinuclear antibody, rheumatoid factor, complement, cryoglobulins, lupus erythematosus prep, antiglomerular basement membrane antibodies
Lung biopsy with special stains and immunofluorescence

possibilities into categories listed in Table 119-2 and provide the information on which further laboratory testing is based (see Table 119-2). Complete blood count, urinalysis, prothrombin time, partial thromboplastin time, platelet count, and studies to quantitate blood volume in the expectorate should be undertaken in every case. Particularly if disorders of the tracheobronchial tree and pulmonary parenchyma are suspected, bronchoscopy should almost always be considered. It may not only establish the diagnosis but also localize the site of the bleeding. This is of potential therapeutic importance if bleeding becomes massive and emergency surgery is required. In order to localize the site of bleeding in more than 90 percent of patients, bronchoscopy should be carried out during the active bleeding. When it is done after bleeding has ceased, accurate location is reduced to approximately 50 percent of the cases. The diagnostic capabilities of the flexible fiberoptic bronchoscope far surpass those of the rigid instrument. In patients with massive uncontrolled hemorrhage, however, the latter is preferred in order to maintain patency of the airway more effectively.

Because the choice of additional laboratory tests depends upon the category of causes, the evaluation of the patient with hemoptysis is considered within the framework of specific clinical situations.

Case 1

A 60-year-old pipefitter with chronic bronchitis who smokes one pack of cigarettes per day presents with increasing cough, sputum production, scant hemoptysis, and a chest radiograph that shows honeycombing localized to the left lower lobe.

Although this information is scant, it provides strong clues for the differential diagnosis. One of the most common causes of hemoptysis is an exacerbation of chronic bronchitis. As defined by the British Medical Research Council, chronic bronchitis is a disorder with chronic recurrent productive cough on most days of at least 3 months a year for at least 2 consecutive years. The importance of this disease as a common cause of hemoptysis has been confirmed in a British study that found chronic bronchitis to be the cause in 17 percent of 324 patients presenting with this symptom. The amount of blood expectorated is usually small, may be associated with exacerbation of cough and sputum production, and relates to mucosal injury due to retained secretions and inflammation. Nevertheless, it would be very wrong to ascribe this patient's hemoptysis to chronic bronchitis without additional investigation.

Pipefitters are exposed to asbestos, and when this is combined with exposure to cigarette smoke, they have a greatly increased risk of bronchogenic carcinoma. Further history, therefore, is needed to determine whether there are local or systemic symptoms indicative of malignancy. The recent onset of hoarseness may point to a vocal cord paralysis caused by mediastinal involvement with tumor. On physical examination, one should look specifically for cervical or axillary lymphadenopathy, the presence of a localized wheeze, hepatomegaly, and clubbing of fingers or toes. Even in the absence of a mass lesion on chest radiograph, the diagnosis of bronchogenic carcinoma cannot be excluded; therefore, sputum cytology and a visual examination of the tracheobronchial tree by flexible fiberoptic bronchoscopy may be necessary.

Other differential diagnostic considerations in this case include a carcinoma of the glottis or larynx or blood arising from an area of bronchiectasis. Bronchiectasis refers to the local dilatation of the bronchial tree caused by distortion of airways by parenchymal scarring. A distorted bronchiectatic airway interferes with the effective clearance of secretions arising from distal lung units. This, in effect, leads to pooling of phlegm, local infection, mucosal ulceration, and hemoptysis. It may be scant, gross, or massive, and it is usually recurrent. More than 90 percent of patients with bronchiectasis show specific abnormalities on radiographs. These range from parallel line markings representing a thickened bronchial wall to cystic changes described as honeycombing, representing destroyed airways ending in blind sacs.

In summary, the differential diagnosis in this patient mainly involves diseases of the tracheobronchial tree itself. Diagnostic tests should be able to help answer two questions: (1) Is the disorder inflammatory, infectious, or neoplastic? (2) What is its anatomic location? Therefore, history, physical examination, radiography or computed tomography of the chest, sputum cytology, and flexible fiberoptic bronchoscopy should be able to provide this information.

Case 2

A 30-year-old Vietnamese immigrant presents with cough, weight loss, night sweats, and a scant amount of blood mixed with sputum.

In this case, the history points to pulmonary infections. Although the incidence of pulmonary tuberculosis has steadily declined in the United States, it is still a major public health problem in Southeast Asian immigrants and is emerging in the immunosuppressed population. A contact investigation, the history of previous positive purified protein derivative (PPD) skin tests, the presence of acid-fast organisms in the sputum, and a chest radiograph compatible with disease involving the upper lung fields are apt to strengthen the clinical suspicion.

Paragonimiasis, a pulmonary parasitic infection related to the ingestion of raw freshwater crabs, is also a strong diagnostic possibility because it is endemic in areas of the Mekong Delta and may be clinically indistinguishable from tuberculosis. The diagnosis can be established by the demonstration of ova and parasites in the sputum and by serologic techniques.

Although both tuberculosis and paragonimiasis may present as cavitary lung disease, hemoptysis, in the presence of a cavitary lung lesion, does not always mean that these diseases are present. Neoplasms, particularly squamous cell carcinoma of the lung, and pulmonary infections due to facultative gram-negative bacilli, *Staphylococcus aureus,* and anaerobes and fungi such as coccidioidomycosis and histoplasmosis may all present with cavitary disease. On the other hand, cavities may become colonized with fungi, particularly *Aspergillus fumigatus.* This organism has a tendency to form fungus balls (rounded densities on chest radiograph) that move freely within the cavity on change of position. Although this form of aspergillosis does not truly represent an invasive infectious process, it does lead to local inflammation and hemoptysis. If a fungus ball causes recurrent gross or massive hemoptysis, surgery is almost always required as definitive treatment.

In summary, the most likely clinical diagnosis is active tuberculosis. At least three adequate sputum samples that are culture-negative for *Mycobacterium tuberculosis* are required in order to exclude the disease. If no other diagnosis is apparent and the chest radiograph shows parenchymal infiltrates or a cavitary lesion, lung biopsy may eventually be required in order to make a diagnosis. Lastly, one should remember that non-tuberculous mycobacterial infections commonly associated with chronic obstructive lung disease may present with hemoptysis in a clinical fashion similar to *M. tuberculosis.*

Case 3

A 35-year-old obese woman who has been taking birth control pills for at least 10 years experiences the sudden onset of dyspnea, chest pain, and hemoptysis 48 hours after a hysterectomy.

Although the differential diagnosis in this case includes postoperative atelectasis or pneumonia as well as blood arising from glottis, larynx, or trachea following a traumatic intubation, this setting is so classic for pulmonary emboli that any other diagnosis must be a surprise. Hemoptysis, the use of birth control pills, and pelvic surgery are all well-identified risk factors for pulmonary emboli. The presence of hemoptysis suggests that hemorrhagic consolidation or pulmonary infarction must have occurred. One should therefore expect a radiographic abnormality such as platelike atelectasis, a peripheral pulmonary infiltrate corresponding to a specific anatomic segment, elevation of the diaphragm consistent with volume loss on the affected side, local oligemia (asymmetry of the bronchovascular markings), or hilar engorgement; rarely will the chest film be normal. Arterial hypoxemia ($PaO_2 < 90$ mm Hg) is common. The diagnosis is confirmed by ventilation/perfusion scanning or pulmonary arteriography. A scan that demonstrates multiple segmental perfusion defects with normal ventilation (ventilation/perfusion mismatch) will establish the diagnosis with greater than 95 percent probability in this clinical setting. A normal perfusion pattern rules out the diagnosis. Particularly when preexisting lung disease is present, however, ventilation/perfusion scans may be difficult to interpret. Under these circumstances, pulmonary angiography should be the definitive test for pulmonary embolism by demonstrating intravascular filling defects or vessel cutoffs.

Case 4

A 40-year-old housewife with a history of rheumatic fever as a child presents with palpitations, shortness of breath, and hemoptysis.

Rheumatic fever and palpitations should strongly suggest a cardiovascular problem. In this particular case, the history of rheumatic fever should alert the physician that mitral stenosis may be present, which when paired with the onset of atrial fibrillation may have led to pulmonary venous hypertension. Sudden increases in pulmonary venous pressure from any cause may lead to pulmonary edema and hemoptysis. In mitral stenosis, hemoptysis can occur for a variety of reasons. Pulmonary edema with some expectoration of frothy, pink, blood-tinged sputum occurs early during the course of the disease. On the other hand, longstanding postcapillary pulmonary hypertension leads to reactive pulmonary hypertension that should protect the lung against hemorrhage from elevated pulmonary venous pressure. Nevertheless, anastomoses between pulmonary and bronchial veins may develop later, causing bronchial vein varicosities that may give rise to bright red hemoptysis. Finally, one should keep in mind that pulmonary infarcts due to thromboembolic disease arising in the legs commonly occur in patients with mitral stenosis and could be the cause of hemoptysis. The diagnosis of mitral stenosis can be made on auscultation of the heart if a loud first heart sound and opening snap and a diastolic rumble with presystolic accentuation are heard. Not infrequently, mitral stenosis is silent, and echocardiography is required to establish the diagnosis.

In the absence of valvular disease, myocardial dysfunction with left ventricular failure may give rise to pulmonary edema and hemoptysis. Pulmonary edema associated with cardiomegaly, the presence of a protodiastolic gallop, systemic hypertension, and electrocardiographic evidence of myocardial ischemia or myocarditis will help uncover the presence of myocardial dysfunction.

In situations in which the diagnosis is less obvious, pulmonary venous hypertension may have to be documented with a right-heart catheterization. Moreover, echocardiography, isotope scanning, and left-heart catheterization with coronary angiography may be useful in further defining the cause of pulmonary venous congestion.

References

Haponik EF, Chin R. Hemoptysis: Clinicians' perspectives. Chest 1990; 97:469.

Irwin RS, Hubmayr RD. Hemoptysis. In: Rippe JM, et al, eds. Intensive care medicine. Boston: Little, Brown, 1985:413.

Lederer DH. Hemoptysis. In: Conn RB, ed. Current diagnosis. 7th ed. Philadelphia: WB Saunders, 1985:17.

Respiratory Failure

Rolf D. Hubmayr, MD

Richard S. Irwin, MD

120

Definition

The respiratory system governs the uptake of oxygen (O_2) and the elimination of carbon dioxide (CO_2). By definition, any disturbance of these tasks can be called respiratory failure. The process of respiration is not confined to movement of gas in and out of the lungs (external respiration), but extends to cellular and subcellular O_2 and CO_2 metabolism (internal respiration). Probably because tests of cellular respiration are generally cumbersome and inadequate, we have come to restrict the term *respiratory failure* to disturbances of external respiration.

The components of the external respiratory system include (1) the respiratory center, which determines the respiratory drive; (2) efferent nervous pathways, which transmit information from the center to the effector organ (i.e., the respiratory muscles); (3) the respiratory muscles (i.e., diaphragm, intercostals, and "accessory" muscle groups); (4) the chest wall (i.e., the rib cage and the abdomen and diaphragm); and (5) the lungs. Because arterial blood gas analysis reflects the function of the external respiratory system, clinically apparent hypoxic respiratory failure is present when the arterial partial pressure of O_2 (PaO_2) is less than 50 mm Hg. Respiratory failure is primarily hypercapnic whenever the arterial partial pressure of CO_2 ($PaCO_2$) exceeds 45 mm Hg.

Etiology

The clinician needs to determine whether respiratory failure is hypoxic or hypercapnic, whether it is acute or chronic, and to what extent the different components of the external respiratory system are responsible for the abnormality in respiration.

Hypoxic Respiratory Failure

In the absence of low atmospheric O_2 tensions, hypoxic respiratory failure is caused by a mismatch of ventilation ($\dot{V}$) and perfusion ($\dot{Q}$). $\dot{V}/\dot{Q}$ mismatch is the principal mechanism whereby lung disease leads to hypoxia (Table 120-1), regardless of whether the primary disturbance is one of the airways, as in asthma; the pulmonary parenchyma, as in the adult respiratory distress syndrome (ARDS); or the pulmonary vasculature, as in pulmonary embolism. When mixed venous (pulmonary artery) blood bypasses the pulmonary parenchyma, it is not oxygenated and a right-to-left shunt exists. This most severe form of $\dot{V}/\dot{Q}$ mismatch occurs with pulmonary arteriovenous malformations or when, in the presence of a patent foramen ovale or an atrial or a ventricular septal defect, sufficient pulmonary hypertension develops to alter the direction of blood flow (Eisenmenger syndrome). Low PaO_2 or hypoxic respiratory failure is therefore seen in diseases of the lung as well as the cardiovascular system with right-to-left shunts. The degree of $\dot{V}/\dot{Q}$ mismatch can be assessed by the calculation of the alveolar-arterial oxygen tension difference, (A-a) PO_2, as discussed in Chapter 115, "Arterial Blood Gases."

One of the more common clinical entities associated with hypoxic respiratory failure is ARDS. Although its causes are many (see Table 120-1), their common pathophysiologic mechanism seems to be the recruitment of inflammatory cells to the lungs, damage to the pulmonary capillary basement membrane leading to the development of capillary endothelial damage and noncardiogenic pulmonary edema, $\dot{V}/\dot{Q}$ mismatch, and severe hypoxemia. It is important to remember that the hypoxemia may precede any radiographic abnormalities by several hours. The

Table 120-1 Common Disorders Associated with Adult Respiratory Distress Syndrome*

Shock
Septic
Anaphylactic
Hemorrhagic
Trauma
Fat embolism syndrome
Central nervous system insult
Head trauma
Subarachnoid hemorrhage
Seizure
Inhalation injury
Smoke
Nitrogen dioxide
Near drowning
Gastric acid aspiration
Drugs
Sedatives (Librium)
Opiates
Uremia
Pancreatitis
High altitude

* This table is not all inclusive.

Pulmonary

$PaCO_2$ is usually decreased and only rises terminally when $\dot{V}/\dot{Q}$ mismatch becomes severe enough to interfere with CO_2 elimination and inspiratory muscle fatigue ensues. The chest radiograph typically shows a diffuse bilateral process that is predominantly alveolar, not unlike that seen in cardiogenic forms of pulmonary edema.

Hypercapnic Respiratory Failure

Hypercapnic respiratory failure is diagnosed by finding a $PaCO_2$ of greater than 45 mm Hg. Because CO_2 elimination is determined by the degree of alveolar ventilation, hypercapnic respiratory failure is not an isolated disorder of the lungs but rather of the external respiratory system as a whole. In the absence of $\dot{V}/\dot{Q}$ mismatch and thus a normal (A-a) Po_2 difference, lung disease is unlikely to be present. Therefore, disorders of respiratory drive, the efferent nervous pathways, and the respiratory muscles and diseases altering the mechanical properties of the chest wall (Table 120-2) should be considered responsible for the decrease in alveolar ventilation and hypercapnia.

When hypercapnia develops in the presence of lung disease (the (A-a) Po_2 difference will be increased), one must conclude that the rise in minute ventilation was insufficient to compensate for $\dot{V}/\dot{Q}$ mismatch and restore an adequate level of alveolar ventilation. In chronic respiratory failure (see Chapter 115, "Arterial Blood Gases"), an adaptive change in ventilatory control allows ventilation to become relatively subnormal at the cost of a higher steady-state $PaCO_2$. At this stage, however, the reserve of the respiratory system to increase ventilation on demand is severely compromised; consequently, a further fall in respiratory drive, a concomitant disorder of the neuromuscular apparatus, or a further decline in lung function (i.e., lower respiratory tract infection) might lead to total decompensation of the system.

Acute hypercapnic respiratory failure, on the other hand, is never the result of adaptive changes but rather indicative that the system is rapidly failing. In this setting, the respiratory muscles play a predominant role. Respiration is an energy-requiring process governed by the principles of energy supply and demand. Whenever energy demand of the inspiratory muscles exceeds the available supply, the muscles become fatigued, ventilation cannot be sustained, and CO_2 retention must occur. The factors leading to inspiratory muscle fatigue are outlined in Table 120-3. Lung disease increases the work of breathing because of the increase in required minute ventilation, changes in timing and length of the respiratory muscle contraction, and the increased load when either airway resistance is high or lung compliance is low. The strength of the inspiratory muscles depends on their length-tension characteristics and therefore lung volume. It is further influenced by atrophy, malnutrition, electrolyte disturbances, or neuromuscular disease. At high lung volume, as can be seen in obstructive lung disease, the diaphragm is flattened and by virtue of its altered geometry may produce an inward motion of the lower rib cage during inspiration. This is inefficient because the major portion of the energy used has gone to distort the chest wall and not to increase lung volume. Lung disease may also influence factors determining the energy available to the inspiratory muscles. Hypoxia and changes in cardiac output may limit O_2 delivery to the respiratory muscles. Furthermore, if the perfusion of respiratory muscles falls during the contraction, as is true for the heart, any change in timing between contraction and relaxation may adversely affect their energy supply.

Table 120-2 Differential Diagnoses of Respiratory Failure

Hypoxic Respiratory Failure
Airway disease
Asthma
Chronic obstructive pulmonary disease
Parenchymal disease
Adult respiratory distress syndrome
Pneumonia (infectious, chemical, etc.)
Trauma
Vascular
Pulmonary embolism
Pulmonary arteriovenous malformation
Pulmonary venous hypertension
Cardiac with right-to-left shunt
Eisenmenger syndrome
Hypercapnic Respiratory Failure in the Absence of Lung Disease
Altered central nervous system drive
Drugs (opiates, barbiturates)
Injury (stroke, tumor, infection, trauma)
Idiopathic
Adaptive response
Abnormal impulse transmission between respiratory center and respiratory muscles
Spinal cord injury (diaphragm paralysis)
Demyelinating disease (amyotrophic lateral sclerosis)
Myasthenia gravis
Drugs
Inspiratory muscle fatigue (see Table 120-3)
Primary (polymyositis)
Secondary due to
Increased work of breathing
Poor efficiency
Electrolyte disturbance (Ca, Mg, K, PO_4)
Malnutrition
Atrophy
Poor perfusion

Diagnostic Approach

Once it has been determined that respiratory failure exists, the history may give clues to the site of the disturbance within the external respiratory system. Although dyspnea may suggest the presence of a respiratory disease, it by no means implies respiratory failure. A good starting point is to ask specific questions to uncover any previous lung disease. The pulmonary disorders that most commonly progress to respiratory failure are chronic obstructive pulmonary disease (COPD), asthma, and interstitial fibrosis. In COPD, the presence of respiratory tract infection, left ventricular failure, or hyperreactive airways may explain any recent deterioration in lung function. In asthma, intermittent

Table 120-3 Factors That Determine Inspiratory Muscle Fatigue

Factors Determining Inspiratory Muscle Energy Demands
Work of breathing
Minute ventilation
Compliance and resistance
Frequency and tidal volume
Strength
Lung volume
Atrophy
Neuromuscular disease
Nutritional status
Efficiency
Factors Determining the Energy Available to the Inspiratory Muscles
Arterial O_2 content
Inspiratory muscle blood flow
Blood substrate concentration
Energy stores (nutrition)
Ability to extract energy sources

episodes of wheezing, cough, and shortness of breath are helpful. Interstitial fibrosis represents a common inflammatory response to a variety of insults to the lung. They range from the inhalation of asbestos, beryllium, and gastric acid to immune-mediated injury in sarcoidosis and rheumatologic and collagen vascular diseases. Drugs that suppress respiratory drive, such as opiates and barbiturates, may be solely responsible for hypercapnic respiratory failure or significantly contribute to failure in patients with preexisting lung disease. Demyelinating processes such as amyotrophic lateral sclerosis or myopathies may ultimately lead to respiratory failure. Mechanical impairment of the thorax, such as that seen in kyphoscoliosis or rarely in ankylosing spondylitis, may reduce the efficiency of the respiratory muscles, increase the work of breathing, and therefore lead to failure.

Although the physical examination cannot replace the blood gas analysis in documenting hypoxemia and hypercapnia, it enables one to suspect impending or acute respiratory failure by observing cardiovascular, ventilatory, and central nervous system (CNS) responses.

The cardiovascular responses to hypoxemia or hypercapnia are increases in heart rate, cardiac output, and systemic vascular resistance resulting in tachycardia and hypertension. Moreover, in the presence of hypoxic vasoconstrictive pulmonary hypertension, which usually accompanies acute respiratory failure, atrial tachyarrhythmias are common. Low cardiac output, hypotension, and bradycardia are also seen, but they signal impending cardiovascular collapse.

Ventilatory responses depend on the etiology of respiratory failure. Patients with abnormalities of respiratory drive and timing related to CNS injury display a variety of breathing patterns depending on the level of CNS function. Apneustic (slow respiration with inspiratory pause) and ataxic (chaotic) breathing are seen with pontine and medullary dysfunction, respectively, and are usually associated with insufficient drive to guarantee gas exchange. Whenever there is inspiratory muscle fatigue, changes in the rate, depth, and pattern of breathing may be observed. Both respiratory rate and tidal volume increase initially. This may be followed by a paradoxic inward motion of the anterior abdominal wall during inspiration. This indicates that the diaphragm fails to contract sufficiently to descend and move the abdominal contents downward, which results in the normal outward motion of the abdominal wall during inspiration. Cyclic changes in breathing patterns with either chest wall or a predominantly abdominal wall motion are another sign of ventilatory compromise. This so-called respiratory alternans represents the cyclic contractions of intercostal and accessory muscles, on the one hand, and the diaphragm, on the other. Presumably, these different muscle groups can alternate in their contribution to the work of breathing and allow each other to "rest." Unless the physician intervenes at this point, tidal volume and frequency may fall and hypercapnia, hypoxia, and acidosis ensue.

In patients with asthma, the use of accessory muscles (sternocleidomastoid, abdominal muscles) and the presence of a paradoxic pulse (>10 mm Hg fall in systolic blood pressure during inspiration) are signs of severe bronchospasm. The intensity of wheezing, however, does not correlate with the degree of airway obstruction. Wheezing may be virtually absent as airflow to and from the lungs decreases during a severe attack.

Hypoxemia, hypercapnia, and acidemia may alter CNS function singly or in combination. As oxygen delivery to the brain declines, higher cortical function is impaired. If the disturbance is severe enough, frank coma can be observed. In the absence of hypoxemia and acidemia, hypercapnia alone can impair consciousness. This most commonly occurs when patients with COPD, who depend on the hypoxic respiratory drive, are given oxygen. Carbon dioxide is a potent cerebral vasodilator; thus, hypercapnia can cause headaches. Before the dysfunction is severe enough to progress to coma, other signs of metabolic encephalopathy such as asterixis (involuntary jerking particularly observed in dorsiflexed hands) may be seen.

Although history and physical examination are helpful, they can only provide clues to the presence of respiratory failure. The physical sign of cyanosis may be absent despite profound hypoxemia. Therefore, blood gas analysis is essential in the evaluation of these patients. It not only identifies and accurately differentiates between hypoxic and hypercapnic failure but also serves to assess the acuteness of the process. (A detailed discussion of these concepts is given in Chapter 115, "Arterial Blood Gases.") Routine blood tests useful in the assessment and management of the patient with respiratory failure are outlined in Table 120-4. A complete blood count will provide information about the granulocyte response to stress and inflammation and is essential in determining the O_2 content of blood. Because arterial O_2 content depends mainly on hemoglobin concentration and its saturation with O_2, the combination of anemia and hypoxemia can profoundly diminish O_2 delivery to tissues. Electrolyte disturbances, most commonly hypokalemia or hypophosphatemia, may be responsible for respiratory muscle weakness and therefore need to be evaluated. Screening tests for associated hepatic or renal failure are of diagnostic, prognostic, and therapeutic value. They may provide clues as to the nature of the underlying illness and influence the choice of drugs based on their pharmacokinetics. Although the correlation between anatomy and function is by no means perfect, a chest radiograph helps to assess the presence and severity of any pulmonary parenchymal disease, evaluate heart size and pulmonary venous congestion, screen for pneumothorax and skeletal chest wall abnormalities, and estimate lung volume.

A number of optional tests help to isolate and differentiate abnormalities of the different components of the external respiratory system. The pressures generated during a maximal inspiratory and expiratory effort against an occluded airway provide a useful estimate of overall respiratory neuromuscular function. Results of the test are expected to be abnormal in patients with neuromuscular disorders or respiratory muscle fatigue. The electromyogram may be useful in the same group of patients. It

Pulmonary

Table 120-4 Tests Useful in the Diagnosis and Management of Respiratory Failure

Essential Tests	
Complete blood count	Potassium
Liver function tests	Chloride
Blood urea nitrogen	Phosphate
Creatinine	Arterial blood gases
Calcium	Chest radiograph
Magnesium	Electrocardiogram

Tests Useful in the Evaluation of

Respiratory drive
- Ventilatory responses to hypoxia and hypercapnia

Neuromuscular function
- Pulmonary function tests (spirometry, lung volumes, maximal mouth pressures, maximal voluntary ventilation)
- Electromyelogram
- Fluoroscopy of the diaphragm

Work of breathing
- Pulmonary function tests
- Compliance and resistance of lung and chest wall

Lung disease
- Routine pulmonary function tests
- Diffusion capacity
- Ventilatory dead space
- Pulmonary shunt
- Right-heart catheterization
- Pulmonary angiography

usually can characterize an abnormality as presynaptic or postsynaptic and thus differentiate between disease of the nervous system and muscle disease.

In the absence of mechanical impairment of the respiratory system, the increase in minute ventilation in response to hypoxia or hypercapnia (CO_2 stimulation test) is a good indicator of central respiratory drive. However, because most patients with respiratory failure display evidence of associated muscle weakness and because their work of breathing is increased, the ventilatory response to hypoxia or hypercapnia must be interpreted with caution.

Pulmonary function tests may help to characterize (restrictive versus obstructive) and quantitate the degree of ventilatory impairment. In COPD or asthma, the degree of obstruction correlates with the increased work of breathing. Furthermore, response to bronchodilators can be tested.

Because cardiovascular dysfunction will aggravate or may be the sole cause of respiratory failure, evaluation of cardiac performance by noninvasive and invasive techniques such as right- and left-heart catheterization may also be required.

References

Cohen CA, et al. Clinical manifestations of inspiratory muscle failure. Am J Med 1982; 73:308.

Lemaire F, Harf A, Teisseire BP. Oxygen exchange across the acutely injured lung. In: Zapol WM, Falke KJ, eds. Acute respiratory failure. Lung biology in health and diseases series. Vol. 24. New York: Marcel Dekker, 1985:521.

Tobin MJ. Respiratory muscles in disease. Clin Chest Med 1988; 9:263.

Wheezing

R. William Corwin, MD

121

Definition

The wheeze is a continuous adventitious sound of the lung caused by the vibrations of narrowed airways, which act much like the uncoupled vibrating reed of a wind instrument. Wheezes are musical sounds classified by their pitch (high and low), complexity (monophonic and polyphonic), duration (long and short), and timing (inspiratory and expiratory). The pitch of a wheeze is determined by the elasticity of the bronchial walls. The pitch is high when an obstruction is rigid and stiff, and it is low when an obstruction is large or flabby. A monophonic wheeze is a single note or several notes that start and stop at different times. Polyphonic wheezes are notes that harmonically start and stop together, much like a musical chord.

Etiology

Differential diagnoses of wheeze are listed in Table 121-1. Stridor is a monophonic inspiratory wheeze caused by a critical narrowing of the extrathoracic upper airway. The loud musical inspiratory wheeze of stridor may be caused by bacterial or viral infection or a toxic inhalation such as smoke, fire, or near drowning. Foreign body aspiration causing partial airway obstruction can produce a stridorous monophonic wheeze. Less common causes of stridor include tumor growth, spasmodic allergic croup, and hysterical forced inspiratory maneuvers that mimic airway obstruction.

A fixed monophonic wheeze implies a partial occlusion of a major lobar bronchus. The most common causes include bronchial stenosis from tumors (malignant or benign), foreign bodies, surgical repairs, granulomatous lesions, and mucous plugging.

Random monophonic wheezes occur in diseases that result in diffuse airway dysfunction. Airways are unpredictably narrowed to near closure by the bronchial spasm of asthma or exacerbation of chronic obstructive pulmonary disease (COPD). A seldom recognized but common cause of expiratory wheezing is extrathoracic upper airway obstruction associated with postnasal drip. The obstruction is probably due to vocal cord edema, but the mechanism of this phenomenon is not well understood.

Sequential inspiratory monophonic wheezes occur in interstitial lung diseases of many etiologies. The wheezing is produced by terminal air units opening late in inspiration and remaining in close contact for a short time.

Expiratory polyphonic wheezes are a sign of widespread obstruction of small airways, which is most often found in asthma and COPD. The compression of many lobar bronchi produces many notes that harmonically stop and start together. The uniform dynamic compression of airways by a single, violent, explosive forced expiration best mimics the polyphonic wheeze of disease.

History

The remote or recent history of wheezing related by the patient or objectively by physical examination is not specific for any particular disease; rather, it signifies airway obstruction. For example, although asthma remains one of the most common causes of wheeze in most clinical practices, of 34 prospectively studied patients with wheeze and a diagnosis of asthma referred to our outpatient department as difficult clinical problems, only 12 (35 percent) had asthma. Even though asthma is a common cause of wheeze, the history of wheeze and asthma alone does not confirm the diagnosis.

To evaluate any wheeze correctly, a detailed review of pulmonary symptoms can be helpful. Because asthma and COPD are probably the most common causes of wheezing, it is logical to continue by directing questions to help support or eliminate these two diagnoses. For asthma, emphasis should be placed on childhood respiratory ailments; symptoms of seasonal atopy; dyspnea with exposure to cold, exercise, aspirin, tartrazine dyes (yellow food dyes), heating, insulations (urea-formaldehyde

Table 121-1 Etiology of Wheezing

Type	Timing	Etiology
Stridor	Inspiratory	Epiglottitis/croup
		Tracheal stenosis
		Upper airway tumor
		Foreign body
		Angioedema
		Spasmodic glottic closure (hysterical stridor)
Fixed monophonic	Inspiratory and expiratory	Bronchial stenosis
		Tumor
		Foreign body
		Intrabronchial granulomata
		Mucous plug
Random monophonic	Inspiratory and expiratory	Asthma
		Chronic obstructive pulmonary disease
		Postnasal drip
Sequential inspiratory monophonic	Inspiratory	Interstitial lung diseases
Expiratory polyphonic	Expiratory	Asthma
		Chronic obstructive pulmonary disease
		Voluntary forced expiratory effort

foam), pets, or hobbies; and swallowing dysfunction. The past and current work history should precisely document work activities and exposures of the patient, and a family history of respiratory ailments should be sought.

For COPD, a smoking history should clearly define the number of years the patient has smoked; the types of smoking, such as pipe, cigars, cigarettes, marijuana, and filtered or nonfiltered cigarettes; and the amount of smoke inhaled. Additionally, information pertinent to other causes of wheeze listed in Table 121-1 must be reviewed. For example, postnasal drip from sinusitis and allergic and nonallergic rhinitis is not an uncommon cause of wheezing (47 percent of cases are serious or difficult clinical problems). This is often suggested by frequent throat clearing, a dripping sensation in the hypopharynx, or a persistent foul taste. Foreign body aspiration is obvious by history except in children, the mentally retarded, or the neurologically impaired, in whom a high index of suspicion is needed. Malignant airway tumors have shorter wheezing histories and are occasionally accompanied by hemoptysis, change in sputum, weight loss, anorexia, hypertrophic osteoarthropathy, and other paraneoplastic symptoms or endocrinopathies. Prior tracheostomy or intubation should suggest the possibility of tracheal stenosis.

Upper airway stridor caused by infection characteristically has a rapid onset, is accompanied by fever, chills, cough, and difficulty in breathing and swallowing, and occasionally is preceded by upper respiratory tract symptoms such as rhinorrhea, earache, or sore throat. In upper airway stridor caused by toxic inhalation, the source of the exposure is important as a prognostic factor, but it rarely changes the immediate aggressive clinical management.

Angioedema of the upper airways is familial or associated with urticaria and is most often related to food ingestions. Spasmodic or hysterical stridor is a diagnosis of exclusion and is characterized by a history of anxiety, hysteria, and depression.

Physical Examination

The physical examination is the absolute criterion for the presence or absence of a wheeze. Using the descriptive terminology of complexity, pitch, location, timing, and duration may help narrow the differential diagnosis and direct the diagnostic evaluation.

Stridor is loud, may be heard without the aid of a stethoscope, occurs during inspiration, and usually indicates advanced extrathoracic upper airway obstruction. Unfortunately, significant extrathoracic upper airway obstruction may occur before stridor is heard. A fixed monophonic wheeze is located in the same area on repeated examination. The wheeze is inspiratory and expiratory, but the timing, pitch, and duration remain unchanged. Random monophonic wheezes are located throughout the chest, come and go on a single examination, and often overlap. The monophonic wheeze heard at the mouth is most often located in large airways; those heard best through the chest wall are more often in the peripheral airways. Sequential inspiratory wheezes are found in the bases of both lungs, occur at the end of inspiration, are short sounds with different pitches and tones, and are frequently reproducible on subsequent breaths. Expiratory polyphonic wheezes are located throughout the lung fields in expiration and span the entire expiratory maneuver. The pitch may rise as end expiration approaches and the point of dynamic compression moves toward smaller airways.

Polyphonic wheezes are strongly correlated with diffuse airway obstruction but are very poor estimates of the amount of obstruction. For example, after an acute asthma attack, more than 50 percent obstruction may remain without wheezing. In contrast, during the acute attack, the cessation of wheezing may indicate incipient respiratory failure. In emphysematous COPD, wheezing is conspicuously absent. This is explained by the distal, small peripheral airway obstruction with very little flow of gas without mucous plugging to form a resonating reedlike apparatus.

Diagnostic Approach

The diagnostic approach to wheezing is guided by the differential diagnosis that is developed from the detailed history, review of systems, and the classification and characterization of the wheeze by physical examination. Table 121-2 lists the tests available for evaluation of the wheezing patient.

Pulmonary function testing is the first step after the history and physical examination and is the most helpful diagnostic tool

Table 121-2 Diagnostic Tests for Evaluation of Wheeze

Pulmonary function tests
- Lung volumes and spirometry with bronchodilator
- Methacholine/carbachol/histamine bronchoprovocation
- Flow-volume loops

Radiographs
- Posteroanterior and lateral chest
- Posteroanterior inspiratory and expiratory chest
- Lateral neck
- Tracheal tomograms

Laryngoscopy or bronchoscopy

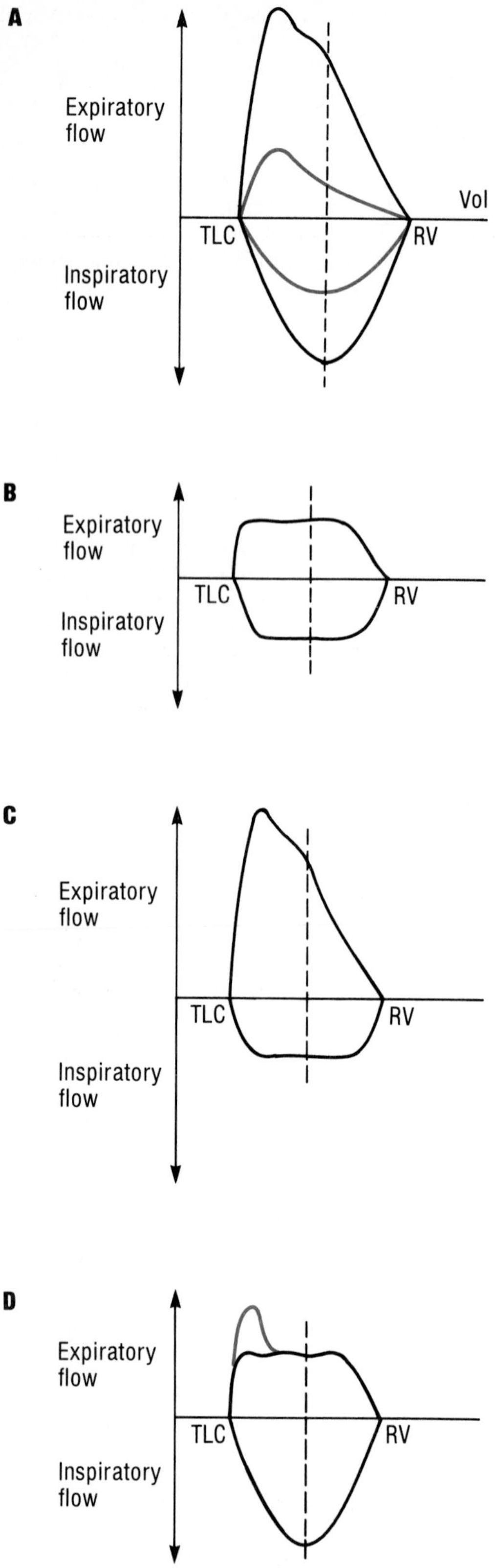

Figure 121-1 Examples of flow-volume loops demonstrating airway obstruction. (**A**) Normal loop (black) with chronic obstructive pulmonary disease (red). (**B**) Fixed intrathoracic or extrathoracic airway obstruction. (**C**) Variable extrathoracic airway obstruction. (**D**) Variable intrathoracic airway obstruction. RV = residual volume, TLC = total lung capacity. (*Adapted from* Crager M. Am J Med 1976; 61:85.)

in the evaluation of the common causes of wheezing. Routine lung volumes will define the restrictive pattern of interstitial lung disease that produces the sequential inspiratory monophonic wheeze. Spirometry with bronchodilators will demonstrate the airflow obstruction of COPD and the reactive airway disease of asthma, which are sources of random monophonic and expiratory polyphonic wheezes. If the pulmonary function test results are normal, but asthma is clinically suspected on the basis of the history, bronchoprovocation with methacholine, carbachol, or histamine will confirm the diagnosis of reactive airways as defined by a decrease of 20 percent in the forced expiratory volume in 1 second (FEV_1). The flow-volume loop "suggests" variable extrathoracic upper airway obstruction if one observes a flattening of the inspiratory loop (Fig. 121-1) or a decrease in the inspiratory or expiratory ratio of 50 percent flow (forced inspiratory flow 50/forced expiratory flow 50) in patients with upper airway edema from toxic inhalations or postnasal drip. Fixed upper airway extrathoracic obstruction (tracheal stenosis) is characterized by flattening of both the inspiratory and expiratory loops (see Fig. 121-1). Unlike lung volumes or spirometry, the flow-volume loop may not be sensitive enough to detect some upper airway disease and is most often helpful if used in combination with the history, physical examination, and other clinical tests.

The chest radiograph is the second step, after pulmonary function testing, in the diagnostic evaluation of wheeze. All older patients who smoke and who have a first diagnosis of expiratory wheeze deserve a posteroanterior-lateral chest radiograph. The chest radiograph will demonstrate obvious mass lesions of tumors, lobar collapse from endobronchial obstruction, mucous impactions, and, in patients with acute asthma or COPD, hyperinflation with flat diaphragms, increased retrosternal airspaces, splayed intercostal spaces, hyperlucent lung fields, and small teardrop heart shadows. The patients with fixed monophonic wheezes occasionally benefit from inspiratory and expiratory posteroanterior chest radiographs. A lobar endobronchial lesion will trap air and cause a persistent hyperinflated lung on the expiratory film. In patients with stridor only lateral neck films are needed to look for a swollen and edematous epiglottis.

If there is reason to suspect a primary tracheal tumor or tracheal stenosis, tracheal tomograms are needed to define the extent of the anatomic abnormality. Additional radiologic techniques such as bronchography or computed tomography may provide additional information in certain circumstances, but they should be done only after thoughtful consideration of the indications and potential information yield.

The final diagnostic test in the evaluation of wheeze is laryngoscopy or bronchoscopy. Fiberoptic laryngoscopy or bronchoscopy yields a direct and detailed examination of the upper airway, trachea, lobar bronchi, and segmental and two to three subsegmental bronchi. In patients with stridor and acute infectious upper airway disease, direct or indirect laryngoscopy is contraindicated except as a part of an intubation procedure done in an operating room with an emergency tracheostomy on standby. Vocal cord edema secondary to postnasal drip may be visualized with either a fiberoptic laryngoscope or a bronchoscope. For fixed inspiratory or expiratory monophonic wheezes, the diagnosis of endobronchial lesions is often not possible without direct examination. A foreign body may be seen and then removed with a fiberoptic bronchoscope, but it is more easily handled with the traditional rigid Jackson-type bronchoscope.

References

Collett PW, Brancatisano T, Engle LA. Spasmodic croup in the adult. Am Rev Respir Dis 1983; 127:500.

Forgacs P. Lung sounds. Philadelphia: WB Saunders, 1983.

Forgacs P. The functional basis of pulmonary sounds. Chest 1978; 73:399.
Hollingsworth HM. Wheezing and stridor. Clin Chest Med 1987; 8:231.
Loudon R, Murphy RLH Jr. Lung sounds. Am Rev Respir Dis 1984; 130:663.
Marini JJ, et al. The significance of wheezing in chronic airflow obstruction. Am Rev Respir Dis 1979; 120:1069.
McFadden ER Jr, Kiser R, DeGroot WJ. Acute bronchial asthma—relations between clinical and physiologic manifestations. N Engl J Med 1973; 288:221.
Pratter MR, Hingston DM, Irwin RS. Diagnosis of bronchial asthma by clinical evaluation—an unreliable method. Chest 1983; 84:42.
Rodenstein DO, Francis C, Stanescu DC. Emotional laryngeal wheezing: A new syndrome. Am Rev Respir Dis 1983; 127:354.

Cyanosis

Joel M. Seidman, MD

122

Definition

Cyanosis, a blue or blue-gray tint to skin, mucous membranes, and nailbeds, may be noticed by the examiner or reported by the patient. The perception of cyanosis depends on the fact that deoxyhemoglobin, which is dark red when viewed directly, takes on a bluish color when viewed in superficial capillaries by light reflected through a translucent layer of epithelium. More specifically, the perception depends on the sensitivity of the viewer, the concentration of deoxyhemoglobin, the thickness and pigmentation of the epithelial layer, the color of the patient's plasma, and, very important, the color and intensity of the lighting used for examination. Each of these factors is discussed in more detail.

Physiology

It has been determined empirically that a minimal deoxyhemoglobin concentration of about 5 g/dl is required before cyanosis is detectable. Few examiners are able to detect cyanosis at a deoxyhemoglobin concentration of 4 g/dl, and one of four examiners will miss even a level of 5 g/dl. In the presence of anemia, 5 g of deoxyhemoglobin will occur with greater desaturation and at a lower arterial oxygen tension (Po_2) than with a normal hemoglobin concentration. Serious degrees of hypoxemia may thus be present in anemic patients before cyanosis is evident. Conversely, the polycythemic patient will exhibit cyanosis, i.e., attain 5 g of reduced hemoglobin, with a lesser proportion of the total hemoglobin unoxygenated, resulting in the appearance of cyanosis at higher oxyhemoglobin saturation (SaO_2) and Po_2. Obviously, deep skin pigmentation may mask the presence of cyanosis, but inspection of the nailbeds and mucous membranes is still useful in darker-skinned patients. Plasma pigments such as bilirubin may alter the color perceived, giving the cyanotic patient a greenish hue.

Bright sunlight is the best lighting source with which to examine a patient in order to detect cyanosis. Incandescent lighting is of mediocre quality. However, the bluish cast generated by fluorescent tubes tends to give a slightly cyanotic tinge to mucous membranes, nailbeds, and lightly pigmented skin even in normal individuals, making the determination of true cyanosis virtually impossible. Therefore, fluorescent lighting should never be used as the light source in a search for cyanosis.

Abnormal hemoglobin molecules, because of different spectral characteristics, cause cyanosis at lower concentration (and thus at higher arterial oxygen saturation). For example, a level of 1.5 g/dl of methemoglobin or 0.5 g/dl of sulfhemoglobin is associated with typical cyanosis.

Conditions that may be confused with cyanosis include carbon monoxide poisoning and argyria. The former leads to the generation of carboxyhemoglobin, which produces a "cherry red" color rather than the blue color of cyanosis. The latter, due to skin deposits of metallic silver (resulting from industrial exposure or from the now largely abandoned use of silver-containing solutions as topical antiseptics), consists of a peculiar slate-gray coloration that, unlike color produced by blood pigment in capillaries, does not blanch on pressure. Patients with polycythemia vera may exhibit a purplish hue called "red cyanosis."

Etiology

The mechanisms of "true" cyanosis, i.e., cyanosis due to desaturation of hemoglobin, are twofold—a decrease in pulmonary venous saturation (central cyanosis) or a decrease in flow through peripheral tissue capillaries with increased oxygen extraction from each volume of blood (peripheral or acral cyanosis). The former may be caused by breathing a hypoxic gas mixture such as might occur at altitudes over approximately 16,000 feet or 5,000 meters; by alveolar hypoventilation, such as occurs in certain forms of chronic obstructive pulmonary disease (COPD) or diseases of the respiratory center of the brain; by severe ventilation/perfusion inequalities, which occur in some patients with COPD or many forms of interstitial lung disease; or by right-to-left shunting, such as in some congenital heart malformations, pulmonary arteriovenous malformations (hereditary hemorrhagic telangiectasia), and with the multiple, small intrapulmonary shunts often seen in hepatic cirrhosis. Hemoglobins characterized by a high P_{50} (the Po_2 at which 50 percent oxygen saturation occurs), i.e., a right-shifted oxyhemoglobin dissociation curve, will have lower saturation at any given oxygen tension. A patient with such a hemoglobin may exhibit cyanosis at a Po_2 that is usually considered normal.

Peripheral cyanosis is seen in diseases characterized by slow flow through capillaries. Low cardiac output states like congestive heart failure or shock are frequently associated with cyanosis. Vascular disease such as peripheral arterial atherosclerosis slows flow to peripheral capillaries, permitting increased extraction. In vasospastic disorders such as Raynaud's phenomenon or diseases characterized by sluggish capillary blood flow, e.g., cryoglobulinemia or other paraproteinemias, cyanosis may occur. All of the peripheral causes of cyanosis are characterized by poor blood flow to skin capillaries, thus causing cool skin temperatures. By contrast, central causes of cyanosis are usually associated with warm skin.

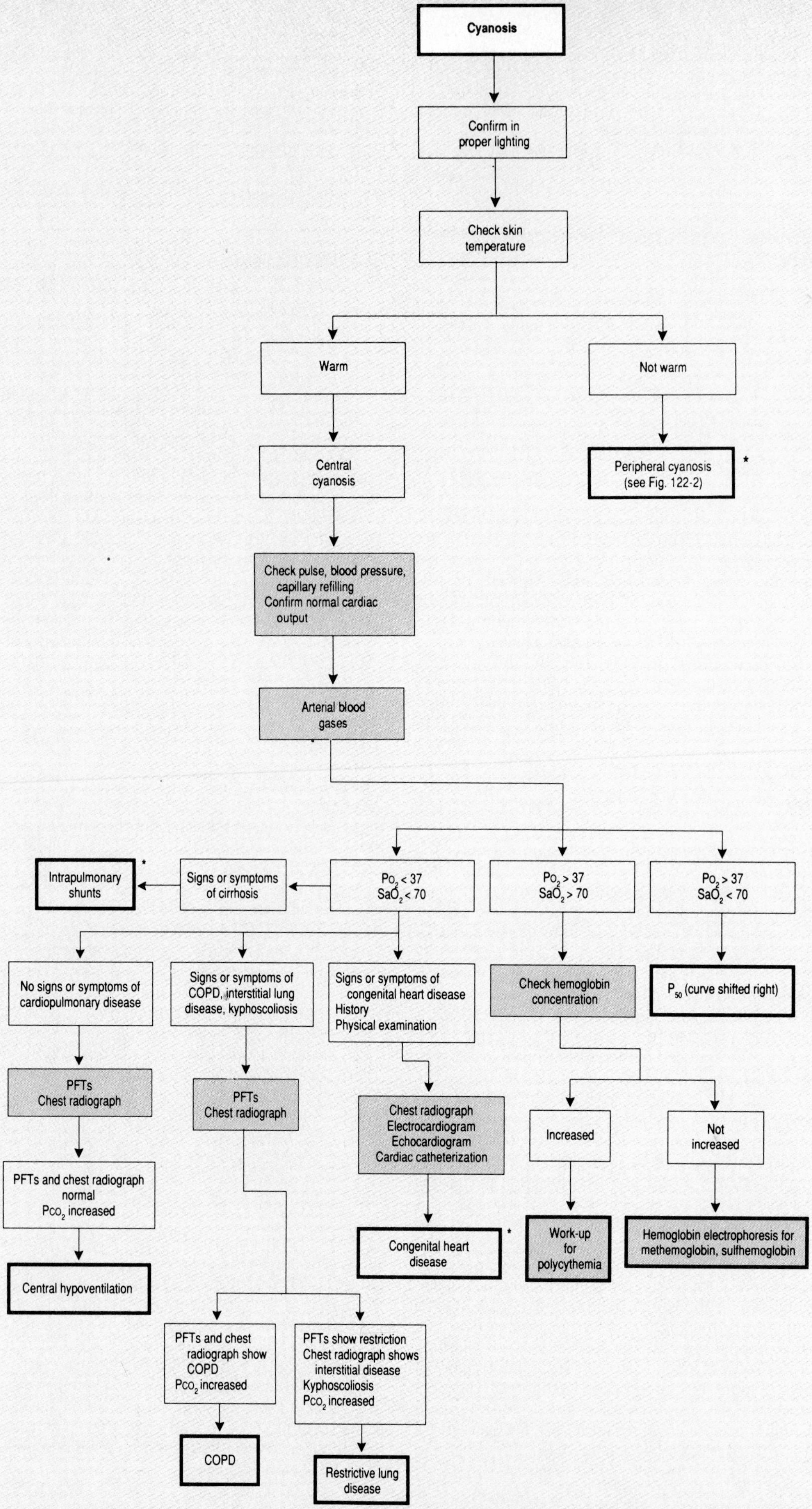

Cyanosis
Confirm in proper lighting
Check skin temperature
Warm
Not warm
Central cyanosis
Peripheral cyanosis (see Fig. 122-2) *
Check pulse, blood pressure, capillary refilling
Confirm normal cardiac output
Arterial blood gases
Intrapulmonary shunts *
Signs or symptoms of cirrhosis
$P_{O_2} < 37$ $SaO_2 < 70$
$P_{O_2} > 37$ $SaO_2 > 70$
$P_{O_2} > 37$ $SaO_2 < 70$
No signs or symptoms of cardiopulmonary disease
Signs or symptoms of COPD, interstitial lung disease, kyphoscoliosis
Signs or symptoms of congenital heart disease
History
Physical examination
Check hemoglobin concentration
P_{50} (curve shifted right)
PFTs
Chest radiograph
PFTs
Chest radiograph
Chest radiograph
Electrocardiogram
Echocardiogram
Cardiac catheterization
Increased
Not increased
PFTs and chest radiograph normal
P_{CO_2} increased
Congenital heart disease *
Work-up for polycythemia
Hemoglobin electrophoresis for methemoglobin, sulfhemoglobin
Central hypoventilation
PFTs and chest radiograph show COPD
P_{CO_2} increased
PFTs show restriction
Chest radiograph shows interstitial disease
Kyphoscoliosis
P_{CO_2} increased
COPD
Restrictive lung disease

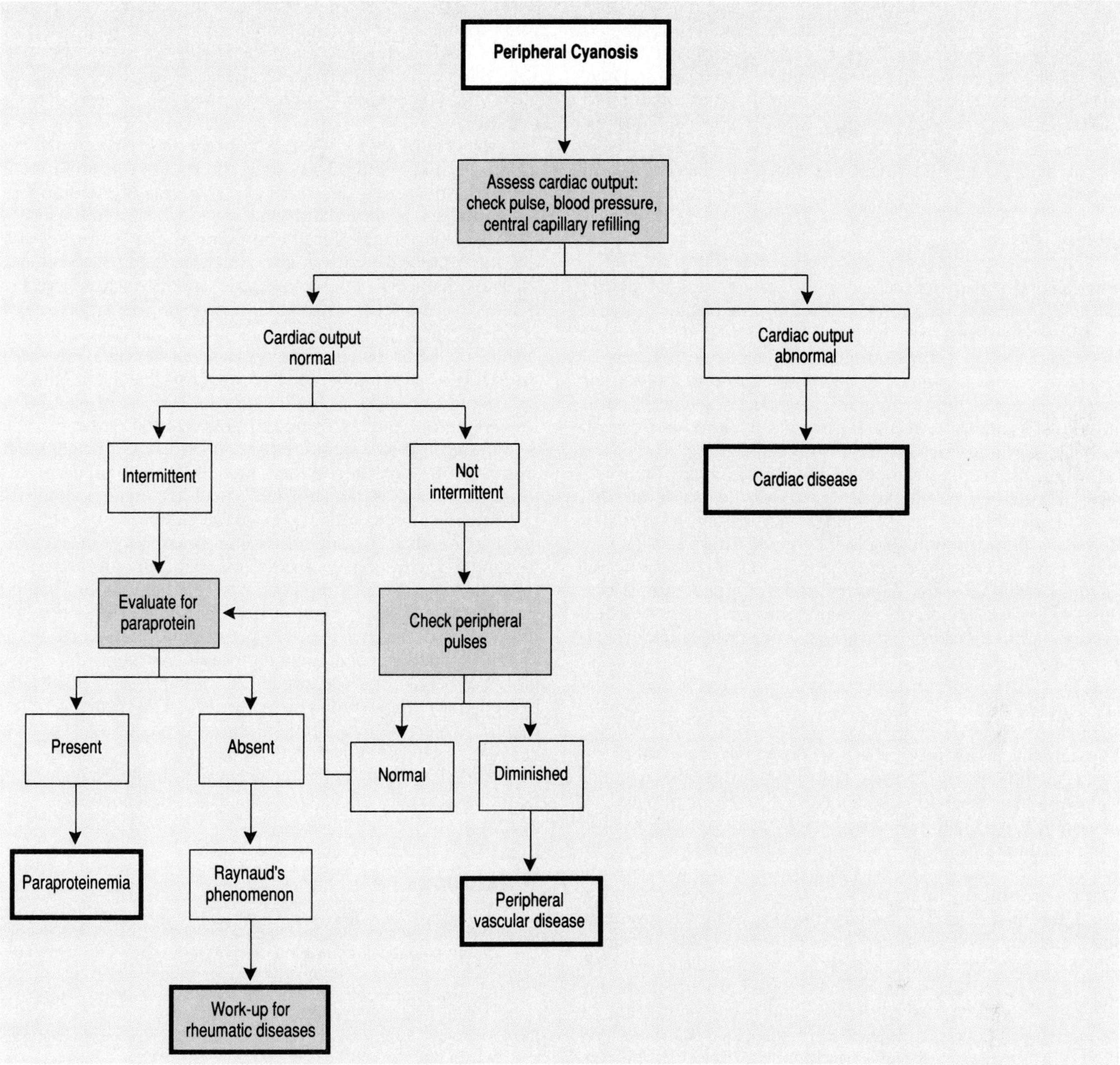

Figure 122-2 Algorithm for the diagnostic evaluation of peripheral cyanosis.

Diagnostic Approach

Physical Examination

When cyanosis is observed or the examiner suspects cyanosis may be present, the examination should proceed under optimal lighting conditions. The hands should receive special attention. The color of unexposed portions of the skin, palms, soles, oral mucous membranes, conjunctival sacs, and nailbeds should be inspected and, if possible, compared with those of a known normal individual. The nailbeds should also be examined for clubbing, the first sign of which is softness or sponginess of the tissues lying deep to the proximal end of the nailplate. Clubbing may be associated with hypoxemia in obstructive and restrictive lung diseases and cyanotic congenital heart disease, among other conditions (see Chapter 116, "Clubbing"). Pulse rate and blood pressure as well as the temperature of the acral skin (finger, toes, ears, nose) should be assessed as a means of judging the adequacy of cardiac output. One should ensure that the cyanotic color blanches on pressure in order to rule out the presence of nonhemoglobin pigments and to observe the speed of capillary refilling as a measure of local blood flow. Comparison should be made with capillary refilling in a central location, such as over the sternum or scapula. The lungs and heart should also be examined carefully for signs of COPD, interstitial lung disease, or murmurs suggestive of congenital heart disease. One should also note any severe chest deformity such as kyphoscoliosis, which could result in hypoxemia and cyanosis. All peripheral pulses should be palpated for signs of vascular occlusive

Figure 122-1 Algorithm for the diagnostic evaluation of central cyanosis. Asterisks (*) indicate conditions that are not improved by oxygen therapy. COPD = chronic obstructive pulmonary disease, PFTs = pulmonary function tests.

disease. The skin, especially over the trunk, should be inspected for telangiectasias, which arise from a central vessel and branch out radially ("spiders"). These are common in cirrhosis and may be markers for similar lesions in the lungs. The lips, tongue, and palmar surfaces of the fingers and toes should be examined for the lesions of hereditary hemorrhagic telangiectasia. These appear as 0.5- to 3-mm bright red, flat spots that blanch on pressure.

History

When taking a history from a cyanotic patient, seek details regarding respiratory symptoms, heart murmurs or other cardiac disease, and arthritis. Ask the patient about a family history of abnormal blood or coloration, and elicit a meticulous history of recent or chronic drug use or chemical exposure, looking for agents (such as nitrates, nitrites, aromatic ring compounds, aniline dyes and drugs, acetanilid, phenacetin, lidocaine, certain sulfonamides) that can oxidize ferrous hemoglobin iron to the ferric iron of methemoglobin or sulfhemoglobin. When cyanosis is confined to the distal aspects of the hands or feet, particularly when it is episodic in its occurrence, a history of Raynaud's phenomenon should be sought. The association of acral cyanosis with exposure to the cold and the occurrence of painful blanching of the digits *prior to* the appearance of cyanosis suggest Raynaud's phenomenon. In such patients, further history should be taken to exclude the presence of underlying rheumatic disease.

Laboratory Tests

The definitive laboratory test is a measurement of arterial blood gases, including pH and P_{CO_2}. Most laboratories also report a value for oxyhemoglobin saturation calculated from pH and P_{O_2}, assuming a normally positioned oxyhemoglobin dissociation curve. Saturation must be determined independently if an abnormal curve is possible. Hemoglobin concentration should also be measured. The response to oxygen therapy may aid in the differential diagnosis, because the cyanosis due to right-to-left shunting, low-flow states, and oxidized hemoglobin generally does not improve with added oxygen. Chest roentgenography helps in the diagnosis of obstructive and interstitial lung diseases as well as cardiac diseases and is complemented by pulmonary function testing (PFT) and electrocardiography (EKG). In rare instances, hemoglobin electrophoresis, protein electrophoresis, echocardiography, peripheral arteriography, or even cardiac catheterization may be needed in order to attain a specific diagnosis. In patients suspected of having Raynaud's phenomenon, serologic studies for rheumatic disease may be helpful.

The general logic of the diagnostic approach is summarized in Figures 122-1 and 122-2. After confirming the presence of cyanosis, one should determine, on the basis of skin temperature, capillary refilling, and vital signs, whether the cause is central or peripheral. Peripheral cyanosis can be further subdivided into local ischemia and generalized poor flow due to cardiac dysfunction. Causes of local ischemia include irreversible occlusive disease, reversible vasospasm, and hyperviscosity of blood due to paraproteinemia. Central cyanosis can be subdivided on the basis of the results of arterial P_{O_2}, SaO_2, and P_{CO_2}. Arterial P_{CO_2} is an index of the adequacy of alveolar ventilation: hypoventilation elevates P_{CO_2}; hyperventilation lowers it. A P_{O_2} low enough to cause a saturation less than 70 percent (about 37 mm Hg) indicates the presence of lung disease or right-to-left shunting. Chest roentgenogram, EKG, PFT, and findings on history and physical examination will usually distinguish among the possible diagnoses easily. A P_{O_2} greater than 37 mm Hg (and SaO_2 greater than 70 percent) implies the existence of an excess of normal hemoglobin (polycythemia) or a hemoglobin that can produce cyanosis at a higher SaO_2 (methemoglobin, sulfhemoglobin). A measurement of hemoglobin concentration will distinguish between these two possibilities, and hemoglobin electrophoresis can document the presence of abnormal hemoglobin molecules and identify the abnormal species. Finally, the presence of cyanosis with P_{O_2} in excess of 37 mm and SaO_2 less than 70 percent defines a hemoglobin with an elevated P_{50}, i.e., a right-shifted oxyhemoglobin dissociation curve.

Note that these conditions are not mutually exclusive; two or more etiologies of cyanosis may exist simultaneously.

References

Braunwald E. Cyanosis. In: Braunwald E, et al, eds. Harrison's principles of internal medicine, 11th ed. New York: McGraw-Hill, 1987:145.

Bunn HF. Disorders of hemoglobin. In: Braunwald E, et al, eds. Harrison's principles of internal medicine. 11th ed. New York: McGraw-Hill, 1987:1524.

Fraser RG, et al. Diagnosis of diseases of the chest. 3rd ed. Philadelphia: WB Saunders, 1988:405.

123 Sputum Production

Joel M. Seidman, MD

Definition

Normally, the tracheobronchial tree produces 100 to 150 ml of mucus per day from goblet cells and mucous glands. This volume, augmented by cellular debris and alveolar fluid, is cleared by ciliary action and coughing to the hypopharynx and swallowed unconsciously. When daily sputum production exceeds usual volumes, there is greater and greater tendency for sputum to be raised to the posterior pharynx and expectorated voluntarily. Whether factors other than volume promote sputum production has not been determined, nor has the exact volume that is abnormal been clearly delineated. However, for the purpose of this discussion, repeated expectoration of sputum should be considered pathologic.

Etiology

Sputum is normally clear and mucoid, with a high content of mucopolysaccharides. The cellular constituents comprise alveolar macrophages and bronchial epithelial cells, with rare lymphoid and polymorphonuclear cells. Increased sputum volume may result from innumerable irritants to the respiratory tract. The common cold and cigarette smoking are probably the leading causes of sputum production. Inflammatory diseases of the pulmonary parenchyma or airways cause the influx of increased numbers of polymorphonuclear cells. These cells release proteolytic, peroxidative enzymes that act on protein constituents, yielding a yellowish or greenish pigment. Eosinophils as well as polymorphonuclear leukocytes are capable of causing yellow or green sputum, so that the color in itself cannot be interpreted as synonymous with infection. Pneumonia, acute and chronic bronchitis, bronchiectasis, lung abscess, and asthma (among many illnesses) may cause purulent sputum. Bronchiectatic sputum classically layers out into an uppermost foamy white layer, a middle opalescent mucoid layer, and a lowermost purulent layer. It may be foul-smelling, and blood streaks may be admixed. Lung abscesses may cause putrid sputum. Cancers of the lung do not usually cause sputum production, although some patients with alveolar cell carcinoma produce copious mucoid sputum. Most primary lung carcinomas shed cells into the sputum and can be detected by exfoliative cytologic techniques.

Diagnostic Approach

Sputum production is a nonspecific sign of disease and should be followed up with appropriate history taking and physical examination, chest roentgenography, and examination of the sputum. A freshly expectorated specimen should be inspected grossly and any odor noted. Using a wooden applicator stick (bent so as to break in a long, sharp, pointed splinter), a pinhead-sized globule of sputum should be teased onto a glass slide, pressed flat under a coverslip, and examined under low power, high power, and oil immersion without stain and using reduced substage lighting. With careful focusing technique, cellular constituents can be discerned and identified.

Squamous cells fill an oil-immersion field; they are multiangular and each has a central nucleus. Plentiful squamous cells should cast doubt on the alveolar source of the specimen. To be labeled as sputum, alveolar macrophages, large (15 to 30 μm) mononuclear cells with various large, irregular inclusion bodies, should be easily found. One may also observe polymorphonuclear leukocytes (multilobed, granules of various size), eosinophils (bilobed, completely filled with uniform, large, refractile granules), and bronchial epithelial cells. Occasionally, motile cilia may be seen. Noncellular constituents such as mucus, refractile Charcot-Leyden crystals (formed from crystallized enzyme from eosinophilic membranes released into the medium), Curschmann's spirals (mucous casts of bronchioles), and bacteria may be observed. Another specimen should be smeared and stained by Gram stain (and other stains as indicated). It is usually of little value to stain or culture a specimen that shows abundant squamous cells on unstained wet mount.

Pneumonias are usually characterized by purulent sputum that contains polymorphonuclear leukocytes and bacteria. Asthma (especially the syndrome of wheezy bronchitis in exacerbation) is frequently associated with purulent sputum, eosinophils, Charcot-Leyden crystals, and occasionally Curschmann's spirals. Clumps of bronchial epithelial cells, called Creola bodies, may also be seen. Influenza and other viral infections may cause shedding of large numbers of bronchial epithelial cells.

Specimens for exfoliative cytologic study and culturing for fungus or tuberculosis should be obtained from the first sputum expectorated on arising. In the case of scant sputum production or for the convenience of outpatients, pooled specimens obtained over several days may be satisfactory. The inhalation of mildly irritating aerosols such as distilled water or hypertonic saline may promote cough and increase sputum production in patients who cannot produce adequate volumes for examination.

References

Chodosh S. Current concepts: Examination of sputum cells. N Engl J Med 1970; 282:954.

Dulfano MJ. The mucous system. In: Sputum: Fundamentals and clinical pathology. Springfield, IL: Charles C Thomas, 1973:3.

Epstein RL. Constituents of sputum: A simple method. Ann Intern Med 1972; 77:259.

Weller PF, Goetzl EJ, Austen KF. Identification of human eosinophil lysophospholipase as the constituent of Charcot-Leyden crystals. Proc Natl Acad Sci 1980; 77:7490.

Solitary Pulmonary Nodule

Marcia K. Liepman, MD

124

The detection of a nodule on the chest radiograph of an asymptomatic person may present a diagnostic dilemma. Diagnosis and management depend on the clinical setting (e.g., presence or absence of symptoms, history of cigarette smoking, environmental exposure, prior illness) and diagnostic and therapeutic options available when the abnormality is noted. A logical approach to management is important. The diagnostic strategy chosen must be individualized. It should optimize the chances of detecting and treating malignancy or other treatable entities and minimize the possibility of an unnecessary thoracotomy.

Definition

A solitary pulmonary nodule (often referred to as a *coin lesion*) is a *single* rounded or oval lesion less than 6 cm in diameter lying *within the lung,* completely surrounded by aerated lung. This definition is sometimes altered in the literature to include only solitary lesions less than 4 cm in diameter. Most authors stress that the borders of the lesion are sharp and that the rest of the pulmonary parenchyma and mediastinum is normal. The patient should be asymptomatic. Once a solitary pulmonary nodule (SPN) is noted on a chest radiograph, it *must* be explained. It is well known that for cancerous nodules the rate of resectability decreases with increasing size of the nodules. Therefore, the major task facing the clinician is to decide when and on whom to operate for SPN.

Signs and Symptoms

The majority of patients with SPN are asymptomatic. The presence of systemic symptoms or hemoptysis in a patient with a history of cigarette smoking who has SPN should strongly suggest malignancy, either primary carcinoma of the lung or metastatic carcinoma. Some patients with metastatic disease from a nonpulmonary primary lesion may not be clinically ill, so a thorough history and physical examination, *including* a thorough review of systems and past medical history, are important.

Etiology

The etiologies of SPN are diverse. The presence of SPN requires an explanation (is it cancer, or not?). Series of patients with SPN have differed in their numbers of benign and malignant lesions. Few features will assure that a lesion is benign. Neither primary lung cancer nor metastatic cancer to the lung is excluded by a patient's asymptomatic status, prior history of tuberculosis or positive skin tests, or flecks of calcium in the lesion on radiograph. Prior radiographs demonstrating that the lesion has been stable for more than 2 years or has been shrinking suggest a benign lesion. Table 124-1 outlines common causes of SPN.

Diagnostic Approach

The diagnostic approach includes four steps: (1) history and physical examination, (2) other noninvasive techniques, (3) invasive techniques, and (4) thoracotomy.

History and Physical Examination

A careful history and physical are mandatory, even though most patients whose pulmonary nodules are truly solitary are asymptomatic. No historical feature can be relied upon to rule out malignancy, but certain features may influence the diagnostic work-up. These include age, smoking history, sex, and prior history of malignancy.

Age. Age correlates directly with an individual's risk of having a malignant coin lesion. Patients less than 35 years of age are at less risk of malignancy, especially if no smoking history is obtained. However, like the other historical factors to be discussed, age alone cannot be relied upon to exclude the presence of malignancy. Close follow-up is indicated in the young patient with a coin lesion, and aggressive intervention is mandatory if malignancy becomes suspect.

Sex. Men are more prone to malignant lesions than women. This may be changing, however, as more women are smoking cigarettes.

Smoking History. The smoking and occupational histories (especially combinations of factors such as smoking and exposure to asbestos) cannot be overemphasized as causative factors in patients with SPN.

Prior History. Prior history of malignancy is an extremely important historical fact in assessing the patient with SPN. The risk of a nodule's being a metastasis varies inversely with the latent period from the primary tumor. Some primary tumors are much more likely to have pulmonary metastases than others. For example, patients with a prior history of sarcoma have a high likelihood of metastatic disease to the lungs as a cause for SPN, whereas SPN in a patient with head and neck cancer is much more likely to be the result of a second primary neoplasm. In a patient whose primary malignancy has been controlled and who develops a new metastatic coin lesion, however, consideration should be given to surgical palliation by resection of the SPN. Many patients can be well palliated, or even cured (25 to 40 percent), by removal of such a solitary metastatic lesion.

Noninvasive Studies

Noninvasive studies are mainly radiologic. The evaluation of the chest radiograph begins with an attempt by the clinician to ascertain the radiographic history of the SPN. Obtaining old chest radiographs is extremely important in the evaluation of the patient with SPN. If such films can be obtained but are not immedicately available, the work-up should be halted until the films can be obtained and reviewed (assuming this can be done in a timely fashion). The rate at which a lesion increases in size, the so-called doubling time, may suggest malignancy; most cancers have doubling times of 5 weeks to 18 months. Those with shorter doubling times are usually benign (inflammatory), and those present and stable for more than 2 years are rarely malignant.

The presence or absence of certain patterns of calcification within a lesion may be of diagnostic significance. The presence of calcium within a lesion does not rule out malignancy. Dense, generalized calcification, laminated calcification, or the so-called popcorn calcification seen in hamartomas may suggest a benign process. Calcification within a lesion alone does not exclude malignancy and is only one feature in a full assessment of SPN.

Finally, fair assurance that the lesion is solitary may be obtained by a computed tomographic (CT) scan of the chest and mediastinum or by whole-lung tomography. These two procedures should be done to assess mediastinal abnormalities as well, if none is apparent on the plain film of the chest.

Table 124-2 outlines the differentiation of benign and malignant nodules.

Invasive Evaluation

None of the historical or noninvasive techniques described is a substitute for a tissue diagnosis. The approach chosen for invasive procedures for diagnosis of any individual patient with SPN should maximize the efficiency of making the diagnosis of cancer and minimize the associated morbidity. The clinician should consider how the results of the procedure will modify the approach to diagnosis and treatment. A suggested algorithm is presented in Figure 124-1. Needless to say, at each step in the

Table 124-1 Incidence of Various Types of Solitary Pulmonary Nodules

Greater than 5%	Less than 1%
Cancer, primary or metastatic	Hematoma
Hamartoma	Infarction
Tuberculoma	Vasculitis
Fungal granuloma	Lymph node enlargement
Artifact (e.g., nipple, skin nodule)	Arteriovenous malformation
1% to 5%	Rheumatoid nodule
Abscess	Sequestration
Lipoid pneumonia	Cyst
Resolving pneumonia	Foreign body
	Fluid ("disappearing tumor")

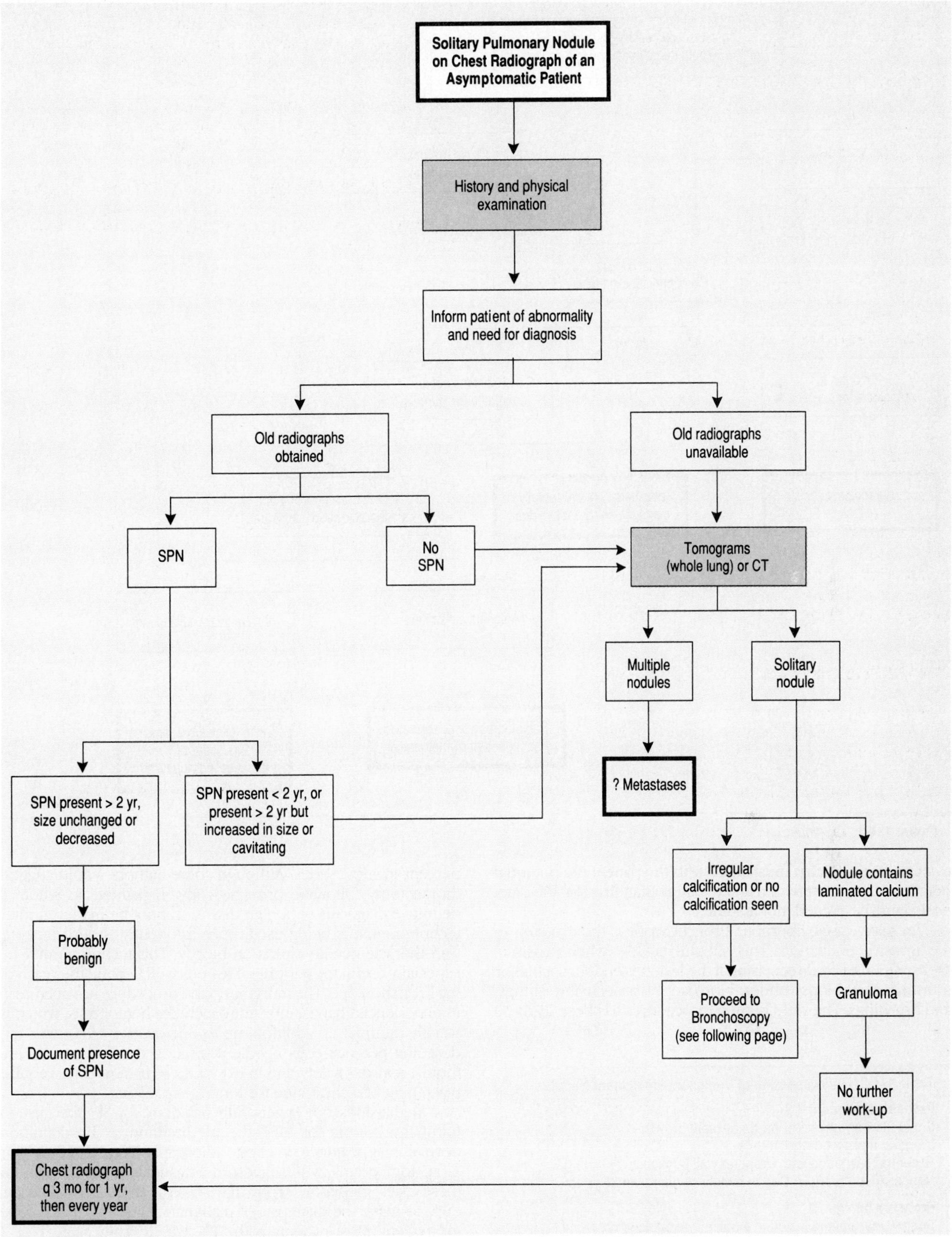

Figure 124-1 Algorithm for the diagnostic evaluation of a solitary pulmonary nodule (SPN). CT = computed tomography.

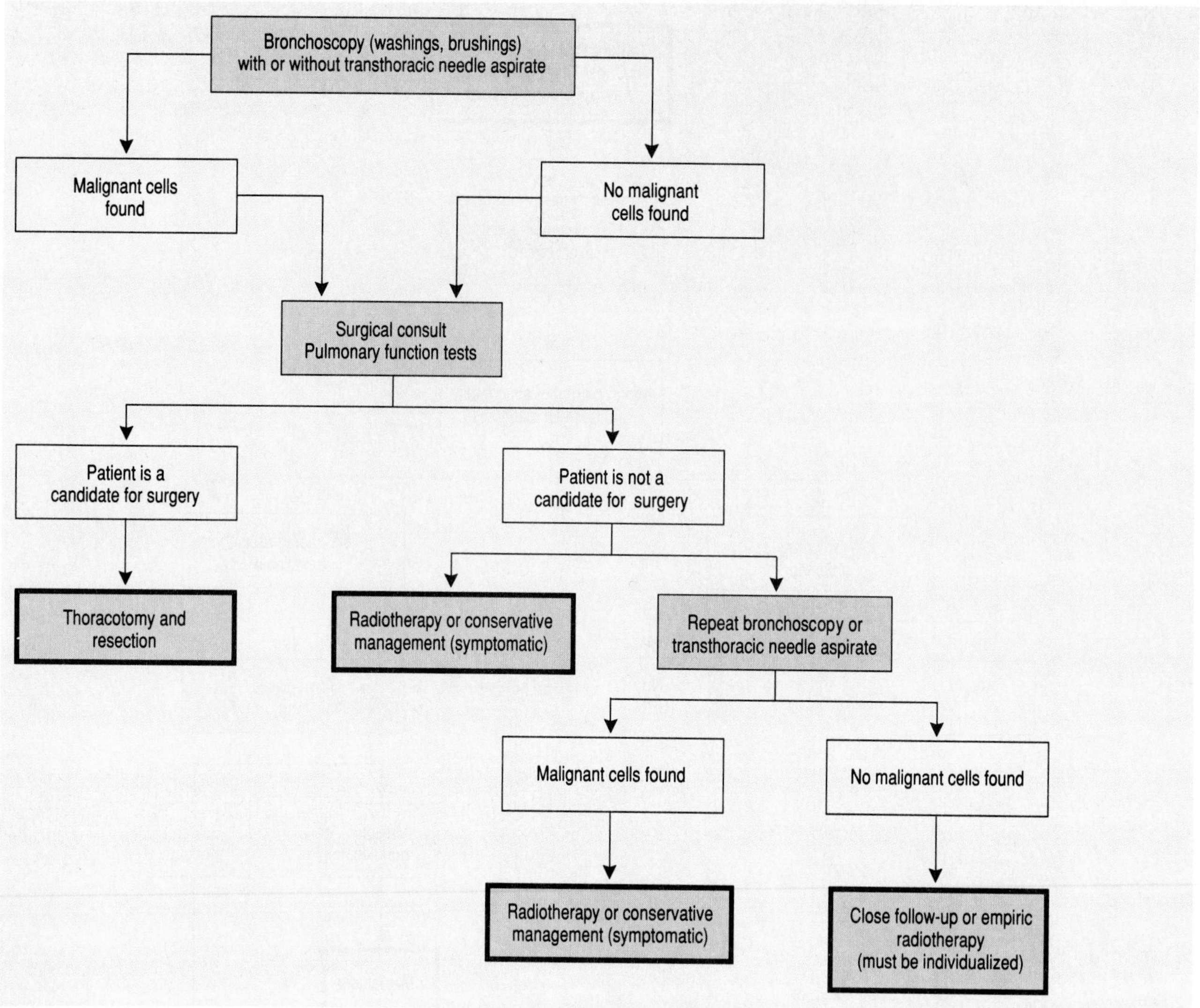

Figure 124-1 *Continued*

evaluation, a clinician must share with the patient the potential outcomes of the evaluation and the understanding that the diagnosis must be proved, not assumed.

In many cases, fiberoptic bronchoscopy is the first step in the invasive evaluation. This should include, when possible, biopsy (guided by direct vision if the lesion is endobronchial or transbronchial biopsy under fluoroscopy), bronchial washings, and brushings. The yield of these procedures has been 25 to 30 percent in most series. Although some authors would suggest thoracotomy following bronchoscopy in patients in whom a definitive diagnosis of benign disease cannot be made, another technique that is being used more frequently is percutaneous transthoracic needle aspiration biopsy. This technique may be especially useful for peripheral lesions well beyond the reach of the bronchoscope. The mortality of the procedure has been zero in experienced hands; morbidity includes hemoptysis, which is usually minimal. In addition, up to one-quarter of patients undergoing percutaneous needle aspiration develop a pneumothorax; approximately one in five of these patients may require placement of a chest tube for lung reexpansion.

Mediastinoscopy is generally not done for SPN because to fulfill the criteria for SPN, the mediastinum is by definition normal in appearance on chest radiograph. Occasionally, CT or x-ray tomograms will suggest mediastinal abnormalities; in these cases, mediastinoscopy may serve as an additional procedure to make the diagnosis of malignancy and to further stage the patient. Most patients with SPN are clinically stage 1 or 2 (according to the American Joint Commission) on the basis of the size of their nodule.

Table 124-2 Differentiation of Benign and Malignant Nodules

Probably Malignant
Serial films show recent origin or rapid growth
Irregular margins of the nodule
Eccentric cavitation with irregular wall thickness
Noncalcified "fuzzy" lesion in a male smoker over 35 yr old
Probably Benign
Sharply marginated lesion in a patient under 35 yr old
Stable appearance on chest radiograph for more than 2 yr
Radiographic appearance characteristic of lesion associated with proven (known) systemic disease
Almost Certainly Benign
Solid or laminated calcification
Stable appearance on chest radiograph for 5 yr
Serial films show evolution characteristic of inflammatory lesion

Thoracotomy

Thoracotomy is the final diagnostic step in patients who are operative candidates and for whom a benign diagnosis is not unequivocally established. Patients whose respiratory status is borderline may require specialized pulmonary function studies to establish their physiologic status for operation. Cooperation between clinician and surgeon is essential here. In experienced hands, morbidity and mortality are very low.

Prognosis

Because 90 to 95 percent of all malignant SPNs are primary lung cancers, and because this special group of lung cancers has a relatively favorable prognosis, motivation for thoracotomy and resection should be high. Carcinomas less than 6 cm in diameter are resectable in over 85 percent of cases, and the 5-year survival rate for cancers less than 2 cm in diameter is 80 percent. Thus, thoracotomy is justified even in high-risk patients.

It cannot be overemphasized that the approach to the patient with SPN must be individualized. A 32-year-old nonsmoking man with a 1-cm nodule may be better served by careful, watchful waiting and follow-up chest radiographs; one should consider invasive therapy only if the size of the nodule increases. Conversely, a 56-year-old female smoker with a 3-cm nodule has a much greater risk of malignancy; with her smoking history, the size of her nodule, and her age, her risk of malignancy is in excess of 50 percent.

The features of any individual case may lead to a more or less aggressive approach by the clinician. The general pessimism associated with the diagnosis and treatment of lung cancer cannot prevail in early, asymptomatic cases of lung cancer, such as those described here. Only an aggressive approach will lead to cure in a certain percentage of these cases.

References

Alexander JC. How best to proceed when x-ray turns up a coin lesion. Your Patient and Cancer 1982; 2:41.

Jackman RJ, et al. Survival rate in peripheral bronchogenic carcinomas up to four centimeters in diameter presenting as solitary pulmonary nodules. J Thorac Cardiovasc Surg 1969; 57:1.

Lillington GA, Stevens GM. The solitary nodule: The other side of the coin. Chest 1976; 70:322.

Meyer TJ. The solitary pulmonary nodule: An aggressive work-up. Postgrad Med 1983; 73:66.

Natale RB. Lung cancer: Establishing the diagnosis. In: Schein PS, ed. Decision making in oncology. Toronto: BC Decker, 1989:66.

Ray JF, et al. The coin lesion story: Update 1976. Chest 1976; 70:332.

Steele JD, et al. Survival in males with bronchogenic carcinomas resected as asymptomatic solitary pulmonary nodules. Ann Thorac Surg 1966; 1:368.

Hematuria

Thomas H. Ebert, MD

Definition

Hematuria is defined as blood in the urine. Microscopic hematuria is blood in the urine that can be seen only under a microscope, whereas macroscopic or gross hematuria is visible to the naked eye (1 ml of blood in 1 L of urine can give the urine a pink tinge). Because everyone excretes some red blood cells in the urine, most experts agree that more than five red blood cells (RBCs) per high-power microscopic field or an absolute excretion rate greater than 2,500 RBCs per minute is abnormal. The clinical patterns of hematuria are as follows: (1) gross (macroscopic) or occult (microscopic), (2) persistent or intermittent, and (3) symptomatic or asymptomatic (painless).

Etiology

Hematuria can arise from any part of the urinary tract. A discrete lesion is almost always responsible for urinary tract bleeding, although such a lesion may be small enough to elude diagnosis in patients with an underlying bleeding diathesis. The bleeding lesion(s) may be microscopic, as in glomerulonephritis, or macroscopic, as in bladder cancer. There is no single "most common" etiology for hematuria because the cause depends so much on age and sex. The most common etiologies in adults are (1) urinary tract infections, (2) ureteral calculi, (3) prostatic disease, (4) carcinoma of the bladder, (5) trauma, and (6) glomerular or other primary renal disease.

History and Clinical Clues

As in all areas of medicine, careful history and physical examination are invaluable to help localize clinical urinary tract bleeding. The other important source of information to localize the site of bleeding is the urinalysis. When taking a history from the patient with hematuria, one must ask about the pattern of the hematuria, the frequency of episodes of gross bleeding, and the relationship of macroscopic bleeding to exercise and infection. For example, bladder trauma may occur in serious runners who develop gross hematuria. Furthermore, patients with some forms of glomerulonephritis, such as IgA nephropathy, may manifest gross hematuria with an intercurrent infection. The person taking the history should also ask the patient if the gross hematuria is present throughout micturition, because patients with urethral lesions may bleed only at the beginning of urination. If a patient has only asymptomatic microscopic hematuria, one must ask how the hematuria was discovered (e.g., on routine urinalysis for a job or school). Many patients with microscopic hematuria have benign, asymptomatic causes; therefore, the hematuria may be discovered serendipitously.

Other pertinent questions in the history should focus on evidence of systemic disease, e.g., weight loss, fever, abdominal or loin (lower abdominal) pain, ureteral colic, frequency and dysuria, joint pain, and hearing loss. Patients with renal cell carcinoma may present with weight loss, fever, and abdominal pain along with hematuria. Certain kinds of bladder or ureteral cancers might present with loin pain or ureteral colic. Renal stones might present with ureteral colic, i.e., pain referred from the kidney down the ureter into the groin. Frequency and dysuria may indicate a urinary tract infection. Joint pain associated with hematuria might be indicative of an immune complex disease or a vasculitis. Hearing loss might be associated with a hereditary renal disease such as Alport's syndrome. The patient's history of drug use, e.g., analgesics, anticoagulants, or drugs whose metabolites turn the urine color, is of interest. Excessive use of analgesics has been associated with analgesic nephropathy resulting in microscopic hematuria and with transitional cell carcinoma of the ureter. The use of anticoagulants may be associated with a prolonged prothrombin time, and a history of easy or excessive bleeding may indicate a bleeding diathesis. Finally, the physician should ask about a family history of renal disease, e.g., deafness associated with Alport's syndrome or recurrent hematuria associated with a family history of IgA nephropathy, a family history of sickle cell disease in blacks, or a family history of subarachnoid hemorrhage in patients with a family history of polycystic kidney disease.

The physical examination should emphasize the blood pressure, evidence of ecchymoses, rash and loin or flank tenderness, and evidence of prostatic hypertrophy or tenderness in older men. In particular, prostatic hypertrophy is a common cause of microscopic hematuria and the most common cause of this condition in urology clinics.

Urinalysis can provide useful information about the source of urinary tract bleeding. The "three-glass test" is an old bedside technique for localizing hematuria. The patient is asked to collect the urine sequentially in three different containers during a single void. If the blood is in the initial container only, it represents bleeding from the urethra; if it is in the second, the bleeding may be from anywhere in the urinary tract; and if it is in the third container only, the bleeding is most likely from the bladder. This test is used infrequently now. Other useful clues when examining the urine with the naked eye are color and the presence of clots. Gross bleeding from a glomerular lesion may be smoky brown because of the presence of methemoglobin from the relatively long exposure of hemoglobin to acid urine. The presence of clots rules out a microscopic glomerular lesion as a source because glomerular bleeding does not clot. Finally, a number of drugs and vegetable dyes give the urine a reddish color when excreted.

Before examining the urinary sediment under a microscope, the examiner should "dipstick" the urine to look for evidence of hemoglobin and to rule out the possibility that a dye or drug metabolite is turning the urine red. Most dipsticks contain benzidine, which reacts with free hemoglobin in the urine. Albuminuria may also be detected with a dipstick and, in combination with hematuria, indicates intrinsic renal disease (significant proteinuria is defined as quantitatively more than 200 mg of protein with microscopic hematuria and more than 300 mg of protein with macroscopic hematuria).

The urinary sediment is examined after the urine is spun for approximately 3 minutes at 3,000 rpm and the supernatant discarded. Again, the company the red cells keep in the urine can help localize the source of urinary tract bleeding. The presence of cellular casts, particularly RBC casts, is diagnostic of intrinsic kidney disease. A cast is formed in tubules from precipitated proteins. These precipitated protein skeletons have either RBCs, white blood cells (WBCs), or epithelial cells attached to them. The presence of RBC casts is diagnostic of glomerulonephritis and vasculitis. Hematuria with pyuria and WBC casts may lead to the diagnosis of renal tubulointerstitial disease. Dysmorphic RBCs indicate that the source of bleeding is glomerular; the dysmorphism is caused when the RBC passes through a rent in an abnormal glomerular basement membrane. RBCs and WBCs in the urine may be associated with urinary tract infections in the kidney, bladder, or prostate.

Diagnostic Approach

The clinician faces two missions in the diagnosis of hematuria: (1) localizing the anatomic site of bleeding and (2) establishing the etiology. As the following paragraphs show, there is a relationship between the anatomy of the genitourinary system and the specific causes of hematuria.

Renal Sources of Hematuria

Glomerular Diseases. Renal glomerular diseases are often divided into those manifested mainly by proteinuria (called "nephrotic" if proteinuria exceeds 3.5 g per 24 hours) and those in which the urinary sediment has evidence of blood and blood casts ("nephritic" disorders). Any glomerular disease may demonstrate nephritic or nephrotic features, but all tend to follow clinical patterns; e.g., IgA nephropathy is more commonly nephritic, whereas minimal change disease invariably has a nephrotic presentation. When systemic vasculitis such as Wegener's granulomatosis is associated with glomerulonephritis, a nephritic sediment is often seen. Finally, accelerated and malignant hypertension characteristically have an "active" urinary sediment with blood cells and proteinuria.

Nonglomerular Diseases. Interstitial nephritis typically shows little proteinuria but rather pyuria and microscopic hematuria. Tumors in the kidney or infarctions in the kidney also can present with hematuria.

Extrarenal Sources of Hematuria

Ureter. In the ureter, calculi, tumors, or infections commonly present with hematuria.

Bladder. Bladder lesions characteristically bleed, and the bleeding can be microscopic or macroscopic. The bladder is sensitive to various toxins, such as cyclophosphamide, and to infectious processes, which often result in at least microscopic hematuria.

Prostate. Any form of prostatic disease may cause hematuria. In general urology clinics, the most common cause of microscopic hematuria is prostatic hypertrophy or prostatitis.

Urethra. Microscopic hematuria occurs in patients with urethral trauma and occasionally in patients with sexually acquired diseases.

Initial Laboratory Tests

These tests should be part of the work-up of any patient presenting with new-onset hematuria. They should at least be employed as stipulated.

1. Urinalysis. Perform urinalysis with careful microscopic examination of the sediment to see what company the red cells keep.
2. Complete blood count. Anemia is characteristic of chronic renal failure, but it is rarely seen with hematuria, even gross hematuria.
3. Prothrombin time, partial thromboplastin time, platelet count, and bleeding time. These should be assessed in a patient with a history of a bleeding diathesis.
4. Hemoglobin electrophoresis. This should be performed in blacks to look for sickle trait (AS), SS, or SC hemoglobin.
5. Urine culture. Use this test to diagnose infection.
6. Serum creatinine. An elevated creatinine level indicates intrinsic renal disease.
7. Electrolytes and calcium. Electrolyte abnormalities may indicate intrinsic renal disease, whereas an elevated calcium level could be seen in renal cancer.
8. Tuberculin skin tests. In genitourinary tuberculosis, the skin test is characteristically positive.

References

Boyd PJR. Hematuria. Br Med J 1977; 2:445.
Pollak VE, Ooi BS. Hematuria. Postgrad Med 1977; 62:115.
Rose BD. Diagnostic approach to the patient with renal disease. In: Pathophysiology of renal disease. 2nd ed. New York: McGraw-Hill, 1987.
Schaeffer AJ, DelGreco F. Hematuria. In: Walsh, PC, et al, eds. Campbell's urology. 5th ed. Philadelphia: WB Saunders, 1986:2342.
West CD. Asymptomatic hematuria and proteinuria in children: Causes and appropriate diagnostic studies. J Pediatr 1976; 89:173.

Azotemia

David M. Clive, MD

126

When disease processes occur in specific organ systems, they may make their presence known through well-recognized signs or symptoms. For example, a patient with peptic ulcer disease may have characteristic epigastric pain. Pneumonia is often diagnosed on the basis of a productive cough and abnormal breath sounds that suggest pulmonary consolidation. In contrast, patients with renal disorders rarely offer the physician substantive clinical clues to localize the problem to the kidney. The symptoms of kidney disease, malaise, pallor, anorexia, and edema, to name a few, are nonspecific and may be subtle, if present at all. The kidney is an organ with diverse functions: maintenance of normal fluid and electrolyte balance, elimination of metabolic wastes, control of blood pressure, activation of vitamin D, and the production of renin and erythropoietin. Renal disease may affect some of those functions more than others, further complicating the diagnostic process.

Definition

Compromise of the kidneys' ability to filter and excrete metabolic waste leads to an accumulation of these substances in the blood. Elevated levels of the nitrogenous wastes, urea and creatinine, termed *azotemia,* are often the heralding signs of kidney disease.

Urea, which is formed in the liver from the deamination of amino acids, is measured as blood urea nitrogen (BUN, normally 8 to 20 mg/dl). Creatinine is a muscle breakdown product with normal circulating levels of 0.5 to 1.5 mg/dl; in general, the larger an individual's muscle mass, the higher the expected normal serum creatinine level. Daily creatinine production occurs at rather fixed rates.

Both of these solutes are filtered and excreted by the kidney. Some reabsorption of urea occurs in the renal tubules, so that urea clearance is less than the true glomerular filtration rate (GFR). The creatinine clearance is slightly greater than the actual GFR (as measured by inulin clearance), because some creatinine is excreted by tubular secretion. In spite of this discrepancy, the creatinine clearance remains a popular clinical method of evaluating renal function.

A geometric relationship has been observed between the GFR and serum creatinine concentration; successive halving of the GFR results in a doubling of the serum creatinine, provided creatinine production continues at a stable rate (Fig. 126-1). It should not be inferred that any two people with the same serum creatinine level have identical GFRs. Older people and people of slight muscle mass *produce* less creatinine on a daily basis. Thus, a 70-year-old woman with a serum creatinine of 1.5 mg/dl will have a lower GFR than a 20-year-old man with the same serum creatinine level.

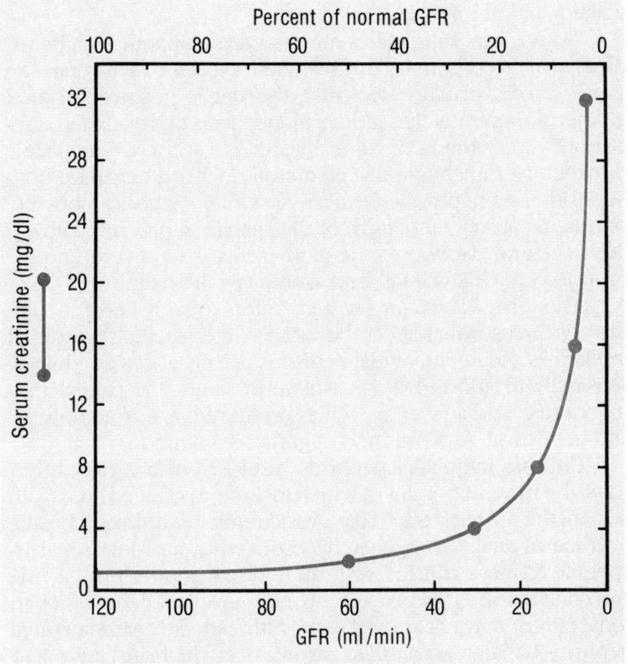

Figure 126-1 Relationship between serum creatinine level and glomerular filtration rate (GFR).

Cockroft and Gault have devised the following formula that estimates creatinine clearance based on age and body mass:

$$C_{Cr} = \frac{(140 - \text{age in yr}) \times W}{P_{Cr} \times 72}$$

where C_{Cr} = creatinine clearance, W = lean body weight in kilograms, and P_{Cr} = plasma creatinine in milligrams per deciliter.

In clinical practice, renal function is commonly assessed by simply following serum urea or creatinine concentrations rather than by calculating the GFR or creatinine clearance. There are two reasons for this. First, measuring the creatinine clearance necessitates collecting a timed (usually 24-hour) urine specimen for quantification of the daily creatinine excretion, because creatinine clearance equals daily creatinine excretion over plasma creatinine. Second, in patients with acute renal failure whose plasma creatinine is changing over the course of the day, interpretation of a 24-hour clearance study is difficult.

Etiology

Tissue catabolism increases ureagenesis, whereas creatinine release is increased in muscle injury. Azotemia generally does not occur in these states unless the patient has diminished renal functional reserve, preventing excretion of the increased burden of nitrogenous waste. Renal failure is the cause, rather than a mere contributor, in most cases of azotemia. It invariably arises during the course of acute and chronic renal failure. It is traditional, and conceptually very useful, to classify azotemia along three major lines: prerenal, renal, and postrenal. The major causes of acute and chronic renal failure are summarized in Table 126-1 and Table 126-2. Each of these causes is considered in the following sections.

Prerenal Azotemia

A brisk renal blood flow must be maintained to sustain a normal GFR; about 20 percent of the cardiac output goes to the kidneys. Reduced renal perfusion means less blood is delivered for filtering; this results in azotemia. This condition, known as prerenal azotemia, can exist in the absence of any intrinsic disease in the kidneys. Patients with hypovolemia secondary to dehydration, hemorrhage, or third spacing of fluid are particularly susceptible to this condition. Prerenal azotemia may also develop in

Table 126-1 Major Causes of Acute Renal Failure

Prerenal
Hypovolemia
Reduced effective circulatory volume (congestive heart failure, liver disease)
Intrinsic
Vasculitis
Malignant hypertension
Acute glomerulonephritis
Acute tubular necrosis syndromes
Toxic (e.g., aminoglycosides, heavy metals)
Intratubular blockade drugs such as methotrexate and acyclovir, acute uric acid nephropathy, tumor lysis syndrome
Radiocontrast nephropathy
Ischemic tubular necrosis
Acute interstitial nephritis
Hypercalcemia
Multiple myeloma
Postrenal
Acute obstructive uropathy (prostatic hypertrophy, nephrolithiasis, tumors, retroperitoneal fibrosis)

Table 126-2 Major Causes of Chronic Renal Failure in the United States
Glomerular disease
Hypertension
Diabetes mellitus
Inherited renal diseases (mainly polycystic kidney disease, and Alport's syndrome)
Chronic interstitial nephritis (including analgesic nephropathy and interstitial disease associated with anatomic abnormalities of the urinary tract)
Chronic obstructive uropathy

patients whose cardiac output is reduced by the hemodynamic alterations of congestive heart failure, cirrhosis, or hypoalbuminemia. This latter group of patients may actually have an expanded extracellular space and gross edema. However, because the "effective circulatory volume" is physiologically reduced in these states, renal perfusion is impaired just as it is in true hypovolemia.

In prerenal azotemia, the concentration of urea in the blood is frequently elevated disproportionately to the serum creatinine. Why does this happen? Reduced renal perfusion results in a low GFR. Flow of filtrate through the nephrons is slow, predisposing to enhanced tubular reabsorption of urea. The degree of urea retention, therefore, is even greater than would be expected solely on the basis of reduced filtration. Because creatinine is not reabsorbed from the nephron, the disparity between urea clearance and creatinine clearance becomes greater. Blood urea/creatinine ratio, normally about 10 : 1, may rise to more than 20 : 1. Elevation of this ratio is not pathognomonic of reduced renal perfusion, however. If urea production is augmented by accelerated catabolism, as is seen in tetracycline and corticosteroid therapy or reabsorption of a hematoma, even though urea clearance has not decreased, blood urea nitrogen levels may rise above normal, especially in patients with antecedent renal insufficiency.

Because renal tubular function is intact in the "prerenal" patient, the kidney can compensate for the perceived volume loss by avidly reabsorbing salt and water. Consequently, a small volume of concentrated, nearly sodium-free urine is excreted. The reduction in sodium excretion is not merely a function of decreased filtration rate, because the *fractional excretion of filtered sodium* (FE_{Na}) is low. This fraction, which represents the amount of filtered sodium not reabsorbed by the tubules, is less than 1 percent in prerenal patients. The fractional excretion of filtered sodium is derived from the following equation:

$$FE_{Na} = \frac{\text{Sodium excretion}}{\text{Filtered load of sodium}}$$

$$= \frac{\text{Sodium excretion}}{\text{GFR} \times P_{Na}}$$

$$= \frac{U_{Na} \times V}{\dfrac{U_{Cr} \times V}{P_{Cr}} \times P_{Na}}$$

$$= \frac{U_{Na} \times P_{Cr}}{U_{Cr} \times P_{Na}}$$

where V = urine volume, U_{Na} = urine sodium concentration, U_{Cr} = urine creatinine concentration, P_{Na} = plasma sodium concentration, and P_{Cr} = plasma creatinine concentration. Creatinine clearance is taken to equal the GFR here.

Water is also conserved by the kidney in these circumstances, with the result that concentrations of unreabsorbed solutes within the tubular fluid increase. The ratio of concentrations of these substances in the urine to those in the plasma provides an approximation of the extent to which the urine is being concentrated. In prerenal azotemia, the urine/plasma creatinine ratio is always high (greater than 40).

Understanding the renal homeostatic mechanisms operative in the "prerenal" state helps to explain its characteristic changes in urine chemistry. These features, a high urine/plasma creatinine ratio, low urine sodium and FE_{Na}, and elevated BUN/creatinine ratio in plasma, are helpful in differentiating prerenal from other forms of azotemia.

Renal Azotemia

Azotemia of this kind is the result of intrinsic damage to the kidney. The list of diseases that produce this kind of damage is too long to permit a thorough overview in this chapter. However, the following general statements are in order:

1. The pathogenesis of renal parenchymal disease includes ischemic, inflammatory, toxic, degenerative, or infiltrative processes.
2. Such processes may reflect primary kidney disease or may be part of an underlying systemic illness (e.g., diabetes mellitus).
3. Renal failure may follow either an acute or a chronic course, depending on the specific etiology.
4. The clinical manifestations of specific renal disorders may vary according to which parts of the nephron are most affected. Thus, the urinalysis features of glomerular disease are generally distinguishable from those of tubulointerstitial disorders.

Diseases of the glomeruli represent the most important causes of chronic renal failure in the United States. When the structural integrity of the glomerulus is damaged, red blood cells and protein escape into the urine. Classically, the glomerulopathies are said to follow two major clinical patterns. *Nephrotic syndrome* is characterized by heavy proteinuria in excess of 3.5 g per day. When such a condition persists, hypoalbuminemia results and, with it, edema. Again, nephrotic glomerular diseases may be either primary (e.g., lipoid nephrosis) or secondary (e.g., diabetic glomerulosclerosis).

Many glomerulopathies present predominantly with hematuria, which constitutes the so-called *nephritic syndrome*. An example of a primary nephritic disorder is poststreptococcal glomerulonephritis. The glomerulonephritis that occurs in association with systemic vasculitis illustrates a secondary nephritic disorder. Not uncommonly, glomerulonephritis may have both nephritic and nephrotic features, as is often seen in lupus nephritis. Whatever the nature of the specific glomerulopathy, if the structural damage to the glomerulus is of severe enough proportions, GFR will fall, and azotemia will result.

The term *interstitial nephritis* refers to a group of inflammatory diseases that affect the tubular interstitial structures of the kidney. Acute interstitial nephritis usually arises as a hypersensitivity reaction to drugs. Not surprisingly, the patient may have a rash and a fever as well as eosinophilia, eosinophiluria, and hematuria. Azotemia and oliguria are common.

Chronic interstitial nephritis results from a variety of insults, the most important of which include anatomic abnormalities in the urinary tract (e.g., vesicoureteral reflux), chronic overuse of analgesic agents, hyperuricemia, and intrarenal ischemia. Kidneys afflicted with these diseases develop scarring and contraction as the processes continue. A slow progression to renal failure may occur over years. Although chronic interstitial nephritis has also been called chronic pyelonephritis, it is not to be confused with infectious pyelonephritis. Acute pyelonephritis never causes azotemia, unless it is superimposed upon preexisting renal insufficiency.

The hallmark of chronic interstitial nephritis is the presence of white blood cells in the urinary sediment (pyuria). Hematuria may occur, but less commonly than in acute interstitial nephritis. White blood cell casts may also be found. The absence of bacteriuria and clinical signs of infection helps to distinguish the disease from acute pyelonephritis, which also presents with pyuria.

Acute tubular necrosis is a tubulointerstitial disease that represents one of the most common causes of acute renal failure, particularly in hospitalized patients. This illness can usually be traced to an episode of renal ischemia or exposure to a nephrotoxin (e.g., an aminoglycoside antibiotic, radiographic contrast agents, or heavy metals). About one-third to one-half of all patients with acute tubular necrosis are nonoliguric. In most patients, the disease runs a course of several days to several weeks.

The diagnosis of acute tubular necrosis usually is not difficult. Owing to the etiology of the syndrome, most patients are hospitalized at the time the disease presents. Eighty percent of patients with this disease have the classic findings of sloughed renal tubular epithelial cells, epithelial cell casts, or muddy brown granular casts in the urinary sediment.

Because hemodynamic alteration is an important etiologic factor in both acute tubular necrosis and prerenal azotemia, differentiating between these two disorders occasionally causes difficulty. The FE_{Na} is useful in this regard. Recall that the FE_{Na} is very low in prerenal azotemia, owing to active sodium reabsorption by the renal tubules. When frank tubular damage has occurred, as in acute tubular necrosis, the tubules can no longer reclaim sodium efficiently and the FE_{Na} is generally high (greater than 1 percent). Urinary concentration is also impaired in tubular necrosis; as a result, urinary osmolality approximates that of plasma and the urine/plasma creatinine ratio is less than 20.

Postrenal Azotemia

Postrenal azotemia is azotemia caused by urinary obstruction. Many lesions can produce obstructive uropathy, including prostatic enlargement, renal stones, infections, and tumors. Obstruction may occur anywhere between the renal collecting system and the urethral meatus. In order for such a lesion to produce azotemia, however, both kidneys must be involved (because, as we know, one functioning kidney is sufficient to maintain a normal GFR) unless the patient has only one functioning kidney at the outset or had underlying renal insufficiency.

The clinical history frequently points to the specific diagnosis in postrenal azotemia. A previous history of nephrolithiasis, pelvic or retroperitoneal malignancy, or prostatism in an azotemic patient makes obstruction the number-one problem to rule out. Finally, renal failure in a newborn infant is probably due to congenital anatomic ureteral obstruction.

When urine output declines precipitously or anuria is present, an obstructive cause is likely. Although urinary obstruction is the most common cause of anuria, these lesions do not invariably cause a decline in urine output. Partial obstruction anywhere in the urinary tract impairs the kidney's ability to concentrate the urine and may even cause polyuria (nephrogenic diabetes insipidus). In complete unilateral obstruction of one ureter, the contralateral kidney will maintain a normal urine output.

The urine chemistry is generally of little use in diagnosing obstructive uropathy. Hematuria is a frequent finding. The presence of large numbers of crystals in the urinary sediment, e.g., uric acid or calcium oxalate, may suggest the presence of an obstructing calculus. Radiographic techniques represent the most important diagnostic tool in evaluating the patient with a possible urinary tract obstruction.

Consequences of Azotemia

By itself, the presence of an elevated BUN level is of little consequence to health. Massive intravenous infusions of urea into the blood stream of healthy animals fail to reproduce the so-called uremic state. More important are the metabolic derangements that accompany azotemia. These derangements arise from reduced homeostatic capacity in the failing kidney and include the following: hyperkalemia, metabolic acidosis, abnormal salt and water metabolism, abnormal calcium and phosphorus metabolism, and uremia.

Hyperkalemia

This is the most immediately life-threatening electrolyte imbalance encountered in renal patients. Note that renal failure is not a cause of hyperkalemia; hyperkalemia merely arises in these patients owing to an inability to respond to a potassium load. Even when GFR is substantially reduced, the kidneys can excrete a large amount of potassium provided that tubular secretion is intact. For this reason, hyperkalemia more often occurs in patients with tubulointerstitial damage caused by renal or postrenal lesions.

Metabolic Acidosis

The kidneys' ability to excrete acid metabolites may be reduced, particularly in parenchymal and obstructive diseases. As with potassium, because acid excretion is largely a tubular function, the degree of acidosis may not always correlate with the degree of impairment of GFR (and thus, the degree of azotemia).

The *anion gap* concept is useful for understanding the pathophysiology of metabolic acidosis in renal failure. The anion gap is simply the extent to which measured cations exceed anions (i.e., bicarbonate plus chloride) in the plasma. The calculation of the anion gap looks like this:

$$\text{Anion gap} = [\text{Na}] - [\text{Cl} + \text{HCO}_3]$$

The normal anion gap, if sodium is the only cation used in the calculation, is 6 to 12 mEq/L; it is 9 to 16 mEq/L if the serum potassium is also counted. It is important to realize that there is no *true* anion gap; the number of cationic and anionic charges in the body *must* be equal. Indeed, when all the unmeasured ionic species present in plasma are accounted for, there is no gap. The anion gap is simply an artifact of the way in which clinical chemistry tests are obtained, but it is extremely valuable in providing clues to the etiology of acid-base disturbances, especially metabolic acidoses.

Metabolic acidoses may be characterized by either a normal or an increased anion gap. The latter case suggests that the acidosis is due to accumulation in the plasma of unmeasured anions. When the GFR is reduced to less than 20 percent of normal, metabolic waste acids are retained in the plasma. The hydrogen ions from these acids titrate the bicarbonate anion to low levels. A patient with advanced renal failure might have a serum bicarbonate level of 16 and an anion gap of 20. Metabolic acids have titrated 8 mEq of bicarbonate per liter of plasma. Each liter of plasma also contains 8 mEq of the unmeasured anionic components of these waste acids (e.g., sulfuric and phosphoric acid), accounting for the increase in the anion gap.

Metabolic acidosis with a normal anion gap also occurs in renal disease and reflects tubular dysfunction in the failing kidney. Bicarbonate may be depleted because the proximal tubules cannot regenerate filtered bicarbonate normally. Alternatively, secretion of hydrogen ions in the distal nephron may be impaired, leading to their retention in the plasma and loss of bicarbonate by titration. With these tubular causes of acidosis, the anion gap remains normal for two reasons: first, no unmeasured anion is being accumulated in plasma; second, the lost bicarbonate is replaced mole for mole by chloride, which is reabsorbed from the nephron in the absence of bicarbonate. For this reason, normal gap metabolic acidosis may also be called *hyperchloremic acidosis*.

Both types of metabolic acidosis may coexist in the azotemic patient. Tubular dysfunction as well as waste acid retention contributes to the acidosis. Hence, the serum bicarbonate is diminished by a greater number of milliequivalents per liter than that by which the anion gap is increased.

Abnormal Salt and Water Metabolism

The ability to maintain a normal serum osmolality in the face of a water load is impaired whenever the GFR is reduced. This is referred to as failure to excrete "free water" and results in hyponatremia when water intake exceeds free-water capacity. Conversely, some renal disorders are characterized by a failure to conserve water. This situation, referred to as nephrogenic diabetes insipidus, is most common in tubulointerstitial disease and in partial obstruction of the urinary tract. Patients with these disorders are prone to dehydration.

The situation is similar with respect to sodium. The patient with pure prerenal azotemia always retains sodium avidly. However, it is wise to think of the patient with other forms of renal failure as having sodium homeostasis, which is "contracted at both ends"; i.e., the kidney can neither increase sodium excretion in response to a sodium load nor conserve sodium avidly during sodium depletion. As a result, such patients are constantly at risk for both fluid overload and hypovolemia.

Abnormal Calcium and Phosphorus Metabolism

The ability of the kidney to excrete phosphorus normally is impaired when the GFR falls to about one-third of normal. As serum phosphorus levels rise, reciprocal decreases in serum calcium levels follow. Secondary hyperparathyroidism may result. In parenchymal renal disease, the hypocalcemic tendency is further aggravated by failure to activate vitamin D. These abnormalities may culminate in metabolic bone disease (uremic osteodystrophy).

Uremia

We have mentioned that azotemia per se is of little consequence to health. We must recall, however, that creatinine and blood urea are only markers for renal function. As they are retained, so too are more toxic metabolites. Accumulation of these endogenous toxins in the body eventually results in uremia. The exact identities of the so-called uremic toxins are not known, although many culprits have been suggested. One cannot deduce on the basis of urea nitrogen and creatinine levels exactly when a patient will become uremic. In general, the syndrome manifests itself at GFRs of less than 10 ml per minute.

Uremia is a multisystem disease with many manifestations (Table 126-3). Advancing uremia brings symptoms of numbness in the extremities, pruritus, nausea, sallow complexion, and mental dysfunction that may lead to seizures, coma, and even death. Dialysis is eventually necessary for survival as well as alleviation of the lesser uremic symptoms.

Diagnostic Approach

A considerable amount of diagnostic information is available to aid in the differential diagnosis of azotemia. In order to identify accurately the etiology of renal insufficiency in any patient, the physician must learn to draw from a wide database. Some components of this database have been discussed in the preceding paragraphs. For the sake of simplicity, they are summarized in the following sections.

History

As mentioned at the beginning of this chapter, the history is not always revealing, but it may furnish important clues.

Acute versus Chronic Azotemia

Does the patient have stigmata of chronic renal failure (pallor, anemia, anorexia)? Is there a history of previous renal problems or diseases that can affect the kidney (e.g., diabetes mellitus or hypertension)?

Differential Diagnostic Clues

Prerenal. Is the patient thirsty? Has weight been dropping daily? Have there been avenues of fluid loss (e.g., diuretic therapy, recent surgical blood loss)? Does the patient have a disorder characterized by ineffective circulatory volume (congestive heart failure, cirrhosis, nephrotic syndrome)?

Renal. Has the patient had an abnormal urinalysis in the past? Has there been exposure to nephrotoxic agents? Is hypertension present? Were any new medications started recently?

Postrenal. Does the patient have a history of nephrolithiasis or genitourinary neoplasia? Has he or she had symptoms of renal colic? Have there been symptoms of urinary hesitancy, frequency, or nocturia? Is the patient known to have only one kidney?

Physical Examination

Differential Clues

Prerenal. Does the patient look dehydrated? Is he or she hypovolemic (is orthostatic hypotension present)? Are stigmata of congestive heart failure or cirrhosis present?

Renal. Is hypertension present? Are there physical signs of systemic diseases that can affect the kidney (e.g., diabetic retinopathy, skin lesions of vasculitis)?

Postrenal. Does the patient have a distended bladder? Is the prostate enlarged?

Laboratory Tests

Remember, azotemia itself is a diagnosis based on a blood test. Other laboratory diagnostic measures are of great use in refining the differential diagnosis of azotemia.

Urinalysis

Prerenal. Is urine very concentrated (high specific gravity, high osmolality)? Are the urine sodium and FE_{Na} low? Is the urine/plasma creatinine ratio high?

Renal. Is proteinuria, hematuria, or pyuria present? Are there renal tubular epithelial cells in the urinary sediment? Are casts present? The presence of red blood cell casts distinguishes the hematuria associated with glomerulonephritis from that of postrenal lesions. Broad and waxy casts suggest that the renal disease is of a chronic nature.

Postrenal. Hematuria may be associated with virtually any lesion that causes obstruction in the genitourinary tract. Crystalluria, if present, may suggest the presence of an obstructing renal calculus.

Table 126-3 Manifestations of Uremia

Cutaneous	**Neuromuscular**
Sallow complexion	Myoclonus
Pruritus	Muscle weakness
Dry skin	Polyneuropathy
Gastrointestinal	Encephalopathy (lethargy, sleep disturbances, seizures, coma, asterixis)
Anorexia	Allesthesia
Nausea	Cramps
Dysgeusia	**Hematologic**
Dyspepsia	Platelet dysfunction
Peptic ulceration, gastritis, duodenitis	Anemia
Cardiovascular	**Endocrine and Metabolic**
Congestive heart failure (probably represents both fluid overload and impaired myocardial performance)	Glucose intolerance
Pericarditis	Hypertriglyceridemia
	Growth retardation
	Gonadal failure, sexual dysfunction, infertility
	Secondary hyperparathyroidism
	Vitamin B deficiency

Blood Tests

Complete Blood Count. The presence of anemia may be a clue to the chronic nature of the renal disease.

Chemistry. As already mentioned, a high BUN/creatinine ratio may help to distinguish prerenal azotemia from other forms of azotemia. In general, abnormalities of the serum electrolytes do not aid greatly in the differential diagnosis of renal failure. The importance of electrolyte determination is rather to detect potentially serious acid-base and electrolyte abnormalities.

Serologic Tests. Certain intrinsic renal diseases, particularly the glomerulonephritides, are associated with serologic abnormalities. Specialized tests include antinuclear antibody (lupus nephritis), cryoglobulin titer (cryoglobulinemia), complement levels (lupus nephritis, membranoproliferative and acute glomerulonephritis). If myeloma kidney disease is a possibility, serum protein electrophoresis or immunoelectrophoresis is indicated.

Imaging Techniques

Abdominal Flat Plate. This is an easily obtained study, but it provides limited information. At best, it tells the clinician that two kidneys are present, and how large they are. If both kidneys are small, azotemia may be chronic in nature. Occasionally, a radiopaque stone may be identified on an abdominal flat plate.

Intravenous Pyelogram. This test can lead to severe renal failure in prerenal patients and patients with intrinsic renal diseases, particularly those associated with diabetic nephropathy or multiple myeloma. It should therefore never be used when either of these conditions is a strong consideration. Furthermore, good imaging cannot be obtained in patients with moderate to severe azotemia (creatinine of 4.0 mg/dl or more). The intravenous pyelogram does offer the best delineation of renal morphology of any imaging technique. It is particularly useful in recognition of hydronephrosis, if performed early in the course.

Renal Ultrasonography. This safe, quick, high-yield procedure is the *first radiologic test that should be ordered in the evaluation of an azotemic patient.* It permits the identification and measurement of both kidneys, and it is a very sensitive technique for detecting obstructive uropathy. Sonography provides almost as much information as intravenous pyelography, with none of the risks; it may be used in severely azotemic patients.

Retrograde Pyelography. This is reserved for patients in whom urinary tract obstruction is strongly suspected. It is generally performed in anticipation of relieving such obstructions (usually by placement of ureteral catheters) as soon as they are identified.

Renal Scanning. These techniques provide a safe means of locating the kidneys and even allow a crude estimation of their functional capacity. Isotopic flow studies may be used to assess the rapidity of uptake of tracer by the kidneys; a delay in uptake helps to substantiate the diagnosis of impaired renal perfusion (whether due to renovascular disease or to impaired hemodynamics). Prolonged retention of radioisotope by the kidneys is suggestive of postrenal obstruction.

Renal Biopsy

This procedure is reserved for patients who are definitely believed to have intrinsic renal disease. The indications for renal biopsy are a matter of some controversy, but the procedure should be considered in the following circumstances: (1) when azotemia is of recent onset and unknown etiology; (2) when there is a possibility that the patient has a renal disease that may require drug treatment (e.g., steroids or cytotoxic drugs); this applies to patients with probable glomerulonephritis, vasculitis, or acute interstitial nephritis; and (3) when the biopsy might be of prognostic importance.

Treatment

The definitive therapy of azotemia rests on recognition of its cause. In patients with pure prerenal azotemia attributable to hypovolemia, restoration of a normal volume will usually suffice to return BUN and creatinine to their normal levels. Any azotemic patient who appears volume-depleted should receive up to 1 L of saline over a 4-hour period as an initial "fluid challenge." This maneuver is of diagnostic as well as therapeutic benefit because rapid response to the fluid challenge will establish that azotemia is due at least in part to prerenal factors. Remember that hypovolemia may complicate intrinsic renal disease and urinary tract obstruction, superimposing a prerenal component on the azotemia caused by these conditions.

Patients with prerenal azotemia due to a functionally contracted vascular volume (i.e., patients with congestive heart failure, cirrhosis with ascites, and nephrotic syndrome) cannot be treated with fluids alone, as this will result in worsening edema and ascites. Although optimization of fluid balance is crucial in these patients, therapy should be aimed at the underlying disorder. Thus, the patient with congestive heart failure may require inotropic and afterload-reducing agents. Occasionally, such patients will have to be kept in a chronically "prerenal" state in order to prevent their ascites and edema from approaching unacceptable levels.

There are few definitive modes of therapy for intrinsic renal diseases. If renal damage occurs as a result of exposure to a drug with allergic or nephrotoxic potential, the offending agent must be withdrawn. As has already been mentioned, steroids may help in the therapy of acute allergic interstitial nephritis. In most forms of acute renal failure, management consists mainly of observation and supportive measures, specifically, maintaining fluid and electrolyte balance while the disease runs its course.

Chronic progressive renal disease is a particularly frustrating problem for the physician, as there may be little opportunity for direct intervention. If hypertension is present, aggressive control may help slow deterioration in renal function. It is hoped that converting enzyme inhibitors, by dilating the efferent arteriole and reducing glomerular capillary pressures, may retard ongoing nephron loss in the chronic phases of parenchymal disease. If current investigation of these agents proves promising, they may gain a regular role in the treatment of progressive renal failure. Limiting dietary protein intake to 0.5 to 1.0 g/kg body weight per day may have similar beneficial effects and also reduces dietary phosphorus restrictions and the use of phosphate binders (e.g., calcium carbonate and aluminum hydroxide). These measures will also help to prevent hypocalcemia, although, in some patients, addition of vitamin D or related substances to the medication regimen may be necessary. If uremia ensues, dialysis or renal transplantation is indicated.

Postrenal acute renal failure requires surgical intervention aimed at relieving the obstruction. Depending on the cause of the obstruction, this may involve either transurethral resection of an obstructing prostate, placement of nephrostomy tubes or ureteral catheters, or removal of stones from the urinary collecting system. Such measures are best performed early to avoid the risk of permanent renal damage.

Recall that the patient with postrenal failure is susceptible to the same abnormalities of fluid and electrolyte metabolism seen with other forms of renal failure, and he or she must be managed accordingly. Careful fluid management is also critical in the period following removal of an obstruction, as some patients experience a massive salt and water diuresis during this phase.

References

Hou SH, et al. Hospital-acquired renal insufficiency: A prospective study. Am J Med 1983; 74:243.

Levinsky NG. Pathophysiology of acute renal failure. N Engl J Med 1977; 296:1453.

Merrill JP, Hampers CL. Uremia. N Engl J Med 1970; 282:953.

Miller TR, et al. Urinary diagnostic indices in acute renal failure. A prospective study. Ann Intern Med 1978; 89:47.

Rose BD. Pathophysiology of renal disease. 2nd ed. New York: McGraw-Hill, 1987.

Proteinuria

David M. Clive, MD

127

The normal adult excretes less than 200 mg of protein in the urine per day. Because almost 10 kg of albumin are presented to the glomeruli every 24 hours, it follows that the kidney must possess an effective mechanism for preferentially filtering and excreting waste molecules while retaining protein and other macromolecules. The ability of the kidney to discriminate in this fashion is crucial to the maintenance of health and internal homeostasis. As we shall see, when the barrier to protein filtration is damaged, there may be serious consequences.

The Filtration Barrier

The glomerular filtration barrier comprises three anatomic components as illustrated in Figure 127-1. A molecule in the plasma passing through a glomerular capillary lumen must cross the endothelial lining of the capillary if it is to be filtered. To do so, it traverses one of the fenestrations in the endothelial cell. Generally speaking, this is easily done by most molecular species. In diseases characterized by endothelial cell swelling or proliferation, e.g., glomerulonephritis or toxemia, the passage of particles may be impeded.

Our reference molecule next encounters the basement membrane, a trilaminar glycoprotein structure on which the endothelial cell rests. This is the most discriminating component of the filtration barrier. Whether a molecule will gain passage across the membrane is a matter of simple molecular biophysics (Fig. 127-2). Larger molecules (especially those greater than 40,000 daltons in weight) encounter greater impedance than smaller ones. Small molecules bound to proteins, or protein molecules bound to each other, will have difficulty negotiating the filtration barrier. Because of peculiarities in their secondary structures, some molecules offer more steric hindrance than other molecules of equivalent molecular weight. Thus, albumin, a fibrillar protein, enters the basement membrane less readily than hemoglobin, a compact globular protein of similar molecular weight but smaller *effective molecular radius*. Lastly, because the basement membrane itself carries a negative charge, it is apt to repel molecules that are negatively charged at urinary pH. This characteristic provides a remarkable degree of selectivity to the glomerular filtration barrier in that two molecules of equal effective molecular radius may have markedly different clearances if their charges differ (Fig. 127-3).

During transit through the basement membrane, molecules are subject to further resistance to passage. This resistance, a form of viscous drag, is proportional to the effective molecular radius, again meaning that fibrillar proteins pass more slowly than globular molecules. Once the particle has cleared the anatomic and electrostatic barriers of the basement membrane, it emerges from between the epithelial cell foot processes and

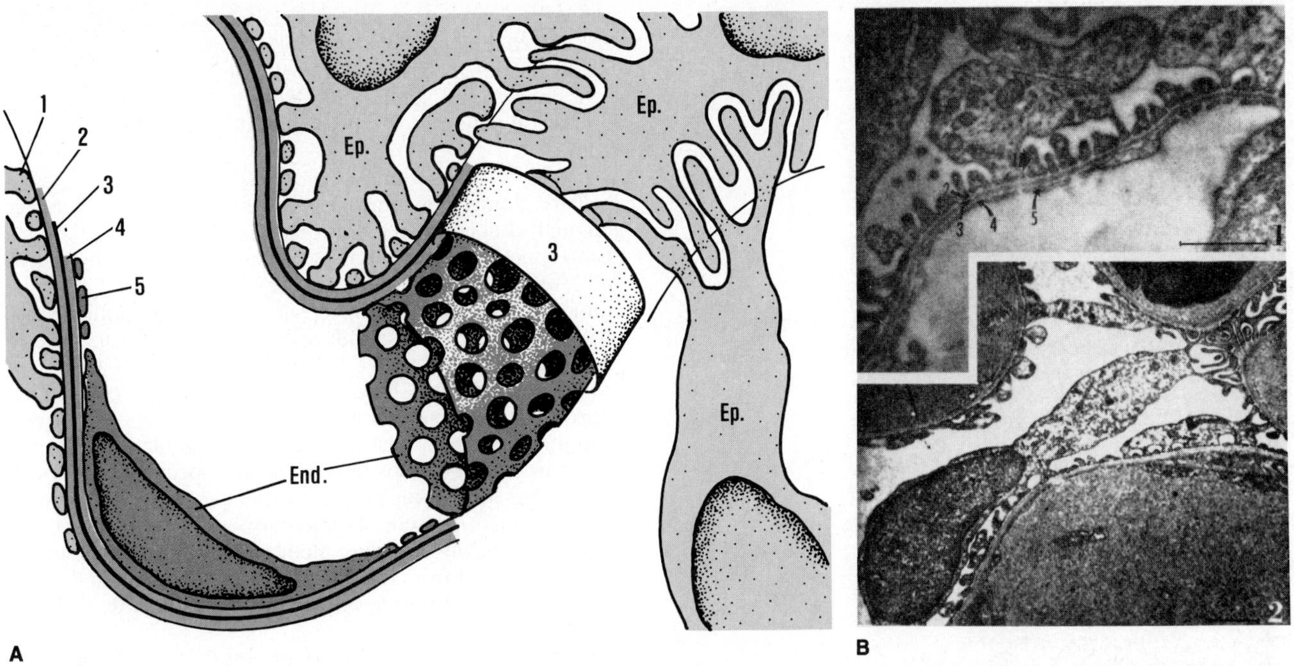

Figure 127-1 (**A**) Diagram of a glomerular capillary loop illustrating the visceral epithelial cells or podocyte (1); basement membrane (2,3,4); and endothelial cell (5). (**B**) Electron micrograph of the same structures illustrated in the drawing, with corresponding numbers (*above*). Another electron micrographic view showing the position of the epithelial cell foot processes on the outer edge of the glomerular basement membrane (*below*). (*From* Pease DC. Fine structures of the kidney seen by electron microscopy. J Histochem 1955; 3:295. Copyright 1955 by Elsevier Science Publishing Co., Inc. Reprinted by permission of the publisher.)

enters Bowman's space, completing its filtration. The foot processes do not offer much of an obstacle. In nephrotic diseases, they are seen to fuse and flatten, but this may represent a consequence of proteinuria rather than a cause.

Filtration Barrier Pathology: The Glomerulopathies

Any disease that destroys the integrity of the filtration barrier can lead to albuminuria. As already stated, the glomerulus must perform two functions: it must serve as a barrier to macromolecules while filtering soluble wastes. It is important to note that both functions may be impaired in glomerular disease. In glomerular diseases, the filtration barrier to proteins may be damaged, allowing proteinuria to occur. At the same time, the glomerular injury may cause thickening of other areas of the basement membrane or even reduction in the available filtration area. In this manner, the creatinine clearance may fall even though the patient has an abnormally high protein clearance.

Not surprisingly, the heaviest proteinuria occurs in diseases in which the pathologic changes center on the glomerulus. The glomerulopathies may follow two clinical patterns of behavior: nephritic or nephrotic. The distinction is not hard and fast; a patient may well display features of both syndromes. However, categorizing diseases along these lines invariably aids in their recognition.

Nephrotic Syndrome

The nephrotic syndrome is defined as albuminuria of at least 3.5 g per day. The presence of nephrotic-range proteinuria virtually establishes the presence of significant glomerular disease. A wide variety of glomerulopathies are capable of evoking the nephrotic syndrome. *Primary nephrotic syndrome* is produced by diseases arising in the kidneys. There are four main types of primary nephrotic disorders.

Minimal change disease (also called nil lesion or lipoid nephrosis) is the most common form of nephrotic syndrome in children; it also occurs frequently in adults. Perhaps the most interesting aspect of this disease is that no distinct histopathologic abnormalities are identified in biopsies of affected patients. The glomeruli appear morphologically normal but clearly have a functional abnormality, because large amounts of albumin are permitted to leak into the urine. It is possible that the central defect in minimal change disease is a loss of the anionic charge from the glomerular basement membrane with a resultant loss of permselectivity.

Although proteinuria may be massive in this disease, albumin is lost in much greater amounts than larger proteins, such as immunoglobulins. We therefore speak of the proteinuria of minimal change disease as being *selective*. Selectivity defines the extent to which the glomerulus retains the ability to discriminate against proteins of higher molecular weight. It is usually expressed as the ratio of clearance of proteins of varying molecular size to that of a reference molecule, usually albumin or transferrin. For a given patient, a graph may be constructed with the molecular weights of test proteins on the abscissa and the clearance ratio on the ordinate (Fig. 127-4). It is apparent that the steeper the angle of the slope (θ) of the regression line, the more selective the proteinuria. This feature is believed to correlate with a favorable prognosis. Indeed, most patients with minimal change nephrotic syndrome will eventually experience a complete remission with corticosteroid therapy.

Membranous nephropathy is the most common form of primary nephrotic syndrome in adults. In this disorder, immune complexes form in the basement membrane. These antigen-antibody complexes incite a low-grade immune response that results in a loss of structural integrity of the filtration barrier. Examination of affected glomeruli reveals extensive thickening of the basement membrane. Although most cases of membranous nephropathy are primary, an identical histopathologic lesion may be seen in association with carcinomas and systemic lupus erythematosus, and following exposure to a wide variety

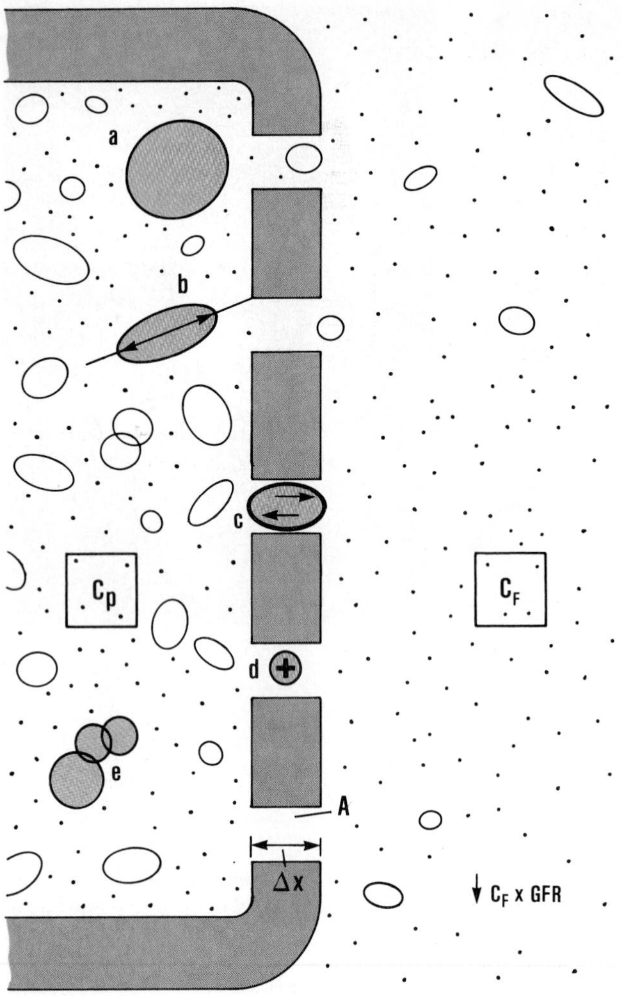

Figure 127-2 Schematic diagram of the filtration barrier illustrating the factors that influence molecular filtration. Molecules and pores of hypothetical size and configuration are shown. (**a**) Molecular dimension hindrance, (**b**) steric hindrance, (**c**) viscous drag, (**d**) electrostatic hindrance, (**e**) protein-protein binding. C_p = concentration of protein in plasma, C_F = concentration of protein in filtrate, A = total pore area, x = pore length. (*From* Heinemann HO, Maack TM, Sherman RL. Proteinuria. Am J Med 1974; 56:71; with permission.)

of drugs. The natural history of idiopathic membranous nephropathy is quite variable. Spontaneous remissions occasionally occur, but persistent nephrosis and progression to chronic renal failure are equally likely. There is some evidence that corticosteroid therapy early in the course of membranous nephropathy may lessen the course of progression.

Another idiopathic nephrotic disorder that affects adults and children is *focal segmental glomerulosclerosis* (FSGS). This is a disease in which portions of the tufts of some glomeruli become hyalinized or scarred. Despite the sporadic involvement of the glomeruli in kidneys with this disease, the prognosis is much poorer than in minimal change disease. Proteinuria is usually less selective, and hematuria is not uncommon. The relationship of this disease to minimal change disease is a matter of current debate, some authorities arguing that focal segmental sclerosis represents a particularly severe form of the same pathologic process. According to this theory, patients whose minimal change disease does not respond to corticosteroids have a high likelihood of "progressing" to focal sclerosis. This contention is difficult to prove because, owing to the focal nature of glomerular involvement, it is possible to miss the sclerotic lesions at the time of renal biopsy. Thus, a patient with true focal sclerosis may initially be thought to have minimal change disease. Syndromes quite similar to idiopathic FSGS have been described in heroin addicts and patients with the acquired immunodeficiency syndrome.

Membranoproliferative glomerulonephritis (mesangiocapillary glomerulonephritis) is mainly a disease of children, although adult cases are occasionally seen. The histopathologic changes include proliferation of endothelial and mesangial cells and extensive deposition of immune complexes throughout the glomeruli. Prognosis is variable, but most commonly the disease progresses slowly to renal failure over a period of years. Investigations are in progress to ascertain whether anticoagulant or antiplatelet drugs may have a role in the treatment of membranoproliferative glomerulonephritis. This concept has arisen from the observation that fibrin thrombi can often be demonstrated in capillary loops of renal biopsy specimens. Although such therapy is the only promising therapeutic development in this disorder at present, its long-term efficacy remains to be proven in controlled studies. Membranoproliferative glomerulonephritis varies from the other primary nephroses in that it is equally likely to present with nephritic features as with nephrotic (see later).

Although it is clear that these diseases are immunologically mediated, their causes remain a mystery. In *secondary nephrotic syndrome,* the glomerulopathy arises as a result of renal involvement by a systemic disease. The most common cause of secondary nephrosis in adults in the United States is diabetes mellitus. Other systemic diseases that can result in nephrotic-range proteinuria include amyloidosis, lupus erythematosus, and toxemia of pregnancy. The glomerular morphology in such diseases may be distinctive, as in renal amyloidosis and diabetic nephropathy, or it may resemble that of the idiopathic nephroses, e.g., in the membranous nephropathy associated with systemic lupus erythematosus. A list of clinical disorders and drugs that can evoke the nephrotic syndrome is shown in Table 127-1.

Nephritic Syndrome

The *nephritic syndrome* is characterized by hematuria and frequently hypertension and azotemia. In these illnesses, hematuria, like the proteinuria of the primarily nephrotic disorders, is

Table 127-1 Major Causes of Secondary Nephrotic Syndrome

Allergy	**Neoplasia**
Insect and reptile venoms	Carcinomas
Plant toxins	Light-chain disease
Pollen	Lymphoma
Infections	Leukemia
Bacterial endocarditis	Melanoma
Ventriculoperitoneal shunt infections	Multiple myeloma
Visceral sepsis	**Others**
Others (tuberculosis, leprosy, malaria, helminths, toxoplasmosis, viruses)	Amyloidosis (primary and secondary)
Drugs	Congestive heart failure (severe)
Captopril	Constrictive pericarditis
Gold salts	Cryoglobulinemia
Heroin ("brown")	Diabetes mellitus
Nonsteroidal anti-inflammatory agents	Goodpasture's syndrome
Penicillamine	Hypertension (accelerated or malignant)
Probencid	Obesity, morbid
Antibiotics	Renal vein thrombosis (see text)
Lithium	Sarcoidosis
	Toxemia of pregnancy
	Vasculitis (most forms)

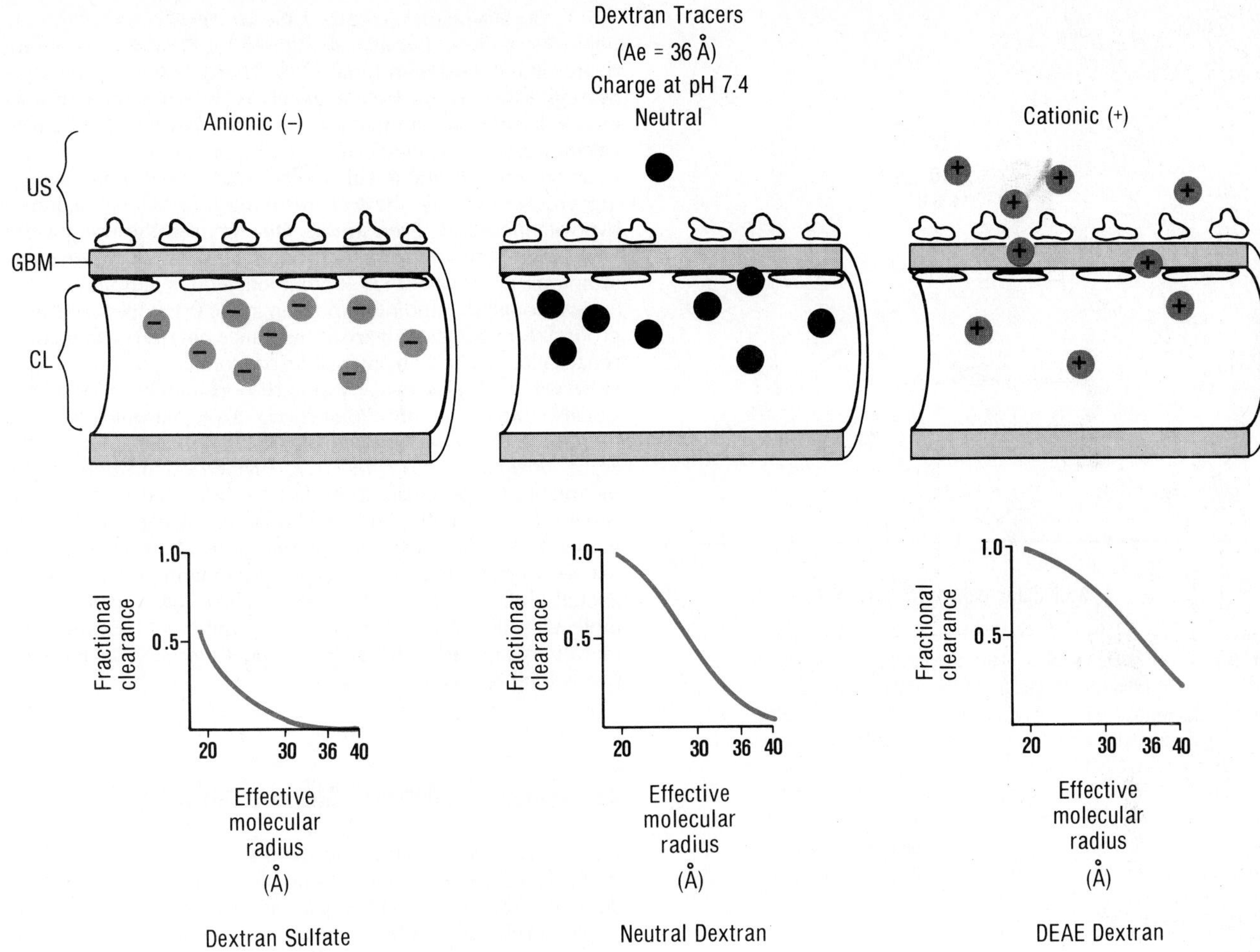

Figure 127-3 Influence of molecular charge on dextran clearance. For a molecule of given size, cationic molecules will be cleared more readily than neutral dextrans, which are in turn cleared more easily than anionic dextrans. In experimental models of nephrotic disease, this permselectivity characteristic is lost. CL = capillary lumen, GBM = glomerular basement membrane, US = urinary space. (*From* Melvin T, Sibley R, Michael AF. Nephrotic syndrome. In: Brenner BM, Stein JH, eds. Pediatric nephrology. New York: Churchill Livingstone, 1984:191; with permission.)

the result of immunologic attack on the glomerulus. Examples of diseases in which nephritic features usually predominate are acute poststreptococcal glomerulonephritis and IgA nephropathy. Systemic diseases may produce secondary glomerulonephritides, as in Goodpasture's disease, vasculitis, bacterial endocarditis, and lupus.

The inflammatory process generating these glomerulopathies is, generally speaking, of a higher grade than that seen in the nephrotic diseases. The urine sediment is more likely to show, in addition to blood, inflammatory cells and cellular casts. However, just as nephrotic disorders can produce nephritic manifestations, 10 to 20 percent of patients with nephritic diseases have nephrotic-range proteinuria.

Consequences of the Nephrotic Syndrome

There are two reasons why excess protein filtration may not adversely affect health. The renal tubules can reabsorb large amounts of filtered protein, catabolize it, and allow the components to be recycled in the systemic circulation. In fact, normal individuals filter and reabsorb large amounts of albumin daily (Fig. 127-5). Furthermore, even when protein filtration outstrips the reabsorptive capacity of the tubular cells, increased hepatic protein synthesis can help maintain a normal serum albumin level in the well-nourished patient. It is only after sustained nephrotic-range urinary protein loss that hypoalbuminemia results, and with it, the major clinical manifestations of the nephrotic syndrome, which are listed in Table 127-2. Some nephrotic patients may excrete only slightly more than 3.5 g of protein per day, whereas in others this figure may approach 60 g. It is to be anticipated that the heavier the urinary protein losses, the more rapidly the symptoms of nephrosis will become apparent.

Edema is the most characteristic clinical feature of nephrosis. The pathophysiology of edema formation in the syndrome is outlined in Figure 127-6. When hypoalbuminemia is severe (usually at serum albumin levels of 2.5 g/dl or less), the reduced plasma oncotic pressure will favor transudation of fluid from the vascular to the interstitial space. Because edema forms at the expense of the plasma volume, the resultant hypovolemia is a stimulus for salt and water retention by the kidney, providing the substrate for further edema formation. Besides interstitial edema, severe nephrosis may be marked by ascites and pleural effusions.

When the serum albumin level approaches 2.5 g/dl, nephrotic patients usually become hyperlipidemic. Elevations in cholesterol concentrations precede hypertriglyceridemia. The reasons for the hyperlipidemia of nephrosis are still debated. It

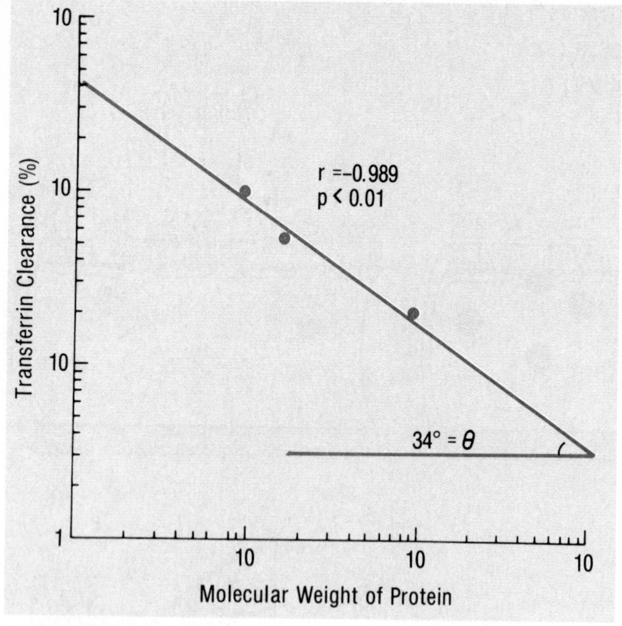

Figure 127-4 Determination of the activity of proteinuria. In this example, the ratios of clearance of three proteins (transferrin, molecular weight = 90,000; IgG, molecular weight = 160,000; and alpha$_2$-macroglobulin, molecular weight = 820,000) to clearance of transferrin are plotted against their respective molecular weights. The angle of intersection between the regression line and the abscissa is a measure of the selectivity of protein excretion. (*From* Sherman RL, Becker EL. Alpha$_2$-macroglobulin and selectivity of protein excretion. Nephron 1971; 8:255; with permission of S. Karger AG, Basel.)

is widely argued that because hepatic protein synthesis is maximally stimulated by hypoalbuminemia, lipoprotein synthesis will be increased as well. It is also possible that lipoprotein lipase deficiency occurs, leading to failure to metabolize lipoproteins normally. Whatever its cause, nephrotic hyperlipidemia may be of severe proportions and quite refractory to dietary or medical treatment.

When levels of lipids are high, they too may spill into the urine. It is characteristic for nephrotic urinary sediments to be loaded with fat globules and fatty casts. Oval fat bodies, which represent lipid-laden phagocytes, may also be seen (Fig. 127-7). Viewed under polarized light, lipid globules have a characteristic "Maltese cross" appearance.

A less frequent but well-described phenomenon in nephrotic syndrome is hypercoagulability. Patients with very heavy proteinuria have a higher than normal incidence of thromboembolic events such as deep venous thrombosis and pulmonary embolism. Renal vein thrombosis, once thought a cause of proteinuria, probably represents a thrombotic complication of preexisting nephrotic disease. The mechanism underlying the hypercoagulability of nephrosis, like that of the hyperlipidemia, is obscure. Hyperactivity of platelets, increased procoagulant synthesis, and urinary antithrombin III and protein S loss have all been suggested.

There is no doubt that patients with nephrotic syndrome are predisposed to infections. Protein depletion generally constitutes an immunocompromised condition; if urinary immunoglobulin losses are heavy, the degree of immunosuppression is considerable. Prior to the advent of corticosteroid therapy, the leading cause of death in childhood lipoid nephrosis was infection.

Hypocalcemia is a common electrolyte abnormality in the nephrotic patient. Because it is rarely of clinically significant degree, it is not listed in Table 127-2. There are two mechanisms through which hypocalcemia may arise. Hypoalbuminemia lowers the bound calcium fraction in plasma. Because the ionized calcium fraction is not affected, patients are rarely symptomatic. In an occasional patient with severe nephrosis, vitamin D binding protein may also be lost, resulting in a state of acquired hypovitaminosis D. Even in this situation, it is the rare patient who develops tetany, seizures, or muscle weakness. When these symptoms arise, vitamin D supplementation is indicated.

Although the finding of protein in the urine may constitute grounds for failing a military or insurance physical examination, renal failure is not an invariable concomitant of proteinuria. However, if the glomerular lesion responsible for protein leakage also impairs the filtration process, azotemia will result. The filtration capability of a glomerulus is expressed mathematically as the *ultrafiltration coefficient* (K_f), which is a function of both the membrane permeability and surface area. If the glomerulus is entirely or partially sclerosed, inflamed, or necrotized, K_f diminishes. In this sense, even though the filtration barrier to macromolecules may be damaged, resulting in proteinuria, the overall ability of the glomerulus to allow passage of smaller molecules like urea and creatinine is hampered. If enough glomeruli are similarly affected, the patient's glomerular filtration rate will be reduced.

Albuminuria Without Glomerulopathy

The preceding paragraphs have focused on albuminuria resulting from changes in the glomerular filtration barrier. There is no doubt that the most prominent proteinuria occurs in the setting of glomerulopathy. Albuminuria may also accompany a wide range of clinical states, not all of which are associated with glomerular pathology. Virtually any form of renal disease, even vascular and tubulointerstitial nephropathies, may cause increased albumin excretion. Although nephrotic-range albuminuria has been reported in nephrosclerosis, nonglomerular diseases will more typically manifest albuminuria of 1 g or less per day.

Proteinuria in nonglomerular renal disease may be explicable in several ways. In tubular nephropathies, there may be impairment of the ability of tubular cells to reabsorb filtered albumin. Secondary glomerular changes may occur in tubulointerstitial disease, perhaps as a result of contiguous interstitial inflammation. Such changes could be responsible for increased albumin filtration.

Recently, a hypothesis has been advanced to explain the mechanism of progression of, and development of proteinuria in, chronic renal diseases. Renal injury, whether a result of immunologic processes, ischemia, infection, surgery, or trauma, decreases the nephron population. The effect of this reduction in renal mass is to place an increased workload on surviving nephrons. Through a series of microcirculatory adaptations, glomerular blood flow and capillary hydrostatic pressure are increased, and the filtration rate in each glomerulus is augmented. Glomeruli undergoing this *hyperfiltration* process are subject to hemodynamic stress, which damages capillary integrity and predisposes to leakage of protein into the urine.

The most important form of injury produced by hyperfiltration is glomerulosclerosis. Indeed, on sequential renal biopsy of animals with different forms of experimental renal disease, glomeruli will be observed to become progressively hyalinized and obsolescent; not surprisingly, the total glomerular filtration rate falls. In progressive reflux nephropathy, a disease characterized by vesicoureteral reflux of urine with ongoing pressure injury and scarring of the renal cortex, secondary glomerular changes may be seen that are histopathologically identical to

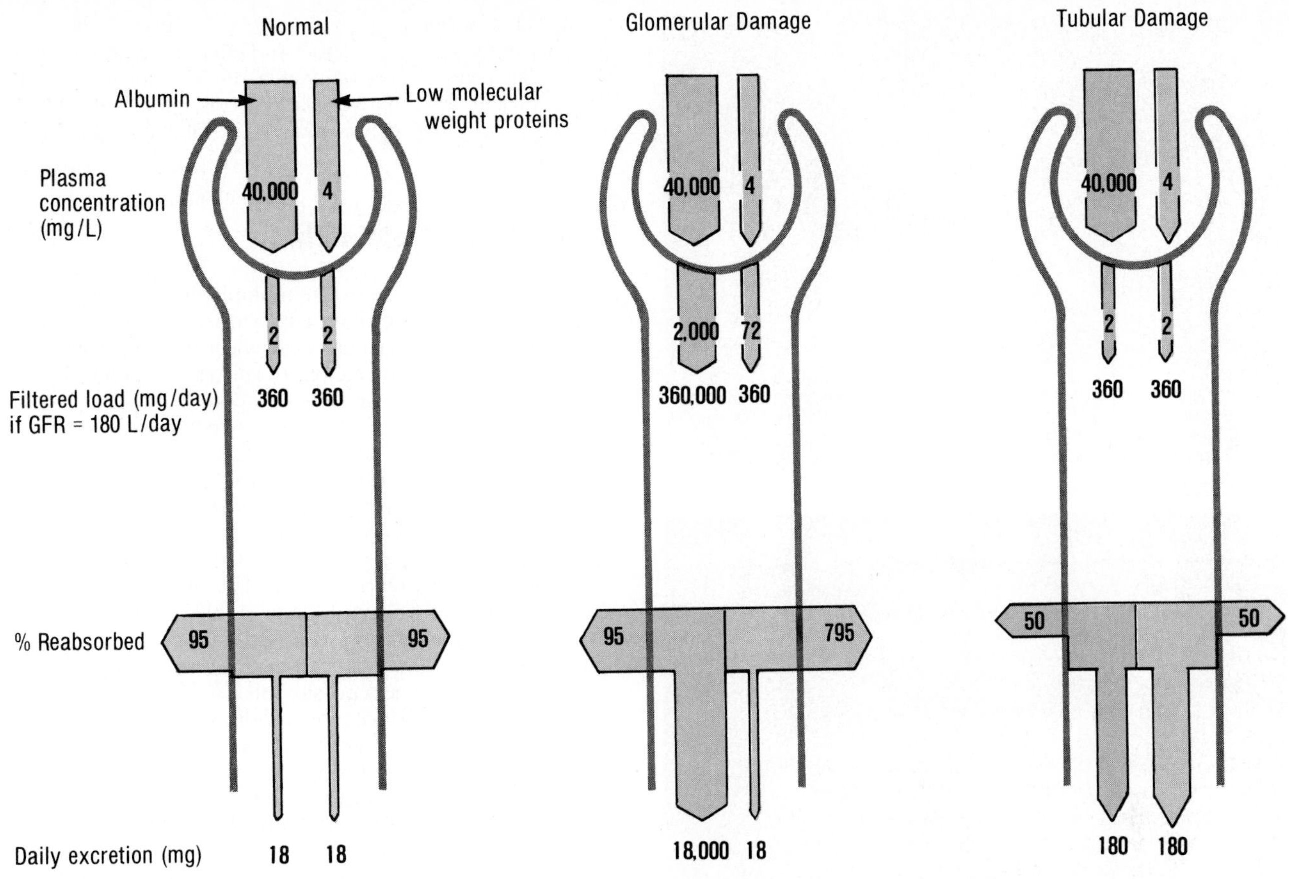

Figure 127-5 Schematic diagram illustrating two basic mechanisms of proteinuria: increased glomerular permeability with normal tubular reabsorption of filtered protein (*center*), and impaired tubular reabsorption of proteins that are normally filtered (*right*). GFR = glomerular filtration rate. (*From* Flynn FV, Platt HS. The origins of proteins excreted in tubular proteinuria. Clin Chim Acta 1968; 21:377; and Heinemann HO, Maack TM, Sherman RL. Proteinuria. Am J Med 1974; 56:71; with permission.)

focal segmental glomerulosclerosis. Patients with this disease commonly develop nephrotic syndrome as their illness progresses, as do patients with idiopathic FSGS.

Transient physiologic alterations may lead to glomerular proteinuria in the absence of anatomic lesions. The course of a febrile illness may be marked by transient proteinuria. This is never of nephrotic magnitude, but it may be sufficient to produce a strongly positive dipstick test. The mechanism responsible for *febrile proteinuria* is unknown, but it probably relates to altered systemic and renal hemodynamics. Vigorous physical activity also may induce mild proteinuria in normal individuals. This phenomenon, which is common in normal individuals, abates within minutes after the completion of exercise. In addition to albumin, "tubular protein" excretion may also increase with exercise.

Severe congestive heart failure and hypertension can increase or cause hemodynamically mediated proteinuria. In malignant hypertension, albuminuria may be of nephrotic magnitude.

Another proteinuric tendency that is occasionally seen in otherwise normal subjects is *orthostatic* or *postural proteinuria*. In this disorder, urinary albumin excretion on the order of 1 to

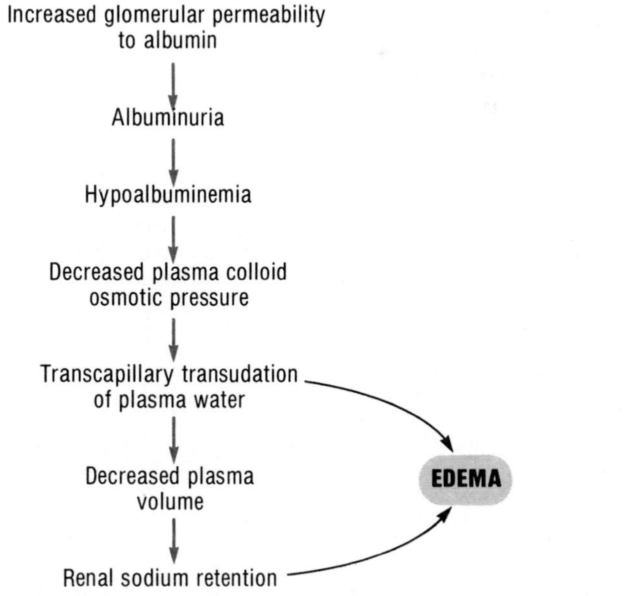

Figure 127-6 Mechanism of edema formation in nephrotic syndrome. Altered capillary Starling forces result from loss of colloid oncotic pressure with consequent transudation of fluid into the interstitium. (*From* Reineck HJ. Mechanisms of edema formation in the nephrotic syndrome. In: Brenner BM, Stein JH, eds. Nephrotic syndrome. New York: Churchill Livingstone, 1982:31; with permission.)

Table 127-2 Complications of Nephrotic Syndrome

Edema	Infections
Hypovolemia	Hypercoagulability
Hyperlipidemia	Hypocalcemia

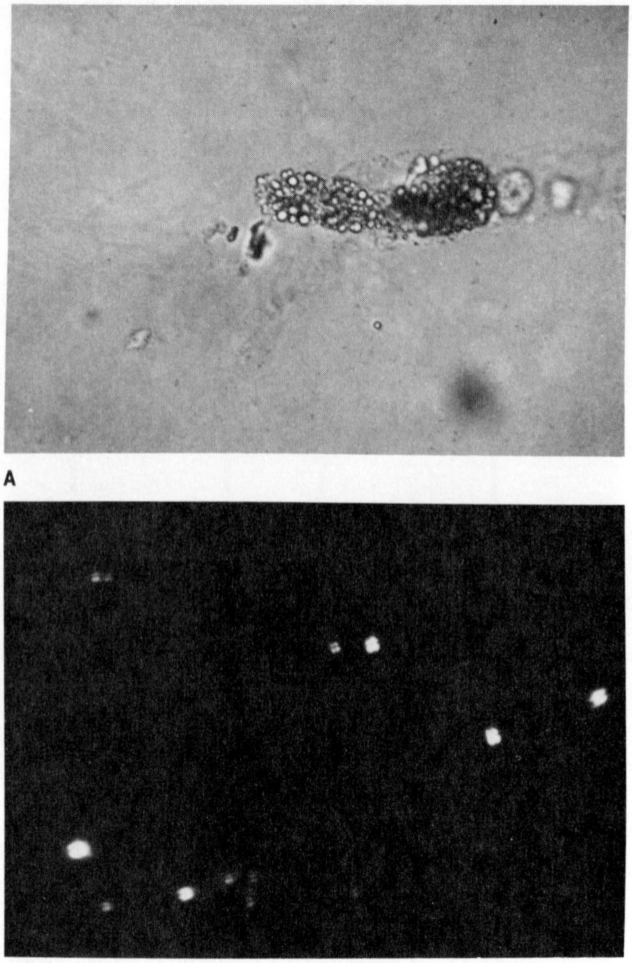

A

B

Figure 127-7 (**A**) Fatty cast in a typical nephrotic urinary sediment. The translucent droplets in the cast are lipid globules. Their varying size helps to differentiate them from red blood cells. (**B**) Appearance of urinary lipid globules under polarized light. Note the characteristic "Maltese cross" appearance.

2 g per day may be seen. If separate collections of diurnally (16 hours) and nocturnally (8 hours) voided urine are made, the diurnal specimen will be found to account for almost all of the total albumin excretion. It has been suggested that upright posture in affected individuals leads to altered glomerular hemodynamics or enhanced permeability. The prognosis for maintenance of renal function in postural proteinuria is excellent.

Tubular Proteinuria

Because albumin is a relatively high molecular weight substance and not freely filterable, its appearance in large amounts in the urine bespeaks glomerular pathology. Not all urinary protein represents albuminuria, however. A number of low molecular weight proteins are normally freely filtered, and it is only tubular reabsorptive capacity that prevents their urinary escape (see Fig. 127-4). Just as albumin is the classic "reference molecule" for glomerular proteinuria, there are two traditional index substances for quantitating tubular proteinuria, lysozyme and beta$_2$-microglobulin.

Lysozyme has a globular structure and a molecular weight of about 14,000 daltons. It is therefore relatively easily filtered, but tubular reabsorption reclaims almost all filtered lysozyme before it can enter the urine. In renal diseases characterized by tubular dysfunction, this reabsorptive capacity is easily exceeded, and lysozymuria and beta$_2$-microglobulinuria result. Virtually all forms of tubulointerstitial renal disease may result in tubular proteinuria. Acute tubular necrosis, interstitial nephritis, and renal transplant dysfunction are probably the most important causes.

Bence-Jones Proteinuria

Paraproteinemic syndromes like multiple myeloma and monoclonal gammopathy are often characterized by production of immunoglobulin light chains in excessive amounts. These light chains, designated as either kappa or lambda depending on their structure, have a molecular weight of about 22,000 and are easily filtered in sufficiently large amounts to overwhelm the reabsorptive capacity of normal tubules. For this reason, urinary light-chain excretion, also known as Bence-Jones proteinuria, has been termed *overproduction proteinuria.*

Myeloma patients with Bence-Jones proteinuria, particularly those excreting large amounts of light chains, are at risk of developing *myeloma kidney disease.* This disorder manifests as acute or subacute, frequently irreversible, renal failure. The pathogenesis is thought to involve intratubular coalescence of light chains ("myeloma cast" formation), with obstruction of nephronal flow. It is also possible that light chains may exert direct toxic effects on renal tubular cells. Volume depletion and radiographic contrast studies further predispose myeloma patients to development of this complication.

Light chains may interact with the kidney in other ways. Two entities characterized by parenchymal deposition of light chains are *amyloidosis* and *light-chain disease.* These disorders may be primary or occur in association with myeloma. Differentiation between these two lesions is based on the ultrastructure of the light-chain aggregates composing the tissue deposits. Glomerular involvement is common and may produce severe albuminuria. Bence-Jones proteinuria is not always present in light-chain disease and amyloidosis.

Tamm-Horsfall Mucoprotein

Tamm-Horsfall mucoprotein is a product of renal tubular cells; as such, it is a normal constituent of the urine. Its major clinical importance is that it comprises the matrix substance of tubular casts; i.e., a cast is simply a mucoprotein cylinder in which are embedded cells, granules, or other elements, and that may be of diagnostic importance in renal disease. Hyaline casts are simply mucoprotein bodies without inclusions. Their presence in the urine does not necessarily denote renal abnormalities, although they may be especially prominent in dehydration, presumably because of the increased concentration of mucoprotein that occurs in these circumstances. It has been suggested that Tamm-Horsfall mucoprotein may figure in the pathogenesis of radiocontrast-induced acute renal failure by interacting with filtered particles of contrast agent in the renal tubules.

Urinary Pigment Proteins

Myoglobin is a heme-containing protein that is liberated into the serum in muscle injury. When the damage is extensive, and plasma myoglobin levels exceed 25 mg/dl, enough of the protein will be filtered to be detectable in the urine, which may be grossly pink-tinged. Because myoglobin will react with the benzidine heme-detecting reagent in dipsticks, the dipstick test for blood will often be strongly positive in the absence of significant hematuria. Occasionally, large amounts of filtered myoglobin coalesce in the tubules, obstructing nephronal flow and producing epithelial cell injury. The combination of dehydration and muscle injury predisposes patients to this condition, which is known as *acute myoglobinuric renal failure.*

Hemoglobinuria rarely, if ever, causes acute renal failure. In order to appear in the urine, the concentration of hemoglobin in serum must exceed 125 mg/dl, because lesser amounts will be entirely bound to haptoglobin, forming a nonfilterable complex. Intravascular hemolysis of sufficient magnitude to produce hemoglobinuria can be seen in transfusion reactions, freshwater drowning, and paroxysmal nocturnal hemoglobinuria.

As in myoglobinuria, when there is free hemoglobin in the urine, there will be a disparity between the degree of dipstick positivity for heme and the number of red blood cells actually observed in the sediment. The disparity, however, merely provides indirect evidence of pigment proteinuria. Furthermore, if the urine sample is not fresh, red blood cells that may have been present will have lysed, mimicking this effect. Urinary myoglobin and hemoglobin are most accurately identified and quantitated through electrophoretic techniques.

Detection of Proteinuria

Any description of the various techniques for detecting and quantifying urinary protein must be organized according to specific types of protein. Albumin is the most abundant protein in normal urine, and, statistically, its excretion is likely to be affected by the most types of renal disease. However, albuminuria is just one type of proteinuria; other urinary proteins must be measured in different ways.

The most common method for detecting albumin in the urine is the dipstick test. The dipstick wafer is impregnated with a pH indicator solution, tetrabromphenol, and an acidic buffer that maintains the pH of the wafer at about 3.0. The ability of albumin molecules to buffer hydrogen ions at this pH can produce a change in the color of the indicator, from yellow, when there is no albumin, to blue-green, when 1 or more g of albumin is present.

The dipstick test is semiquantitative; i.e., it provides only an approximation of the albumin concentration rather than a direct quantitative measurement. For this reason, it is customary to grade the dipstick color change on a scale of 0 to 4+, as is done with diabetic glycosuric test tablets. Although it is feasible that urinary pH could affect the degree of positivity of a dipstick test for protein, this is rarely a significant factor.

Another semiquantitative technique for detecting albuminuria is the addition of sulfosalicylic acid to urine in a test tube. Acidification of the urine results in protein denaturation, and the amount of turbidity that results is a function of the albumin content of the specimen. If the urine remains transparent, no albumin is present. If the urine can be read or seen through, it is scored as 1 to 3+, depending on the degree of difficulty in distinguishing a printed page behind the specimen. A 4+ specimen is too turbid to see anything through, and usually corresponds to 2 or more g of protein. Obviously, urine that is cloudy before the acid is added may give a false-positive result.

The concentration of albumin in an acid-precipitated urine specimen can be measured more accurately by the biuret and Lowry methods, in which the actual quantitation is done through spectrophotometry. This is the usual technique for the clinical measurement of albumin in 24-hour urine specimens. Semiquantitative techniques should be thought of as screening tests for proteinuria; in patients who are found to have proteinuria or renal disease, a 24-hour urine collection is the only way to establish the degree of the protein-losing tendency.

Although they are not detected by standard dipsticks, Bence-Jones proteins will precipitate in response to acidification with sulfosalicylic acid. An unusual feature of Bence-Jones proteins is their thermal behavior. When virtually any mineral acid or acidic buffer solution is added to the urine specimen, which is then heated to approximately 60°C, the light chains will precipitate. This technique is appealing because of its historical significance: it was the manner in which urinary light chains were first detected 140 years ago. However, Bence-Jones proteins are more accurately identified and measured by urinary electrophoresis. This method is also useful in quantitating the excretion of the pigment and tubular proteins. Precise characterization of urinary immunoglobulins and light chains is accomplished using urinary immunoelectrophoretic techniques.

Diagnostic Approach

When albuminuria is discovered, the history and physical examination assume paramount importance in helping the clinician establish whether the condition is a manifestation of primary renal disease or a systemic process affecting the kidney secondarily. Heart failure and organ enlargement may represent amyloidosis. A history of diabetes mellitus in a patient with proteinuria should raise suspicion of diabetic glomerulosclerosis; if proliferative retinopathy is present, this suspicion is strengthened. Licit or illicit drug use should be noted (see Table 127-1). A history of recent infection, particularly streptococcal pharyngitis or cellulitis, may also prove significant.

Occasionally, the patient denies any previous history of renal disease at the time proteinuria is found; in others, the abnormal urinalysis represents part of a longstanding problem. It is useful to question patients as to whether they have been told of protein in the urine during health screening for the military, for school, or for insurance purposes. Hypertension may reflect renal disease; if the patient is known to be hypertensive, an attempt should be made to establish its time of onset relative to that of the proteinuria. Especially in women, systemic lupus erythematosus enters the differential diagnosis of proteinuria. Accordingly, the patient should be questioned for the presence of other symptoms of lupus, e.g., cutaneous rashes and photosensitivity, alopecia, and joint pains.

The extent of albuminuria should be determined with a 24-hour quantitation. If the patient is edematous, chances are that nephrotic-range proteinuria will be recorded. If the daily albumin excretion is 1 g per day or less and the patient is otherwise healthy, postural proteinuria should be ruled out with separate daytime and nighttime collections. Other reversible factors augmenting albumin excretion should be minimized, if possible, prior to the collection; these include fever, hypertension, and vigorous exercise.

Examination of the urine sediment will help differentiate between glomerulopathies of the nephrotic type and the nephritic disorders. Indeed, urinalysis is the first and most important laboratory test in the diagnosis of proteinuria. Serologic tests are useful in ruling out specific diseases; e.g., antinuclear antibodies should be sought if there is a possibility of lupus. Complement levels help in the diagnosis of immune-complex renal diseases like lupus nephritis, poststreptococcal glomerulonephritis, membranoproliferative glomerulonephritis, and the glomerulonephritis of bacterial endocarditis. A positive antistreptolysin-O titer in a person with proteinuria and hematuria in the setting of a recent streptococcal infection suggests the diagnosis of acute poststreptococcal glomerulonephritis.

Renal imaging techniques are of little use in the evaluation of proteinuria. Renal biopsy is usually required to provide an exact histopathologic diagnosis, the only exceptions being, as already mentioned, patients in whom proteinuria is clearly the result of a well-recognized systemic disease. Because relatively few nephropathies are amenable to definitive therapy, questions are frequently raised regarding the value of establishing an exact tissue diagnosis. We currently recognize three main indications for renal biopsy (the reader is cautioned that other authors may entertain other views): (1) to establish the etiology of renal disease for which the use of potentially toxic medications is contemplated; this would include most cases of adult idiopathic nephrotic syndrome in which there are equal chances for the presence of a steroid-treatable or -resistant lesion; (2) to evaluate the extent of renal parenchymal injury and help formulate a prognosis; and (3) to aid in the diagnosis of acute renal failure of uncertain etiology.

As a general rule, if the patient has signs of chronic renal disease, e.g., anemia and reduced renal size, the potential gain from renal biopsy is small. Furthermore, biopsy is technically more difficult under these circumstances. Percutaneous biopsy technique is satisfactory for the diagnosis of most forms of renal disease. Open (surgical) biopsy is preferred when anatomic considerations make percutaneous stick unwise, as in patients with ectopic or anomalous kidneys, or when an especially large tissue sample is required to ensure diagnosis of focal pathologic processes.

Because most of the commonly used proteinuria screening tests are sensitive only to albumin, glomerular diseases are more likely to be detected early in their course than are nonalbuminuric syndromes. Thus, in tubulointerstitial disease, the finding of tubular proteinuria is more likely to be a secondary observation made after the diagnosis has been established. Although myeloma has been diagnosed following the detection of asymptomatic Bence-Jones proteinuria, it is more common to look for light chains in the urine of a patient in whom the diagnosis of myeloma is already entertained.

When asymptomatic nonalbuminuric proteinuria is discovered, the work-up should proceed in the fashion outlined previously. The identity of the urine protein should be ascertained with electrophoresis. Systemic diseases that can affect the kidney must be ruled out; if they are a strong diagnostic possibility, the work-up must be tailored appropriately. For a patient with Bence-Jones proteinuria, for example, serum protein electrophoresis and bone marrow biopsy have priority over renal biopsy.

Treatment

Patients with albuminuria due to glomerular disease can be managed with both definitive and supportive therapy. Definitive therapy refers to measures that can be taken to treat the underlying disease. When nephrotic syndrome arises as a manifestation of a systemic disease, the underlying disorder should be treated. For example, in nephrotic syndrome associated with diabetes or neoplasia, therapy should be aimed at those diseases rather than at the renal lesion per se. Nephrotic syndrome due to drugs will frequently regress following withdrawal of the offending agent.

When one speaks of definitive therapy of primary glomerulopathies, one is referring mainly to steroids and cytotoxic agents. Minimal change disease responds favorably to corticosteroids; a regimen of 1 to 2 mg prednisone per kilogram of body weight given orally on alternate days for about 8 weeks is commonly used now, and will induce a remission of proteinuria in the majority of patients. A similar regimen is used for membranous nephropathy. Although the results are less favorable than in minimal change disease, there is some evidence that if prednisone is administered early in the course of the illness, the chance of progression to renal insufficiency may be diminished. Patients with minimal change disease who relapse in spite of repeated courses of prednisone may derive additional benefit, not the least of which is diminution of the steroid dose required to control proteinuria, by the addition of chlorambucil or cyclophosphamide to the regimen. Clinical trials of adjunct chlorambucil therapy in membranous disease are under way. There are no convincingly effective regimens for either of the other primary nephroses, membranoproliferative disease or focal segmental glomerulosclerosis.

Not all primary nephritic disorders are treatable, either. Rapidly progressive, crescentic glomerulonephritis is now widely treated with corticosteroids or cyclophosphamide alone or in combination. There are a number of accepted regimens. Sometimes, as in the case of Goodpasture's syndrome, plasmapheresis may be added to the therapeutic protocol. In the literature, the response rates have varied according to the specific disease entity, the stage of the disease at the time of initiation of treatment, and the reporting center. There is no definitive therapy for IgA nephropathy; this disease runs a variable course, with some patients experiencing no ill effects after decades of illness and others suffering a rapid progression to end-stage renal failure. Poststreptococcal acute glomerulonephritis is also not treatable, but the majority of patients have a short course marked by complete recovery.

As has been said of secondary nephrotic syndrome, when nephritis occurs in the setting of primary extrarenal disease, as in the glomerulonephritis of bacterial endocarditis, or vasculitis, definitive therapy should be targeted at the underlying disease.

Supportive therapy is treatment that does not induce a cure or remission, but rather is meant to ameliorate the severity of the symptoms. For patients with heavy proteinuria and edema, supportive measures include dietary sodium restriction and diuretic use. Diuretics decrease renal tubular sodium reabsorption, thus interrupting the role of the kidney in the formation and perpetuation of edema. The rationale for sodium restriction is similar. An important point to remember is that the nephrotic, hypoalbuminemic patient may have hypovolemia, and because diuretics work by increasing the excretion of filtered sodium, they may induce further volume depletion. Dizziness, hypotension, and weakness may be signs of overdiuresis in the nephrotic patient. In very hypoalbuminemic patients, the severity of these complaints often precludes the effective control of edema.

When renal failure accompanies proteinuria, diuretics may be ineffective in preventing sodium retention. In this situation, dialysis may be useful not only for fluid removal but also as a means of treating electrolyte imbalance and uremia. Dialysis may be employed on an interventional or maintenance basis, as the patient's particular illness mandates. Interim dialysis is indicated when acute renal failure occurs with any of the disorders discussed in this chapter. Patients with myoglobinuric renal failure usually achieve a complete recovery, although they may require supportive dialysis for several weeks. If myoglobinuria is diagnosed before renal shutdown occurs, intravenous fluid administration is encouraged in order to maximize urinary flow rates and reduce the chance of intratubular protein coagulation.

Treatment of Bence-Jones proteinuria depends on whether or not multiple myeloma is present; if this is the case, the correct approach is chemotherapy. If radiographic contrast studies are necessary, the myeloma patient should undergo the study while diuresing, the rationale being the same as that for preventing myoglobinuric renal failure. Renal failure remains a leading cause of death in patients with multiple myeloma. However, many patients with myeloma kidney disease can be supported for years with dialysis.

References

Brenner BM, Meyer TW, Hostetter TH. Dietary protein intake and the progressive nature of kidney disease: The role of hemodynamically mediated glomerular injury in the pathogenesis of progressive glomerular sclerosis in aging, renal ablation, and intrinsic renal disease. N Engl J Med 1982; 307:652.

Heinemann HO, Maack TM, Sherman RL. Proteinuria. Am J Med 1974; 56:71.
Melvin T, Sibley R, Michael AF. Nephrotic syndrome. In: Brenner BM, Stein JH, eds. Pediatric nephrology. New York: Churchill Livingstone, 1984:191.
Perry MC, Kyle RA. The clinical significance of Bence-Jones proteinuria. Mayo Clin Proc 1975; 50:234.
Reineck HJ. Mechanisms of edema formation in the nephrotic syndrome. In: Brenner BM, Stein JH, eds. Nephrotic syndrome. New York: Churchill Livingstone, 1982:32.
Renkin EM, Robinson RR. Glomerular filtration. N Engl J Med 1974; 290:785.
Rose, BD. Pathophysiology of renal disease. 2nd ed. New York: McGraw-Hill, 1987.

Hyperuricemia

Ann Gateley, MD

128

Definition

Hyperuricemia can be defined simply as an excess of uric acid in the serum. In most laboratories, the normal uric acid level as determined by the colorimetric method is less than 7 mg/dl in men and postmenopausal women, and less than 6 mg/dl in premenopausal women.

Etiology

Uric acid is the end product of purine degradation. Elevated uric acid levels can be due to overproduction of uric acid, underexcretion of uric acid, or a combination of both processes. Overproduction, found in 20 percent or less of patients with hyperuricemia, can occur with increased biosynthesis of uric acid and increased turnover of tissue nucleic acids. Much less frequently, an increased intake of purine precursors can result in hyperuricemia. The kidney completely filters, then alternately reabsorbs and secretes uric acid along the length of the nephron. Therefore, underexcretion can result from a reduction of glomerular filtration, decreased tubular secretion, or increased tubular reabsorption of uric acid. A combined disorder of urate metabolism can occur when two conditions that affect uric acid balance coexist.

History and Physical Examination

Often, hyperuricemia is an asymptomatic finding on multiphasic screening tests; the patient offers no complaints, and the physical examination does not reveal any stigmata of uric acid excess. However, a number of clinically important conditions are associated with elevated uric acid levels: acute gouty arthritis, chronic or tophaceous gout, and uric acid renal stones. Of these, acute gouty arthritis is the most common clinical sequela of uric acid excess.

Because men have higher uric acid levels than premenopausal women, and because it generally takes at least 30 years of sustained hyperuricemia before clinical gout occurs, men over the age of 40 and postmenopausal women are affected much more commonly than premenopausal women. During an acute gouty arthritis attack, the patient complains of a swollen, hot, tender joint, classically the metatarsal joint of the great toe (podagra). Ninety-eight percent of gout sufferers will have podagra at some time. The patient may have a low-grade fever as well. The gouty attack most often has its onset in early morning; without treatment, it generally lasts 5 to 7 days. Between attacks, the patient's joints are asymptomatic. If the patient has a series of severe untreated attacks, however, peripheral joints may be destroyed. Subcutaneous deposits of uric acid (tophi) may appear, classically about the affected joints and bursae as well as the pinna of the ear.

Other Clinical Considerations

Patients whose excretion of uric acid is above normal (hyperuricosuria) are at risk for uric acid nephrolithiasis. Two-thirds of these patients are hyperuricemic. Uric acid stone formers represent a small fraction (about 10 percent) of patients with nephrolithiasis. If such a stone passes through the genitourinary tract, the patient may complain of intense pain radiating from the flank to the testicle or groin. The patient may be unable to lie still and may experience nausea and vomiting. On physical examination, costovertebral angle or flank tenderness may be elicited, and the laboratory data may reveal increased uric acid or hematuria.

Hyperuricemia greater than 1.5 to 2 standard deviations above the mean in either the symptomatic or asymptomatic patient should prompt consideration of the possible mechanisms. The elevation could represent artifact from interference of other reducing substances with the colorimetric method (e.g., ascorbic acid or hyperglycemia). Increased nucleic acid turnover leading to overproduction of uric acid can be seen in hematologic or lymphoproliferative malignancies, extensive crush injuries, and psoriasis. Common problems in renal excretion of uric acid can be found with (1) decreased filtration, as seen in dehydration and renal insufficiency, and (2) competition for proximal tubular secretory sites by weak organic acids (e.g., low-dose salicylates, thiazide diuretics, lactic acid, and ketoacids). These mechanisms are helpful to keep in mind in the evaluation of patients with hyperuricemia.

To date, there is little evidence to justify uric acid lowering therapy in asymptomatic patients in order to prevent gouty arthritis, urate renal disease, or other associated states, such as cardiovascular disease. Acute gout, if it occurs, can be treated promptly and safely with anti-inflammatory agents. Additionally, renal and cardiovascular disease do not appear to have an increased incidence in hyperuricemic patients as compared with normouricemic patients.

It was once believed that asymptomatic hyperuricemia predisposed to renal insufficiency by inducing a form of chronic interstitial nephritis called urate nephropathy. Recent studies have shown that the only hyperuricemic patients who are at risk for urate nephropathy are those few with a history of prolonged lead exposure. Such patients generally have hypertension and recurrent gouty arthritis ("saturnine gout").

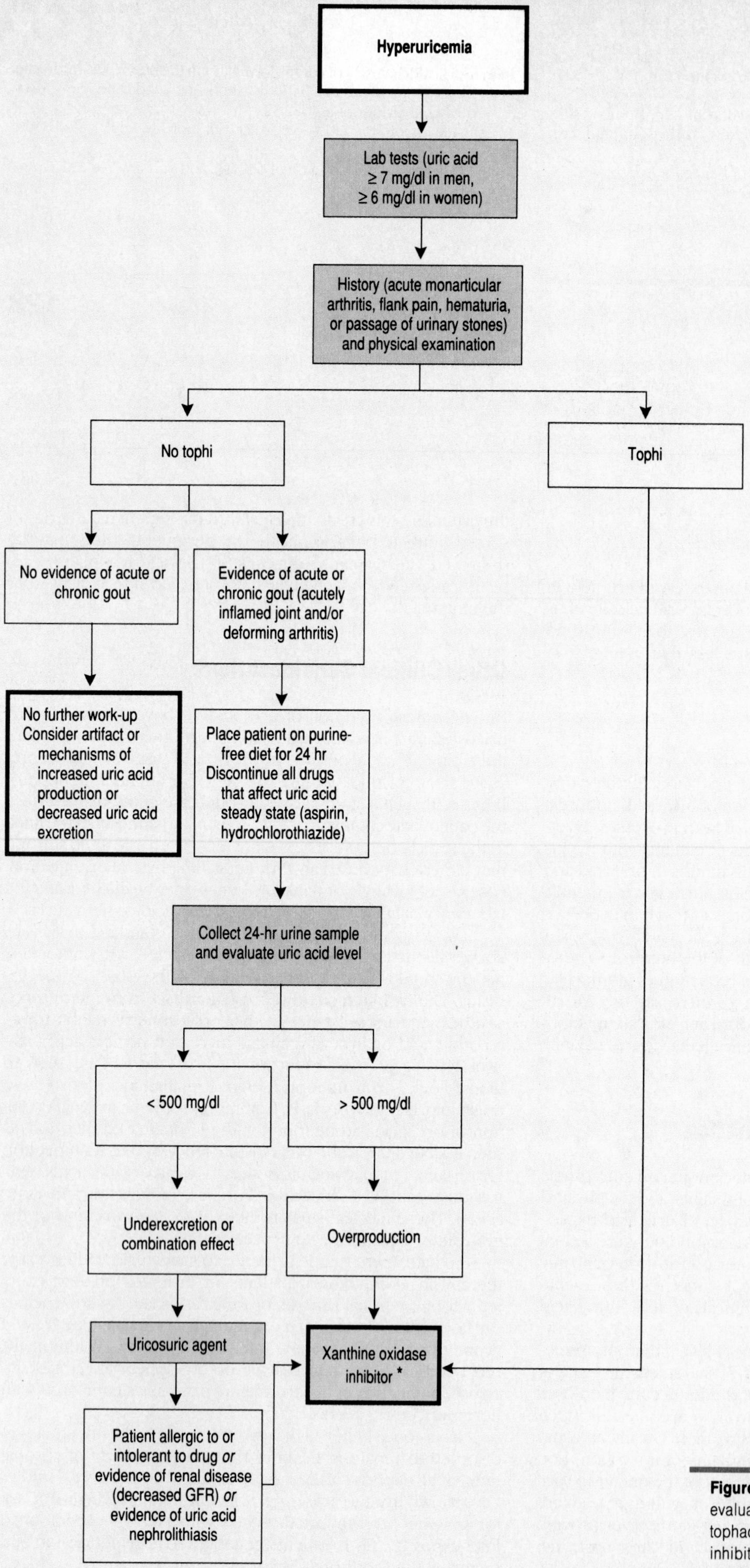

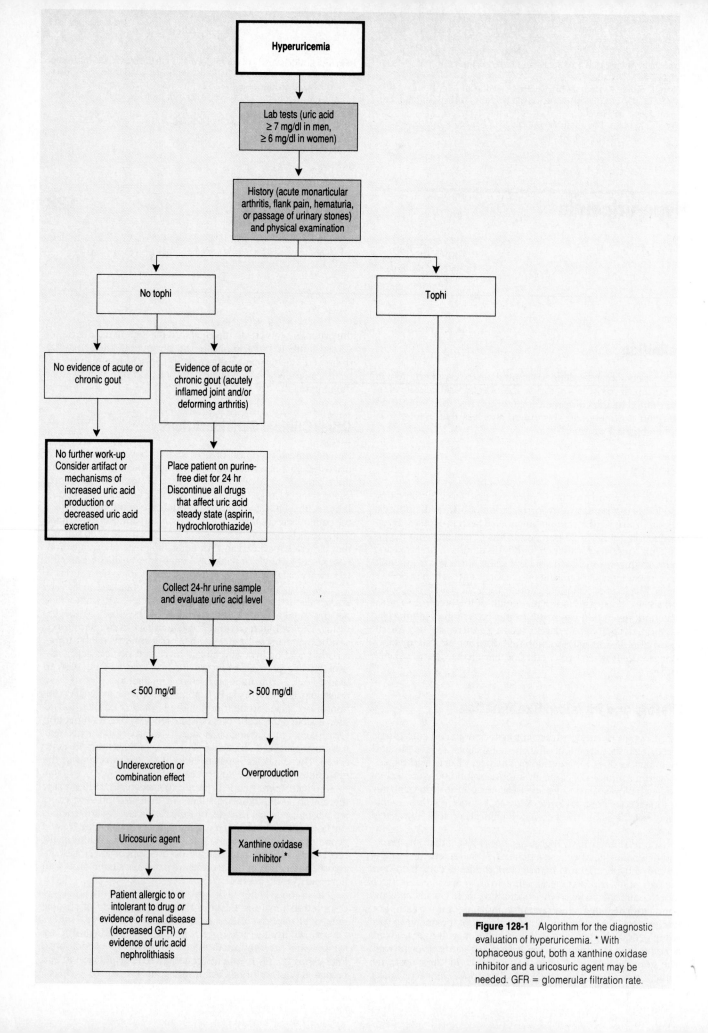

Figure 128-1 Algorithm for the diagnostic evaluation of hyperuricemia. * With tophaceous gout, both a xanthine oxidase inhibitor and a uricosuric agent may be needed. GFR = glomerular filtration rate.

Diagnostic Approach

Although the asymptomatic hyperuricemic patient need not be evaluated, hyperuricemia should be addressed when patients present with gouty arthritis or urate nephrolithiasis. First, one must determine the cause of the elevated uric acid level: oversecretion, underexcretion, or both? To do this, the patient must be placed on a purine-free diet for at least 24 hours. All medications that affect uric acid steady state (e.g., aspirin, diuretics) should be discontinued. At least one 24-hour urine collection should be made. Because the amount of uric acid produced in 24 hours approximates that excreted in 24 hours, a urine uric acid level greater than 500 mg (or 750 mg on a normal diet) implies overproduction, whereas less than 500 mg suggests normal production with undersecretion or a combination effect.

It should be emphasized that during an acute gouty attack, the sole purpose of therapy is relief of symptoms, not lowering of uric acid. This relief is achieved with anti-inflammatory agents or colchicine. The choice of therapy for interval or chronic gout depends on the 24-hour uric acid determination. For underexcretors, except those with renal insufficiency, uricosuric agents are appropriate. For overproducers, an inhibitor of uric acid synthesis, such as allopurinol, is used. In severe tophaceous gout, both a uricosuric agent and a uric acid synthesis inhibitor may be needed because of the large pools of uric acid sequestered subcutaneously.

An algorithm for the diagnostic approach to hyperuricemia is presented in Figure 128-1.

References

Becker MA. Gout: Pathogenesis of hyperuricemia. In: Schumacher HR, ed. Primer on the rheumatic diseases. Atlanta: The Arthritis Foundation, 1988:195.

Boss GR, Seegmiller JE. Hyperuricemia and gout. N Engl J Med 1979; 300:1459.

Cahill GF. Gout. In: Rubenstein E, Federman DD, eds. Scientific American medicine. New York: Scientific American, 1983; IV:1.

Duffy WB, et al. Management of asymptomatic hyperuricemia. JAMA 1981; 67:2215.

Fessell WJ. Renal outcomes of gout and hyperuricemia. Am J Med 1967; 67:1133.

Hall DW, Vroom DH. Uric acid. In: Walker HK, Hall WB, Hurst SW, eds. Clinical methods. Boston: Butterworth, 1980.

Thompson CS, Weinman EJ. Acute and chronic hyperuricemic nephropathy. In: Bayless TM, Brain MC, Cherniack RM, eds. Current therapy in internal medicine. Toronto: BC Decker, 1987:1074.

Wyngaarden B, Kelly WM. Gout. In: Stanbury JB, et al, eds. The metabolic basis of arthritic disease. New York: McGraw-Hill, 1972:889.

Kidney Stones

James L. McGuire, MD

129

Definition

Renal lithiasis, also called nephrolithiasis or urolithiasis, is the clinical condition caused by the formation and movement of stones within the urinary tract. Several types of stones have been identified, based on chemical composition and opacity by radiographs. Intensive research into the mechanisms of stone formation has resulted in an expanded medical evaluation for most patients. These investigations have led to advances in the metabolic and surgical approaches to kidney stones. A brief description of the acute disease provides a necessary foundation for the metabolic work-up of the patient with renal lithiasis.

Stones as a Urologic Problem

Kidney stones are usually dramatically symptomatic. An obstructing stone in the ureter may result in the most exquisite pain encountered in clinical medicine. It is usually described as a sharp colicky pain in the flank with radiation to the groin, testicle, or tip of the urethra.

Depending on the site of obstruction in the kidney or ureter, nephrolithiasis can mimic other intra-abdominal problems, especially when associated with nausea and vomiting. Stones in the right ureteropelvic junction may lateralize to the right upper quadrant and be confused with symptomatic gallstones, especially when the pain is colicky. Lower ureter obstruction may enter into the differential diagnosis of testicular pain, dysuria, frequency, and inguinal hernias. Occasionally a stone may be painless and is discovered during an evaluation of hematuria, urinary tract infection, or rarely, uremia.

The acute clinical episode usually resolves with the spontaneous painful passage of the stone, surgical removal of the stone by several urologic procedures, or stone destruction by extracorporeal shock waves (lithotripsy). Removal of stones through the urethra can often be accomplished by specialized stone baskets and loops passed through the cystoscope. When high-grade obstruction persists, several surgical options exist. Direct removal through a flank incision or percutaneous nephrostomy is usually successful. The recent introduction of lithotripsy has spared many patients from surgical procedures. The kidney stone, obtained either surgically or by straining the urine during spontaneous passage, is then sent for chemical analysis.

Types of Kidney Stones

Four main stone types are found by chemical analysis. The most common is calcium oxalate, although calcium can also crystallize with phosphate. Uric acid stones are radiolucent on plain radiographs and are often seen in patients who have gout. Struvite or infection stones are formed in urine infected with urea-splitting bacteria (usually *Proteus* species), which generate the alkaline milieu conducive to the precipitation of magnesium, phosphate, and ammonia. Finally, cystine stones are the result of a renal tubular defect that allows large amounts of cystine to be excreted. This supersaturation results in precipitation of this type of stone.

Diagnostic Approach

History

The detailed history of the patient with recurrent stone formation can often provide strong pathogenetic clues. In calcium oxalate nephrolithiasis, a dietary history is critical.

Intake of calcium-containing foods such as cheese, milk, and ice cream is especially dangerous to the patient with an inherited tendency to hyperabsorb calcium from the small intestine. Dietary sodium plays an important role in renal calcium excretion. High salt intake almost uniformly results in hypercalciuria on the basis of renal tubular handling of sodium and calcium.

Urinary volume is a direct function of fluid intake. The lower the volume, the higher the concentration of potential stone-forming substances in the urine. It is surprisingly common to elicit a history of very low urine output in patients with renal lithiasis. Estimation of fluid intake can be approximated by asking the number of standard glasses (10 oz) or equivalent cans of cola (12 oz) consumed daily. The amounts of coffee, tea, and juices can be determined in a similar fashion. It is appropriate, therapeutically, to expect patients with stones to excrete urinary volumes in excess of 2 L daily. This may require a daily intake of 3 L of fluid.

Little is known about the relative contribution of dietary oxalate to the calcium oxalate stone diathesis. A history of ingestion of oxalate-rich foods, especially spinach, rhubarb, tea, or high doses of vitamin C (converted to oxalate), may be a significant risk factor for stone formation.

Uric acid and its urate salts play a central pathogenetic role in both calcium oxalate and pure uric acid stones. A previous personal or family history of gout should be sought. Other risk factors for abnormal urate excretion include obesity, salt ingestion, and myeloproliferative disorders.

Bacterial infections of the urinary tract predispose to stone formation, especially if anatomic variants of the urinary system, which predispose to stasis, are present. As mentioned earlier, chronic infection with *Proteus* or other urea-splitting organisms is essential for struvite stone formation.

It is important to ask about medication. Chronic antacid therapy containing high amounts of absorbable calcium may predispose to calcium stone formation. Long-term antibiotic therapy, used to suppress urinary tract infections, or known antigout medicines may suggest struvite or uric acid stones, respectively.

The prior urologic history is equally important. For each stone episode, the presentation, site, side involved, and type of stone must be delineated. The resolution of the episode by spontaneous passage, instrumentation (cystoscopy), operation (e.g., ureterolithotomy), or lithotripsy is recorded. Any residual stones, anatomic abnormalities, or persistent urinary tract infections are, of course, risk factors for subsequent stone symptoms. Several types of renal disease predispose to nephrolithiasis, including medullary sponge kidney and polycystic kidney disease.

A family history can provide etiologic clues in all types of stones. The hyperabsorption of calcium from the small intestine in patients with calcium oxalate nephrolithiasis is inherited in an autosomal dominant pattern. The abnormalities of dibasic amino acid transport in patients with cystine stones typically show an autosomal recessive inheritance. Certain types of congenital anomalies of the urinary tract may give rise to chronic infections due to urostasis. This may be important in struvite stone formation. Finally, as discussed earlier, a history of gout may suggest either pure uric acid or calcium oxalate stones with a uric acid nidus.

Physical Examination

The physical examination of the patient with kidney stones is influenced by the clinical setting. During the acute attack, emphasis is placed on a careful evaluation of the abdomen, flanks, inguinal area, and genitalia. The demonstration of lateralized tenderness over the costovertebral angle with radiation to the flank is a key physical finding.

When the pain is predominantly abdominal, the physical examination is often nonspecific in differentiating kidney stones from other intra-abdominal problems. Localization of pain to one quadrant helps to narrow the diagnostic possibilities. The presence of nausea and vomiting with or without audible bowel sounds is usually not helpful in the differential diagnosis. If no abnormal findings can be ascertained in areas of maximal discomfort, the examiner should consider the possibility of a referred cause of pain. Thus, a normal examination of the genitalia or inguinal region in the presence of pain may suggest a kidney stone.

The physical examination during the metabolic evaluation of renal lithiasis often focuses on the extra-abdominal manifestations. A search for chronic arthritis involving the great toe at the metatarsophalangeal joint may suggest gout, especially if uric acid deposits (tophi) are found in the subcutaneous tissue of the ear or the extensor surface of the elbow. Chronic hypercalcemia or primary hyperparathyroidism may rarely present as calcium deposits in the eye called band keratopathy. A search for a goiter suggestive of hyperthyroidism is occasionally helpful in patients with calcium oxalate stones. Finally, careful attention to the bone structure may reveal a metabolic bone disease such as osteoporosis, osteomalacia, or rarely, osteitis fibrosa cystica generalisata.

Flank pain may still be elicited by palpation or percussion long after the resolution of a stone episode, especially if other stones remain. Obviously, scars from surgical incisions in the flanks should be noted.

Radiographic Evaluation of Stones

The plain radiograph of the abdomen, which emphasizes *k*idneys, *u*reters, and *b*ladder (KUB), is obtained in all patients with suspected nephrolithiasis. The presence of a radiopaque object in the region of the kidney or bladder should prompt further laboratory (urinalysis) and radiographic studies, such as an intravenous pyelogram (IVP). Remember that some stones are radiolucent (uric acid) and are not found on KUB films.

The IVP is critical to both the diagnosis and management of stones. First, it determines the anatomy of the urinary system. Second, delayed excretion or absence of contrast medium may suggest the site of the obstructing stone. Third, the IVP allows localization of stones suspected on KUB film to within or outside the urinary tract. Fourth, the finding of a defect in the pyelographic figure, coupled with obstruction, is consistent with a radiolucent stone. Finally, the IVP can monitor stone passage and position during the acute attack. Renal ultrasonography can provide a useful adjunct to IVP in the assessment of urinary tract obstruction and may be a necessary alternative in patients with contraindications to intravenous pyelography.

Laboratory Tests

During the acute attack, the presence of gross or microscopic hematuria on urinalysis coupled with a positive IVP establishes the diagnosis of renal lithiasis. The serum creatinine level and/or the blood urea nitrogen level may reveal functional impairment of the kidney, i.e., obstructive uropathy. Similarly, the presence of a urinary tract infection, established by urine culture, may be important both etiologically and therapeutically.

The metabolic evaluation begins with the stone analysis. A

number of excellent stone laboratories can identify the relative amounts of the primary constituents of the stone.

Calcium-containing stones necessitate extensive but straightforward laboratory assessment to determine the primary pathogenetic mechanism of stone formation. Blood is obtained for calcium, phosphate, uric acid, alkaline phosphatase, creatinine, and parathyroid hormone (PTH). These values rapidly screen for hyperparathyroidism (hypercalcemia and PTH level), metabolic bone disease (alkaline phosphatase), hyperuricemia, and existing renal disease (creatinine).

A 24-hour urine collection for calcium, creatinine, uric acid, citrate, pH, oxalate, and volume on a random diet is probably the most important test in patients with calcium kidney stones. The demonstration of hypercalciuria (more than 250 mg of calcium in 24 hours) is a pivotal determination (Figure 129-1). A low urinary volume can be readily determined. Volumes less than 1 L per day may aggravate the degree of urinary supersaturation in patients with stones. Uric acid levels higher than 600 mg daily are considered abnormal with respect to stone formation. Most patients with calcium oxalate nephrolithiasis show pH values greater than 6.5. Finally, urinary citrate levels below 320 mg daily may predispose to stone formation by loss of urinary inhibitor activity.

Idiopathic hypercalciuria has been divided into two categories: that due to overabsorption of dietary calcium from the gut, and that due to excessive renal leaking of filtered calcium. A convenient way to assess the relative contribution of intestinal calcium absorption or renal leaking of calcium is a second 24-hour collection. A diet of low calcium (no cheese, milk, ice cream) and low sodium (no salt added) is given for 7 days prior to and including the day of collection. If the urinary calcium becomes normal or drops dramatically (greater than 100 mg) as a result of the diet, this suggests a component of absorptive (intestinal) hypercalciuria. A persistence of high calcium excretion in a patient who is adhering to a diet is consistent with a renal (leak) hypercalciuria.

The finding of hyperuricosuria (greater than 600 mg daily) has pathogenetic implications in calcium oxalate nephrolithiasis because uric acid crystals represent a potential nidus for calcium salt crystallization. Urinary uric acid excretion is best determined on a random outpatient diet. Hyperuricosuria may be associated with hypercalciuria or may be the only abnormality detected in the urine of the calcium stone former.

The time-honored treatment of forcing fluids to promote urinary flow in patients with stones is based on the premise that supersaturation of the stone-forming constituents will be minimized. Recent studies using physicochemical determinations on the urine uphold this theory. Therefore, low urine volumes must be viewed as a possible risk factor.

Urinary oxalate values are within normal limits (less than 40 mg) in almost all patients with calcium oxalate stones. The relative importance of the oxalate moiety to stone formation is being debated. Patients who have had intestinal bypass for obesity and patients with chronic inflammatory bowel disease may exhibit marked hyperoxaluria (usually greater than 100 mg) and recurrent calcium stones. The hyperoxaluria is a reflection of increased intestinal oxalate absorption.

Renal tubular acidosis may present with calcium kidney stones. The findings of hyperchloremic acidosis and hypokalemia associated with elevated urinary calcium and pH should

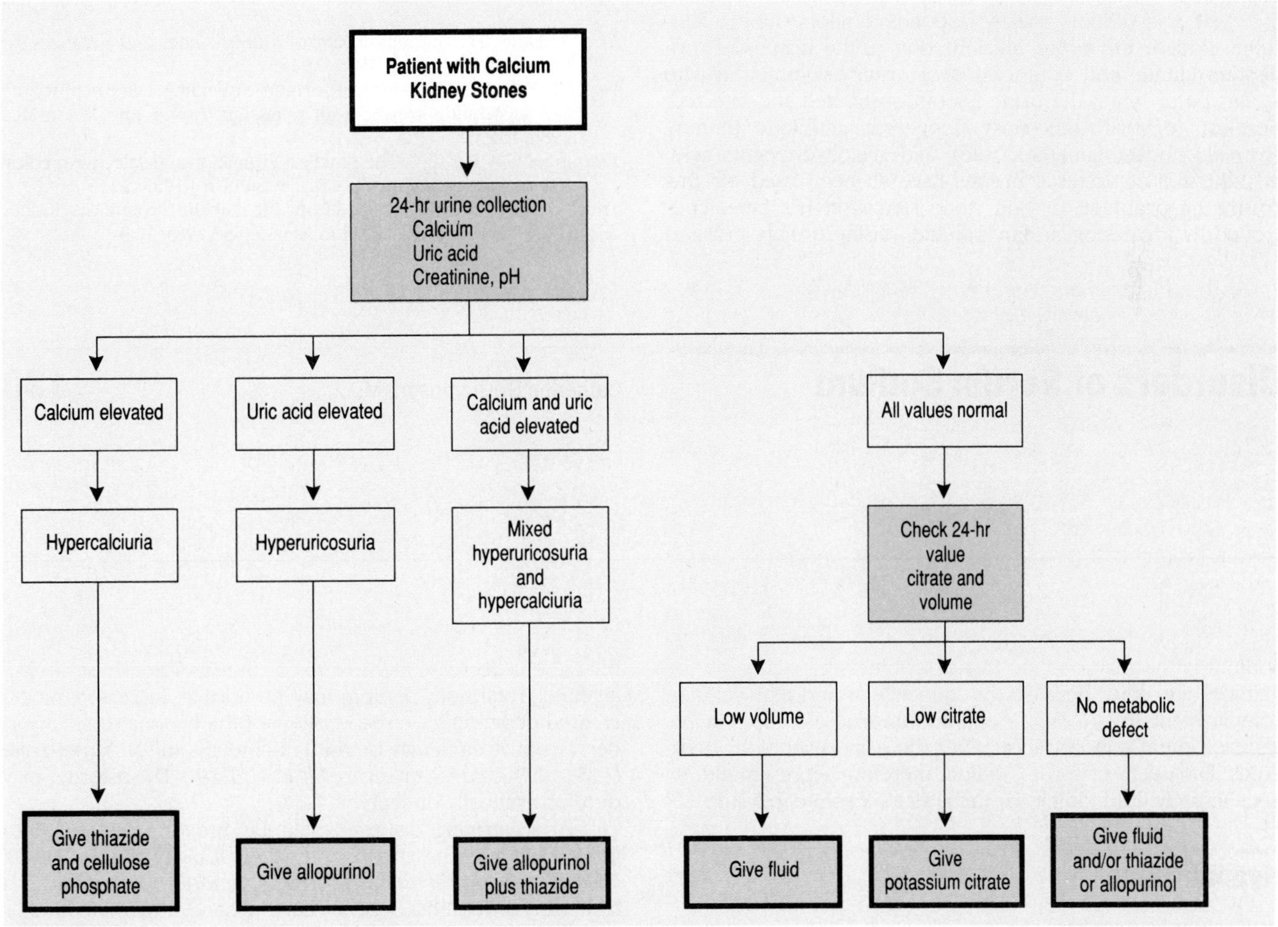

Figure 129-1 Algorithm for the urinary work-up of the patient with calcium kidney stones.

suggest this condition. Patients with renal tubular acidosis may also have hypocitraturia.

The laboratory values in patients with pure uric acid stones usually reflect the abnormal urate metabolism. Hyperuricosuria and a low urinary pH are characteristic. Hyperuricemia is almost uniformly found.

Normal 24-hour urine chemistries are reported in most patients with struvite (infected) stones despite the participation of magnesium, phosphate, and sometimes calcium. The presence of a high urinary pH and a positive culture for *Proteus* or other urea-splitting bacteria are characteristic.

Patients with cystine stones have cystinuria on the basis of a defect in renal tubular reabsorption. A low urinary pH is usually found.

Discussion of Stone Types: Implication for Therapy

The most important diagnostic clue for the clinician is the stone itself. The analysis of uric acid, struvite, or cystine rapidly defines the laboratory investigation and subsequent therapy.

The most conservative forms of management are often the best, and this is the case with nephrolithiasis. *Regardless of stone type, all patients should be encouraged to maintain a high urine volume.* Dietary modification is safe and may be beneficial, particularly for patients shown to have the absorptive form of hypercalciuria. These patients should be instructed to avoid calcium-rich foodstuffs. All patients with hypercalciuria should restrict dietary sodium. Many experts recommend limiting dietary protein as well, which can be shown to reduce calcium excretion.

Uric acid lithiasis usually responds to allopurinol (a xanthine oxidase inhibitor), alkalinization of the urine with potassium citrate, and optimization of urinary volume. Struvite stones occur when the urine is both obstructed and infected. Surgical removal, lithotripsy, long-term antibiotic therapy (trimethoprim-sulfamethoxazole), and acetohydroxamic acid, an inhibitor of bacterial urease, have all been used for this frustrating problem. Cystine stone formation has been controlled by increasing urinary volume, raising urinary pH, and administering penicillamine. Alpha-mercaptopropionylglycine (Thiola) has recently shown promise in this stone type.

The finding of a calcium-containing kidney stone should prompt a complete metabolic evaluation. The demonstration of either hypercalciuria or hyperuricosuria in most patients, coupled with new techniques of urinary physical chemistry, has resulted in well-defined subsets of stone formers. Therapy, based on a demonstrated defect, has greatly reduced calcium-stone formation.

Thiazide diuretics are effective in most patients with hypercalciuria (renal and absorptive) because of their hypocalciuric effects. Cellulose phosphate can bind intestinal calcium and may become the specific therapy for absorptive hypercalciuria.

Allopurinol is dramatically effective in the group of patients with hyperuricosuric calcium oxalate nephrolithiasis. The inhibition of uric acid synthesis may stop stone formation completely in this group.

Patients with recurrent kidney stones due to primary hyperparathyroidism are considered candidates for surgical parathyroidectomy.

Patients found to have low urinary volumes or no metabolic defect at all usually benefit from increasing urinary flow. If stone formation continues, allopurinol or thiazide may be arbitrarily added with surprising effectiveness. Some patients who have low urinary citrate levels will benefit from potassium citrate therapy.

The specific conditions of renal tubular acidosis and intestinal hyperoxaluria may respond to corrective therapy directed at the acidosis or intestinal bypass, respectively.

References

Coe FL, Parks JH. Pathophysiology of kidney stones and strategies for treatment. Hosp Pract 1988; 23:185.

Pak CYC, Fuller C. Idiopathic hypocitraturic calcium-oxalate nephrolithiasis successfully treated with potassium citrate. Ann Intern Med 1986; 104:33.

Preminger GM, Pak CYC. The practical evaluation and selective medical management of nephrolithiasis. Semin Urol 1985; 3:170.

Smith L. Medical treatment of idiopathic calcium urolithiasis. Kidney (National Kidney Foundation Newsletter) 1983; 16:9.

Disorders of Serum Sodium

Catherine S. Thompson, MD

130

Sodium is the major solute that determines the osmolarity of extracellular fluid. Because the intracellular and extracellular compartments are in osmotic equilibrium, true alterations in the serum sodium concentration affect the osmolarity of all body fluids. Disorders of serum sodium therefore represent alterations in body fluid tonicity or in the ratio of solute to water.

Hyponatremia

Hyponatremia is defined as a serum concentration of sodium less than 135 mEq/L. The presence of hyponatremia, however, does not necessarily imply a reduced total body sodium content but rather a decrease in the *ratio* of solute to water in extracellular fluid. Total body sodium may be normal, increased, or decreased depending on the etiology of the hyponatremic disorder. Hyponatremia may be mild (125 to 134 mEq/L), moderate (115 to 124 mEq/L), or severe (<115 mEq/L). The disorder may develop gradually or acutely.

Hyponatremic disorders can be broadly classified into three categories based on body fluid tonicity (Table 130-1). *Isotonic hyponatremia,* also termed *pseudohyponatremia,* is a laboratory artifact that occurs when the concentration of lipid or protein in serum is markedly increased.

Hypertonic hyponatremia is observed in cases of severe hyperglycemia (>500 mg/dl) or mannitol infusion and occurs

Table 130-1 Hyponatremia: Relation to Serum Osmolarity

	Measured Na^+	Measured osmolarity
Isotonic hyponatremia (pseudohyponatremia)	Low	Normal (285–295 mOsm/kg)
Hypertonic hyponatremia	Low	High (>300 mOsm/kg)
Hypotonic hyponatremia	Low	Low (<280 mOsm/kg)

because of osmotically driven water movement from the intracellular to the extracellular space. *Hypotonic hyponatremia* is the most significant of the three categories because of its clinical sequelae. Cell swelling is the pathologic hallmark of these hypotonic states and is the result of water movement into the intracellular space. Clinically, central nervous system findings predominate in hypotonic hyponatremias and include confusion, lethargy, seizures, and coma. In general, the most severe symptoms and signs are observed in acute-onset or severe ($Na^+ < 115$ mEq/L) hyponatremia.

Hypotonic hyponatremias can occur in a variety of settings and may involve diverse pathophysiologic events. However, these disorders can be subclassified into three major groups based on the state of the patient's extracellular volume: hypovolemic, hypervolemic, and isovolemic.

Hypovolemic hyponatremia occurs as a consequence of significant renal or extrarenal sodium and water loss. Patients typically demonstrate signs of extracellular volume depletion such as hypotension, orthostasis, or tachycardia. Their loss of solute (sodium) exceeds their free-water loss. The problem can be compounded in those patients who continue to ingest large amounts of free water.

Any clinical condition that is characterized by fluid and electrolyte loss can induce hypovolemic hyponatremia. Examples include vomiting, diarrhea, and heavy perspiration. It should be pointed out that if water intake is not maintained, *hyper*natremia may result instead.

Diuretics are a major cause of hypovolemic hyponatremia and the major iatrogenic cause of hyponatremia. There are several mechanisms through which diuretics can lower the serum sodium concentration, including hypovolemic stimulation of antidiuretic hormone (ADH) release; impaired delivery of filtrate to the distal nephron, leading to reduced free water excretion; and urinary sodium loss disproportionate to water loss.

Thiazides are the diuretics most commonly implicated in hyponatremia, because the ratio of sodium loss (natriuresis) to water loss (diuresis) is higher with these agents than with loop diuretics. The latter promote free-water excretion. Extracellular volume status may not be perceptibly reduced in patients with thiazide-induced hyponatremia, making it difficult to distinguish this entity from the syndrome of inappropriate antidiuretic hormone secretion (SIADH). The presence of hypokalemia or a hypochloremic alkalosis may be a clue to the diuretic-related etiology in these cases.

Hypervolemic hyponatremia can develop in association with severe congestive heart failure, cirrhosis with ascites, or nephrosis. Affected individuals have increased total body sodium and water and are usually edematous. Inappropriate retention of sodium and water by the kidney is common to all of these disorders. *Isovolemic hyponatremic* conditions are characterized by decreased renal excretion of free water. SIADH is included in this group of disorders that are mediated by excessive activity of ADH on the renal collecting ducts.

SIADH is not an uncommon disorder; it most often occurs in association with chronic intrathoracic diseases like tuberculosis, with neoplasms, or as a result of medications (e.g., narcotics, cyclophosphamide, vincristine).

Diagnostic Approach

The diagnostic approach to the patient with hyponatremia can be simplified by excluding the isotonic and hypertonic variants of the disorder (Fig. 130-1). This is easily accomplished by obtaining a serum osmolarity and glucose level. Hyponatremia associated with normal serum osmolarity (285 to 295 mOsm/kg) qualifies as "pseudohyponatremia" and is usually caused by excessive serum proteins or lipids. Because tonicity is not affected, this condition has no physiologic significance and requires no additional evaluation. Hypertonic hyponatremia can be detected by elevated serum osmolarity (>300 mOsm/kg) and is most often the result of hyperglycemia. The serum sodium concentration falls by approximately 1.6 mEq/L for each 100 mg/dl increment in the serum glucose concentration. The serum sodium in these cases will return to normal with correction of the hyperglycemia.

Hypotonic hyponatremia should be approached initially with a complete history and physical examination. The patient should be questioned about medications, a known cardiac, liver, or renal disease, and the presence of diarrhea or vomiting. The dietary intake of sodium and water should also be estimated. The physical examination provides information regarding the extracellular volume status of the patient and in many cases allows for separation of these disorders into the hypovolemic, isovolemic, and hypervolemic categories. The vital signs, cardiopulmonary examination, and the presence of peripheral edema or ascites provide clues that help to distinguish these entities.

The laboratory evaluation of the hyponatremic patient should include serum osmolarity, creatinine, urea nitrogen and uric acid levels, and simultaneous urine osmolarity and sodium concentration. The utility of these determinations is outlined in Table 130-2.

Treatment

The treatment of hypotonic hyponatremia depends upon the severity of the disorder, the underlying cause, and the magnitude of the associated neurologic symptoms. Prompt correction of hyponatremia that has developed *acutely,* and is associated with neurologic *dysfunction,* is imperative. Conversely, slower correction of longstanding hyponatremia, regardless of its severity, is indicated in the patient with minimal neurologic impairment.

Hypovolemic hyponatremia is best managed with repletion of the extracellular fluid volume and treatment of the underlying causes of excess sodium and water loss. Normal saline (0.9 percent) is most often used, although hypertonic saline (3 percent) can be infused with caution if the hyponatremia is severe. However, the goal of correction should be a serum sodium level of about 125 mEq/L after the first 24 to 36 hours with a rate of rise in sodium of only 1 mEq/L per hour, particularly if the hyponatremia is subacute or chronic. Exceeding this rate of correction may place the patient at risk for neurologic deterioration with central nervous system demyelination.

Hypervolemic hyponatremia is best managed by means of controlled diuresis using loop diuretics combined with restriction of sodium and water intake. Individuals with severe renal dysfunction may require dialysis if they are resistant to diuretics.

Isovolemic hyponatremic patients typically respond to free-water restriction or, in more severe cases, infusion of saline combined with intravenous loop diuretics, which effect a free-water diuresis. Chronic SIADH often can be managed with a liberal salt diet and oral diuretics combined with free water restriction.

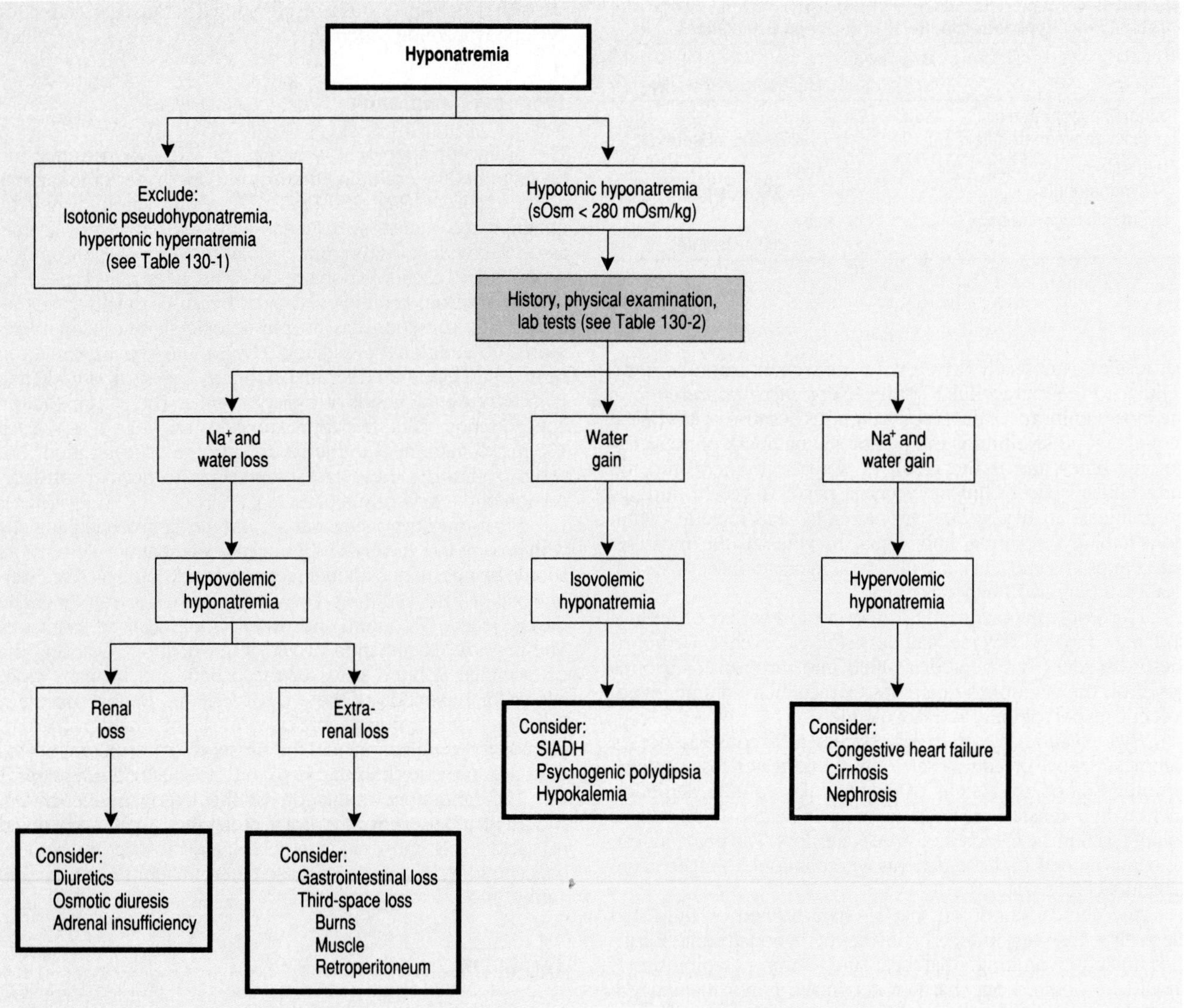

Figure 130-1 Algorithm for the diagnostic evaluation of hyponatremia. SIADH = syndrome of inappropriate antidiuretic hormone secretion.

Hypernatremia

Hypernatremia is defined as a hypertonic syndrome associated with elevation of the serum sodium concentration to 145 mEq/L or higher. An increase in the ratio of solute (Na^+) to water in body fluids and an elevation in the serum osmolarity (>300 mOsm/kg) are common to all hypernatremic disorders. An inability to ingest sufficient free water to preserve normal body fluid osmolarity is a universal finding in all these disorders; it may be the result of an inability to communicate thirst, lack of access to water, or even altered thirst drive. Despite the often marked increase in serum sodium concentration, however, the *total* body sodium content may be reduced, normal, or increased depending on the cause of the hypernatremic condition.

The pathologic hallmark of the hypernatremic disorders is cell shrinkage. Clinically, this is manifested by central nervous system signs such as confusion, lethargy, seizures, or coma. The

Table 130-2 Laboratory Evaluation of Hypotonic Hyponatremia

	Urine Na^+ (mEq/L)	Urine osmolarity (mOsm/kg)	BUN (mg/dl)	Uric acid (mg/dl)
Hypovolemic hyponatremia (nonrenal)	<20*	>300	High	Normal to high
Hypovolemic hyponatremia (renal origin)	>20	Usually equal to serum osmolarity	High	Normal to high
Isovolemic hyponatremia (SIADH)	>20, usually >40	>Serum osmolarity†	Normal to low	Low
Hypervolemic hypernatremia	<20, often <10*	>Serum osmolarity	Normal to high	Normal to high

Abbreviations: BUN = blood urea nitrogen, SIADH = syndrome of inappropriate antidiuretic hormone secretion.

* Diuretics may cause a urine Na^+ level >20 mEq/L.

† In SIADH, depending upon the severity of the defect, urine osmolarity may be less than, equal to, or greater than the osmolarity of serum. The urine osmolarity is *always* inappropriately high for the degree of hypotonicity of the serum, i.e., higher than that of maximally dilute urine (60–80 mOsm/kg H_2O).

clinical presentation in hypernatremic patients depends on the severity of the hypertonic state and the rapidity of its development. Chronic hypernatremic states can be relatively asymptomatic as compensatory mechanisms restore brain cell volume toward normal.

Hypernatremic states can be classified into three categories based on the volume status of the patient. *Hypovolemic hypernatremia,* the most common, results from combined losses of sodium and water. Renal, mucocutaneous, or gastrointestinal losses of hypotonic fluid generate the disorder, and an inability to ingest adequate amounts of free water perpetuates the problem. Renal loss of volume most commonly results from an osmotic diuresis associated with hyperglycemia, as occurs in hyperglycemic, nonketotic coma. An elevated urine sodium level and isotonic urine are typical. Conversely, extrarenal losses of volume result in a low urine sodium level and an increased urine osmolarity, reflecting the kidney's tendency to conserve water and sodium appropriately.

Isovolemic hypernatremia occurs in the setting of pure free-water loss from either a mucocutaneous or a renal source. The most common cause of this type of hypernatremia is nephrogenic or central diabetes insipidus, which leads to a significant free-water diuresis. An inability to ingest an adequate amount of free water to preserve normal body fluid osmolarity is common to these conditions. These individuals usually lack signs of intravascular volume depletion because free-water loss occurs mainly at the expense of the intracellular space. Vascular volume is preserved until the deficit of free water becomes severe. The urine osmolarity in these cases is usually low (<200 mOsm/kg). Extrarenal losses of free water from skin or lung occur in hypercatabolic, febrile states and can cause similar degrees of hypernatremia. Affected individuals have an elevated urine osmolarity (>300 mOsm/kg) that reflects the kidney's conservation of water.

Table 130-3 Laboratory Evaluation of Hypernatremic Disorders

	Urine Na^+ (mEq/L)	Urine osmolarity (mOsm/kg)
Hypovolemic hypernatremia (nonrenal loss)	<20	Concentrated, >300 mOsm/kg
Hypovolemic hypernatremia (renal loss)	>20	Concentration equals or exceeds that of serum. Glycosuria may be present.
Isovolemic hypernatremia (renal loss)	<20	Dilute, usually <150 mOsm/kg
Isovolemic hypernatremia (nonrenal loss)	<20	Concentrated > 300 mOsm/kg
Hypervolemic hypernatremia	>20	Concentrated relative to serum osmolarity

Hypervolemic hypernatremia is almost exclusively an iatrogenic disorder that occurs in ill, hospitalized patients. The disorder is characterized by pure solute (Na^+) gain due to excessive infusion of hypertonic saline or sodium bicarbonate. Salt poisoning has also occurred in individuals receiving enteric tube feedings. The urine sodium level is typically elevated, and the urine is concentrated.

Diagnostic Approach

The hypernatremic patient may be unable to provide an accurate history owing to alterations in mental status. Information regarding thirst, ingestion of food and water, urinary output, medications (specifically diuretics and laxatives), and known diseases

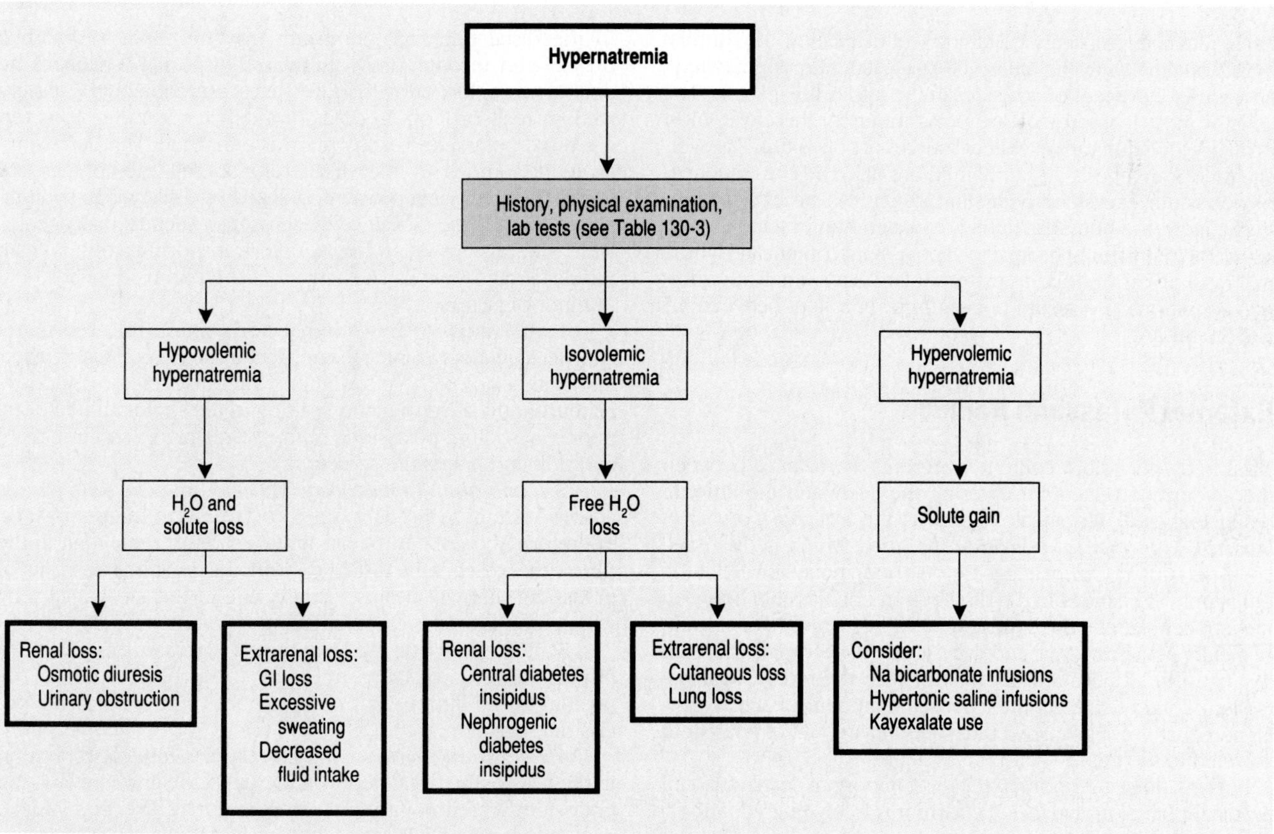

Figure 130-2 Algorithm for the diagnostic evaluation of hypernatremia. GI = gastrointestinal.

such as diabetes mellitus or diabetes insipidus may need to be obtained from a third party. The physical examination, which should emphasize vital signs, mucosal moisture, and skin turgor, allows for an assessment of fluid volume status. Neurologic function must also be carefully appraised.

The laboratory determinations that are helpful in the hypernatremic patient include serum osmolarity, electrolytes, creatinine, urea nitrogen level, urine sodium level, and urine osmolarity. These tests assess the severity of the hypertonic syndrome and allow for easy differential diagnosis of the underlying cause of the hypernatremia (Table 130-3).

Prompt and appropriate treatment of the hypernatremic patient is critical, particularly when the serum osmolarity exceeds 340 mOsm/kg. An assessment of the free-water deficit is often helpful as a guide to therapy. The hypovolemic patient with hypernatremia typically has significant intravascular volume depletion and is best managed with infusion of isotonic saline (0.9 percent) until volume is restored. Hypotonic fluids can then be administered to replete the free-water deficit. The serum sodium concentration should fall no faster than 1 mEq/L per hour, particularly in cases of hypernatremia present for several days or weeks. Rapid correction of the serum sodium can lead to life-threatening cerebral edema. Individuals with pure free-water losses should be treated with hypotonic fluids. Individuals with central diabetes insipidus benefit from replacement therapy with vasopressin analogues. Salt-poisoned individuals can be treated with hypotonic fluids and loop diuretics. Refractory cases may require emergent dialysis, particularly when associated with renal failure.

An algorithm for the diagnostic approach to the patient with hypernatremia is presented in Figure 130-2.

References

Andreoli TE. Disturbances of fluid volume, electrolyte, and acid-base balance. In: Wyngaarden JB, Smith LH, eds. Cecil textbook of medicine. 18th ed. Philadelphia: WB Saunders, 1988:528.

Arieff AI. Osmotic failure: Physiology and strategies for treatment. Hosp Pract 1988; 23:173.

Narins RG. Therapy of hyponatremia: Does haste make waste? N Engl J Med 1986; 314:1573.

Snyder NA, Feigal DW, Arieff AI. Hypernatremia in elderly patients: A heterogenous, morbid, iatrogenic entity. Ann Intern Med 1987; 107:309.

131 Disorders of Serum Potassium

Catherine S. Thompson, MD

David M. Clive, MD

Potassium is the most abundant intracellular cation. The human body contains approximately 3,000 to 4,000 mEq of potassium, and all but 2 percent of it resides in the intracellular space. The cells of most living things are potassium-rich; therefore, most ordinary foodstuffs are excellent sources of potassium. The average American ingests 70 to 100 mEq per day. The consequences of potassium excess or potassium deficit can be catastrophic. Fortunately, the body has tightly regulated homeostatic mechanisms for maintaining normal total potassium content and a normal ratio of intracellular to extracellular potassium. Under normal conditions, the serum potassium level is kept between 3.5 and 5.0 mEq/L.

External Potassium Balance

Total body potassium content represents the balance between the amount of potassium entering the body and the amount being excreted. We speak of this as the *external potassium balance*. The *internal potassium balance,* which is discussed later, pertains not to changes in total body potassium content, but simply to changes in the distribution of potassium between the intracellular and the extracellular space. Of the 70 or so mEq of dietary potassium ingested daily, about 80 percent is excreted through the kidneys and the rest of it in the feces. Stool potassium content reflects the minuscule amount of dietary potassium that is not absorbed plus a certain amount of potassium secreted in the gut.

The kidney, therefore, is the most important determinant of external potassium balance. Potassium is freely filtered, and 90 percent of it is reabsorbed before the distal nephron (i.e., the cells of the late distal tubule and early cortical collecting duct). In the distal nephron, potassium may be either reabsorbed or secreted through active tubular transport mechanisms. In potassium-replete or overloaded states, secretion outweighs potassium reabsorption. In potassium-deficiency states, however, net distal potassium reabsorption is enhanced. The potassium-secreting pumps in the distal tubular cell membranes are powered by ATP in a process catalyzed by the enzyme sodium-potassium ATPase. Some of these pumps secrete hydrogen as well as potassium ions while countertransporting sodium from tubular lumen to cell. The activity of the pumps depends on a number of factors:

1. *Aldosterone.* This adrenal hormone is released in response to extracellular volume depletion or potassium overload. Either one of these conditions will cause release of aldosterone from the adrenal gland, leading to the stimulation of distal nephron sodium-potassium pumps, enhancing sodium reabsorption and potassium secretion.

2. *Luminal sodium delivery.* The sodium-potassium pumps absorb sodium as fast as it can be delivered to the pump sites. Therefore, the greater the amount of sodium remaining in the filtrate that reaches the distal nephron, the greater the amount of potassium that will be lost. This is one of the mechanisms by which loop diuretics cause potassium wasting.

3. *Urine flow rate.* By definition, the greater the volume of filtrate delivered distally, the lower the concentration of potassium in the filtrate. This enhances the gradient favoring potassium secretion.

4. *Potassium overload.* Increased potassium concentration in the cells of the distal nephron increases the gradient favoring potassium secretion into the lumen, and may directly stimulate sodium-potassium ATPase activity in these cells.

5. *Alkalosis.* Alkalosis causes potassium to shift from the

extracellular space into the intracellular space, which enhances the gradient for potassium excretion.

Nontubular factors influence the rate at which filtered potassium will be excreted. Important among these is the presence in the urine of nonreabsorbable anions. These are negatively charged molecules (e.g., bicarbonate, penicillin) that cannot be reabsorbed from the nephron and therefore obligate the concomitant loss of a cation in order to preserve electroneutrality.

Internal Potassium Balance

As mentioned earlier, there is a tremendous disparity between the large amount of potassium present inside the cell and the relatively scanty amount in the extracellular fluid. In the equilibrium state, one would expect that this large gradient would be obliterated by passive diffusion of potassium out of the cells. The fact that this does not happen is attributable to the existence in cell membranes of sodium-potassium countertransporting pumps. These extrude three sodium ions from the cell for each two potassium ions transported into the cell. The extent to which nonkidney cells are under the influence of aldosterone is a matter of some debate.

The following physiologic influences affect the distribution of potassium between cells and extracellular fluid:

1. *Plasma pH.* Acid-base disturbances, particularly metabolic disturbance, have a significant effect on the serum potassium concentration. In metabolic acidosis, for example, excess hydrogen ions from the plasma enter the cells to be buffered by intracellular proteins; this process leads to a shift of potassium into the external extracellular space. In metabolic acidosis, the serum potassium level may rise 0.5 mEq/L for every 0.1 drop in the serum pH. The reverse is true in metabolic alkalosis.

2. *Beta-adrenergic hormones.* These hormones favor movement of potassium into cells through mechanisms that are poorly understood but probably involve stimulation of sodium-potassium ATPase. Beta-adrenergic blockers (e.g., propranolol) blunt this effect.

3. *Alpha-adrenergic hormones.* These hormones exert the opposite effect of beta-adrenergic hormones; i.e., they mitigate cellular uptake of potassium.

4. *Hyperosmolar states.* Sudden increases in plasma osmolarity, e.g., hyperglycemia, pull water from the intracellular space into the extracellular space, and potassium follows via a "solvent drag" effect.

5. *Insulin.* Insulin renders cell membranes more permeable to potassium, leading to enhanced uptake. The insulin deficiency of diabetes, plus the hyperglycemic osmotic effect mentioned previously, enhance the predisposition of the diabetic patient to hyperkalemia.

6. *Cell membrane defects.* In disorders that render the cell membrane abnormally permeable to potassium, e.g., the so-called kalemic paralyses, spontaneous hyperkalemia and hypokalemia may arise. Similarly, trauma or toxicity to cells may lead to leakage of potassium into the extracellular space.

The external potassium balance exerts its effects on the serum potassium level over a long time (days to weeks). The internal arm, however, is critical in buffering the body against minute-to-minute swings in the serum potassium level. Its effectiveness is evidenced by the rapidity with which a 50-mEq potassium load, absorbed quickly from the gut after a large meal, is translocated into the cellular compartment.

Because such a small percentage of total body potassium resides in the serum, and because various factors can alter this percentage, the serum potassium concentration is not always an accurate indicator of body potassium balance and must be interpreted with caution. Small decrements in the serum potassium concentration often reflect a major deficit of total body potassium. Conversely, redistribution of a minute fraction of intracellular potassium into the extracellular space may cause a significant rise in the serum potassium level without a major change in body potassium content.

Hypokalemia

Etiology

The causes of hypokalemia are listed in Table 131-1. Hypokalemia usually arises through some disorder in the external potassium balance. Dietary deficiency of potassium is uncommon in American society. Generally, it is seen only in chronically ill and malnourished people or in alcoholics.

Any state characterized by metabolic alkalosis leads to enhanced potassium excretion through the mechanisms cited earlier. In addition, metabolic alkalosis lowers serum potassium through the internal balance mechanism by promoting potassium uptake into cells.

Hypokalemia is not uncommon among medical patients being treated with diuretics. The potassium losses are attributable to the increased distal delivery of sodium, which occurs as a result of the renal tubular actions of the diuretic. The metabolic "contraction" alkalosis, which these medications engender, also contributes to potassium wasting.

Disorders characterized by glucocorticoid or mineralocorticoid excess, e.g., Cushing's syndrome, Conn's syndrome, and Bartter's syndrome, are also causes of potassium loss. In these cases, kaliuresis is driven by the mineralocorticoid effects of the hormones on the tubular cells and by the metabolic alkalosis that occurs in these physiologic states.

The major effects of hypokalemia are on electrically excitable cells, particularly skeletal and cardiac muscle cells. Muscle weakness is common in severe hypokalemia, and rhabdomyolysis may actually occur. Marked hypokalemia produces characteristic electrocardiographic changes. Cardiac arrhythmias are the most dangerous complication of hypokalemia. Hypokalemia has effects on the kidney itself. In potassium-deficient states, the kidneys lose the ability to concentrate urine, leading to polyuria (i.e., nephrogenic diabetes insipidus).

Diagnostic Approach

The patient with hypokalemia should be questioned about dietary ingestion of potassium and the use of medications, includ-

Table 131-1 Causes of Hypokalemia

Reduced potassium intake
Renal losses
Tubular defects (renal tubular acidosis)
Metabolic alkalosis
Diuretics
Mineralocorticoid excess
Edematous disorders
Bartter's syndrome
Magnesium deficiency
Filtered, nonreabsorbable anions
Leukemia
Extrarenal losses
Vomiting, nasogastric suction
Losses from large intestine
Biliary drainage
Profuse sweating

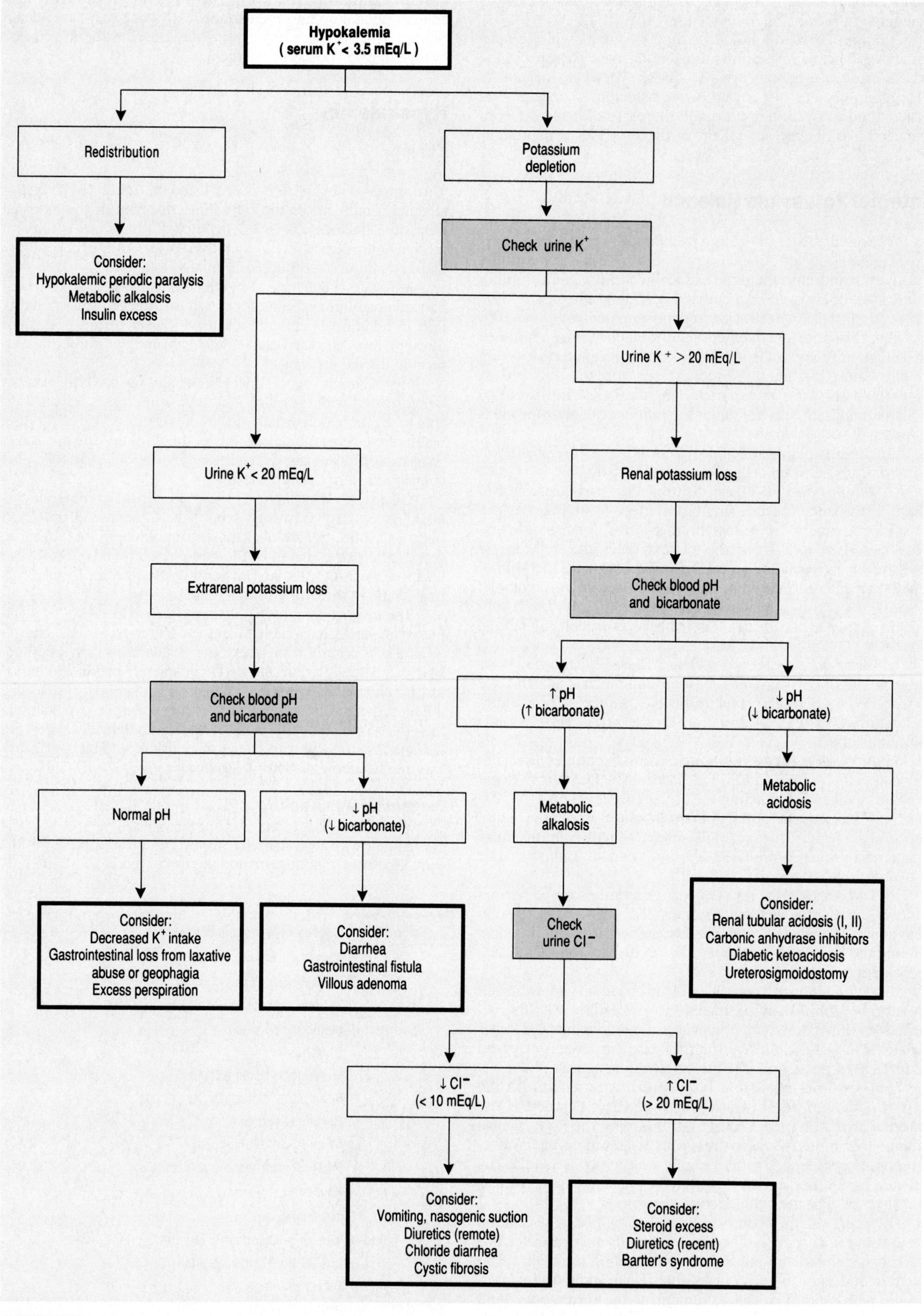

Figure 131-1 Algorithm for the diagnostic evaluation of the patient with hypokalemia.

ing diuretics or laxatives, that can cause potassium depletion. Symptoms such as vomiting or diarrhea or a family history of hypokalemia are additional important features. The physical examination provides clues if the patient has signs of volume depletion (hypotension or tachycardia) or if it detects the presence of gastrointestinal fistulae, a nasogastric drainage tube, or ureterosigmoidostomy.

The initial laboratory assessment of the hypokalemic patient includes an electrolyte profile, blood pH, and urine electrolytes (urine sodium, potassium, chloride). Serum aldosterone and renin levels are occasionally helpful. An algorithm for the approach to the hypokalemic patient, shown in Figure 131-1, divides the disorders on the basis of urine potassium, blood pH, and urine chloride.

Treatment

Adequate treatment of hypokalemia caused by true body potassium depletion requires identification of the underlying cause of the disorder and then specific interventions to replete potassium stores (Table 131-2). Volume depletion should be corrected in hypokalemic individuals with excessive gastrointestinal fluid losses, and medications that aggravate hypokalemia, specifically diuretics, should be discontinued. In most cases, potassium repletion can be accomplished with oral potassium supplements. In patients with severe hypokalemia (potassium < 2.5 mEq/L) or in patients with cardiac arrhythmias referable to hypokalemia, intravenous repletion is indicated. In these cases, potassium salts should be administered no faster than 10 to 20 mEq per hour, paying close attention to cardiac rhythm and serum potassium concentration.

Hyperkalemia

The causes of hyperkalemia are outlined in Table 131-3. Eating a potassium-rich diet is unlikely to provoke hyperkalemia because of the extraordinary capacity of the kidney to dispose of excess potassium. However, the combination of renal insufficiency plus a normal or high potassium intake may lead to hyperkalemia; this is a constant concern in patients with kidney diseases. Diets must be modified accordingly. Other disorders of external potassium balance leading to hyperkalemia include glucocorticoid and mineralocorticoid deficiency (i.e., Addison's disease and hypoaldosteronism). The pathophysiology of these disorders is the exact reverse of that mentioned in connection with the hormone excess states.

Hyperkalemia arises not infrequently as a result of perturbations in the internal mechanism of potassium balance. Metabolic acidosis, as mentioned previously, can provoke hyperkalemia through transcellular shifting of potassium stores. Tissue necrosis or toxic injury to cells can also cause leakage of potassium into the extracellular space. As already mentioned, deficiency with or without hyperglycemia can lead to impaired cellular potassium uptake.

Hyperkalemia is potentially the most rapidly lethal of all electrolyte disturbances. The normal function of electrically excitable cells depends on maintaining the critical difference between the resting membrane potential and the threshold potential for "firing." The resting potential is determined mainly by the potassium potential difference across the cell membrane (i.e., the Nernst potential):

$$V_k = -61.5 \log \frac{[Ki]}{[Ko]}$$

where V_k = potassium potential, [Ko] = extracellular potassium concentration, and [Ki] = intracellular potassium concentration. One can appreciate that a given change in the extracellular potassium concentration has a tremendous impact on this potential difference. Electrocardiographic changes may be seen when the potassium concentration in the plasma rises to 6 mEq/L or higher (see Fig. 131-2). With further increases in serum potassium concentrations, cellular irritability and eventually lethal arrhythmias will develop.

Diagnostic Approach

The patient with hyperkalemia should be questioned closely about dietary intake of potassium, including the use of salt substitutes (KCl). A number of drugs, including potassium-sparing diuretics, beta-adrenergic blockers, nonsteroidal anti-inflammatory agents, and angiotensin-converting enzyme inhibitors, can aggravate a hyperkalemic tendency in certain patients. A history of prior renal disease or recent reduction in urinary output is also important.

The laboratory assessment of the hyperkalemic patient should include serum electrolytes, creatinine, blood urea nitrogen, and determination of acid-base status. Additional tests such as aldosterone and renin levels may provide information regarding renal tubular disorders that lead to hyperkalemia. "Spurious" hyperkalemia can be excluded by obtaining a plasma potassium level, which will be normal if the hyperkalemia is the result of cell lysis after the blood specimen is obtained. An algorithm outlining an approach to the patient with hyperkalemia is presented in Figure 131-2.

Treatment

The treatment of hyperkalemia exploits both the internal and external pathways of potassium disposition (Table 131-4). Internal mechanisms are the fastest acting; i.e., one can engender shifts of potassium into cells more quickly than one can remove potassium from the body. Thus, insulin and alkalinizing agents (sodium bicarbonate) are rapidly administered to patients with life-threatening degrees of hyperkalemia. Calcium salts may also be administered because these have a membrane-stabilizing effect, although they do not engender potassium movement in and of themselves. To reduce total body potassium stores, ion-

Table 131-2 Treatment of Hypokalemia

Acute
IV replacement (potassium chloride or potassium phosphate) ≤ 20 mEq/hr or 200 mEq/day
Chronic
Increased dietary supply (citrus fruits, etc.)
Oral solutions (potassium chloride, potassium citrate)
Oral tablets (avoid enteric-coated preparations)
Potassium-sparing agents (spironolactone, triamterene)

Table 131-3 Causes of Hyperkalemia

Increased Excretory Load
Dietary excess
Iatrogenic
Tissue breakdown
Reduced Excretory Ability
Acute and chronic renal failure
Mineralocorticoid insufficiency
Hyporeninemic hypoaldosteronism
Potassium-sparing diuretics
Renal tubular defects (acute interstitial nephritis, transplant kidney)
Transcellular Potassium Movement
(Metabolic) acidosis
Exercise
Endocrine abnormalities (diabetes mellitus)
Periodic paralyses
Drugs (succinylcholine, digitalis, etc.)
Osmolar load

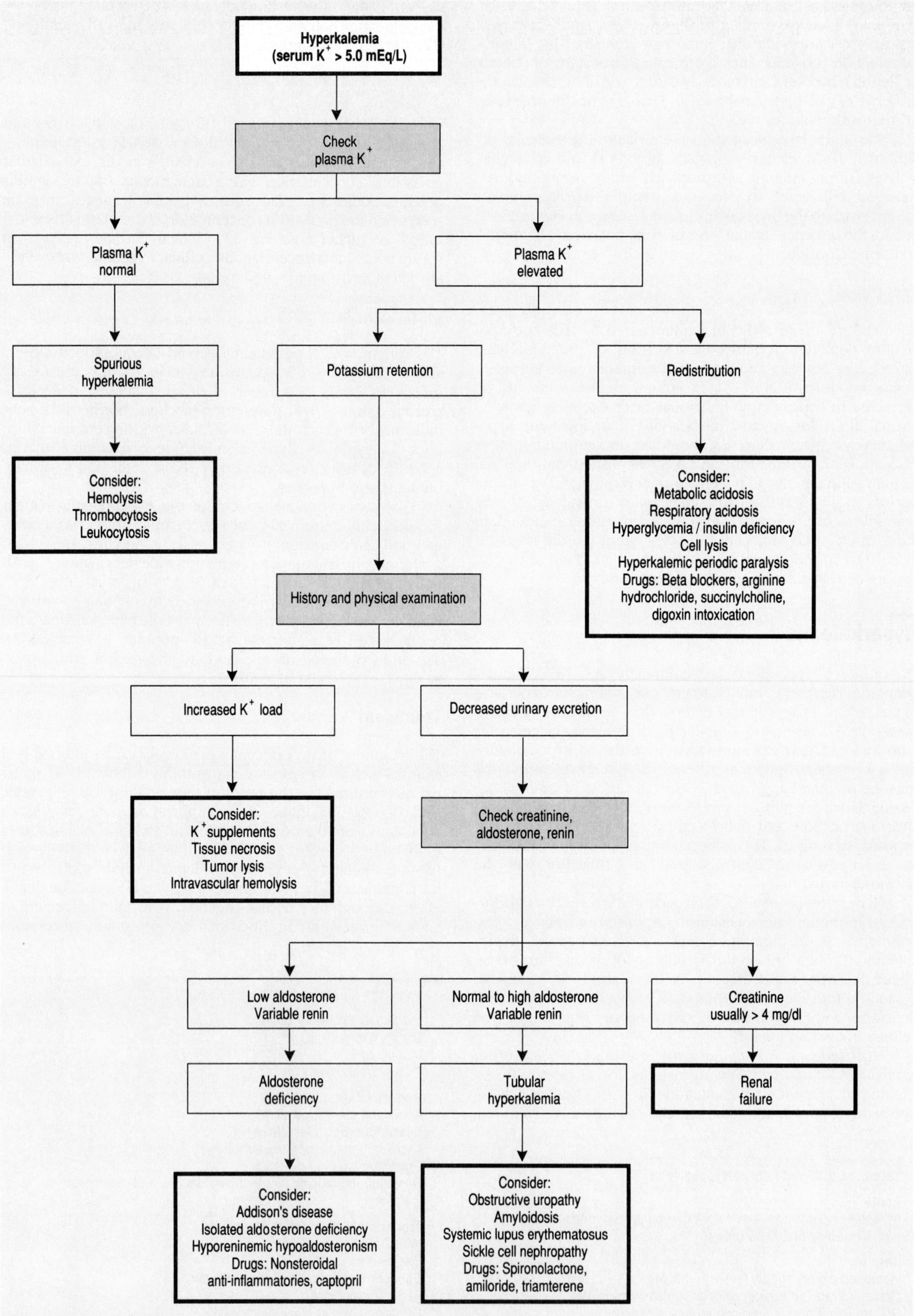

Figure 131-2 Algorithm for the diagnostic evaluation of the patient with hyperkalemia.

Table 131-4 Treatment of Hyperkalemia

Drug	Dose	Time of onset	Duration of action	Mechanism
Calcium gluconate	1 amp, 10% solution	1–5 min	30–120 min	Membrane stabilization
$NaHCO_3$	1–2 amp (bolus)	5–10 min	2 hr	Redistribution
Glucose/insulin	50 g dextrose, 10 units regular insulin	Rapid	Variable	Redistribution
Sodium polystyrene sulfonate resin (Kayexalate)	15–30 g orally or rectally	10–60 min	As long as continued	Increased excretion
Mineralocorticoid replacement	For specific indications	—	—	Increased excretion
Dialysis	For severe hyperkalemia	—	—	—

exchange resins like sodium polystyrene sulfate (e.g., Kayexalate) are introduced into the gastrointestinal tract. These absorb potassium from the gut and release, in exchange, a sodium molecule. For hyperkalemic patients with renal insufficiency, emergent dialysis may be required.

References

Brown RS. Extrarenal potassium homeostasis. Kidney Int 1986; 30:116.

Cox M, Sterns R, Singer I. The defense against hyperkalemia: The roles of insulin and aldosterone. N Engl J Med 1978; 299:525.

DeFronzo R. Hyperkalemia and hyporeninemic hypoaldosteronism. Kidney Int 1980; 17:118.

Gabow PA, Peterson LN. Disorders of potassium metabolism. In: Schrier RW, ed. Renal and electrolyte disorders. 3rd ed. Boston: Little, Brown, 1986:207.

Goldfarb S, et al. Acute hyperkalemia induced by hyperglycemia: Hormonal mechanisms. Ann Intern Med 1976; 84:426.

Rose BD. Clinical physiology of acid-base and electrolyte disorders. 3rd ed. New York: McGraw-Hill, 1989.

Stein JH. Hypokalemia: Common and uncommon causes. Hosp Pract 1988; 23:55.

Tannen RL. Potassium disorders. In: Kokko JP, Tannen RL, eds. Fluids and electrolytes. Philadelphia: WB Saunders, 1986.

Valtin H. Renal dysfunction: Mechanisms involved in fluid and solute imbalance. Boston: Little, Brown, 1979:89.

Adolescent Medicine, Geriatric Medicine, Behavioral Medicine

III

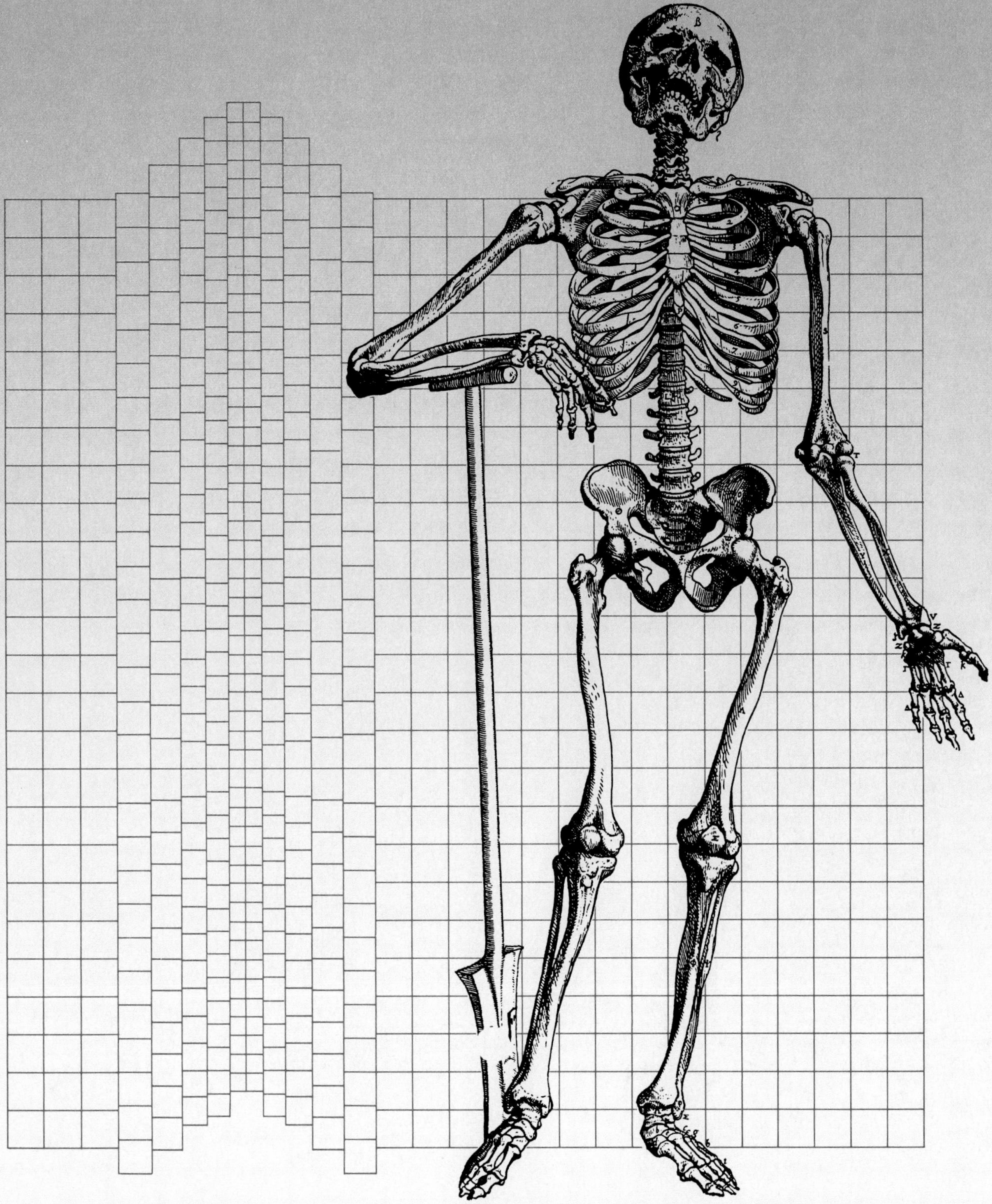

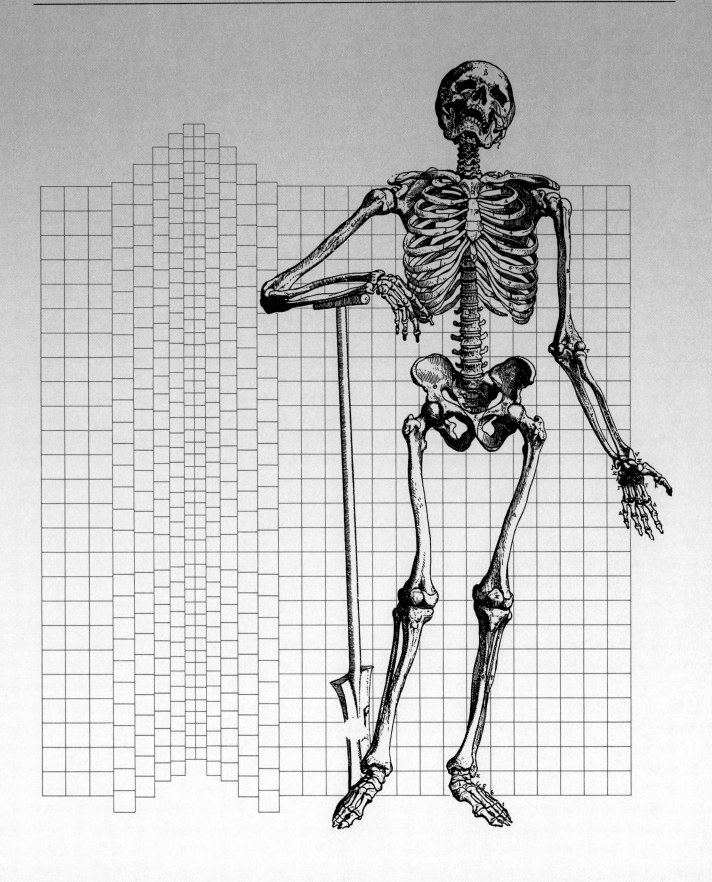

Adolescent Medicine

Sarah L. Stone, MD

132

Caring for adolescents is a challenge. Adolescents differ from adults in that neither physical nor psychological maturation has been completed. Because of their continually changing bodies and intellect as well as the nature of their medical problems, adolescents are unique. Physicians caring for adolescents need to be competent in the art of the medical interview. They must be aware of the physical, intellectual, and social issues of adolescence. Finally, they need to be familiar with the health-maintenance issues that are unique to the adolescent population.

Interviewing the Adolescent

Certain skills are essential in conducting the medical interview with adolescents. At the beginning of the interview, it is important to survey the problems so that the adolescent will be able to talk about *all* the issues he or she wants to address. Adolescents often have psychosocial issues they want to discuss, and they will be reluctant to talk about them immediately; therefore, after the adolescent describes his or her reason for coming, simply ask, "Is there anything else?" Continue asking this until the adolescent says that there is nothing more he or she wants to discuss. Learn to tolerate periods of silence during the normal interview and give the adolescent adequate time to formulate an answer after a question is asked.

Be aware of body language and the image you project. A nonjudgmental and supportive attitude is vital. It is important not to be too authoritarian; however, it is also important not to project yourself solely as a friend. In a relationship with a physician, adolescents need more than friendship; they need an adult whom they respect and from whom they can seek advice. Finally, it is important to be flexible. If an adolescent is not interested early in the interview in elaborating on the history of the present illness or his or her social history, go on to the review of systems or physical examination; often the adolescent will "open up" and provide information later in the interview.

Working with Patients and Parents

Adolescent health care involves a relationship among three people: the adolescent, the practitioner, and the parent or guardian. As in pediatrics, the parent needs to be involved. Frequently, the parent is genuinely concerned, and with difficult problems such as substance abuse or eating disorders, a supportive family is often essential in getting an adolescent through treatment. However, adolescents have a right to confidential health care. A practitioner can care for adolescents effectively only if they can be assured that they can talk about difficult problems such as sexuality and substance abuse with confidentiality.

Practitioners need to communicate with both the parents and the adolescent sometime during the medical interview. It is most helpful to meet with the adolescent and the parents initially. At that time the rules regarding confidentiality should be made clear to both patient and parents. The adolescent should then be interviewed and examined without the parents present. During the interview, again stress the issue of confidentiality. After the physical examination, you can meet with both the adolescent and the parents to review any recommendations that the adolescent agrees can be discussed with the parents present.

Legal Issues

In general, minors need parental consent to obtain health care. The age of majority in most states is 18 years. Emancipated minors, generally defined as minors who are in the armed services, who have married, or who are completely financially independent and living away from home, do not require parental consent. Many states make specific exceptions and grant confidential treatment without parental consent for problems such as drug abuse, sexually transmitted diseases, or contraception. Most states honor the court decision in the Supreme Court vs. Planned Parenthood of Central Missouri, which upheld an adolescent's right to an abortion; however, some states may require that the court decide whether a minor is mature enough to make that decision.

Health Maintenance

Growth and Development

Adolescence is a time of tremendous growth and development. Weight gain during puberty accounts for 50 percent of adult body weight, and height gain during this time accounts for 15 percent of adult height. In addition, the development of secondary sexual characteristics is a major change that occurs during puberty. Adolescents frequently have questions about when they will start growing, when they will stop growing, and whether or not their individual sexual development is normal. To answer these questions and assess abnormal development, the physician must be familiar with sexual maturity ratings and the normal ranges of physical growth among adolescents. Height, weight, and sexual maturity ratings should be recorded annually in adolescents.

Physical Growth

During adolescence there is a rapid acceleration in the rate of growth, followed by a deceleration in the rate, the adolescent growth spurt. The adolescent growth spurt occurs, on average, over a 24- to 36-month period. Within this growth spurt, there is a period when the rate of growth is at a maximum. This maximum rate within the growth spurt is termed the *peak height velocity*. During this year of peak height velocity, a boy will grow 7 to 12 cm in height and a girl will gain 6 to 11 cm in height. The peak height velocity occurs, on average, 2 years earlier in girls; the age at the time of peak height velocity is approximately 12 years in girls and 14 years in boys. The peak height velocity can also be correlated with the sexual maturity rating (SMR). The time of most rapid growth generally occurs earlier in sexual development for girls (SMR-2) than it does for boys (SMR-4).

There is a seasonal variation in the height spurt, with maximal increase in height during the spring and summer. Therefore, growth velocities should be evaluated over a 6- to 12-month period. Weight gain during adolescence peaks during the growth spurt.

Sexual Maturity

Physicians need to be familiar with the SMRs for adolescents. These can be used to predict onset of menarche and ejaculation, to identify abnormal changes in puberty, and to assure the adolescent that he or she is normal. SMRs are descriptive ratings developed by Tanner, based on breast and pubic hair development in girls and on pubic hair and development of the genitalia in boys (Fig. 132-1 to 132-3). Onset of menarche generally occurs at SMR-4 (mean age 12.5 years) and ejaculation generally begins in young men at SMR-3.

Immunizations

Immunizations are an essential part of adolescent health care. Immunization status should be part of the problem list on the initial visit with the adolescent, and a primary series should be given if there is no proof of immunization. Not all states require immunizations for school attendance; therefore, a significant number of adolescents are at risk for communicable diseases. Rubella occurs commonly in adolescents, and the peak incidence of mumps has shifted from children aged 5 to 9 years to the adolescent age group. Mumps infection can result in severe orchitis in adolescent boys.

Tetanus

A primary series should be given in unimmunized adolescents. This consists of two doses of diphtheria-tetanus at least 1 month apart, followed by a booster 8 to 12 months later. Diphtheria-tetanus boosters are recommended routinely every 10 years; thus, the first booster generally is given at age 14 to 16. Diphtheria booster should be given at the time routine tetanus boosters are given; however, pertussis vaccination is not recommended after the age of 7 because of the incidence of serious side effects with immunization. Tetanus booster should also be given if the patient sustains a dirty wound and has not received a booster in the previous 5 years.

Polio

If unimmunized, adolescents should receive two doses of trivalent oral polio live vaccine 6 weeks apart, followed by a booster in 8 months. Oral polio vaccine is not recommended for persons over the age of 20; these people should receive inactivated vaccine.

Measles

Primary measles immunization consists of a single dose of live-attenuated vaccine. Some groups are now recommending a booster at age 6 or age 12. Individuals vaccinated before 1968 should be revaccinated because they may have been vaccinated with an inactivated vaccine. This vaccine can be given once as the measles-mumps-rubella (MMR) vaccine.

Mumps

Primary immunization with mumps vaccine should be given to susceptible individuals, which include the following groups: (1) individuals who have not had physician-diagnosed mumps; (2) individuals without documentation of vaccination after 12 months of age; and (3) individuals without laboratory evidence of immunity. Immunization can be given alone or as the MMR vaccine.

Rubella

Primary immunization should be given if there is no documentation of vaccination after the age of 12 months or no laboratory evidence of positive serology. If an adolescent is *pregnant,* this is an *absolute contraindication to giving the vaccine,* and young women should be advised to avoid pregnancy for 3 months after vaccination.

Counseling on Health-Maintenance Issues

Preventive screening for the common medical problems of adolescence is essential. Health maintenance in the adolescent is not simply obtaining an immunization history and assessing the rate of development. Practitioners need to be aware of the common causes of morbidity and mortality in adolescents and address these issues during the visit. The three most common causes of death in adolescence are accidents, homicide, and suicide. Many of these deaths are drug- or alcohol-related. The question of drug use, risk of suicide or accidents, and issues regarding sexuality need to be addressed with adolescents on a yearly basis.

Sexual History

Teenage sexuality constitutes a tremendous problem in the United States. The pregnancy rate for teenagers in the United States is the highest in the developed world. Approximately 1 million teenaged girls get pregnant every year. Besides the medical problems, there are tremendous economic implications to teenage sexuality. Adolescent mothers are more likely to require state and federal aid and are also much less likely to finish high school than those who delay child bearing. Teenagers often wish

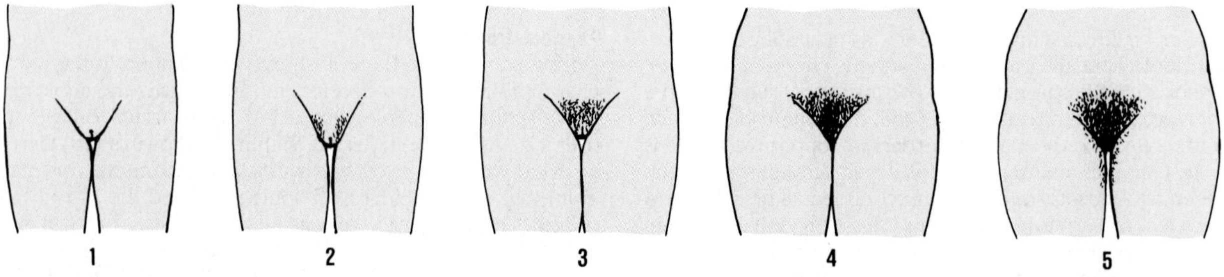

Figure 132-1 Female pubic hair development. Sexual maturity is indicated by numbers 1 through 5: (**1**) prepubertal; no pubic hair; (**2**) straight hair extends along the labia and, between ratings 2 and 3, begins on the pubis; (**3**) pubic hair has increased in quantity, is darker, and is present in the typical female triangle but in smaller quantity than in the adult; (**4**) Pubic hair is more dense, curled, and adult in distribution but less abundant than in an adult; (**5**) abundant, adult-type pattern; hair may extend on to the medial aspect of the thighs. (*From* Daniel WA Jr, Paulschock BZ. A physician's guide to sexual maturity. Darien, CT: Patient Care Publications, 1979; with permission.)

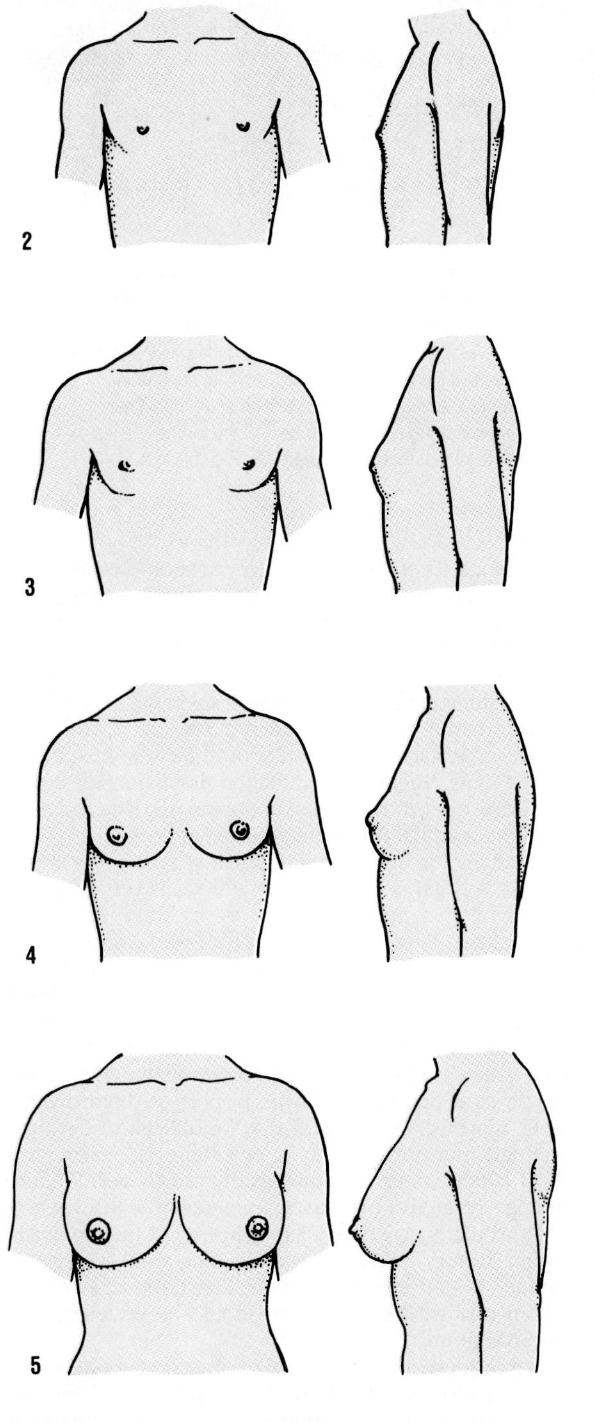

Figure 132-2 Female breast development. Sexual maturity is indicated by numbers 1 through 5: (**1,** not shown) prepubertal; elevations of papilla only; (**2**) breast buds appear; areola is slightly widened and projects as a small mound; (**3**) enlargement of the entire breast with no protrusion of the papilla or of the nipple; (**4**) enlargement of the breast and projection of areola and papilla as a secondary mound; (**5**) adult configuration of the breast with protrusion of the nipple; areola no longer projects separately from remainder of breast. (*From* Daniel WA Jr, Paulschock BZ. A physician's guide to sexual maturity. Darien, CT: Patient Care Publications, 1979; with permission.)

to talk with their physicians about these problems, but in fact the issues are rarely discussed.

The problems of adolescent sexuality underscore the necessity of interviewing the adolescent alone and assuring confidentiality. Young people should be asked if they have ever had sexual intercourse or are engaged in heavy petting that might lead to pregnancy or a sexually transmitted disease. Asking teenagers if they are "sexually active" is often misleading. Teenagers may presume this to imply that they are promiscuous or presume the question to mean only whether they have had sex in the previous week. It is very important, therefore, to be direct and explicit. Adolescents who are not sexually active should be supported for their decision. All adolescents, regardless of their sexual activity, should be counseled about the importance of birth control and preventing sexually transmitted diseases.

Sexually active teenagers should be encouraged to use condoms to protect against sexually transmitted diseases, even if they are using another method of birth control. Female adolescents require a yearly pelvic examination if they are sexually active or have symptoms of abdominal pain or vaginal discharge, or if they request it.

Depression

Suicide is one of the leading causes of death among adolescents. The overall incidence among adolescents has increased by over 200 percent in the last three decades. It has been estimated that for every completed suicide among adolescents, there have been 50 to 200 attempts.

Most adolescents who attempt suicide have been seen by a primary care physician in the 3 months prior to the suicide. The high prevalence of these behaviors and the fact that adolescents at risk are frequent users of the medical system place primary care physicians in a pivotal role in prevention of this devastating problem.

Eliciting a history of depression from the adolescent can be a challenge. Adolescents are often less able to articulate their feelings of depression. They are more impulsive, and this impulsive behavior can be further exacerbated if they are using drugs. Therefore, changes in an adolescent's behavior are very important in attempting to assess depression. Behaviors associated with adolescent depression are listed in Table 132-1. Drug abuse is an important concomitant of depression. Drugs may be used by the adolescent in an attempt to treat the depression, or conversely, drugs may precipitate the depression. If drug abuse is suspected, it is essential to think of depression also.

Behaviors that are manifested as changes in family relationships or changes in behavior at school must be assessed over time. A student who is receiving all C grades is performing adequately for an average student, but this can be a cause for concern if it represents a significant change in performance from the previous year. Adolescents with physical illnesses or disabilities also have a higher rate of suicide attempts; primary care physicians should therefore be especially vigilant with the chronically ill adolescent.

Nutritional History

During adolescence, young people gain 50 percent of their adult weight and 50 percent of their skeletal mass. Adolescents are particularly vulnerable to nutritional problems because of large energy needs during this time of rapid growth as well as their consumption of "fast foods." The incidence of obesity among adolescents is estimated at 20 percent, and a significant number of female adolescents have some symptoms of bulimia nervosa. Iron-deficiency anemia is also common among adolescents.

A brief nutritional assessment should be done on the initial visit. This can include a 24-hour diet recall of a typical day, asking the adolescent if he or she feels the diet is adequate and if he or she has particular concerns about the diet. Female adolescents

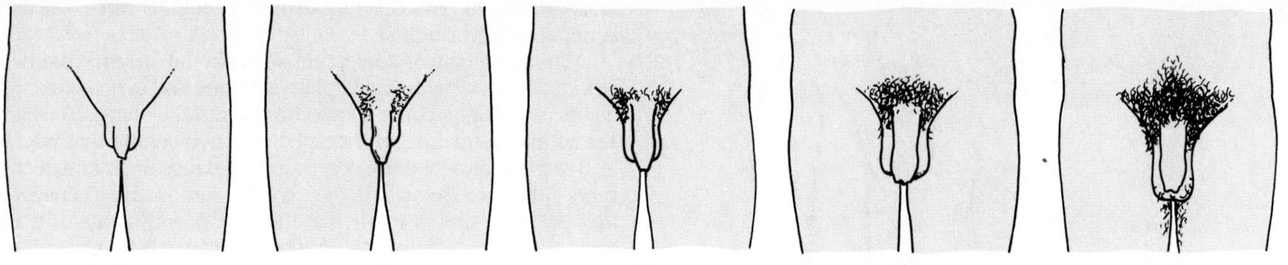

Figure 132-3 Male genital and pubic hair development. Sexual maturity is indicated by numbers 1 through 5 (note that ratings for pubic hair and for genital development can differ in a given boy at any given time, as pubic hair and genitalia do not necessarily develop at the same time): (**1**) prepubertal; no pubic hair, genitalia unchanged from childhood; (**2**) light, downy hair develops laterally and becomes dark, penis and testes may be slightly larger, and scrotum becomes more textured; (**3**) pubic hair has extended across the pubis, testes and scrotum are further enlarged, and penis is larger, especially in length; (**4**) more abundant pubic hair with curling, testes resemble those of an adult, penis has become larger, and scrotum is darker; (**5**) adult quantity and pattern of pubic hair, now present along the inner borders of the thighs; the testes and the scrotum are adult in size. (*From* Daniel WA Jr, Paulschock BZ. A physican's guide to sexual maturity. Darien, CT: Patient Care Publications, 1979; with permission.)

should be asked whether they are trying to lose weight and, if so, by what type of diet.

Drug Use

The prevalence of drug use among adolescents is astonishing. In a 1986 survey (Johnston et al, 1989), 58 percent of high school seniors reported illicit drug use at some time in their lives, and 4.8 percent of high school seniors reported using alcohol daily. No medical illness among this age group approaches this prevalence. It is therefore essential for physicians to elicit a thorough history of drug use in adolescent patients. Knowledge of drug use among family members or friends of the patient is particularly worrisome because exposure to people who use drugs makes adolescents more likely to use drugs. Other signs and symptoms that may indicate drug use in the adolescent include failing grades, increasing truancy in school, withdrawal from friends and family, and neglect of personal hygiene.

Table 132-1 Behaviors Associated with Adolescent Depression

Drug use
Withdrawal from family
Doing poorly in school
Loss of interest in personal hygiene
Loss of interest in friends and social life
Eating problems

Common Problems

Sports Physicals

Participation in sports is very important for many adolescents. With a greater number of sports being offered in high schools, the risk of injuries is increasing. Physicians are often asked to perform preparticipation sports physicals on adolescent athletes. The purpose of the preparticipation sports physical is to identify the adolescent who is at risk for injury and make recommendations to prevent those injuries. These recommendations may simply be advice on proper stretching prior to practice, or they may include recommending that an individual not participate in certain sports. Injuries to the musculoskeletal system are the most common, and cardiovascular complications are the most serious. Therefore, particular attention should be paid to these two systems during the preparticipation sports physical.

The medical history should include any history of previous injuries, any ongoing medical illness, history of allergies, use of medication, and any history of loss of consciousness or dizziness, palpitations, or fainting with exercise. In addition, ask about any family history of sudden death.

The physical examination should include height, weight, and vital signs. A general examination should include evaluation of the head, eyes, mouth, chest, abdomen, and skin and examination of the inguinal canal and genitalia in boys.

Examination of the cardiovascular system is very important. Although sudden death in young athletes is very rare, when it does occur it is most often due to structural cardiovascular abnormalities. Functional murmurs are very common and may occur in up to 25 percent of young athletes. Functional murmurs are always systolic and are usually grade 1 to 2 (on a scale of 6) in intensity. Diastolic murmurs should always be evaluated further.

The most common cardiovascular cause of sudden death in young athletes is hypertrophic cardiomyopathy. The most common physical finding with hypertrophic cardiomyopathy is a systolic murmur; therefore, it may be difficult to distinguish a pathologic murmur from an innocent one. However, the murmur of hypertrophic cardiomyopathy usually gets louder with standing or Valsalva maneuver. Adolescents with hypertrophic cardiomyopathy may have a family history of sudden death or a personal history of dizziness or fainting with exercise. If the examiner is concerned about the diagnosis of hypertrophic cardiomyopathy, the adolescent should be evaluated with an echocardiogram.

A thorough musculoskeletal examination is essential in the preparticipation sports physical. The purpose of the musculoskeletal exam is to (1) identify any previous injuries and assess them for further injury potential, (2) identify present injuries or abnormalities (sprains, Osgood-Schlatter disease), (3) identify any ligamentous laxity and assess for injury potential, and (4) evaluate overall level of physical conditioning. Recommendations for musculoskeletal evaluation are listed in Table 132-2.

Common Sexually Transmitted Diseases

In 1989, the Centers for Disease Control reported 204,023 cases of gonorrhea among teenagers aged 15 to 19. It is thought that this figure represents approximately 10 to 20 percent of the actual cases. Sexually transmitted diseases are an enormous problem. The majority of such diseases occur in adolescents and

Table 132-2 Orthopedic Screening Examination

Athletic activity (instructions)	Observation
Stand facing examiner	Acromioclavicular joints, general habitus
Look at ceiling, floor, over both shoulders; touch ears to shoulders	Cervical spine motion
Shrug shoulders (examiner resists)	Trapezius strength
Abduct shoulders 90 degrees (examiner resists at 90 degrees)	Deltoid strength
Full external rotation of arms	Shoulder motion
Flex and extend elbows	Elbow motion
Arms at sides, elbows flexed 90 degrees; pronate and supinate wrists	Elbow and wrist motion
Spread fingers, make fist	Hand or finger motion and deformities
Tighten (contract) quadriceps, relax quadriceps	Symmetry and knee effusion, ankle effusion
"Duck walk" four steps (away from examiner with buttocks on heels)	Hip, knee, and ankle motion
Back to examiner	Shoulder symmetry, scoliosis
Knees straight, touch toes	Scoliosis, hip motion, hamstring tightness
Raise up on toes, raise heels	Calf symmetry, leg strength

Reprinted with permission from *Sports Medicine: Health Care for Young Athletes.* Copyright © 1983 American Academy of Pediatrics.

young adults. In addition to the initial problem of the infection, long-term problems, including pelvic inflammatory disease, infertility, and acquired immunodeficiency syndrome (AIDS) infections, exist. Common sexually transmitted diseases in adolescents include *Chlamydia trachomatis, Neisseria gonorrhoeae,* and herpesvirus infections. Other less common sexually transmitted diseases are reviewed in detail elsewhere (Neinstein, 1984).

Gonorrheal cervicitis in young women may present with lower abdominal pain or purulent vaginal discharge, but most often it is asymptomatic. Young men may have dysuria or a purulent penile discharge, or they may be asymptomatic. Anorectal and pharyngeal infections also occur and may or may not be symptomatic. Examination of the cervix may be normal with gonorrheal infections; often, however, the cervix is inflamed and a mucopurulent cervical discharge exists. Endocervical discharge may reveal gram-negative diplococci. The presence of intracellular gram-negative diplococci in the endocervical discharge is highly suggestive of gonorrhea; such patients should be treated. Definitive diagnosis of gonorrhea is made by a positive culture on Thayer-Martin medium or its equivalent. Adnexal tenderness, fever, or pain on cervical motion suggests pelvic inflammatory disease, and in-patient treatment should be considered. Because of recent penicillin-resistant strains, current recommendations for the treatment of gonococcal cervicitis include the following: ceftriaxone, 125 to 250 mg intramuscularly once, or amoxicillin, 3 g orally once, plus probenicid, 1 g orally once. Many patients with gonorrhea have concomitant chlamydial infections; therefore, they should also be treated presumptively for chlamydia. Sexual contacts should be treated, and the patient should receive follow-up cultures to ensure effective treatment.

Infections caused by *Chlamydia trachomatis* are the most common sexually transmitted disease in adolescents. This disease has had a tremendous impact among female adolescents because of the resultant pelvic inflammatory disease and infertility. Young women with chlamydial cervicitis may have a purulent vaginal discharge but are often asymptomatic. Young men are usually symptomatic with dysuria or a penile discharge. Diagnosis is made by culture of the endocervix in women, or of the urethra in men. Tissue culture is considered the "gold standard" for diagnosis. This method has the greatest specificity of all diagnostic methods; the major disadvantages are the cost and complexity of the test. Antigen detection methods by fluorescence antibody and enzyme immunoassay are also available. Recommended treatment is doxycycline hyclate, 100 mg orally twice a day for 7 days, or erythromycin, 500 mg four times a day for 7 days. Because 10 to 20 percent of women with gonorrhea or chlamydia go on to develop pelvic inflammatory disease, sexually active female adolescents should be cultured for gonorrhea and chlamydia annually.

After an incubation period of 2 to 20 days, herpesvirus infection presents as single or multiple painful vesicles in the genital area. Several days after presentation, the vesicles rupture and leave a shallow ulcer that lasts approximately 2 weeks. The lesions are often quite painful, and the infection may be accompanied by systemic signs such as fever, malaise, and headache. Dysuria and urinary retention may also occur. After the initial infection, the virus remains in the sensory neurons of the involved area; therefore, the infection may recur. Symptoms of a recurrent infection are similar to the initial infection but less severe. Duration of symptoms is generally 5 to 7 days. Oral acyclovir, 200 mg five times daily for 5 days, given when symptoms appear, is effective in decreasing the duration of viral shedding and the duration of the lesions.

Infectious Mononucleosis

Mononucleosis, which is caused by the Epstein-Barr virus, is a common infection among adolescents. It is particularly common among middle-class people, as they are more likely to be protected from early exposure to the virus and thus do not develop immunity. Infection in younger children is likely to present as a flu-like illness and will not manifest the symptoms seen in adolescents and adults.

The incubation period for mononucleosis is 30 to 50 days. Following this, a prodrome occurs that includes symptoms of fatigue, malaise, and headache. Patients may then develop fever, adenopathy, and pharyngitis. Hepatomegaly and splenomegaly can also occur.

Diagnosis is made by assessing the clinical symptoms, the white blood cell count, the differential count, and the presence of heterophile antibodies. Adolescents with infectious mononucleosis usually have greater than 50 percent lymphocytosis on the white blood cell count, with atypical lymphocytes accounting for 10 to 20 percent of these cells. Heterophile antibody tests, the most common of which is the Monospot test, are also usually positive.

There is no specific treatment for the Epstein-Barr virus. Treatment of mononucleosis consists of bed rest, fluids, and analgesics. Occasionally, the pharyngitis from mononucleosis may be severe enough to cause airway obstruction or dehydration secondary to severe odynophagia. If patients develop these complications, steroid therapy can be used. Patients may develop a concomitant streptococcal pharyngitis, which should be treated. Other complications from mononucleosis are rare. The most serious complication is splenic rupture, which may occur if significant splenomegaly exists. Therefore, adolescents should not participate in contact sports for 6 weeks after the diagnosis of infectious mononucleosis, or longer if the spleen is still palpable. Complications such as hepatitis, pericarditis, mild hemolytic anemia, pneumonitis, or proteinuria are rare.

Acne Vulgaris

Acne vulgaris affects approximately 80 percent of all teenagers. It is one of the most common reasons for office visits by adolescents. Because of the adolescent's concern about body image, the problem of acne can be devastating to a young person, and physicians should not underestimate the problem.

Acne vulgaris is a result of the effect of hormones and bacteria within the pilosebaceous units. Hormones cause an increase in the amount of sebum within these units. Concomitantly, the bacterium *Propionibacterium acnes* breaks up the fats in the sebum to produce free fatty acids. Subsequent inflammation within the glands produces acne, which is manifested by open or closed comedones (blackheads and whiteheads, respectively), papules (reddened palpable lesions resulting from inflamed, obstructed follicles), nodules (a confluence of pustules that forms an abscess), and sometimes scarring.

A brief history is important in the evaluation of acne. Certain medications, including phenytoin, steroid preparations, isoniazid, and oral contraceptives, may exacerbate acne. It is also important to ascertain what over-the-counter preparations the adolescent may have already tried. Acne can be exacerbated by stress, the onset of menses, and pressure on the skin (leaning the face on the hands). Acne is not exacerbated by eating chocolate or fatty foods. Acne is also not caused by dirt; washing the face twice a day with mild soap is adequate.

Treatment

Topical medications are indicated for mild to moderately severe acne. Benzoyl peroxide, 5 to 10 percent solution, can be used once or twice daily. This can cause peeling and irritation; therefore, initial therapy should be 5 percent solution once daily. Topical antibiotics are also helpful and can be used in conjunction with benzoyl peroxide. Patients may apply antibiotic ointment in the morning and benzoyl peroxide at night. A third topical agent that can be effective is tretinoin. This must be used with caution, as it can be irritating to the skin and can result in a heightened sensitivity to sunlight.

Systemic antibiotics should be reserved for individuals with severe acne or those who are unresponsive to topical agents. Tetracycline or erythromycin, 500 to 1000 mg in two divided doses daily, can be used initially; this dose can be tapered after 4 to 6 weeks.

Adolescents need to be educated about how to use the medicines, and this can take time. Furthermore, they need to understand that therapy is not effective overnight; treatment takes weeks, and because the topical agents may be irritating, the acne may look worse for 3 to 4 weeks before it begins to improve.

Birth Control

Fifty percent of teenagers 15 to 19 years old are sexually active. *All* teenagers should be counseled about birth control. Teenagers who have not had sexual intercourse should be supported for their decision and encouraged to consult a physician *before* they have sexual intercourse. Sexually active teenagers should be educated about the birth control methods available.

When comparing effectiveness of different methods of birth control, it is important to distinguish use effectiveness from theoretical effectiveness. Use effectiveness is defined as the average number of pregnancies observed over a 1-year period in a cohort of 100 women using a particular method of birth control in a typical fashion. Theoretical effectiveness is the lowest observed number of pregnancies that occur in 1 year in 100 women using the method correctly and consistently 100 percent of the time. Statements in the following section refer to the use effectiveness.

Condoms have the advantage of being inexpensive, easy to use, and easily available. They also provide important protection against sexually transmitted diseases; therefore, they are often recommended for the adolescent. When they are used alone, however, the use effectiveness is approximately 2 to 20 pregnancies per 100 woman-years. When condoms are used in conjunction with a spermicide, the effectiveness is significantly improved.

The diaphragm is a rubber cap that fits inside the vagina and covers the cervix. Users place spermicidal jelly in the cap and then place the cap over the cervix prior to intercourse. Effectiveness is similar to that of condoms. Diaphragms have the advantage of being very safe and a female-controlled method of contraception. However, they do require fitting by a physician. Also, the adolescent must be comfortable placing the diaphragm and must be motivated to use it consistently.

Oral contraceptives are a frequently chosen method of contraception for adolescents. They are very effective and have little risk of serious side effects in healthy adolescents. Adolescents need explicit, written instructions when beginning oral contraceptives. They need to understand that they have to take the pill daily for effectiveness, and they need instructions on what to do if they have breakthrough bleeding, miss periods, or miss a pill.

Women using contraceptives may experience minor side effects such as nausea, slight weight gain, breakthrough bleeding, acne, and breast tenderness. If the adolescent experiences breakthrough bleeding during the first 3 months and is taking the pills correctly, she can simply be reassured. If breakthrough bleeding continues after 3 months, consider switching to a pill with higher progestin content.

Amenorrhea may occur with use of oral contraceptives. If the adolescent has not taken every pill, she should be evaluated for pregnancy; however, it is unlikely that pregnancy has occurred if the adolescent has missed only a single dose. If the amenorrhea persists, switch to an oral contraceptive with a higher progestin content.

Serious risks of oral contraceptives include an increase in cardiovascular mortality and venous thromboembolic disease. These risks are higher in individuals who smoke, and are highest for women over the age of 35. The risk of these serious side effects is negligible for healthy, nonsmoking women under the age of 30.

Absolute contraindications for oral contraceptives include a history of thromboembolic disorder, cerebrovascular accident, impaired liver function, and malignancy of the reproductive system. Practitioners should take precaution and consider alternative methods when prescribing oral contraceptives to women with hypertension, migraine headaches, or diabetes.

Adolescents beginning oral contraceptives should be seen in 1 to 2 weeks for a blood pressure check and a pill count and in 3 months to review any problems or questions and to check the blood pressure. They can then be followed every 6 months.

Summary

Physicians in adolescent medicine must be excellent communicators. It is necessary to be patient and willing to let the adolescent speak in order to get adequate information from the patient. Caring for adolescents also requires attention to the unique causes of morbidity and mortality among this population. Physicians need to be familiar with issues of growth and development, as well as the problems of drug use, sexually transmitted diseases, and depression, which frequently occur in adolescence.

References

Berman AL. Adolescent suicide: Issues and challenges. Semin Adolesc Med 1986; 2:269.

Chlamydia trachomatis infections: Policy guidelines for prevention and control. MMWR 1985; 34(3S):53S.

Johnston LD, O'Malley PM, Bachman JG. Drug use, drinking and smoking: National survey results from high school, college and young adult populations. Washington, DC: U.S. Department of Health and Human Services, Public Health Service. DHHS Publication No. (ADM) 89-1638, 1989.

Jones EF, et al. Teenage pregnancy in developed countries: Determinants and policy implications. Fam Plann Perspect 1985; 17(2):53.

McAnarney ER, Hender WR. Adolescent pregnancy and its consequences. JAMA 1989; 262:74.

Maron BJ, Roberts WC, McAllister HA. Sudden death in young athletes. Circulation 1980; 62:218.

Medical Letter 1988; 30(757):5.

Neinstein LS. Adolescent health care: A practical guide. Baltimore: Urban & Schwarzenberg, 1984.

Nettleman MD, Jones RB. Cost-effectiveness of screening women of moderate risk for genital infections caused by *Chlamydia trachomatis.* JAMA 1988; 260:207.

Rapp CE. The adolescent patient. Ann Intern Med 1983; 99:52.

Reichman RC, et al. Treatment of recurrent genital herpes simplex infections with oral acyclovir. JAMA 1984; 251: 2103.

Slap GB. Normal physiological and psychological growth in the adolescent. J Adolesc Health Care 1986; 7:135.

Stadel BU. Oral contraceptives and cardiovascular disease. N Engl J Med 1977; 305:672.

Tanner JM, Falkner F, eds. Human growth. 2nd ed. New York: Plenum Press, 1986.

Zelnik M, Kantner JF. Sexual activity, contraceptive use and pregnancy among metropolitan-area teenagers: 1971–1979. Fam Plann Perspect 1980; 12:231.

Physiologic Alterations of Aging

Roger B. Hickler, MD

Lynn Li, MD

The physiologic alterations of aging have major clinical implications, predisposing the patient to untoward and unique reactions to even minor stress and to modified or masked manifestations of serious medical disorders. Age-related, functional changes are distinguished from pathologic processes by the presence of *each* of the following characteristics: intrinsicality, universality, progressiveness, and deleteriousness.

Theories of Aging

Two basic genetic mechanisms have been advanced to provide the molecular basis for these physiologic decrements: (1) those that are intrinsically programmed and (2) those that are randomly derived. Intrinsically programmed mechanisms imply the predetermined "switching off" of certain genes that control the further division of important cell types, leaving them in the "postmitotic" state, e.g., neurons, muscle cells, certain endocrine cells, and thymic immunocytes; this inability to replicate renders the associated organ system particularly vulnerable to progressive attrition. Randomly derived mechanisms refer to accumulative, random damage to the DNA-RNA protein-synthesizing system due to mutagens (both intrinsic, as in the form of destructive, oxidative "free radicals," and extrinsic, as in the form of ultraviolet radiation). Limited intrinsic ability of the cell to "neutralize" mutagens or to keep pace with nucleic acid damage through its DNA repair mechanism has been correlated with shortened longevity. These are prominent postulates, linking intrinsic and random genetic events to the aging process. Age-related structural changes in organs and tissues are "post-translational" in nature and could, to a major extent, be the direct or indirect consequence of such alteration of nucleic acid function. These changes include tissue damage (e.g., cell wastage and "cross linkage" of both structural and functional proteins) and accumulation of nonfunctional substances (e.g., lipofuscin pigment in postmitotic cells, and extracellular amyloid).

It is emphasized that there is no single or conglomerate physiologic "marker" of chronologic age, and that different physiologic functions deteriorate to very different extents in the same individual and between individuals. However, N.W. Shock (1984) does cite work relating decreased probability of survival in apparently healthy individuals to the degree of unfavorable alteration in the following cluster of physiologic variables: pulmonary function (forced expiratory volume in 1 second and vital capacity), systolic blood pressure, serum protein concentrations, and certain estimates of neurologic integrity (reaction time, "tapping rate"). Some of the clinically most relevant functional changes with age are summarized according to the major organ systems.

Nervous System

Cerebral blood flow decreases by 20 percent and brain weight by 10 percent with advanced old age. This is associated with the loss of neurons, selective for the cerebral (20 percent loss) and cerebellar (25 percent loss) cortex and for the pigmented cells of the brain stem. In nonwasted areas, the "aging" pigment, lipofuscin, accumulates. Degenerative changes in the ultrastructure of surviving cells are extensive, including a loss of mitochondrial DNA. A loss of dendritic connections is seen in cortical pyramidal cells, leading to decreased synaptic interactions. The predilection for this change to occur in the Betz cells of the motor cortex has relevance for the exaggerated antigravitational tone (stiffness) of the elderly. Neurofibrillary tangles appear, occluding the neuronal cytoplasmic space, along with senile plaques (necrotic foci of amyloid-rich material); both of these degenerative changes, when present in great excess, are the hallmark of Alzheimer's dementia. Conduction velocity decreases by 10 percent in peripheral nerves and is associated with a reduction in nerve fibers (34 percent loss in vestibular nerve); taste buds decrease by 64 percent. These anatomic changes have been associated with significant alterations in neurotransmitters in the human brain with aging. There is a reduction in content of and synthetic capacity for dopamine in the basal ganglia, which has direct relevance to the problem of Parkinson's disease. There is a highly selective loss of choline acetyltransferase activity (essential for acetylcholine synthesis) in areas of the forebrain (hippocampus and neocortex), which has a relevance to the problem of Alzheimer's disease, and a large decrease in the norepinephrine content of the hindbrain.

The total of these changes accounts for the commonly observed neurologic status of the very old, which includes presbycusis, decreased sense of smell and taste, reduced psychomotor activity and reaction time, flexed posture, decreased vibratory sense, loss of fine coordination, absent "ankle jerks," and susceptibility to confusion (particularly with stress).

Cardiovascular System

Between the ages of 30 and 80 years, individuals in our society who are apparently healthy show (on average, but with wide variation) the following linear hemodynamic changes: 40 percent fall in cardiac output (30 percent in cardiac index), attended by a 14 percent increase in mean arterial pressure, giving a calculated 90 percent increase in total peripheral resistance (TPR). This reduction in blood flow is considerably greater than the reduction in lean body mass with aging; therefore, it is indicative of a decreased perfusion per unit weight of highly metabolizing tissues. The disproportionate increase in the systolic component of the arterial pressure in the latter decades reflects the additional effect of progressive aortic stiffening (loss of compliance) at that time. Both the increased TPR and decreased compliance augment the vascular input impedence. This factor plus the increased "inertance" imposed by the greater volume of aortic blood (relating to the age-related increase in aortic circumference) increase the left ventricular workload. These changes contribute to a 25 percent increase in left ventricular wall thickness and reduced stroke volume with advancing age. In the elderly, resting left ventricular ejection fraction (LVEF) and heart rate are unaltered, while stroke volume is decreased. With exercise, however, the elderly fail to show the rise in LVEF or degree of increment in heart rate and stroke volume (and, therefore, cardiac output) as shown by the young; arteriovenous oxygen difference widens. Baroreceptor sensitivity, as determined by heart rate response to changes in aortic pressure, is diminished in old age, and cardiac rate (pacemaker) response to sympathetic stimulation (isoproterenol or plasma norepinephrine concentration) is diminished. Clearly, it is necessary to redefine "normality" in old age to determine whether or not the various indices of cardiac performance are indicative of disease.

Respiratory System

Progressive stiffening of the chest wall over a lifetime increases the work of breathing on average by 20 percent or more. Structural changes in the lung include a diminution of elastic tissue in the alveolar ducts and alveoli, destruction of alveolar septa (decreasing alveolar surface area by 30 percent), loss of capillary area, and calcification of bronchial cartilages. Between the ages of 20 and 60 years, although total lung capacity remains constant, residual volume on average increases by 18 percent at the expense of vital capacity, and functional residual capacity increases by 17 percent at the expense of inspiratory capacity. By age 80, vital capacity decreases by 50 percent, lung distensibility (compliance) increases, and elastic recoil decreases. This, in conjunction with muscle weakness and chest wall stiffness, leads to a reduction in the various measures of airflow, including forced vital capacity, forced expiratory volume in 1 second, and maximum breathing capacity (60 percent reduction by age 80). Alveolar diffusing capacity decreases, probably because of loss of capillary bed. As a consequence of these changes, and reflective of ventilation/perfusion aberrations, arterial oxygen tension decreases from 90 mm Hg at age 30 to 75 mm Hg at age 80. Further, these changes contribute to the 70 percent reduction in maximum oxygen uptake and maximum work rate observed by the eighth decade.

Gastrointestinal System

With normal aging, salivary gland secretions diminish and amplitude of esophageal peristalsis decreases. The prevalence of esophageal hiatal hernia is relatively low below the age of 30 (10 percent) but increases dramatically after age 60 (60 percent). It is usually asymptomatic but may account for reflux symptoms in a small fraction of individuals. Impaired production of gastric juice leads to hypochlorhydria and hyposecretion of intrinsic factor and can produce vitamin B_{12} malabsorption. Frank atrophic gastritis is prevalent and can cause delayed gastric emptying. Minor reductions in small intestinal function are evidenced by flattening of the D-xylose absorption curve and lower serum levels of vitamins B_{12} and C. Lower levels of 1,25-dihydroxy vitamin D_3 are equated with poorer calcium absorption. Hepatic microsomal dysfunction accounts for slower biotransformation of certain lipid-soluble drugs, and a diminished rate of albumin synthesis leads to a moderate depression in serum concentration. Results of standard liver function tests are not abnormal. Pancreatic function is unimpaired. Colonic transit time is normal, and constipation is not part of normative aging. The prevalence of diverticulosis increases from 8 percent below age 60 to 40 percent above age 70 and has been related to the lack of bulk and fiber in the refined diet our society favors. Minuscule vascular ectasia of the right colon may appear in the elderly and account for the majority of unexplained gastrointestinal bleeds.

Kidneys and Bladder

Between the ages of 40 and 80 years, progressive renal shrinkage is evidenced by a 20 percent reduction in weight, associated with the loss of some 40 percent of the glomeruli. This may be a consequence of ischemic atrophy, secondary to extensive hyalinization of the cortical glomerular tufts. Associated functional changes are a reduction in renal blood flow and glomerular filtration rate by 50 percent and a slight increase in the filtration fraction. Serum creatinine concentration fails to increase despite the associated 30 percent reduction in its clearance because of the concurrent reduction in lean body mass. Associated renal tubular alterations are an increase in the concentration of blood glucose at which glycosuria will appear and a loss of urinary concentrating capacity (maximum specific gravity at age 40 is 1.030; at age 60, 1.026; and at age 90, 1.023, on average).

Nocturia is reported by 60 to 70 percent of elderly persons. Urinary incontinence occurs in approximately 20 to 40 percent of persons over 65 years of age and is largely related to diminished central nervous system inhibition effect, neuromuscular changes of the bladder, and obstruction of the bladder necks, in association with a decreased bladder capacity and increased residual urinary volume. Asymptomatic urinary tract infection, present in 20 percent or more of individuals over the age of 70 years, has been regarded as a relatively benign finding in most instances.

Endocrine System and Metabolism

Menopause is initiated by failure of ovarian secretion of estrogens and progestins. Low plasma levels of these hormones lead to atrophic changes in the uterus, vagina, and mammary glands and marked increases in pituitary secretion of gonadotropins, such that plasma follicle-stimulating hormone (FSH) may increase by 15-fold and luteinizing hormone (LH) by threefold. A much smaller and more gradual increase in circulating gonadotropins has been reported in men of advancing age as evidence of testicular failure, although evidence for declining serum testosterone levels is conflicting. The regular occurrence of prostatic hypertrophy in old men has been related to increased prostatic binding of dihydrotestosterone. In general, the relationship of hypothalamic-pituitary (neuroendocrine) changes to the aging process is a subject of great importance that is under intensive investigation at this time.

Fasting blood sugar increases on average by 5 mg/dl per decade after the age of 50, but it should not normally exceed 140 mg/dl. Fasting hyperglycemia is indicative of frank diabetes. The 1-hour and 2-hour serum levels after a glucose load become increasingly elevated. This age-related decrease in carbohydrate tolerance is related to a decrease in peripheral response to insulin rather than to a failure of insulin secretion, and it should not be mistaken for diabetes.

Plasma concentrations of growth hormone, thyrotropin, and corticotropin are unaltered by age. Adrenal secretion of cortisol and androgen in response to corticotropin and thyroid secretion of thyroxine in response to thyrotropin are diminished in old age. With the exception of adrenal androgen, however, this phenomenon is not reflected in a lower plasma concentration of adrenal and thyroid hormones, which have a lower rate of metabolic turnover in the elderly.

Musculoskeletal System

After age 40, bone mass decreases by 5 to 10 percent per decade, accelerating five- to sevenfold in women after menopause until the seventh decade, when it returns to the premenopausal rate.

This acceleration derives from a combination of increased bone resorption and decreased formation. It is clearly related to low estrogen levels, which lead to a potentiation of parathormone-induced calcium removal from bone and reduction of skin and renal elaboration of 1,25-dihydroxy vitamin D_3 (reducing intestinal calcium absorption). This physiologic senile osteopenia becomes clinical osteoporosis, predisposing to fractures (particularly hip and vertebral) in women whose bone mass is relatively low to begin with (i.e., at the time of menopause). Although patients with osteoporosis have a normal rate of bone formation, their bone resorption rate is more than double that of normal individuals. This may relate to the finding of low levels of 1,25-dihydroxy vitamin D_3 in elderly, osteoporotic patients.

Elderly persons show a decrease in the number and bulk of selected muscle fibers, with fibrous replacement of this "postmitotic" tissue. The extent to which this age-related loss of power can be minimized by physical conditioning is conjectural.

Immune and Hematopoietic Systems

By midlife, the thymus gland has lost 90 percent of its original mass; this is associated with a progressive fall in serum concentration of the thymic hormone thymopoietin, which becomes undetectable by the age of 60. In vitro studies of thymic lymphocytes (T cells) from the elderly show the following functional alterations: (1) decreased maturation, as evidenced by diminished capacity to bind sheep erythrocytes and increased capacity to bind autologous erythrocytes; (2) significant increase in the number of helper-inducer T cells; (3) impaired proliferative response to mitogens (plant lectins); and (4) decreased production and binding of the protein interleukin-II, which stimulates a T-cell proliferation. It is not difficult to postulate from these and other related deficiencies to the increased susceptibility of the elderly to malignancies, infections, and autoimmune phenomena.

In the healthy elderly, iron absorption is normal and stores are high, although serum levels and red cell uptake are depressed, but red cell parameters should not be below those of the young. According to one study of the elderly, 70 percent of subjects with a hemoglobin level of less than 12 g/dl or a hematocrit value less than 35 percent had an identifiable pathologic cause for their anemia.

References

Finch CE, Hayflick L, eds. Handbook of the biology of aging. New York: Van Nostrand Reinhold, 1985.

Rowe JW, Kahir RL. Human aging: Usual and successful. Science 1987; 237:143.

Shock NW. Normal human aging: The Baltimore Longitudinal Study of Aging. Washington, DC: U.S. Department of Health and Human Services. NIH Publication No. 84-2450, 1984.

Timiris PS, ed. Physiological basis of geriatrics. New York: Macmillan, 1988.

Hypertension and Cardiovascular Disease in the Elderly

134

Roger B. Hickler, MD

Lynn Li, MD

One of the most common and important tasks facing the clinician is that of management of the elderly patient with elevated blood pressure and cardiovascular disease. Nearly 50 percent of all individuals over 65 years of age have hypertension, defined as a blood pressure (BP) higher than 160 mm Hg systolic and/or higher than 95 mm Hg diastolic. This is the most potent, prevalent, and preventable contributing factor to cardiovascular disease because of its powerfully accelerating effect on atherosclerosis. Strokes and heart attacks account for more than 50 percent of all deaths in the elderly, the rate for both more than doubling with each successive decade after middle age. The death rate from coronary artery disease is nearly five times that for stroke. Although atherosclerotic events are still the leading cause of death in the aged, the mortality rate has shown a remarkable 25 percent decline during the past decade in the United States. This highly encouraging trend is largely attributable to advances in antihypertensive therapy. Thus, it behooves the clinician to have a perspective that integrates aging, hypertension, and atherosclerosis in terms of pathophysiology, risk, and management.

Classification of Geriatric Hypertension

The common phenomenon of a disproportionate elevation of systolic pressure in the hypertensive elderly patient relates to the late-life superimposition of aortic stiffening onto an increased peripheral vascular resistance. When this mechanism is the most striking factor in the hypertension, it is called *predominant systolic hypertension,* defined as a BP higher than 160 mm Hg systolic but less than 95 mm Hg diastolic. In extreme examples, the diastolic BP is less than 85 mm Hg, in which instances the term *isolated systolic hypertension* is applied. Otherwise, the term *diastolic hypertension* is used when the diastolic BP is higher than 95 mm Hg, irrespective of the degree of systolic elevation. Etiologic mechanisms for diastolic elevation in the elderly are the same as in the young, representing "essential" hypertension in at least 90 percent of instances. All of the rare endocrine forms have been found in the elderly and should be considered when de novo or suddenly accelerating hypertension occurs in the aged. Of these, renovascular disease is by far the most common.

Epidemiology

In population studies in our society, but not in certain nonindustrialized societies, there is a progressive rise in systolic and diastolic pressure up to the age of 55 years, at which time diastolic pressure levels off; this probably correlates with our penchant for high dietary salt intake. However, systolic pressure continues to rise at an increasingly steep rate from middle years until advanced old age. These trends correlate precisely with the known incidences of both "diastolic" and "systolic" hypertension. Thus, the incidence of diastolic hypertension (diastolic higher than 95 mm Hg) reaches a peak of 15 to 20 percent in whites and over 30 percent in blacks by age 55. In contrast, the incidence of isolated systolic hypertension is quite low up to age 55 but then increases sharply and progressively throughout the remainder of life. It peaks by the eighth decade: 30 percent in whites and 40 percent in blacks. Thus, more than half of all cases of geriatric hypertension are of the "predominant" or "isolated systolic" variety. When both systolic and diastolic hypertension are summed for the elderly, one reaches the extraordinary finding that approximately 40 percent of whites and more than 50 percent of blacks over 65 years of age have a BP that places them at a decidedly increased risk for morbid and mortal cardiovascular events.

Pathophysiology

Elevated systolic or diastolic pressure or *both* are reflective of an increased peripheral vascular resistance (PVR). To the extent that systolic pressure is *disproportionately* elevated in geriatric hypertension, the additional factor of loss of aortic compliance has been superimposed. Normally, 50 percent of the cardiac stroke volume is stored in the aorta during systole. If aortic inelasticity were the only factor in the systolic elevation, mean arterial pressure would not change and diastolic pressure would actually decrease. Thus, to keep diastolic pressure from falling in the face of a progressively stiffening aorta, PVR must increase, which, in turn, will augment the degree of systolic elevation. Therefore, even in "isolated" systolic hypertension, with diastolic BP in the range of 80 to 85 mm Hg, there must be an element of increased PVR. This has important implications for antihypertensive therapy in geriatric hypertension, in which the usual classes of drugs have been shown to be effective, irrespective of the predominance of the systolic component in the hypertension.

Risk of Geriatric Hypertension

With respect to diastolic hypertension, the Framingham Study established that elderly individuals of both sexes (aged 65 to 74 years) with BPs higher than 160/90, as compared with BPs lower than 140/90, experience an approximate threefold increase in cardiovascular mortality, which is comparable to that for the younger groups. Even more impressive were the findings in borderline diastolic hypertension (BP 140/90 to 160/95). In comparison with normotensive individuals (BP less than 140/90) of corresponding ages, the increase in cardiovascular mortality in the *younger* groups was relatively small (less than twofold), whereas in the old group (65 to 74 years), it was more than doubled; it was greatest in elderly women. This should dispel the myth that hypertension, particularly of a mild degree and in women, is better tolerated by the aged.

With respect to isolated or predominant systolic hypertension, which is peculiar to the geriatric age group, the findings are comparable to those cited for diastolic hypertension. There is a two- to threefold increase in cardiovascular events (myocardial infarction, angina pectoris, and strokes) in elderly patients with a systolic BP greater than 160 mm Hg and diastolic BP less than 90 mm Hg in comparison with those patients whose BP was less than 140 mm Hg systolic and less than 90 mm Hg diastolic. Kannel et al, in their prospective Framingham data, found a two- to fourfold increase in stroke rate with isolated systolic hypertension (systolic BP greater than 160 mm Hg, diastolic BP less than 95). From their findings (including an analysis of indirect brachial arterial pulse recordings), it appeared that systolic pressure elevation predisposed to stroke, independently of arterial rigidity and more predictably than diastolic pressure level.

Efficacy of Therapy for Geriatric Hypertension

With respect to diastolic hypertension, the Veterans Administration Cooperative Study established that the incidence of strokes and congestive failure in men over 60 years of age was one-quarter as frequent with treatment of diastolic levels of 105 to 114 mm Hg and one-third as frequent with treatment of diastolic levels of 90 to 104 mm Hg. The more recent HDFP Study demonstrated unequivocally the benefits of aggressive, as opposed to casual, treatment of mild diastolic hypertension (average of 101 mm Hg); mortality in the older patients (60 to 65 years) was reduced by 16 percent (comparable to that for *all* ages). The isolated finding that there was no difference in mortality among white women between the two treatment groups simply seems to reflect the fact that lowering of maximum BP had already been achieved with the less aggressive management program. Further, the latter study showed for the first time a significant reduction (by 45 percent) in deaths from coronary events with aggressive therapy.

With respect to isolated or predominant systolic hypertension, there is a prospective trial in progress, the Systolic Hypertension in the Elderly (SHEP) trial, that will settle the question of treatment benefit. In the mean time, the subject remains controversial. However, the consensus of the experts is that judicious and gentle treatment of BP levels above 180 mm Hg to no lower than levels in the range of 150 to 160 mm Hg can, in most instances, be accomplished readily and safely with at least a strong possibility of reducing the incidence of untoward cardiovascular events. This can be achieved without undue depression of diastolic pressure. The theoretical basis for the benefit of systolic lowering argues that the inordinate systolic elevation is more than just an innocent "marker" of vascular sclerosis, contributing *directly* (1) to the tendency to strokes (as indicated by the Framingham data) and (2) to myocardial work (which would predispose to ischemia and its potential consequences of failure, arrhythmia, angina, and infarction). With respect to the latter, the higher intramural tension developed by the left ventricle to generate an elevated pressure in systole *does* indicate increased work and myocardial oxygen requirement. Isolated systolic hypertension is associated with a higher incidence of ischemia and infarction and a twofold increase in coronary mortality rate.

Treatment and the Cerebral Circulation

A major concern in treating geriatric hypertension has been the potential for precipitation of cerebral ischemic events. Clearly, agents that cause excessive postural hypotension are to be avoided. Short of that, the available data do not bear out this concern. Although "cerebral autoregulation" is shifted to a higher level in hypertension (i.e., cerebral blood flow starts to decrease at a higher level upon graded pressure reduction), there is still a wide margin for aortic pressure reduction before cerebral flow is compromised. Further, on prolonged treatment, this abnormality tends to correct itself. Although the Hypertension-Stroke Cooperative Study Group failed to show a reduction for the total group in rate of stroke recurrence upon treatment of associated hypertension after a stroke had occurred, for the "over 70" population, reduction in recurrence rate, along with a decreased rate of congestive failure, was clearly demonstrated. Further, the treatment was well tolerated by this vulnerable group. The *degree* of hypertension control is related positively to reduced stroke recurrence rate. Cerebral hemodynamics improved in terms of reduced vascular resistance and increased flow upon treatment of hypertension in patients with known cerebrovascular disease.

References

Carb JD. Detection and treatment of hypertension in older individuals. Am J Epidemiol 1985; 121:371.

Hickler RB. Aging and hypertension. In: Hemodynamic implications of systolic pressure trends. J Gen Am Geriatr Soc 1983; 31:421.

Kannel WB, et al. Systolic blood pressure, arterial rigidity, and risk of stroke. The Framingham Study. JAMA 1981; 245:1225.

Sowers JR. Hypertension in the elderly. Am J Med 1987; 82(suppl 1B):1.

Drug Use by the Elderly

Roger B. Hickler, MD

Lynn Li, MD

135

Nearly one-third of all prescription drugs in the United States are purchased by the elderly (over 65 years of age), who comprise less than 12 percent of the population. The estimated average, per capita number of drugs taken by the noninstitutionalized elderly is three to four (half of which are "over the counter"), and the average number taken by institutionalized elderly is five or more. The main determinant of this polypharmacy is the accumulation of multiple chronic disabilities in the aged. This leads to *continuous* medication with *multiple* agents. The most frequently prescribed drug classes in the elderly are cardiovascular (digitalis, diuretics, antihypertensives), psychotropic (sedatives, hypnotics, antidepressants, antipsychotics), and analgesic medications.

Adverse drug reactions in hospitalized patients vary from 3 percent in younger patients (aged 20 to 29 years) to 21 percent in older patients (aged 70 to 79 years), a sevenfold increase in incidence. One factor causing this is the polypharmacy in the elderly, which increases the likelihood of untoward drug-drug reactions. The number of adverse drug reactions in one survey increased progressively by tenfold when the *number of drugs* taken simultaneously increased from one to 20. Other factors are medication errors and altered pharmacokinetics and pharmacodynamics as a consequence of the physiologic decrements of aging. Drugs most frequently cited in adverse drug reactions in the aged are the frequently utilized diuretics and psychotropics; drugs with the greatest risk of producing an adverse drug reaction in the aged (reactions per prescription) are antihypertensives, anti-Parkinsonian agents, psychotropics, and digitalis (Table 135-1). A compilation of statistics indicates that adverse drug reactions complicate approximately 15 percent of hospital stays and almost double the length of such stays, causing an estimated 30,000 deaths and 1.5 million (3 to 5 percent of total) hospital admissions per year in this country, at an annual cost of 1 to 3 billion dollars.

Altered Pharmacokinetics in the Elderly

Alterations directly attributable to the aging process that, in specific instances, have been shown to modify the plasma concentration of active drug to a significant degree involve the following parameters: absorption, plasma protein binding, volume of distribution, hepatic metabolism, and renal excretion. Steady-state plasma concentration of drugs (Css) on any given regimen is directly proportional to the drug's "half-life" ($T_{1/2}$) and inversely proportional to drug distribution volume (V_d) and drug clearance (Cl). Thus, Css is proportional to dose/Cl and to dose $\times$ $T_{1/2}/V_d$. From this, it is derived that $T_{1/2}$ is proportional to V_d/Cl.

Absorption

On theoretical grounds, several age-related gastrointestinal changes could affect drug absorption. These include hypochlorhydria, reduced splanchnic blood flow (by 40 to 50 percent), and reduced intestinal motility and number of absorbing cells. However, there is little evidence that altered absorption is a major concern.

Much more important is altered absorption from drug-drug interactions, as in all patients; e.g., antacids (Ca^{++}, Mg^{++}, Al^{++}) can chelate tetracyclines in the gut; cholestyramine can bind fat-soluble vitamins, thyroxine, and aspirin; anticholinergics can slow gastric emptying and absorption rate (e.g., tricyclic antidepressants can slow uptake of L-dopa and phenylbutazone).

Plasma Protein Binding

Plasma albumin concentration falls with advancing age by 15 to 20 percent, leading to a decreased protein binding of certain drugs that bind preferentially to albumin. This allows a greater fraction to be "free" or active, and pertains to warfarin, phenytoin, phenylbutazone, tolbutamide, and meperidine. This phenomenon can triple the plasma concentration of active meperidine with a given dose between the ages of 20 and 80 years. Equally important, certain drugs that bind avidly to plasma proteins in general (e.g., salicylates, phenylbutazone, sulfonamides, and thiazides) can displace less tightly bound drugs and thus produce potentially hazardous (free) levels of the latter. For example, an elderly diabetic person taking tolbutamide may become hypoglycemic when an intercurrent urinary tract infection is treated with a sulfonamide.

Volume of Distribution

Age-related alterations in body fat and water composition can affect the distribution of certain drugs to a major degree. On average, between the ages of 20 and 80 years, body fat as a proportion of total body weight increases by 35 percent, whereas lean body muscle mass and total body water decrease

Table 135-1 Common Side Effects of Psychotropic Drugs

Generic name (brand name)	Sedation	Anticholinergic effects	Postural hypotension	Extrapyramidal effects
Antidepressants				
Tricyclics				
Tertiary amines				
Amitriptyline hydrochloride (Elavil)	5+	6+	3+	
Doxepin hydrochloride (Sinequan)	5+	4+	3+	
Imipramine hydrochloride (Tofranil)	3+	3+	3+	
Secondary amines				
Nortriptyline hydrochloride (Aventyl, Pamelor)	3+	2+	2+	
Desipramine hydrochloride (Norpramin)	1+	2+	2+	
Others				
Maprotiline hydrochloride (Ludiomil)	3+	2+	3+	
Amoxapine (Asendin)	3+	2+	3+	1+
Trazodone hydrochloride (Desyrel)	3–5+	1+	3+	
Fluoxetine hydrochloride (Prozac)	2+	1+	1+	1+
Antipsychotics				
Chlorpromazine hydrochloride (Thorazine) 10–100 mg/day	3+	2+	3+	2+
Thioridazine hydrochloride (Mellaril) 10–100 mg/day	3+	3+	3+	1+
Acetophenazine maleate (Tindal) 10–60 mg/day	2+	1+	2+	3+
Trifluoperazine hydrochloride (Stelazine) 4–20 mg/day	2+	1+	2+	3+
Thiothixine hydrochloride (Navane) 1–20 mg/day	2+	1+	2+	3+
Haloperidol (Haldol) 0.25–6.0 mg/day	1+	1+	1+	4+

by 17 percent; plasma volume decreases by 8 percent. For water-soluble drugs (e.g., ethanol, lithium carbonate) this can lead to a higher concentration because the volume of distribution is contracted. For lipid-soluble drugs it can lead to a greater distribution volume (V_d) and, therefore, longer duration of action ($T_{1/2}$) (e.g., benzodiazepines and phenothiazines). The extraordinary three- to fourfold increase in V_d for diazepam between the ages of 20 and 80 years, and the consequent equivalent increase in its $T_{1/2}$, is a phenomenon of major concern for this often-utilized drug in the geriatric population.

Hepatic Metabolism

The age-related reduction in hepatic mass, blood flow (by 40 percent), and microsomal (biotransforming) enzyme activity can lead to a major reduction in the clearance rate of a number of relatively nonpolar, often highly protein bound, lipid-soluble agents that are "cleared" mainly by the liver. The liver "clearance" involves a transformation into more polar, highly ionized metabolites that can be excreted by the kidney. The age-related effect is a prolonged $T_{1/2}$ and higher Css with multiple dosing.

The effects of aging on drug metabolism are complex and depend on the precise pathway by which a drug is metabolized in the liver. For drugs that are extensively cleared on a "first-pass" basis (i.e., propranolol, lidocaine, nitrates, and the tricyclic antidepressants) that are dependent on liver blood flow for their clearance, the decreased liver size and blood flow will lead to higher serum levels. The liver enzyme metabolism of drugs can be divided into two phases. The first, or preparative, phase of drug metabolism, which depends on liver microsomal enzyme activity, decreases most significantly with aging. Thus, drugs that undergo hepatic oxidation, hydroxylation, and phosphorylation, including the long-acting benzodiazepines (diazepam, chlordiazepoxide, and flurazepam) and theophylline, tend to have a very prolonged $T_{1/2}$ in the elderly. On the other hand, the second phase of drug metabolism (conjugation, acetylation, and glucuronidation) is much less affected by aging. Drugs such as short-acting benzodiazepines (oxazepam, temazepam, and lorazepam) show the least age-related increase in Css and therefore are preferable to the long-acting ones in geriatric practice (Table 135-2).

Equally important in the elderly is alteration of level of microsomal enzyme activity by one drug, which alters the metabolism of another drug. For example, phenobarbital can induce an increased metabolism of coumadin, and allopurinol can inhibit the hepatic degradation of 6-mercaptopurine, both of which could lead to serious consequences.

Renal Excretion

Perhaps the most important single pharmacokinetic consideration in the elderly is the inexorable and progressive regression in renal excretory capacity over a lifetime. This amounts to a 40 to 45 percent decrease in renal blood flow and an associated 30 percent reduction in creatinine clearance. Because muscle mass is also reduced, the elderly do not show any corresponding increase in serum creatinine concentration when creatinine clearance is reduced. A formula was derived from empirical data to estimate creatinine clearance, taking into account the patient's age and body weight. This obviates the need to collect a 24-hour urine sample for creatinine clearance calculation.

$$\text{Cl creatinine} = \frac{(140 - \text{age}) \times \text{body wt (kg)}}{72 \times \text{serum creatinine}}$$

Drugs that are primarily cleared by renal excretion (gener-

Table 135-2 Benzodiazepine Pharmacokinetics

Generic name (common brand)	Geriatric doses (mg)	Time to peak concentration (hr)	Half-life in young (hr)	Half-life in elderly (hr)
Flurazepam hydrochloride (Dalmane)	15	0.5–1.5	40–100	40–150 (active metabolite)
Diazepam (Valium)	2–5	1–2	24	75
Chlordiazepoxide hydrochloride (Librium)	5	—	10	18–30
Oxazepam (Serax)	7.5–20	2–4	7–10	7–10
Temazepam (Restoril)	15	2.3	11	10
Lorazepam (Ativan)	0.5	2.0	12	12
Triazolam (Halcion)	0.125	1.4	2.6	3.3
Alprazolam (Xanax)	0.25	1.1	12.4	12

ally the more polar and water-soluble agents) will show an increase in Css (and prolonged $T_{1/2}$) on any given dose schedule proportional to the reduced creatinine clearance. In the very elderly, it is a good rule of thumb to *halve* the usual dose of potentially toxic drugs (particularly those with a narrow therapeutic margin of safety). Important examples of such renally excreted drugs are (1) most antibiotics (e.g., aminoglycosides, sulfonamides, penicillins, and nitrofurantoin), and (2) many cardiovascular drugs (e.g., digoxin, procainamide, methyldopa, and thiazide diuretics). Digoxin toxicity in the elderly is frequently missed because so many of its symptoms are attributed to "old age" (e.g., fatigue, visual complaints, muscular weakness, nausea, anorexia, dizziness).

Altered Pharmacodynamics in the Elderly

The term *pharmacodynamics* refers to altered receptor sensitivity to a drug at a given plasma level. The elderly's *increased* receptor sensitivity to psychoactive drugs, coumadin, and analgesics is well described. Thus, a "therapeutic level" of benzodiazepines can cause adverse effects. For a smaller number of drugs, the elderly exhibit a *decreased* receptor sensitivity. Important examples are beta-adrenergic agonists (isoproterenol) and antagonists (propranolol) and insulin.

Recommendation

Given the vulnerability of the elderly to adverse drug effects and the high frequency with which they occur, it behooves the physician to conduct critical drug review at regular intervals and to stop any unnecessary drugs. If a drug is truly necessary, abide by the principle "start low, go slow."

References

Avorn J. Medications and the elderly. In: Rowe JW, Besdine RW, eds. Geriatric medicine. 2nd ed. Boston: Little, Brown, 1988:114.

Everett DE, Avon J. Drug prescribing for the elderly. Arch Intern Med 1986; 146:2392.

Montamat SC, et al. Management of drug therapy in the elderly. N Engl J Med 1989; 321:303.

Vestale RE. Clinical pharmacology. In: Andres R, Bierman EL, Hazzard, WR, eds. Principles of geriatric medicine. New York: McGraw-Hill, 1985:424.

136 Mental Changes in the Elderly

Merle R. Ingraham, MD

Mental, emotional, and behavioral changes in the elderly are commonly observed in both normal aging and in aging that is attended by maladaptive and disease processes. The point at which normal aging becomes abnormal aging may not be easily determined for a variety of reasons. Some of these reasons include the great individual differences in the personalities, defense mechanisms, and coping styles of a heterogeneous elderly population.

The aged cannot be viewed stereotypically in any particular way. Nonetheless, society, including physicians, has tended to adopt mythical stereotypes that easily allow the presence of mild mental changes such as a little confusion or memory failure to be viewed either as normal in an old person, when diagnostic suspicion ought to be aroused, or catastrophized into a more serious disease process such as dementia, when no such condition exists. Some of the mild mental changes can be attributed to the threshold phenomenon, in which an elderly person may be functioning well at one moment but less well at the next, depending upon fatigue, time of day, presence or absence of stimuli, use of drugs, and the status of digestion, elimination, cardiorespiratory function, and diverse psychological, physiologic, sociologic, and environmental factors.

It is probable that in no other population is it as important as in the elderly to consider not just the biologic changes but all of these other changes to make an accurate assessment. Diagnosis is a highly dynamic process. For these reasons, the physician is encouraged to take a generous amount of time in deriving a complete history, which is not always easy to achieve because of slower-thinking and slower-responding older patients and because of richer and more complex histories in general. The physician is also encouraged to be patient with older persons who may make light of their symptoms, feeling that others are "more needy" of the physician's valuable time. Older persons may underreport their symptoms, and the symptoms that may be pressing and urgent in other age groups may present more mildly. The need for collateral interviewing of family members and home health personnel is therefore obvious.

The healthy younger-old patient may not differ much from his middle-aged counterpart, but the unhealthy older patient may challenge the most astute clinician by the multiplicity of disease processes, altered presentations, and psychosocial and iatrogenic disturbances. It can be very difficult to tease out, weigh, and interpret symptoms for establishing diagnostic formulations.

In a textbook in which common symptoms are highlighted, it is important for the reader to understand that multiple symptoms may coexist and that they often derive from organic, functional, or socioenvironmental sources to a greater degree than those symptoms do in younger persons. The diagnosis of a primary psychiatric disorder in the elderly is often a process of exclusion of other conditions, and an accurate assessment of the symptoms of mental changes in the elderly behooves a global appreciation of many factors.

Two of the most commonly encountered mental changes in the elderly are depression and paranoia. However, the general considerations and diagnostic approaches subsumed in a discussion of these conditions apply in the mental changes of hypochondriasis and the relatively uncommon mania of the elderly.

Depression

Definition

Depression may be a normal affect of everyday life. "Blue Mondays" and "Sunday downs" are common experiences felt by many of us. Depression may also be a symptom of other conditions, or it may be an illness in its own right. Existential depression may occur in any age group and, although painful, may not lead to any treatment intervention. "Normal pessimism/depression" of the elderly is not a depressive illness. The patient may use synonyms for depression such as "downer," "blahs," "slowing up," "give up," "going off my feed," and "senile," especially when reduced mental alertness is conspicuous.

It is often important to differentiate between depressive neurosis (dysthymic disorder) and major depression (major affective disorder) because of the different treatment and risk considerations attending these disorders. For example, although suicide rates are high among depressed elderly persons in general, the rates soar in psychotically depressed old men.

The phenomenon of grieving is included in the symptom of depression. This, too, may be observed to vary in its severity and pervasiveness along a continuum ranging from normal grieving to delayed and pathologic grieving and treatable melancholia. People vary widely in their ability to overcome grief.

A popular conceptual differentiation is that of endogenous and nonendogenous depressions because of the treatment considerations that apply to each.

Etiology

Depression is the most common mental change in the elderly. It is estimated that 38 percent of people over age 65 will experience a severe depression at some point. Reactions to losses of loved ones, sense of usefulness, work, home, pets, and possessions are frequent triggers of depression. The perceptions of Neugarten (1970) regarding the various stresses encountered and their diminished severity if occurring at appropriate times of life are useful.

A wide variety of biologic disorders may cause depression. Especially common are viral disorders, hypo- or hyperthyroidism, anemia, cancer, parkinsonism, electrolyte imbalance, and the aftermath of surgery or trauma.

Drugs, especially some antihypertensive agents, steroids, and anticancer agents, also may cause depression.

Dementing illness may provoke depression, especially when the patient is aware of his or her brain failure. Faulty nutrition, inadequate stimuli, and diminished general health, especially failing organs of special senses, may cause depression.

Endogenous depression is thought to be due to both biogenetic factors and stress, resulting in changes in the hypothalamic-pituitary-adrenal axis.

Finally, depression may accompany other mental disorders, whether it is caused by them or not. Schizophrenia, schizoaffective disorder, manic depressive illness, and character disorders such as chronic depressive and borderline personality disorders may have depression as a major manifestation. Some argue that the schizophrenic patient is more likely to suffer anhedonia, an inability to experience pleasurable feelings, than to suffer depressive affect, but the differences may be very difficult to determine.

Diagnostic Approach

In diagnosing mental and emotional disorders, a most important recommendation is to feel with the patient. Trust your gut. An empathic response is helpful for diagnosing, establishing a relationship, and treating the patient. This feeling can be especially helpful in differentiating dementia from depression with cognitive impairment.

While identifying your feeling responses, however, you must gather a careful history, noting the presence of previous depressive disorders in the patient and kin and trying to identify precipitating events. A drug profile history should be taken, not only to identify those iatrogenic depressions possibly associated with antihypertensive drugs or steroids or a host of others, but also to identify those drugs used in the past that may have been successful in the treatment of depression. Such information regarding a successful drug treatment may weight your current assessment in the direction of an endogenous depression. A history of the successful use of electroconvulsive treatment would achieve the same diagnostic goal. It can never be overstated in the assessment of a depressed person that the physician should look for the loss. Often this will be the loss of a person on whom the patient has grown dependent or the loss of a role that fed his or her self-esteem. The elderly patient may conceal a loss for private reasons, downplay it, or deny it, making the interviewer's task more difficult.

Deriving a history from a depressed person may be time-consuming because of psychomotor retardation, delusions of worthlessness, and poverty of ideas. Some elderly present with a surrogate symptom like a sore foot rather than confess their depressed state and risk being considered "mental." It is often imperative to solicit information from family, friends, neighbors, or caretakers to obtain significant clues. In the differentiation of dementia and pseudodementia associated with depression, e.g., it is important to know whether the cognitive failure came on insidiously, as with dementia, or abruptly, as is more common with pseudodementia. The patient may be unable to give you this information. Getting a sense of the premorbid personality while in the presence of a depressed person may be impossible without collateral data.

It is also useful to conceptualize the depressed elderly from several perspectives: cognitive, vegetative, social, and emotional. Depressive illness will usually exhibit a pervasive disturbance in each of these dimensions. The patient will be slow in thinking and have trouble with memory (especially short-term memory), attention, concentration, and comprehension. He or she will also often worry excessively and obsess. Vegetatively, the patient will have low energy, anorexia, constipation, lack of interest in sex, diurnal mood shift (feels worse in the morning), early awakening (assuming the patient has not been sleeping since early the previous night or is not suffering from prostatism). He or she may be fixated on some part or function of the body. The presence of paresthesias, unexplained neurologically, may suggest the diagnosis. Socially, the depressed person is withdrawn, helpless, self-deprecatory, and evidencing little interest in former friends or activities. He or she may feel hopeless and demoralized. Self-care may be neglected, and increasing dependency upon others may be seen. The mood is, of course, depressed, but there may be less tearfulness in the elderly patient than in the younger depressed patient. Be sure to ask a depressed patient whether he or she has thought of suicide and, if so, whether a plan to commit suicide has been made.

When taking the history of the depressed person, note the content of what is said as well as the manner in which it is said. The pseudodementia patient may complain much more bitterly about diminished cognitive abilities than the patient with irreversible dementia. A useful differential guide is that of C. E. Wells (1979).

The physical examination is important in order to rule in or rule out any one of several conditions that contribute to the depression. The greater agitation of the depressed elderly may be noted. A chest examination may reveal pneumonia in the absence of a febrile response and thus explain the apathetic or depressed affect. Signs of physical neglect or unusual injuries may confirm your suspicion of suicidal behavior. Obvious neurologic signs of intracranial neoplasm or frontal release and two-point simultaneous touch signs of organic brain disease can be checked. The tremor, rigidity, and difficulty in getting out of a chair and walking of Parkinson's disease are but a few examples of physical diagnostic clues that should be sought. The odor of alcohol may arouse a line of questioning. According to Simon et al (1968), 28 percent of 526 consecutive patients over 60 years of age who were admitted to their psychiatric facility had serious alcohol problems.

Except as an additional means of diagnosing organic illness, which might be contributing to depression, laboratory and psychological testing instruments are more often corroborative than definitive. No test will absolutely identify an organic versus a "functional" disorder. Chemistry screens, the usual hemogram, urinalysis, chest radiograph, and electrocardiogram are in order. In the differential diagnosis of dementia, additional studies such as erythrocyte sedimentation rate, B_{12} and folate levels, electrolytes, thyroid tests, calcium level, and computed tomography scan of the head may be necessary. One laboratory test that appeared to be useful occasionally in the difficult differential diagnosis of the depressed person has been the dexamethasone suppression test. Nonsuppressors are much more likely to suffer from an endogenous depression (Guirtsman et al, 1982). The value of the dexamethasone suppression test has become controversial recently, especially in the elderly. However, a mini mental status examination such as the FROMAJE test (Libow and Sherman, 1981; Table 136-1), if used regularly, can be very helpful as part of the diagnostic approach.

The use of psychostimulants to assist in the diagnosis of medically ill, apathetic patients in whom depression might be easily masked by concomitant physical illness is reported by Hackett (1978) and others.

Table 136-1 Psychological Assessment: FROMAJE Test

Function: "Do you need at-home support?"

Reasoning: "Do you know the meaning of the proverb 'a stitch in time saves nine'?"

Orientation: "Do you know the day, date, year, where you are, your own name?"

Memory: "Do you remember which president was assassinated, was in a wheelchair, where you were born, where you were yesterday, three object names in 5 minutes?" Distant/Recent/Immediate

Arithmetic: "Can you count from 1 to 10, from 10 to 1, subtract 7 from 100?"

Judgment: "Would you know what to do if there were a fire in your wastebasket, if you found a stamped, addressed envelope?"

Emotional state: "Do you feel sad, cry, fear for the future?"

From Libow LS, Sherman FT. A rapidly administered, easily remembered mental status evaluation: FROMAJE. In: The core of geriatric medicine. St. Louis: CV Mosby, 1981:85.

Paranoia

Definition

Paranoia may be defined as the presence of ideas ranging from suspiciousness to persecutory delusions, sometimes accompanied by grandiosity.

Etiology

Paranoid states are second only to depressive states in the elderly. When many people age, they lose confidence in themselves as they witness increasing frailty, loss of a work-role identity, advent of one or more chronic illnesses, and loss of friends, family members, and power. Although it is not inevitable and depends upon adaptive capability and basic ego strength, many elderly become diminished, socially withdrawn, and isolated. Under these circumstances, the phenomenon of paranoid thinking may occur, especially in older women, for reasons that are undetermined. The usual psychiatric explanation lies in the unconscious projection by the patient of hostile feelings onto the environment. Other dynamics often contribute to the paranoia. One is the sensory deprivation that applies when the older person loses his hearing or visual acuity. A high percentage of paranoid elderly suffer bilateral deafness (Cooper et al, 1974). Sensory deprivation occurs with social isolation as well, and most paranoid conditions of the elderly are found among lonely, depressed, seclusive people.

Old age is also a time when persons can more easily get caught up in a sick role. Such persons are inadvertently reinforced by caretakers for being sick as they develop a body focus, turn inward, and substitute pills for people and affection. Depending on how angry with their plight they may be, they may develop frank paranoia or an irritating hypochondriasis. Depending on how needy for affiliation they may be, they may present with a litany of organic symptoms (the organ recital) or develop an overt depressive stance, clinging anxiously to their doctors and demanding care.

The meaning of symptoms in the elderly is more richly determined by the psychological development of the individual and his or her unique mental mechanisms, fixations, and style, and warrants interpretation. The paranoid symptom may express a depressive disorder, a functional psychosis, a personality disorder, an organic mental disorder, or none of these. Paranoid symptoms often attend the elderly alcoholic. In the male alcoholic who is especially concerned with waning sexual interest and erectile dysfunction (these concerns are probably compounded by his use of alcohol), the paranoid phenomenon may take on delusional jealousy features, with bitter and humiliating accusations regarding his spouse's presumed infidelity. Conjugal paranoia need not occur in the matrix of alcohol abuse, however. It is a poorly understood, albeit very disruptive, symptom complex. Alcoholic withdrawal phenomena such as paranoia and hallucinations of terrifying, persecutory animals and people are no strangers to the elderly.

The elderly person who has the beginning of dementia, with its attendant memory impairment, finds it easier to blame others for stealing his personal items than to acknowledge or remember misplacing them himself. Psychological regression often accompanying organic mental disorders may produce an obsessional concern about money and bowel functions. Hoarding and suspiciousness may become troublesome to the patient and to the family. Patients with advanced organic mental syndromes often manifest inflexibility and paranoia. Toxic deliria, frequently associated with drugs, also may provoke acute paranoia.

The persistence of a paranoid personality or paranoid schizophrenia into old age is mentioned for completeness, but these possible diagnoses ought not to be the first ones considered when paranoid ideation is found. Another psychiatric syndrome is paraphrenia (involutional paranoia), comprising persecutory ideation to the degree of delusional thinking in an otherwise clear-minded older person who has no evidence of organic brain disease and none of the other affective or cognitive changes of schizophrenia. It is possible that our diagnostic tools are not refined enough to identify organic lesions, however, and paraphrenia may be an organic delusional syndrome.

Finally and sadly, concern that one may be evicted from one's home or sent to a nursing home, that the doctor considers one to be a nuisance, that one's home may be broken into, or that one may be mugged on the street may have a generous basis in reality.

Diagnostic Approach

Much of what has been written about the approach to the depressed patient continues to apply. The paranoid patient presents, if at all, as an angry, aloof individual who often believes he or she has been coerced into coming (often true). Such a patient resists a warm, friendly approach, and the doctor is better advised to adopt a firm, business-like manner, displaying little anxiety and an economy of touching. The paranoid person's spatial bubble is likely to exceed that of the examiner's; it is wise to take this into account and to give the patient room and not crowd him. With the agitated, threatening, extremely paranoid person, it may be wise never to position yourself between the patient and the means of egress from the examining room. The felt needs by the physician to consider such tactics are diagnostic in themselves.

Other physical signs of diagnostic value are paranoid headlights (a startled appearance with sclera showing all about the iris) and avoidance of eye contact or suspicious side glances. Such patients are also excessively preoccupied with intercom and dictating equipment and hypodermic paraphernalia. They may insist on seeing what you are writing about them in their record, and some can be observed attending to auditory hallucinations. Certain statements by the patient have high diagnostic value, e.g., "You know what I'm thinking!"

An assessment of hearing and visual acuity is vital. The usual laboratory screening, including thyroid function studies, is recommended, because myxedema madness is a paranoid manifestation. The physical examination may have to be modified initially if it is to include rectopelvic examinations, because of the paranoid patient's usual sexual anxiety and fear of hurtful penetration. If possible, perhaps at a subsequent appointment, such examinations should be done, because paranoiacs also may have rectal or uterine cancer.

The history is an important means of obtaining evidence of long-term paranoia versus more recent paranoia; it is also an integral part of developing a diagnosis. The drug history is very important because numerous products can produce an organic mental syndrome that presents as paranoia in the elderly.

References

Blazer D. Depression in the elderly. N Engl J Med 1989; 320:164.

Cole J, Barrett J. Psychopathology in the aged. New York: Raven Press, 1980:19, 145.

Cooper AF, et al. Hearing loss in paranoid and affective psychosis in the elderly. Lancet 1974; 2:851.

Guirtsman H, Gerner R, Sternbach H. The overnight dexamethasone suppression test: Clinical and theoretical review. J Clin Psychiatry 1982; 43:8.

Hackett TP. The use of stimulant drugs in general hospital psychiatry [audiotape]. Glendale, CA: Audio-Digest Foundation, 1978.

Hodkinson HM. Common symptoms of disease in the elderly. 2nd ed. Oxford: Blackwell Scientific Publications, 1980:21.

Libow LS, Sherman FT. A rapidly administered, easily remembered mental status evaluation: FROMAJE. In: The core of geriatric medicine. St. Louis: CV Mosby, 1981:85.

Neugarten B. Adaptation and the life cycle. J Geriatr Psychiatry 1970; 4:71.

Simon A, Epstein LJ, Reynolds L. Alcoholism in the geriatric mentally ill. Geriatrics 1968; 23:125.

Wells CE. Pseudodementia. Am J Psychiatry 1979; 136:895.

Whitehead JM. Psychiatric disorders in old age. Haverhill, Suffolk: Lowe, Brydone, 1974:23.

Vision Problems in the Elderly

Lynn Li, MD

137

Definition

Decrease in visual acuity usually signifies a major medical problem. Although lenticular opacification occurs in about 60 percent of people over 65 years of age, the majority of elderly persons continue to have useful vision throughout their lives. The elderly do not expect to have perfect vision, but they are concerned with preservation of functional vision to maintain independence in daily activities such as keeping house, pursuing hobbies, and socializing. For that purpose, the field of vision may be more important than the acuity of central vision.

A survey of 1,000 elderly residents of nursing homes in New York City showed that 70 percent of them had "good to useful vision" (15/15 to 15/40). Another 15 percent had "fair to adequate vision" (15/50 to 15/70). Only 15 percent had "poor vision" (15/100 or less) or "very poor vision" (15/200 or less). About 1 percent had no light perception.

In the United States, a person is considered legally blind if central vision is 20/200 or less in the better eye with correction and/or if peripheral vision is of 10-degree angle or less in both eyes on perimetry. The legally blind person should be registered by the Commission for the Blind in his or her home state to receive assistance such as low-vision aids and seeing eye dogs.

Diagnostic Approach

History

The physician should actively inquire about visual loss because the elderly tend to minimize symptoms and there is a common prejudice that poor eyesight is part of normal aging ("ageism"). The elderly may also blame poor eyesight on their eyeglasses.

When a patient does report visual loss, it is important to find out exactly what is meant—whether it is monocular or binocular, sudden or gradual in onset, transient or recurrent, or accompanied by pain. It is also important to inquire about any other associated systemic symptoms. For example, transient hemiparesis is often associated with amaurosis fugax; headache, fatigue, and malaise are associated symptoms of temporal arteritis. Sometimes a complaint of visual loss really means a visual field cut. In such a case the character of the field cut often suggests the location of the lesion and the diagnosis. For example, compression or inflammation of the optic nerve will cause central scotoma, whereas opacity within the media (cornea, lens, and vitreous) may cause generalized constriction of the visual field. Lesions compressing the optic chiasm result in bitemporal hemianopsia, whereas lesions further posterior in the optic tract will result in homonymous field cuts in both eyes.

A complete medication list must be obtained. Tricyclic antidepressants and other agents with anticholinergic effects can dilate the pupil to induce glaucoma. Chronic systemic steroid therapy may induce cataracts and glaucoma in susceptible people. The primary care physician often has to make tradeoffs, balancing therapeutic needs of the patient with a systemic illness against the risk to the patients' ocular system.

Physical Examination

Examination of the eye to evaluate visual loss in the elderly should include the following tests:

1. *Visual acuity.* Central macular vision should be tested using a standard eye chart (i.e., Snellen chart) with the patient wearing his or her own eyeglasses. Looking through a pinhole puts everything in relative focus. If a pinhole can improve vision, there is probably a refractive error, which is correctable by eyeglasses. Peripheral visual fields should be assessed by confrontation.

2. *Pupillary reflex.* Direct and consensual constrictive response to light should be tested. Afferent pupillary defect (Marcus-Gunn pupil) is detected by the "swinging flashlight test": A light is repeatedly and rhythmically swung back and forth between the two eyes; when light is brought in front of the eye with a relative optic nerve defect, both pupils dilate. When light is brought in front of the other eye, both pupils constrict. This is found in optic nerve damage, i.e., from glaucoma or ischemia.

3. *Extraocular motion.* Conjugate motion in all six directions should be tested.

4. *Intraocular pressure by Schiotz tonometry.* Pressure less than 21 mm Hg is generally considered normal. Higher intraocular pressure may not be associated with optic nerve damage, but lower pressure measurements do not exclude glaucoma (normal-pressure glaucoma).

5. *Funduscopic examination by direct ophthalmoscopy.* The pupils can be dilated with two drops of 0.5 percent short-acting tropicamide solution in each eye if intraocular pressure measurement is normal and there is no other obvious risk of inducing acute angle-closure glaucoma. If the fundus cannot be seen, there may be opacity in the media, such as cataract or vitreous hemorrhage. If the fundus can be seen, careful attention should be directed toward the optic nerve head and macula for swelling, hemorrhage, or exudate. Lesions in these two areas cause central visual disturbances.

Differential Diagnosis

The major causes of visual loss in the elderly that a primary care physician is likely to see are cataracts, glaucoma, age-related macular degeneration, amaurosis fugax, and temporal arteritis (Table 137-1).

Cataracts

Aging is the main cause of cataracts. Most patients over 50 years of age have some degree of opacification of the ocular lens, although vision is not necessarily impaired. Less common causes are ocular injury or surgery, juvenile diabetes mellitus, and corticosteroid therapy.

Decreased visual acuity is the major symptom. Patients commonly complain of unclear vision and say it seems as if they are looking through a screen. The blurred vision could almost be wiped away like dirt on eyeglasses or mucus in the eyes. A seemingly strange phenomenon of improved near vision may develop in early stages of nuclear cataracts. As the nucleus hard-

Table 137-1 Etiology of Visual Loss in the Elderly

Ocular
Cataract (up to 60%)
Age-related macular degeneration (up to 30%)
Glaucoma (5–10%)
Retinal detachment
Vascular disorder
Central retinal vein occlusion
Central retinal artery occlusion
Ischemic optic neuropathy
Diabetic retinopathy (up to 7%)
Systemic
Transient ischemic attack/amaurosis fugax
Temporal arteritis
Optic nerve compression

ens, the patient becomes more nearsighted, so that although the distant vision is blurred, near vision may improve and reading no longer requires eyeglasses for the first time. The patient may report better vision indoors than outdoors. This is because in posterior subcapsular cataract, conditions that cause the pupil to constrict (such as bright lights) force the image to go through the cataract. Patients should be cautioned against night-time driving because lights from oncoming cars can be diffusely scattered by the cataract, virtually blinding the cataractous driver.

On examination, the visual acuity is decreased and not correctable by pinhole. The pupillary reaction should be normal. Direct ophthalmoscopic examination may show specks of gray against the red reflex, or the cataract may be so dense that no red reflex can be seen. Slit-lamp examination is necessary to delineate the exact location and therefore the type of cataract. Nuclear and cortical types are more commonly associated with aging and usually progress slowly. The posterior subcapsular type is more common in younger people and more debilitating owing to its central location. Figure 137-1 presents diagrams of nuclear, cortical spoke, and posterior subcapsular cataracts.

Surgical removal is indicated when the patient desires it because the cataract is interfering with his or her lifestyle. An intraocular lens implant can be successfully implanted in a majority of patients at the time of cataract extraction, allowing a rapid return of normal vision. This is the most common eye operation performed today and is usually done in day surgery.

Age-Related Macular Degeneration

Age-related macular degeneration (ARMD), which causes loss of central visual acuity, affects up to 30 percent of the elderly

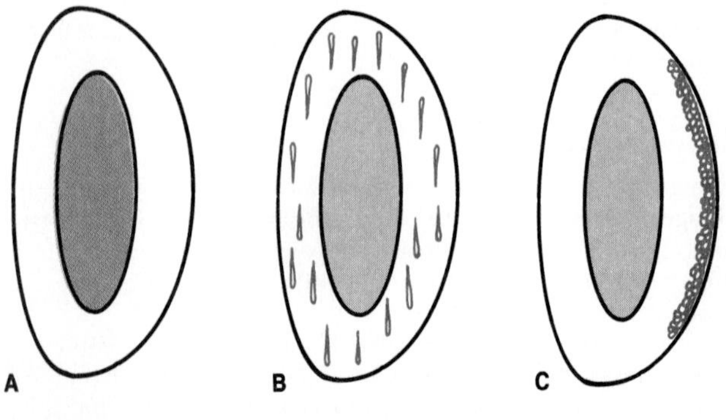

Figure 137-1 Types and locations of cataracts. (**A**) Nuclear cataract. (**B**) Cortical spoke cataract. (**C**) Posterior subcapsular cataract.

population and is the leading cause of legal blindness in the geriatric group in the United States.

The process starts with degeneration of Bruch's membrane, the layer between the retinal pigmented epithelium and choriocapillaries, which allows ingrowth of choroidal vessels beneath the retina. Leakage of fluid and blood from the new vessels has a predilection for the macula and causes severe central visual loss. In the so-called atrophic or dry form, scattered drusen (yellowish-white spots) and hyper- or hypopigmentation are seen on the fundi. In the wet or neovascular form, hemorrhages and exudates from the new vessels eventually form dense scars over the macula (disciform scars).

Both forms are associated with drusen and can coexist in a given patient. The majority (90 percent) of patients with ARMD present with the dry form. There is no effective therapy, but low-vision aids are helpful. It is important to reassure the patient that the chance of remaining independent in daily living activities is good because peripheral visual fields are usually preserved in this condition.

The other 10 percent of patients with ARMD present with the wet form, which is characterized by choroidal neovascularization. The visual loss is rapidly progressive, but it can be controlled by laser photocoagulation, which abolishes the choroidal neovascularization if detected early. The sudden hemorrhage or exudation is signaled by distortion of vision (metamorphopsia). The patient may notice while reading with one eye that parts of words are missing, or notice that the straight line of a door frame looks crooked. All patients at risk for ARMD should be instructed to test vision in each eye daily by looking at a straight object or by using an Ansler grid card. If new distortion is noted, this patient should be seen urgently by an ophthalmologist for fluorescein angiography and possible laser therapy.

Laser photocoagulation can ablate the neovascular membrane and prevent visual loss. However, up to 60 percent of patients treated with lasers have recurrence of neovascularization, so they must be followed closely.

Glaucoma

Glaucoma is a condition in which elevated intraocular pressure damages the optic nerve, resulting in loss of peripheral fields and finally loss of central vision. It is almost always due to decreased outflow of aqueous humor from the anterior chamber (anatomy of the anterior chamber is illustrated in Figure 137-2). Glaucoma is the second leading cause of blindness in the United States; 1 million people in the United States are estimated to have glaucoma without knowing it. There are two major types of glaucoma: acute angle-closure glaucoma and chronic open-angle glaucoma.

Acute Angle-Closure Glaucoma

Acute angle-closure glaucoma is caused by obstruction of aqueous humor outflow by closure of the angle between the cornea and the root of the iris, thereby blocking access to the outflow canal (Fig. 137-2B). It presents dramatically with severe deep ocular pain that is often associated with nausea and vomiting. The eye is red, with a hazy cornea and a poorly dilated or nonreactive pupil. Vision may be extremely blurred or may be completely lost. The patient is often over 60 years old and has a strong family history because the anatomic predisposition is genetic.

An attack may be provoked by prolonged periods of darkness in which the pupils are dilated. Exposure to drugs that dilate the pupils, such as anticholinergics, which are used to treat Parkinson's disease, depression, or gastrointestinal upsets, can precipitate attacks. On palpation, the globe is very hard because the pressure may be in the range of 50 to 90 mm Hg, as opposed to a normal range of 10 to 20 mm Hg. This is an emergency, and the patient should be referred immediately to an ophthalmologist for medication and possible surgery.

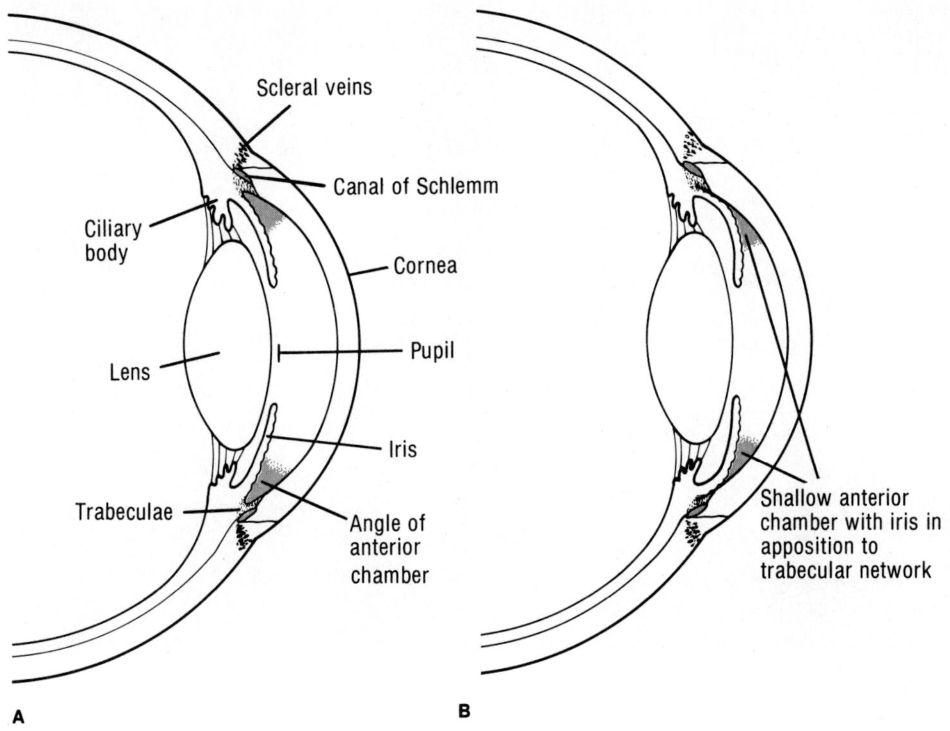

Figure 137-2 Anatomy of the anterior chamber. (**A**) Normal chamber. (**B**) Angle-closure glaucoma.

Chronic Open-Angle Glaucoma

In open-angle glaucoma, the access to the canal is open but microscopic defects in the tissue of the canal itself interfere with the aqueous drainage (Fig. 137-2A).

Data from the Framingham Heart Study showed the prevalence of chronic open-angle glaucoma to be 5 percent for the age group 65 to 74 years and 7 percent for the age group 75 to 85 years. Frequently, there is a positive family history. Both topical and systemic corticosteroids may induce glaucoma in genetically susceptible individuals. Prior surgery or trauma to the eye is another predisposing factor. In chronic open-angle glaucoma, the intraocular pressure rises *gradually* to the range of 30 to 50 mm Hg. Because of the gradual nature of the disease, the patient is often asymptomatic until a peripheral visual field cut develops. In the elderly, a peripheral cut is often unnoticed until central vision is affected.

Chronic glaucoma can be detected only by periodic intraocular pressure measurement, visual field testing, and ophthalmoscopic examination. The fundi show nasal displacement of the vessels and vertical enlargement of the cup (cup-to-disk ratio becomes greater than 0.5) and pallor of the disk (Fig. 137-3). The ophthalmoscopic examination is more important than tonometry because changes can occur at normal intraocular pressure. Therefore, in the geriatric population, regular screening for chronic glaucoma is obligatory. The treatment is initially medical. The next step is laser trabeculoplasty. The presumed mechanism is to burn small scars in the trabecular meshwork. As the scars retract, they pull open the adjacent collapsed and closed meshwork. If the patient continues to lose visual fields after laser trabeculoplasty, surgery to create a fistula from the anterior chamber to the subconjunctival space is the definitive treatment.

Amaurosis Fugax

Fleeting monocular blindness resulting from transient ischemic attack of the retina is most often (80 to 90 percent) due to microembolization of cholesterol, fibrin, or platelets from the internal carotid arteries to branches of the ophthalmic artery. In the geriatric population, temporal arteritis must also be considered.

The history is very dramatic: the patient often reports that suddenly a shade has been pulled down over one eye and that this sensation lasts a few minutes and then clears completely. The patient usually is older than 50 and has other conditions related to arteriosclerosis such as high blood pressure, diabetes, angina, or history of cerebral ischemia, or is a cigarette smoker.

On physical examination the ipsilateral carotid artery may have decreased upstroke or a bruit, and there may be other signs of arteriosclerosis elsewhere in the body such as bruits, abdominal aortic aneurysm, or absence of distal arterial pulses. Funduscopic examination should include a careful search for fragments of refractile cholesterol emboli (Hollenhorst plaque) or whitish platelet emboli in retinal arteries, especially near the bifurcations.

Amaurosis fugax, like hemispheric transient ischemic attack, is a warning sign of impending stroke or permanent retinal damage. Some patients may never have another attack, others will have many more attacks, and up to 16 percent will become blind or suffer strokes.

Temporal Arteritis

Giant cell arteritis is a systemic vasculitis that affects the elderly exclusively. Characteristically, systemic symptoms of fever, malaise, weight loss, headache, arthralgia, and proximal myopathy (polymyalgia rheumatica) precede ocular involvement. However, such complaints are frequently ignored, especially by the elderly. Therefore, sudden, profound loss of vision in one or both eyes may be the presenting symptom. This is a true emergency, because optic nerve infarction in the other eye often follows a few days after the attack in the first eye. Infarction of the coronary and the vertebral artery systems is a well-known complication. A high degree of suspicion for this not uncommon and

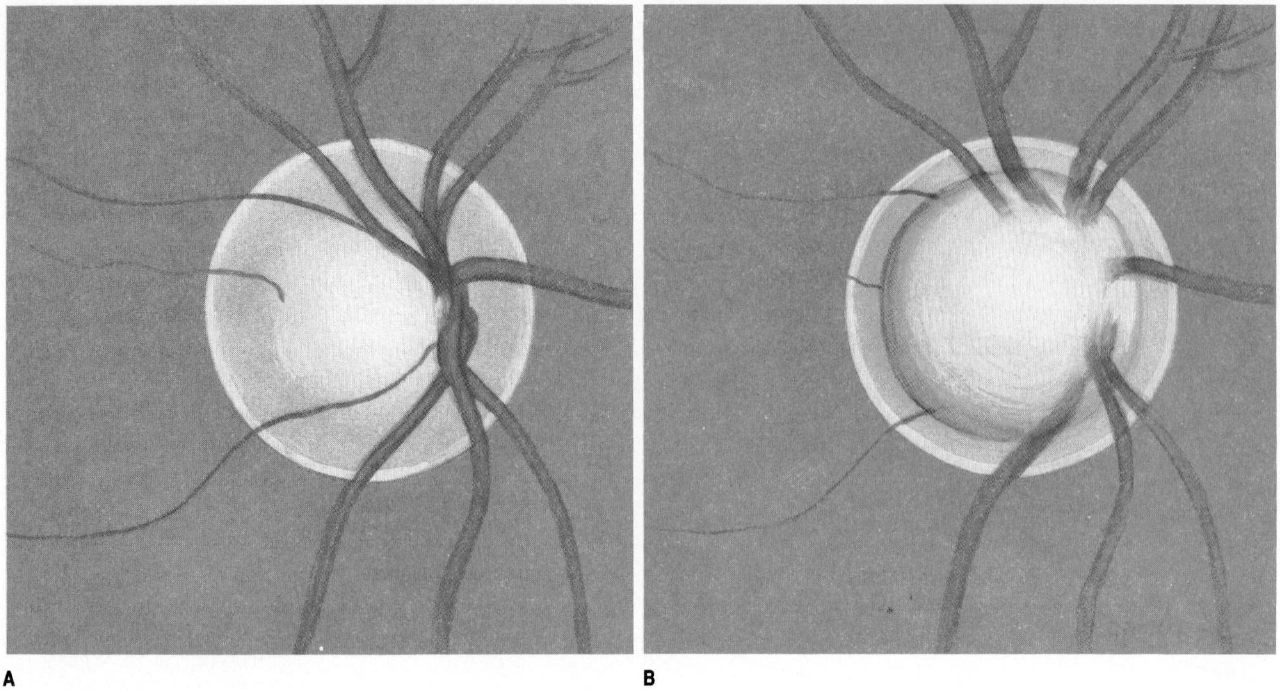

Figure 137-3 (**A**) Normal optic disk of the right eye. (**B**) Glaucomatous disk of the right eye.

devastating geriatric illness is the key to diagnosis. A history of claudication of the masseter muscles, facial pain, or tender scalp is another suggestive symptom.

Ocular pathology includes ischemic optic neuropathy (40 to 50 percent), central retinal artery occlusion (5 to 10 percent), and rarely retinal ischemia (amaurosis fugax). Ophthalmoplegia (15 to 50 percent) and cortical blindness (rare) can be seen as a result of involvement of intracranial vessels.

Ischemic optic neuropathy is infarction of the optic nerve head due to local vascular occlusion. It can cause sudden painless visual loss or gradual visual deterioration over a few days. It is most often due to vasculitis, but it may also be caused by arteriosclerosis. The optic nerve head may look swollen, pale, yellowish or even whitish, or it may appear normal.

Central retinal artery occlusion is usually due to arteriosclerosis or vasculitis. It causes sudden, profound loss of vision. Initially, the retinal arteries look narrowed and devoid of blood, and the veins look slightly dilated with segmentation. A few hours later, a cherry red spot may be seen at the macula. This is because only the fovea (supplied by the choroidal artery) is spared and has normal red retinal color. The rest of the retina is edematous and pale. About 2 days later, signs of optic atrophy begin to develop.

In temporal arteritis the superficial temporal arteries are abnormal on palpation, ranging from pulseless, hard cords to minimal arterial wall thickening; in either case, they may be tender. There may be ptosis or abnormal extraocular motion. The fundi may appear normal or may show disk swelling, cherry red spots, or optic atrophy, depending on the pathology and the stage of the disease.

Typical laboratory abnormalities are a striking elevation of the Westergren sedimentation rate, usually to the 80 to 120 range, and an anemia of chronic disease.

Definitive diagnosis is made by biopsy of the temporal arteries. It shows multinucleated giant cells, plasma cells, and lymphocytes infiltrating the intima and media. Thrombosis may occur in the inflamed arteries. Because it is a segmental disease, it is important to get a large (4 to 5 cm) segment, and bilateral biopsies are often needed before the diagnosis can be established.

Administration of high doses of corticosteroids may avert visual loss in the second eye, but recovery of vision in the involved eye is extremely rare. In the appropriate clinical setting, high-dose corticosteroids should be started without delay when this diagnosis is suspected, before development of ocular symptoms. The temporal artery biopsy can be done either just before or shortly afterward. The histologic findings will not revert in the first few days. Maintenance steroids should be continued for 1 to 5 years, depending on the clinical picture and sedimentation rate. It is hoped that this will prevent development of blindness, but such an outcome cannot be assured.

References

Bienfang DC. Ophthalmologic problems. In: Branch W, ed. Office practice of medicine. 2nd ed. Philadelphia: WB Saunders, 1987:1137.

Brewer SS, Singerman LJ. Vision loss in age-related maculopathy: Primary care referral guide. Geriatrics 1987; 42:99.

Capino DG, Leibowitz HM. Age-related macular degeneration. Hosp Pract 1988; March 30:23.

Kahn C. Visual disorders. In: Libow LS, Sherman FT, eds. The core of geriatric medicine. St. Louis: CV Mosby, 1981:207.

Leighton DA. Aging of the eye. In: Brocklehurst JC, ed. Geriatric medicine and gerontology. 3rd ed. New York: Churchill Livingstone, 1985.

Vaughan D, Asbury T, Cook R. General ophthalmology. 11th ed. Los Altos, CA: Lange Medical Publications, 1986.

Wray SH. Disturbances of vision and ocular movements. In: Braunwald E, ed. Harrison's principles of internal medicine. 11th ed. New York: McGraw-Hill, 1987:70.

Musculoskeletal Pain in the Elderly

David F. Giansiracusa, MD

Janice C. Hitzhusen, MD

138

Definition

Musculoskeletal disorders in the elderly may present as pain localized to joints, to structures around joints, to muscles, or to bone; as weakness, stiffness, or diffuse body aching; or as systemic (constitutional) symptoms such as fatigue, fever, weight loss, depression, and malaise. Common musculoskeletal problems in the elderly are listed in Table 138-1.

Diagnostic Approach

History

Obtaining a detailed history of the patient's complaints is the first and often the most important part of the evaluation of musculoskeletal problems. Obtaining an accurate history may be difficult and time-consuming in an elderly patient for several reasons. Older people may feel that the aches and pains that they experience are to be expected with aging and may not volunteer these complaints. They may feel that a physician would also discount these complaints as part of the aging process. The elderly patient's multiple medical problems may confound the patient and physician. Older people may experience memory deficits and may forget specific aspects of their musculoskeletal pain as well as confuse the chronology of their symptoms. Finally, many elderly patients present with symptoms that are vague and nonspecific and not necessarily classic for a specific disease.

Pain is the most frequent complaint. History taking should attempt to elicit the location, character, intensity, type of onset, duration, course, frequency (intermittent, persistent, progressive, or improving), and associated symptoms.

Localization of the pain to the joint(s), structures around the joint(s) (periarticular region), muscles, or bones, or establishing that the pain is referred or generalized, may help to establish a differential diagnosis as listed in Table 138-1.

The character of the pain may also help to define the disorder. Acute inflammatory processes such as gouty arthritis, pseudogout, and a septic joint tend to cause severe pain at rest as well as during movement of the joint. The pain associated with more chronic inflammatory diseases of joints such as rheumatoid arthritis and polymyalgia rheumatica tend to be dull and aching in character and associated with stiffness after periods of inactivity. In contrast, structural problems such as osteoarthritis, lumbar spinal stenosis, and fractures, as well as obstructive peripheral vascular disease, characteristically cause more pain during activity such as standing, walking, or use of the affected part than during periods of rest.

Because intensity and severity of pain are so subjective, these aspects are often difficult to quantitate. One way to assess the degree of pain is to identify and characterize functional impairment or disability that results from the pain. After questioning the patient about general functional limitations, the physician should ask about performing specific activities of daily living (ADL) such as standing, walking, climbing and descending stairs, dressing, eating, bathing, washing and grooming, getting out of bed, and standing from a chair. The mnemonic ADEPT, which stands for *A*mbulation, *D*ressing, *E*ating, *P*ersonal hygiene, and *T*ransfers, may remind the examiner when assessing an individual's functional status. Inquiries regarding the patient's ability to perform such tasks as combing hair, turning keys, door knobs, or water taps, holding playing cards, pulling zippers, and buttoning garments not only help to assess functional capabilities but also identify problems that may be helped by specific therapeutic intervention and use of assistive devices.

In attempting to identify a cause of a disability by history (as well as during the physical examination), the examiner must try to distinguish (1) limitations due to pain from those due to (2) true muscle weakness, (3) mechanical musculoskeletal abnormalities, (4) lack of effort due to depression or poor cooperation, and (5) lack of ability to hear or understand the questions.

The nature of the onset as well as the subsequent course of a musculoskeletal problem may help to define the disorder. For example, the history of acute, episodic pain, swelling, and erythema of the base of the great toe that resolves over 5 to 10 days, with or without treatment, in a middle-aged man is consistent with gouty arthritis, whereas the history of slowly progressive pain, joint deformity, and loss of motion without signs of inflammation of a weight-bearing joint is indicative of osteoarthritis. The acute onset of joint pain and swelling in an individual with a chronic articular disease such as rheumatoid arthritis or osteoarthritis should always raise concern of joint sepsis. Similarly, the acute onset of bone pain in an individual with a chronic disorder such as osteoporosis or Paget's disease of bone should raise concern of a fracture or a malignant lesion.

At times, the symptoms that are associated with musculoskeletal pain may be more significant to the patient and more indicative of the underlying disorder than the musculoskeletal pain itself. For example, malaise, depression, and stiffness in the muscles of the neck, shoulders, and pelvic girdle may be the most predominant symptoms in elderly individuals with polymyalgia rheumatica, rheumatoid arthritis, hypothyroid myopathy, and even osteomalacia. In patients with polymyositis, proximal muscle weakness is a much more common and severe symptom than is pain. The presence of fever, chills, and sweats in the patient with musculoskeletal pain mandates a careful search for joint sepsis. More important, it is not uncommon for the elderly individual with a septic joint to present with more subtle symptoms and findings than the severe pain, muscle spasm, swelling and erythema, fever, and leukocytosis that usually characterize septic arthritis in younger individuals. Because septic arthritis may rapidly cause joint damage as well as even jeopardize the life of the individual, one should have a high index of suspicion of joint sepsis in the elderly individual who presents with joint pain and swelling. Joint effusions should be aspirated, and the joint fluid should be examined by Gram stain and cultured for aerobic as well as anaerobic bacteria, fungus, and mycobacteria. Because most cases of joint sepsis are due to hematogenous seeding, blood cultures and a search for a primary source of infection such as pneumonia or urinary tract sepsis should be performed, as well as a careful examination of the skin to look for a portal of entry.

Table 138-1 Common Musculoskeletal Disorders in the Elderly

Pain Localized to Joints
Osteoarthritis
Rheumatoid arthritis
Crystal-induced arthritis:
- Gouty arthritis
- Pseudogout (calcium pyrophosphate dihydrate)
- Hydroxyapatite crystal arthritis

Septic arthritis

Periarticular Pain
Bursitis
Tendonitis

Muscular Pain
Viral syndromes
Polymyalgia rheumatica
Fibrositis (fibromyalgia syndrome, myofasciitis)
Muscle cramps
Myalgias as a component of systemic lupus erythematosus
Muscle pain, cramping, or fatigue with exercise (claudication)
Obstructive peripheral vascular disease
Lumbar spinal stenosis
Polymyositis/dermatomyositis (uncommonly)

Bone Pain
Fractures
Osteoporosis
Osteomalacia
Osteomyelitis
Malignancy metastatic to bone
Paget's disease of bone

Diffuse Pain and Aching
Osteomalacia
Hypothyroidism
Polymyalgia rheumatica
Rheumatoid arthritis
Depression

Physical Examination

The major objectives of performing the physical examination in the elderly patient with rheumatic complaints are to search for evidence of (1) muscle pain (polymyalgia rheumatica) and weakness (polymyositis), (2) periarticular problems (bursitis and tendonitis), (3) structural joint disease (osteoarthritis), (4) inflammatory joint disease (rheumatoid arthritis, gout, pseudogout, spondylitis), (5) bone disease (Paget's disease of bone, osteoporosis, fractures), and (6) systemic connective tissue disease such as systemic lupus erythematosus and vasculitis. The physical evaluation of the elderly patient consists of a thorough general physical examination as well as a detailed examination of the muscles, joints, bones, skin, and neurologic system. Because peripheral vascular disease and vasculitis may present as musculoskeletal pain, a detailed vascular examination should also be performed.

Physical assessment of complaints referable to muscles includes (1) inspection for atrophy, (2) palpation for tenderness and muscle mass, (3) evaluation of passive motion to assess muscle tone for such findings as cog-wheel rigidity, suggestive of Parkinson's disease, and gagenhalten (resistance to movement), which may occur in demented individuals, (4) formal muscle strength testing (see Chapter 93, "Limb Pain and Weakness"), and (5) identification of discrete tender points in the muscle as a result of bursitis or trigger points. Trigger points tend to occur in fairly stereotypic locations (see section on soft-tissue rheumatism). An attempt must be made to distinguish true muscle weakness from a poor effort due to pain or failure to understand the examiner's requests.

The presence of bursitis and tendonitis is suggested on examination by the identification of localized tenderness in the anatomic region of the bursa or tendon as well as pain that is greater during active than passive motion. Specific maneuvers that stress the tendon(s) in question without moving the joint may also be helpful. The most common tendons involved are the supraspinatus tendon at its insertion onto the humeral tuberosity, the bicipital tendon on the anterior aspect of the shoulder, the extensor and abductor tendons of the thumb overlying the radial styloid, flexor tendons of the fingers, and the Achilles tendon. The bursae that most commonly cause pain are the subacromial (subdeltoid) bursa of the shoulder, the olecranon bursa on the tip of the elbow, the trochanteric bursa, which overlies the greater femoral trochanter and causes lateral hip pain that may radiate down the anterior or lateral thigh to the knee, and the anserine bursa, which is located along the medial aspect of the leg several centimeters inferior to the knee joint.

The findings of structural joint disease may include bone overgrowth and joint instability and malalignment, limited joint motion, joint deformity, crepitance on joint motion, joint effusion, and muscle atrophy.

In contrast, inflammatory joint disease is generally manifested by prominent warmth, erythema, swelling, tenderness, and effusion. Loss of joint motion and pain on motion may be seen as a result of structural as well as inflammatory joint disease.

Bone disease is suggested by skeletal deformities such as an accentuated thoracic kyphosis as seen in individuals with osteoporotic vertebral body compression fractures, bowing and enlargement of long bones, which are manifestations of Paget's disease of bone, and shortening and external rotation of the leg as occur with femoral neck fractures. The bones should also be percussed for tenderness.

Manifestations of systemic involvement due to such disorders as giant cell arteritis, systemic vasculitis of the polyarteritis variety, extra-articular rheumatoid disease, and systemic lupus erythematosus may present with positive physical findings owing to involvement of multiple organ systems. As such, a thorough general examination with specific attention to the vascular system should be performed, including assessment of peripheral arterial pulses as well as a search for arterial tenderness, nodularity, bruits, and ischemic changes.

Laboratory Tests

The interpretation of laboratory data in the evaluation of the etiology of musculoskeletal pain in an elderly person must be viewed in terms of normal laboratory changes in this population.

Erythrocyte Sedimentation Rate. The mean erythrocyte sedimentation rate (ESR by Westergren or Wintrobe method) rises with each decade of life. This rise does not seem to be related to sex or race. Forty percent of people over 50 years of age have an ESR greater than 20 mm per hour. The ESR of an older person may be greater than 30 mm per hour, but a result greater than 40 mm per hour should be considered abnormal.

Antinuclear Antibodies. The antinuclear antibodies (ANAs) in elderly people are most commonly directed against nucleic acid histone. They typically produce a homogeneous or diffuse immunofluorescent pattern. Three percent of people aged 16 to 50 years have a positive ANA. Sixteen percent of people aged 60 to 91 years have a positive ANA. The titer is usually low (1:16 or less).

Rheumatoid Factor. Rheumatoid factor, an immunoglobulin, usually immunoglobulin M (IgM) which binds to immunoglobulin G (IgG), has been found to be elevated in 1 to 3 percent of people younger than age 65 and 16 percent of people aged 65 to

103 who are healthy. Half of these have a titer of 1:80 or less; 20 percent have a titer of 1:160 or greater.

Gamma Globulin. With advancing age, changes occur in B- and T-lymphocyte function that alter the gamma globulin concentration. Immunoglobulin A (IgA) remains relatively unchanged, whereas IgG and IgM decrease, an overall relative hypogammaglobulinemia. A clone of lymphocytes may produce homogeneous immunoglobulin that produces a characteristic M spike (M component) on serum protein electrophoresis. IgG and IgM migrate in the gamma globulin region, whereas IgA is contained in the beta globulin region. Monoclonal immunoglobulin disorders may be due to benign or malignant conditions. A serum M component IgG concentration of less than 2 g/dl or an IgM M component of less than 1 g/dl suggests a benign process, particularly if levels remain unchanged. A malignant monoclonal gammopathy is suggestive of the presence of Bence-Jones proteinuria, hypoalbuminemia, plasmacytosis of more than 20 percent with increased numbers of atypical and immature forms on bone marrow aspiration or biopsy, a progressive increase in the quantity of the monoclonal immunoglobulin, and a progressive decrease in the other immunoglobulin classes.

Serum Protein. Total serum protein and albumin levels are slightly lower in the older age groups.

Common Disorders in Elderly Patients That Cause Musculoskeletal Pain

Osteoarthritis

Osteoarthritis is the most prevalent of the diseases that present as musculoskeletal pain in the elderly. Autopsy studies demonstrate the degenerative changes of osteoarthritis as early as the second decade and in 90 percent of individuals by 40 years of age. Radiographic changes of osteoarthritis have been identified in the weight-bearing joints of 85 percent of people by the age of 75, although *only* 25 to 30 percent are symptomatic. The large weight-bearing joints—the knees, hips, and spine—are the most common sites of involvement. Pain initially occurs with weight bearing and use of the affected joint and is relieved with rest. With disease progression, pain may occur at rest and may interfere with sleep. Stiffness occurs after inactivity and tends to resolve after several minutes of motion, in contrast to the profound morning stiffness that frequently occurs in patients with rheumatoid arthritis. Osteoarthritis of the digits (distal and proximal interphalangeal joints of the fingers, carpometacarpal and interphalangeal joints of the thumb, and the metatarsophalangeal joints of the great toes) is much more common in women than in men. Pain in these joints is less common than is "knobby" deformity of the joint and angulation of the digit. However, some individuals experience significant pain, tenderness, erythema, and swelling during initial phases of involvement (so-called inflammatory osteoarthritis).

Physical examination may reveal bony enlargement of the distal interphalangeal and proximal interphalangeal joints as well as flexion contractures and deviation of the phalanges. A squared appearance of the thumb may result from osteoarthritic changes of the carpometacarpal joint. Audible and palpable crepitance with motion, restricted active and passive range of motion, irregular bony enlargement of the joint, joint instability due to ligamentous laxity, joint effusion, and quadriceps atrophy may be found on examination of the osteoarthritic knee. The patient with osteoarthritis of the knee or hip often walks with a limp (so-called antalgic gait). The physical findings often elicited in the patient with osteoarthritis of the cervical spine or lumbar spine are loss of motion and pain on motion of the affected part of the spine and paraspinous muscle tenderness and spasm. Neurologic deficits, specifically weakness or sensory loss and pain, may be present as a result of nerve root compression, which is commonly due to osteophytes of lumbar facet and intervertebral joints.

The radiographic appearance of osteoarthritis includes joint-space narrowing, sclerosis and cysts in the bone beneath the articular cartilage (subchondral bone), and bone spurs (osteophytes). The weight-bearing aspects of the affected joints tend to demonstrate the most severe changes. In the spine, loss of the normal spinal curves, intervertebral disk-space narrowing, sclerosis of vertebral margins, osteophytes, joint-space narrowing and sclerosis of the posterior (apophyseal) joints, and subluxation may be seen.

The laboratory evaluation of the patient with osteoarthritis is generally normal. Synovial fluid has noninflammatory characteristics, including fewer than 2,000 white blood cells per cubic milliliter, a predominance of mononuclear cells, and a good mucin clot. Cartilage fragments may also be seen on synovial fluid analysis.

Pseudogout

Calcium pyrophosphate arthropathy due to the deposition of calcium pyrophosphate dihydrate (CPPD) in articular cartilage occurs in 5 percent of adults. The radiographic appearance of abnormal deposition of calcium salts has been noted to increase with increasing age, and by the ninth decade is present in 25 to 30 percent of individuals. The CPPD crystal deposition most commonly occurs in the fibrocartilage of the menisci and symphysis pubis, the articular cartilage of the knees, and the triangular cartilage of the wrists. Pain presents in several ways. Monarticular pain, the most common presentation, is called pseudogout because of its resemblance to an acute gouty attack. Individuals are asymptomatic between attacks. The other presentations resemble other arthritides and are appropriately called pseudo-osteoarthritis, pseudorheumatoid arthritis, and pseudoneuropathic arthritis. Pseudogout may present as pain, swelling, erythema, restricted joint motion, and effusion of either a single or multiple joints. The knee and wrist are the most frequently affected joints.

A definite diagnosis of acute pseudogout requires identification of CPPD crystals in synovial fluid or cartilage biopsy specimens by x-ray diffraction or the presence of typical radiographic articular chondrocalcinosis and the identification by polarized microscopy of rhomboid or rectangular positively birefringent crystals from the synovial fluid. Biopsy during an acute attack reveals proliferation of synovial cells, vascular congestion, fibrinous exudate, and leukocytes in the tissues. The finding of inflammatory synovial fluid with CPPD crystals within leukocytes does *not* necessarily mean that the crystals initiated the joint inflammation. Pyogenic arthritis and acute gouty arthritis may also present in this way. Synovial fluid analysis should always include Gram stain, culture, and examination under polarizing light. Metabolic diseases associated with CPPD deposition are hyperparathyroidism, hemochromatosis, diabetes mellitus, hypophosphatasia, Wilson's disease, and hypothyroidism, although aging is the most common condition associated with the deposition of CPPD crystals in articular structures.

Rheumatoid Arthritis

Approximately 10 percent of patients with rheumatoid arthritis experience the onset of their disease after age 60. Seventy-five percent of these individuals have a disease course identical to that in younger patients, i.e., pain and stiffness of the proximal interphalangeal, metacarpophalangeal, metatarsophalangeal, wrist, knee, elbow, ankle, or shoulder joints in a symmetric distribution, with malaise, fatigue, or aching poorly localized to the joint. The other 25 percent have a more acute onset and severe constitutional symptoms: anorexia, weight loss, malaise, depression, severe morning stiffness, a lesser degree of female preponderance, and a greater frequency of shoulder and cervical involvement, which may suggest the diagnosis of polymyalgia rheumatica.

Physical examination may reveal soft-tissue swelling, warmth, tenderness, pain on motion, joint effusions, muscle atrophy, joint contractures, and restricted joint motion. Loss of joint motion may be the result of joint effusions, splinting due to joint pain, muscle spasm, and contractures of articular connective tissue (joint capsule, tendons, ligaments, and muscle). Ulnar deviation of the fingers, hyperextension of the proximal interphalangeal joints associated with flexion of the distal interphalangeal joints (so-called swan-neck deformity), and flexion contractures of the proximal interphalangeal joints associated with hyperextension of the distal interphalangeal joints (so-called boutonnière deformities) are characteristic deformities. The combination of synovitis of the metacarpophalangeal joints, ulnar deviation of the fingers, atrophy of the interosseous muscles of the hands, and synovitis of the wrists with soft-tissue swelling over the dorsum of the wrists is a presentation that is quite specific for rheumatoid arthritis.

Radiographs of rheumatoid joints may reveal joint effusions, soft-tissue swelling, periarticular and diffuse demineralization, diffuse joint-space narrowing indicative of cartilage loss, and bony erosions and cysts (see Fig. 89-5, page 382).

Laboratory evaluation generally reveals elevation of the ESR, C-reactive protein, and gamma globulins. Rheumatoid factor is found in approximately 75 percent of individuals with rheumatoid arthritis. Synovial fluid from involved joints is characteristically inflammatory, with white blood cell counts ranging from 12,000 to 50,000 cells/ml^3, generally with a predominance of polymorphonuclear leukocytes, poor viscosity, a poor mucin clot, and protein levels greater than 4 g/dl. Cultures for microorganisms are negative.

Systemic Lupus Erythematosus and Drug-Induced Lupus-Like Syndromes

Although idiopathic systemic lupus erythematosus (SLE) occurs most commonly in women during the child-bearing years, approximately 12 percent of individuals who develop SLE do so after age 50; approximately half of these are men. Initial symptoms may be nonspecific and include weight loss, fatigue, and myalgias. Chest pain due to pericarditis and pleuritis is often a predominant symptom. Other manifestations are joint pain and inflammation, skin rashes, sun sensitivity, hair loss, mouth and nasal ulcers, digital vasospasm (Raynaud's phenomenon), seizures, organic brain syndromes, psychiatric disturbances, renal disease (specifically glomerulonephritis), and hematologic disorders, including hemolytic anemia, thrombocytopenia, leukopenia, and production of antibodies to one's own tissues, such as ANAs. (See section on laboratory tests in this chapter and Chapter 96, "Laboratory and Radiographic Abnormalities in Rheumatic Diseases.")

Because elderly patients are more likely than younger individuals to be treated with medications such as antiarrhythmics (procainamide, quinidine, and beta-blockers), which may be associated with the development of drug-induced lupus-like syndromes, this disorder should be considered in the differential diagnosis of joint pain or other lupus-like symptoms. Pleuritis and pericarditis are more common, while renal and central nervous system involvement is less common in drug-induced lupus-like syndromes than in idiopathic SLE.

Gout

Gouty arthritis is primarily a disease of middle-aged men and postmenopausal women. Elderly individuals of both sexes have increased presence of conditions such as renal disease, chronic diuretic therapy, and diseases associated with accelerated cell proliferation such as hemolytic anemia, lymphomas, and leukemias, which increase the urate pool and thus the likelihood of developing gouty arthritis.

Gouty arthritis usually presents as acute arthritis of the first metatarsophalangeal joint (joint at the base of the great toe), the instep of the foot, the ankle, or the knee. The wrist and finger joints may be involved less commonly. Simultaneous involvement of multiple joints, so-called polyarticular gouty arthritis, occurs more commonly in the elderly individual than in younger patients. The diagnosis is established by joint aspiration and identification under the polarized microscope of needle-shaped, negatively birefringent monosodium urate crystals within synovial fluid leukocytes. The synovial fluid should also be examined by Gram stain and cultured to exclude the concurrent presence of joint sepsis.

Elderly individuals, particularly women with renal insufficiency who are receiving thiazide diuretics, may develop tophaceous gout in the absence of previous histories of acute gouty arthritis.

Soft-Tissue Rheumatism (Fibrositis, Bursitis, and Tendonitis)

Soft-tissue rheumatism, also termed nonarticular rheumatism and periarthritis to denote disorders involving structures around but not within the joint, includes fibrositis (also called fibromyalgia and the myofasciitis syndrome), tendonitis, and bursitis. These problems are common in the elderly and need to be distinguished from diseases of joints, muscles, and bones.

Patients with fibrositis typically present with aching and stiffness of the neck, back, shoulders, and hips. The pain is aggravated by cool, damp weather, fatigue, and emotional stress and is relieved with heat, relaxation, and a warm, dry climate. Physical examination characteristically reveals areas of discrete tenderness in the soft tissues in stereotypic locations in the posterior and anterior neck muscles, trapezial ridges, rhomboid muscles, lumbar paraspinous muscles, upper buttocks, and distal medial thighs. The periarticular shoulder areas, costochondral junctions, epicondyles, anserine bursal, and femoral trochanteric regions may also be sources of pain and tenderness (Fig. 138-1). Firm palpation of these regions causes local discomfort as well as pain that may radiate for some distance, such as down the arm and up the neck, in the case of the tender point in the trapezial ridge, thereby acquiring the name "trigger points." Laboratory studies are characteristically normal.

The tendons that most commonly become inflamed as a result of repetitive trauma or an associated connective tissue disease are the supraspinatus tendon at its insertion onto the greater humeral tuberosity under the acromion, the bicipital tendon in the bicipital groove along the anterior aspect of the shoulder, the abductor and extensor tendons of the thumb along the radial aspect of the wrist, and the Achilles tendon. Pain due to tendonitis is characteristically aggravated by active motion more than during passive motion, by active resistance, and by direct palpation of the inflamed site. For example, the pain of supraspinatus tendonitis is aggravated by abduction of the shoulder against resistance while reaching behind to put an arm in a coat or shirt sleeve and by lying on one's side during sleep. Pain due to bicipital tendonitis is aggravated by flexion of the elbow and shoulder against resistance of carrying objects. The pain due to inflammation of the extensor and abductor tendons of the thumb, so-called DeQuervain's tenosynovitis, is aggravated by grasping objects and ulnar deviation of the wrist while the thumb is held in the closed fist, the so-called Finkelstein sign.

The bursae that most frequently become inflamed and cause pain in elderly individuals are the subacromial (subdeltoid), the olecranon bursa overlying the extensor surface of

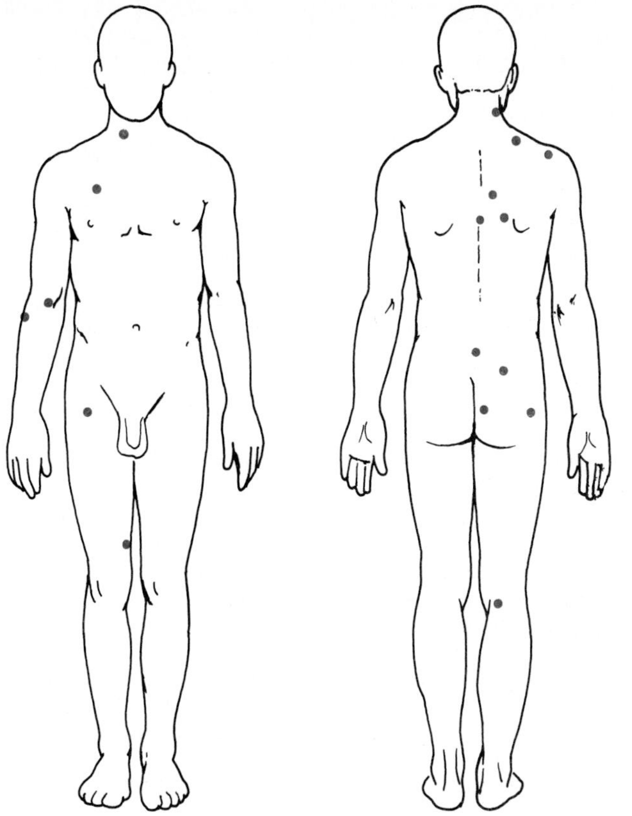

Figure 138-1 Fibrositic tender points.

the elbow, the trochanteric bursa located over the greater femoral trochanter on the lateral aspect of the hip, and the anserine bursa, which is located just below the knee on the medial surface of the tibia. Bursitis may be due to repetitive traumatic injury, inflammatory rheumatic disorders such as rheumatoid arthritis and gout, or an infectious process. Anserine bursitis is particularly common in women with osteoarthritis of the knee. Like supraspinatus tendonitis, the pain due to subacromial bursitis is aggravated by lying on the affected shoulder and by abduction and rotation of the shoulder. Osteoarthritis of the joint between the distal end of the clavicle and the acromion, the so-called acromioclavicular joint, is another common cause of shoulder pain that is aggravated by abduction in the elderly individual. However, the tenderness in this problem is located on the top of the shoulder at the anatomic site of the acromioclavicular joint rather than in the lateral shoulder area of the subacromial region. Olecranon bursitis, which is often due to leaning on the elbows, is particularly common in bed-bound patients who move themselves with their elbows. Often discrete swelling and sometimes a bursal effusion are found on examination. Owing to the proximity of the olecranon bursa to the skin, infection due to direct introduction of bacteria through the skin may occur. In contrast, the trochanteric bursa is a deep structure that is located over the lateral and posterior aspect of the greater femoral trochanter under the abductor muscles of the hip. Pain due to trochanteric bursitis is typically aggravated by lying on the affected side, which may interrupt sleep, and by activities that require forceful contraction of the hip abductors, such as standing and climbing stairs. The pain frequently radiates down the lateral and anterior thigh to the knee. The pain may be so severe as to interfere with walking. A discrete area of tenderness over the greater femoral trochanters can usually be identified on examination, as can aggravation of pain during resisted abduction of the hip. The hip motion is usually normal, or internal rotation may be limited owing to the presence of osteoarthritis in the hip joint.

Polymyalgia Rheumatica and Giant Cell Arteritis

Polymyalgia rheumatica occurs almost exclusively in individuals over 50 years of age and has a peak incidence in individuals in their mid-sixties. Polymyalgia rheumatica typically manifests as aching in the muscles of the neck, shoulders, and pelvic girdle, and is often associated with profound morning stiffness, which may be confused with rheumatoid arthritis. Fatigue, lethargy, anorexia, weight loss, malaise, apathy, and depression are common associated symptoms. The muscles are frequently tender on examination, but profound weakness is not a clinical feature. ESRs typically are elevated, with ESRs by Westergren method often in the range of 50 to 80 mm per hour. A normochromic, normocytic anemia is a frequent laboratory finding. In contrast to inflammatory muscle problems (polymyositis), muscle enzymes, electromyographic studies (EMGs), and muscle biopsies in patients with polymyalgia rheumatica are normal.

Approximately 15 percent of individuals with polymyalgia rheumatica also have giant cell (temporal) arteritis. This form of vasculitis affects medium and large arteries and most commonly involves the branches of the external carotid artery. The vertebral, common carotid, and subclavian arteries and even the aorta and its abdominal branches may be affected. Like polymyalgia rheumatica, giant cell arteritis occurs more frequently in women than men and is a disorder of elderly individuals. In addition to the muscular symptoms of polymyalgia rheumatica, the individual with giant cell arteritis may present with headache, scalp pain, visual disturbances, and jaw pain with chewing due to vascular inflammation, as well as profound constitutional symptoms, including malaise, fatigue, apathy, weight loss, depression, and fevers. Scalp and temporal artery tenderness, nodularity, and diminished arterial pulses may be found on physical examination. Detailed visual field and visual acuity testing should be performed to evaluate for visual impairments. Funduscopy should include inspection for retinal infarctions, hemorrhage, cotton wool patches, and blurring and pallor of the optic disk. A detailed examination of the peripheral vascular tree should be performed that includes palpation of peripheral pulses for arterial pulsations and tenderness, auscultation for bruits, and examination for ischemic changes. Laboratory abnormalities in patients with giant cell arteritis characteristically include markedly elevated ESRs (often over 100 mm per hour by the Westergren method), elevation of other acute-phase proteins such as C-reactive protein and alpha globulins, elevation of alkaline phosphatase, and normochromic, normocytic anemia. Biopsies of the superficial temporal artery (a procedure which can be done under local anesthesia) typically reveal disruption of the internal elastic lamina, infiltration by histiocytic giant cells, lymphocytes, plasma cells, and fibroblasts, and thrombosis in the vessel lumen at the site of inflammation.

Osteoporosis

Clinical osteoporosis is the state of too little bone mass that can result in bone fracture. Because the maximal skeletal mass is less in women than men and because skeletal loss with aging is greater in women than men, osteoporosis is primarily a disease of postmenopausal women.

Osteoporosis may present as a painless loss of height and development of an exaggerated kyphosis (forward bend of the thoracic spine) due to compression fractures of vertebral bodies or as acute pain associated with fracture, most commonly of a vertebral body(ies), femoral neck, or distal forearm (Colles' fracture), after minimal trauma. Pain from collapsed thoracic and lumbar vertebrae may radiate to the chest and may be confused with pain due to coronary artery disease or to the discomfort of reflux esophagitis, common medical problems in the elderly. Coughing, sneezing, and straining may exacerbate the back pain. The pain due to vertebral compression fractures tends to subside over the course of a few months. Between fractures, the individual is generally pain-free. However, back deformities may result in chronic back pain due to paraspinous muscle spasm and mechanical stress on ligaments, muscles, and joints of the back.

In the United States, the incidence of hip fractures among white women increases fourfold every decade after the age of 50 years. Elderly people who have sustained a femoral neck fracture are 20 times more likely to fracture the other hip. The mortality rate within the first 6 months after sustaining a femoral neck fracture is approximately 20 percent. Falls are the leading cause of accidental death in the elderly.

Osteoporosis is often noted incidentally on chest radiographs as diffuse demineralization and vertebral compression fractures. Generally, 50 percent of skeletal mass must be lost before demineralization may be apparent on plain radiographs. Osteoporotic vertebral body compression fractures generally have an anterior-wedge appearance that produces the dorsal kyphosis. Such fractures most commonly occur in the mid-thoracic to mid-lumbar regions. Compression fractures in the cervical and upper thoracic regions and posterior vertebral body wedging are unusual in osteoporosis and may be due to other processes such as infection, metastatic tumor, or multiple myeloma.

Laboratory evaluation of age-related osteoporosis includes normal calcium, phosphate, and alkaline phosphatase levels. (The alkaline phosphatase level may be elevated in the presence of a healing fracture.) Parathyroid hormone and vitamin D measurements may be helpful. Measurement of bone mineral content may now be quantitatively performed by dual-photon densitometry (absorption) and computed tomographic techniques.

Loss of bone mass may be due to a number of (1) endocrine diseases, such as hyperthyroidism, hyperparathyroidism, and Cushing's syndrome; (2) metabolic diseases, including chronic renal failure, chronic liver disease, and calcium and vitamin D malabsorption; (3) drugs, including glucocorticosteroids, long-term heparin therapy, anticonvulsants, and alcohol; and (4) multiple myeloma, leukemia, lymphoma, and malignancy metastatic to bone. Clinical data and laboratory studies should be scrutinized for evidence of these secondary causes of osteoporosis.

Paget's Disease of Bone

Paget's disease of bone is rare before age 40 but increases progressively with age thereafter. Although Paget's disease of bone causes chronic, aching pain in only 10 percent of affected individuals, the fact that 3 percent of the overall population and 10 percent of individuals in their eighties have the disease makes this form of bone disease a fairly common cause of musculoskeletal pain in elderly individuals. The disease most commonly affects the spine, femur, skull, and pelvis. Bowing of the long bones of the legs and enlargement of the skull are typical deformities. Hearing loss, dental problems, visual impairment, headache, and neck pain may result from involvement of the head. Involvement of the pelvis and leg bones predisposes to osteoarthritis.

The cardinal laboratory finding is elevation of the alkaline phosphatase level, which may be increased as much as 20-fold, reflecting increased osteoblastic (bone formation) activity, which is also demonstrated by increased areas of activity (so-called hot areas) on bone scans.

Ninety-five percent of patients with Paget's disease are diagnosed in the asymptomatic state by an incidental finding of an elevated alkaline phosphatase level or radiographic appearance of coarse trabecular markings, increased bone size, and a thickened cortex due to periosteal new bone formation. In contrast to the decrease in bone density of osteoporosis, Paget's disease of the spine may feature a homogeneous increase of vertebral body density (ivory vertebra), central vertebral body osteopenia with thickening of vertebral margins, and coarsening of central vertebral trabeculae. The affected vertebral bodies may have increased thickness without disruption of the cortex in contrast to the manifestations of metastatic disease of the spine. The involved femur bows laterally, and the radiograph may demonstrate the radiolucent appearance of an advancing wedge of osteopenia, the border between normal and pagetic bone. Cystic-appearing lesions may also develop in weight-bearing bones at sites of active bone resorption. The skull radiograph may feature well-demarcated areas of osteopenia, osteoporosis circumscripta, in the frontal, parietal, or occipital area. The cortex may appear thickened, and the base of the skull may flatten (platybasia). When the pelvis is involved, osteoblastic areas resemble the lesions of prostatic cancer metastatic to bone. Paget's disease, however, thickens the pelvic brim and widens the pubic and ischial rami. Also helpful in distinguishing Paget's disease of bone from prostatic cancer metastatic to bone is the finding of elevated prostatic fractions of acid phosphatase and prostatic specific antigen in metastatic prostatic cancer and normal levels in the man with Paget's disease of bone. Osteoarthritis of the hip (medial joint-space narrowing) and knee may manifest secondary to pagetic disease of the pelvis.

References

Bennett RM. Fibrositis. In: Kelley WN, Harris ED, Ruddy S, et al, eds. Textbook of rheumatology. 3rd ed. Philadelphia: WB Saunders, 1989:541.

Giansiracusa DF, Kantrowitz FG. Rheumatic and metabolic bone diseases in the elderly. Lexington, MA: The Collamore Press, 1982.

Kantrowitz FG, Giansiracusa DF. Rheumatic disease. In: Rowe JW, Besdine RW, eds. Geriatric medicine. 2nd ed. Boston: Little, Brown, 1988.

Kay M, et al, eds. Aging, immunity, and arthritic disease. Aging series. Volume II. New York: Raven Press, 1980.

Schumacher HR Jr, Klippel JH, Robinson DR, eds. Primer on the rheumatic diseases. 9th ed. Atlanta: The Arthritis Foundation, 1988.

Sheon RP, Moskowitz RW, Goldberg VM. Soft tissue rheumatic pain. Philadelphia: Lea & Febiger, 1987.

Swezey RL, Spiegel TM. Evaluation and treatment of local musculoskeletal disorders in elderly patients. Geriatrics, January 1979:56.

Discharge Planning for the Older Patient

Sandra A. Hall, RN, MSN

Deborah Wexler, MSW

Rosalie S. Wolf, PhD

139

Definition

Discharge planning is the process of coordinating posthospitalization, health, and supportive services to meet patient needs and facilitate maximal functioning. Effective discharge planning is critical with older patients. They are likely to have multiple chronic health problems and slower recovery rates after acute illnesses or injuries. Discharge planning should begin on the day of admission.

Principles of Discharge Planning

The following are the principles of discharge planning:

1. Assess the patient's status in the following areas: physical/medical, cognitive/emotional, functional, social, economic, and environmental.

2. Use a team approach. Consult with the nurse, social worker, physical therapist, occupational therapist, nutritionist, psychiatrist, and other professionals as appropriate.

3. Beware of ageist stereotypes. Most older people are alert and manage well at home with minimal or no assistance. The patient's overall ability to function, when not acutely ill, is more important than the diagnosis.

4. Make sure that the patient can hear you. Note that people with hearing loss sometimes may appear confused or paranoid.

5. Involve the patient (if competent) and family, as well as other significant people, including the community social workers, visiting nurses, and neighbors. Make sure that all decision makers have adequate information. Family conferences can be helpful. Be aware of family dynamics, issues, and problems.

6. Do not assume that the family will provide all or most of the patient care. Family members may be unavailable (because of work or other responsibilities) or unwilling or unable (physically or emotionally) to help. They may need training, assistance, or relief in order to provide care.

7. Consider not only the needs and desires of the patient and family but also financial constraints and the availability and eligibility criteria of services and facilities in the patient's geographic area.

8. Realize that nursing home placements, as well as plans for in-home services, may require filling out forms, receiving approval, and waiting for beds or other services.

9. Plan for the "least restrictive" environment. Allow the patient as much independence as is safely possible.

10. Do not be surprised if the patient or family is reluctant or refuses to go along with the team's discharge plan. It often takes time for people to agree to placement or in-home services, even if this is clearly the only safe option. The patient or family may *never* agree to your plan. If the patient is competent, or if a family member has guardianship, there is little you can do except express your professional opinion. If you are really concerned about the patient's safety, consult a lawyer or adult protective service agency.

Patient Assessment for Discharge Planning

Before decisions about posthospitalization care are made, a comprehensive, multidimensional patient assessment is necessary. The following is a guide.

Medical and Physical Assessment

In addition to your routine history and physical examination, consider the type and amount of discomfort or incapacitation the patient will sustain on discharge, any restrictions on activity, and the likely consequences and complications of treatment. Keep in mind the patient's (and family's) understanding of the feelings about the diagnosis, prognosis, and treatment plan.

Consider the need for continued medical supervision or treatment. How often will the patient need to see a physician or other care providers? How are medications to be administered (e.g., orally or intravenously)? How often? Can they be administered by the patient? By the family? Is a nurse needed to administer medications or monitor their use?

Is physical, occupational, or speech therapy needed? What is the goal (e.g., return to baseline, maintain present level of functioning, improvement)? What is the patient's rehabilitation potential? How often are services needed? How long will they be needed?

Will the patient need a cane, walker, wheelchair, brace, commode, hospital bed, respirator, or oxygen? For how long? Will the patient leave with any of the following: a new colostomy or tracheostomy, intravenous or tube feedings, a decubitus ulcer, any open wound sites or infected areas, an unstable medical condition, diarrhea, constipation, or incontinence? What kind of care is needed? How often? For how long?

Does the patient maintain adequate nutrition? If not, are any of the following needed: dental care, diet counseling, monitoring, help with meal preparation?

Cognitive and Emotional Assessment

Check the patient's orientation, memory, ability to reason, and use of good judgment. Is he or she alert or confused? If confused, is this an acute or chronic problem? Is cognitive loss mild or severe? How does it affect the patient's ability to function? Is the patient able to remember appointments, take medications, cook, manage money, communicate, and the like?

Is the patient cooperative or combative? Does he or she wander, fall frequently, exhibit extreme restlessness or inappropriate behaviors? If left unattended, would the patient constitute a danger to him- or herself or others? (Consider safety in cooking, smoking, driving, and so forth.) Is the patient competent to make decisions for him- or herself? If incompetent, in which areas? Does he or she have or need a guardian?

Has the patient experienced any recent or unresolved losses? Does he or she have any problems with sleeping, change of appetite or mood? Does he or she look sad, complain of loneliness or dissatisfaction with life? Is the patient depressed or

Table 139-1 Community Resources for the Elderly

Type	Service description	Service providers	Service payment
Home health	Nursing services involve case assessments, development of care plans, administration of medications and treatments, and monitoring of vital signs and education Rehabilitation services (including physical, occupational, and speech therapies) are offered in the home to help patients achieve and maintain maximum functioning	Visiting nurse association Home health agencies Public health department Rehabilitation organizations	Medicare, if medically necessary (must meet requirements) Medicaid, if patient income eligible and service deemed appropriate Sliding fee scale Fee for service
Home care	Personal care worker assists with personal care, such as bathing, hair washing, shaving, dressing Homemakers assist older people with light housekeeping tasks, meal preparation, shopping, errands, and management of money; provide emotional support and escort service Chore services (heavy household cleaning and yard work) are available in some localities	Family agencies (e.g., Catholic Charities) Home health agencies Home care and homemaker organizations	Medicaid, if patient income eligible and service deemed appropriate Title XX if client income eligible State support if client income eligible Sliding fee scale Fee for service (not covered by Medicare)
Day care	Day health programs provide a supervised environment for elders with some loss of physical and/or mental functioning but who are reasonably independent in their activities of daily living; nursing, medical, and rehabilitative services are offered in addition to recreation and socialization	Nursing homes Senior centers Hospitals Social service agencies Councils on aging	Medicaid, if patient income eligible and service deemed appropriate Sliding fee scale Fee for service
Family care, foster care (adults)	Applicants must meet financial eligibility criteria, be mostly alert, and require minimal to moderate assistance with activities of daily living	Nonprofit social service	Medicaid
Home communication systems	A unique communi-call system provides emergency notification through computer relay and transmitter for persons living alone and at risk because of health; *not* recommended for the confused or demented	Regional hospitals Home care agencies and visiting nurse associations can make referrals to system	Low cost; at times available through prearranged programs
Casework counseling, crisis intervention, protective services	Older persons and their families are offered assistance with the emotional and practical problems associated with aging. Each community has an agency designated to investigate elder abuse and neglect, offer appropriate services (counseling and concrete help), and initiate legal action as needed.	Local legal service agencies	No fee charged by social service agencies; other providers accept Medicare, Medex
Information and referral	Information services about community programs, benefits, and facilities, as well as advocacy and support assistance in the resolution of problems involving the above, are available to elders	Senior service programs Town/city senior programs	
Legal services	Special elder advocacy units provide legal assistance and consultation to senior citizens and their families	Local legal service agencies	No fee for senior citizens

Table 139-1 (*Continued*)

Type	Service description	Service providers	Service payment
Nutrition	Home-delivered meals (Meals-on-Wheels) are available for the homebound who are unable to prepare their own meals and who have no assistance (family or homemaker) present during the day; meals are provided at noontime, Monday through Friday Congregate meal sites provide noontime meals for those who can get out but find it difficult to prepare meals and/or do not wish to eat alone; meals are available Monday through Friday; van transportation is often provided	Senior centers Organizations serving older adults Churches Nursing homes Hospital	Donations
Transportation	Transportation is available for Medicaid recipients with doctor's letter stating they cannot use public transportation owing to physical disability. It should be used for medical appointments only, and is available to home care clients. A limited number of trips are available per month for appointments, errands, and social activities. Van services are available for medical appointments, shopping, and social activities.	Regional transit authorities Private transportation organizations Senior centers Elder service agencies	Medicaid, if client income eligible State and federal subsidization Donations Fee for service
Visually impaired program	Program provides home visits for visually impaired and newly blind, information and referral, advocacy, transport, various homemaker services, and large assortment of personal, household, recreational, communication, and visual items for the visually impaired and blind	State Commission for Blind (must be certified legally blind) Private associations for blind	Medicaid Private pay
Rehabilitation	An intensive therapeutic program is provided. Patients must have good potential for rehabilitation and require at least two skilled rehab services (physical, occupational, speech therapies) on a daily basis per physician's orders.	Rehabilitation hospitals Rehabilitation clinics Outpatient physical therapy, occupational therapy, speech therapy located in acute care hospitals	Medicare Medex Medicaid Private insurance Fee for service
Mental health care, alcoholism treatment (outpatient)	Home visits are available for assessments and ongoing treatments; services are also available to patient's family. Note that for alcohol/drug detox programs, the client must make *initial* and *daily* phone calls while waiting for an opening in order to show commitment to treatment.	Nonprofit family/social service agencies Community mental health centers, and geriatric mental health clinics and outreach services Private practitioners Outpatient psychiatric alcoholism treatment Community health education and self-help groups (e.g., Alcoholics Anonymous)	Medicare Medex Medicaid Private insurance Private pay Sliding fee
Social services	Casework and counseling are available to assist older people and their families with some of the emotional and psychological problems associated with aging Protective services offer assistance to older adults who have limited mental, emotional, and physical functioning, which may result in harm or hazard to themselves or others Friendly visiting and senior companion programs provide volunteers to visit isolated home-bound or nursing home elders on a regular basis	Family social service agencies Senior service programs Community mental health centers	Medicaid, if client income eligible and services deemed appropriate Medicare, if medically necessary Title XX, if client income eligible State-subsidized services Sliding fee scale

Table 139-2 Long-Term Care Facilities for the Elderly

Type	Service description	Service providers	Service payment
Level 1	Offers skilled rehabilitative *services* 7 days/week, including intensive physical, occupational, and speech therapy, and nursing care; for patients with qualified rehabilitation potential; short-term service only	Skilled nursing facility	Medicare, Title XVIII eligibility, if patient meets rigid rehabilitation potential eligibility requirements 3-day hospital stay required
Level 2	Offers total nursing care in relation to five ADLs: bathing, feeding, dressing, ambulation, bladder/bowel; for patients with debilitating illnesses and those who, with a program of intensive restorative care, may regain some areas of independence in relation to five areas of ADLs	Skilled nursing facility	Medicaid, Title XIX eligibility, if patient is income eligible and service deemed appropriate Private pay
Level 3	Offers nursing care in relation to bathing, feeding, dressing, ambulation, bladder/bowel with minimum to moderate assistance; for patients who may or may not require assistance in all five areas of ADLs; therapeutic services also available	Intermediate care facility	Medicaid, Title XIX eligibility, if patient is income eligible and service deemed appropriate Private pay
Level 4	Offers protective supervision; for patients who do not require medical or nursing care	Rest home Retirement home Personal care home	Medicaid, Title XIX eligibility, if patient income eligible and service deemed appropriate Private pay
Chronic care	Offers at least weekly physician visits in addition to skilled nursing and regular intervention by therapists and technicians; for patients who require intermittent intravenous lines and respirators, and whose debilitating condition is expected to continue for some time	Chronic disease hospital	Medicaid, Title XIX eligibility, if patient is income eligible and service deemed appropriate Private pay
Respite care	Offers temporary nursing home placement for patients in order to provide temporary relief to family caretakers; category available in limited number of states	Skilled nursing facility Intermediate care facility Rest home In-home caregivers	Medicaid Private pay

Abbreviation: ADLs = activities of daily living.

anxious? If so, is this an acute or chronic problem? How severe is it, and how does it affect the patient? Is this problem being treated? Does the patient threaten or talk about suicide? Have there been any suicide attempts in the past? Does the patient have a past psychiatric history?

Does the patient hallucinate or exhibit marked behavioral or thought disorder? Is this a new or old problem? Is it being treated? Does the patient have a drinking problem?

Finally, consider any other problems or information reported by patient, hospital staff, family, neighbors, or community caregivers.

Functional Assessment

Assess the patient's ability to manage activities of daily living (toileting, bathing, eating, dressing, grooming, communicating, ambulating, climbing stairs, using a wheelchair or walker, and transferring from bed to chair) and instrumental activities of daily living (using the telephone, shopping, preparing meals, doing household chores and laundry, taking medications, handling money, getting around—driving, using buses or taxis).

Social, Economic, and Environmental Assessment

Where, and with whom, does the patient live? Is this arrangement satisfactory to the patient? The family? How much help is the family willing and able to provide? Is this adequate? Is other help available from friends or neighbors? Is anyone available in case of emergency?

Are there any family problems or issues that might affect patient care at home (e.g., alcoholism, depression, marital problems)? Does the patient or family seek intervention? Does the family need some relief from patient care? Has the patient been neglected or abused (physically or psychologically) at home? Has there been any material abuse (mishandling of money or property)? Have any social service or home health agencies been involved?

What health insurance does the patient carry? What kind of care and how much is covered? Does the patient have the financial resources (income, savings, help from family) to cover living expenses? Are any health care costs not covered by insurance? If so, does he or she qualify for assistance from governmental or private agencies?

Are there any health or safety hazards at home or in the neighborhood? Does the home have heat, hot water, and cooking facilities? Is there an accessible bathroom? Are there many stairs to be negotiated? Is there adequate room for a hospital bed or for using a walker?

Is the patient socially involved or isolated? Is the patient involved in activities he or she finds satisfying?

Community and Institutional Resources

After the multidimensional assessment of the individual is completed, the results are reviewed with the patient and the family and a decision is made whether the patient can be discharged to a home environment or whether institutional care will be required. In most localities, there is an array of services for the elderly that can be organized to help maintain the older person at home, either for a limited convalescent period or for continuous long-term care. Some of the most frequently utilized programs, along with the types of providers and methods of payment, are presented in Table 139-1. The various levels of institutional care, kinds of facilities, and reimbursement and payment mechanisms are described in Table 139-2.

References

Gello JJ, Reichel W, Andersen L. Handbook of geriatric assessment. Rockville, MD: Aspen Publishers, 1988.

Getzel GS, Mellor MJ. Gerontological social work practice in the community. New York: Haworth Press, 1985.

Hooyman NR, Lustbader W. Taking care: Supporting older people and their families. New York: The Free Press, 1986.

Matteson MA, McConnell ES. Gerontological nursing: Concepts and practice. In: Monk A, ed. Handbook of gerontological services. New York: Van Nostrand Reinhold, 1985.

Williams TF. Assessment of the geriatric patient in relation to needs for services and facilities. In: Reichel W, ed. Clinical aspects of aging. Baltimore: Williams & Wilkins, 1983:543.

Behavioral Medicine

Anxiety

Jonathan S. Rothman, MD

Definition

Anxiety is a human emotion that occurs in all individuals in response to a perceived threat, loss, or stress. Anxiety can be adaptive in preparing the individual emotionally and physically to perform well. In the medical setting, anxiety is a typical response to the threat of illness and hospitalization. Anxiety is classified as a psychiatric disorder when its severity and persistence impair mental, physical, and social functioning. The state of anxiety is accompanied by physical symptoms and signs that contribute to the individual's distress (Table 140-1).

Synonyms for anxiety are fear, panic, dread, terror, apprehension, tension, nervousness, and stress.

Differential Diagnosis

Normal Anxiety

Anxiety can be a normal human emotional response in situations of apparent or unconscious threat. Medical hospitalization raises risks of illness, pain, abandonment, and separation. Situations in which we are asked to perform something new or to risk embarrassment often lead to anxious feelings.

Example. B.Z. is a 28-year-old single white male medical student. On the first morning of his medicine clerkship, he awoke at 4 AM. Unable to fall back asleep, he was feeling anxious and worrying whether he would know enough to be able to deal with the clerkship. He could not eat breakfast and had diarrhea. He noted feeling tense and had a dry throat and sweaty palms. After his first day he calmed down, and these feelings did not recur until the start of his surgical clerkship.

Primary Psychiatric Disorder

Certain states of anxiety are classified as primary because the symptoms follow the course of a separate illness without being secondary to another problem. The anxiety disorders most commonly seen in medical practice are panic disorder, agoraphobia, simple phobia, and generalized anxiety disorder.

Panic Disorder (Anxiety Neurosis)
Panic disorder occurs in 2 to 3 percent of the population. Its onset is usually in early adulthood, with a predominance in women. It is characterized by sudden, severe episodes of panic in conjunction with at least four of the symptoms listed in Table 140-1. Panic disorder may occur with or without agoraphobia.

Example. T.C., a 22-year-old single black female coed, reports a 2-month history of sudden episodes of dizziness, terror, hyperventilation, and tremulousness. The first episode occurred at the hairdresser. Since then, she has had two to three episodes each week.

Agoraphobia
Individuals with agoraphobia fear being in situations from which escape is thought to be difficult. Agoraphobics may fear being alone, being in crowds, or being in enclosed spaces. Such individuals may end up restricting themselves to the house. Agoraphobia is commonly associated with panic disorder.

Example. Recall T.C., who continued to have panic attacks and gradually became afraid to walk on campus alone, go to the movies, ride in cars or buses, or do anything if she felt there was a barrier to getting to the university dispensary. The mere mention of class led her to anxiously anticipate the walk across campus or sitting in a crowded lecture hall. She began to restrict herself to her dormitory room and eventually dropped out of college.

Simple Phobia
Simple phobias are persistent, specific, irrational fears of an object, activity, or situation. The patient is compelled by fear to avoid the phobic object at all costs. Patients are aware that the anxiety is irrational but cannot convince themselves to change their beliefs.

Example. D.M. is a 35-year-old white male lawyer with a successful practice. He has not been to the doctor since age 21 when he fainted after having a venipuncture for routine lab work. Since then, the image of a needle makes him extremely anxious. He cannot see a needle on television without experiencing acute anxiety. He understands rationally that there is nothing to fear and that the pain is minimal. He is seen by a physician because his wife is pregnant and he wants to be present at the birth of his child. The obstetrician has told him that his wife will have an intravenous needle in her arm during the delivery.

Generalized Anxiety Disorder
This is a chronic state of excessive or unrealistic anxiety associated with a number of symptoms indicating motor tension, autonomic hyperactivity, vigilance, and scanning behaviors. Patients with generalized anxiety disorder may describe themselves as "uptight," "stressed," or "nervous." Such patients relate to everything in their lives in an anxious manner.

Example. T.N. is a 68-year-old white woman with six children. Her husband is an alcoholic. She says she is "nervous about everything all the time." She comes to her internist frequently and calls each week worrying about every ache and pain as a sign of serious illness. She commonly complains of muscle aches, dry mouth, sweaty palms, and difficulty falling asleep.

Anxiety Secondary to Medical Illness

Anxiety may be a psychophysiologic presentation of an underlying medical disorder. Table 140-2 lists some of the medical conditions that may have anxiety as a manifestation.

Table 140-1 Symptoms and Signs of Anxiety

Symptoms	Signs
Dizziness or faintness	Pallor, cold extremities
Chest pain, pressure	Flushing
Paresthesias	Diaphoresis
Nausea or abdominal pain	Dilated pupils
Hyperventilation or shortness of breath	Tremor
Palpitations or rapid heart rate	Elevated blood pressure
Trembling or shaking	Tachycardia
Sweating	Tachypnea
Choking	Urinary frequency
Feelings of depersonalization or derealization	
Flushes or chills	
Fear of dying	
Fear of losing control or going crazy	

Table 140-2 Physical Causes of Anxiety-like Symptoms

Cardiovascular
Angina pectoris, arrhythmias, congestive heart failure, hypertension, hypovolemia, myocardial infarction, syncope, valvular disease, shock, myocardiopathy

Dietary
Caffeinism, monosodium glutamate, vitamin deficiency

Medications
Antipsychotics, anticholinergics, digitalis, sympathomimetics, bronchodilators, antihypertensives

Hematologic
Anemias

Immunologic
Systemic lupus erythematosus

Metabolic
Cushing's disease, pheochromocytoma, hyperthyroidism, hypoglycemia, hypocalcemia, porphyria, hyponatremia, hypoxia, carcinoid

Neurologic
Encephalopathies, central nervous system tumor, seizures, vertigo, central nervous system infection, subdural hematoma

Respiratory
Asthma, chronic obstructive pulmonary disease, pneumothorax, pulmonary embolism

Example. W.P. is a 30-year-old married white female leather stitcher who takes birth control pills. Her birthday was 4 days ago. Three days ago, she experienced the sudden onset of acute panic, hyperventilation, and tremor. She was seen in the emergency room and given the diagnosis of panic disorder. Today she returns with similar symptoms. On physical examination, her respirations are 35, her pulse is 110, her lungs are clear to auscultation, and there is a tenderness to palpation in her right thigh. Lung scan reveals multiple pulmonary emboli.

Diagnostic Approach

The anxiety symptoms that commonly accompany medical illness or stressful life events may be managed simply by giving people the opportunity to talk about their concerns. For patients for whom this is not sufficient, the administration of benzodiazepines in low doses for short periods of time may be useful. For severe, persistent anxiety symptoms, a thorough psychiatric evaluation is necessary. In people with accompanying medical illness, it is important first to rule out the medical illness or medication as the etiology. It may be difficult to differentiate these complaints of anxiety from a primary anxiety disorder. Too often the clinician depends solely on minor tranquilizers to alleviate the patient's symptoms without trying to understand the underlying cause of the anxiety.

References

Klein DF, Rabkin JG, eds. Anxiety: New research and concepts. New York: Raven Press, 1981.

Krystal JH, et al. Anxiety disorders. In: Lazare A. Outpatient psychiatry: Diagnosis and treatment. Baltimore: Williams & Wilkins, 1989:416.

Marks I, Lader M. Anxiety states. Anxiety neurosis: A review. J Nerv Ment Dis 1973; 156:3.

Sheehan DV, Ballenger J, Jacobson G. Treatment of endogenous anxiety with phobic, hysterical and hypochondriacal symptoms. Arch Gen Psychiatry 1980; 37:51.

Psychosis

Steven A. Adelman, MD

Definition

Psychosis is the most extreme and dangerous of all mental aberrations. Psychosis is a clinical syndrome, not an illness. This means that individuals who are psychotic may be suffering from any one of a number of different illnesses. Some of the conditions that cause psychosis are organic; others are psychiatric. A person who is psychotic is someone who is *grossly* out of touch with reality.

Gross impairment in reality testing is not always easy to detect. Certain individuals are openly and dramatically psychotic. Others may work hard at concealing their difficulties from outside observers. In order to determine whether or not an individual is psychotic, one must observe him or her carefully and ask questions designed to elicit the person's psychotic symptoms.

Features of Psychosis

Hallucinations

Hallucinations are sensory perceptions that are not caused by actual stimulation of the senses. When someone hears, sees, smells, tastes, or feels something that is not actually there, that person is hallucinating. Hallucinations differ from illusions, which are mistaken perceptions of real sensory stimuli. Hallucinations that signify psychosis seem very real and typically do not diminish over brief periods of time.

The most common form of hallucination is the auditory hallucination. Psychotic patients with auditory hallucinations often complain of hearing voices which repeatedly utter statements that disturb or hound them. The voice may command an individual to take an action (a command hallucination). Auditory hallucinations may consist of sounds other than voices. The other types of hallucinations are generally less common than auditory hallucinations. Visual hallucinations may consist of organized images, such as objects or people, or disorganized images, such as colors, dots, or flashes of light. These hallucinations involving the sense of sight are most frequently seen in the organic psychoses. A well-known example of a visual hallucination is the vision of kaleidoscopic colors experienced by an individual who has ingested a hallucinogenic drug such as LSD or mescaline.

Hallucinations of taste (gustatory hallucinations) are rare and generally consist of unpleasant tastes. Hallucinations involving smell (olfactory hallucinations) are also rare. Individuals who complain of certain pungent smells, like burnt rubber or oranges, may be suffering from temporal lobe epilepsy, an organic condition that frequently mimics some of the psychiatric causes of psychosis.

Tactile hallucinations involve the sense of touch. Intoxicated alcoholics who are "drying out" often experience a squirming sensation beneath their skin known as formication. Somatic hallucinations involve the perception of experiences within the body that are thought not to be attributable to an actual physical illness. Somatic hallucinations, no matter how outlandish, always warrant a thorough medical evaluation to rule out the existence of an underlying physical condition that might be at the root of the patient's complaints.

Delusions

Another common manifestation of psychosis is the delusion. Delusions are firmly held beliefs that fly in the face of reality as it is perceived by individuals other than the individual harboring the delusion. Like hallucinations, delusions are just one manifestation of psychosis, and delusions are present in a variety of organic and psychiatric illnesses. Delusions and hallucinations frequently coexist and reinforce one another.

Delusions have been subdivided into a number of categories based on their content. One of the most familiar types of delusions is the persecutory delusion. People with delusions of persecution believe that they are being plotted against, attacked, or fooled. Delusions of persecution occur in a variety of psychotic disorders. Grandiose delusions involve an exaggerated sense of one's intelligence, significance, or power. Delusions of jealousy focus on the belief that one's sexual partner is unfaithful. Bizarre delusions are distinguished by their striking implausibility; an example is one person's belief that a duck and an elephant both lived inside of him.

Individuals with nihilistic delusions are convinced that certain aspects of the real world simply do not exist. The Capgras syndrome is a specific type of nihilistic delusion in which a person believes that the people he or she knows have been replaced by identical strangers. Delusions of poverty comprise the belief that one is, or is about to become, materially destitute. The delusion of poverty is most characteristic of psychotic depression, and individuals harboring such a delusion are sometimes so convinced of their hard times that they attempt suicide. Delusions of being controlled consist of the belief that one's thoughts, words, or actions are dictated by forces outside of oneself. People with delusion of reference believe that the course of external events focuses on or refers to them, often in a negative way. When a false referential belief is held with less conviction than a delusion, it is labeled an idea of reference.

Other Signs of Psychosis

Hallucinations and delusions indicate a disturbance in the *content* of the psychotic person's thoughts. Some psychotic individuals also have disturbances in the process of thinking. These latter disturbances are referred to as thought disorder or thought pathology, and frequently coexist with the disturbances of thought content described previously. In some psychotic individuals, however, extreme signs of a thought disorder may be the only indication that they are psychotic.

The presence of a thought disorder is frequently detected in a psychotic person's speech patterns. The most striking example is incoherent speech, sometimes referred to as "word salad." Made-up words, known as neologisms, are sometimes a feature of the psychotic's speech patterns. Clinicians should always keep in mind that disturbances of speech may represent a neurologic problem (such as a stroke) masquerading as a mental disorder.

Other speech patterns indicating that someone has a thought disorder and may be psychotic include loosening of associations and flight of ideas. In speech characterized by loose associations, individual phrases and sentences appear to make sense. However, the connections between the phrases and sentences are tenuous and vague. When speech demonstrates flight of ideas, there is a shifting from topic to topic, and the connections between various parts of the monologue are usually discernible. Such speech is usually rapid-fire and has a pressured, uninterruptible quality.

There are several other features of speech that suggest the presence of thought disorder. Poverty of speech refers to the sparse verbal productions of some psychotic patients. Poverty of content of speech describes speech that is normal in amount but conveys almost no information owing to its vagueness. Blocking occurs when the speaker stops talking because the train of thought is suddenly lost. Echolalia is the tendency to repeat or mimic the words of another person. Perseveration, a related concept, refers to the propensity for the speaker to refer repeatedly to a single word or phrase. Clanging has to do with wordplay that is determined by sound rather than meaning. Taken alone, none of these aberrations in speech constitutes a profound enough impairment in reality testing to represent psychosis. However, if present in conjunction with other signs that suggest the existence of psychosis, they fortify the clinical determination of a psychotic state.

Concrete thinking signifies the loss of the ability to think abstractly. People who think concretely answer questions literally and are unable to explain the meaning of familiar proverbs. Overinclusive thinking, illogical thinking, and autistic thinking are all indicative of a thought disorder and may signify the presence of psychosis. Overinclusive thinking involves the usage of a single thought or concept as a means of explaining or understanding phenomena that would appear to most people to be unrelated or disconnected. The term *illogical thinking* is self-explanatory. Autistic thinking refers to a person's intense preoccupation with himself. These subtle disorders of thinking do not, by themselves, represent a significant enough impairment in reality testing to warrant automatically being equated with psychosis.

The determination that an individual is psychotic is most readily made when hallucinations or delusions are present. Disorders of thinking may be independent of, or coexist with, hallucinations and delusions. A third type of disturbance sometimes present in psychotic people is abnormal behavior. Like thought disorder, abnormal behavior is most reliable as an indicator of psychosis when it is accompanied by other psychotic signs and symptoms. Two abnormalities of behavior that are suggestive of psychosis are catatonic behavior and bizarre behavior.

The word *catatonic* generally refers to behavior in which movement is slowed, reduced, or absent. Some catatonic patients lie still and let their bodies go limp when an attempt is made to move them. Others maintain an entirely rigid posture. Sometimes a strange or inappropriate posture may be maintained for long periods of time. In catatonic waxy flexibility, the person's body remains in whatever position it is "molded" into. Some catatonic patients appear stuporous or comatose. The rigidity and motoric slowing that sometimes occur as side effects of antipsychotic medications have been confused with catatonia. It is important to rule out medical, neurologic, and drug-related problems before labeling an individual "catatonic."

Bizarre behavior is sometimes seen in cases of severe psychosis. Bizarre behaviors, such as eating excrement, underscore the profound alterations in reality testing that constitute psychosis. In the remaining portion of this chapter, the various disorders that cause psychotic states are described.

Etiology

The discussion of the many causes of psychosis will take place in a manner that resembles the actual thought processes of a sophisticated clinician performing the initial evaluation of a psychotic person. It is important that anyone evaluating a psychotic patient go about the evaluation in a systematic fashion, considering different possible causes for the patient's psychosis.

The sequence of possible causes of psychosis presented in this chapter is hierarchical in nature; i.e., the types of psychosis early in the sequence have features that are also found in the psychoses described later in the sequence. The reverse is not true. One should begin thinking about a psychotic patient's diagnosis by considering the more inclusive causes of psychosis first, as this minimizes the chances of making the wrong diagnosis.

Organic Psychoses

Before a patient's psychosis is attributed to another etiology, the possibility of an organic cause needs to be thoroughly considered and ruled out. The term *organic* is used here to refer to disorders caused by a temporary or permanent dysfunction of the brain. The causes of organic mental disorders include several degenerative brain diseases, a variety of medical illnesses, and use of and withdrawal from psychoactive drugs such as alcohol, marijuana, amphetamines, and heroin. The major categories of organic causes of psychosis are listed in Table 141-1, with representative causes in each category.

One may determine that a patient's psychotic symptoms have an organic cause in one of two ways. The first way is to recognize that the patient is suffering from a disorder known to cause brain dysfunction. A delusional patient with Huntington's disease (an illness known to cause psychotic symptoms) is an example. The second means of determining that psychotic symptoms are caused by an organic process is to look carefully at the mental status findings that accompany the hallucinations and delusions. When psychotic symptoms are accompanied by additional abnormalities suggesting that a patient is either delirious or demented, the cause of the psychotic symptoms is usually the underlying organic disorder causing the patient's delirium or dementia.

Delirium is an acute disturbance in a patient's level of consciousness, marked by disorientation, confusion, inattention, and a rapidly waxing and waning time course. Dementia refers to the more gradual fall-off in cognitive abilities seen in elderly persons afflicted with any one of a number of different dementing processes (e.g., Alzheimer's disease, hypothyroidism, and

Table 141-1 Organic Causes of Psychosis

Autoimmune Disease	Systemic lupus erythematosus
Degenerative Diseases	Huntington's chorea, Parkinson's disease
Infectious Diseases	Acquired immunodeficiency syndrome, herpes simplex (encephalitis)
Metabolic Diseases	Hepatic encephalopathy, porphyria
Neoplastic Diseases	Primary brain tumors, meningiomas, brain metastases (e.g., lung, breast)
Neurologic Diseases	Multiple sclerosis, strokes, seizure disorders (temporal lobe epilepsy), Wilson's disease
Toxic	Medications (bromocriptine, L-dopa), drug intoxication (cocaine, marijuana), drug withdrawal (alcohol)

normal pressure hydrocephalus, to name just a few). The following two examples illustrate how psychosis may be related to delirium and dementia.

An intern was called to the emergency room to evaluate a 45-year-old man who had vivid visual hallucinations of green and red demons who were taunting him. Mr. Brown was agitated and did not know the date or the name of the hospital. His temperature, blood pressure, and pulse were elevated, and he was sweating profusely. Mr. Brown's wife reported that her husband was a heavy drinker who had gone on the wagon 2 days earlier. The intern concluded that he was suffering from alcohol-withdrawal delirium, also known as delirium tremens ("DTs").

In this case, psychotic symptoms (visual hallucinations) were accompanied by a clouded state of consciousness (not knowing the date or the name of the hospital) and by other signs of alcohol withdrawal. Making the correct diagnosis permitted the institution of proper therapy and saved Mr. Brown's life.

Another example illustrating the importance of determining which additional mental status changes accompany psychotic symptoms considers Mrs. Green, a 75-year-old woman. Mrs. Green was brought to the physician by her grandson, who explained, "Grandma started to forget things last year so I figured she was getting senile. But now she seems to be going crazy—she claims that every night a man crawls into her window, tries to kill her, and leaves. We live on the 10th floor." The physician found that Mrs. Green had a severely impaired memory along with her persecutory delusion. Her medical evaluation revealed that she had clinical hypothyroidism. After 4 months of treatment with thyroid hormone, Mrs. Green's memory returned to normal and her delusion disappeared.

This case demonstrates that psychotic symptoms in the elderly may be the result of an underlying medical condition that causes dementia. In each of these examples, the organic etiology of the psychotic symptoms was suggested by their coexistence with signs of delirium and dementia, respectively. Some organic psychoses, however, appear as pure psychoses, unaccompanied by other mental status changes that point to an organic cause. This is frequently the case in drug-induced psychosis. Drugs can induce syndromes marked by any combination of delusions, hallucinations, and mood alteration.

Individuals with drug-induced psychotic states may appear to have a manic psychosis, schizophrenia, or paranoid disorder. Therefore, it is extremely important to determine the likelihood of drug abuse in any newly psychotic individual. Along with a careful history and physical examination, toxicologic analysis of a person's blood or urine may be very helpful in diagnosing a drug-induced psychosis. Making such a determination has important implications for both the short-term and long-term treatment of the newly psychotic person. Although most drugs of abuse can cause psychotic states, cocaine, amphetamines ("speed"), and phencyclidine ("PCP" or "angel dust") are especially well known for their propensity to cause psychotic symptoms.

Brief Reactive Psychosis

When a person reacts to a very stressful event by becoming psychotic for a short time, this form of psychosis is known as brief reactive psychosis. By definition, in brief reactive psychosis, the psychotic symptoms last no more than a month. In most cases of this condition, the psychotic symptoms subside within a few days of their onset. Often the psychotic symptoms are accompanied by confusion and disorientation, along with rapid shifts in mood. Because of the clouding of consciousness (confusion and disorientation) that accompanies brief reactive psychosis, individuals with this disorder sometimes resemble those with organic psychosis. Thus, the diagnosis of brief reactive psychosis should be deferred until organic causes of psychosis (especially substance abuse) are ruled out.

The most common situation causing brief reactive psychosis is military combat. Traumatic battlefield situations frequently lead to brief self-limited psychotic episodes in soldiers. When removed from the dangerous and stressful situations of battle, such soldiers frequently come to their senses in a few days. In civilian life, loss of a loved one and natural disasters are the most familiar precipitants of brief reactive psychosis.

Mood Disorders with Psychotic Features (Psychotic Depression and Manic Psychosis)

The two predominant mood disorders are major depression and bipolar disorder. The latter disorder also goes by the more familiar name of manic-depressive illness. The hallmark of the two disorders is a disturbance in mood. The mood of an individual suffering from a major depressive episode is often described as depressed, sad, low, or blue. The predominant mood of a manic-depressive depends on which phase of the illness is manifest. The manic-depressive may be depressed, elated and euphoric, or hostile and irritable, or have a changeable mood that rapidly fluctuates among all of these. It has been estimated that up to one-third of patients suffering from either of these major affective disorders become psychotic.

When assessing a psychotic patient, it is important to look for evidence of a mood disturbance. Individuals with mood disorders frequently undergo alterations in their patterns of sleeping, eating, and motor behavior. When psychosis coexists with the signs of a mood disturbance, this has important implications for the patient's treatment and course, because such patients have a better prognosis than do schizophrenics.

It is sometimes difficult to decide whether or not a patient's psychosis is due to an underlying mood disorder. When the psychotic symptoms precede the mood disturbance, making the diagnosis of a simple mood disorder becomes a complicated matter. Examining the content of a patient's hallucinations and delusions may prove helpful in confirming the diagnosis of a mood disorder with psychotic features. When the flavor of the patient's psychotic symptoms is in keeping with the disturbance of mood, then the diagnosis is most secure. Depressed patients often have delusions that center on themes of guilt, sin, poverty, physical decay, and deserved persecution. Manic patients often exhibit flight of ideas in their speech, and those who are euphoric may have delusions of grandeur, believing that they possess special abilities or that they have been elected by God to perform a special task. It is important to stress, however, that the presence of delusions that are not in keeping with the patient's mood disturbance does not eliminate the possibility of a mood disorder with psychotic features. The case of Joe, a 20-year-old college student with manic-depressive illness, illustrates many of the important points about psychosis accompanying a mood disorder.

Joe, an honors student, stopped attending class and failed all his sophomore courses. His roommate, noting that Joe had a strange look in his eyes and sometimes seemed to talk to himself, took him to the student health service. There Joe revealed the delusion that God was communicating with him through a computer terminal. The incorrect diagnosis of schizophrenia was made. The evaluating physician had neglected to assess Joe for a mood disturbance. When Joe was hospitalized, he was noted to be sad and tearful, unable to sleep through the night, and uninterested in food. Joe's diagnosis was changed to major depression with psychotic features. Joe was treated with a combination of antidepressant and antipsychotic medications. He improved rapidly, and was discharged after 5 weeks in the hospital. After a short time, the antipsychotic medication was discontinued. Two weeks later, Joe began to behave erratically. After staying up for 3 days straight, he withdrew all his money from the bank and started throwing dollar bills off the campus bell tower. Chased by the police, he ran naked through the campus shouting gibberish and was finally subdued and rehospitalized after jumping into an icy duck pond. On readmission, Joe demonstrated pressured speech, flight of ideas, grandiose delusions, and a mood that was intermittently irritable and expansive. At this point, it was clear that Joe was in the throes of a manic episode and that he suffered from manic-depressive illness. Following appropriate treatment, he returned to school, where he has done well for 1 year with no recurrence of symptoms.

The case of Joe illustrates the very important point that diagnosis rests on the course of the patient's symptoms over time, as well as on the patient's mental status at a given point in time. As Joe was observed over a period of a month, the intermittent quality of his symptoms and his fluctuations in mood emerged, and the diagnosis of manic-depressive illness could be made with a high degree of certainty.

Schizophrenia

Schizophrenia is a complex mental illness that has at times been mistakenly equated with the clinical syndrome of psychosis. Psychotic symptoms are the central feature of the active phase of schizophrenia. Traditionally, bizarre delusions such as being able to broadcast one's thoughts, having thoughts inserted or withdrawn from one's mind, or being controlled by an outside force have been considered most characteristic of schizophrenia. Other psychotic symptoms seen in the active phase of schizophrenia include the following: delusions and hallucinations with jealous or persecutory content; delusions with somatic, religious, nihilistic, or grandiose themes; auditory hallucinations; disordered thinking; and behavior that is bizarre or catatonic. In relating to other people, schizophrenics may seem zombie-like or socially inappropriate.

In addition to the psychotic symptoms of the active phase, schizophrenics also manifest deterioration in their ability to get along with other people, to care for themselves, and to function appropriately at home, work, or school. When an individual displays such deterioration for more than 6 months and has at one time been actively psychotic, the diagnosis of schizophrenia can be made. The diagnosis is valid only when the symptoms cannot be attributed to an organic mental disorder or to a mood disorder.

Schizophrenia is classified into the following five types: (1) disorganized type, in which incoherence predominates and delusions are absent; (2) catatonic type, marked by the presence of catatonia; (3) paranoid type, in which hallucinations and delusions with themes of jealousy and persecution predominate; (4) undifferentiated type, in which psychotic symptoms are prominent but do not fit neatly into any of the other types; and (5) residual type, in which active psychotic symptoms, once present, no longer exist.

Some individuals have a history of acting withdrawn, odd, or suspicious prior to developing the severe symptoms that qualify them for the diagnosis of schizophrenia. In some cases the deterioration of functioning precedes the active phase of the illness by months or even years; in other cases, the first evidence of any dysfunction is the sudden eruption of an acute psychotic state. Schizophrenia is rarely, if ever, cured entirely. Schizophrenics often have recurrent episodes of acute psychosis in the course of a lifetime. Their overall level of functioning may remain marginal or progressively deteriorate. The treatment of schizophrenia is both complicated and controversial, generally involving the use of medication to control the acute symptoms and some combination of psychotherapy and environmental stabilization to help schizophrenic individuals cope with their long-term deficits.

Miscellaneous Causes of Psychosis or Psychotic-like States

The major causes of psychosis have been outlined previously. The following disorders are either less clearly defined or less prevalent than the organic psychoses, mood disorder psychoses, and schizophrenia.

Schizophreniform Disorder. This is the diagnosis made when the clinical picture resembles schizophrenia, except that the duration of symptoms is less than 6 months. A patient with schizophreniform disorder whose symptoms persist longer than 6 months is then rediagnosed as schizophrenic. The category of schizophreniform disorder is a useful one because it encourages clinicians to reserve the diagnosis of schizophrenia for patients whose symptoms are truly long-standing.

Schizoaffective Disorder. This is a vaguely defined diagnostic category that is reserved for patients whose disorders have features of both schizophrenia and a mood disorder. For example, some individuals may appear initially to have a classic psychotic depression, but they may remain chronically psychotic and dysfunctional long after the disturbance of mood is gone. A surprisingly large number of patients do seem to fall into this in-between diagnostic category.

Delusional (Paranoid) Disorders. When a person's only symptom is a nonbizarre delusion (most commonly, with paranoid content), the diagnosis of delusional disorder is made. The diagnosis is excluded if either hallucinations or a mood disturbance is prominent. In shared paranoid disorder (also known by the colorful name of "folie a deux"), the delusion or delusional system is shared by more than one individual.

Postpartum Psychosis. Women frequently become sad and depressed after delivering a baby. Some go on to have a full-blown episode of major depression, and some of these depressed mothers become psychotic. Most, but not all, postpartum psychoses are caused by depression. Some cases of postpartum psychosis may be due to organic factors, bipolar disorder, a schizophreniform disorder, or unknown causes. Like the general category of psychosis, it is a syndrome and not a specific disorder.

Factitious Psychosis and Malingering. Malingering refers to the voluntary feigning of psychosis in order to achieve a discernible goal. An example of malingering is the conscious mimicking of hallucinations and delusions by a military inductee intended to prevent his being sent into a combat unit. Some patients in mental hospitals who are not psychotic appear to mimic the psychotic symptoms of other patients with no apparent goal in mind. This is known as factitious psychosis, detected when there is an intermittent and inconsistent quality to the psychotic symptoms.

Treatment

Psychosis is a serious and potentially dangerous state of mind. Psychotic individuals act unpredictably and are prone to harm both themselves and other people. Any psychotic individual should be evaluated by a psychiatrist, and most newly psychotic people should be hospitalized.

A detailed description of the treatment of psychosis goes beyond the scope of this text. Making the proper diagnosis of a psychotic state is the most important step in determining the appropriate form of treatment. When an organic cause for psychosis is determined, treatment of the underlying organic condition follows. In the treatment of mood disorder psychoses, one employs drugs that correct mood disturbances, such as lithium and the various antidepressant drugs. The mainstay of treatment for most psychotic states is the antipsychotic (neuroleptic) medications. Along with the appropriate medications, a safe and stable environment and psychotherapy are invaluable in helping the psychotic person to regain and maintain the ability to perceive reality accurately.

References

Cummings JL, Benson DF. Dementia: A clinical approach. Boston: Butterworth, 1983.

Cummings JL. Organic psychoses. Psychiatr Clin North Am 1986; 9:293.

Kendler K. Demography of paranoid psychosis (delusional disorder): A review and comparison with schizophrenic and affective illness. Arch Gen Psychiatry 1982; 39:890.

Lipowski ZJ. Transient cognitive disorders (delirium, acute confusional states) in the elderly. Am J Psychiatry 1983; 140:1426.

Lipowski ZJ. Delirium. Springfield, IL: Charles C Thomas, 1980.

Manschreck TC. Schizophrenic disorders. In: Lazare AL, ed. Outpatient psychiatry: Diagnosis and treatment. Baltimore: Williams & Wilkins, 1989:510.

Manschreck TC. The paranoid syndrome and delusional (paranoid) disorders. In: Lazare AL, ed. Outpatient psychiatry: Diagnosis and treatment. Baltimore: Williams & Wilkins, 1989:526.

Manschreck TC, Petri M. The paranoid syndrome. Lancet 1978; 2:251.

Massion AO, Benjamin S. Manic behavior. In: Lazare AL, ed. Outpatient psychiatry: Diagnosis and treatment. Baltimore: Williams & Wilkins, 1989:256.

Nasrallah HA, Weinberger DR, eds. The neurology of schizophrenia. Amsterdam: Elsevier, 1986.

Neale JM, Oltmanns TF. Schizophrenia. New York: John Wiley & Sons, 1980.

Pope HG, Lipinski JF. Diagnosis in schizophrenic and manic-depressive illness. Arch Gen Psychiatry 1978; 35:811.

Depression

Steven A. Adelman, MD

142

Definition

The term *depression* means different things to different people. Depression is a type of mood usually described by words like "sad," "blue," "down in the dumps," and "depressed." Depression is also the name given to one of the most prevalent mental disorders. What is sometimes confusing is that the term *depression* applies to several different mental disorders. Consequently, the statement that someone is "suffering from depression" has many possible meanings and conveys very little information.

People with depressed mood frequently manifest a number of related emotional and physical disturbances. Psychiatrists refer to the entire constellation of problems known to accompany depressed mood as the *depressive syndrome.* The first section of this chapter describes the depressive syndrome in detail. Each of the disorders described in the section on differential diagnosis of depression is discussed with regard to the depressive syndrome and its unique identifying characteristics. The final portion of this chapter focuses on the treatment of depressive disorders.

The Depressive Syndrome

The depressive syndrome is rarely, if ever, present in its entirety. Rather, it is a constellation of possible abnormalities, some of which are found in any person suffering from a depressive disorder. As suggested previously, a prevailing mood described by words like "blue," "sad," or "low" is a central feature of the depressive disorders. In some individuals, this mood varies predictably during the day; often it is lowest upon awakening, with gradual improvement during the course of the day. Psychiatrists apply the term *diurnal mood variation* to such regular fluctuations in mood.

It is surprising that not all people suffering from depressive disorders complain of disturbances in mood. Some complain of "not feeling right"; others appear depressed without voicing any complaints about their moods, feelings, or thoughts. In addition to assessing a person's mood, the clinician who is attempting to determine the presence or extent of a depressive syndrome needs to focus on a number of additional areas. These include appearance, behavior, feelings, thought process, and thought content.

Appearance

The following description delineates the characteristic appearance of an individual with a depressive syndrome.

Mr. Blue, who was middle-aged, looked like a haggard old man. He was unshaven and his clothes appeared too big for him. His hair had not been combed or washed for days. Mr. Blue wore a glum expression on his face. He frequently burst into tears, seemingly over nothing. His movements were slowed—getting up for a drink of water was a tremendous undertaking. Mr. Blue spoke in a monotone and had very little to say.

The slowed movements of the depressive syndrome are referred to as psychomotor retardation. Some depressed individuals manifest a form of hyperactivity referred to as psychomotor agitation. These individuals appear tense and nervous and often pace anxiously while wringing their hands.

Behavior

The individual with a depressive syndrome behaves as though he or she has lost interest in the usual activities of living. Frequently, he or she withdraws from friends and family. At work, the individual is less motivivated and productive. Previously pleasurable pursuits are frequently dropped as interest in hobbies, sports, and community activities is lost. The person's sex drive diminishes; consequently, sexual activity decreases, often to a standstill.

Disturbances of appetite and sleep, when present, are important components of the depressive syndrome. The depressed individual may lose interest in food and consequently suffer a significant loss of weight. However, some depressed individuals experience increases in appetite and gain weight.

Like the appetite disturbances, the disturbances of sleep associated with the depressive syndrome are variable. The most familiar sleep disturbance is early morning awakening. Depressed people frequently complain of waking up in the early morning and finding it either impossible or quite difficult to fall back to sleep. Some depressed people have difficulty getting to sleep; some have insomnia predominantly in the middle of the night. In some individuals with depressive syndromes, the major sleep disturbance is oversleeping. These people find themselves needing as much as 4 or 5 hours of sleep per night more than they typically require.

Feelings

In addition to feelings of depression, individuals with a depressive syndrome experience a number of other unpleasant feelings. They frequently describe feeling tired and listless. They can be overwhelmed by anxiety and irritability. Feelings of fear, guilt, hopelessness, and helplessness are also common.

Many people with depressive syndromes feel physically ill. The terms *somatic complaints* and *somatic preoccupations* refer to the bodily concerns of certain depressed people. Physical complaints in the absence of any detectable medical problems are frequently a clue to the existence of a depressive syndrome in the elderly.

Thought Process

People with depressive syndromes tend to have difficulty thinking. Their thoughts are muddled. They have trouble concentrating. They are distractable, indecisive, and sometimes even forgetful. Depressed people typically brood and ruminate about trifles and often blow things up out of proportion.

Thought Content

In addition to disturbances in the process of thinking, the depressive syndrome is also marked by characteristic abnormalities in thought content. Depressed individuals usually suffer from low self-esteem and harbor thoughts of self-reproach. They think a lot about sin, evil, death, and suicide. Researchers estimate that as many as 15 percent of individuals with major depression actually succeed in killing themselves.

When the depressed individual's thinking and appreciation of reality are grossly impaired, the depressive syndrome includes psychotic features. The coexistence of mood disturbances and psychosis is discussed at length in Chapter 141, "Psychosis." Psychiatrists have found that psychotically depressed people are a greater suicide risk than depressed people who are not psychotic. Furthermore, the treatment of psychotic depression is more complex than the treatment of nonpsychotic forms of depression.

Differential Diagnosis

The order in which the depressive disorders are discussed in this section parallels the kind of thought process employed by a psychiatrically sophisticated clinician who is sytematically evaluating an individual with a chief complaint of depression. The first causes of depression to consider are medical and neurologic illnesses that engender a clinical state resembling major depression. When a physical cause for depression is not apparent, the psychiatrist then looks for evidence of a major depressive episode. It is appropriate to attribute a person's complaints of depression to other disorders only after physical illness and a major depressive episode have been considered and ruled out. This rationale ensures that serious disorders that sometimes respond dramatically to treatment are never overlooked.

Organic Mood Syndrome (Depressed)

When a depressive syndrome emerges in the context of a physical disorder, the diagnosis of an organic mood syndrome is made. A wide variety of organic processes can cause depressive syndromes. Organic mood syndromes range from mild cases, with subtle depression of mood as the only feature, to severe cases, with psychomotor retardation, sleep and appetite disturbances, suicidal thoughts, and psychosis all present. An organic mood syndrome may appear identical to a major depressive episode, with the only distinguishing characteristics being the underlying organic etiology. There are numerous causes of organic mood syndromes. Examples of each of the major categories are listed in Table 142-1.

This listing of causes of the organic mood syndrome is incomplete. Within each of the major categories listed, there exist many other conditions that have been associated with depressive syndromes. It is of crucial importance that health professionals assessing an individual whose chief complaint is "depression" keep in mind that organic conditions should always be considered before ascribing the "depression" to any other cause. The following example is a case in point.

Mrs. Black was a 55-year-old housewife who gradually lost interest in sex over a 2-month period. This disturbed her husband greatly, and he and Mrs. Black together sought the help of a marriage counselor. Despite weekly meetings in which the Blacks and their counselor discussed marital and sexual issues at great length, Mrs. Black's interest in sex continued to wane. She became apathetic about her appearance and lost interest in housework. After several months of unsuccessful counseling, she was referred to a psychiatrist for evaluation of her increasing dysfunction and presumed depression. The psychiatrist was certain that Mrs. Black manifested several features of a depressive syndrome. In taking a careful history, he discovered that a few weeks before Mrs. Black's interest in sex had begun to diminish, her general practitioner had started her on propranolol for hypertension. Knowing that this is one of the antihypertensive medications associated with depression, the psychiatrist contacted her physician, who agreed to switch Mrs. Black to another

Table 142-1 Conditions Causing an Organic Mood Syndrome (Depressed)

Drugs	Certain antihypertensives, steroids, oral contraceptives, benzodiazepines, alcohol
Endocrine Disorders	Adrenal insufficiency (Addison's disease), hypothyroidism
Neurologic Disorders	Brain tumors, strokes, multiple sclerosis, Wilson's disease, Alzheimer's disease
Infectious Diseases	Influenza, mononucleosis, infectious hepatitis, acquired immunodeficiency syndrome
Cancer	Pancreatic, lung, leukemia, lymphoma
Autoimmune Disorders	Systemic lupus erythematosus, rheumatoid arthritis
Nutritional Deficiencies	B_{12} deficiency (pernicious anemia), folate deficiency
Blood Electrolyte Disturbance	Hypocalcemia, hyponatremia

drug. Within 2 weeks she began to perk up, and her interest in sex returned.

This case demonstrates the importance of taking a medication history and of always considering the possibility of organic causes of the depressive syndrome. Marital counseling, psychotherapy, and even treatment with antidepressants all miss the mark if an underlying organic cause of a depressive syndrome goes undetected. As is the case in all of medicine, one rarely makes a diagnosis that one does not first consider.

Major Depression

As noted previously, clinicians should consider and rule out the possibility of an organic mood syndrome before making the diagnosis of any other type of depressive disorder. In practice, this is often accomplished by requiring depressed people, especially those over 50 years old, to undergo a thorough medical evaluation before making a referral to a psychiatrist or instituting psychiatric treatment. When organic causes of depression have been ruled out, one proceeds to determine whether or not the nature and duration of the depressive syndrome qualify it as a major depressive episode.

A major depressive episode exists when an individual has experienced at least five of the following nine depressive symptoms almost continuously for at least 2 weeks:

1. Depressed mood
2. Disturbed appetite or change in weight
3. Disturbed sleep
4. Psychomotor retardation or agitation
5. Loss of interest in previously pleasurable activities; inability to have fun; diminished sex drive
6. Loss of energy, fatigue
7. Feelings of guilt, worthlessness, and self-reproach
8. Difficulty in concentrating and thinking clearly
9. Morbid or suicidal thoughts or actions

Major depressive episodes are defined in terms of these nine symptoms because psychiatrists have discerned that they frequently cluster together in certain individuals who tend to be seriously depressed. Hence the term *major depressive episode*. Major depressive episodes occur in the context of three related mood disorders: major depression (single episode), recurrent major depression, and bipolar depression (also known as the depressed phase of manic-depressive illness).

These three disorders are related, and tend to occur in members of the same family. Episodes of bipolar depression are similar to episodes of major depression. The diagnosis of bipolar depression can be made only when an individual has a previous history of a manic episode (described in Chapter 141, "Psychosis").

The following case history illustrates many of the salient features of major depression.

Brad was 22 years old when he first consulted a psychiatrist. While Brad was growing up, his mother suffered from recurrent episodes of major depression and had to be hospitalized on three occasions. Several months after her last hospitalization, she became profoundly depressed and killed herself. Brad was 17 at the time. Five years later, Brad decided to ascertain what his chances of getting depressed would be.

In their first meeting, Dr. Hall and Brad agreed that thus far in his life he had not suffered from a major depressive episode. The family history revealed that Brad's maternal uncle was a manic-depressive and that several cousins on that side of the family were alcoholics. Dr. Hall explained, "Alcoholism, manic-depressive illness, and major depression often run together in families. You have a strongly positive family history of mood disorders. The risk that any male will develop a mood disorder is about 10 percent. For a woman, the risk is closer to 20 percent. A positive family history like yours increases that risk by a factor of two or three. Overall, I'd say your chances of developing major depression are close to one in three. Remember, the onset of major depression is often not until the thirties or forties." Brad was somewhat encouraged by the news that the odds were in his favor.

At the age of 30 Brad returned to Dr. Hall and complained of feeling depressed. Several weeks earlier he had been passed over for a promotion at work. Within a few days, Brad noted that he was having trouble sleeping through the night. At times he burst into tears over nothing. He was crestfallen about not getting promoted. He noticed that he was losing track of important details at work. Brad agreed to go and see a psychiatrist after his family doctor was unable to find a physical cause for his 15-pound weight loss.

Dr. Hall treated Brad's major depression with antidepressants and supportive psychotherapy. Within 3 weeks Brad was starting to feel a bit better, and after 10 weeks he felt almost completely better. Brad asked Dr. Hall what his chances were of having further episodes of major depression. He replied, "About half of all people who have an episode of major depression go on to have one or more additional episodes. About a quarter of people with major depression have frequent recurrences, like your mother. Discontinuing your antidepressant might increase the risk of a recurrence. We should keep all this in mind before deciding to stop your medicine."

After more than a year on medication, Brad and Dr. Hall agreed to taper the dosage of the antidepressant gradually. Brad continued to feel good, and the medication was finally stopped. He lived and worked happily and productively for another 5 years until his wife noted that something was wrong. Brad had stopped smiling. He began to toss and turn at night. He lost interest in food, sex, and bowling. When Brad started questioning whether or not life was worth living, his wife urged him to return to Dr. Hall. Unlike the first episode of major depression, this episode was not preceded by a precipitating stressful event.

Brad's second major depressive episode again responded to treatment. Subsequently, Brad has continued both to take medications and to meet with Dr. Hall on a monthly basis for supportive psychotherapy. Brad and Dr. Hall have agreed that ongoing treatment is preferable to the risk of recurrent depression.

This example demonstrates the clinical features of a classic case of recurrent major depression. Precipitating events sometimes precede a major depressive episode; often they do not. Major depression does not always respond to treatment as straightforwardly as in Brad's case. Furthermore, in as many as 30 percent of cases of major depression, psychotic features complicate the clinical picture.

Other Causes of Depression

A sizable proportion of individuals who seek professional help with complaints of depression do not suffer from either an organic mood syndrome or major depression. Most of these people fit into one of the three categories discussed in the following sections.

Uncomplicated Bereavement

Also known as grief reaction, uncomplicated bereavement is the normal experience of sadness and depression felt by someone reacting to the loss of a loved one. Many features of the depressive syndrome appear in bereavement, most typically loss of appetite and sleep. Profound loss of functioning, suicidal thoughts, and psychosis do not usually accompany bereavement. Uncomplicated bereavement and major depression seem to exist on a continuum. When the death of a loved one precipitates an extensive depressive syndrome that does not simply run its course and remit spontaneously, it is wise to diagnose the condition as a major depression and to prescribe treatment accordingly. Sigmund Freud's idea about the psychological causes of depression stem from his observation that "mourning" (bereavement) and "melancholia" (major depression) bear a striking resemblance to one another.

Adjustment Disorder with Depressed Mood

Some people react maladaptively to stressful life events by developing a depressed mood. When this disturbance in mood is not accompanied by a sufficient number of features of the depressive syndrome to warrant the diagnosis of a major depressive episode, the diagnosis of an adjustment disorder with depressed mood is made. The kinds of stresses that provoke adjustment reactions include moving, leaving home, getting married, marital discord, divorce, occupational problems, and physical illness. In some cases of chronic illness, the distinction between an organic mood syndrome and an adjustment disorder with depressed mood is difficult to make, and perhaps is not of much significance. The utility of this diagnostic category is that it identifies a group of mildly depressed people for whom psychosocial forms of treatment are of more use than antidepressant medication. The following case illustrates the principal features of an adjustment disorder with depressed mood.

Ms. Green was a successful 32-year-old hairstylist who sought help 6 weeks after her husband abruptly left her to live with another woman. Ms. Green complained that her husband had dealt her a low blow, and that ever since his departure she had felt like "two cents" and could not keep from crying herself to sleep at night. Ms. Green was not suicidal or psychotic, and she did not manifest the disturbances of sleep, appetite, energy level, or concentration characteristic of a major depressive episode. The diagnosis of an adjustment disorder with depressed mood was made, and Ms. Green was referred for psychotherapy. After several weeks of exploring and coming to terms with her feelings of betrayal, anger, loss, and guilt, Ms. Green started to feel better.

As noted, the key features of an adjustment disorder with depressed mood are the presence of a clear-cut stressor and the absence of sufficient symptoms to warrant diagnosis of a major depressive episode. In the past, adjustment disorder with depressed mood has gone by the names of *reactive depression, situational depression,* and *depressive reaction.*

Dysthymic Disorder

People who feel chronically depressed and unhappy for at least 2 years, without manifesting the extensive depressive syndrome of a major depressive episode, qualify for the diagnosis of dysthymic disorder. This disorder is often associated with an underlying maladaptive personality structure. Some individuals with dysthymic disorder come from families in which mulitple family members are afflicted with mood disorders. In these cases dysthymic disorder may be a forme fruste of major depression.

Treatment

Careful identification of a depressive disorder leads the clinician to choose the most appropriate form of treatment for a specific individual with a specific disorder. A detailed description of the treatment of depression goes beyond the scope of this text. The following will help orient the reader to current trends in the treatment of depressive disorders.

Organic Mood Syndrome

As mentioned previously, the first step in treating an organic mood syndrome is to identify and treat the underlying organic condition. When symptoms of a depressive syndrome persist in the face of optimal treatment of the underlying condition, other therapeutic modalities are frequently useful. When the residual picture resembles a major depression, it should be treated as such, with a combination of psychotherapy and antidepressant medication. In the case of a chronic debilitating physical illness like cancer, support groups for both the patient and his or her family are very helpful. Organizations that share the task of coping with a chronic illness, such as hospices, visiting nurse associations, and homemaker services, help to alleviate the burden of depression felt by chronically ill people and their families.

Major Depression

Before undertaking a program for treating a major depressive episode, psychiatrists attempt to make certain that the depressed person has no history of mood elevations (mania or hypomania). When the psychiatrist elicits a history of mood elevations, treatment of the major depressive episode usually includes the use of lithium in addition to antidepressants and psychotherapy. Antidepressants and psychotherapy are the mainstays of treatment for major depression.

Antidepressants work by causing biochemical changes in the brain that reverse the symptoms of the depressive syndrome. The antidepressants are effective in doing so in about 80 percent of the cases of major depression. Most antidepressants begin to work only after the depressed person has taken the medication consistently for at least 2 or 3 weeks. Sometimes the response comes as late as 6 to 8 weeks after the onset of treatment, one of the major drawbacks of antidepressant treatment.

When people with major depression fail to respond to an adequate trial of an antidepressant (defined as 6 to 8 weeks of treatment at a high enough dose), switching to an antidepressant from another chemical group can lead to a response. In cases of major depression with psychotic features, the combination of antidepressants with antipsychotic medications leads to the best outcome. Severe depressions that do not respond to medication are often cured by electroconvulsive therapy. Despite its unfavorable image conveyed by the media, electroconvulsive therapy is a safe and effective means of alleviating severe, treatment-resistant depressions.

Drug treatment of depression is by itself inadequate. The emotional experience of a major depressive episode is so difficult and uncomfortable that some form of psychological support and guidance is an essential component of a comprehensive treatment program for the individual suffering from major depression. Various types of psychotherapy have been used to treat patients with major depression. Cognitive therapists tend to utilize task-oriented techniques such as mood monitoring and re-educating the depressed person to correct his negativistic, self-reproachful thinking. Psychoanalytically oriented therapists probe into the past as they attempt to understand and interpret the depressed person's sadness. Psychopharmacologists reassure the person suffering from major depression that he has a treatable illness that will take some time to go away. Despite these differences in technique, most clinicians who treat individuals with major depression favor an approach that is fundamentally supportive and empathic.

For seriously depressed people who are either suicidal, psychotic, or unable to care for themselves at home, hospitalization is frequently necessary. Most people hospitalized for a "nervous breakdown" probably suffer from a profound case of major depression. Ideally, the psychiatric hospital or ward is a safe place where treatment can be rapidly instituted. In conjunction with medication and psychotherapy, group meetings and rehabilitation activities help the individual with major depression to regain his or her interests, self-esteem, and social skills.

When the symptoms of major depression have resolved, how much longer does treatment need to continue? For both psychotherapy and antidepressant medication, the answer is at least several months. The psychotherapy will typically focus on processing the miserable experience of going through a major depression, learning to face and readjust to the demands of the world, and gaining insight into the circumstances that led up to the major depressive episode.

Continuing treatment with antidepressant medication maintains the symptoms of the depressive syndrome in remission. It is safest to begin tapering the dose of antidepressants 6 to 12 months after the symptoms have entirely cleared. Most individuals with major depression will not experience an immediate recurrence of symptoms when this is done. For those who do, and for people who have a history of frequent episodes of recurrent major depression, chronic maintenance on antidepressants may be preferable to the risk of repeated episodes of disabling major depression. There are no known long-term cumulative side effects of chronic antidepressant treatment.

Other Depressive Disorders

Many people who suffer the loss of a loved one find that bereavement support groups and bereavement counseling help to facilitate the process of mourning. When bereavement is complicated by persistent, incapacitating symptoms of major depression, psychotherapy and antidepressants are definitely indicated (see Chapter 175, "Bereavement and Grief"). The treatment of choice for adjustment disorders with depressed mood is psychotherapy. Brief psychotherapy, lasting a few weeks to a few months, may suffice in helping an individual to understand, cope with, and overcome the stressful life event that has precipitated the adjustment disorder. For individuals who desire to change a longstanding pattern of reacting maladaptively to stress, more extensive psychotherapy is necessary. Long-term psychotherapy is also the treatment of choice for the chronic feelings of depression characteristic of dysthymic disorder.

Summary

As in all of medicine, the successful treatment of the depressive disorder requires that the therapy, both pharmacologic and psychological, be tailored to fit a carefully made diagnosis. Adherence to the thorough diagnostic approach outlined in this chapter minimizes the chances of overtreating or undertreating a given depressive disorder. Depression is one of the most common problems for which people seek the help of physicians. A variety of effective therapies for the treatment of the depressive disorders is readily available.

References

Akiskal HS, et al. Chronic depressions. Part 1. Clinical and familial characteristics in 137 probands. J Affective Disord 1981; 3:297.

Barreira PJ. Depression. In: Lazare AL, ed. Outpatient psychiatry—diagnosis and treatment. Baltimore: Williams & Wilkins, 1989:252.

Barreira PJ, Lazare L. Mood disorders. In: Lazare AL, ed. Outpatient psychiatry—diagnosis and treatment. Baltimore: Williams & Wilkins, 1989:362.

Hall RCW, et al. Physical illness presenting as psychiatric disease. Arch Gen Psychiatry 1980; 37:989.

Keller MB, et al. Recovery in major depressive disorders. Arch Gen Psychiatry 1982; 39:905.

Keller MB, et al. Relapse in major depressive disorder. Arch Gen Psychiatry 1982; 39:911.

Lingjaerde O. The biochemistry of depression. Acta Psych Scand 1983; 302(suppl):36.

143 Hypochondriasis

Barry Ginsberg, MD

Jonathan S. Rothman, MD

The fundamental feature of hypochondriasis is the patient's preoccupation with having a serious disease despite a negative physical evaluation. A characteristic of the doctor-patient relationship that is central to hypochondriasis is that any effort by the doctor to demonstrate the absence of pathology or to remove symptoms is countered by "illness-claiming behavior." Patients with hypochondriasis will not relinquish the sick role. A hypochondriacal patient often "doctor shops," and sometimes the patient's existence seems to be organized around the illness and obtaining medical care. Iatrogenic problems such as medication addiction and surgery-related pathology may complicate the picture.

Although there may be evidence of major problems in other aspects of the patient's life, it is usually difficult to interest these patients in anything but their medical status. The disorder occurs in both sexes. The age of onset for men is most commonly in the thirties; for women, it is in the forties. Past experience with organic illness in a family member and psychosocial stress are predisposing factors. A related condition called somatization disorder is characterized by a multiplicity of symptoms in various systems over time. Somatization disorder is seen predominantly in women and has its onset in the teens and early twenties.

Hypochondriacal patients may present particular problems for the beginning doctor. The trainee's efforts to master the information and technique of medicine may heighten the frustration experienced when encountering a patient who insists upon remaining ill. The negative emotional reaction of the physician to the hypochondriac provides a helpful clue in diagnosis. If acted upon without examination, however, this reaction may preclude proper investigation and management of the patient's condition.

Differential Diagnosis

Undiagnosed Physical Illness

Despite unremarkable physical examination and negative laboratory studies, an early or subtle physical illness may be present. A premature diagnosis of hypochondriasis may render the physician less alert to late-developing signs of illness, particularly if he adopts a reductionistic notion of illness as either in the mind *or* in the body. Hypochondriacal complaints are sometimes elaborated upon real organic disease.

Somatization Disorder

Whereas hypochondriasis is characterized by preoccupation with having a specific serious illness, the hallmark of somatization disorder is multiple complaints in multiple organ systems. Patients qualify for the diagnosis of somatization when they complain of *13 or more* symptoms in the following five categories: gastrointestinal, pain, cardiopulmonary, neurologic, and sexual. Somatization disorder begins before age 30.

Conversion Disorder

Patients with this disorder experience the sudden onset of a seemingly physical symptom in reaction to a clear-cut psychological stressor. The specific symptom may have a symbolic meaning that clarifies the nature of the psychological conflict (e.g., a teenage girl who sees her father with his mistress experiences a sudden onset of hysterical blindness).

Reactive Hypochondriasis

In a setting of stress and new information, bodily sensations formerly dismissed as trivial may be redefined as suggestive of illness. This phenomenon is seen in patients who have had a recent close brush with cancer or other major illness; they may subsequently interpret minor physical changes as signs that they now have the feared disease. A similar phenomenon is sometimes referred to as "medical student's disease"; previously ignored sensations or signs are redefined as being diagnostic of recently studied (but imperfectly understood) illness. This condition is differentiated from hypochondriasis in that these patients respond to reassurance when appropriate investigation proves negative, whereas hypochondriacs characteristically remain unconvinced or offer a new complaint.

Depression

Hypochondriasis and depression often coexist. Patients primarily suffering from depression, however, tend to seek medical help less often and less insistently; their hopeless attitude and lack of initiative often extend to their physical problems. Other features of depression such as appetite and sleep changes, mood disturbance, and depressive thought content are usually present. The primarily depressed patient often elicits feelings of sympathy and concern from the doctor rather than the frustration typical of the doctor's relationship with the hypochondriac. Hypochondriacs may become depressed; in such cases, the physical complaints clearly antedate the onset of depressive symptoms (see Chapter 142, "Depression").

Panic Disorder

Panic attacks are characterized by the sudden onset of intense anxiety, and symptoms may include (among others) shortness of breath, dizziness, palpitations, tachycardia, sweating, and chest pain. Not surprisingly, patients with panic disorder sometimes mistakenly believe that they are having a heart attack, and they may remain concerned despite the absence of cardiac disease. Panic attacks are quite treatable; thus, psychiatric consultation is recommended when this disorder is suspected (see Chapter 140, "Anxiety").

Malingering

These patients feign illness for specific gains such as lessened criminal or financial responsibility or transfer from jail to hospital. These patients can be differentiated from hypochondriacs by the presence of such circumstances. They also differ, although less visibly, in that they are aware of the falseness of their claims to illness, in contrast to hypochondriacs, who believe that they are actually ill and need medical care.

Factitious Disorder with Physical Signs

Patients with factitious disorder intentionally produce or feign physical symptoms in order to assume the sick role. They lack the external incentivies seen in malingering. A wide and astounding array of symptoms has been reported, often resulting from self-inoculation with contaminated material. These patients tend to suffer from severe personality disorders.

Psychosis

Somatic delusions occasionally accompany psychosis. Whereas the hypochondriac may be able to concede the possibility that his belief that he is ill is unfounded, the psychotic patient with somatic delusions is absolutely convinced that the symptoms are real. Somatic delusions typically coexist with other symptoms suggesting a psychotic disorder (see Chapter 141, "Psychosis").

Etiology

The hypochondriac's paradoxical affinity for illness may be better appreciated by considering the underlying psychodynamics. Unconscious wishes that are consciously unacceptable because they are embarrassing, frightening, or painful may be expressed indirectly via more acceptable channels. The "patient role" affords an opportunity for the individual to receive wished-for care, attention, and a relationship with a doctor without having to acknowledge these wishes, because physical illness is seen in our culture as something that happens *to* a person, for which the person is not responsible. Unacceptable dependency needs have most often been hypothesized to motivate the illness-claiming behavior, but other needs have been identified as well. These include a need for another person to bolster a defective sense of self (without the relationship with the doctor, the patient would feel intolerably empty and disconnected) and anger (the illness causes other people to suffer and make sacrifices for the patient). Thus, the doctor's attempt to "cure" the patient of his symptoms or to demonstrate to the patient that he does not have an illness and therefore should relinquish the patient role are far from welcome. It is important to be aware, however, that the hypochondriac does not consciously elect to manipulate the situation; rather, he experiences a sense of discomfort that is explained to himself as well as to the physician in the acceptable terms of a legitimate need for medical care.

Diagnostic Approach

Most hypochondriacal patients have seen a number of doctors; this is particularly so at tertiary-care medical centers. The patient often communicates to a new doctor his disappointment with previous caregivers and his confidence that his new care will be better. When this resonates with the beginning doctor's own aspirations, the early interaction will be smooth, even interesting and gratifying. Unfortunately, this increases the mutual disillusionment that subsequently occurs when the patient's complaints prove groundless; at that point, the most compassionate doctor will become frustrated and ultimately will face a choice between unappealing alternatives. The physician may decide to insist that the patient is not ill despite his complaints, and perhaps tell him that his problems are "all in his head," which is certain to alienate the patient. Or the physician may feel that he should press on beyond the limits of appropriate work-up in an effort to find *some* legitimate organic diagnosis. Most physicians are justifiably uncomfortable with this alternative as well.

The proper approach to the hypochondriacal patient involves balanced attention to the patient's physical and emotional pathology. Initially, the work-up proceeds appropriate to the patient's complaints. When the characteristically frustrating interaction occurs (usually when initial examination and tests are negative), a change in stance is indicated: the physician begins to consider that the patient may have an emotional need to be ill and that, in addition to the emotional pathology that is present, physical illness may also occur.

Although psychiatric consultation may be useful in diagnosis, these patients generally refuse or do poorly with psychiatric referral; they insist that their problems are medical, not psychiatric. Proper management by the primary physician is therefore fundamental. If the patient's claim to the sick role is granted rather than challenged, the doctor's attention can focus on diagnosis and treatment. As investigation proceeds, the legitimacy of the patient's hospitalization or need for follow-up appointments should not be challenged. Negative test results should be presented in the context of worrisome illnesses being ruled out, rather than evidence that no "real" illness exists. When a diagnosis of hypochondriasis is appropriate, long-term management is similar: the doctor cannot expect to "cure" the patient, but can minimize the patient's need to prove how ill he is, support his functioning despite his symptoms, and detect organic illness should it occur.

References

Adler G. The physician and the hypochondriacal patient. N Engl J Med 1981; 304:1394.

Dubovsky SL. Psychotherapeutics in primary care. A hypochondriacal patient. New York: Grune & Stratton, 1981:152.

Kenyon FE. Hypochondriacal states. Br J Psychiatry 1981; 129:1.

Lazare AL, ed. Outpatient psychiatry—diagnosis and treatment. Baltimore: Williams & Wilkins, 1989.

Lipsitt DR. Medical and psychological characteristics of "crocks." Psychiatry Med 1970; 1:15.

Reaction to Illness

Barry Ginsberg, MD

Jonathan S. Rothman, MD

144

A patient's emotional reaction to illness and hospitalization may at one extreme go unnoticed, or at the other extreme be so dramatic that medical treatment is interrupted. Examples of the latter include the patient who responds to a heart attack with dangerous demonstrations of physical and sexual prowess, and the patient who makes endless demands.

The response to illness of any given patient is determined by many factors. These include the new social role of being a patient, as well as the nature of the illness. These stresses will be understood and responded to in the context of the patient's premorbid personality. More specifically, areas of "sensitivity" or unresolved inner conflict may be brought up by illness and "patienthood." Illness may heighten the patient's usual ways of dealing with (or defending against) unpleasant feelings, sometimes to a pathologic degree. All these factors need to be explored in order to understand the patient's individual reaction so that a successful management approach can be devised.

Becoming a patient, particularly a hospitalized one, forces an individual to become much more dependent than usual. He or she also must cede control over many decisions, even very important ones. The patient must be able to trust relative strangers. Abilities that have been a source of pride and self-esteem may be gone; even early childhood foundations of self-esteem such as sphincter control may be lost. The temporary nature of some changes makes them somewhat easier to accept; a person with chronic disease can be expected to have more difficulty and must deal with permanent losses.

The nature of the illness is important not only in terms of how sick (or in danger of dying) the patient feels, but also sometimes in terms of specific meanings. For example, a patient with breast cancer may have a different emotional reaction than one with lung cancer, based on the personal meaning of the affected organ and specific disease process. A particular illness may have a less obvious personal meaning derived from the patient's previous experience, such as when a relative has had the same disease.

The patient's personality is another major factor. Bibring and Kahana (1964) have described seven personality "types" and the inner meaning that illness and hospitalization are apt to carry for each. They note that few patients manifest a pure single type, and that each represents a "normal" personality trait heightened by stress. The more common presentations are summarized briefly as follows:

1. For the dependent, overdemanding person who fears abandonment and helplessness and wishes for boundless interest and care, illness increases the intensity of both the fears and the wishes. This patient may therefore cling to the doctor. This type of patient is also prone to becoming depressed and angry when needs for care are not met.

2. The person who characteristically deals with anxiety by being controlled, orderly, and intellectualized may perceive illness as implying a loss of control; he or she is apt to redouble efforts to take charge and tightly control all aspects of care.

3. For people in whom the issue of sexual attractiveness and competence is unresolved, illness may be especially threatening. The patient who does cartwheels out of bed after a heart

attack is likely to be in this category. The illness is perceived by the patient as a personal defect, implying weakness or unattractiveness. To ward off these feelings, the individual may go to extraordinary and inappropriate lengths to demonstrate his or her attractiveness and strength.

4. The self-sacrificing or masochistic person is apt to find illness oddly gratifying. Despite complaints, the individual seems reluctant to give up the illness; it is a visible sign of his or her burden.

5. The narcissistic person, whose grandiosity reflects inner self-doubt, is likely to react to the "insult" of illness by a combination of idealizing some caregivers (this patient needs to believe that he or she is at the "best" hospital, treated by the "best" specialist) and criticizing any imperfection in others.

Diagnostic Approach

Managing the patient's emotional reaction to illness requires perhaps as much skill as managing the illness itself; as a physician, you will need some interviewing ability, an understanding of common human conflicts, an ability to examine rather than act on personal feelings as they arise in relation to the patient, and sufficient flexibility to alter your management style to fit the patient. Although a psychiatric consultation may help with these tasks, various emotional reactions are such a regular feature of patient care that referring the patient for psychiatric treatment is usually not indicated.

Whether or not the patient's emotional reaction has caused problems, the patient should be given the opportunity to discuss his or her illness and care in an open-ended way. Your task is to listen as well as to inform: listen for indirect and direct reflections of the patient's emotional reaction. For example, does the patient seem to cling to your every remark? If you find yourself getting irritated when it seems difficult to terminate the interview, consider this as data supporting dependency as an important issue for the patient, and begin to plan the patient's management accordingly. Is there a grandiose quality to the patient's spontaneous comments? Should you find that you are feeling inflated (or possibly devalued) by the patient, this may be a narcissistic patient whose sense of vulnerability is defended against by entitlement.

Management

The following general guidelines may help you decide on the proper management style for a patient. These should not be adopted automatically; it is important to interview and understand each individual patient. Management of the patient whose illness brings up primarily dependency issues should involve communicating to the patient the staff's readiness to care for him or her while *nonpunitively* setting limits should the patient's demands become excessive. The controlling, orderly person usually responds well to a precise, scientific, medical approach. This patient will usually need to be informed in some detail about his or her illness; decision making may need to be shared more than usual with this patient. The patient who demonstrates his or her own attractiveness and strength, fearing inadequacy and humiliation, may need to be assured of your appreciation, within reasonable and professional boundaries. These patients may need to discuss their fears repeatedly; these should be acknowledged, but the patient should be reminded of the actual outlook. The patient who wishes to suffer does not respond well to reassurance; this patient is more likely to appreciate an acknowledgment of his or her difficult struggle. The narcissistic patient's sense of entitlement (to special treatment) should not be directly challenged; rather, it should be acknowledged and then channeled into entitlement to the very best medical care, the details of which should be negotiated with the patient. It must be reemphasized that the proper management style cannot be "prescribed" without understanding the meaning of the illness to the individual patient.

References

Bibring G, Kahana R. In: Zinberg N, ed. Psychiatry and medical practice in a general hospital. New York: International Universities Press, 1964.

Groves JE. Taking care of the hateful patient. N Engl J Med 1978; 298:883.

Lazare A, Eisenthal S. Clinic/patient relations. I: Attending to the patient's perspective. In: Lazare A, ed. Outpatient psychiatry—diagnosis and treatment. Baltimore: Williams & Wilkins, 1989:125.

Nemiah JC. Foundations of psychopathology. New York: Oxford University Press, 1961.

Strain JJ, Grossman S. Psychological care of the medically ill. New York: Appleton-Century-Crofts, 1975.

145 Assessment of the Suicidal Patient

Steven A. Adelman, MD

Linda G. Peterson, MD

Suicide is one of the leading causes of death for individuals under 45 years of age. It also accounts for increasing numbers of deaths with every decade of life for elderly men. Seventy percent of people who take their lives have had contact with a physician within the 90 days preceding their deaths. Suicide is a significant hazard for individuals who suffer from any of the following common conditions seen in general medical or general psychiatric practice: chronic physical illness, alcoholism, drug abuse, and depression. Thus, the detection, assessment, and management of the suicidal patient are essential skills for all practicing physicians.

Physicians learn that a patient is suicidal both directly and indirectly. Patients may communicate verbally that they are thinking of hurting or killing themselves, or that they have already attempted to do so. A reticent patient's recent attempt may be detected on physical examination (e.g., scars on the wrists or neck) or with laboratory tests (e.g., acidosis from an aspirin overdose, or hepatic dysfunction from an acetaminophen overdose). In many cases, changes in a patient's demeanor, behavior, or mental status will prompt the physician to wonder if the patient is suicidal.

The astute clinician pays close attention to a number of subtleties that may indicate that a patient is thinking of ending his or her life. Does the patient sound or look depressed, despondent, helpless, or hopeless, or feel that he or she is a burden or embarrassment to his or her family? Is the patient overwhelmed by a recent personal loss? Is the patient concerned about putting affairs in order? Is he or she behaving as though this is a final appointment? Is the patient making innuendoes such as, "I'll show them!"? If the answer to any of these questions is "yes," a more detailed assessment is in order.

Beginning clinicians sometimes worry that questions about suicidality will prompt self-destructiveness in a patient who was not previously suicidal. There is no evidence to indicate that this actually happens. On the contrary, the risks of ignoring or minimizing signals suggesting suicidality are great. The very fact that the suicidal patient is being evaluated by a physician indicates some ambivalence about the patient's intentions to end his or her life. A physician who ignores the cues indicating that someone is suicidal is giving that person the following message: "I don't care about you enough to find out what is really bothering you." This message may aggravate feelings of hopelessness, depression, and low self-esteem, which may increase the likelihood that the patient will attempt suicide. So whenever a patient's words, behavior, physical findings, or laboratory findings suggest the possibility of suicidality, it is crucial to pursue a more thorough assessment.

Assessment and management of the suicidal patient is one of the most stressful and difficult tasks faced by physicians. An important principle that helps to make this task bearable is, *whenever possible, involve other people.* Talking to members of the patient's social support system (relatives, friends, coworkers) is crucial in determining the seriousness of the patient's intentions. Furthermore, a decision not to hospitalize a suicidal patient may depend upon knowledge of the strength and extent of the social support system.

In addition to involving people who know the patient, involve other health professionals who are comfortable evaluating suicidality. Primary care physicians may consult one another or elect to refer the patient to a psychiatrist. Psychiatrists themselves may consult colleagues or elect to have a patient evaluated by an emergency mental health service. Unless you are fully comfortable evaluating a suicidal patient alone, you should never attempt to do so. Reviewing your evaluation on the phone with a trusted colleague may be all that is necessary to confirm that your assessment and plans are appropriate for the particular situation at hand.

Once you become aware that a patient is suicidal, a methodical evaluation is in order. Assess the degree of lethality by focusing specific questions on the suicidal thoughts: Are these passing thoughts or persistent ones? When do they occur? Are the thoughts getting stronger, or do they seem to be diminishing? Has a specific plan been considered? What is the plan? Do the means exist to carry out the plan? How much determination is there to carry out the plan? Lethality is greatest when the individual has persistent thoughts involving a lethal plan that is readily available. The availability of firearms is particularly worrisome.

In addition to assessing the lethality of the patient's plan, carefully consider the presence or absence of specific risk factors that correlate with the likelihood of completed suicide. Demographic statistics indicate that men are at greater risk than women; adolescents and elderly persons are at greater risk than others; and Protestants are at greater risk than Jews, who are at greater risk than Catholics.

Specific questions to determine risk should be pursued: Is there a history of previous suicide attempts (40 percent of those who kill themselves have a history of previous attempts)? Is the patient depressed, psychotic, or impulsive? Is there a history of drug or alcohol abuse? Is there a history of recent psychiatric hospitalization? Does the person suffer from a significant chronic physical illness, or has he or she recently been diagnosed with a serious condition such as acquired immunodeficiency syndrome (AIDS) or cancer? Has a loved one recently died or committed suicide? Has the individual recently retired or lost his or her job or suffered another humiliating change in status? Does the person live alone and/or have a poor social support system? Each answer of "yes" to these questions increases the risk of actual suicide.

The determination of risk factors helps to establish the degree of perturbation. Patients who are at highest risk are those who manifest both significant lethality and significant perturbation. An example of a very high risk patient would be a 60-year-old man suffering from systemic lupus erythematosus who is currently psychotic as a result of high-dose steroid treatment. He believes he is being followed by the FBI and hears voices telling him to kill himself before he is arrested. When asked about a plan, he informs the physician that he has a loaded revolver in his glove compartment. The patient is both highly perturbed and very lethal, and is clearly a candidate for immediate psychiatric hospitalization, either voluntary or involuntary.

Because of the organic psychosis, such a patient is clearly not competent to make the decision to end his own life. The issue of competence becomes problematic in the case of a 40-year-old college professor diagnosed with AIDS who states he intends to end his life because he knows his days are numbered and is fed up with the pain of recurrent opportunistic infections. Although physicians are obligated to "do no harm" and to work actively to preserve life, the decision whether or not to force involuntary treatment on a seemingly competent yet suicidal person with a terminal illness clearly raises complex ethical dilemmas, the resolution of which clearly lies beyond the scope of this chapter.

The approach to assessing the suicidal patient just outlined may be applied equally well both to patients who are contemplating suicide and to those who have recently made an attempt. In both cases, the goal of the physician is to keep the patient alive and to engage the patient in a treatment situation that is likely to diminish the likelihood of self-destructive actions. Depending on the extent of the patient's perturbation and the degree of lethality, immediate stabilization may require a single outpatient session, an emergency room evaluation, referral to a psychiatrist, or immediate psychiatric hospitalization. The appropriate intervention is the one that diminishes the patient's suicidality in a way that reassures doctor, patient, and members of the social support system that suicidal actions are highly unlikely. One can be comfortable with a decision *not* to hospitalize a suicidal patient when all parties involved have agreed upon a clear-cut plan of action in the event that the patient's suicidal thoughts worsen.

It is probable that most physicians will lose patients to suicide in the course of a career with tens of thousands of patient contacts. When a significant doctor-patient relationship has existed, attending the patient's funeral and meeting with surviving relatives may help both the physician and the family come to terms with the terrible loss. Thus, in addition to learning to detect, assess, and manage suicidality, physicians may play a crucial role in helping people cope with the loss of a loved one by suicide.

References

Abrams HS, Moore GI, Westervelt FB Jr. Suicidal behavior in chronic dialysis patients. Am J Psychiatry 1971; 127:1199.

Bassuk EL, Schoonover SC, Gill AD, eds. Lifelines: Clinical perspectives on suicide. New York: Plenum Press, 1982.

Maltsberger JT. Suicide risk: The formulation of clinical judgement. New York: New York University Press, 1986.

Motto JA. Suicide risk factors in alcohol abuse. Suicide Life-Threatening Behav 1980; 10:230.

Peterson LG, Bongar B. The suicidal patient. In: Lazare A, ed. Outpatient psychiatry—diagnosis and treatment. Baltimore: Williams & Wilkins, 1989.

Pokorny AD. Suicide rates in various psychiatric disorders. J Nerv Ment Dis 1964;139:499.

Alcoholism

Abigail Adams, MD

Edward L. Goldberg, MD

146

Epidemiology

Alcoholism and alcohol abuse are common problems, with a lifetime prevalence rate of 10 to 15 percent. Approximately two-thirds of the adults in a physician's practice drink alcohol, and about half of these patients drink heavily at times. Of this latter group, more than one-third may be categorized as alcoholics or alcohol abusers (Sixth Special Report to US Congress, 1987). One-fifth of our health care dollars are spent for alcohol-related illnesses. More than 20 percent of the admissions to general hospitals are complicated by alcohol abuse or alcoholism. In spite of the enormous health care consequences, however, physicians fail to make a diagnosis and to intervene in more than 9 out of 10 cases.

There are many reasons why physicians fail to recognize alcoholic patients. They stem from the mixture of myths and misinformation about alcoholism and from the fact that people with alcohol problems sometimes deny their reliance on alcohol. In contrast to common misconceptions, clinicians should keep in mind the following: (1) most alcoholics hold jobs and are married, (2) alcoholics commonly consume beer, and (3) alcoholics are usually *not* difficult patients, but they often have more medical problems (Hill, 1983).

By definition, the alcoholic is *out of control* with respect to his or her drinking. Often the alcoholic will not seek treatment voluntarily. It commonly takes a warning by a physician or other health professional of the effects on health or a crisis at home or work to persuade the alcoholic to enter treatment.

In most cases, alcoholism is *not* just a symptom of some underlying personality disorder or mental illness. This mistaken notion of "secondary alcoholism" implies that treatment will be directed toward an underlying psychiatric condition. Alcoholism generally should be thought of as a primary disorder for which treatment is not only readily available but also highly successful.

Definitions

The essential feature of alcoholic drinking is a repetitive and often inconsistent loss of control over drinking. If one looks at alcohol abuse and alcoholism as two linked stages in a continuum of alcoholic drinking, the American Psychiatric Association's DSM III-R criteria for abuse and alcoholism (dependence) are probably the most useful definitions:

Abuse requires three of these criteria:

1. The individual either (a) continues use despite knowledge that alcohol is causing social, occupational, or physical problems, or (b) shows recurrent use in situations in which alcohol is hazardous.
2. Symptoms have been present for 1 month or longer.
3. The individual does not meet criteria for alcohol dependence.

Dependence requires three of the following:

1. The individual drinks more than he or she means to, *often*.
2. The individual is unsuccessful at cutting down.
3. Much time is spent thinking about getting a drink, or when the next drink will be taken.
4. There are frequent ill effects from intoxication or withdrawal (absence from work, being drunk or hung over during work).
5. The individual gives up important nondrinking activities.
6. The individual continues to drink even though it causes problems in family or with health.
7. A tolerance for alcohol has developed (e.g., the individual has an alcohol level of 150 with no signs of intoxication, or is awake with an alcohol level of 300).
8. The individual has physical withdrawal symptoms.
9. The individual takes substances to relieve withdrawal symptoms.

In summary, the DSM III-R criteria for dependence on alcohol include all of the criteria for alcohol abuse plus the evidence for physical or psychological dependence. Both DSM III-R definitions highlight the essential feature of alcoholic drinking, which is *loss of control.* For alcohol abusers, it is more inconsistent; for the alcoholic or alcohol-dependent person, it is constant, often involves daily drinking, and tends to involve physical addiction.

Time Course of Alcohol-Related Problems

The detailed DSM III-R criteria *allude* to quantity and frequency of alcohol intake (development of tolerance), but it is clear that quantitating the amount and frequency of drinking is not enough to get at the nature of someone's relationship to alcohol. Nonetheless, it is still useful to look at how quantity of alcohol intake and frequency of drinking can affect patients over time.

Longitudinal studies on alcohol usage, abuse, and dependence demonstrate that alcoholism is a process that often evolves over *years.* Vaillant (1983) has studied cohorts of alcoholic patients over a decade and, on the basis of this research, describes three linked stages in the time course of alcoholism. These stages confirm the chronic nature of alcohol problems, suggest that heavy drinking places a patient at higher risk for development of alcoholism, and offer clinicians a time line that has implications for prognosis and treatment.

Vaillant describes *Stage I* as heavy social drinking and *not* abusive or alcoholic drinking. This includes usual daily use of more than 6 oz of 80-proof liquor (or four 12-oz beers or four 5-oz glasses of wine). This pattern of alcohol usage may persist over a lifetime. It may never cause adverse symptoms or be associated with loss of control. However, a percentage of those in Stage I will evolve, imperceptibly, into the second stage of Vaillant's time line. This evolution usually occurs over less than 10 years, and Stage II is called alcohol abuse.

Vaillant defines *Stage II* as the recurrent intake of 10 oz or more of 80-proof liquor (or wine/beer equivalent) in 24 hours. Typically affecting patients 25 to 35 years old, it includes the social, medical, or legal complications often associated with this level of alcohol use, including drunken driving, marital difficulties, gastritis, sleep disturbances, and hypertension.

At some point in their lives, 10 to 15 percent of all Americans may reach this level of usage. Estimates are that one-third revert back to Stage I, and one-third progress to Stage III. One-third remain in Stage II, with its associated morbidity affecting the abusive drinker, his or her family, and society at large.

Stage III is manifested by alcohol dependence and is often called "late-stage alcoholism." Vaillant's data found that most Stage III alcoholics spent roughly 10 years drinking "abusively" (Stage II) before progressing to Stage III. Thus, the Stage III drinker is typically over age 35. He or she may meet all the DSM III-R criteria for alcohol dependence with daily drinking, constant loss of control over drinking, withdrawal symptoms, morning drinking, a history of hospitalization for detoxification, and medical complications of alcoholism. Estimates are that this stage is reached by 5 to 10 percent of all adult Americans. In Vaillant's data, one-third of those at Stage III met with premature death. Even in this group of late-stage alcoholics, however, Vaillant found that stable abstinence was finally achieved in greater than one-third of the cases.

Vaillant's linked stages or "natural history" of alcoholism is useful because it allows us to see the chronic nature of many alcohol problems. This is a disease whose course may be measured in decades. Vaillant's work gives us a framework with which to evaluate our patients and a database that suggests that at no stage is the process irreversible.

Disease Concept

Is alcoholism a disease or just a set of bad behaviors? This issue has been debated in different forms since the 1800s. A recent court case in which a veteran's claim that his alcoholism was a service-related medical disability was disqualified indicates that the controversy over the disease concept remains unresolved.

Certainly, there is evidence that genetic factors may play a role in half of all alcoholics and that genetically susceptible individuals may have a different physiologic response to alcohol. It has also been shown that women become intoxicated with lower per-body-weight doses than men. Because much data remain to be collected regarding the biology of alcoholism, debates over the disease concept are unproductive.

The concept of alcoholism as a chronic disease can be a useful paradigm. It allows us to use familiar medical techniques to establish a diagnosis, initiate treatment, and institute long-term follow-up to monitor its long course (Clark, 1981).

The essential feature of alcoholic drinking is intermittent, recurrent, or constant loss of control. This qualitative difference between alcoholic or abusive drinking and "normal" drinking is addressed by the disease concept. It provides a useful construct for patients that (1) helps explain their repetitive self-destructive behavior (the disease concept implies that there are factors present other than simply personal irresponsibility, e.g., "We may not understand it, but some people react differently to drinking"); (2) offers an outline for continuing management (there is help once a diagnosis is made); and (3) reinforces that they must take responsibility for their disease and behavior.

Intervention

All studies support the increased success rate seen with early intervention in alcoholism. The trick is to diagnose the alcohol problem *early,* when the patient is still "asymptomatic."

Screening

Early alcohol abuse is picked up by behavioral signs and symptoms, not by laboratory or physical examination data. Therefore, the clinician's focus must be on the history, e.g., presenting complaints, family history, family life, marriage, and job status. Common presenting conditions associated with early alcohol abuse include high blood pressure, sleep disturbances, gastritis, fatigue, depression, marital discord, and work problems.

Because of the extremely high prevalence of alcohol problems (1.5 times higher than hyperglycemia, for which we commonly screen), all patients should be screened. Although laboratory tests are a very poor screening technique (increases in mean corpuscular volume, gamma-glutamyltransferase, and high-density lipoproteins have sensitivities of only 25 to 40 percent [Harp and Spickard, 1987]), standardized screening questions are quite effective when combined with routine medical histories. Here are two examples that are short, easy to remember, and highly sensitive and specific:

CAGE Questionnaire: Two out of four positive answers give 85 percent sensitivity and 95 percent specificity (Harp and Spickard, 1987)

C Have you ever tried to *cut* down on your drinking?
A Have you ever been *annoyed* by someone's criticism of your drinking?
G Have you ever felt *guilty* about your drinking?
E Have you ever needed an *eye-opener* to settle you down the morning after drinking?

Two Questions: Two positive answers give 91.5 percent sensitivity and 90 percent specificity (Cyr and Wartman, 1988)

1. Have you ever had a drinking problem?
2. When was your last drink? (positive = less than 24 hours)

These screening questionnaires are effective because they get at *how* alcohol is being used and not just at how much. They give us insight into how the patient feels about his or her alcohol usage and whether or not it is causing problems for the patient.

Some additional factors that increase a patient's risk and that should alert the physician to screen more carefully include the following:

1. A first-degree relative with an alcohol problem or alcoholism (this increases the risk approximately fourfold)
2. An urban or hospital-based practice setting
3. Patient occupation or social network that (a) makes alcohol freely available throughout the workday, (b) includes social pressure to drink from coworkers or friends, or (c) provides high job stress with frequent separation from normal work or family routines

In summary, the physican who is armed with the knowledge of risk factors, common presenting conditions, and effective screening techniques should be prepared to uncover *early* problems with alcohol. Remember, research suggests that education alone may serve as an effective early intervention.

Making the Diagnosis

A successful 40-year-old businessman sits across from you. He is here for a check-up and complains of fatigue, which he attributes to stress. On examination, his blood pressure is elevated at 150/95 and the patient reveals that his father "had a problem with alcohol." This businessman has tried to cut down on his drinking in the past, especially after fights with his wife. He doesn't think he drinks much more than his friends. He admits to having four or five drinks daily. It helps him relax and get to sleep. He is getting irritated by your questions.

What clues you in to the diagnosis of alcohol abuse in this case? To strengthen the diagnosis, you need to focus on collecting additional data in three areas:

1. Loss of control. This patient describes unsuccessful attempts at cutting down. You need to know more about what this was like for him.

2. Adverse effects on health, marriage, or work. The patient is telling you that he is "stressed out, tired" and that he can't sleep well—all are hallmarks of heavy alcohol usage. His blood pressure elevation may well be secondary to heavy alcohol usage.

3. Evidence of dependence or addiction. The patient admits to significant daily usage. You need to know more about any increased usage. Was he drinking less 3 years ago? Does he feel upset if he can't have a drink to relax? Does he have other ways to unwind? Is there any evidence of the alcohol withdrawal syndrome?

As you collect these data, it is critical that you approach the issue as a concerned and nonjudgmental clinician. As you question him, be supportive and educative. For example, you might say, "Most patients don't realize that alcohol taken after supper can interfere with restful sleep. This has been shown in sleep lab testing. I am concerned for your health."

Remember, the patient with an alcohol problem is often humiliated by his or her reliance on alcohol. The combination of shame and dependence may produce reactions of angry denial. This may interfere with taking a complete history, but the reaction itself is highly suggestive of an alcohol problem.

Although alcohol abusers may underestimate alcohol intake, they are usually accurate in describing the extensive problems caused by excessive drinking (Society of General Internal Medicine, 1988).

Presenting the Diagnosis

The key to a fruitful discussion lies in your ability to sympathetically convey your concern for the patient and about his or her alcohol usage. The diagnosis can be presented with whatever degree of certainty has been established by the interview. If you are uncertain as to the existence of an alcohol problem, it may be prudent to share your questions with the patient.

Use specific examples that illustrate the issue of loss of control. Whenever possible, link the adverse effects of alcohol to the patient's presenting complaint or medical problem (e.g., hypertension, fatigue). Try to elicit what the patient's understanding of alcoholism is. Does he or she understand the nature of the disease? Is the disease concept clear? Educating the patient about alcohol abuse and alcoholism as a disease helps to increase patient participation in treatment (Sixth Special Report to the US Congress).

This kind of discussion may be difficult for the patient. The clinician must acknowledge and empathize with the feelings stirred up by discussion of a patient's problem with alcohol. It is extremely important to provide a sense of hope and support. Alcohol problems are highly treatable. You might say, for example, "Anyone would find it difficult to talk about these issues. I only bring them up because in my experience, I know they are important and I am concerned for you. We can sort these things out, and there are ways to treat every alcohol problem" (Society of General Internal Medicine, 1988).

Treatment

Treatment must be patient-centered and as explicit as possible. Although setting realistic treatment goals requires an individualized approach, two general rules of thumb apply to treatment plans:

1. Make ample use of Alcoholics Anonymous (AA). AA is a self-help group that is readily available, free, educational, and therapeutic. Although no well-controlled studies have documented the efficacy of AA, indirect evidence supports its effectiveness.

2. Develop a referral network that includes clinicians and programs that specialize in alcohol rehabilitation. Although intervention by the primary care physician may resolve mild alcohol problems, a specialized approach is usually necessary for more serious problems.

Using the severity of the drinking problem as a guide, various patient-centered treatments can be outlined.

Case 1. After the diagnosis of "problem drinking" is presented to the 40-year-old businessman, the patient responds with resistance. He's not sure he has any problem. You might suggest to the patient that he attend five AA meetings in the next 2 weeks. These would be "open" AA meetings, which are educational and open to the public and to nonalcoholics. Suggest that the patient return to dicuss the meetings. In order to clarify the issue of "loss of control," you could challenge the patient to limit his intake to no more than two drinks per 24-hour period, without exceptions. If the patient is unable to control his drinking to the agreed-upon amount, there is evidence for loss of control. If he maintains control, his ability to continue doing so should be monitored regularly.

Case 2. A later-stage alcohol problem is uncovered in a 50-year-old man who is alcohol-dependent. He is drinking daily and is aware of the damage it is doing to his marriage and job performance. The physician collaborates with an alcohol specialist who will help with the following: (1) designing an appropriate detoxification plan and (2) engaging the patient in a long-term rehabilitation program. Once the initial alcohol withdrawal symptoms have passed (3 to 5 days), longer-term rehabilitation is an absolute necessity. This includes learning about alcoholism and learning new coping mechanisms to prevent relapse. Rehabilitation may involve a time-limited in-patient program, long-term outpatient alcohol counseling, and a significant commitment to AA.

When you decide that a patient requires specialized treatment, it is *not* sufficient to say, "Go find yourself some help." Instead, you should play an active role in the referral process. You should familiarize yourself with AA and with specific alcohol rehabilitation programs. Patients are likely to follow the recommendations of knowledgeable physicians who are themselves engaged in the referral and treatment process.

To summarize, alcohol abuse and alcoholism are different points on a lengthy continuum. Establishing the diagnosis and engaging the patient in alcoholism treatment require time and patience on the part of the physician, who plays a central role in the treatment process even when alcohol counselors or specialists are involved.

Clinical Pharmacology and Pathophysiology of Alcohol

Absorption and Metabolism

Alcohol is absorbed readily across much of the gastrointestinal mucosa. Most alcohol is absorbed from the small bowel. Absorption from the gastric mucosa does occur, but it is affected by the presence or absence of food. In healthy adults, absorption is completed 2 to 6 hours after ingestion. Metabolism of alcohol occurs primarily via the hepatic enzyme system, alcohol dehydrogenase being the most important enzyme present. The elimination of alcohol is linear except at lower serum levels (Naranjo and Sellers, 1986). This averages out to an effective elimination rate of 1.5 oz of 80-proof liquor (12 oz of beer or 5 oz of wine) over 2 hours. As the alcohol blood level falls to below 20 mg/dl, the rate of elimination slows. The exact pharmacokinetics will vary with body size (volume of distribution) and concurrent food intake (Hawkins and Kalant, 1972).

The legal limit for driving drunk in most states is a blood alcohol concentration of 100 mg/dl. However, the risk of being in a traffic accident is increased at blood alcohol concentrations of 50 mg/dl, a level produced by as little as 2 to 3 oz of 80-proof liquor on an empty stomach (Fifth Special Report to the US Congress).

Review by Systems

Acute Central Nervous System Effects

Alcohol has its primary effects on the central nervous system (CNS). Both structure and function are eventually impaired, with the initial alteration occurring at the neuronal membrane level. Alcohol is a CNS depressant or anesthetic, but when taken in low to moderate doses, it can selectively depress inhibitory nerve cells, producing a stimulatory effect.

Alcohol Intoxication. Alcohol intoxication is defined as the impairment of motor performance and depression of mental function. Early on, there is mood elevation, garrulous speech, and even aggressive behavior, which coincides with depression of inhibitory centers. Body sway is the most sensitive marker for acute intoxication and may occur in nontolerant individuals with blood alcohol levels as low as 50 mg/dl.

The spectrum of alcohol intoxication extends from the mildly intoxicated patient to the patient who dies in coma from respiratory depression. The usual lethal dose is 450 to 500 mg/dl, and unresponsive patients at this blood level should be considered for hemodialysis. For the usual mild case of intoxication there is no special therapy, and observation appropriate for the clinical setting is all that is necessary (Fifth Special Report to the US Congress).

Development of Tolerance. Chronic consumption of alcohol produces an adaptation at the neuronal level that is manifested by alcohol tolerance (Sixth Special Report to the US Congress). Chronic heavy alcohol users can tolerate greater amounts of alcohol (higher blood alcohol levels) without major signs of intoxication. The occasional drinker may have slurred speech at a blood alcohol level of 100 mg/dl, whereas a chronic alcohol abuser may appear alert and fully functional with an alcohol level greater than 150 mg/dl.

Alcohol Withdrawal Syndrome. Alcohol tolerance and physical dependence are distinct effects of alcohol ingestion, but they are closely linked in that the presence of tolerance in a patient can necessitate or permit the consumption of alcohol in amounts that can lead to physical dependence.

The alcohol-dependent patient will experience the alcohol withdrawal syndrome as his or her blood alcohol level falls. This may begin with mild tremulousness even as the patient cuts down on his or her intake. The spectrum of withdrawal ranges from tremulousness to death from alcohol withdrawal delirium (delirium tremens, or "DTs"). The most common form of alcohol withdrawal is characterized by tremulousness or "the shakes." This usually begins 12 to 24 hours after the last drink and is accompanied by tachycardia, facial flushing, and irritability. In severe cases, there is slight confusion, inattentiveness, and auditory hallucinations.

Seizures ("rum fits") may accompany alcohol withdrawal and typically occur within 48 hours of withdrawal. These are usually generalized seizures that often occur in bursts of two to six seizures at a time. The postictal state may blend into the initial confusion of the delirium tremens, and roughly one-third of untreated seizures progress to delirium tremens. Seizures should be treated with intravenous phenytoin if there is a history of epilepsy and if the seizures are recurrent, prolonged, or associated with respiratory problems. Alcoholics with a previous history of seizure disorder should be treated with prophylactic phenytoin during alcohol withdrawal.

Delirium tremens is the extreme form of the withdrawal syndrome. It is most common in patients with a long history of severe, chronic alcoholism. It occurs 24 to 72 hours into withdrawal and is characterized by hallucinations, agitated confusion, and markedly increased sympathetic discharge. The patients have tremor and are profoundly agitated, diaphoretic, and tachycardic. Delirium tremens usually lasts 72 hours and in the past has been associated with a mortality rate of up to 15 percent. Hyperthermia and hypotension are predictors of a fatal outcome. Recent advances in monitoring for medical complications have lowered the mortality rate to under 10 percent. Associated complications such as electrolyte disturbances (hypokalemia, hypomagnesemia, and acidosis), aspiration pneumonia, hepatic failure, pancreatitis, and gastrointestinal bleeding contribute to the persistently high mortality rate (Naranjo and Sellers, 1986).

There are over 125 published regimens for the treatment of alcohol withdrawal, but most physicians today use either chlordiazepoxide or diazepam, for they have a wide margin of safety and are easy to administer. Underlying medical disease (i.e., pancreatitis, pneumonia) must be vigorously treated. If delirium tremens is present, intravenous diazepam is indicated. The patient must be monitored for respiratory depression, as 5 mg of diazepam is given intravenously every 5 minutes until the patient is appropriately sedated. Large doses (50 to 100 mg) are not unusual in these patients. Beta-blockers and clonidine have been added to several withdrawal treatment strategies but do not appear to be as effective as benzodiazepines in suppressing the progression to delirium tremens (Kraus et al, 1985).

Chronic Central Nervous System Damage

Wernicke's Encephalopathy. *Wernicke's encephalopathy* is one manifestation of alcohol's effects on the CNS. The patient presents with generalized confusion, ophthalmoplegia, nystagmus, ataxia, and associated peripheral neuropathy. If untreated, it may be fatal. When treated with thiamine, ophthalmoplegia disappears, the confusion clears, and the ataxia improves. Conversely, glucose given to an alcoholic who is not first treated with thiamine can precipitate Wernicke's encephalopathy.

Korsakoff's Psychosis. *Korsakoff's psychosis* may persist as a chronic encephalopathic state even after the acute Wernicke's abnormality clears. The cause of Korsakoff's psychosis is unknown. Severe amnesia is part of the clinical picture and frequently leads to confabulation in an attempt to cover gaps in memory. The patient cannot remember or learn, and few make a significant recovery.

Peripheral Neuropathy

Peripheral neuropathy occurs with chronic excessive alcohol usage. The B-vitamin deficiencies seen in alcoholic patients can contribute to the polyneuropathy present. Alcohol-associated polyneuropathy is distal, symmetric, and involves both sensory and motor systems. Patients complain of pain, paresthesias, and weakness. Examination reveals loss of touch, position, vibration, and distal (ankle) deep tendon reflexes. Abstinence and vitamin replacement are associated with improvement in 4 to 6 months (Eckardt et al, 1981).

Musculoskeletal Effects

Myopathies are seen in approximately one-third of all alcoholics. A myopathy may present as only subacute progression of weakness, muscle wasting, and asymptomatic elevations of muscle enzymes. However, following an episode of heavy drinking, one can see *acute* alcoholic myopathy (alcoholic rhabdomyolysis) with marked elevations of creatine phosphokinase and aldolase, painful and tender muscles, and myoglobinuria. In severe cases, the patient must be hydrated intravenously and closely monitored for the development of acute tubular necrosis (Eckardt et al, 1981).

Skeletal abnormalities are produced by alterations in calcium metabolism, and there is an increased risk for fractures and osteonecrosis of the femoral head. The exact mechanism is not known, but moderate to heavy drinking appears to increase the risk of developing osteoporosis (Van Thiel et al, 1982).

Endocrine Effects

Direct toxicity to the testes, ovaries, pituitary, and hypothalamus results in decreased estrogen and testosterone production, loss of libido, and impotence. With the development of liver disease and altered estrogen metabolism, feminization occurs in men. In some of these cases the prognosis is good. For example, in men without severe testicular atrophy, abstinence from drinking will reverse alcohol-associated sexual dysfunction within 3 to 4 months. However, for others who have chronically used alcohol, the impotence may persist even after cessation (Van Thiel et al, 1982).

Cardiac Effects

Alcohol has multiple effects on the cardiovascular system. Alcoholic cardiomyopathy usually occurs in those who have been alcoholics for more than 10 years. Right ventricular heart failure is the most common presentation, but there are no specific findings on examination or laboratory testing to differentiate alcoholic cardiomyopathy from the other possible causes of heart disease. Small amounts of alcohol have been shown to impair cardiac function in patients with congestive heart failure.

Arrhythmias occur with even moderate alcohol usage. "Holiday heart" refers to the phenomenon of cardiac irritability seen in susceptible patients with otherwise normal cardiac function. Both atrial and ventricular arrhythmias have been recorded (Ettinger et al, 1978). Moderate amounts (2 to 5 oz of hard liquor) have also been shown to raise blood pressure, increase pulse in healthy patients, and produce exercise-associated ischemia in patients with established coronary artery disease. It is reasonable to advise patients with cardiovascular disease to limit alcohol intake to 2 oz of hard liquor daily (Klatsky et al, 1977; Orlando et al, 1976).

Hematologic Effects

Alcohol affects the hematopoietic system. Production of red blood cells is decreased after weeks of heavy drinking. The mean corpuscular volume may be elevated secondary to ill-defined but direct effects of alcohol. Hypersegmented polymorphonuclear leukocytes, decreased reticulocyte count, and hyperplastic bone marrow suggest folic acid deficiency.

Chronic heavy alcohol usage will also decrease bone marrow production of white blood cells and alters their function, making the patient more susceptible to infection.

Thrombocytopenia may be severe and is secondary to decreased bone marrow production, decreased platelet survival, hypersplenism, or folic acid deficiency. Platelet counts that were lowered by the direct marrow-suppressive effects of alcohol will begin to rise 2 to 3 days after cessation of drinking (Hebert, 1980).

Gastrointestinal Effects

Alcohol contributes to gastrointestinal tract problems, Mallory-Weiss syndrome (esophageal tear), esophageal varices, erosive gastritis, gastroduodenal ulcers (especially in combination with aspirin), diarrhea due to motility disorders, malabsorption syndrome, and both acute and chronic pancreatitis.

The effects of alcohol on the liver are well studied. Early injury to the liver causes a reversible fatty liver that improves with cessation of alcohol. With progressive damage, there is a wide spectrum of alcoholic hepatitis ranging from mild disease to fulminant liver failure. Hepatomegaly is present in over 75 percent of patients with alcoholic hepatitis; roughly half present with jaundice, ascites, and spider angiomata. A hallmark of this disease is that the aspartate aminotransferase (AST, formerly SGOT) is greater than the alanine aminotransferase (ALT, formerly SGPT), a reversal of the pattern found in viral hepatitis. Elevations of the bilirubin and alkaline phosphatase levels are also present. Liver biopsy can confirm the diagnosis by well-established histologic criteria, but biopsy is most useful when the etiology is in doubt (e.g., positive hepatitis B serology, elevated ferritin level).

With supportive therapy, which includes administration of fluids, correction of electrolytes, and replacement of magnesium, phosphorus, and vitamins, more than 80 percent of patients with alcoholic hepatitis recover. A poor prognosis is suggested by a prolonged prothrombin time, decreased albumin, the presence of ascites, and, most important, by continuation of drinking.

More than half of patients with alcoholic hepatitis who cannot stop drinking progress to cirrhosis. Cirrhosis occurs despite adequate nutrition. It is defined histologically by the presence of fibrosis and the destruction of the normal architecture of the liver. The disruption of blood flow that follows this destruction produces the subsequent portal hypertension and hepatocellular dysfunction. The clinical presentation may include features associated with alcoholic hepatitis. Complications specific to end-stage cirrhosis are due to portal hypertension and late-stage hepatic dysfunction: hepatic encephalopathy, varices, splenomegaly, and ascites (Pimstone and French, 1984).

Hepatic encephalopathy produces an altered mental status that ranges from lethargy to profound confusion or coma. It occurs in liver failure from any cause but is most commonly seen secondary to long-term alcohol usage. The precise etiology of hepatic encephalopathy is still under study, but it appears linked to the inability of the liver to detoxify metabolites generated from the intestines. Ammonia is one such metabolite, and arterial levels are usually elevated but do not always correlate with the degree of encephalopathy. They may be normal. In the brain, ammonia is metabolized to glutamine, and cerebrospinal glutamine may also be elevated in hepatic encephalopathy (Pimstone and French, 1984).

Nutrition

One gram of alcohol provides 7 kcal of energy. Few vitamins or minerals are associated with this. Alcoholism is the most common cause of vitamin and trace mineral deficiency in the United States. The major deficiencies are folic acid, thiamine, magnesium, and phosphate.

Cancer Risks

Mouth and Pharynx. The use of tobacco is probably the most important factor in causing cancer of the pharynx and larynx, but tobacco and alcohol appear to act synergistically. Data show that the risk of cancer of the mouth and pharynx more than doubles when alcohol is used heavily (approximately three to four mixed drinks per day). The heavy drinker who smokes increases this risk of oral cancer by more than tenfold. Laryngeal cancer is more strongly associated with tobacco usage, but alcohol usage elevates this risk even further.

Esophagus. Cancer of the esophagus is linked to heavy alcohol usage. It is also associated with tobacco usage, diet, and lye ingestion. Heavy alcohol usage is reported to produce a risk 20 times that found in the nondrinker (Rothman, 1980).

Primary Cancer of the Liver. Seventy to ninety percent of hepatomas in the United States occur in cirrhotic patients. The cirrhosis is usually due to alcoholism. Liver cancer usually occurs about 2 to 8 years after the onset of cirrhosis and usually occurs in livers with large hyperplastic nodules. Cessation of drinking does not protect one from hepatoma once these nodules form. Alcohol may act as a cocarcinogen with chronic hepatitis B infections (Ohnishi et al, 1982).

Fetal Alcohol Syndrome

Fetal alcohol syndrome may occur in 40 percent of children born to alcoholic mothers. These children have facial abnormalities, mental retardation, microcephaly, poor motor coordination, and genitourinary and cardiovascular abnormalities. Eighty percent are below the third percentile in height and weight. In addition, there is an increased incidence of stillbirths and infant deaths. Because even moderate use of alcohol during pregnancy may increase the risk of mild aspects of this syndrome, it is advisable for pregnant women to use alcohol rarely or abstain completely (Eckardt et al, 1981).

References

Clark WD. Alcoholism: Blocks to diagnosis and treatment. Am J Med 1981; 71:275.

Cyr M, Wartman S. The effectiveness of routine screening questions in the detection of alcoholism. JAMA 1988; 259:51.

Eckardt M, Harford TC, Kaelbert CT. Health hazards associated with alcohol consumption. JAMA 1981; 246:648.

Ettinger PO, et al. Arrhythmias and the "holiday heart": Alcohol associated cardiac rhythm disorders. Am Heart J 1978; 95:555.

Fifth Special Report to the US Congress on Alcohol and Health. Adverse social consequence of alcohol use and alcoholism. Washington, DC: United States Department of Health and Human Services. DHHS Publication No. ADM 84 1291, 1984.

Harp JT, Spickard WA. Alcoholism: Early diagnosis and intervention. J Gen Intern Med 1987; 2:420.

Hawkins RD, Kalant H. The metabolism of ethanol and its metabolic effects. Pharmacol Rev 1972; 24:67.

Hebert V, ed. Hematologic complications of alcoholism. Semin Hematol 1980; 17:83.

Hill PS. Alcoholism: Images, impairments, interventions. Postgrad Med 1983; 74:87.

Klatsky AL, et al. Alcohol consumption and blood pressure: Kaiser-Permanente. N Engl J Med 1977; 296:1194.

Kraus ML, et al. Randomized clinical trial of atenolol in patients with alcohol withdrawal. N Engl J Med 1985; 313:905.

Naranjo CA, Sellers EM. Clinical assessment and pharmacotherapy of the alcohol withdrawal syndrome. In: Recent developments in alcoholism. New York: Plenum Press, 1986.

Ohnishi K, et al. The effect of chronic habitual alcohol intake in the development of liver cirrhosis and hepatocellular carcinoma: Relation to hepatitis B carriage. Cancer 1982; 49:672.

Orlando J, et al. Effect of ethanol on angina pectoris. Ann Intern Med 1976; 84:652.

Pimstone NR, French SW. Alcoholic liver disease. Med Clin North Am 1984; 68:39.

Rothman KJ. The proportion of cancer attributable to alcohol consumption. Prev Med 1980; 9:174.

Sixth Special Report to the US Congress on Alcohol and Health. Psychobiological effects of alcohol. Washington, DC: United States Department of Health and Human Services, DHHS Publication No. ADM 87 1519, 1987:55.

Sixth Special Report to the US Congress on Alcohol and Health. Epidemiology. Washington, DC: United States Department of Health and Human Services, DHHS Publication No. ADM 87 1519, 1987:6.

Society of General Internal Medicine. Faculty development course in substance abuse education. Barnes HN, Bigby J, course directors. Boston: Brigham and Women's Hospital, January 1988.

Spencer H, et al. Chronic alcoholism: A frequently overlooked cause of osteoporosis in men. Am J Med 1986; 80:393.

Spitzer R. Diagnostic and statistical manual of mental disorders. 3rd ed rev. Washington, DC: American Psychiatric Association, 1987.

Vaillant GE. The natural history of alcoholism. Cambridge, MA: Harvard University Press, 1983.

Van Thiel DH, Gavaler JS, Saryhvi A. Recovery of sexual functioning in abstinent alcoholic men. Gastroenterology 1982; 84:677.

Cigarette Smoking

Judith K. Ockene, PhD

147

Definition

Epidemiologic investigations have demonstrated a direct relationship between dosage of cigarette smoking (i.e., number of cigarettes smoked, depth of inhalation, and duration of smoking) and the degree of risk of premature death or disability. Even so-called light smokers (less than 20 cigarettes per day) are at an increased risk for disease when compared with ex-smokers or people who never smoked. Epidemiologic investigations have also shown that cessation of cigarette smoking has a definite benefit. Cessation is related to a significant decrease in the premature development of smoking-related diseases and death from those diseases in smokers who have not yet become ill. Likewise, individuals who have already developed a smoking-related disease have a decreased chance of dying from it or of the disease progressing if they stop smoking. As the length of time free from cigarettes increases, the risk of disease or death continues to decrease until, after about 10 to 15 years, it eventually reaches that of the nonsmoker. The risk of dying from coronary heart disease decreases rapidly after cessation, whereas the risk of dying from lung cancer decreases more slowly. Benefits of quitting are seen even after many years of heavy smoking.

Approximately 30 percent of adult Americans (32 percent of men and 27 percent of women) smoke cigarettes regularly (US Department of Health and Human Services, 1989). This rate represents a significant decrease for men since the publication of the first Surgeon General's Report on Smoking and Health in 1964, when 50 percent of men were cigarette smokers, but only a small decrease for women, for whom the prevalence of cigarette smoking was 34 percent in 1964. By 1987, nearly half of all living adults who ever smoked had quit. More than 90 percent of the 30 million smokers who gave up cigarettes between 1964 and 1982 did not use an organized program to help them stop smoking, and most smokers who continue to smoke state that they prefer to stop without the aid of a formal smoking-cessation program. It is with this group that the physician can have a major impact. Seventy-five percent of the adult population has at least one contact per year with a physician, with the average yearly number of contacts being five per adult; thus, the physician as educator, facilitator, or counselor has the potential to be a powerful agent for smoking cessation. Individuals probably think more seriously about their health and smoking's effect on it when they are in a physician's office or a hospital than at any other time. This opportunity for health promotion with smokers, ex-smokers, or would-be smokers should not be overlooked.

Almost any intervention strategy for cessation can be effective, given a commitment to cessation by both the smoker and the physician. As a supportive authority figure and role model, the physician can promote cessation of cigarette smoking in every smoking patient by direct intervention or by encouraging and reinforcing the use of smoking control treatment programs. Consistent and enthusiastic intervention by physicians can achieve at least one of the following: (1) motivation of the patient to decide whether he or she is willing to make an effort to stop smoking or helping the patient toward a time when cessation may be possible, (2) reduction of smoking, (3) immediate cessation, (4) support and reinforcement of cessation programs in which the smoker is already involved, and (5) maintenance of cessation.

Physiologic Effects of Cigarette Smoke

The health consequences and symptoms of smoking have been attributed to the many noxious substances found in cigarette smoke. The lighted cigarette is separated into gas and particulate phases. Carbon monoxide, found in the gas phase, develops a strong bond with hemoglobin, causing smokers to lose as much as 15 percent of the oxygen-carrying capacity of their red blood cells, depending on how much they smoke. The loss of this oxygen can have a major effect on the heart and circulatory system and may be the major causal factor for the increased risk that cigarette smokers have for coronary heart disease. Although levels of tar and nicotine have declined in cigarettes manufactured in recent years, the level of carbon monoxide has not decreased.

Inhaled along with carbon monoxide in cigarette smoke are other toxic gases such as acrolein, hydrogen cyanide, ammonia, hydrogen oxide, and nitrogen oxide, all of which have been shown to produce toxic effects. These gases are most immediately responsible for coughing and narrowing of the bronchial tubes after inhalation. They also paralyze the action of the cilia, and if this is allowed to continue over a long period of time, the cilia can die and the mucus-secreting membranes will thicken. With the bronchi and bronchioles narrowed and the alveoli strained by prolonged pressure, carbon dioxide may be retained, possibly resulting in chronic obstructive pulmonary disease.

The total particulate matter consists primarily of nicotine, water, and "tars" and ranges from 0.2 to 9.0 percent of the weight of the "mainstream" smoke drawn from the puffing end of the cigarette. Tar includes total particulate weight minus water and nicotine, and it has decreased in cigarettes manufactured in the United States from an average of 39 mg per cigarette to 17 mg. Nicotine content has also decreased from 2.5 mg to 1.1 mg. Tar includes many of the toxic organic compounds related to those found in the gas phase, with the nonvolatile N-nitrosamines including organ-specific carcinogens and the aromatic amines also including human carcinogens. The smoke from the burning end of the cigarette, "sidestream" smoke, contains considerably higher amounts of the carcinogenic aromatic amines than does mainstream smoke, and it has been implicated as having significant disease-producing effect on individuals in the smoker's environment.

The nicotine in the particulate phase causes the release of catecholamines, epinephrine, and norepinephrine, which cause an increase in heart rate, blood pressure, cardiac output, oxygen consumption, coronary blood flow, arrhythmias, peripheral vasoconstriction, and mobilization and utilization of free fatty acids. Thus, nicotine and carbon monoxide produce the major adverse effects with regard to coronary heart disease. In addition to chronic disease and death, additional symptoms of cigarette smoking include morning cough, shortness of breath, fatigue, sputum production, hoarseness, increased pulse and blood pressure, and skin and teeth stains.

In summary, the constituents of cigarette smoke in both the gas and particulate phases have been found to affect almost every organ of the body and to cause excess mortality and morbidity of all of the major diseases. The symptoms of smoking are often obvious, and the more the physician is able to relate these effects to smoking, the greater the likelihood that the smoker will be motivated to attempt cessation.

Etiology

Cigarette smoking is a complex behavior pattern that, like most behavior patterns, is affected by psychosocial and physiologic factors and goes through a sequence of stages. During the initiation phase, individuals start experimenting with cigarettes, generally before they are 20, and then move into the transition phase, in which environmental, psychological, and physiologic factors influence their becoming smokers or nonsmokers. The sequence then proceeds through the stages of maintenance (of the habit), cessation, and maintenance of cessation. Because relapse occurs at very high rates among those who have stopped smoking (often as many as 70 to 80 percent return to smoking within 1 year), the maintenance of the cessation phase is also a transition phase that influences whether a smoker becomes a permanent ex-smoker or a recidivist who returns to the old behavior of smoking.

In each stage, different motives, needs, and environmental factors are operating to determine whether an individual will move into the next stage. Initiation of smoking is strongly associated with social forces, or forces extrinsic to the individual, e.g., peer pressure, as well as with psychological variables such as self-esteem, status needs, and other personal needs. The sociologic variables that are so important during the formation of the habit seem to play a minor role in the maintenance stage once smoking has become part of the lifestyle of the individual. As the habit continues, it becomes more and more tied to psychological and physiologic needs and becomes an intrinsic part of the person's life, having many functions. Cessation and maintenance of cessation are affected by a combination of social, psychological, and physiologic variables that act on and within the individual. Treatment approaches must reflect the differences in the factors that determine who will become a smoker, who will maintain the habit, who will be able to discontinue it, and who will maintain abstinence for an extended period. When working with a young patient who is starting to smoke, one's approach is not the same as when working with a man who has been smoking for the last 30 years. Different approaches are also indicated for the 30-year smoker who has never stopped smoking and smokes 40 non-filter-tipped cigarettes per day as compared with the 30-year smoker who has stopped in the past without difficulty and is smoking 20 low tar and nicotine cigarettes per day.

Diagnostic Approach

In contrast to most medical problems, in which a differential diagnosis lists possible causes of the symptoms, in the case of cigarette smoking the goals are to diagnose the factors maintaining the problem behavior, to assess the patient's past experiences with smoking cessation, and to understand his or her support system, strengths, and resources.

A proper evaluation not only provides a basis for treatment

but also is a valuable intervention tool. A patient-controlled counseling approach using a sequence of "guided questions" can be effectively implemented and takes only a few minutes of each visit. This approach permits the physician to initiate intervention with the patient and assist the patient in making the decision to stop smoking and in developing a cessation plan. Diagnosis and treatment are interwoven and cannot be separated easily.

As a first step, the physician can ask the smoker if he or she is aware of the *effects of smoking on his or her health*. During the physical examination, feedback of findings pertinent to smoking is an effective way to personalize the effects of smoking. Time should be allowed for the patient to ask questions and arrive at independent conclusions about the implications of the information provided. The physician's knowledge of physiology and the pathogenesis of disease affords powerful leverage that must be used skillfully in order to educate patients without frightening them unnecessarily. Arousing anxiety can have a negative effect unless potential solutions to the problem addressed can be explored.

After exploring and discussing the health consequences of smoking on the individual smoker, the next step is to foster his or her *awareness of the value of cessation*. Smokers often rationalize that the damage has been done and that there is little value in quitting.

Assessment of a smoking patient also necessitates a determination of other risk factors that act synergistically to cause coronary heart disease, chronic obstructive pulmonary disease, and cancer. For example, the smoking patient who has other coronary risk factors, such as hypercholesterolemia and hypertension, is at an even greater risk of coronary heart disease than the smoker without these other risk factors. This risk is greater than just the additive effect of each risk factor. Similarly, when coupled with exposure to asbestos and some other occupationally encountered substances, smoking greatly increases the smoker's risk of cancer of the lung when compared with smokers who are not exposed to these substances. The magnitude of the combined risk for disease is dependent on the levels of the risk factors. Feedback to the patient regarding the effect of the combination of risk factors on his or her health may increase efforts to stop smoking and maintain long-term cessation.

Finally, it is important to determine whether an individual believes that he or she is capable of making the specified change. There is little value in attempting a change that both the patient and physician believe is headed toward failure, as failure will then likely occur. Knowing the patient's past experiences with the sought-after change (or other changes if the patient has never stopped smoking) is useful and important in helping the patient make the present change. This knowledge can provide an understanding of the patient's strengths and resources as well as information about how to deal with problems that may arise.

The following is a series of "guided" questions that could be used for assessment and intervention:

1. How do you feel about being a smoker? (Eighty percent of smokers indicate that they want to stop smoking.)
2. What are your reasons for wanting to stop smoking? (The best reasons for cessation are the smoker's reasons.)
3. Have you ever stopped smoking before? (Eighty percent of smokers have.) When? Why?
4. What was your experience the last time you stopped? (Some smokers say, "It was terrible. . . ." With that statement, it is important to help the smoker recount the exact experience and remember the positive aspects.)
5. How did you stop? (This question helps the smoker develop ideas for stopping now.)
6. Why did you return to smoking? (Answers to this question help to illustrate that in many cases a particular event or thought triggered the return to smoking.)
7. Could you handle the same problem today without cigarettes? How? (This question alerts the smoker to the idea that he or she can prepare and have available alternative mechanisms for handling stress, depression, or anger.)

For the smoker who never stopped smoking or who had a difficult time throughout the entire cessation experience, other questions may be helpful, e.g., "What changes have you made with other habits?" "How?" "Why?"

The final questions in this series of guided questions might be the following:

8. Have you thought about stopping smoking now?
9. Do you think you can stop now?
10. How? (It is important for the smoker to come up with the "how.") It is at this point that a plan for change can be developed.

Some smokers can easily develop their own strategies for cessation and stop on their own without further help from the physician; they need only to decide that the benefits of cessation outweigh the disadvantages and that they can stop smoking. These patients should be encouraged to stop smoking and given whatever support is requested. Other smokers may require a persistent expenditure of their own effort as well as effort and support from those individuals available to help them. Therefore, it is essential not to expect that all patients will stop smoking immediately after the initial discussion. Cessation for most is a continuing process and not a single event. There is no right way to stop smoking. It is important for each smoker to develop a personalized, appropriate method. With the use of questioning and feedback, physicians can facilitate the choice of a particular approach to cessation. With the more difficult smoker, the aforementioned series of steps can be accomplished over a few visits, allowing the physician to utilize effectively the time that is available for diagnosis and intervention.

Patients who are not ready for cessation may benefit from keeping a record of their smoking that facilitates examination of when, why, and how much is smoked as well as the circumstances that surround the behavior (Figure 147-1). Each cigarette is recorded before it is smoked, and its importance is rated on a scale of 1 to 5. Recording forces smokers to become aware of each cigarette; the result is often a decision to do without one cigarette that otherwise would have been smoked almost without thinking. This procedure can aid the physician and smoker in developing a treatment plan for cessation as well as in producing a fairly rapid reduction in the number of cigarettes smoked. The smoker can be instructed to omit cigarettes given a rating of 5 (least important). Smokers who are willing to develop a step-by-step program, who adhere to it, and who expect it to help them to make the desired change are the most successful in their attempts to change.

At the end of the first visit with the potential nonsmoker, an appointment for the next visit should be made with the specific goal of follow-up for smoking cessation. This is analogous to scheduling a follow-up visit with a hypertensive patient. A follow-up letter in which the physician expresses the strong hope and expectation that the smoker has taken some action on what was decided in the first visit is also good reinforcement. The same sequence is helpful in the in-patient setting.

Some smokers eventually stop smoking after taking the time to think over the information they have been given to assess their smoking needs. Others prefer to taper, going through a gradual retraining process. Insistence upon immediate cessation, when the patient is not ready, may result in failure for both patient and physician. Often small successes are necessary before the patient feels confident that complete cessation is possible.

There are other important factors for the physician to keep in mind when determining a treatment approach. Smokers who have stopped in the past and relapsed are often able to stop successfully when they try again. In general, smokers who are

DAILY SMOKING RECORD

Name: ______________________________ Date: __________

	Time	Place	Activity	With Whom	Need* Rating
1.					
2.					
3.					
4.					
5.					
6.					
7.					
8.					
9.					
10.					
11.					
12.					

*Estimate how much you need the cigarette on a scale of 1 to 5.
1 = very important (cannot do without), 5 = least important (can do without).

Figure 147-1 Example of a daily smoking record.

smoking fewer cigarettes are more successful than heavier smokers. Thus, even for the smoker who cannot stop smoking, reduction in the number of cigarettes smoked can represent a step toward eventual cessation. The more support a smoker is able to receive, the greater the likelihood for success. Available evidence suggests that physicians can have a major impact on the cigarette smoking behavior of their patients. For many smokers, this can be accomplished with minimal intervention and a small investment of time. The first and most important step is to question your patients about their smoking behavior and patterns and then listen to their answers.

References

Fagerstrom KO. Effects of number of follow-up sessions and nicotine gum in physician based smoking cessation. Presented at Fifth World Conference on Smoking and Health, Winnipeg, Canada, July 14, 1983.

Glynn TJ, Marley MW. How to help your patients stop smoking. Washington, DC: US Department of Health and Human Services, Public Health Service, National Cancer Institute. NIH Publication No. 89-3064, 1989.

Greene HL, Goldberg RJ, Ockene JK. Cigarette smoking: The physician's role in cessation and maintenance. J Gen Intern Med 1988; 75–87.

Ockene JK, et al. A psychosocial model of smoking cessation and maintenance of cessation. Prev Med 1981; 10:623.

Schwartz JL, Dubitzky M. Requisites for success in smoking withdrawal. In: Borgatta EF, Evans RR, eds. Smoking, health and behavior. Chicago: Aldine, 1968.

US Department of Health and Human Services. The health consequences of smoking: 25 years of progress. Rockville, MD: DHHS Publication (CDC) 89-8411, 1989.

US Department of Health and Human Services. The health consequences of smoking: The changing cigarette: A report of the Surgeon General. Public Health Service. Washington, DC: DHEW Publication No. (PHS) 81-50156, 1981.

US Department of Health and Human Services. Vital and Health Statistics. Physician visits: Volume and interval since last visit. United States, 1980. Hyattsville, MD: DHHS Publication (PHS) 185-1572, 1983.

Wilson DG, Johnston N, Sicuvella J. Randomized clinical trial of supportive follow-up for cigarette smokers in a family practice. CMAJ 1982; 126:127.

Substance Use Disorders

Judith Eaton, MD

Jonathan S. Rothman, MD

148

Psychoactive substance *dependence* is a cluster of symptoms that indicate that the person has impaired control of substance use and continues use despite the knowledge of impairment in physical, psychological, social, or occupational functioning. The user usually recognizes that the use is excessive or causes problems or impairment, but he or she is unable to control the use. A great deal of the user's time is spent in obtaining and using the substance. Frequent intoxication or withdrawal symptoms occur when the person should be fulfilling major role obligations at work, school, or home. The symptoms must be present for at least 1 month.

Psychoactive substance dependence syndrome includes, but is not limited to, physical tolerance and withdrawal symptoms. Tolerance means that increasing amounts of substance are required to produce the desired effect. Withdrawal means that a specific syndrome appears when the substance is reduced or stopped. Substances are often taken repeatedly to avoid the withdrawal symptoms.

The term *substance abuse* is used to describe a pattern of maladaptive use that does not meet criteria for psychoactive substance dependence. Substance abuse involves persistent use that occurs with the individual's knowledge that recurrent social, occupational, or physical problems may be caused by use of the drug, e.g., driving while intoxicated. The diagnosis of substance abuse often applies to people experimenting with drugs or to those who have occasional binges.

There are three different groups of people with substance use disorders. These are differentiated mainly by the types of substances used and the lifestyle that results:

1. The "hard-core junkie" uses mostly opiates or solid cocaine freebase ("crack") and is usually heavily involved in criminal activities in order to support his or her expensive drug habit. The procurement process in itself becomes an exciting way of life that may be as difficult to abandon as the substance.

2. The young "experimenter" is acting in response to peer pressure. He or she is by no means committed to a drug-using lifestyle but is searching for identity. The problems he or she encounters are usually quite accidental, such as inadvertent overdoses. The "experimenter's" drugs of choice are more likely to be hallucinogens and cannabis.

3. The "nice junkie" is a middle- to upper-class person whose lifestyle appears to be normal (e.g., housewife, business person, physician), but who typically becomes addicted to tranquilizers, barbiturates, amphetamines, or cocaine. Such individuals are not involved in criminal behavior; thus, their addictions go unnoticed (or are frequently covered up by families or colleagues) for a long time, thereby delaying entry into treatment. Their drugs of abuse are medically more dangerous than the opiates. Cocaine abusers may need to add some criminal activities to support the extremely high cost of this addiction.

Etiology

A definitive etiology of substance use disorders is not known. Different theories have been proposed, and probably all factors contribute to varying degrees in each individual. Psychoanalytic theory sees the substance abuser as one who handles strong sexual and aggressive feelings in a passive manner by avoidance rather than by active coping. Behavioral theories explain drug-taking behavior as a way of avoiding withdrawal symptoms or as a way to handle unpleasant affects and situations. Addicts who have been "clean" for long periods may experience withdrawal symptoms when returning to old neighborhoods. Drug craving may also be a learned response.

Physiologically, the opiate receptors and naturally occurring opiate-like substances, endorphins, may be involved. There appears to be a feedback mechanism whereby the body's own endorphins are shut down when external opiates are introduced. It may be that for some, once this external substance is removed, the natural system does not return to functioning and there is a deficiency. It is possible that some opiate abusers may have a naturally occurring endorphin deficiency that antedates their history of substance abuse.

Finally, overprescription of addictive medications by physicians has been invoked as a cause of substance use disorders. It is rare that patients being treated with narcotics for pain relief remain addicted unless there are complicating personality factors. However, problems such as chronic back pain may lead to iatrogenic narcotic addiction. A greater problem is the prescription of medications by physicians to try to solve the difficulties of everyday living. A patient's expectation that there is a pill to eliminate every unpleasant feeling may be reinforced by a physician who believes that he or she has the power to provide relief for all conditions. This faulty *system* contributes to substance use disorders.

Opioid Abuse and Dependence

Opioids are analgesics such as morphine, heroin, meperidine (Demerol), methadone, hydromorphone (Dilaudid), oxycodone (Percodan), and codeine. They are highly addictive physiologically and are characterized by the rapid development of tolerance and a distinct withdrawal syndrome. Opioids cause a pleasant euphoria in addition to relieving pain. They are usually taken orally or intravenously. Heroin is a totally illegal drug in this country (except for federal research centers) and is sold on the street cut with products such as quinine and sugar. The dose a user receives is therefore always variable.

Clinical Presentation

Acute Intoxication. Acute intoxication produces flushing and itching of the skin, nausea and vomiting, euphoria, "nodding" (short naps with head nodding), pupillary constriction, decreased respiratory rate, and decreased body temperature.

Overdose. An overdose usually is manifested by pinpoint pupils, slow periodic respirations, unresponsiveness, bradycardia, hypotension, hypothermia, and decreased to absent reflexes. Death is usually due to respiratory arrest, which is immediately reversible by 0.4 mg of intravenous naloxone, a narcotic antagonist. Heroin addicts sometimes present in the emergency room with acute pulmonary edema, which is frequently fatal. It is not clear whether this is a reaction to the heroin itself or to one of the substances with which it is cut, e.g., talc, sugar.

Withdrawal Syndrome. Opioid withdrawal syndrome is like a rather unpleasant case of flu. Symptoms may include craving, nausea, vomiting, muscle aches, lacrimation or rhinorrhea, pupillary dilation, piloerection or sweating, diarrhea, yawning, fever, or insomnia. Addicts who have used intravenous heroin daily for as little as 3 weeks will experience withdrawal symptoms if they curtail usage. The opioid withdrawal syndrome is usually greatly exaggerated by hospitalized addicts, who hope to attain more narcotic to eliminate it. All withdrawal treatment should be based on physical signs and symptoms rather than on subjective reports. It is not a life-threatening predicament. Subjective symptoms include restlessness, yawning, and marked insomnia. Objective signs to be watched are blood pressure, heart rate, increased temperature, and dilated pupils.

The diagnosis of opioid abuse may be made by history alone. Physical examination usually shows the result of intravenous drug use, such as "tracks" or scars along major veins, e.g., antecubital, hand and wrist, neck, penile; tattoos in the same areas to hide tracks; phlebitis and punched-out ulcers in the same area; and abscesses and edema of hands from use of unclean needles. Associated illnesses are commonly found. Virtually all active narcotics users have elevated liver function test results, especially aspartate aminotransferase and lactate dehydrogenase, and these may persist for months even in the absence of active hepatitis. Jaundice may be present, but it is unusual unless there is hepatitis. Murmurs may be present, indicative of bacterial or fungal cardiac infections. Tuberculosis, tetanus, and malaria have been found in addicts. Serology for syphilis is often positive, sometimes falsely so, and this may persist. Ulcers are common, as is extremely poor dental care. These are more apt to become problems after narcotic use has stopped and pain is unmasked. In women, amenorrhea and menstrual irregularities are common. There usually is also a history of social problems including arrest, history of prostitution, an antisocial lifestyle, poor marital adjustment, and violence. In this high-risk population, there may be the presence of human immunodeficiency virus (HIV) infection or symptoms of acquired immunodeficiency syndrome (AIDS) or AIDS-related complex.

Narcotic addicts often present to emergency rooms and outpatient clinics in search of narcotics. They may skillfully mimic a variety of symptoms ranging from renal colic to acute otitis media. Their fear of withdrawal symptoms and immersion in a lifestyle devoted to the procurement of drugs make addicts demanding and devious in all treatment settings. They should never be given narcotics except for medically necessary conditions, and treatment of the addiction per se should be confined to specialized facilities such as detoxification centers, drug rehabilitation programs, methadone maintenance clinics, and long-term therapeutic communities.

Stimulant Abuse and Dependence

Amphetamines

Amphetamines are used by all three types of addicts. They may be abused intravenously for an acute high or "rush," or orally on a more chronic basis. They produce a feeling of well-being, reduce fatigue, and increase energy. They also markedly reduce appetite.

Acute Intoxication. Acute amphetamine intoxication is marked by flushing; increases in temperature, blood pressure, and heart rate; tremor; agitation; excitement; anxiety; panic; anorexia; insomnia; logorrhea; and moodiness. The picture is one of a "speeded-up" person who is talking and moving a great deal with either anxiety or euphoria out of proportion to the situation. Fighting, grandiosity, hypervigilance, and impaired judgment are all common manifestations of amphetamine intoxication.

Complications. Amphetamine overdose causes extreme hypertension, which may be associated with convulsions, tetany, hyperpyrexia, cerebrovascular accidents, arrhythmias, coma, and death.

Medical problems associated with amphetamine use are the same as those with narcotics if they are used intravenously (hepatitis, AIDS, abscesses, and so forth). Necrotizing angiitis is more common with amphetamine use. Malnutrition and exhaustion may occur with chronic use.

A paranoid psychosis may also occur with amphetamine abuse. This resembles the acute functional psychoses (mania, schizophrenia) and usually can be differentiated from them by history and by its rapid resolution.

Withdrawal. The symptoms of amphetamine withdrawal include lethargy, fatigue, disturbed sleep, agitation, depression, nightmares, anxiety, and irritability. Intense hunger, violence, and confusion may also be seen.

Cocaine

Cocaine produces an intense euphoria of rapid onset. Cocaine powder may be snorted intranasally or injected intravenously; the freebase preparation ("crack") is smoked or inhaled.

Acute Intoxication. Acute intoxication produces stimulation and an intense craving for more cocaine. There may be irritability and anxiety. Paranoid psychoses may ensue rapidly (and repeatedly with each use). There are often tactile hallucinations with feelings of bugs crawling under the skin (formication). This may persist long after the drug is discontinued. There may be tachycardia, elevated blood pressure, pupillary dilation, perspiration or chills, and nausea or vomiting.

Complications. Overdose produces seizures and cardiac or respiratory arrest. Often cocaine is used with heroin, so respiratory depression may also be present. Cocaine withdrawal is similar to amphetamine withdrawal. Chronic use of cocaine leads to decreased eating and sleeping. Concentration is also decreased. The nasal mucosa and septum may deteriorate owing to irritation.

Because of the intense pleasure it produces, cocaine is highly addictive. What was once considered a harmless "high-class sport" has become an extremely expensive addiction with much criminal activity needed to support it.

Sedative-Hypnotic or Anxiolytic Dependence

The depressants include barbiturates, benzodiazepines, and other sedative-hypnotics such as methaqualone and chloral hydrate. These are used either to produce a high by experimenting drug users or to relax from excessive amphetamine use. The clinical use of some of these compounds is to reduce anxiety. Because they are available by prescription, their abuse may be well hidden until the dependent individual is admitted to the hospital for a seemingly unrelated medical problem. When these compounds are abruptly discontinued, a withdrawal syndrome that includes life-threatening seizures may ensue. Of all these compounds, the barbiturates are the most highly addicting. Unexplained trauma and accidents are sometimes associated with secretive barbiturate abuse. Physicians must maintain a high index of suspicion for sedative-hypnotic and anxiolytic dependence in order to prevent life-threatening withdrawal seizures.

Acute Intoxication. Acute intoxication looks like drunkenness without the odor of alcohol on the breath. There is slurred speech, poor judgment, emotional lability, and often hostility, quarreling, and violence. Nystagmus may be present, as are a positive Romberg's sign, hypotension, and decreased superficial reflexes.

Complications. Because barbiturates cause short-term memory loss (especially when combined with alcohol), "inadvertent" accidental overdoses are common. The clinical picture is of marked central nervous system depression and coma.

Withdrawal. Withdrawal from barbiturates is medically dangerous and should be treated in a hospital as an emergency. There is anxiety, weakness, sweating, and insomnia. Seizures may ensue with delirium and cardiovascular collapse. Benzodiazepines may produce a similar syndrome with a somewhat longer time course.

Hallucinogens

The hallucinogens include lysergic acid diethylamide (LSD), tetrahydrocannabinol (THC), phencyclidine (PCP), and others. The most commonly used hallucinogen is PCP, or "angel dust," an anesthetic agent used legally only in veterinary medicine. Drugs sold on the streets as mescaline or THC often turn out to be PCP, which is very prevalent. Any acute intoxication of the type described below should be considered PCP intoxication and so treated, unless proved otherwise by toxic screen.

Acute Intoxication. Acute intoxication produces euphoria and/or anxiety. There may be fearfulness, confusion, a blank stare, and agitation. There may be self-destructive behavior, belligerence, and hallucinations, both auditory and visual. There may be depersonalization. Physical manifestations include dysarthria, ataxia, and muscular rigidity of face and neck. There may be nystagmus, increased blood pressure or heart rate, numbness to pain, seizures, or hyperacusis.

Complications. Overdosage initially manifests as a state of further excitement, subsequently leading to anesthesia. There is agitation, clonic jerking of the extremities, opisthotonic posture, stupor with eyes open, seizures and status epilepticus, increased blood pressure (especially systolic), and vomiting. Nystagmus—horizontal, vertical, and rotary—may be present. Then coma may ensue. Acute psychosis may result from PCP use. The person stares into space, has posturing and echolalia, sleep disturbance, depression, paranoid ideation, and behavioral disturbance, including violence. There is potential for serious harm to self or others in this state. Chronic PCP abuse leads to dulled thinking, confusion, and decreased concentration. It does not produce physiologic dependence; there is no withdrawal syndrome.

Less medically dangerous substances include the other hallucinogens and marijuana. Acute LSD intoxication produces alterations in mood, perception, and thinking, visual disturbances, and pseudohallucinations. "Bad trips" may be frightening and produce dangerous behavior briefly. Flashbacks or chronic deterioration into psychosis may be long-term sequelae. There is no physical dependence and no withdrawal syndrome.

Marijuana can occasionally produce an acute panic reaction. This usually occurs in an anxious person who is fearful of or ambivalent about the use of the drug. It responds to reassurance. Occasional psychotic episodes have resulted from marijuana use. Long-term effects of marijuana continue to be debated. There is no physical withdrawal syndrome, but psychological dependence occurs in some people.

Summary

A high index of suspicion of drug use should be maintained for all types of patients. Unexplained physical and mental states can often be acute or chronic intoxication or withdrawal phenomenon. The history is often unreliable. Toxicology screens are helpful but take time for results to be available. Most drug users (all types) mix substances, so polydrug abuse (including alcohol) is the rule, not the exception.

Mild substance use disorders respond much better to treatment interventions than do severe ones. For this reason, physicians should focus their efforts on prevention, early identification, and aggressive early intervention. In this way the horrific medical consequences of drug abuse described in this chapter can be significantly reduced.

References

Galea R, Lewis B, Baker L. AIDS and IV drug abusers: Current perspectives. Baltimore: National Health Publishing, 1988.

Kaplan HI, Sadock BJ. Comprehensive textbook of psychiatry. 5th ed. Baltimore: Williams & Wilkins, 1989.

Kosten TR, Kleber HD. Psychoactive substance use disorders: Drug abuse. In: Lazare A, ed. Outpatient psychiatry: Diagnosis and treatment. Baltimore: Williams & Wilkins, 1989:488.

Pickens RW, Heston LL, eds. Psychiatric factors in drug abuse. New York: Grune & Stratton, 1979.

Spitzer RL. Diagnostic and statistical manual of mental disorders. 3rd ed rev. Washington, DC: American Psychiatric Association, 1987.

Wilfred BB. Drug abuse: A guide for the primary care physician. Chicago: American Medical Association, 1981.

Principles of Behavioral Change

149

Cheryl L. Albright, PhD, MPH

John W. Farquhar, MD

The risk factors for coronary heart disease (i.e., smoking, hyperlipidemia, obesity, hypertension, hyperglycemia, sedentary living) are present in a large proportion of the adults seen by primary care physicians. The purpose of this chapter is to present a six-step method that physicians can use to help their patients make lifestyle changes that will affect these risk factors and reduce premature morbidity and mortality. This method is described in detail elsewhere (Farquhar, 1987), but it has been reformulated in this chapter to meet physicians' needs in the new and important field of clinical preventive medicine.

Six-Step Method for Behavioral Change

Promoting behavioral change on the part of patients is something that physicians do commonly, but it may not be so labeled. When a physician treats a patient who has an infection, the behavior sought is compliance to the medication regime and perhaps attention to nutrition and rest. However, problems such as diabetes and hypertension require considerable change in nutrition and exercise to achieve weight control, for example. The methods discussed in this chapter are intended to provide a system for aiding patients in making simple or complex changes in behavior.

This section describes a procedure that has, at its core, the standard clinical progression of diagnosis, treatment, and follow-up (Table 149-1). However, psychosocial concepts or strategies such as self-efficacy, contracts, self-monitoring, and stimulus control often are not introduced into this scheme. There is no fixed rate for progression through the steps, nor is there any limitation on recycling back through previous steps (using different strategies). It is critical that they not be viewed as rigid or linear, because changes in internal (i.e., patient motivation) and external forces (i.e., the environment) may keep some patients in one step longer, or a relapse will lead to recycling through previous steps.

The steps are derived from the findings of several scientists in the field of cognitive-behavioral psychology (Bandura, 1969, 1977a, 1977b, 1978; Lazarus, 1971; Mahoney, 1974a; Mahoney and Thoresen, 1974; Thoresen and Mahoney, 1974; Meichenbaum, 1977). Over the last 30 years, numerous studies have found the strategies derived from these psychologists to be extremely effective in achieving behavior change both in research and in clinical settings (Meyer and Henderson, 1974; Hersen et al, 1977; Davidson and Davidson, 1980; Stunkard et al, 1980; Braunstein and Toister, 1981; Hersen and Bellack, 1985; Crouch et al, 1986; Kaplan, 1986; Sheridan and Winogrond, 1987). Also, researchers in the fields of health psychology, public health, health education, community health, social ecology and medicine have used similar strategies as components in their intervention programs.

Although use of the entire six-step method with every patient is neither appropriate nor warranted, physicians will find the conceptual framework of the steps and the strategies specified within each step to be useful in changing a wide range of health behaviors.

Acknowledgments. The authors want to thank the faculty and trainees of the Stanford Faculty Development Program for their contributions concerning the application of the six-step method in primary care settings.

Step 1: Identify the Problem

The first step is analogous to the diagnostic step in traditional medical terminology. It involves assessing the patient's risk factors and his or her knowledge and attitudes about the behaviors linked to those risk factors. This assessment (or risk appraisal) can occur during any routine office visit by using short patient questionnaires. Information is needed on both the patient's health-damaging behavior and the history behind that behavior (e.g., number of years patient has smoked, previous attempts to change). The following questions can be used as a guide for obtaining this information:

1. What does the patient do? (Do you smoke? Do you exercise regularly? Do you limit your intake of dietary fat and cholesterol?)
2. What does the patient know about the problem?
3. Has the patient tried to change the behavior in the past?
4. What does the patient believe might inhibit change? What are his or her major barriers to changing?

As with any diagnostic process, the physician usually must go beyond the interview to make the diagnosis. For many health-damaging behaviors, the clinical examination provides much of the information necessary to recommend changes in health habits (e.g., weight, blood pressure, distribution of body fat). However, additional laboratory tests are often required to quantify the patient's risk level, especially measurement of total blood cholesterol or lipoprotein subfractions for risk of coronary heart disease. The National Cholesterol Education Program (NCEP) recently recommended that all adults over the age of 20 be screened for total cholesterol, and that all adults should strive to keep their total cholesterol below 200 mg/dl and their low density lipoprotein (LDL) cholesterol below 130 to 160 mg/dl, depending on the presence of other risk factors (see Chapter 19, "Elevated Serum Cholesterol"). In addition to obtaining these laboratory values, a brief screening questionnaire on dietary fat and cholesterol is needed. Examples of questions that take only a few minutes include the following: (1) How many egg yolks (visible) do you eat in a week? (2) How many meatless, eggless, cheeseless meals do you eat in a week? (3) Of those meals when you don't eat meat, how many per week consist of fish or chicken? Patients eating more than two to three eggs a week, fewer than 10 to 12 vegetarian meals a week, or more red meat than chicken or fish should be considered candidates for the six-step method addressing nutritional issues (an early and often simple way of achieving a prudent diet is to move toward vegetarian breakfasts).

Once the physician has identified a behavior to be changed, he or she should state directly that this behavior is harmful to the patient's present or future health, and that modifications in this behavior must be made. The physician should neither attempt to frighten the patient into changing nor equivocate. A key feature of step 1 is that the physician should give the patient the opportunity to talk about the problem and any perceived barriers to changing. In so doing, the physician will obtain information

Table 149-1 Six-Step Method for Behavioral Change

Traditional medical terminology	Six-step method
Diagnosis	1. Identify the problem
	2. Build commitment and confidence
	3. Increase awareness
Treatment/prescription	4. Develop and implement action plan
Follow-up prescription	5. Evaluate the action plan
Maintenance	6. Maintain change and prevent relapse

needed to determine readiness and therefore how rapidly to proceed, or even whether to proceed (e.g., smokers may need to consider the issues before they are "ready" to quit).

Given awareness of the physician's belief that a particular behavior is harmful and requires changing, the patient almost always holds secret reservations or "belief barriers" regarding (1) the reason for change (i.e., he or she may not believe the link between cholesterol and heart disease), (2) his or her ability to change, or (3) the effort or inconvenience involved in making such a change. These barriers need to be confronted and countered by the methods described in the next step.

Step 2: Create Confidence and Commitment

This step involves building the patient's commitment and confidence by expanding the clinical interview to incorporate counseling that assesses the patient's barriers to change and provides responses or counterarguments to these barriers. The patient must be asked, "What are your real thoughts on if and how you can change?" and "What are your secret fears about how tough it is going to be to change?"

Changing patients' beliefs about themselves can usually be accomplished by focusing on specific barriers, e.g., statements such as "I can't lose weight. I love to eat!". This statement allows the physician to introduce exercise as an additional avenue for weight loss. An open line of communication between patient and physician is important in order to build confidence.

Given frank and honest answers by the patient, physicians can provide specific counterarguments to their barriers. Smokers who are discouraged by past failures can benefit from knowing that most people try to quit three or four times before finally succeeding. The patient who says he cannot reduce cholesterol or fat in the diet because all of his favorite foods are "bad" for him will be aided by being told that he is not being asked to give up his favorite foods all at once, but to reduce them gradually. Also, the physician can add that he or she enjoys the flavors of low-fat, low-cholesterol foods (personal testimony from physicians is very effective in stimulating a patient's interest and motivation).

In developing counterarguments, the physician should move the patient away from externally based responses. For example, if the barrier is "I really like steak, and I don't want to stop eating it," an "external" counterargument is "My wife is really going to be mad at me if I don't lower my cholesterol." A better internally based counterargument would be "I know I can cut back on how often I eat steak, and I would like to try some new recipes for fish and chicken."

Once counterarguments have been made and the patient commits to changing a behavior, the physician can finalize the discussion and reinforce the importance of the change by having the patient sign a contract to begin working on a particular behavior. Contracts are written summaries of the agreed-upon course of treatment and are particularly effective in building commitment. An example of such a contract is as follows: "Dr. Smith and I agree that I should eat a more heart-healthy diet. I agree to lower my intake of saturated fat and cholesterol over the next 2 to 3 months. To begin, I will record my food intake for 3 days, and I will return in 1 week." In diet-change programs, the return visit should include the person who prepares most of the meals. As seen in this example, the contract can also be used as an introduction to step 3, which includes keeping a record of the targeted behavior.

Step 3: Increase Awareness of Behavior

Step 3 leads to increasing a patient's awareness of his or her behavior patterns through self-observation. The easiest way to do this is with a diary that lists factors such as what occurred, where it occurred, who was present when it occurred, and why it occurred or how the patient felt just prior to the action. The diary is part of the database for treatment. It is *not* used as an outcome variable but to determine the internal and external precursors to the behavior that often act as cues for the behavior. The diary will also help to identify barriers to change or problems for possible relapse. Once identified, these issues can be incorporated into goal setting and environmental changes needed in the treatment plan.

A sample food diary is provided in Table 149-2. Notice that the individual eats in response to stress, often does other things while eating, and has accumulated many conditioned eating responses to external cues (e.g., watching television).

Step 4: Develop and Implement the Action Plan

In traditional medical terminology, the action plan is analogous to the prescription or treatment plan. It is here that a plan establishing specific goals for change and strategies for achieving them are developed. Several strategies can be used, such as teaching new information and skills to the patient, helping the patient set short-term goals, teaching the patient how to restructure thoughts, helping the patient eliminate environmental stimuli for the behavior, encouraging the patient to provide incentives to change the behavior, incorporating support to change from the patient's family and friends, and finally, making a behavioral prescription that explicitly describes what the patient will do to accomplish his or her goals. Not all of these strategies will be appropriate for every patient or every problem. They should be considered as treatment options for testing with a particular patient and problem. However, the power and efficacy of these strategies cannot be appreciated unless the physician uses them actively with a variety of patients. It is also important to negotiate with patients to develop "individualized" treatment plans that are reasonable to them. Definitions and examples of the preceding strategies are discussed in the sections that follow.

New Information

Many patients lack information needed to change their behavior. The physician can provide this in several ways: (1) verbally or through written materials, or (2) by referring the patient to other health professionals (such as dietitians) for information or counseling. Many physicians use a combination of the two, depending on their own time and resources and on the patient's needs and desires. If the physician chooses to use patient education materials or referrals, he or she should be familiar with the information provided in those resources and be sure that it agrees with what he or she is telling the patient. In the case of referrals, it is important for physicians to determine (1) whether the patient actually went to see the person he or she was referred to, (2) what that person told the patient to do, and (3) whether the patient understood what the person recommended (i.e., did the patient know exactly what to do when he or she left the office?).

Some examples of the nutritional information that patients need are as follows: both dietary fat and cholesterol contribute

Table 149-2 Example of Food Diary

NAME: John Doe — DATE: 10/12/90

Time of day	What did I eat?	Where?	Time spent eating	What else did I do while eating?	How did I feel?
7:30 AM	Coffee with sugar, three slices bacon, two eggs, whole milk	Kitchen table	10 min	Talked to wife and watched TV	Sleepy
8:30 AM	Coffee, sugar, cream	Office desk	3 min	Worked	Frustrated, rushed
10:30 AM	Coffee, sugar, cream, glazed doughnut	Office	5 min	Worked	Mad at boss
12:00 noon	Lunch: chopped sirloin, buttered vegetables, roll with butter, chocolate cake	Restaurant	35 min	Talked (lunch conference)	Focused on business discussion, worried about new deal
2:45 PM	Coffee, sugar, cream	Office	10 min	Worked	Rushed
3:30 PM	Soft drink	Delicatessen	5 min	Talked to friend	Tired and depressed
6:00 PM	Nibbled cheeses and crackers, had two cocktails	Family room	30 min	Watched TV news	Wanted to forget job
6:30 PM	Dinner: steak, baked potato with sour cream, ice cream	Dining room	20 min	Talked to family	Upset with son
7:00 PM	Cookies, milk	Bedroom	5 min	Watched TV	Worried about work

to serum cholesterol; all the cholesterol in eggs is in the yolk; chicken skin contains high amounts of fat; and all meats and animal products contain cholesterol, whereas plants are free from cholesterol (although palm and coconut oils are extremely high in saturated fat). The word "hydrogenated" means that the oil has been artificially saturated, thus increasing its deleterious effect on serum cholesterol relative to that of nonhydrogenated oils. The last example can be used as a way of introducing the patient to new skills, e.g., how to read food labels. Ingredients are listed on a product's content disclosure in descending order by volume; thus, the first item listed is the main ingredient, with the next being proportionally smaller, and so on. Many breakfast cereals that are advertised as having oat bran do not list it as the main ingredient.

Voluntary health agencies, such as the American Cancer Society, the American Lung Association, the American Heart Association, and numerous others, have patient education materials that provide patients with facts, helpful tips, recipes, and even classes on how to change risk behaviors. Physicians should investigate these materials and have them readily available to give to patients.

Proximal (Short-Term) Goals

How should goals be set? Is the goal "I will lose 10 pounds in the next 3 months" as good as "I will take a 15-minute walk before dinner every day during the next week"? No, the second is easier to achieve and can be monitored more directly (Did you take your walk today?) than the vague and distal goal of losing 10 pounds in a certain period of time (Bandura and Simon, 1977). The key to setting proximal goals is to make them target *specific* behaviors that are *realistic* and *achievable* by the patient. Thus, the principle of gradualism is important; the patient should not be allowed to set too many goals or to decide to make large changes in the beginning. The patient who is changing his or her diet should change one to two meals a day for a few weeks, preferably breakfast or lunch, rather than making strict restrictions for every meal. Breakfast is the meal over which most people have the greatest individual control, and it is an easier target for beginning diet change.

Cognitive Restructuring (Self-Talk)

Patients need to reprogram their "inner voice" or "internal dialogue" so that it will be productive and not destructive (Goldfried and Davidson, 1976; Mahoney and Mahoney, 1976). An example is substituting constructive for destructive thoughts, such as "Hey, I lost half a pound this week!" for "People think I'm a fat slob; I'll never lose all this weight." Another example of constructive thinking is to cope with mistakes by saying "That's OK. I'll do better tomorrow" rather than "I blew it. I might as well finish the whole cookie jar." Constructive thoughts are not to be viewed as excuses for slips but as a method for refocusing the patient away from negative thoughts that discourage or depress the patient.

Many negative cognitions are based on previous failures to change behavior. If step 1 or 2 uncovers several previous failed attempts at change, the physician should ask the patient how he or she felt immediately after failing and what the patient said to himself or herself. If the patient reports only negative thoughts, the patient should be reassured that he or she now has an ally and coworker (the physician) who will help find ways of increasing the chances for success. The patient should not spend time on self-criticism for minor indiscretions, but instead should decide what to do differently next time.

Stimulus Control

Physicians can help patients change the immediate environment to facilitate change. The diary information is very helpful in finding specific environmental stimuli or cues that initiate the behavior. Diaries of overweight patients may reveal a snacking pattern while watching television. The solution is to eat only at the kitchen table. Smokers should remove cigarettes, ashtrays, and perhaps alcohol from the house, because they can be cues to smoke.

Research in behavior therapy often calls for more drastic methods of changing environmental stimuli, such as placing high-calorie foods on the top shelf of the pantry, storing high-fat foods in aluminum foil to "block them from sight," and changing chairs that are commonly used while smoking. Not having high-calorie, high-fat foods in the house is clearly another way to avoid eating them.

Incentives

Incentives involve creating awards for accomplishing goals. It is usual for physicians to think the patient's satisfaction at improving health is a sufficient incentive, but research in behavior therapy has shown that explicit "rewards" can greatly enhance performance and stimulate continued change (Mahoney, 1974b; Mahoney et al, 1973). Patients tend to punish themselves for failing, and not to reward themselves for success. Incentives should not be tied only to the final goal (i.e., cholesterol under

200 mg/dl or loss of 10 pounds); they should be linked to proximal goals. Rewards work best when closely linked in time to the behavior rather than to the final outcome. One patient may want to set her incentive as buying a new dress if she loses 10 pounds; however, she should be encouraged to reward herself for completing her goal of walking 15 minutes a day for 2 weeks (regardless of whether any weight was lost during this time). Immediate "process" rewards can be given repeatedly, such as a single flower for the home or office (especially good for ex-smokers), a phone call to a friend in another town, or a magazine not often purchased.

Incentives must be appropriate to the final goal (e.g., the reward for weight loss should not be a chocolate cake). They should be pleasurable, readily available, given repeatedly, or revised upon accomplishment (e.g., the patient can establish a hierarchy of rewards for progressive improvement in the action plan). Rewards, of course, include attention; a telephone call from the office nurse with encouragement will often yield surprising benefits at a follow-up visit.

Behavioral Prescription or Contract

A behavioral prescription is a written contract that is specific about what the patient will be doing in the next few days or weeks to achieve the proximal goal. It is both convenient and effective that this contract be written on a blank prescription pad. The text can be brief, such as "I will switch five out of seven breakfasts to meatless, eggless, cheeseless, nonfat-milk meals." Both the physician and the patient should sign the agreement. The patient can post it on the refrigerator door or the bathroom mirror, where he or she will see it daily. The date of a return visit can also be on the contract.

For smokers, the behavioral prescription should specify a quit date. Recent studies found that smokers who set a quit date were four times more likely to make a quit attempt than those who did not set a quit date (Cummings et al, 1989). After obtaining a commitment to cessation, the physician should help the patient set a quit date within a reasonable time. An optimal period is 1 to 2 weeks later or when a vacation period allows freedom from stress in the critical week after quitting. Following the quit date, the patient should have a return visit within 2 to 4 days, when any withdrawal symptoms or effects of nicotine polacrilex (if prescribed) can be checked.

Social Support

Enlisting support from friends, relatives, and coworkers will assist the patient in the action plan. For dietary change, a spouse or friend should be included, especially if this person prepares the meals. As mentioned in step 2, ideally this person accompanies the patient on the visit when the action plan is discussed, and should be enlisted to assist the patient with revised menus and be reassured that changes will be relatively easy and often less costly.

There is a tendency for patients (especially ones who do not normally prepare meals) to transfer all the responsibility for their diet to a spouse or partner who prepares the food. Thus, the patient may not learn the information necessary to stay on the diet and may relapse when the "cook" cannot prepare or select the food.

A second caveat concerns the "nag effect." Perhaps the spouse has been trying to change the patient's behavior for months or even years. If it is evident that the spouse has been "nagging" the patient to change, the physician can educate the support person about the type of support needed. Tips on how to give feedback include "Don't say don't." Frame advice positively, e.g., "Let's have fruit for dessert," instead of "You can't have ice cream." Reward small successes and offer ways to avoid temptations to relapse rather than belittling the patient for slips.

When possible, the spouse also should be enlisted to change the behavior under scrutiny, because separate lives under the same roof lead to dissonance. If this is not possible, at least the spouse needs to agree not to sabotage the patient's efforts. This is crucial if the spouse continues to smoke after the patient quits. The two should agree to have "nonsmoking" areas within the house (with the patient selecting as "smoke-free" those rooms where he or she has had the strongest urges to smoke). The smoking spouse must agree to restrictions on lighting up, leaving cigarette packs around the house, and so forth. Clearly, ex-smokers who live with smokers should be followed more closely, given their higher risk for relapse.

Step 5: Evaluate the Plan

Step 5 involves evaluating the plan of action shortly after its initiation. In the typical medical model, this step encompasses the follow-up after treatment. In the six-step behavior change process, step 5 can span as little as 2 to 3 days or as long as 2 to 3 months. We define it as the period when the patient is working actively on the action plan. Such evaluations often lead to modified goals (e.g., if the patient's choices for breakfast are too difficult to change, he or she could try changing lunches).

At the follow-up visit 1 to 3 weeks after the start of the action plan, the patient should be praised (rewarded) for making progress even if only small steps have been taken. Small successes build confidence for the more difficult steps to follow. The focus should be on benefits associated with change and solutions to any difficulties. Solutions might include modifying old goals, adding new goals, changing social support providers, and, most important, returning to previous steps to work on building the patient's confidence or increasing his or her awareness of the cues to behavior.

Obviously, patients taking medications that are used in combination with behavioral changes need to be evaluated for side effects, compliance to the regimen, and attitudes toward the medication. Patients often perceive drugs as "magic bullets" that obviate the need for lifestyle changes. In clinical preventive medicine, most drugs will accomplish their purpose only if the patient also makes substantial changes in lifestyle. The use of nicotine polacrilex to assist with smoking cessation is a good example. Patients should *not* use the medication until they stop smoking completely; even with its use, they must learn to deal with the social, environmental, and mental cues to smoke by progressing through the six steps.

Step 6: Maintain Change and Prevent Relapse

Once the patient has successfully changed behavior with resulting losses in weight, lower LDL cholesterol, or better fitness, the task then is to maintain or retain such achievements and to prevent relapse to earlier behavior patterns. For many behaviors, the training and skill required for maintenance is often greater than that needed to bring about the original change.

Eventually, when new behaviors and lifestyle are well accepted and self-rewarding, patients no longer perceive that they are "on a diet" or "working on quitting." When this occurs, the likelihood of relapse is decreased. Therefore, many patients will need to expend considerable effort to maintain or further their progress. Many of the behavioral skills used to change the original behavior can be modified slightly for use in relapse prevention. The physician must help the patient anticipate circumstances that put him or her at high risk for relapse and teach the patient how to deal (both cognitively and behaviorally) with those situations. Common high-risk situations include trips, parties, guests, stressful life events, crises at work, bars (for smokers), and restaurants. No one can avoid making occasional slips; however, a "slip does not equal a fall." The patient should not feel overwhelmed with guilt. Only a complete return to previous behavior patterns should be considered a full relapse, and the patient should start anew with step 1.

As in step 4, there are specific strategies physicians can recommend their patients use to maintain a "status quo" and prevent relapse. Incentives reinforce newly acquired behaviors and encourage maintenance of those behaviors. Small incentives like flowers, sugarless mints, special fruit, special activities, or just time for oneself are good choices. At this point, incentives can apply to a particular period of maintenance. For example, the ex-smoker may prevent relapse by celebrating the number of days, weeks, or months he or she has remained abstinent. The money saved each month by not smoking (about $35 for a pack-a-day smoker) may be used as a monthly reward to buy something "extra."

It is important for patients to enlist support for long-term maintenance. This support may come from those who assisted them during the initial phases of change (steps 1 through 4). A logical source of continued support is also from individuals who recently changed a similar behavior. Finding someone the patient can exercise with, eat lunch with, and take nonsmoking breaks with at work will support his or her commitment to maintenance, and might provide a new social network in which he or she can discuss successes and problems with people who have "been there." The organization with the most sophisticated structure specifically designed to provide such support is Alcoholics Anonymous.

The patient must anticipate future stresses that can induce relapse. The patient needs instruction not only on what to do but on what to think (i.e., self-talk) and what to say to the persons involved in the situation. Patients should be encouraged to write a list of high-risk situations (e.g., a reunion or a party) and practice aloud their responses to them (Donovan and Marlatt, 1988). They can be told it's like a fire drill, in which practicing what to do avoids panic under stress (Lazarus, 1978).

It is important to follow successful patients for reasons beyond relapse prevention. Persons who have changed one behavior often covertly or inadvertently start working on changing another, offering opportunities for a renewed physician role. Also, many treatment strategies produce beneficial changes in multiple endpoints. For example, the patient who has lost weight may have also reduced blood pressure or cholesterol level. Physicians need to point out these concurrent benefits to the patient and support continued efforts to maintain those changes or embark on more progressive changes if warranted (e.g., once LDL cholesterol is below 160 mg/dl, begin working to reduce it to 130 mg/dl).

Summary

It is critical to realize that a patient's progress through the six-step method is not static or in one direction, but *cyclical.* Patients can cycle through one or more of these steps a number of times, each time revising goals and behaviors and building on prior experience. It will take more than one or two office visits to move a patient through the first few steps. In working with patients who are ready to change, the first five steps can often be accomplished in three visits, with steps 1 and 2 combined in one visit that ends with the contract and the patient's agreement to do a diary. The second visit would encompass steps 3 and 4, in which the treatment plan is developed and strategies for implementing it are specified. The third visit would address step 5, in which the patient's experiences with the plan are evaluated and brainstorming solutions to problems or revising goals can take place, if necessary. Ideally, another visit is important to review maintenance or relapse issues or to cycle patients back into a previous step.

These six steps have been used in the Stanford Faculty Development Program, an ongoing national training program for primary care and internal medicine faculty and residents. Significant changes occurred in clinical practices relevant to cholesterol management, nutrition, and smoking cessation. Physicians' self-confidence to address preventive medicine issues with patients was also significantly increased. In addition to this program, the National Cancer Institute and the US Preventive Services Task Force have recently published guidelines on physician counseling for smoking cessation and other risk behaviors that incorporate many of the strategies discussed in this chapter (Glynn and Marley, 1989; Report of the US Preventive Services Task Force, 1989). Finally, in order to familiarize themselves with the six-step method, physicians can experiment by using it to change their own health habits. This experience would provide them with a knowledge regarding use of such strategies and would also help avoid the consequences of the old adage, "Do as I say, not as I do."

References

Bandura A. Principles of behavior modification: An integrative approach. New York: Plenum Press, 1969.

Bandura A. Social learning theory. Englewood Cliffs, NJ: Prentice Hall, 1977a.

Bandura A. Self-efficacy: Toward a unifying theory of behavior changes. Psych Rev 1977b; 84:191.

Bandura A. The self-system in reciprocal determinism. Am Psychol 1978; 33:344.

Bandura A, Simon KM. The role of proximal behavior intentions in self-regulation of refractory behavior. Cognitive Ther Res 1977; 1:177.

Braunstein JJ, Toister JP. Medical applications of the behavioral sciences. Chicago: Year Book Medical Publishers, 1981.

Craighead LW. A problem-solving approach to the treatment of obesity. In: Hersen M, Bellack AS, eds. Handbook of clinical behavior therapy with adults. New York: Plenum Press, 1985.

Crouch M, et al. Personal and mediated health counseling for sustained dietary reduction of hypercholesterolemia. Prev Med 1986; 15:282.

Cummings SR, et al. Training physicians in counseling about smoking cessation. Ann Intern Med 1989; 110:640.

Davidson PO, Davidson SM. Behavioral medicine: Changing health lifestyles. New York: Brunner/Mazel, 1980.

Donovan DM, Marlatt GA. Assessment of addictive behaviors. New York: Guilford Press, 1988.

Farquhar JW. The American way of life need not be hazardous to your health. Reading, MA: Addison-Wesley, 1987.

Glynn TJ, Marley MW. How to help your patients stop smoking. Washington, DC: United States Department of Health and Human Services, Public Health Service, National Cancer Institute, NIH Publication No. 89-3064, 1989.

Goldfried MR, Davison GC. Clinical behavior therapy. New York: Holt, Rinehart & Winston, 1976.

Hersen M, Bellack AS, eds. Handbook of clinical behavior therapy with adults. New York: Plenum Press, 1985.

Hersen M, Eisler RM, Miller PM. Progress in behavior modification. Vol 5. New York: Academic Press, 1977.

Kaplan SJ. The private practice of behavior therapy. New York: Plenum Press, 1986.

Lazarus AA. Behavior therapy and beyond. New York: McGraw-Hill, 1971.

Lazarus AA. In the mind's eye. New York: Rawson, 1978.

Mahoney MJ, Moura NJ, Wade TC. Relative efficacy of self-reward, self-punishment, and self-monitoring techniques for weight loss. J Consult Clin Psych 1973; 40:404.

Mahoney MJ. Cognition and behavior modification. Cambridge, MA: Ballinger, 1974a.

Mahoney MJ. Self-reward and self-monitoring techniques for weight control. Behav Ther 1974b; 5:48.

Mahoney MJ, Mahoney K. Permanent weight loss. New York: Norton, 1976.

Mahoney MJ, Thoresen CE. Self-control: Power to the person. Monterey, CA: Brooks/Cole, 1974.

Meichenbaum DH. Cognitive behavior modification: An integrative approach. New York: Plenum Press, 1977.

Meyer AJ, Henderson JB. Multiple risk factor reduction in the prevention of cardiovascular disease. Prev Med 1974; 3:225.

Report of the National Cholesterol Education Program Expert Panel on Detection, Evaluation, and Treatment of High Blood Cholesterol in Adults. Arch Intern Med 1988; 148:36.

Report of the US Preventive Services Task Force. Guide to clinical preventive services. Baltimore: Williams & Wilkins, 1989.
Sheridan DP, Winogrond IR. The preventive approach to patient care. New York: Elsevier, 1987.
Stunkard AJ, Craighead LW, O'Brien R. Controlled trial of behavior therapy, pharmacotherapy, and their combination in the treatment of obesity. Lancet, November 15, 1980; 1045.
Thoresen CE, Mahoney MJ. Behavioral self-control. New York: Holt, Rinehart & Winston, 1974.
Wilson GT. Cognitive factors in lifestyle changes: A social learning perspective. In: Davidson PO, Davidson SM. Behavioral medicine: Changing health lifestyles. New York: Brunner/Mazel, 1980.

Delivering Bad News

Harry L. Greene, MD

150

One of a physician's most difficult tasks is the responsibility of delivering bad news. The physician must convey the diagnosis clearly and adequately while providing support and hope, and keeping himself or herself separate from the cause. The physician is only the bearer of the news, not its instigator.

If we take as an example the diagnosis of cancer (it might as easily be end-stage cardiomyopathy, inoperable three-vessel coronary disease, amyotrophic lateral sclerosis, or a 90 percent third-degree burn), we can give some guidelines for managing the news.

The diagnosis of cancer can be a painful and frightening experience for both patient and physician. The physician knows that the news will be traumatic to the patient. It is incumbent upon the physician to attempt to reduce this trauma, provide support, and begin to set a constructive and realistic framework for solving or softening the problem. The person to deliver the news should be the patient's primary physician or the one with whom there is greatest rapport.

Naturally, there is no one "right" way to approach every patient, but a few basic principles gained from talking to patients and their families who have been through the process can be applied to each situation to facilitate a more "therapeutic" interaction. Delivery of bad news begins before the biopsy diagnosis is known. When discussing the possibilities, cancer should be mentioned if appropriate. It is important at this time to gain an understanding of what the patient's knowledge of cancer is and what it means to him or her. Many patients will have had a family member or close friend with cancer. The patient's perception will be colored by that experience. For example, the patient who states, "My mother had ovarian cancer; they operated and said they couldn't get it out, and she died in 3 weeks" will have a perception of cancer that is different from that of the patient who says, "My cousin had Hodgkin's disease, received chemotherapy and radiation therapy and was sick during therapy, but has been normal for the past 9 years."

It is also important to know what the patient's support structure is like and whether or not the patient would like another person present when information about the diagnosis is received. Never assume that the patient wants another person present; always follow the patient's lead. The deliverer of bad news should have maximal knowledge about the diagnosis, its natural history and prognosis, and all reasonable treatment options. This, coupled with a thorough knowledge of the patient and his or her social situation, will allow you to answer questions factually, sympathetically, and realistically.

Appropriate setting and proper timing are crucial considerations. If possible, the patient should be alert, not recovering from the effects of anesthesia or under sedation or heavy analgesia. He or she should be comfortably appointed and not in an awkward or uncomfortable position. Select the time so as not to be rushed, but avoid delays that cause the patient to agonize for hours before learning the news, or worse, learn it inadvertently from a nursing assistant, lab tech, or escort person, or by reading his or her own chart. The news should come in person and never by telephone. So much is conveyed through nonverbal communication that it is hard to comfort him or her adequately by telephone. An occasional patient learns of the diagnosis by calling in for a laboratory result. Office and lab personnel must be cautioned against this practice, for it is the physician's task to share painful truths with the patient. Bad news should be delivered only by those who are able to deal with all of its ramifications. The personnel present for this meeting should be minimal, including caregivers with whom the patient feels comfortable and who will serve to help support him or her after the news, i.e., primary nurse. This is not a teaching moment and should not be done in the context of routine ward or teaching rounds.

For the person inexperienced in delivering bad news, it is helpful to rehearse or mentally role play in order to anticipate the questions that will follow. Prior thought will prevent damaging errors in syntax that, no matter how well intended, can be painful and difficult to correct. It is important to remember that reaction to bad news may be quite varied; e.g., the patient may be stunned and unable to hear further information, or he or she may experience anger, denial, doubt, and emotional decomposition. Certainly each of these reactions requires a different set of responses on the part of the physician.

Most patients will be somewhat stunned upon hearing bad news. They become distracted by consideration of its impact on their life and why they might be affected, and they experience a plethora of feelings and thoughts that significantly limit the amount of information that can be given after the initial news. In addition to providing limited information, the physician must be concise and speak in the patient's own language, paying careful attention to the degree of comprehension. Avoid terms like *benign, malignant,* and *lymphatic spread* unless these are carefully defined for the patient. This is not an appropriate time for an extensive course in medical terminology. Unfamiliar terms only add to the patient's sense of isolation and frustration.

Table 150-1 A Protocol for Delivery of Bad News: Guidelines for the Clinician

Background
1. Establish an honest and caring relationship with all patients.
2. Through cancer screening done during health maintenance visits, patients can learn about cancers that can be cured.
3. The physician can learn who the significant people are in a patient's life.
4. If cancer is a reasonable possibility during the work-up of a problem, share that information with the patient.

Once a cancer diagnosis is confirmed:

Preparation
1. Set up an appointment as soon as possible.
2. Allow adequate time.
3. Ask if the patient would like to bring someone along. Never assume that the answer is yes; some people prefer to be alone.
4. Try to use a quiet office; avoid the examining room, recovery room, and the telephone, if possible.
5. Know your material, i.e., curability, treatment, prognosis, referral sources, and support systems.

Disclosure
1. Give simple information.
2. Determine what cancer means to the patient.
3. Use clear, careful, and sensitive language. Avoid medical terminology or jargon.
4. Provide more information as requested.
5. Ask questions to assess understanding.
6. Be alert for sensory overload and cognitive shutdown.
7. Realize that you may need to go through all of these steps again if the patient isn't hearing you.

Adjusting to the Patient's Responses
1. Allow for sensory overload and cognitive shutdown.
2. Be aware of unshared meanings, and be ready to define terms as needed.
3. Read nonverbal communication.
4. Use exploratory questions (i.e., What is your understanding of what I tried to say? What does what I said mean to you?).
5. Encourage questions from the spouse or significant other, if present.

Follow-up
1. Allow for second opinions and expedite them, when reasonable.
2. Don't rush the patient to treatment, but have a treatment plan ready if requested.
3. Assist in setting up appointments.
4. Identify other support systems.
5. Set the time and place for your next meeting.
6. Offer telephone contact with you as needed.
7. Encourage writing questions down ahead of time and bringing them to the next visit.
8. Give written materials, and write down key dates and instructions.
9. If the diagnosis was given during the day to a hospitalized patient, try to see the patient again before you leave for the night.

Demeanor and Attitude
1. Emphasize your care and support.
2. Stress quality of life and ability to manage symptoms if these are concerns.
3. Create an atmosphere of hope tempered with realism.
4. When appropriate, encourage the patient to attend to the unfinished business of life (e.g., wills, unresolved conflicts with family).

Following the initial shock, many patients describe concerns about pain, suffering, family reaction, fears of abandonment, and death. The physician should view such concerns as acceptable; at the same time, these concerns may be softened by stressing hope wherever appropriate, assuring pain control if it is raised as an issue, and promising continued care and support. This is a time, within the realm of honesty, to accentuate the positive. A very simple discussion of what to do next is appropriate. This is not the time for detailing all the effects of chemotherapy, radiation therapy, and the like. This can follow later, when the mind is less overwhelmed. The initial meeting should include an offer to explain the situation to the patient's family or significant others as he or she wishes, and a time for answering questions. Be cognizant of the patient's religious beliefs and encourage support and help from clergy when indicated.

Many patients spend the entire night after receiving such news awake, agonizing over unanswered questions. If you are able to do so, it is worthwhile to visit the patient again in the early evening to follow up on any new questions and alleviate anxiety before the loneliness of the night. For some patients, this second visit may be a more appropriate time to discuss in greater detail the plans for further therapy or palliation. This second visit also gives a very clear message that you care about the patient and that you will continue to provide support. Before leaving, set a time for the next meeting, instruct the patient to write down any questions, and make clear how you can be reached in the interim, if necessary.

Subsequent visits can deal in more detail with crucial issues such as prognosis, treatment options, hospital support systems, future plans, lifestyle change, need for or interest in second opinions, "why me" issues, and the "contagiousness" of cancer, all common concerns in cancer patients.

Sometime during these visits, you should again attempt to gauge the patient's impression of the situation. A simple question like "What is your understanding of the cancer that you have, and how is it affecting your life?" allows an appraisal of the patient's impression of the disease. The patient's answer will highlight misconceptions to be dealt with and unrealistic concerns to be alleviated. Don't be afraid to ask your colleagues how you might improve future interactions. By following the guidelines mentioned, you can provide some needed therapy in a very challenging situation. Table 150-1 presents general guidelines to be used when thinking about delivering a difficult diagnosis.

References

Goldberg RJ. Disclosure of information to adult cancer patients: Issues and update. J Clin Oncol 1984; 2:948.

Lazare A. Three functions of the clinical interview. In: Lazare A, ed. Outpatient psychiatry: Diagnosis and treatment. Baltimore: Williams & Wilkins, 1989:153.

Lazare A. Shame and humiliation in the medical encounter. Arch Intern Med 1987; 147:1653.

Lazare A, Eisenthal S. Clinician/patient relations. I. Attending to the patient's perspective. In: Lazare A, ed. Outpatient psychiatry: Diagnosis and treatment. Baltimore: Williams & Wilkins, 1989:125.

Lazare A, Eisenthal S, Frank A. Clinician/patient relations. II. Conflict and negotiation. In: Lazare A, ed. Outpatient psychiatry: Diagnosis and treatment. Baltimore: Williams & Wilkins, 1989:137.

Rodabough T. The minister as death counselor: A typology of role enactments. Pastoral Psychol 1981; 30:89.

Oral Cavity; Ears, Nose, and Throat; Gynecology

IV

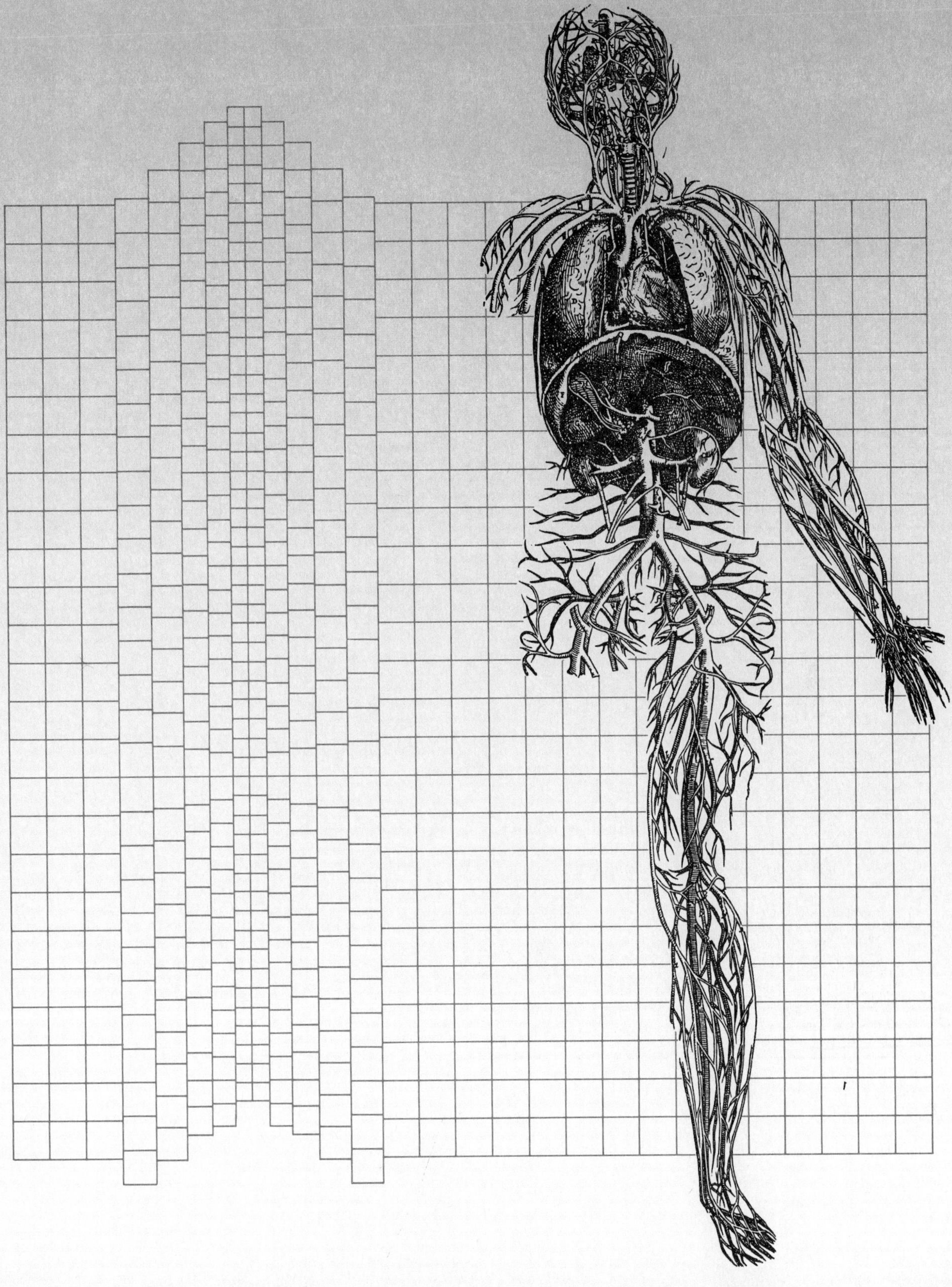

Oral Cavity

Mouth Pain

Joseph M. Kelly, DDS

Katherine L. Kahn, MD

Definition

Pain is the usual symptom of diseases involving the oral cavity. Extension of mouth pain beyond the oral cavity is common and often presents as orofacial pain.

Etiology

The causes of mouth and orofacial pain can be grouped into diagnostic categories. In order of frequency, these categories are (1) dental and periodontal disease, (2) mucosal lesions and ulcerations, (3) myofascial and temporomandibular joint pain, (4) vascular headaches, and (5) neurogenic pain.

Dental and Periodontal Disease

Dental and periodontal disease are the most common causes of mouth pain. Tooth decay (caries) leads to irritation of the nerve (pulpitis) and a sensitive tooth that is aggravated by cold and sweets. Eventually pulpal necrosis occurs. Trauma to the tooth with or without fracture of the crown or root can also cause pulpal necrosis. The crown becomes dark gray. Bacteria enter the necrotic pulp through the open carious lesion in the tooth or from the blood stream. The inflammatory reaction at the apex of the root and in the surrounding bone results in a periapical abscess. The pain is a throbbing toothache that is aggravated by heat, pressure while chewing, and lying down. A traumatized tooth with a necrotic pulp may develop a periapical abscess years after the initial trauma. Extension of the infection through the alveolar bone to the periosteum results in an alveolar abscess with the swelling in the mucobuccal fold. Release of the pressure at the apex of the tooth at this time often decreases the pain. Further extension of the infection into the adjacent soft-tissue planes can result in facial, submandibular, or sublingual cellulitis and an elevated temperature. Extension of the infection into the floor of the mouth and tissue planes in the neck results in a clinical condition referred to as Ludwig's angina.

Periodontal disease results from local irritants around the teeth and gums such as calculus, plaque, and food debris. Gingivitis causing mild discomfort can become acute necrotizing gingivitis (Vincent's infection) if oral hygiene is poor. Gingivitis may progress to periodontitis with bone loss, loose teeth, and periodontal abscesses. Systemic diseases such as diabetes can exacerbate the condition.

In teenagers and young adults, infection around erupting wisdom teeth is common. Food debris trapped under the gingival tissue covering the erupting crown results in a pericoronitis.

Mucosal Lesions and Ulcerations

Mucosal lesions and ulcerations of infectious or traumatic origin are a common cause of mouth pain. A source of mouth pain in children is herpetic gingivostomatitis; in adults, canker sores (aphthous ulcers), erosive lichen planus, candidiasis under dentures, geographic tongue (glossitis migrans), glossodynia, and neoplasms; and in the elderly, atrophic mucosa.

Myofascial Pain and Temporomandibular Joint Pain

Myofascial pain and temporomandibular joint disorders are extremely common causes of orofacial pain in adults.

Temporomandibular joint disorders are characterized by pain, limitation on opening and closing, clicking or grating, and pain on palpation directly over the joint. Causes include acute trauma, chronic microtrauma from malocclusion, clenching habits or night grinding, as well as various arthritides such as rheumatoid arthritis.

Clicking in the temporomandibular joint is common in young people and is due to anterior displacement of the cartilaginous disk in front of the condyle. When the mouth is opened wide, the condyle moves onto the disk with a loud pop. Most cases are asymptomatic, but some are painful as a result of the condyle riding on the sensitive retrodiscal tissues. Permanent dislocation of the disk limits opening and is very painful initially.

Myofascial pain is a cause of orofacial pain more frequently in adult women. In many cases, it is associated with or indistinguishable from muscle tension headache. Many of the patients also have neck and shoulder pain. When the muscle pain or spasm is in the muscles of mastication, there is pain on opening and chewing. This type of pain may also lead to or be associated with joint discomfort or damage. It usually responds to dental splint therapy. Referred muscle pain and trigger points are frequently present in this syndrome.

Vascular Headaches

Vascular headaches may involve the orofacial region, particularly the maxilla. Patients with myofascial pain frequently have a history of vascular headaches.

Neurogenic Pain

Neurogenic pain such as trigeminal neuralgia, characterized by severe paroxysms of pain, occurs primarily in the elderly. It usually follows the maxillary or mandibular branches of the trigeminal nerve and may be attributed to dental problems.

Diagnostic Approach

The history of orofacial pain frequently indicates the source of the problem. The essential elements of the history include the onset, location, duration, and character of the pain as well as factors that increase or decrease the symptoms.

Onset

Recent onset of pain is characteristic of dental or acute periodontal problems. Patients tend to seek immediate treatment. The dental problems causing pain include pulpitis, abscessed teeth, periodontal abscesses, and pericoronitis of erupting teeth. Infections or traumatic lesions of the oral mucosa such as aphthous ulcers, herpetic gingivostomatitis, and Vincent's infection present with a history of sudden onset of pain.

Chronic longstanding and recurrent pain over months or years is characteristic of myofascial and temporomandibular joint pain as well as vascular and muscle tension headaches. Longstanding painful mucosal conditions include lichen planus and denture irritation.

Location

Pain may be localized to individual teeth, gingiva, and specific areas of oral mucosa or generalized throughout the upper or lower jaw, and may include both sides. Toothaches and abscessed teeth are always unilateral; however, the pain can be referred to the opposing jaw on the same side. Generalized bilateral mouth pain occurs in most infectious processes involving the oral mucosa. Atrophic mucosa in the elderly causes bilateral burning mouth pain.

As in many neurologic and headache syndromes, duration and character of the pain are very specific in many dental conditions. Sharp localized pain of short duration involving a tooth is suggestive of pulpitis, particularly if the pain is aggravated by cold liquids or sweets. Teeth with nerves exposed by either decay or trauma also are painful when cold air is inhaled. Constant pain of recent onset that is limited to several adjacent teeth and gums usually is due to a tooth with a necrotic pulp or to periodontal infection.

Throbbing pain around a tooth, if it is increased when chewing, drinking hot liquids, or lying down, indicates pulpal necrosis or periapical abscess. When a patient is lying in bed at night, the increased cranial pressure markedly increases the pain from an abscessed tooth. Swelling over the jaw indicates an acute alveolar abscess. The patient usually states that the toothache diminished at the same time the swelling developed.

Recent onset of pain in the mouth involving the gingiva in a localized area may be caused by mucosal lesions such as canker sores, pericoronal irritation around an erupting tooth, periodontal infection, or traumatic lesions. Generalized pain throughout the mouth is not likely to be of tooth origin.

History of upper respiratory tract infection and generalized pain in the upper teeth suggests sinusitis.

Sudden and recurrent uncomfortable swelling in the preauricular or submandibular area suggests blocked salivary ducts, particularly if eating exacerbates the swelling and pain.

Chronic, recurrent throbbing orofacial pain that is not associated with chewing or eating and has no obvious physical findings requires a review of the patient's history for headaches. Many patients with jaw pain, myofascial pain, and temporomandibular joint problems also have a history of migraine or tension headaches.

Constant burning pain in the mouth and tongue occurs in the elderly as a result of mucosal atrophy. Ill-fitting dentures can irritate or aggravate the problem. These patients are also likely to develop monilial infection under the denture.

Physical Examination

Clinical examination of the mouth requires adequate lighting, a mouth mirror or a tongue depressor, and gloves. Careful inspection of the mouth, palpation of the oral tissues, and percussion of the teeth are necessary. Following inspection of the oral cavity, a gloved finger should be placed high up in the vestibule and the entire vestibule palpated both medially and laterally. By sliding the finger over the roots of the teeth, any tender or swollen areas are readily identified.

Percussion is done by tapping individual teeth with a mirror handle or tongue depressor. Functional movements of the mandible should be observed and the temporomandibular joint evaluated.

Limited opening may indicate the following:

1. Infection, such as pericoronitis of a third molar, may be causing spasm in the muscles of mastication.
2. Temporomandibular joint dysfunction or trauma to the joint limits opening. Pain on palpation over the joint directly anterior to the tragus of the ear confirms the diagnosis.
3. Myofascial pain with muscle spasm can be determined by palpating the masseter and temporalis muscles for tenderness and spasm.

Clicking may be produced by a displaced cartilaginous disk in front of the condyle, which prevents full opening until the condyle slips onto the disk, allowing full opening and producing a clicking in the process.

Deviation on opening may be caused by internal joint dysfunction or pathology, which causes the jaw to deviate to the same side.

Decayed teeth, lost fillings, or large new fillings are potential sources of pain. Discolored teeth with a dark gray hue usually have a nonvital pulp. The teeth in the area of pain should be tapped with the handle of a mirror or tongue depressor. Both upper and lower teeth should be percussed on the side being examined. If increased pain results from percussing a particular tooth, a periapical abscess is probable.

Gingivitis gives an inflamed puffy appearance to the crestal margin of the gingiva. Vincent's infection produces generalized mouth pain, a fetid odor, markedly inflamed gingiva, and gray necrotic papillae between the teeth. Pericoronitis is inflammation of the tissue over an erupting tooth, most often the lower wisdom tooth. In young adults, the inflamed pericoronal tissue can become infected from food debris under the pericoronal flap, resulting in limited opening, difficulty in swallowing, tenderness in the submandibular area, and a fever. Localized swelling around one or two teeth at the crest of the ridge is usually due to a periodontal abscess.

Periapical abscesses are determined by palpating the vestibule around the jaw with a gloved finger. As the finger passes along the roots of the teeth, the swollen, tender area in the mucobuccal fold is easily felt. Tenderness and swelling in the floor of the mouth can be the early stages of a cellulitis that may become Ludwig's angina. This serious infection causes a swelling in the floor of the mouth and submandibular spaces bilaterally. There is marked trismus. The tongue and floor of the mouth are raised. The airway may become obstructed, and a tracheostomy may be required. Hospitalization and intravenous antibiotic therapy are routinely needed.

Examination of the tongue and oral mucosa requires both careful inspection and palpation. The various lesions and ulcerations are discussed in Chapter 152, "Lesions of the Mouth."

Trigeminal neuralgia is a severe pain of short duration in older patients. The pain follows the anatomic distribution of one of the branches of the trigeminal nerve. If the intraoral and extraoral tissues are palpated, a trigger zone will usually be found. Very light stimulation of the trigger area such as washing the face will initiate a spasm of pain. Patients with an intraoral trigger zone often assume a head-down position, which allows saliva to flow out of the mouth. The patients refuse to swallow or talk because these actions set off spasms of pain.

Swelling and pain in the preauricular and mandibular angle area are characteristic of parotitis. Saliva flow from the parotid (Stensen's) duct should be checked by retracting the cheek with the thumb and milking the gland by sliding the fingers from the gland forward. A cloudy or purulent discharge is present in suppurative parotitis, a condition usually found in elderly debilitated patients. In viral parotitis the saliva is clear. Blockage of the duct by mucous plugs or salivary stones prevents the flow of any saliva. Salivary stones are more common in the submaxillary duct. They can be felt with bimanual palpation, i.e., the finger of one hand palpating the floor of the mouth and the fingers of the other hand beneath the jaw pressing up the floor of the mouth.

Physical examination will be negative in most cases of neuralgia, various headaches, and referred pain. In rare instances jaw pain may be the presenting symptom of myocardial ischemia or infarction.

Laboratory Tests

When pulpitis, pericoronitis, or periapical, alveolar, or periodontal abscesses are suggested on the basis of history and physical examination, radiographs are required to confirm the diagnosis. Periapical intraoral radiographs, orthopanographic films, and hematologic studies are indicated if mucosal lesions suggest a systemic condition. See Chapter 152, "Lesions of the Mouth."

References

Bell WE. Orofacial pains. 4th ed. Chicago: Year Book Medical Publishers, 1989.

Bell WE. Temporomandibular disorders. 3rd ed. Chicago: Year Book Medical Publishers, 1990.

Heyck H. Headache and facial pain. Chicago: Year Book Medical Publishers, 1981.

Lesions of the Mouth

152

Joseph M. Kelly, DDS

Katherine L. Kahn, MD

Definition

The lesions of the mouth discussed in this chapter are defined as localized changes in the mucosa of the lips, tongue, gingiva, and remaining oral cavity. The oral lesions are grouped on the basis of their gross clinical appearance—white lesions, red lesions, pigmented lesions, vesicles, or ulcerations (Table 152-1). Some lesions will present a combination of those clinical characteristics. Swellings and tumors are covered in Chapter 153, "Tumors and Swellings in the Mouth."

Etiology

White lesions result from changes in the mucosa that block out the normal pink color of the mucosa. The main difference between mucosa and skin is that mucosa lacks the secondary skin structures—hair follicles, sebaceous glands, and sweat glands in the corium. The corium below the epithelium of the mucosa is much thinner than the thick connective tissue of the dermis layer of the skin. Finally, the lack of pigmentation and a minimal or absent cornified layer of the oral mucosa allows the blood in the highly vascular underlying tissues to show through. Although severe anemia produces a generalized pale mucosa, white lesions are contrasted from the surrounding tissues because there are changes in the mucosa itself.

White lesions are due to increases in the thickness of the mucosa, particularly the keratin layer, necrosis and destruction of the mucosa, or the presence of foreign material over the mucosa. Blood clots in the oral cavity become gray in color over time as the saliva washes out the red blood cells, leaving the fibrin clot.

Increased keratin, or hyperkeratosis, due to chronic mechanical or chemical irritation produces white lesions as seen in nicotinic stomatitis, mucobuccal fold lesions in snuff users, and chronic cheek biting and buccal occlusal line lesions.

Necrosis of mucosa from thermal, chemical, or traumatic injury leaves a grayish white surface. A common chemical burn is found in the mucobuccal fold of patients with toothaches who have placed aspirin tablets next to the tooth to relieve the pain.

Fungal infections from *Candida albicans* produce white areas on the tongue and oral mucosa.

Red lesions result from increased vascularity under the mucosa generally due to inflammation. Loss of a portion of the epithelial layer or atrophy of the mucosa changes the mucosa from pink to red. Often red lesions are bordered or crossed by white areas, as in geographic tongue and lichen planus.

Pigmented lesions in the oral cavity may result from melanin deposits, ingestion of certain drugs or heavy metals, or traumatic tattoos, particularly amalgam filling material incorporated in the gingiva. Varicosities and hemangiomas produce discoloration beneath the mucosa. Pigment-producing fungi can cause discoloration on the surface of the mucosa, as in black hairy tongue. This latter condition is not uncommon after prolonged use of certain antibiotics.

Hormonal changes may cause increased pigmentation. Addison's disease causes marked melanin deposits in the mucosa of the mouth and lips. Peutz-Jeghers syndrome consists of oral melanosis and intestinal polyposis.

Hereditary factors account for oral pigmentation in a number of ethnic groups.

Vesicles are blister-like lesions that can arise within the epithelium (intraepithelial) or below the epithelium (subepithelial). Large vesicles are referred to as bullae. These lesions may be caused by viruses, allergic reactions, or other immunologic disorders.

Ulcerations refer to the total loss of overlying epithelium and sometimes may be found as a secondary lesion following the rupture of a vesicle, the primary lesion. Infections, trauma, and neoplasms all may cause ulcerations.

Vesicular lesions and ulcers of viral origin include primary herpetic gingivostomatitis, herpes labialis, herpes zoster, chickenpox, herpangina, measles, and hand, foot, and mouth disease.

Vesicular lesions and ulcers of immunologic, allergic, or unknown origin include recurrent aphthous ulcers, erythema multiforme, Behçet's syndrome, Stevens-Johnson syndrome, pemphigus vulgaris, benign mucous membrane pemphigus, allergic stomatitis, and Reiter's syndrome.

Ulcerations not usually associated with vesicles include acute necrotizing gingivitis (Vincent's infection), traumatic ul-

Table 152-1 Lesions of the Mouth

White lesions	Pigmented lesions	Ulcerative or vesicular lesions
Acute Onset	**Acute Onset**	**Infectious**
Trauma	Trauma (local hematoma)	Acute herpetic gingivostomatitis
Chemical (aspirin)	Coagulopathy (hematoma)	Recurrent herpes labialis
Thermal	Drug ingestion	Herpes zoster
Mechanical	Tranquilizer	Chickenpox (varicella)
Subacute, Chronic, Recurrent	Birth control pill	Measles (rubella)
Local candida infection (thrush)	Antimalarial	Infectious mononucleosis
Systemic candidiasis*	Leukemia*	Primary syphilis
Lichen planus	Idiopathic thrombocytopenic purpura*	Secondary syphilis
Nicotinic stomatitis	**Subacute, Chronic, Recurrent**	Gonorrhea*
Leukoplakia	Addison's disease*	Tuberculosis*
Squamous cell carcinoma	Peutz-Jeghers syndrome*	Histoplasmosis*
Systemic lupus erythematosus*	Heavy metal intoxication	Dermatologic
Sjögren's syndrome*	Bismuth	Erythema multiforme (Stevens-Johnson)*
Wegener's granulomatosis*	Mercury	Behçet's syndrome*
Fordyce's spots	Lead	Mucous membrane pemphigoid
	Osler-Weber-Rendu* (hereditary hemorrhagic telangiectasia)	Pemphigus vulgaris
	Black hairy tongue	**Neoplastic**
	Amalgam tattoo	Squamous cell carcinoma
	Varicosity	Acute leukemia*
	Angiomas	Lymphosarcoma*
	Hairy leukoplakia†	Non-Hodgkin's lymphoma
	Nevi	**Miscellaneous**
		Trauma
		Recurrent aphthous stomatitis

* Usually associated with systemic symptoms or signs.
† May precede the development of AIDS.

cers, erosive lichen planus, various bacterial lesions and stomatitis, infectious mononucleosis, leukemias, and neoplasms.

Dental fistulae ("gum boils") are due to constant drainage from a chronic periapical abscess. They appear as small, raised lesions on the gingiva adjacent to the root of an abscessed tooth. A drop of pus can often be expressed from the lesion. Normally, they are asymptomatic because no pressure builds up at the apex of the abscessed tooth.

Differential Diagnosis

The differential diagnosis of oral lesions requires a general knowledge of primary oral diseases and conditions, as well as an awareness of secondary oral manifestations of systemic diseases. A large percentage of systemic infections as well as metabolic, nutritional, and endocrine disorders will at some stage produce oral changes. The following represent only the more common conditions producing oral lesions.

Hyperkeratosis, leukoplakia, and carcinoma in situ can only be differentiated by histologic examination. Most present as painless lesions, usually in older men who smoke pipes or cigars. Snuff held in the mucobuccal fold of the mouth will also cause hyperkeratosis. Nicotinic stomatitis from pipe smoking eventually leaves the palate covered with hyperkeratosis and multiple red pinpoint openings of the palatal mucous glands, which are contrasted against the white background. Ulceration in the center of any of these lesions is highly suggestive of squamous cell carcinoma.

Lichen planus is found most often on the mucosa of the cheek. Here the lesion presents as a lattice-work arrangement of white lesions, or Wickham's striae. Cutaneous lesions occur on the flexor surfaces of the wrists, arms, and legs. The reported incidence varies widely from 30 to 70 percent. Erosive, atrophic, and ulcerative forms of the condition occur frequently on the tongue and are usually painful. The condition is slightly more prevalent in women and has periods of remission or exacerbation that may be related to psychogenic factors.

White sponge nevus (pachyderma oralis, congenital leukokeratosis, leukoedema exfoliativum mucosae oris) is a congenital disturbance of the oral mucosa. Several members of a family may have the condition. The buccal mucosa often appears parboiled.

Primary herpetic gingivostomatitis is the initial lesion of a young adult or more commonly a child with herpesvirus infection. Fever and lymphadenopathy precede the vesicular eruption, which involves the entire oral mucosa, lips, and marginal gingiva next to the teeth. Recurrent infection in later years may occur as herpes labialis (cold sores) or recurrent herpetic stomatitis.

Hand, foot, and mouth disease and herpangina are caused by coxsackie A viruses. The former occurs mostly in children. Small vesicles in the oral mucosa, palate, tongue, and pharynx quickly change to ulcers. Lesions around the parotid duct opening cause facial pain. Similar lesions occur on the palmar surfaces of the hands and the soles of the feet. Herpangina lesions are limited mostly to the soft palate and pharynx. Laboratory culture and identification of coxsackie A virus is more reliable than serology.

Chickenpox (varicella) usually begins with a maculopapular rash that starts on the trunk and spreads to the face and the scalp. On occasion, lesions may be found on the hard and soft palate before the skin rash appears. Clinical episodes of herpes zoster represent reactivation of a varicella virus. It may follow the distribution of the trigeminal nerve and involve the oral mucosa and the skin. The Ramsay-Hunt syndrome is herpes zoster infection with lesions of the soft palate, tongue, external auditory meatus, and sometimes the facial nerve, causing unilateral facial palsy.

Clinically, measles starts with the symptoms of a common cold but on the second or third day, Koplik's spots appear on the buccal mucosa opposite the molar teeth. The bluish white pinpoint spots are surrounded by a dark red border.

Infectious mononucleosis results from infection with the Epstein-Barr virus. It is common in young adults. The classic signs of fever, pharyngeal inflammation, and lymph node enlargement (particularly posterior cervical nodes) are often preceded by clusters of fine petechial hemorrhages at the junction of the hard and soft palate. Some patients with infectious mononucleosis present with fever, lymphadenopathy, and unilateral pericoronitis around an erupting wisdom tooth.

Recurrent aphthous ulcers (canker sores) are of unknown etiology and occur in three forms: minor aphthous ulcers, major aphthous ulcers, and herpetiform ulcers. Minor aphthous ulcers account for 80 percent of recurrent aphthous ulcers. These lesions, which are more common in women, are the typical canker sores that occur in the 10- to 40-year-old age group. They are rarely found in keratinized mucosa such as the palate and gingiva. The lesions heal in less than 14 days without scar. Major aphthous ulcers (Sutton's aphthae, periadenitis mucosa necrotica recurrens) usually present as a single, very large, painful canker sore–like lesion that may involve both keratinized and nonkeratinized mucosa. The lesions heal slowly over weeks, leaving a scar. Herpetiform ulcers occur as a large number (up to 100) of painful pinhead-sized lesions throughout the oral cavity. Serologic studies are negative for herpes simplex virus.

Erythema multiforme is a mucocutaneous disease of immunologic origin that is often seasonal and most commonly affects young adults. The oral lesions are present in more than 50 percent of cases and characteristically result in crusted, painful bleeding lesions of the lips. Stevens-Johnson syndrome involves the conjunctiva as well as the oral cavity and skin.

In pemphigus vulgaris, which appears to be an autoimmune disease, oral bullae precede the skin lesions in more than 50 percent of cases. Because the bullae rupture quickly, leaving a nonspecific ulcer, diagnosis is often delayed until skin lesions appear. Pemphigus vegetans is another variant that frequently has oral lesions as the initial symptom. Benign mucosal pemphigoid and bullous pemphigoid cause subepithelial bullae, which last longer than the suprabasilar bullae of pemphigus. Nearly all patients with benign mucosal pemphigoid have oral lesions; less than one-third of patients with bullous pemphigoid have oral lesions, however. Desquamative gingivitis is common in benign mucous membrane pemphigoid.

Contact allergy may occur in the mouth, with vesicles giving rise to mucosal ulcers. Allergic rhinitis may cause mouth breathing, which will result in anterior maxillary hyperplastic gingivitis.

Reiter's syndrome may produce painless oral lesions in addition to the classic triad of arthritis, conjunctivitis, and urethritis. These are small, raised, red lesions with a white circinate border resembling circinate balanitis. The incidence of oral lesions has been reported to be as high as 48 percent.

Candidiasis is a term applied to a variety of clinical conditions caused by the fungus *Candida albicans.* Predisposing factors for the fungus include the use of antibiotics, steroids, and chemotherapy and the presence of debilitating diseases or malnutrition. It is frequently present in patients with acquired immunodeficiency syndrome (AIDS). Clinically, the classic pearly or bluish-white patches are found on the palate, buccal mucosa, and tongue. These can be scraped off, leaving an erythematous base. Another form of candidiasis is the atrophic type, which presents as a more painful red and inflamed mucosa. This is frequently seen under dentures, involving the palate, and may be associated with angular cheilosis.

Thermal, chemical, and mechanical injuries to the oral mucosa can cause white lesions due to necrosis of the tissue. Aspirin burn is a common lesion seen in the vestibule of the mouth resulting from the patient's placing aspirin tablets next to a painful tooth. Denture sores appear as grayish ulcerations at the peripheral border of the denture.

Traumatic tattoos, particularly from amalgam filling materials, appear as bluish lesions on the gingiva near teeth with amalgam fillings or where teeth have been extracted.

Hemangiomas and varices appear as bluish lesions or swollen veins on the floor of the mouth, the ventral surface of the tongue, or the labial mucosa. Lingual varices are common in the elderly. Hairy tongue is due to overgrowth of filiform papillae in the posterior dorsum of the tongue. The color can vary from creamy white to brownish black, depending on the type of chromogenic organism present. It occurs often with prolonged antibiotic therapy.

Diagnostic Approach

The first diagnostic objective is to determine whether the lesion(s) is a localized oral condition(s) or whether it represents a systemic problem with oral manifestations. The second objective is to determine whether the lesion is acute, chronic, or recurrent.

Systemic symptoms with multiple bilateral lesions suggest that the oral lesions are the manifestation of a systemic condition. If the patient gives a history of malaise, fever, sore throat, gastrointestinal symptoms, swollen glands, or other mucocutaneous lesions, the oral lesions should be examined and should provide a clue to the probable diagnosis. The physical examination then can concentrate on detecting those findings suggested in the differential diagnosis. Oral lesions are found in herpetic gingivostomatitis, herpangina, measles, chickenpox, infectious mononucleosis, hand, foot, and mouth disease, erythema multiforme, and Reiter's syndrome. Candidiasis is often present in young patients with AIDS and elderly debilitated patients with malignancies or diabetes. The appropriate lab tests should be ordered based on the physical findings. Localized oral lesions without systemic symptoms may be new or recurrent painful lesions such as aphthous ulcers or denture sores. Chronic painful lesions may include lichen planus or neoplastic growths. Careful history and oral examination provide the diagnosis in most cases. In the case of potential neoplasms, a biopsy will be necessary.

Fordyce's granules are ectopic sebaceous glands found bilaterally in the buccal mucosa of a large percentage of adults. They appear as numerous small, light yellow spots and are asymptomatic.

References

Greenspan D, Greenspan JS. Oral mucosal manifestations of AIDS. Dermatol Clin 1987; 5:733.

Greenspan D, et al. Relation of oral hairy leukoplakia to infection with the human immunodeficiency virus and the risk of developing AIDS. J Infect Dis 1987; 155:475.

Haverkos HW, Drotman DP. Prevalence of Kaposi's sarcoma among patients with AIDS. N Engl J Med 1985; 313:1518.

Jones JH, Mason DK. Oral manifestations of systemic disease. 2nd ed. Philadelphia: WB Saunders, 1990.

Klein RS, et al. Oral candidiasis in high-risk patients as the initial manifestation of the acquired immunodeficiency syndrome. N Engl J Med 1984; 311:354.

Newman MG, Nisengard R. Oral microbiology and immunology Philadelphia: WB Saunders, 1988.

Pindborg JJ. Atlas of diseases of the oral mucosa. 4th ed. Philadelphia: WB Saunders, 1986.

Quinnan GV, et al. Herpes virus infections in the aquired immunodeficiency syndrome. JAMA 1984; 252:72.

Robertson PB, Greenspan JS. Oral manifestations of AIDS. Proceedings of Symposium, January 18–20, 1988, San Diego. Littleton, MA: PSG, 1989.

Tumors and Swellings in the Mouth

Katherine L. Kahn, MD

Joseph Kelly, DDS

153

Definition

Tumors and swellings in the mouth include a clinical spectrum ranging from infections and trauma to benign and malignant neoplasms. The tumors and swellings may arise from within the maxillary or mandibular bone, from soft tissue over these bones, or from the soft tissues of the tongue, cheeks, and lips.

Etiology

The majority of swellings in the mouth are due to inflammatory or infectious processes. Acute and chronic trauma also account for many swellings. Benign growths and cysts are relatively common; malignant tumors are far less frequent, except in certain high-risk groups. Swellings that arise in the maxillary or mandibular bone are most often due to dental infection or cysts of dental origin. Swellings arising in the gingiva around the teeth are usually due to periodontal disease. Elsewhere in the mouth, benign tumors arise from the mucosal epithelium or from the mucous and salivary glands. Chronic intraoral trauma such as denture irritation or cheek biting causes swelling and mucosal ulcerations. Young children given local anesthesia for dental treatment may chew the numb lip or cheek, causing significant tissue injury.

A dental alveolar abscess, which develops from a tooth with a necrotic pulp, is the most common acute inflammatory swelling in the mouth. It is an infection of mixed organisms at the apex of the tooth root that spreads through the nearby bone cortex, causing an inflamed swelling of the overlying periosteum and soft tissue. The extent and severity of the swelling depend upon the virulence of the organism and upon host resistance. Some periapical abscesses break through the bone cortex and the overlying gingiva, resulting in a draining dentoalveolar fistula. These "gum boils" usually persist and periodically drain a few drops of purulent material. Otherwise, they tend to be relatively asymptomatic.

Dental infection occasionally causes osteomyelitis in the normal healthy patient. If the patient is immunocompromised or has had radiation therapy to the head and neck, osteomyelitis or radio-osteonecrosis is common. Chronic swelling of the mandible with multiple cutaneous fistulae suggests actinomycosis, a less common infection of the jaw.

Swellings arising within the maxilla and mandible are usually caused by cysts or tumors. Generally, these are of odontogenic origin. A nonvital tooth does not always produce an active infection or abscess. The inflammation may stimulate odontogenic epithelial remnants to produce a periapical cyst. Children may develop a bluish swelling over the site of an erupting tooth, an eruption cyst. This arises from the follicle around the developing crown. In older patients with unerupted and impacted teeth, the follicle may give rise to relatively large odontogenic cysts. The developing dental tissue within the bone may give rise to benign odontomas. These encapsulated masses contain rudimentary teeth or tooth-like structures. Ameloblastoma is a relatively rare odontogenic tumor that is locally invasive; over time, it can become very large and destroy the mandible.

Cysts within the mandible and maxilla usually fill with fluid. They cause expansion of the bone cortex and eventually may perforate the cortex. The overlying mucosa then becomes bluish in color. The fluid nature of the cyst can often be noted on palpation. Cysts may occur at developmental suture sites, e.g., globulomaxillary and incisive canal cysts in the maxilla.

Swellings around the gingiva are usually secondary to periodontal infection. Food debris causes plaque formation between the teeth and beneath the gingiva. The inflammatory process results in bone resorption around the roots of the teeth and the formation of pockets between the gingiva and the root. Localized swellings and periodontal abscesses can develop as sequelae. Gingival inflammation leads to hyperemic changes and gingival hyperplasia. Systemic problems can further affect the gingiva. During pregnancy, an inflammatory granuloma can occur on the gingiva, known as a "pregnancy tumor." Epileptic patients using hydantoin have an exaggerated degree of gingival hyperplasia that can cover the teeth. Hyperemic, inflamed gingiva is common in uncontrolled diabetes, and severe gingival changes may occur in leukemia. Bone loss from periodontal disease eventually loosens the teeth, causing repeated periodontal abscesses and, in some cases, exfoliation of the teeth. Hyperparathyroidism loosens the teeth and gives rise to giant cell tumors within the bone. These "brown tumors" can extrude through the tooth sockets. Longstanding external bone overgrowth (exostosis) is common in the mandible and maxilla. Bilateral bone protuberances on the lingual side of the lower jaw are called mandibular tori. These hereditary growths occur in 7 percent of the white population. They often have a cauliflower shape and are covered with normal mucosa. Palatal tori are similar overgrowths found in the midline of the palate. Systemic conditions may cause bone swelling or enlargement, as in Paget's disease of bone, fibrous dysplasia, acromegaly, and maxillary enlargement in children with Mediterranean anemia.

Malignant tumors in the mandibular and maxillary bones are rare. The malignancies that do occur in the mandible include osteosarcoma, chondrosarcoma, and fibrosarcoma, and Burkitt's tumor, which usually involves the mandible. Malignant tumors in the maxilla tend more often to develop from the sinus epithelium or the minor salivary glands in the palate. Metastatic spread to the mandible can occur, e.g., from breast or prostate.

Swellings and tumors arising in the soft tissue of the lips, tongue, cheek, and floor of the mouth are not usually dental in origin. These arise from either the mucosal epithelium or the mucous and salivary glands.

Sudden swellings in the floor of the mouth can be due to the lingual extension of a dental infection from a lower molar tooth or extension of a pericoronal infection around an erupting wisdom tooth. The submaxillary gland may become blocked with a stone (sialolith) in the duct, causing swelling in the floor of the mouth and swelling in the gland below the mandible. The mucous and sublingual salivary glands can become blocked and form a large bluish soft swelling called a ranula. Blockage of the mucous glands in the lips causes a similar type of swelling known as a mucocele. Both of these cysts can be ruptured, releasing a clear, thick mucus. Hypertrophy of sublingual gland tissue may also give rise to swelling in the floor of the mouth. Lipomas and dermoid cysts can cause swelling in the floor of the mouth. The roof of the mouth may be the site of a swelling due to dental infection. Otherwise, benign and malignant neoplasms of the minor salivary glands must be considered.

Papillomas and fibromas of the oral mucosa of the cheeks, lips, and tongue are very common. Edentulous patients tend to develop overgrowth of fibrous tissue, epulis fissuratum, around the alveolar ridges as a result of ill-fitting dentures. These may appear as folds of inflamed fibrous tissue in the vestibule of the mouth along the borders of the ill-fitting denture. Enlargement of the tuberosities at the posterior end of the edentulous maxillary ridge is common under dentures.

The tongue can be the site of a lymphangioma, which has a localized, swollen, pebbled appearance. Hemangiomas also occur in the tongue; they are purple in color and have the same pebbled appearance as a lymphangioma. Enlargement of the tongue occurs in amyloidosis, hypothyroidism, and Down syndrome. Small purple hemangiomas are common on the lip, and varicosities occur in the floor of the mouth and under the tongue in older patients. Lymphadenitis is common in the submandibular region. Malignant tumors arising in soft tissue of the oral cavity are usually epidermoid (squamous cell) carcinoma and are found in patients with a history of pipe or cigar smoking and tobacco or snuff use. The major and minor salivary glands are also the sites of malignant tumors.

Diagnostic Approach

The history in a patient with a mouth swelling or tumor should focus on the duration of the swelling, the presence of associated local or systemic symptoms, and the relevant past medical history. Sudden onset of swelling usually indicates inflammatory, traumatic, or infectious conditions or soft-tissue cysts. Recurrent swellings usually have the same list of differential diagnoses as sudden-onset swellings. Rarely are recurrent swellings due to neoplasms. Long-term swellings indicate chronic infection, inflammation, cysts (particularly in bone), or neoplasms. Progressive enlargement of a chronic swelling suggests tumor.

Pain and tenderness overlying a swelling suggest an inflammatory or infectious process. A history of a toothache or gum problems suggests a dental origin for the swelling. Nontender swellings occur with cysts and benign and malignant neoplasms. Increased swelling over a salivary gland when eating is characteristic of salivary duct blockage. Fever, joint pain, fatigue, and bruising are among the symptoms suggesting a systemic illness. Many systemic diseases have oral manifestations. Swollen, bleeding gums are common in leukemia. Generalized periodontal disease is found in uncontrolled diabetes. Swelling of the jaw from central giant cell tumors occurs in hyperparathyroidism. Swollen salivary glands occur in systemic lupus erythematosus and Sjögren's syndrome, whereas swollen tongue can result from amyloidosis. Intraoral lesions of Kaposi's sarcoma have been found in patients with acquired immunodeficiency syndrome (AIDS).

The past medical history may provide important clues to the etiology of oral swellings. A previous history of malignancy increases the possibility of metastatic lesions to the jaw. Radiotherapy in the head and neck can cause osteoradionecrosis. Chemotherapy with lowered host resistance increases the chance of oral infection. Hydantoin therapy for seizures usually causes gingival hyperplasia. The prolonged use of a pipe, cigar, or snuff increases the risk for epidermoid (squamous cell) carcinoma. Alcoholism further increases the risk of malignancy.

Physical Examination

The physical examination of a swelling or tumor in the mouth should determine the location of the swelling or tumor, and the size, character, and appearance of the lesion. Localization of the swelling narrows the diagnostic possibilities.

Swelling in the tongue, lips, or cheeks, with no involvement of tissue over the mandible or maxilla, usually means nondental origin. Palpation with a gloved finger over the bone adjacent to the teeth will detect swelling that originates below the periosteum. Most swellings from dental infection elevate the tissue in this area. Sudden painless swellings on the floor of the mouth are usually the result of salivary gland blockage or ranula. Abscessed teeth and pericoronitis from erupting wisdom teeth cause swelling in the floor of the mouth and are usually accompanied by pain on limited opening of the mouth. Long-term swellings on the floor of the mouth are likely to be neoplastic. Swelling characterized by a tender, red, inflamed mucosa suggests infection and inflammation. An indurated, ulcerated lesion with a whitish or reddish border is typical of epidermoid carcinoma. A ranula appears as a bluish soft swelling in the floor of the mouth. A clear mucocele or a bluish hemangioma is common in the lip, tongue, or palate. Nontender soft or firm growths with normal overlying mucosa usually are papillomas or fibromas. Freely movable, tender, firm masses in the submandibular area are usually due to lymphadenitis or submaxillary sialadenitis. Bimanual palpation of the floor of the mouth with one finger inside and the other hand outside is helpful. The submaxillary gland can be best palpated in this way. The flow of saliva can be observed by milking the duct with the finger. Cloudy saliva indicates infection. Hard, asymptomatic protuberances over bone with overlying normal mucosa may be exostosis or bony tumors.

Dental abscesses come from within the bone and must elevate the periosteum to appear externally. Palpation intraorally can determine the intrabony origin of a swelling. Swellings below the mandible may be fixed to the jaw or bone or freely movable. A freely movable mass below the jaw may be a lymph node, soft-tissue cyst, submaxillary gland, or soft-tissue tumor. The swelling is fixed to the inferior border of the mandible; it may originate within the bone or be a soft-tissue mass adherent to the jaw. A careful examination for neck and supraclavicular nodes should be done in all patients as part of the physical examination. Where indicated, evaluations of the pharynx and vocal cords may be warranted.

Laboratory Tests

Radiographs of the teeth are warranted in any patient with a dental infection. Any patient with swelling presumed to arise from bone should have radiographs of the jaw (preferably orthopanographic).

References

Schluger S, et al, eds. Periodontal diseases. Philadelphia: Lea & Febiger, 1989.

Williams RC. Medical progress: Periodontal disease. N Engl J Med 1990; 322:373.

Hearing Loss

James P. Hughes, MD

Definition

Partial or complete loss of hearing is one of the most common complaints for which patients present to the physician's office. It may be described as a sensation of fullness, blockage, or pressure. A hearing loss of more than 25 decibels at any of the speech frequencies (500, 1,000, or 2,000 Hz) is considered abnormal, but a loss of lesser degree may also indicate significant underlying pathology, particularly in children. Hearing losses are traditionally classified as (1) conductive, involving the outer or middle ear up to the oval window; (2) sensorineural, indicating a lesion to the organ of Corti or the central pathways; and (3) combined (Fig. 154-1).

Diagnostic Approach

History

An attempt should be made to determine the onset, progression, and severity of the hearing loss. Associated factors should be identified if possible. The loss may result from acoustic or physical trauma, exposure to ototoxic drugs, change in atmospheric pressure, or excessive physical activity. A previous history of similar loss or a family history of deafness is worthy of note.

Associated otic symptoms such as pain, drainage, vertigo, or tinnitus should be recorded. Inquiry should be made regarding a recent upper respiratory tract infection or viral syndrome. Because certain conditions are related to specific types of hearing loss (pregnancy and otosclerosis, nasopharyngeal carcinoma and serous otitis media), a brief review of systems is indicated. The length and complexity of the history should be guided by the nature of the complaint, the patient's age, and other clinical factors such as those noted previously. A patient who has had recurrent cerumen impactions may simply require cleaning of the external auditory canal; no further evaluation will be necessary if the hearing is restored to its previous level. Other patients will require extensive work-up and diagnostic testing (e.g., in the case of idiopathic sudden sensorineural hearing loss).

Physical Examination

A careful inspection of the postauricular area for scars or tenderness, followed by examination of the pinna, should be done first. The otoscope may be inserted after the auricle has been pulled laterally to line up the cartilaginous and bony auditory canals. Ordinarily, most or all of the tympanic membrane can be visualized (Fig. 154-2). Although the "light reflex" (the light reflection from the anterior inferior quadrant of the tympanic membrane) is a common finding, its absence is of limited diagnostic value. The character of the tympanic membrane, its thickness, and whether there is fluid present behind the drum are of far greater significance. A lesion of the tympanic membrane, such as a perforation, may affect the transmission of sound to the inner ear, resulting in a conductive hearing loss. If the drum is dehiscent, one can appreciate the character of the mucous membrane of the middle ear cleft and, at times, ossicular discontinuity can be identified.

Although an audiogram is required for adequate evaluation of most types of hearing loss, two common screening tests are the Weber and Rinné tests, which are illustrated in Figure 154-3. For the Weber test, a tuning fork of the proper frequency (at least 256 Hz) is held on the midline of the forehead or on the central incisor teeth. Sound will not lateralize to either ear in normal patients or patients with equal sensorineural loss (Fig. 154-3A). In patients with unilateral or bilateral but asymmetric hearing loss, however, the sound will lateralize (appear louder in one ear). With a conductive hearing loss, the tuning fork is heard better in the ear with the hearing deficit. In a sensorineural loss, the tuning fork sound is heard louder in the ear opposite the hearing deficit. Some patients will have deafness with both sensorineural and conductive components, making interpretation of the test results difficult. Prior ear disease or surgery should also be taken into consideration.

To distinguish whether the abnormal (lateralized) Weber test is a result of a conductive or sensorineural deficit, the Rinné test is helpful. In the Rinné test, the tuning fork is used to compare the sensitivity over the mastoid tip with that obtained by holding the tuning fork opposite the external auditory canal (Fig. 154-3B). The tines of the fork should be held vertically and with the nearest tine approximately 1 cm from the external auditory meatus. The tuning fork is normally heard louder by air conduction than by bone conduction. This is called a "positive" Rinné and can be found in patients with normal hearing and those with sensorineural hearing loss. In the case in which bone conduction is greater than or equal to air, a conductive loss in excess of 20 to 25 dB is likely present. Because sound is transmitted through the skull with minimal loss of acoustic energy, it is important to mask the nontested ear. This is usually done by rubbing the ear or, preferably, with a Barany noise box. Besides their utility as screening tests, the Weber and Rinné tests are valuable for checking the validity of the audiogram.

Audiologic Evaluation

Following the physical examination, any patient who is thought to have a hearing loss should be referred for audiologic evaluation to confirm the loss and determine its degree. Occasionally, more than a routine audiogram will be required. It may be necessary to perform tympanometry with or without stapedial reflex testing or other diagnostic tests, particularly if a retrocochlear lesion is suspected. This determination is usually made by the otologist after review of the audiogram.

Occasionally, objective audiologic testing will be required. This is suitable for patients who are either unable or unwilling to cooperate. One such test is the brain-stem evoked response audiogram. Sound is used to stimulate the cochlea, and the electronic response is recorded from the scalp. After background electrical activity has been averaged out by computer, a central response can be identified. This technique can be used to get an accurate assessment of hearing loss in infants, particularly those who are considered at high risk for hearing loss. It is also useful in determining the likelihood of retrocochlear dis-

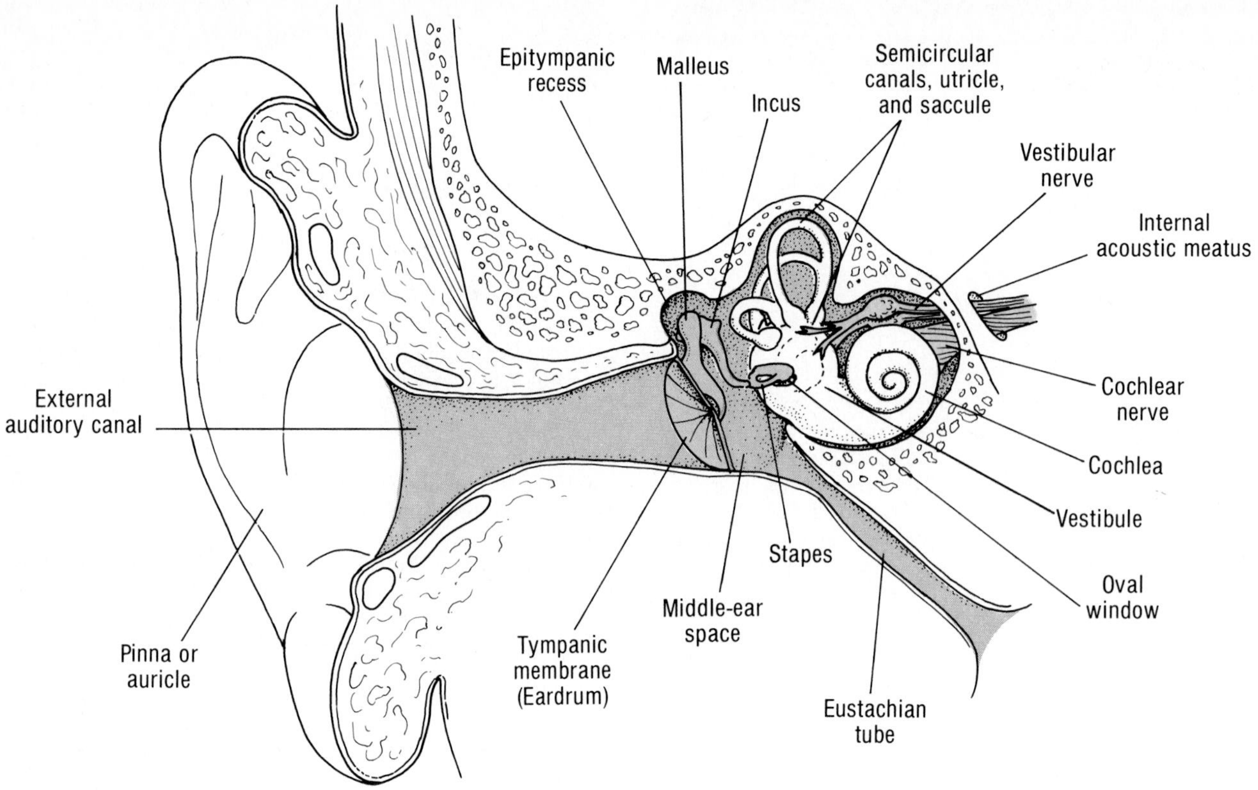

Figure 154-1 Anatomy of the ear.

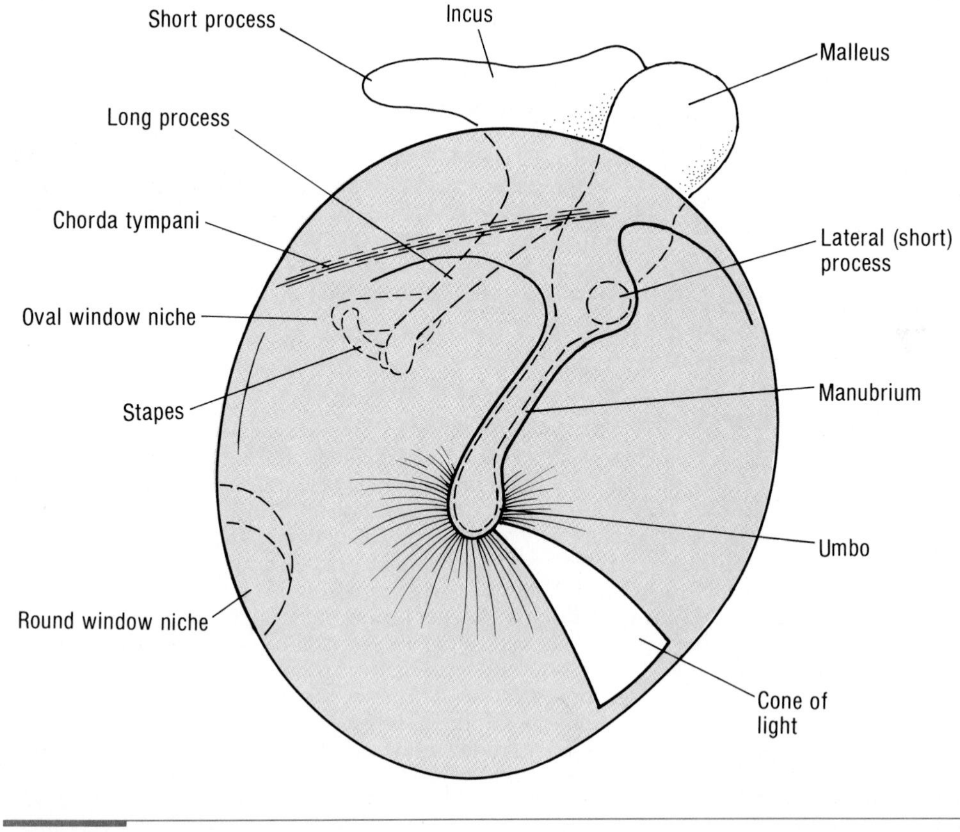

Figure 154-2 The tympanic membrane.

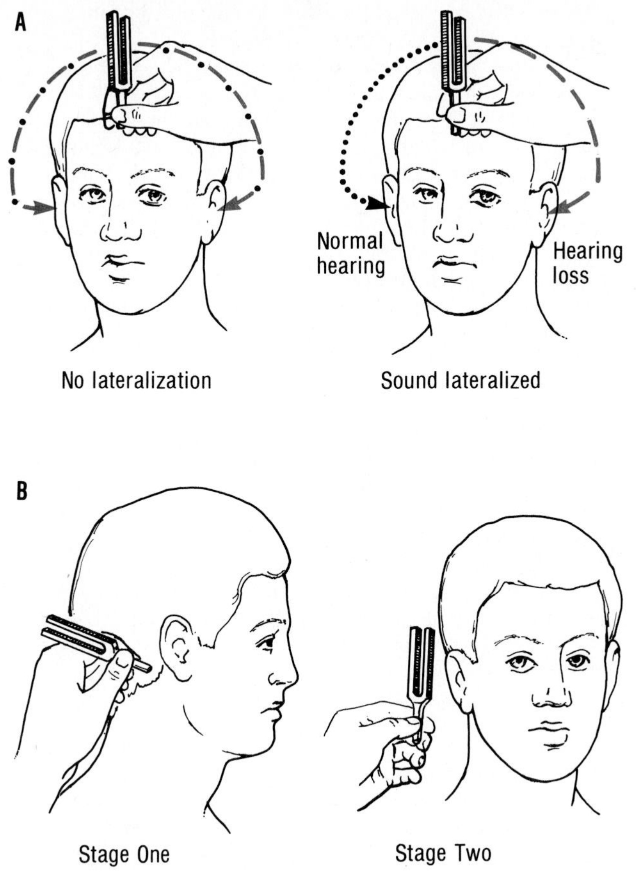

Figure 154-3 Screening tests for hearing loss. (**A**) The Weber test. *Left,* Sound does not lateralize to either ear in persons with normal hearing or those with bilateral, symmetric conductive or sensorineural hearing loss. *Right,* The tuning fork is referred to the side of hearing loss in conductive disease (*dashed arrow*) or to the side opposite the hearing loss in sensorineural disease (*dotted arrow*). (**B**) The Rinné test. If air conduction is greater than bone conduction, significant conductive loss can be ruled out; the problem is generally sensorineural disease. If bone conduction is greater than air conduction, conductive disease on the side of the hearing loss is suggested.

ease, such as cerebellopontine angle tumors or other posterior fossa lesions.

Radiologic Evaluation

Radiographs are sometimes indicated to identify lesions of the middle-ear space and mastoid and also to evaluate congenital or acquired abnormalities of the inner ear and internal auditory canal. Routine mastoid views have largely been replaced by computed tomography or magnetic resonance imaging; nonetheless, they are still useful for rapid screening to rule out suppurative mastoid disease or lytic lesions. Because of the number of studies available and the rapid development in x-ray technology, the choice of a specific test should be made after consultation with the radiologist or the otologic consultant.

Vestibular Function

An electronystagmogram (ENG) may be used to establish the integrity of vestibular function and to evaluate the vestibular portion of the eighth cranial nerve.

Differential Diagnosis

Table 154-1 lists common causes of hearing loss, which may be classified as sensorineural or conductive.

Sensorineural Hearing Loss

Sensorineural hearing loss is caused by lesions of the cochlea, auditory nerve, central pathways, or auditory cortex.

A congenital sensorineural hearing loss is one that has existed from the time of birth. It may or may not be hereditary. Many genetic types of deafness have been defined and may occur alone or in combination with other abnormalities. Some of the more common types of congenital deafness that may be seen in adults are listed in Table 154-2. Nongenetic types of congenital hearing loss may be associated with fetal ototoxins (Thalidomide), maternal viral infections (rubella, cytomegalovirus, and mumps), prematurity, Rh incompatibility, and birth trauma.

Traumatic hearing loss may be classified as acoustic, physical, or barotrauma. Acoustic trauma is a common cause of hearing loss. Recent interest by government and regulatory agencies in the problem of occupational noise exposure has led to extensive monitoring of the degree of acoustic trauma to which workers are exposed. Although efforts have recently been made to prevent injury from acoustic trauma by use of hearing protection such as ear muffs and ear plugs, many middle-aged patients and most older workers have not had the benefit of this protection. Significant high-tone sensorineural hearing losses are commonly seen in patients exposed to a lifetime of excessive noise. Along with the history of exposure to industrial noise, care should be taken to inquire about other types of noise exposure, such as gunfire, chainsaws, power tools, loud music, firecrackers, and the like. Even small portable radios used with headphones have enough acoustic energy to cause significant hearing impairment.

Table 154-1 Common Causes of Hearing Loss

Sensorineural	Conductive
Congenital	External auditory canal
Genetic	Atresias
Nongenetic	Cerumen impaction
Traumatic	Exostosis
Acoustic trauma (noise-induced)	Otitis externa
Physical trauma (concussion)	Foreign bodies
Barotrauma	Cholesteatoma
Toxic	Tumors
Presbycusis	Middle ear
Idiopathic	Tympanic membrane
Meniere's disease	Atrophy
Sudden sensorineural hearing loss	Sclerosis
Autoimmune disease	Myringitis
Cerebellopontine angle tumors	Perforation
Acoustic neuroma	Effusions
Meningiomas	Serous
Primary cholesteatoma	Purulent
Infections	Hemorrhagic
Viral	Ossicular problems
Mumps	Congenital
Measles	Traumatic erosions
Varicella	Otosclerosis
Adenovirus	Tuberculosis
Cytomegalovirus	Cholesteatoma
Bacterial	Tumors
Spirochetal syphilis	Benign (glomus tympanicum)
Meningitis	
Vascular	Malignant (carcinoma)

Table 154-2 Common Types of Congenital Deafness in Adults

Condition	Characteristics
Aplasias	
Michel's deformity	Demonstrates a total lack of development of the inner ear; very rare; results in total hearing loss
Mondini's dysplasia	Demonstrates flattening of the cochlea with only 1½ turns; may retain some hearing potential
Schiebe aplasia	Deformity primarily involves the membranous rather than the bony labyrinth
Alexander aplasia	Characterized by the lack of development of the cochlea duct and generally demonstrates some residual hearing
Degenerative	
Waardenburg's syndrome	Results from a dominant gene and is characterized by unilateral or bilateral hearing loss, white forelock, hypertelorism, and heterochromia iridium
Alport's syndrome	A dominantly transmitted syndrome that may begin in early adolescence and is characterized by bilateral symmetric hearing loss associated with progressive glomerulonephritis
Pendred's syndrome	Involves as many as 10% of the cases of recessive hereditary deafness and is associated with a goiter and defective iodine metabolism
Jervell and Lange-Nielsen syndrome	Characterized by congenital bilateral severe deafness in association with prolongation of the Q-T interval and occasionally sudden death
Usher's syndrome	Moderate to severe sensorineural hearing loss associated with progressive retinitis pigmentosa

Physical trauma involving direct insult to the skull and temporal bone may result in significant sensorineural hearing loss. The extent of the hearing loss is highly variable and depends upon the degree of force and its point of impact. The greatest loss occurs at the frequency of 4 kHz. Losses are most frequently sensorineural, but they may be conductive or combined if injury to the external ear canal, tympanic membrane, or ossicular chain has occurred. Temporal bone fractures are classified as (1) longitudinal, paralleling the long axis of the petrous temporal bone, or (2) transverse, in which the fracture line is perpendicular to the long axis. The majority of longitudinal fractures are caused by lateral blows to the skull. Although the facial nerve is injured in approximately 20 percent of longitudinal fractures, the inner ear is frequently spared. Transverse fractures are more likely to violate the internal auditory canal or bony labyrinth, resulting in permanent sensorineural loss. Occasionally, hearing loss may follow a surgical procedure of the ear.

Barotrauma, including rupture of the membranes of the inner ear secondary to pressure change, is a well-documented cause of sudden hearing loss that may be sensorineural, conductive, or combined. The history should include any exposure to a major change in pressure. This is most commonly associated with significant physical exertion or activities such as scuba diving. Clinically, the patient may develop hearing loss or vertigo. Patients who have previously undergone inner ear surgery, such as stapedectomy, are at increased risk.

Many pharmacologic agents have ototoxic side effects. The drugs most frequently implicated are the aminoglycosides such as streptomycin, gentamicin, tobramycin, and amikacin. Other drugs and chemicals that cause hearing loss include diuretics, such as ethacrynic acid and furosemide, and many of the heavy metals, including cisplatin, that are used in chemotherapy. Salicylates, which are well-known causes of tinnitus, occasionally will also cause a sensorineural loss. In the case of the aminoglycosides, the ototoxic effect may occur after only a few doses or may even present as a delayed hearing loss after the medication has been discontinued. Sensorineural loss has also been observed with chemotherapeutic agents.

Presbycusis

Presbycusis, or hearing loss associated with aging, is the most commonly diagnosed hearing loss in the older age group. The exact etiology is unclear and may be related to the chronic acoustic trauma to which people are exposed during their lifetimes. Schuknecht identified four varieties of presbycusis based on morphologic changes noted in the cochlea on histologic examination of decalcified temporal bones. Although the majority of elderly individuals with sensorineural loss suffer from presbycusis, other possible diagnoses should be excluded.

Idiopathic

Meniere's disease or syndrome refers to hearing loss associated with vertigo. This syndrome is characterized by severe episodic vertigo associated with a roaring tinnitus and sensorineural hearing loss. The syndrome may involve either the labyrinthine or cochlear portions of the inner ear and manifests as either fluctuating dizziness or fluctuating hearing loss. In such cases, the unaffected portion of the inner ear frequently becomes involved at a later date.

Sudden sensorineural hearing loss is an abrupt loss of hearing that occurs in less than 24 hours. Many etiologies have been postulated, e.g., viral infection, vascular accident secondary to vasospasm, thrombosis, or a hypercoagulation state. Sudden sensorineural hearing loss is a medical emergency, and the patient should be referred to an ear, nose, and throat specialist as soon as possible.

Many of the diseases that are thought to be autoimmune in nature (systemic lupus erythematosus, scleroderma, arteritis, and others) may include hearing loss in their symptom complex.

Tumors involving the cerebellopontine angle or retrocochlear area may produce sensorineural hearing loss. The most frequent lesions of this area are acoustic neuromas (a schwannoma, usually of the superior vestibular nerve), meningiomas of the base of the skull, and primary cholesteatomas. These lesions should always be considered in a differential diagnosis of hearing loss, particularly if the speech discrimination is poor or if other neurologic signs or symptoms accompany the hearing loss.

Like most organ systems, the auditory complex is vulnerable to assault from a multitude of infective organisms. In most cases, the clinical picture will suggest the source or nature of the infection. In some cases, however, the primary infection may be subclinical (viral) or the otic manifestations may be delayed (tertiary syphilis, late congenital syphilis).

Late congenital syphilis may present with severe bilateral asymmetric hearing loss in otherwise healthy adults. This should be considered in any unexplained sensorineural hearing loss. One classic physical finding is Hennebert's sign, in which dizziness and nystagmus are provoked by negative pressure on pneumatic otoscopy. The diagnosis is usually confirmed by a positive fluorescent treponemal antibody absorption test. Attention should be given to the possibility of other central nervous system involvement. This is one of the few sensorineural hearing losses that may respond to medical therapy.

Meningitis is a frequent cause of sensorineural deafness in children, and it may occur in adults. Viral meningitis is much less likely to provoke a significant hearing loss than bacterial meningitis.

Vascular sources of deafness have been postulated for many years. Owing to its lack of collateral circulation, the inner ear is particularly vulnerable to any interruption in blood supply. Ischemia due to capillary sludging, vascular spasm, or even frank hemorrhage is a likely etiology for hearing loss, particularly in patients with a history of hypertension or previous vascular disease.

Conductive Hearing Loss

Conductive hearing losses include those lesions that effect blockage of the sound transmission from the auricle to the vestibule of the inner ear.

Ear canal lesions are common causes of significant hearing loss. Atresias of the auricle or the external auditory canal are easily diagnosed on physical examination. Any obstructing lesion of the external auditory canals such as cerumen, exostosis, foreign body, canal cholesteatoma, or tumor can generally be identified without difficulty. Occasionally, inflammatory disease of the external auditory canal, such as an external otitis, may affect the sound transmission.

Middle ear pathology, including any change in the position or character of the tympanic membrane, may result in hearing loss. The tympanic membrane may be atrophic, sclerotic, or perforated. A perforation of the eardrum allows sound to reach the middle ear and round window membrane, creating a dampening effect on the excursion of the basilar membrane. This dampening effect, along with the impaired vibration of the tympanic membrane, will cause a hearing loss of varying degree, depending on the size and location of the perforation. Effusions of the middle ear will also hamper the sound transmission by dampening the vibration of the tympanic membrane and ossicular chain. The effusion may be serous, purulent, or hemorrhagic. If the middle ear space is partially pneumatized, the dampening effect will be less severe. Lesions that affect the ossicles will also depress hearing. Traumatic injury to the delicate middle ear ossicles is a relatively frequent sequela of head trauma. Occasionally, erosion of the ossicles will occur with cholesteatomas and chronic otitis media. One of the more common diseases affecting the ossicles is otosclerosis, a disease of the bony labyrinth. Foci of new bone growth can be demonstrated histologically in the cochlea and at the anterior edge of the oval window. This new bone growth causes ankylosis of the stapes, with a resultant conductive hearing loss. This hereditary disease generally presents in middle age, is commonly bilateral, and occurs approximately twice as frequently in women. Otosclerosis is frequently exacerbated at the time of pregnancy.

Tuberculosis is an uncommon disease today, and middle ear involvement is a rarity. It does occur in children and is thought to be derived from contamination of the eustachian tube. The classic physical finding is multiple perforations of the tympanic membrane. The tuberculosis lesion creates a profound deafness with relatively little pain.

The cholesteatoma is a skin-lined cyst filled with epithelial and keratin debris. Although occasionally cases of primary cholesteatomas of the temporal bone are described, the cholesteatoma is usually derived from a retraction pouch or perforation of the tympanic membrane, generally as a sequela of chronic eustachian tube dysfunction. The retraction pouch usually extends from the pars flaccida or the posterosuperior portion of the tympanic membrane. The cyst may initially be small, but it will gradually increase in size, causing bone destruction by pressure necrosis and enzymatic lysis of bone. Cholesteatomas may erode the bony labyrinth, resulting in sensorineural deficit. The physical findings suggesting a cholesteatoma may be subtle; therefore, crusts covering the tympanic membrane should be removed in order to evaluate the drum surface adequately.

Lipodystrophies are extremely rare causes of hearing loss. Occasionally, the temporal bone may be involved with Letterer-Siwe disease, Hand-Schuller-Christian disease, or histiocytosis X. These lesions must be confirmed by a biopsy.

Although benign tumors of the ear are relatively rare, one unusual type, the glomus tumor, is worthy of note. Glomus tumors are derived from the glomus bodies on the tympanic branch of the glossopharyngeal nerve (glomus tympanicum) and from the jugular bulb (glomus jugulare). They are referred to as chemodectomas, or nonchromaffin paragangliomas, and, although benign, may create significant damage by local extension. They frequently are manifested by hearing loss or pulsatile tinnitus. Any mass lesion behind the tympanic membrane requires otologic referral.

Malignant tumors, other than epidermoid carcinomas of the auricle and external canal, are quite rare. Frequently the exact site of origin of the tumor of the ear cannot be determined because of the extent of spread by the time the diagnosis is made. The prognosis is largely determined by the degree of tumor involvement and any evidence of nodal or distant spread.

Carcinoma metastatic to the temporal bone, although also relatively rare, most frequently may be derived from primary renal cell carcinomas, bronchogenic carcinomas, and adenocarcinomas. Occasionally, meningiomas or intracranial neoplasms will invade the temporal bone. Less frequently, a primary malignancy of the nasopharynx may involve the temporal bone directly or via the eustachian tube.

References

Adams GL, Boies LR Jr, Hilger PA. Fundamentals of otolaryngology. 6th ed. Philadelphia: WB Saunders, 1989.

DeWeese DD, et al. Textbook of otolaryngology. 7th ed. St. Louis: CV Mosby, 1987.

Glasscock M III. Shambaugh's surgery of the ear. 4th ed. Philadelphia: WB Saunders, 1987.

Goodhill V. Ear diseases, deafness and dizziness. New York: Harper & Row, 1979.

Paparella MM, Meyerhoff WL. Sensorineural hearing loss, vertigo and tinnitus. Baltimore: Williams & Wilkins, 1981.

Paparella MM, Shumrick DA. Otolaryngology. 2nd ed. Philadelphia: WB Saunders, 1980.

Schuknecht HF. Pathology of the ear. Cambridge, MA: Harvard University Press, 1974.

Nose Bleed (Epistaxis)

James P. Hughes, MD

155

Definition

The word *epistaxis,* derived from the Greek words *epi,* meaning "upon," and *stazin,* a "drip," is the term most frequently used to indicate bleeding from the nose. This common disorder is usually easily controllable; however, it may be serious and even life-threatening if the bleeding comes from a major vessel. The nose is a frequent site of bleeding owing to the vulnerability of the anterior septal vessels and to its generous blood supply. The nose is supplied by branches of both the external and internal carotid arteries (Fig. 155-1). Epistaxis is generally classified as anterior, in which the bleeding comes from the anterior nasal septum, or posterior. Although an anterior bleeding site is usually easily identified and dealt with, posterior bleeding poses a much more difficult management problem. Posterior epistaxis is ordinarily controlled by packing the entire nose from the nostrils to the choanae.

Etiology

Although nasal bleeding most frequently occurs as a result of local factors relating to the anatomy and physiology of the nose, it may herald an underlying systemic disorder. In approximately 25 percent of cases, the etiology is not discovered.

The most frequent local causes of bleeding are drying and crusting of the nasal septum secondary to low humidity, local trauma, or acute inflammation from an upper respiratory tract infection. Bleeding following a nasal fracture or surgery of the nasal bones or septum is extremely common and usually self-limiting. Less frequently, the bleeding may derive from a foreign body or a perforation of the nasal septum. Rarely, bleeding may result from telangiectasias of the nasal septum (Osler-Weber-Rendu syndrome) or from tumors of the nose.

Hypertension is classically associated with posterior nosebleeds, which are most commonly seen in the older age group. Increased venous pressure (e.g., mitral stenosis) may also be a factor in the development of epistaxis.

Underlying blood dyscrasias may predispose to recurrent epistaxis. Clotting disorders occasionally occur that may be spontaneous, drug-induced, related to vitamin deficiency, or associated with advanced liver disease. Epistaxis may indicate drug-induced thrombocytopenia in patients receiving chemotherapy.

Figure 155-2 outlines etiologies of epistaxis.

Diagnostic Approach

A brief history will usually give an indication of the site of bleeding. Anterior epistaxis is most frequently seen in the winter and is associated with low humidity. Patients who pick, scratch, or vigorously blow their noses are particularly susceptible to nosebleeds. Frequently, the patient with an upper respiratory tract infection will traumatize the anterior nasal septum, disrupting the septal vessels. Patients should be queried regarding the use of anticoagulants or antiplatelet drugs, specifically aspirin or aspirin-containing compounds. A history of liver disease may also be relevant. Occasionally, an acute blood dyscrasia will result from a drug reaction and manifest with thrombocytopathy or thrombocytopenia. Patients with a family history of epistaxis may have nosebleeds as the only sign of hereditary hemorrhagic telangiectasia (Osler-Weber-Rendu syndrome). Vasospasm and soft-tissue necrosis with bleeding may occur with chronic use of cocaine.

Physical Examination

Careful examination of the nose should be performed in an attempt to identify the site of bleeding. Anterior bleeding is seen in the younger population and can be visualized easily if the proper instruments are available. Anterior bleeding is generally a result of local trauma and is usually of limited degree. Posterior bleeding, on the other hand, is seen in an older age group and occurs more frequently in patients with hypertension. It may be recurrent. Posterior epistaxis deserves consultation with an ear, nose, and throat specialist and usually will necessitate anteroposterior packing of the nose.

Unless there is evidence of excessive blood loss or postural hypotension, the patient may be placed in the upright position. For adequate management and treatment of the nosebleed, the following equipment must be available:

1. Nasal speculum
2. Bayonette forceps
3. #7 Frazier suction tip
4. Headlight or head mirror

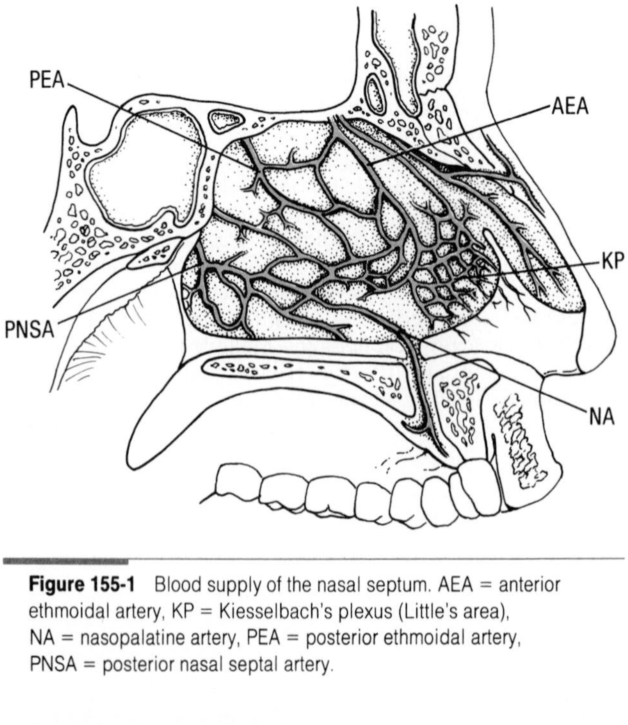

Figure 155-1 Blood supply of the nasal septum. AEA = anterior ethmoidal artery, KP = Kiesselbach's plexus (Little's area), NA = nasopalatine artery, PEA = posterior ethmoidal artery, PNSA = posterior nasal septal artery.

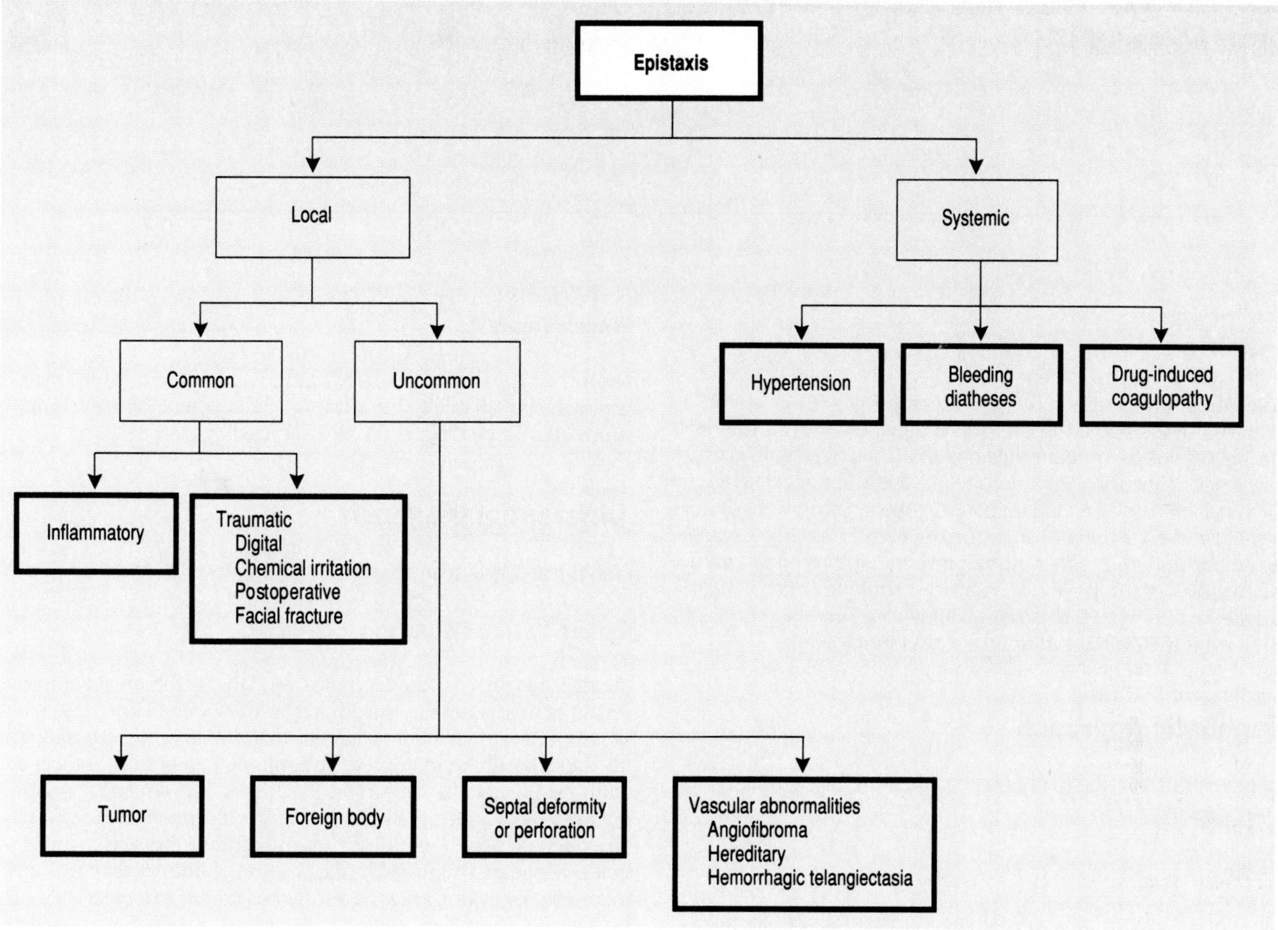

Figure 155-2 Etiologies of epistaxis. Note that in approximately 25 percent of cases of epistaxis, the etiology is unknown.

5. Topical anesthetics and topical vasoconstrictors (phenylephrine, lidocaine, cocaine)
6. Cotton
7. Silver nitrate sticks or an electrocoagulation unit
8. Wall suction or a suction machine

Initially, clear the nose of all clots and debris by instructing the patient to blow the nose forcefully. After the nose has been cleared, the speculum can be introduced to provide adequate visualization. In the event that the bleeding has stopped, forceful noseblowing or straining may provoke the bleeding to recur so that the bleeding site can be identified. With the speculum in one hand and suction in the other, clear all the fresh blood until the source of the bleeding can be identified. Once the vessel is identified, a topical anesthetic combined with a vasoconstrictor should be used to provide hemostasis. Cocaine is an ideal choice because it has both pharmacologic effects. After hemostasis has been achieved, the bleeding point can be cauterized with silver nitrate. If the bleeding is persistent or the site of origin cannot be identified, otolaryngologic consultation is indicated. In most cases, a posterior bleed can be controlled with an anteroposterior pack. Failing that, other procedures, such as ligation of the internal maxillary or ethmoid arteries, may be required.

Laboratory Tests

Hemoglobin and hematocrit levels are of value if the bleeding appears to have been significant. Unless the patient has a previous history of bruising or excessive bleeding, it is unlikely that screening tests for coagulopathy, such as prothrombin time, partial thromboplastin time, platelet counts, or bleeding time, will be of value. Such tests should generally be reserved for patients who are strongly suspected of having an underlying bleeding disorder or who fail to respond to initial management. For patients with recurrent bleeding, more extensive evaluation, including radiographs and direct examination of the nasopharynx, may be necessary to rule out an underlying source of the bleeding, such as tumor.

References

Baron BC. Epistaxis. In: Gates GA, ed. Current therapy in otolaryngology–head and neck surgery-4. Philadelphia: BC Decker 1990:277.

Culbertson MC Jr. Epistaxis. In: Bluestone CD, Stool SE, eds. Pediatric otolaryngology. 2nd ed. Philadelphia: WB Saunders, 1989.

Davis WE, Epistaxis. In: Holt GR, et al, eds. Decision making in otolaryngology. Toronto: BC Decker, 1984:30.

Hoarseness

James P. Hughes, MD

156

Definition

Hoarseness or change in the vocal quality is the most common symptom of laryngeal disease. It is a nonspecific symptom and can be provoked by many lesions that interfere with normal anatomy or function. The etiology may be a physical change in the vocal cords due to inflammation, tumor, ulceration, denervation, or even a functional disturbance. Traditionally, hoarseness of more than 2 weeks' duration in an adult requires careful examination of the larynx by indirect technique (mirror exam) to rule out the possibility of malignancy. This chapter deals solely with the evaluation of hoarseness in the adult.

Diagnostic Approach

An algorithm for the diagnostic evaluation of hoarseness is shown in Figure 156-1.

History

A complete history will usually suggest possible etiologies for the hoarseness. Note the onset, duration, and character of the voice change. Have the episodes of hoarseness been recurrent? What is the quality of the voice between attacks? When was the last time the voice was considered perfectly normal? It is sometimes helpful to confirm the onset and severity of this symptom with other family members, because the patient may not be conscious of a gradual but progressive voice change. Other factors that are associated with chronic vocal change such as occupation, smoking history, abuse of alcohol, previous surgery, exposure to toxins or fumes, and vocal overuse or abuse should be noted.

Physical Examination

External examination of the larynx can be accomplished by palpation of the laryngeal cartilage; note any abnormal mass or tenderness. Loss of laryngeal crepitus should be recorded because this sign may indicate a retrocricoid lesion. The larynx is grasped and gently pushed backward while being moved from side to side. There should be a definite roughness as the larynx moves against the vertebral bodies. Internal examination of the larynx should be performed next. Indirect visualization of the vocal cords can be accomplished with a laryngeal mirror. The patient is asked to open the mouth widely while the examiner grasps the extending tongue with the left hand and places the warmed laryngeal mirror against the soft palate. In most cases, the epiglottis, aryepiglottic folds, valleculae, pyriform sinuses, arytenoids, and both true and false cords can be visualized clearly. It may be necessary to have the patient phonate a high-pitched E to bring the true cords fully into view. Occasionally, topical anesthesia or light sedation is required. If the patient is unable to tolerate the indirect examination, fiberoptic visualization or direct laryngoscopy under general anesthesia can be done.

Radiography

With the rapid advances in imaging technology, a multitude of studies are available to the clinician. Selection of the appropriate study should be deferred to the laryngologist.

Differential Diagnosis

Table 156-1 lists many common etiologies of hoarseness.

Inflammatory Causes

Acute Laryngitis. Acute laryngitis is probably the most common cause of hoarseness in the adult. It is most often associated with an upper respiratory tract infection and may be severe enough to cause partial or complete aphonia. It is generally associated with significant discomfort in the throat and laryngeal region. Symptoms of lower respiratory tract involvement such as cough are often present. On indirect examination of the larynx, there is generalized erythema with mild edema of both vocal cords and occasionally minor areas of submucosal hemorrhage.

Epiglottitis. Epiglottitis in adults is seen much less frequently than in children. The initial symptoms are the same as in any pharyngitis; however, they progress rapidly to severe throat pain with inability to swallow secretions. There is generally a partial upper airway obstruction that may progress to complete obstruction secondary to supraglottic edema. The diagnosis is made by the appearance of the epiglottis on the lateral neck radiograph. Direct examination of the epiglottis should be avoided if there is concern about the security of the airway. Depending on the degree of epiglottic swelling and stridor, the patient may be closely observed if personnel are immediately available who can perform an emergency intubation or tracheostomy. Frequently, intubation in the operating room under controlled conditions is preferred (see also Chapter 158, "Sore Throat").

Diphtheritic Laryngitis. Diphtheria, caused by *Corynebacterium diphtheriae,* is a rare cause of laryngitis in the United States today. The presenting symptoms are generally moderate. The involvement of the larynx is characterized by hoarseness with, occasionally, a croupy cough. The larynx is covered with a grayish white membrane. There may be associated symptoms of generalized systemic illness and other physical findings in the oral cavity and pharynx consistent with diphtheria. When the diphtheritic membrane is removed, the surface bleeds freely.

Chronic Conditions

Chronic Laryngitis. Chronic laryngitis implies a longstanding (several weeks or more) inflammatory reaction of the laryngeal tissues. It is generally associated with vocal overuse, smoking, and the use of alcohol. Hoarseness is a hallmark of chronic laryngitis. In contrast to acute laryngitis, pain is generally mild or absent. Recurrent insult to the larynx may result from bronchopulmonary disease with chronic cough and resultant trauma to the vocal cords. The true cords are thick and reddened, and the inflammation may extend to involve the false cords and supraglottic larynx. In adults with a history of tobacco use or excessive use of alcohol, a direct examination with biopsy under general anesthesia is usually indicated.

Contact Ulcer. The point at which the vocal cord attaches to the vocal process of the arytenoid cartilage may occasionally become ulcerated from excessive use or misuse of the voice, particularly during an attack of acute inflammatory laryngitis. This may result in granuloma formation. These lesions can be unilateral or bilateral. Primary symptoms of contact ulcers are hoarseness and pain, which may radiate to the ear.

Vocal Cord Polyps. Polyps of the vocal cords frequently involve the middle portion of the vocal cord and may be unilateral or bilateral. They may be associated with underlying allergic disorders or hypothyroid state.

Vocal Nodule. The vocal nodule, or "singer's node," is usually bilateral and is situated at the junction of the anterior and middle thirds of the vocal cords. It may be associated with vocal dysfunction and is frequently seen in patients who use their voices professionally, e.g., singers.

Pachyderma. Pachyderma of the larynx is a rare entity that demonstrates hyperplasia of the cornified layers of the epithelium in the interarytenoid area and occasionally on the posterior portions of the vocal cords. There is no evidence of dyskeratosis. The lesion is not premalignant. It must be differentiated from tuberculosis or malignant lesions.

Hyperkeratosis. *Keratosis* or *hyperkeratosis* is the term used to denote a group of epithelial lesions that may involve the larynx. Hoarseness may be the only symptom. The mucosa is similar in appearance to that of chronic laryngitis, and the lesion is thought to be secondary to smoking, vocal abuse, and contact irritants such as alcohol. These white lesions are sometimes referred to as leukoplakia and are considered premalignant. Differentiation from carcinoma in situ or invasive carcinoma must be made by biopsy.

Laryngitis Sicca (Atrophic Laryngitis). Laryngitis sicca is characterized by hoarseness of the voice. On indirect examination, there is a marked crusting and mild irritation of the throat. The crust adheres to the posterior commissure of the larynx and produces a chronic cough. Histopathologically, there is atrophy of the mucosa and the mucosal glands with moderate fibrosis.

Tuberculosis. Tuberculous laryngitis is usually secondary to active pulmonary involvement. Hoarseness is usually present. The cough is sometimes productive of blood-streaked sputum. Pain may be referred to one or both ears. The lesion is usually situated posteriorly in the larynx on the interarytenoid fold. The diagnosis is made by chest radiograph and a high level of suspicion. Direct laryngoscopy with biopsy to rule out malignancy may be necessary.

Mycotic Granulomas. Mycotic involvement of the larynx is rare. In the southern United States, histoplasmosis has been documented to involve the larynx. Candidiasis also may be seen as a complication of chemotherapy or an altered immune state. It is characterized by white patches on bright red mucous membrane.

Reaction to Radiation Therapy. Significant hoarseness with marked edema of the vocal cords and supraglottic larynx may occur as a complication of radiation therapy to the region. This may lead to almost total aphonia. Marked edema following radiation therapy for a malignancy of the larynx raises suspicion of persistent disease.

Trauma

Internal Trauma. Intubation for even relatively brief periods of time may result in significant injury to the vocal cord mucosa. This acute injury generally resolves with conservative management, but occasionally it may result in permanent cicatricial damage. One well-recognized entity is the intubation granuloma, which appears over the vocal process of the arytenoid and may reach considerable dimensions. Nasogastric tubes are also associated with inflammatory change in the area of the cricoid, the arytenoids, and cricoarytenoid joints. They may cause hoarseness, pain, chondritis, and even subglottic stenosis.

Irritants such as smoke or chemicals may cause temporary or permanent damage to the larynx. All patients should be questioned about possible exposure to irritants.

External Trauma. Blunt or penetrating trauma to the neck may cause a wide variety of laryngeal injuries, many of which will result in hoarseness. A mild blow to the neck may result in hemorrhage in the glottic and supraglottic larynx. More severe force may fracture the larynx or result in contusion of the recurrent laryngeal nerve. Although it may be possible to make the diagnosis of a fracture on physical examination and with the laryngeal mirror, in most cases direct examination under general anesthesia will be required.

Postsurgical. Multiple endoscopic and external procedures are available for diagnosis and treatment of laryngeal lesions. Occasionally, hoarseness will be seen as a complication or side effect of a surgical procedure.

Neurogenic Causes

Vocal Cord Paralysis. Disturbance of the innervation of the larynx can cause various vocal changes, depending on which nerve is involved. The larynx is supplied by two branches of the vagus nerve. The first, the superior laryngeal branch, provides innervation to the cricothyroid muscle through its external

Table 156-1 Common Etiologies of Hoarseness

Inflammatory	**Trauma**
Acute	Internal
Acute laryngitis	External
Epiglottitis	Surgical
Diphtheria	**Neurogenic**
Chronic	Vocal cord paralysis
Chronic laryngitis	Unilateral
Contact ulcers	Bilateral
Polyp	**Neoplasms**
Nodules	Benign
Pachyderma	Malignant
Hyperkeratosis (leukoplakia)	**Systemic diseases**
Atrophic laryngitis (sicca)	Allergic reactions
Granulomas	Angioedema
Tuberculosis	Anaphylactic reactions
Scleroma	Arthritis
Sarcoidosis	Hypothyroidism
Wegener's granuloma	Uremia
Syphilis	Blood dyscrasias
Mycotic infections	Amyloidosis
Monilial	Agranulocytosis
Histoplasmosis	
Benign mucous membrane pemphigoid	**Functional voice disorders**
Reaction to radiation therapy	**Central disorders**

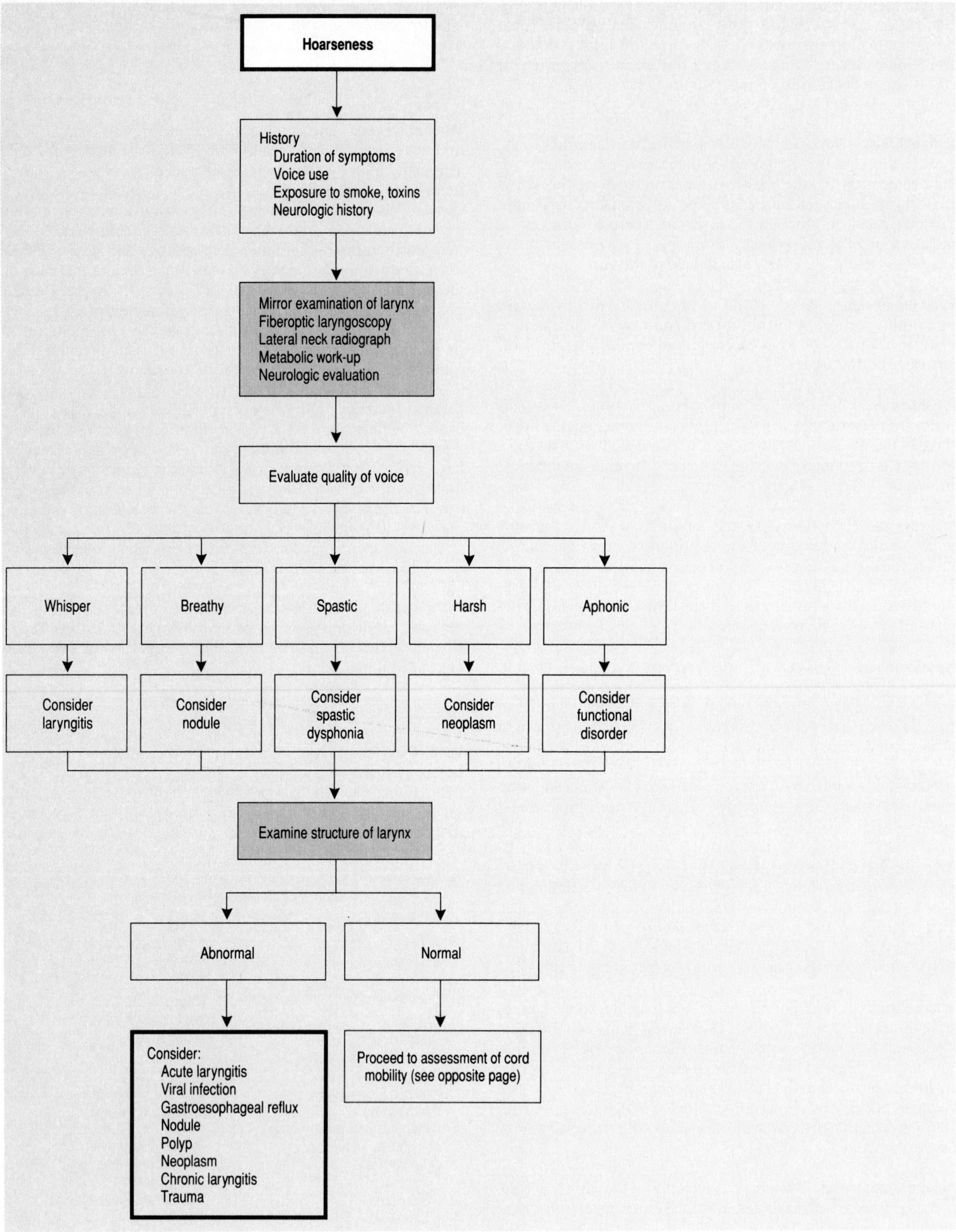

Figure 156-1 Algorithm for the diagnostic evaluation of hoarseness. (Modified from Holt GR, et al, eds. Decision making in otolaryngology. Toronto: BC Decker, 1984.)

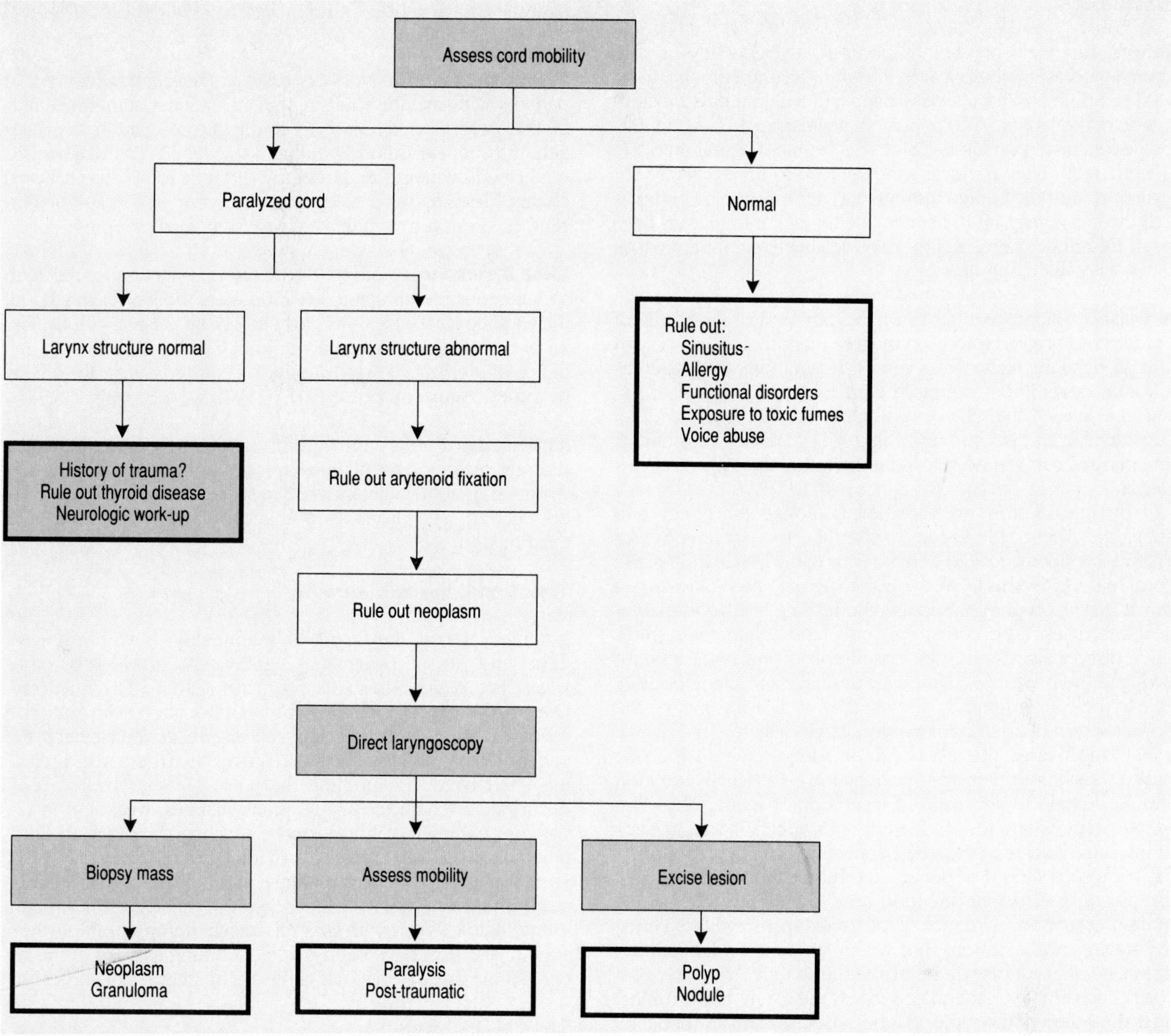

Figure 156-1 *Continued*

branch and sensation to the laryngeal membranes via the internal branch. The recurrent laryngeal nerve is the second branch of the vagus, which loops deep in the neck, around the subclavian artery on the right side, and around the aortic arch on the left. Interruption of the superior laryngeal nerve will result in a change in the position of the vocal cord, with a deviation of the posterior commissure and a change in the pitch of the voice. There is generally limitation of the dynamic vocal range. The diagnosis can usually be made by indirect examination. Dysfunction of the recurrent laryngeal nerve may result in a more severe problem. If the recurrent laryngeal nerve is involved on only one side, the vocal quality will depend on the position of the paralyzed cord. If the cord is in a median position, there will usually be no significant airway problem, because the opposite mobile cord can abduct normally. The voice may be normal if the functioning cord can compensate and reach the immobile cord. If the paralyzed cord is in a lateral position, however, there will be escape of air and significant hoarseness. This produces a "breathy" quality to the voice. If both vocal cords are paralyzed and in a median or paramedian position, the voice will usually be satisfactory; however, the airway can be significantly compromised, particularly with exertion or upper respiratory tract infections.

In a unilateral vocal cord palsy, the left recurrent laryngeal nerve is more frequently involved owing to its location. The nerve is more likely to be compromised by an aortic aneurysm, dilatation of the left atrium secondary to mitral stenosis, or involvement of mediastinal nodes with metastatic carcinoma. Other possible causes of unilateral cord palsy are toxins and neuropathy, such as those caused by diabetes or viral infections. Bilateral paralysis is relatively uncommon. In approximately 15 to 20 percent of cases, the etiology of vocal cord paralysis cannot be determined.

Diagnostic evaluation for vocal cord palsy should include a general history and physical examination of the head and neck, including indirect examination of the vocal cords. Particular attention must be paid to vocal cord position and motion. Position of the arytenoids should also be noted. The work-up may also include complete blood count, urinalysis, chest radiograph, skull radiographs, computed tomography, cervical spine films, barium swallow, glucose tolerance test, and a thyroid scan. Selection of specific tests must be individually determined.

Neoplasms

Benign. Laryngeal papillomas occur most frequently in children but occasionally appear in the adult. They are thought to be viral in origin and have a classic appearance on indirect examination of the larynx. They appear somewhat verrucous and may be pedunculated or sessile. Biopsy is required. Papillomas frequently recur after removal and may lead to upper airway obstruction. Multiple benign tumors (e.g., neurofibromas, granular cell myoblastomas, chondromas, adenomas) of the larynx have been described; however, they are relatively uncommon. The diagnosis usually requires biopsy.

Malignant. Malignant tumors of the larynx are almost all of epidermoid origin. Lesions on the free margin of the vocal cord will produce hoarseness as a very early symptom. Pain is generally not a prominent symptom with early involvement. If the lesion is in the subglottic or supraglottic larynx, it may grow to considerable size prior to becoming symptomatic. Occasionally, an enlarged cervical node will be the initial sign of a laryngeal tumor.

Laryngeal lesions are classified as supraglottic, glottic, and subglottic. The glottic lesion involves the true vocal cord and extends for not more than 1 cm inferior to the free margin of the vocal fold. Below this level, the lesions are subglottic and carry a much graver prognosis. Supraglottic lesions involve the laryngeal ventricles, false cords, epiglottis, and aryepiglottic folds. They carry a significantly increased risk of metastatic disease owing to their increased lymphatic drainage and silent location. Pain in the ear, particularly provoked by swallowing, may be the first symptom of an occult laryngeal carcinoma.

In most cases, the larynx can be adequately visualized by indirect technique (mirror examination). Particular attention should be paid to any areas of ulceration or leukoplakia. The exact extent of any lesion, including its superior and inferior limits, must be assessed. Likewise, any impairment of motion of the vocal cord should be documented at the time of the indirect examination. Particular attention must be paid to the cervical nodes because any evidence of metastatic spread will influence the staging of the lesion. Biopsy can be done under indirect vision, but in most cases general anesthesia with direct laryngoscopy is preferable to adequately assess the extent of the tumor. After the extent of the tumor has been defined and any nodal or distant metastatic disease evaluated, the tumor can be staged by the TNM system.

Systemic Diseases

Allergic Reactions. Vocal change secondary to edema of the larynx may be a result of recurrent angioedema or true anaphylaxis. Initial hoarseness may progress rapidly to stridor or complete upper airway obstruction.

Arthritis. Involvement of the cricoarytenoid joint has been estimated to occur in as many as 25 percent of patients with rheumatoid arthritis. The classic symptoms are hoarseness, a weak voice, and pain aggravated by swallowing. Ankylosis of the cricoarytenoid joint must be differentiated from laryngeal paralysis by direct examination and palpation of the joint. Ankylosis may also be found in patients who have been intubated for prolonged periods.

Hypothyroidism. The vocal cords are frequently involved in patients with hypothyroidism, and hoarseness sometimes may be the presenting symptom. On indirect examination, the cords generally appear diffusely dull and thickened. The diagnosis is confirmed by measurement of thyroid function. The vocal cord changes may respond to thyroid replacement therapy or may require surgical treatment, such as vocal cord stripping.

Blood Dyscrasias. Clotting disorders may be associated with spontaneous bleeding into the mucosa of the larynx and that of the vocal cords. The lesions are hemorrhagic or ecchymotic. The vocal cord mobility is usually unimpaired, and there is no evidence of ulceration. No treatment is required unless the airway becomes compromised.

Amyloidosis. Primary amyloidosis of the larynx is manifested by discrete lesions. The plaques are generally less than 1 cm in diameter, but they may increase in size and cause partial airway obstruction. The diagnosis is made by biopsy and histologic examination.

Functional Voice Disorders

Not infrequently, the laryngeal examination is within normal limits and yet the patient has significant hoarseness or other vocal disturbance. These disorders are described as functional. One of the more common types is phonation with the false cords. In this disorder, called dysphonia plicae ventricularis, the patient closes the false vocal cords over the true cords, occluding the larynx and muffling the voice. Other types of vocal disturbances characterized by pitch changes, weakness in the voice, or complete aphonia may be psychogenic in origin. Spastic dysphonia is associated with an interrupted, stuttering type of vocal pattern. It is seen in patients who use their voices excessively and may progress in severity until the speech is virtually unintelligible. Along with general speech therapy, multiple therapeutic attempts have been made, including surgery of the recurrent laryngeal nerves, all with varying degrees of success.

Central Disorders

Various distortions of speech and voice pattern may occur with central nervous system lesions. Among these are cerebral palsy, parkinsonism, and bulbar paralysis. Some speech patterns are pathognomonic, such as the scanning speech of multiple sclerosis.

References

Blacklow RS, Catlin FI. MacBryde's signs and symptoms. Philadelphia: JB Lippincott, 1983:112.

DeWeese DD, Saunders WH. Textbook of otolaryngology. 7th ed. St. Louis: CV Mosby, 1988.

Schaefer SD. Hoarseness. In: Holt GR, et al, eds. Decision making in otolaryngology. Toronto: BC Decker, 1984:36.

Tinnitus

James P. Hughes, MD

157

Definition

Tinnitus is derived from the Latin word *tinnire,* meaning "to ring." It is generally used to refer to any sound heard in the ears or head. This symptom can be evidenced in the normal adult, or it may be a harbinger of serious underlying pathology. Virtually all adults have experienced tinnitus at one time or another, and approximately 6.4 percent of the population, or over 7 million people, complain that the tinnitus is severe. Tinnitus was mentioned in the writings of Hippocrates several hundred years before Christ. Beethoven was also noted to have complained of tinnitus in association with his progressive deafness. A distinction is occasionally made between tinnitus aurium and tinnitus cerebre. In tinnitus aurium the sound is identified in one or both ears, whereas in tinnitus cerebre the sound is diffusely present in the head and cannot be localized to either ear. Both types may coexist. Tinnitus cerebre may be due to organic or functional disease and requires medical and neurologic evaluation. This chapter deals exclusively with otogenic tinnitus.

Etiology

Owing to the ubiquitous and nonspecific nature of this symptom, attempts to identify discrete etiologies have been difficult. Over the years, many researchers have postulated theories for tinnitus generation. Although histologic studies have demonstrated areas of pathology of the inner ear, such as loss of hair cells and neuron population, none of these have definitely been related to the presence of tinnitus. Most frequently, tinnitus results from an abnormality of the inner ear, the eighth cranial nerve, central auditory pathways, or the cerebral cortex.

Differential Diagnosis

Tinnitus has been divided into two types: (1) subjective, in which the sound can only be heard by the patient, and (2) objective, when the sound is also audible to the examiner (Table 157-1).

Subjective Tinnitus

In the vast majority of cases, tinnitus is subjective and reflects a lesion of the auditory pathway. Tinnitus can be defined in terms of its character, periodicity, pitch, loudness, and maskability. None of these parameters, however, have been particularly useful from a diagnostic standpoint. Although lesions of the external ear canal (such as cerumen impaction) and middle ear lesions (such as otosclerosis) may be etiologic, many individuals have evidence of the same pathology without experiencing tinnitus. Moreover, surgical correction of an otosclerotic lesion or removal of cerumen does not always eliminate the tinnitus. The tinnitus that follows acoustic trauma is frequently transient. Certain drugs may cause tinnitus. Some of the most frequent offenders are anti-inflammatory agents such as salicylates and indomethacin. Ototoxic antibiotics, especially the aminoglycosides, will provoke tinnitus in association with hearing loss or vertigo. Multiple medical diseases have been reported to be related to tinnitus, among which are diabetes, hyperthyroidism, hypothyroidism, and vascular or hematologic diseases. Head injuries and certain central nervous system lesions such as viral neuropathies, multiple sclerosis, and acoustic neuromas have been related to the development of tinnitus. Of note, approximately 50 percent of the patients who have undergone resection of acoustic neuromas with transection of the vestibulocochlear nerve still experience tinnitus. Glomus tumors, an uncommon lesion of the middle-ear space and mastoid, are reported to cause a pulsatile tinnitus. Some factors that appear to exacerbate or aggravate tinnitus are stress, fatigue, smoking, and allergens.

The evaluation of the patient with tinnitus is somewhat controversial and must be tailored to each patient's presentation. A complete medical history and otologic evaluation should be performed. Inquiry should be made regarding noise exposure, a family history of tinnitus, drug usage, and prior ear disease or surgery. Associated symptoms of otalgia, headache, dizziness, vertigo, or hearing loss are sought in an attempt to localize the problem to the ear or the central auditory apparatus. Symptoms of diabetes and thyroid disease or other endocrinopathy should be noted. Basic audiologic testing should be performed if the symptom persists after apparent sources of the tinnitus have been corrected. Audiologic testing should include air and bone testing and speech discrimination tests. In cases of unilateral tinnitus, a more detailed work-up is indicated.

Table 157-1 Common Etiologies of Tinnitus

Subjective
- External and middle ear
  - Cerumen
  - Perforated tympanic membrane
  - Ossicular discontinuity
  - Otitis media (serous or acute)
  - Otosclerosis
  - Glomus tumors
- Inner ear
  - Presbycusis
  - Post-traumatic (physical, acoustic, or barotrauma)
  - Viral neuropathy
  - Ototoxins
  - Meniere's disease
- Central nervous system
  - Acoustic neuroma
  - Cerebellopontine angle tumors
- Nonotic causes
  - Multiple sclerosis
  - Head injury
  - Endocrinopathies
    - Diabetes mellitus
    - Hypo- or hyperthyroidism

Objective
- Muscular
  - Contraction of stapedius, tensor tympani, or palatal muscle
  - Patulous eustachain tube
- Vascular
  - Transmission of heart tones
  - Atrioventricular malformation

Objective Tinnitus

Objective tinnitus, which can be heard by the examiner, can best be elicited by placing the bell of the stethoscope over the patient's ear or attaching the tubing of the stethoscope to an ear mold. The character of the tinnitus may give some clue to its etiology. One of the more frequent types is a clicking sound that may be present in one or both ears. This is caused by spasm of the palatal musculature. On examination of the palate, it is possible to note an actual spasm of the palate synchronous with the clicking. A similar clicking sound can be produced by spasm of the stapedius or tensor tympani muscles. Occasionally, the patient will sense a whistling or blowing tinnitus that may be noted to be synchronous with respiration. The patient will usually also admit to autophony, which is the sensation of an echo of the patient's voice in the ear when speaking. This symptom is derived from a patulous eustachian tube and frequently is improved when the patient lies down or develops an upper respiratory tract infection. Occasionally, patients with temporomandibular joint disease complain of a clicking sound that is related to opening and closing the jaw. Such patients may notice tinnitus from the muscular spasm in the area of the ear associated with exacerbation of temporomandibular joint dysfunction. Vascular bruits may cause tinnitus that is usually pulsatile in character and synchronous with the heart beat. Sound may also radiate from a narrowed carotid artery or an arteriovenous communication in the area of the ear. One cause of nonpulsatile tinnitus is a venous hum from the jugular vein. This can be eliminated by compression of the vein.

Control of Symptoms

Multiple medications, such as steroids, antibiotics, vitamins, hormones, vasodilators, and others, have been used to attempt to control or limit tinnitus. No satisfactory treatment has yet been achieved. Currently, lidocaine injection, biofeedback, and masking are under clinical trial. Lidocaine injection carries with it substantial risk and is probably not warranted. Biofeedback has been successful in eliminating the tinnitus in approximately 30 percent of the patients who have tried it; of the remaining 60 percent, 30 percent feel that the tinnitus may be slightly improved, and 30 percent notice no change. Because this symptom is completely subjective, statistical validity is lacking. Masking the tinnitus may simply require playing a radio or tape recorder at night, when the tinnitus is most troublesome. During the day, a hearing aid will frequently provide some masking effect if there is an associated hearing loss. If not, a tinnitus masker, worn like a hearing aid, may be used. Early success rates are on the order of 35 to 50 percent, but this percentage diminishes with time.

Multiple surgical procedures have been used in the past to attempt to alleviate the tinnitus. If there is a specific lesion such as otosclerotic focus, its correction may provide relief of the tinnitus.

References

Anderson RG. Tinnitus. In: Holt GR, et al, eds. Decision making in otolaryngology. Toronto: BC Decker, 1984:14.

DeWeese DC, et al, eds. Textbook of otolaryngology. 7th ed. St. Louis: CV Mosby, 1987.

Goodhill V. Ear diseases, deafness and dizziness. New York: Harper & Row, 1979.

Paparella M, Meyerhoff W. Sensorineural hearing loss, vertigo and tinnitus. Baltimore: Williams & Wilkins, 1981.

Paparella MM, Shumrick DA. Otolaryngology. 2nd ed. Philadelphia: WB Saunders, 1980.

Proceedings of the First International Tinnitus Seminar. J Laryngol Otol V. 95(suppl):81.

Sore Throat

Thomas H. Winters, MD

158

Definition

Sore throat, the most common symptom of pharyngitis, is pain or discomfort secondary to inflammation in the posterior oropharyngeal or nasopharyngeal area, especially on swallowing. The anatomic structures involved include tonsils, peritonsillar bed, uvula, posterior palate, and nasopharynx. Sore throat is one of the five most common problems seen by the primary care physician. Forty million people seek medical care each year for sore throats.

Etiology

Sore throats are most commonly caused by infectious agents and occasionally by noninfectious agents. The goal for the clinician is to differentiate infectious etiologies from noninfectious etiologies, and treatable causes from nontreatable causes. Viruses are the prototype for nontreatable causes of sore throat, while bacteria are responsible for most treatable causes. Table 158-1 lists the treatable infectious causes of sore throat in adults.

Respiratory viruses are the most common cause of sore throat, accounting for 35 to 50 percent of sporadic (epidemic) presentations. Rhinovirus and coronavirus are the major viruses causing pharyngitis. The Epstein-Barr virus is the cause of sore throat in only 5 percent of adults. Despite this low incidence, the most common symptom of clinically apparent infectious mononucleosis is sore throat. Cytomegalovirus, herpes simplex, adenovirus, parainfluenza, influenza, coxsackie A, and respiratory syncytial virus are other respiratory viruses that can cause pharyngitis. Occasionally, infection with poliovirus, varicella-zoster, measles virus, rubella virus, and hepatitis virus can present as a sore throat before there is evidence of systemic disease.

Group A beta-hemolytic *Streptococcus pyogenes* is the most common bacterial agent associated with sore throat, accounting for 10 to 15 percent of sore throats in adults and 20 to 40 percent of sore throats in children. Because acute rheumatic fever, the most dreaded complication of group A streptococcal infection,

Table 158-1 Treatable Infectious Causes of Sore Throat	
Streptococcus pyogenes	Spirochetes and *Fusobacterium*
Haemophilus influenzae	*Mycoplasma pneumoniae*
Neisseria gonorrhoeae	*Neisseria meningitidis*
Corynebacterium diphtheriae	*Francisella tularensis*
Candida albicans	*Chlamydia trachomatis*

can be prevented by appropriate use of antibiotics, identification of the organism is indicated. Interestingly, the severity and prevalence of acute rheumatic fever have been decreasing since the beginning of the century, even before the discovery of penicillin.

Acute glomerulonephritis, another nonsuppurative complication of streptococcal infection, does not seem to be prevented by antibiotics. Other streptococci (groups B, C, and G) cause sore throat, especially in epidemic settings. They rarely cause the suppurative sequelae and do not cause the nonsuppurative sequelae of acute rheumatic fever or acute glomerulonephritis.

Infection with the organism *Mycoplasma pneumoniae* can present as a sore throat prior to the development of pneumonia, although pneumonia is the most common manifestation of infection. In young adults with sore throat, *M. pneumoniae* is the cause about 5 to 10 percent of the time. The clinical diagnosis of *M. pneumoniae* pharyngitis can only be made when there is concomitant bullous myringitis, bronchitis, or classic *Mycoplasma* pneumonia. Recent information indicates that *Chlamydia trachomatis* may be an important pharyngeal pathogen. Twenty percent of patients with pharyngitis had serologic evidence of *C. trachomatis* infection in a preliminary study.

Neisseria gonorrhoeae colonizes the pharynx of approximately 20 percent of homosexual men presenting with genital infections. Colonization of the pharynx offers a reservoir for the spread of gonorrhea, which may be manifested by sore throat, adenopathy, or any of the other manifestations of gonorrhea infection. Gonorrhea accounts for about 1 percent of throat infections in a general medical practice, but the incidence seems to correlate with orogenital sexual practices. This emphasizes the value of taking a sexual history when developing a differential of diagnostic possibilities.

Haemophilus influenzae, Neisseria meningitidis, and *Francisella tularensis* are rare but treatable causes of bacterial pharyngitis in adults. Spirochetes and *Fusobacterium* can cause gingivitis or trench mouth (Vincent's infection), infections that are manifested by sore throat, mouth ulcers, and foul breath. *Treponema pallidum* can cause pharyngitis with either primary or secondary syphilis. In the immunocompromised host, *Candida* is a common cause of pharyngitis.

Noninfectious causes of sore throat include trauma secondary to heat, sharp objects, inhalation of irritants such as smoke, and other chemicals. Occupational exposures to irritative solvents, gases, or smoke set up an inflammatory state that may predispose to infection. Allergies and postnasal drip are common causes of sore throat. Dehydration, reflux esophagitis, subacute thyroiditis, monomyelocytic leukemia, Waldeyer's ring from non-Hodgkin's lymphoma, and psychological factors are other noninfectious causes of sore throats.

Diagnostic Approach

The goal in evaluating a sore throat is to differentiate infectious from noninfectious etiologies, and then those conditions that require specific treatment from those that do not. The history, physical examination, and proper use of laboratory facilities often contribute to determining the approach to people with infectious sore throats. If no infectious symptoms or signs are evident, a pursuit of allergic, occupational, or irritative causes is essential.

History

It is important to determine a history of rheumatic fever, because patients who have had rheumatic fever are definitely at increased risk for its recurrence (certain of these patients should have suppressive therapy; see Chapter 81, "Prophylaxis Against Rheumatic Fever and Endocarditis"). If a family member, particularly a school-aged child, has documented streptococcal throat infection, the patient's likelihood of having the disease is increased. Historical information about the patient's practicing fellatio and being at risk for gonorrhea exposure is helpful for the clinician who must decide the value of obtaining a culture for *N. gonorrhoeae.*

Physical Examination

An infectious cause is suggested by symptoms such as fever, runny nose, cough, swollen glands, or rash, and by a family history of the same symptoms. Signs suggesting an infectious etiology include fever, tonsillar exudate or erythema, enlarged lymph nodes, and scarlatiniform rash. Unfortunately, these symptoms are nonspecific. A sore throat in conjunction with bad breath is somewhat specific for infection with spirochetes or *Fusobacterium.*

When an infectious etiology is suspected, the clinically important task is to distinguish beta-hemolytic streptococcal infection from other etiologies. Streptococcal pharyngitis can be treated and thus prevent the nonsuppurative sequelae of rheumatic fever and the suppurative complications of peritonsillar cellulitis and abscess, parapharyngeal or retropharyngeal abscess, otitis media, and sinusitis. The goal is to identify and treat in a cost-effective manner the person with streptococcal pharyngitis, sparing unnecessary antibiotics, cost, and patient inconvenience. Accurate diagnosis of non-group A streptococcal infection is also valuable, particularly when the sore throat portends the development of a serious and sometimes systemic illness, e.g., diphtheria, tularemia.

The symptoms and signs associated with *S. pyogenes* infection include fever, sore throat, anterior cervical adenopathy, abdominal pain, headache, fiery red tonsils with an exudate, and scarlatiniform rash. Approximately 56 percent of adults (15+ years old) who have a combination of tonsillar exudate, swollen anterior cervical lymph nodes, history of fever, and lack of cough will have a throat culture positive for *S. pyogenes.* Except for the rash, which feels rough and appears as multiple punctate papules around hair follicles, the symptoms and signs of streptococcal disease lack specificity. Approximately 65 percent of patients with viral pharyngitis and 40 percent of those with *Mycoplasma* infection can have pharyngeal exudate, which is indistinguishable from the exudate of streptococcal infection. Unfortunately, there is no constellation of signs and symptoms that allows a clinician to differentiate easily between nonstreptococcal infection and *S. pyogenes* infection. Figure 158-1 is a guide to the diagnosis and treatment of *S. pyogenes* pharyngeal infection.

Irregular white patches of exudate overlapping shallow pharyngeal ulcers are characteristic of *Candida* infection. This is most common in diabetic and immunocompromised patients.

Common cold viruses often cause mild pharyngitis, rhinorrhea, cough, or occasional anterior cervical adenopathy, but usually no fever. Influenza virus causes a more severe sore throat with headache, myalgia, fever (101 to 103°F), and cough.

The finding of a pseudomembrane on physical examination suggests diphtheria. Ulcerations and dark gray membranes apparent on inspection of the posterior pharynx in conjunction with foul anaerobic breath suggest *Fusobacterium* and spirochetal infections.

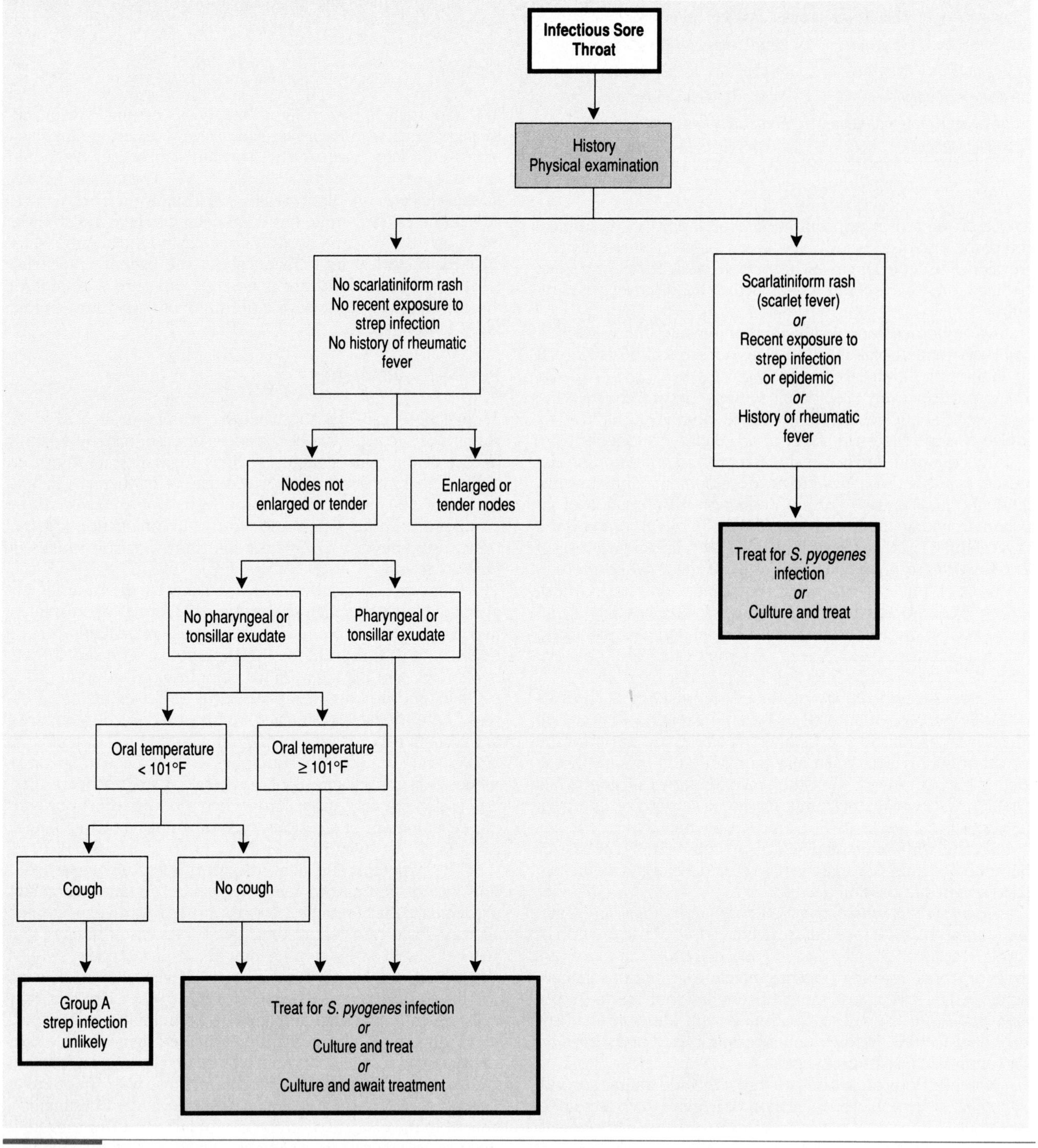

Figure 158-1 Algorithm for the diagnosis and treatment of a patient with *Streptococcus pyogenes* pharyngeal infection.

Laboratory Tests

The patient with pharyngitis, petechiae of the palate, diffuse adenopathy (posterior auricular, axillary, inguinal), and splenomegaly requires further laboratory investigation with a complete blood count and differential and a heterophile antibody (Monospot) test to detect infectious mononucleosis (Fig. 158-2).

In the clinical arena, the throat culture remains the gold standard for identifying *S. pyogenes* infection, because immunologic studies take 1 to 3 weeks to demonstrate an antibody rise. The sensitivity of a single throat culture is 70 percent in people with severe pharyngitis secondary to *S. pyogenes*. Rapid determination of group A streptococcus antigen on throat swab is available in the physician's office within 10 minutes with acceptable sensitivities and specificities. Selective use of these tests augments the clinical approach to diagnosis of a sore throat, thus improving management by decreasing short-term morbidity and inappropriate use of antibiotics.

Unfortunately, a positive throat culture cannot differentiate between the 5 to 20 percent of adults who are pharyngeal streptococcus carriers and those adults with true infection. The use of the culture does, however, generally eliminate antibiotic use in people with negative cultures. An exception to this is made by treating patients with a negative culture if they have a history of known rheumatic fever, exposure to a community outbreak of *S. pyogenes* disease, or a scarlatiniform rash.

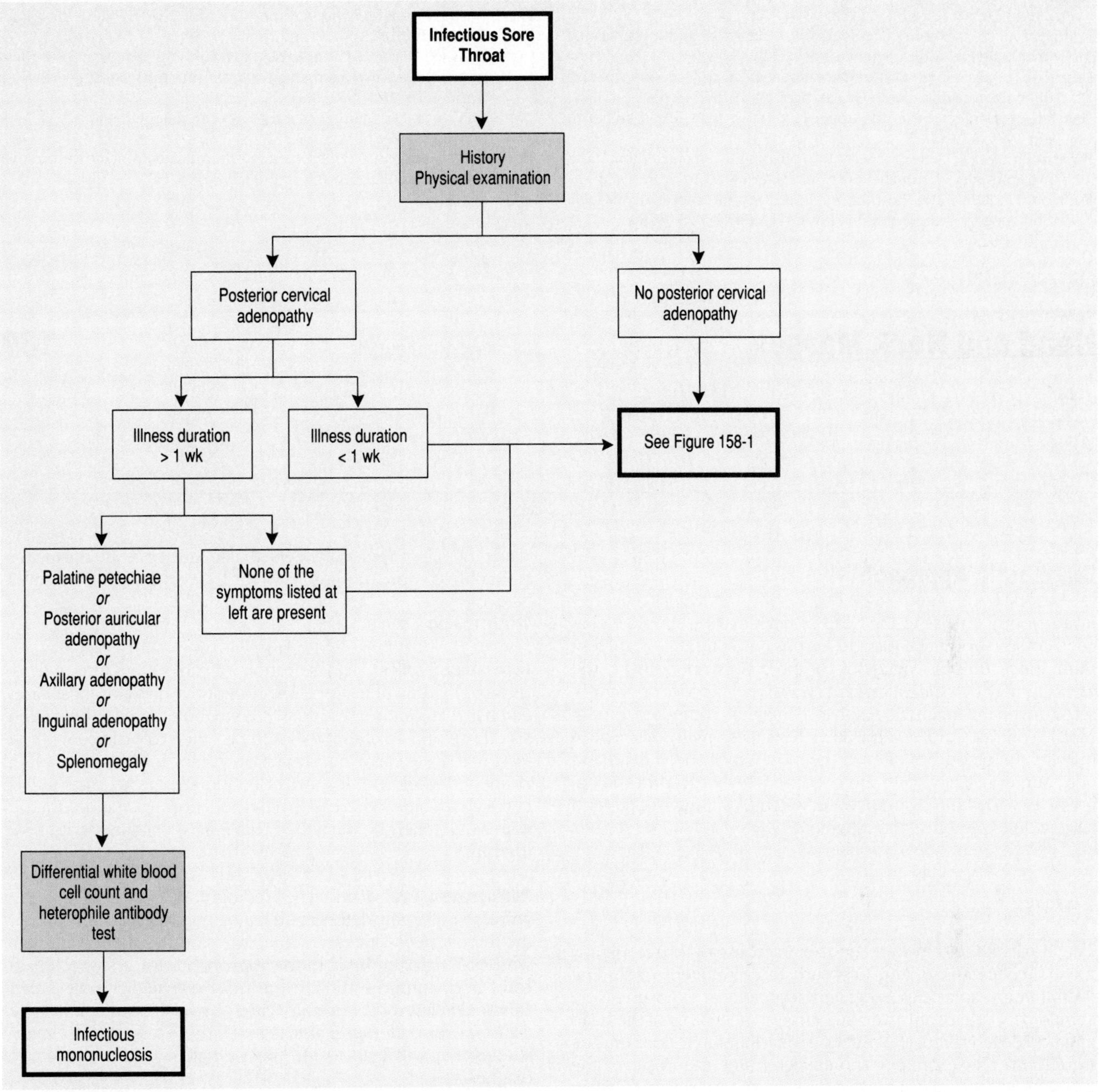

Figure 158-2 Algorithm for the diagnosis of infectious mononucleosis.

A throat culture is best performed by visualizing the posterior pharynx and rubbing a sterile swab over the tonsils, exudate, and posterior pharynx. Gram stain or quantification culture of a pharyngeal exudate is not reproducible and cannot be reliably used for identification of streptococcal throat infection. A crystal violet smear of a pharyngeal exudate on a necrotic ulcer should be done if *Fusobacterium* or spirochetal infection is suspected. One will see nonsporulating moderate-sized gram-negative rods or loosely wound spirilla on the crystal violet smear. If diphtheria is suspected, a throat culture should be obtained and plated on Loeffler's medium. A complement fixation test for *Mycoplasma* is indicated if sore throat and cough are persistent symptoms. A *Candida* infection can be documented by culture or less expensively by a potassium hydroxide (KOH) smear of an exudate, which will show yeast buds or pseudohyphae.

Because culture and serologic determination of *M. pneumoniae* and *C. trachomatis* are not readily available or cost-effective, a clinical diagnosis of each should be considered in a patient with fever, prolonged cough, and sore throat who does not have group A streptococcus or mononucleosis infection.

References

Aronson MD, et al. Heterophil antibody in adults with sore throat. Ann Intern Med 1982; 96:505.

Bisno AL. Therapeutic strategies for the prevention of rheumatic fever. Ann Intern Med 1977; 86:494.

Centor RM, et al. Throat cultures and rapid tests for diagnosis of group A streptococcal pharyngitis. Ann Intern Med 1986; 105:892.

Centor RM, et al. The diagnosis of strep throat in adults in the emergency room. Med Decision Making 1981; 1:239.

Gerber MA. Comparison of throat cultures and rapid strep tests for diagnosis of streptococcal pharyngitis. Pediatr Infect Dis J 1989; 8:820.

Komaroff AL. A management strategy for sore throat. JAMA 1978; 239:1429.
Komaroff AL, et al. Serologic evidence of chlamydial and mycoplasmal pharyngitis in adults. Science 1983; 222:927.
Lehrer JF, et al. Recognition and treatment of allergy in sinusitis and pharyngotonsillitis. Arch Otolaryngol 1981; 107:543.
Levy ML, et al. Infections of the upper respiratory tract. Med Clin North Am 1983; 67:153.
Pantell RH. Cost effectiveness of pharyngitis management and prevention of rheumatic fever. Ann Intern Med 1977; 86:497.
Perlman PE, Ginn DR. Respiratory infections in ambulatory adults: Choosing the best treatment. Postgrad Med 1990; 87:175.
Stollerman RH. Global changes in group A streptococcal diseases and strategies for their prevention. Chicago: Year Book Medical Publishers, 1982:373.
Tompkins RK, Burnes DC, Cable WE. An analysis of the cost effectiveness of pharyngitis management and acute rheumatic fever prevention. Ann Intern Med 1977; 86:481.
Walsh BT, et al. Recognition of streptococcal pharyngitis in adults. Arch Med 1975; 135:1493.
Wood RW, et al. An efficient strategy for managing acute respiratory illness in adults. Ann Intern Med 1980; 93:757.

159 Head and Neck Masses

James P. Hughes, MD

Diagnostic Approach

Evaluation of a mass in the head or neck may be simple (sebaceous cysts, superficial parotid lesions) or complex (recurrent skull base tumors, metastatic lesion). Correspondingly, the work-up may be straightforward (excisional biopsy) or complicated, involving magnetic resonance imaging, computed tomography, contrast studies, and other tests. Lesions in this region may tax the resources of even the most experienced head and neck surgeon. Therefore, the decision whether to proceed aggressively or with reassurance and watchful waiting will depend largely on experience and judgment.

History

The history should include age, sex, race, use of tobacco in any form, alcohol abuse, and exposure to carcinogens, including radiotherapy, solar exposure, and occupational exposure. Note should be made of any previous surgery in the area of the head and neck; even removal of minor-appearing skin lesions may be significant. The examiner should determine the onset of the mass, its growth or fluctuation in size, the presence of other masses locally or elsewhere, and whether the lesion is painful or tender. If an infectious process is suspected, inquiry should be made regarding exposure to areas where specific organisms might be endemic. Depending on the location of the lesion, it may be appropriate to inquire about other regional symptoms such as dysphagia, odynophagia, hoarseness, epistaxis, facial pain, and so forth.

Physical Examination

A complete head and neck examination should be done next. This must include evaluation of the scalp, eyes, ears, nose, and throat. Indirect examination of the nasopharynx and larynx should also be accomplished. The tonsillar fossae and tongue base should be palpated, and the floor of the mouth should be examined by bimanual palpation.

The lesion itself should be characterized in terms of its size, position, tenderness, consistency, and mobility. Note should be made of other regional masses. The presence of fluctuance, pulsation, compressibility, and a thrill or bruit should be noted.

Diagnostic Tests

Laboratory Studies. The selection of laboratory tests will be dictated by the clinical presentation of the mass. In most cases, extensive laboratory testing will contribute little to the diagnosis. Therefore, an attempt should be made to order only those tests that are clearly indicated. For instance, a complete blood count and Monospot test might be indicated with acute diffuse cervical adenitis, whereas thyroid function tests and a thyroid scan would likely be warranted with a mass contained within the thyroid.

Radiographic Evaluation. The radiographic studies indicated will also be largely determined by the clinical picture. A mass in the thyroid necessitates a radioactive isotope scan of that organ, whereas angiography is more appropriate for a suspected carotid body tumor. Although the most effective overall patient care is delivered by a primary care physician, the regional specialist is ordinarily better able to select those tests and laboratory studies that will lead to the most efficient, and cost-effective, diagnosis.

Following the aforementioned diagnostic tests, it may be necessary to proceed with endoscopy of the esophagus, pharynx, and tracheobronchial tree and, on occasion, direct examination with biopsy of the nasopharynx under anesthesia. Familiarity with the metastatic pathways and lymph node drainage for head and neck lesions is essential for the work-up and diagnosis of head and neck lesions. Knowledge of specific nodes and node groups may give an indication of the site of the primary lesion. For example, posterior cervical node involvement may represent metastatic carcinoma from the nasopharynx, whereas involvement of the Delphian node may herald carcinoma of the thyroid. Finally, if the preceding tests do not reveal a primary lesion, it may be necessary to perform biopsy by needle aspiration, needle-core biopsy, or excisional biopsy.

Differential Diagnosis

Table 159-1 lists many common causes of head and neck masses.

Table 159-1 Head and Neck Masses

Inflammatory Conditions	**Neoplasms**
Cellulitis	*Benign*
Adenitis	Salivary gland
Bacterial	Thyroid
Viral	Carotid body tumors
Deep neck abscess	Glomus jugulare
Mumps	Neurogenic tumors
Thyroiditis	Fibroma
Bezold's abscess	Lipoma
Tuberculosis	Chordoma
Actinomycosis	*Malignant*
Sarcoidosis	Metastatic carcinoma
Ludwig's angina	Thyroid tumors
Tularemia	Salivary gland
Rubella	Fibrosarcoma
Infectious mononucleosis	Liposarcoma
Diphtheria	Rhabdomyosarcoma
Brucellosis	Systemic
Cat scratch disease	Lymphoma
Sialadenitis	Hodgkin's disease
Syphilis	Metastatic disease from a distant primary
Toxoplasmosis	
Wegener's granulomatosis	
Congenital Masses	**Miscellaneous**
Midline	Traumatic
Thyroglossal duct cyst	Spontaneous hemorrhage
Lingual thyroid	Laryngocele
Dermoids and epidermoids	Diverticulum of the esophagus
Teratomas	Vascular aneurysm
Lateral	Muscle rupture
Branchial cleft cysts	
Cystic hygroma	
Hemangioma	

Inflammatory Conditions

Cellulitis and Adenitis. Acute inflammation of the neck may present with diffuse soft-tissue swelling or discrete adenopathy. Cervical adenitis is an extremely common finding in association with upper respiratory tract infection and is most frequently of viral origin. Adenopathy may persist for prolonged periods after resolution of the infection. Bacterial involvement may be a secondary complication of viral adenitis or a primary infection. The most common etiologic organisms are *Streptococcus* and *Staphylococcus.* Bacterial cervical adenitis may localize or resolve with or without the aid of antibiotic therapy. At times the nodes will become fluctuant, reflecting abscess formation that may extend to the deep neck spaces. Deep neck infections are generally characterized by edema and induration. Fluctuance is usually difficult to appreciate owing to the depth of the infection. Specific signs and symptoms depend on which of the potential deep spaces is involved. For example, Horner's syndrome is seen if the lesion involves the sympathetic trunk; hoarseness may indicate involvement of the vagus; spiking temperatures are characteristic of thrombophlebitis of the jugular vein; and bleeding from the pharynx or external auditory canal may herald major vessel involvement. Such infections may have a catastrophic outcome if appropriate steps are not taken to provide drainage of the abscess cavity.

Mumps. Mumps is a relatively common acute inflammatory disease of the salivary glands and most frequently involves the parotid gland. The lesion is characterized by pain, swelling, and tenderness. The course of the disease is usually benign, but it may be associated with significant complications such as orchitis or deafness. The differential diagnosis includes sialadenitis of other etiologies. The white blood cell count in mumps generally reveals a lymphocytosis.

Thyroiditis. Inflammatory disease of the thyroid is uncommon and can be divided into three types. Acute bacterial thyroiditis is generally associated with marked pain and swelling; on occasion, upper airway compromise may occur. There is an associated leukocytosis. Bacterial thyroiditis usually responds to antibiotics, but occasionally surgical drainage is required. Subacute thyroiditis (De Quervain's) is thought to be viral in origin. It is associated with a poor uptake of radioactive iodine and elevated thyroxine and triiodothyronine levels. Although it usually responds to aspirin and heat, occasionally steroids and thyroid replacement are indicated. Chronic thyroiditis is associated with either a lymphocytic infiltrate, as seen in Hashimoto's disease, or a fibrous infiltrate, which is characteristic of Riedel's struma. The diagnosis is made by measuring the antibody titers.

Bezold's Abscess. Rarely, a chronic infection of the mastoid will dissect anteriorly and may present as an abscess in the digastric space just under the mandible. This has been named a Bezold's abscess.

Tuberculosis. Although the condition is relatively uncommon today, patients still present with tuberculous adenitis. The nodes are frequently matted together. Cervical involvement is thought to be secondary to hematogenous seeding from a pulmonary primary. The diagnosis is suspected if there is a history of contact with a person who is actively infected or of exposure to a region where tuberculosis is endemic. The diagnosis can be confirmed with chest radiograph, gastric washings, or culture of the node or draining sinus tract. If the nodes are fluctuant, they will require incision and drainage combined with medical therapy. If the adenopathy fails to resolve, surgical excision may be necessary. Involvement of the neck with atypical mycobacteria is more common than *Mycobacterium* tuberculosis. With this organism, the nodes are less likely to be matted. Several groups of atypical mycobacteria have been identified. Skin testing generally confirms the diagnosis in the presence of a negative purified protein derivative test. The treatment involves resection of the involved nodes.

Actinomycosis. Actinomycosis is an uncommon fungal infection that is usually associated with previous dental infection or recent dental surgery. The infection may involve the salivary glands or the cervical nodes, and localized abscesses commonly form draining cutaneous sinus tracts. The diagnosis is generally made on the basis of a smear that reveals "sulfur granules" and by culture. The treatment is long-term penicillin therapy.

Rubella. Rubella is a common viral infection that is generally characterized by its systemic symptoms. The most frequent involvement of the cervical nodes is manifested by the suboccipital and postauricular node swelling and tenderness.

Infectious Mononucleosis. Infectious mononucleosis produces one of the most impressive examples of cervical adenopathy. The adenitis is characteristically associated with systemic symptoms such as sore throat, fatigue, and temperature elevation. The spleen and liver are often enlarged. The diagnosis is made by the preponderance of lymphocytes on the complete blood count with usually at least 10 to 15 percent atypical forms. The diagnosis can be confirmed by measuring the heterophile antibodies or by a Monospot test. Treatment is primarily symptomatic.

Diphtheria. Diphtheria is a relatively rare disease today, but it must be considered in a differential diagnosis for any patient with acute throat infection. There is characteristic cervical adenopathy and relatively severe systemic symptoms, including headache, nausea, vomiting, and toxemia. The temperature is generally moderately elevated. There may be a characteristic firm gray membrane covering the tonsils. When the membrane is removed, the tonsils bleed freely. The diagnosis can be confirmed with culture. Specific diphtheria antitoxin must be used to neutralize the circulating toxin.

Cat Scratch Disease. The exact etiology of cat scratch disease has not been confirmed, but it is thought to be viral. The lesion produces a granulomatous involvement of local nodes that is generally multiple. There is usually a history of exposure to cats, but a specific history of cutaneous injury cannot always be documented. Skin tests are difficult to obtain, and the diagnosis is primarily one of exclusion.

Syphilis. The incidence of sexually acquired diseases continues to increase. Although a history of exposure frequently cannot be obtained, a possible spirochetal etiology for cervical adenopathy must be considered in any patient presenting with one or more tender neck nodes.

Congenital Masses

Thyroglossal Duct Cysts. Thyroglossal duct cysts occur relatively commonly in children and young adults. The thyroid gland develops from the foramen cecum at the base of the tongue and descends into the anterior neck region during the first trimester of fetal development. The developmental path is intimately involved with the hyoid bone and usually has no external communication. Along the epithelial tract, remnants of tissue may present as cysts or functional thyroid. Most cysts appear before 20 years of age. They are generally asymptomatic but may increase in size, particularly with upper respiratory tract infections. Occasionally, surgical drainage of an infected cyst is necessary, but definitive therapy requires excision of the entire cyst and tract to the base of the tongue.

Lingual Thyroid. Lingual thyroid is residual thyroid tissue at the base of the tongue that has failed to descend into the neck in normal embryologic development. This may represent the only functioning thyroid tissue; therefore, a thyroid scan should be done prior to surgical extirpation of the lesion. Any midline mass at the base of the tongue should be considered of possible thyroid origin. This lesion should not be confused with the normal lingual tonsils, which may achieve considerable size but are lateral and usually symmetric.

Dermoids and Epidermoids. Dermoid and epidermoid cysts are generally found in the midline and are relatively superficial. The epidermoid cyst contains only squamous epithelium and cheesy debris, whereas dermoid cysts contain other skin structures such as hair follicles and sweat glands.

Teratomas. Teratomas are derived from three germ layers. They may contain tissue representing muscle, bone, fat, cartilage, or neural tissue. They generally appear during the first year of life and may or may not be symptomatic, depending on location. They are rarely malignant.

Branchial Cleft Cysts. The branchial cleft cyst represents a remnant of the fifth branchial arches and associated pouches and grooves. The branchial cyst may present as a painless mass at any age and occurs with equal frequency in men and women. When the cyst has an associated fistula or sinus tract, the path of the tract depends upon the arch from which the cyst has been derived.

It is important to be familiar with the embryology of the first five arches and the structures that are derived from them. First branchial cleft cysts are found above the hyoid bone. They may have an internal opening in the external auditory canal and be associated with otorrhea. This tract is closely approximated to the facial nerve. If an external opening exists, it will be found beneath the angle of the mandible. The second branchial sinus tract opens internally in the area of the tonsillar fossa and externally along the anterior border of the sternocleidomastoid muscle. The tract passes over the ninth and twelfth cranial nerves and between the external and internal branches of the carotid artery. The third branchial cleft sinus opens internally in the area of the lower lateral hypopharynx, and the tract is superficial to the hypoglossal nerve and deep to the glossopharyngeal nerve. Its tract runs posterior to both branches of the carotid artery before entering the hypopharynx through the area of the thyrohyoid membrane. Fourth branchial cleft anomalies have not been demonstrated.

Cystic Hygroma. Cystic hygromas are derived from a large lymphatic sac in the neck of the embryo. Frequently, they are present at birth, and all are evident by the second year of life. The lymphatic tissue does not communicate with the remainder of the lymphatic system and therefore accumulates fluid and increases in size. They may be demonstrated to transilluminate. Cystic hygromas tend to have multiple processes intimately involving the other structures of the area. This lesion may be fatal if the upper airway is compressed as a result of swelling or hemorrhage within the cyst.

Neoplasms

Any of the tissues of the head or neck may develop benign or malignant neoplasms. Each organ may be associated with tumors derived from its respective cell type. Although a full description of all tumors is beyond the scope of this chapter, a few of the more common lesions are mentioned.

Benign

Salivary Gland Lesions. Most of the tumors derived from the major salivary glands are benign. Lesions derived from minor salivary glands, however, have a high incidence of malignancy. The majority of salivary gland tumors occur in the parotid gland; of these, approximately 75 to 80 percent are benign. The most common benign parotid tumor is the mixed tumor or pleomorphic adenoma. Another common tumor is papillary cystadenoma lymphomatosum, or Warthin's tumor, which is generally seen in men 45 years of age or over and is frequently bilateral.

Carotid Body Tumors. The carotid body tumor is a nonchromaffin paraganglioma derived from the carotid body, a chemoreceptor situated at the carotid bifurcation. These uncommon tumors are generally not functional and are found in middle-aged and older patients. They may be multiple. The lesion usually presents as a firm, painless mass in the neck. It is slow growing and is frequently associated with a bruit. Carotid body tumors are usually benign and radioresistant. The characteristic angiogram demonstrates a tumor blush in the area of the carotid bifurcation, separating the internal and external carotid arteries—the "lyre sign."

Neurogenic Tumors. Neurogenic tumors include the neurilemomas derived from the nerve sheath and neurofibromas. The tumor may present as a single nodule or in multiple locations, such as in von Recklinghausen's disease. Occasionally, a malignant variant may be seen.

Thyroid Tumors. Most thyroid tumors are found to be benign. However, the suspicion of malignancy is increased with factors such as previous irradiation, rapidity of growth, invasion of the

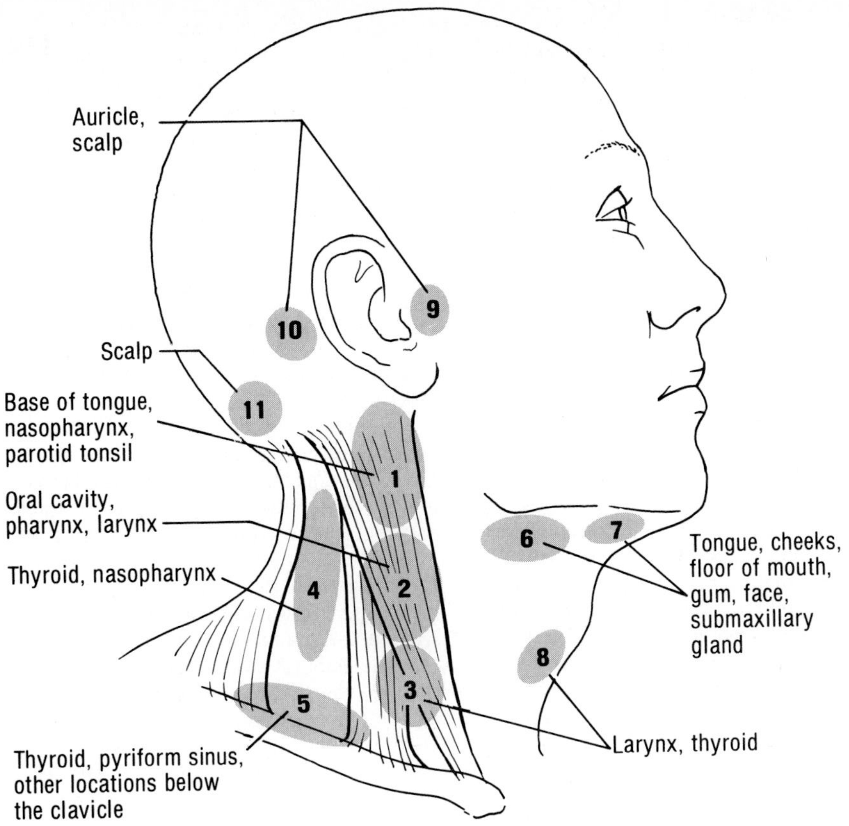

Figure 159-1 Metastatic lymph node sites in primary cancer of the head and neck. Labels indicate the site of the primary cancer. Lymph node groups are identified by number as follows: (*1*) superior jugular chain, (*2*) middle jugular chain, (*3*) inferior jugular chain, (*4*) posterior triangle, (*5*) supraclavicular (left—Virchow's node), (*6*) supramandibular (*7*) submental, (*8*) cricothyroid (Delphian node), (*9*) preauricular, (*10*) postauricular, and (*11*) occipital.

skin, trachea, or esophagus, paralysis of the recurrent laryngeal nerve with vocal cord palsy, and family history of thyroid cancers. Malignant nodules usually scan "cold"; i.e., they do not pick up the radioactive iodine tracer used for thyroid scanning.

Malignant

Primary Malignancies. Malignant tumors can be derived from any of the aforementioned organs or any of the tissues of the head or neck. The clinical picture will vary widely, depending on the organ or area involved. The work-up is directed at specific lesions that are suspect from the clinical presentation.

Metastatic Nodes. Progressive cervical adenopathy in an adult must be regarded as evidence of malignancy until proved otherwise. Approximately 80 to 85 percent of metastatic cervical nodes are derived from a primary tumor in the head or neck. Distant neoplasms account for slightly less than 10 percent of the metastatic nodes, and primaries of unknown origin account for the remaining 5 percent. In some cases the primary lesion is never discovered, even at autopsy. By far the most frequent primary malignancy is of epidermoid (squamous) origin. Every attempt must be made to identify the site of the primary tumor prior to violating the neck. Occasionally, aspiration or core-needle biopsy will be required to establish the cell type. This is usually not associated with an increased risk of spread of the tumor. Incisional or excisional biopsy without definitive therapy of the neck, however, is associated with a marked increase in morbidity and mortality. It is essential that the physician be familiar with the lymphatic drainage of the head and neck so that the most likely primary site can be investigated (Fig. 159-1).

Miscellaneous

Hematoma. Injury to the neck, either from blunt trauma or from sudden movement, may result in a vascular injury or, occasionally, stripping of the sternocleidomastoid muscle from its insertion. This will lead to hematoma formation. Patients who receive anticoagulant therapy are at increased risk for spontaneous bleeding into the soft tissues of the neck.

Laryngocele. The laryngocele, a sac-like dilation of the laryngeal ventricle, may present as a mass in the neck. This diagnosis can generally be confirmed with anteroposterior and lateral radiographs of the neck. This mass is seen in glass blowers and musicians who play wind instruments.

Diverticulum. Zenker's diverticulum of the cervical esophagus may present as a neck mass, usually on the left side. The patient may give a history of progressive dysphagia and occasionally bring up previously eaten undigested food. On physical examination, crepitus may be identified over the neck mass.

Muscle Rupture. Weight lifters, who can tear neck muscles while lifting, may have a scarred muscle remnant that presents as a lump in the occipital region. There is usually a history of a sharp pain, and some patients hear an audible snap at the time of rupture.

Vascular Masses. An aneurysm of the carotid artery may rarely present as a neck mass. There is frequently a characteristic bruit or flow murmur. Occasionally, it is difficult to differentiate an aneurysm from a vessel that is simply tortuous. Diagnosis can be confirmed by arteriography.

References

Adams GL, Boies LR Jr, Hilger PA, eds. Fundamentals of otolaryngology. 6th ed. Philadelphia: WB Saunders, 1989.

DeWeese DD, et al, eds. Textbook of otolaryngology. 7th ed. St. Louis: CV Mosby, 1987.

Earache

George H. Eypper, MD

160

Causes of pain in the ear may be divided into two groups: (1) primary, in which the pathologic process is in the same location as the perceived pain, and (2) secondary, or referred, in which the pathologic process is not in the ear at all.

Neuroanatomy

The fact that it is possible for pain to be referred to the ear is due to the complex neuroanatomy of the organ. General somatic afferent pain fibers from the external ear, external auditory canal, and external tympanic membrane are carried by cranial nerves V3, VII, IX, and X, as well as by the greater auricular and lesser occipital nerves, both of which contain fibers from spinal nerves C2 and C3. General visceral afferent pain fibers from the middle ear, medial tympanic membrane, most of the mastoid air cells, and the posterior end of the eustachian tube are carried by the tympanic nerve, a branch of cranial nerve IX. General visceral afferents from parts of some mastoid air cells are carried by the meningeal branch of V3. Approximate innervation of the external ear is shown in Figure 160-1.

A discussion of the courses and interconnections of these nerves is beyond the scope of this text, and the interested reader is referred to the reference by Williams and Warwick. The cell bodies of the general somatic afferent pain fibers of cranial nerves V3, VII, IX, and X supplying the external ear are located in the gasserian, geniculate, superior petrosal, and jugular ganglia, respectively, and all send their central connections to the spinal nucleus of V. In this respect, all the general somatic afferent pain fibers from the ear may be considered to be part of the trigeminal system.

Other structures innervated by general somatic afferent pain fibers that comprise parts of V3 are the anterior two-thirds of the tongue, the lower teeth and gums, the mucous membrane within the cheek, the skin over the lower face and chin, the dura of the middle cranial fossa, and the temporomandibular joint. Pathologic processes involving these structures occasionally produce pain that is perceived as coming at least in part from the ear.

The cell bodies of the general visceral afferent pain fibers of cranial nerve IX that supply the middle ear are found in the inferior petrosal ganglion and send their central connections to the caudal part of the nucleus of the tractus solitarius. Thus, these pain fibers may be regarded as part of the vagal system, which also carries general visceral afferent pain fibers from the posterior one-third of the tongue, the mucous membranes of the uvula, soft palate, posterior pharyngeal wall from the eustachian tube to the tip of the epiglottis, the lateral pharyngeal wall and the tonsillar region (all IX), and from the lower pharynx, larynx, trachea, and upper esophagus (X). Pathologic processes in these regions may also produce pain that is perceived as coming from the ear.

History and Physical Examination

A diagnosis can usually be made after a careful history and physical examination. During the history, it is wise to ask the

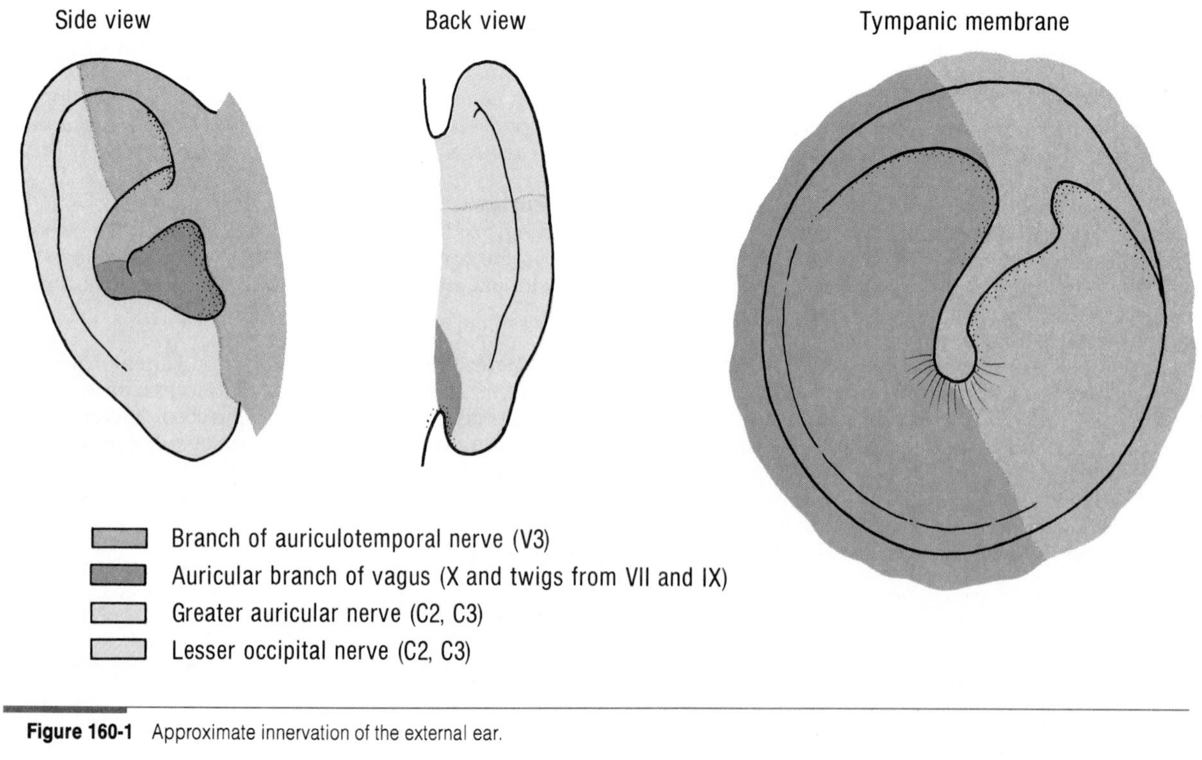

Figure 160-1 Approximate innervation of the external ear.

patient to localize the pain by outlining or pointing to the exact region that hurts.

A thorough review of systems should include questions about the following symptoms:

1. Ears: discharge, swelling, ulceration, deafness, tinnitus, vertigo, trauma, prior surgery, prior infection
2. Nose and sinuses: facial pain, discharge, nosebleed
3. Mouth: toothache, ulceration, soreness of mouth or tongue, difficulty chewing
4. Throat: hoarseness, sore throat, dysphagia, hemoptysis
5. Neurologic: headaches, diplopia, facial weakness, changes in taste sensation, impaired equilibrium
6. General: fever, chills

The auricle and mastoid process should be carefully palpated and examined visually. Hearing should be tested and the external canal and tympanic membrane examined. Palpation of a normal-looking canal with a tightly wound cotton-tipped wire applicator may produce tenderness, allowing localization of early neoplasm. This done, the examiner must not forget to palpate the temporomandibular joint as the patient opens and closes the mouth. The nose, mouth, and throat should be inspected carefully. The teeth, especially the lower molars, should be tapped individually with a tongue blade to elicit tenderness. If the patient is cooperative, the tonsillar fossa may be palpated for evidence of a tender styloid process, and structures in the floor of the mouth may be palpated bimanually between index fingers placed under the chin and on the floor of the mouth. The sinuses should be transilluminated and palpated for tenderness. The neck should be examined carefully for nodes, tenderness, bruits, and thyromegaly. Finally, the cranial nerves should be examined.

Differential Diagnosis

In the child, most ear pain is caused by local processes, usually suppurative otitis media or otitis externa. Otitis media is rare in adults; furunculosis, otitis externa, and referred pain become common. In old age most ear pain is referred, often from the teeth, temporomandibular joint, or degenerative joint disease of the cervical spine: True otitis media in an adult requires referral to an otolaryngologist to rule out the possibility that a pharyngeal tumor is causing eustachian tube blockage.

The reader is encouraged to examine the patient and then refer to Table 160-1, which is divided into sections based on the

Table 160-1 Lesions That Cause Otalgia

Lesion	Subjective findings	Objective findings	Comments
Lesions Visible on the Auricle			
Furuncle	Pain, especially on manipulation of auricle	Tender on manipulation; visible pustule	Most common cause of ear pain
Acute otitis externa of auricle	Pain, swelling, weeping of external ear	Red, tender, oozing, crusting lesions; pustules often present; if tympanic membrane visible, may be red; landmarks present; lymphadenopathy, fever sometimes present	*Staphylococcus aureus* is most common organism; eczema, seborrheic dermatitis, contact dermatitis, psoriasis may be predisposing factors, but seen alone they cause itching, not pain
Infected sebaceous cyst	Tender lump behind ear	Tender nodule, sometimes red, fluctuant, or pointing in skin behind lobule	Common
Trauma	History of trauma	Abrasions, laceration, hematoma; parts of ear may be severed completely from the head	Preserve severed parts in iced saline for subsequent reattachment
Perichondritis	Severe pain, followed by redness, swelling; history of burn or trauma to same area 3–5 wk earlier	Red, warm, swollen, tender auricle with intact skin; sparing of lobule	Diabetes mellitus may be predisposing factor; high incidence of recurrence
Frostbite	History of cold exposure; onset of pain with rewarming	Erythema, weeping vesiculation on helix, lobule	Never rub with snow; avoid radiant heat and surgical debridement
Chondrodermatitis (nodularis chronica helices)	Pain localized in nodule on helix	Grayish firm nodule, size of pea on free edge of auricle; exquisitely tender	Uncommon
Relapsing polychondritis	Fever, ear pain, pain in nose, hoarseness, joint pain	Red, warm, tender, swollen auricles bilaterally with intact skin; sparing of lobule; may have scleritis, arthritis	Rare; elevated erythrocyte sedimentation rate; respiratory stridor may herald tracheal obstruction and should be considered an emergency
Herpes zoster oticus (Ramsay Hunt syndrome)	Pain, often overshadowed by facial weakness; sometimes with vertigo, hearing loss, altered taste, hyperacusis, rash in ear	Vesicular eruption in external auditory meatus, concha, skin of crease behind ear, and sometimes ipsilateral anterior tongue; peripheral facial weakness; sometimes with sensorineural hearing loss, decreased lacrimation, loss of taste on ipsilateral anterior two-thirds of tongue	Rare; herpes zoster of cranial nerves V, VII, IX, or X; Tzanck smear of scrapings of base of vesicle shows eosinophilic intranuclear inclusions and multinucleated giant cells; may be followed by postherpetic neuralgia

Table continues on following page

Table 160-1 *(Continued)*

Lesion	Subjective findings	Objective findings	Comments
Lesions Visible in the External Canal			
Acute otitis externa of external canal	Pain, discharge, decreased hearing or sensation of blockage if canal swollen shut	Tender with traction on auricle or pressure on tragus; patient may refuse to allow otoscope exam; canal is swollen, inflamed; tympanic membrane may be red, but landmarks are visible, and it is mobile on pneumatic otoscopy; lymphadenopathy common	Causative organisms are *Pseudomonas aeruginosa, Proteus vulgaris, Staphylococcus aureus,* and *Streptococcus;* predisposing factors same as for acute otitis externa of auricle
Furuncle in external canal	Pain, especially on manipulation of ear	Tender with pressure on tragus; pustule visible with otoscope exam	Common
Foreign body	Pain; sometimes drainage, tinnitus; sometimes asymptomatic	Foreign body readily visible	May require much skill to remove without damage to canal and tympanic membrane
Malignant otitis externa	Severe ear pain, usually in an elderly diabetic or immunosuppressed patient	Granulation tissue at junction of bony and cartilaginous canals; pain on manipulation of ear; tympanic membrane may be intact; development of cranial neuropathy portends poor prognosis	Rare; lethal unless quickly and properly treated; causative organism almost always *Pseudomonas aeruginosa,* which causes necrotizing vasculitis and spreads rapidly to periauricular soft tissue and to mastoid, eroding bone
Keratosis obturans (cholesteatoma of external auditory canal)	Pain from erosion of bony canal; sometimes deafness, otorrhea	Pearly white glistening mass deep in canal	Associated with bronchiectasis, sinusitis; rare
Cancer of external canal	Pain may be early, intense, out of proportion to physical findings; sometimes otorrhea, bleeding, hearing loss	Localized growth, which must be biopsied	Basal cell, squamous, or adenoid cystic carcinoma; rare
Lesions Visible on Examination of the Tympanic Membrane			
Acute suppurative otitis media	Severe throbbing pain in ear, hearing loss, fever; possibly nausea, vomiting, dizziness; onset of otorrhea coincides with decrease in pain (perforation of the tympanic membrane relieves middle-ear pressure, decreasing the pain)	Diffusely red tympanic membrane, immobile to pneumatic otoscopy, either bulging or without visible landmarks; perforated if otorrhea present; conductive hearing loss; usually tender mastoid; diffusely red tympanic membrane without bulging and with landmarks visible is an unreliable sign	*Pneumococcus, Branhamella catarrhalis,* group A streptococci most common organisms; *Haemophilus influenzae* common in young children; predisposing factors: young age (short, horizontal eustachian tube allows entry of organisms), upper respiratory infection or allergy (both cause eustachian tube swelling with mechanical blockage), cleft palate (causes functional eustachian tube obstruction, or "floppy tube"), pharyngeal tumor (adults)
Bullous myringitis	Malaise and headache followed by fever, myalgias, sore throat, then cough and earache, which may be severe	Inflamed tympanic membrane and adjacent canal with bullae that are sometimes hemorrhagic; inflamed throat; pulmonary crackles frequently occur	Symptom complex due to *Mycoplasma pneumoniae* infection; chest film may show infiltrate
Secretory (serous) otitis media	Hearing loss, feeling of fullness; usually painless, but sometimes associated with brief episodes of pain, especially on sneezing, blowing nose	Amber, dull, retracted tympanic membrane; incus not visible; immobile to pneumatic otoscopy; a fine black horizontal line represents an air-fluid level in middle ear; sometimes air bubbles seen through tympanic membrane	Predisposing factors same as noted above for suppurative otitis media; middle ear effusion usually sterile; adults with secretory otitis media must be referred to an otolaryngologist for exam and possible biopsy to rule out pharyngeal cancer

Table 160-1 (*Continued*)

Lesion	Subjective findings	Objective findings	Comments
Acute mastoiditis	Failure to respond to therapy for suppurative otitis media; persistent ear pain; slowly increasing purulent discharge	Usually tympanic membrane is perforated, with purulent drainage in external canal; sometimes sagging of posterosuperior bony canal; tender mastoid process	Radiographs of temporal bone show clouding of mastoid air cells caused by their failure to drain through perforated tympanic membrane; requires treatment by otolaryngologist to prevent potentially lethal complications
Complications of acute mastoiditis, chronic otitis media, chronic mastoiditis	See symptoms of acute mastoiditis; chronic otitis media and mastoiditis characterized by hearing loss and intermittent painless discharge over months to many years, without fever; in this setting, onset of unexplained fever, earache, ipsilateral headache (especially if relieved at times of ear drainage), vertigo, or symptoms referable to ipsilateral cranial nerves may represent an emergency	See signs of acute mastoiditis; permanent perforation (sometimes difficult to see) of the tympanic membrane and conductive hearing loss are the hallmarks of chronic otitis media and mastoiditis; presence of a white, shiny, opalescent mass in the middle ear or canal represents a cholesteatoma; fever, fluctuance over the mastoid process, abnormal exam of ipsilateral cranial nerves VI–XI, cerebellar signs, or focal seizures may signify life-threatening infection; a mass in the middle ear may represent cancer	Pain in this setting may represent infection eroding into the central nervous system, a cholesteatoma (debris from abnormal squamous epithelialization of the middle ear cavity), eroding bones of the middle ear, or cancer of the middle ear; although all are exceedingly rare, their importance lies in their devastating consequences. Immediate otolaryngology consultation is mandatory; CT of temporal bone is test of choice
Barotrauma	Pain on rapid descent in airplane; usually associated with sleeping in a semirecumbent position	Tympanic membrane that is amber and retracted, ecchymotic, or bluish, signifying blood in the middle ear	Relatively common
Concussion	Severe pain, partial deafness after proximity to an explosion, after a slap on the ear, or after a fall while water skiing without earplugs; tinnitus, vertigo may occur	Rupture of tympanic membrane, conductive hearing loss	Consult otolaryngologist
Temporal bone fracture	History of trauma	Bluish discoloration of tympanic membrane (signifies blood in middle ear), or blood oozing through torn tympanic membrane; obvious fracture of superior bony canal sometimes seen; hearing loss; sometimes facial nerve paralysis, cerebrospinal fluid otorrhea, or postauricular ecchymosis	Uncommon; obtain radiographs of temporal bone
Lesions Causing Pain Referred to the Ear			
Dental pain	Pain poorly localized to posterior jaw, ear	Pain reproduced by tapping affected tooth with tongue depressor	Causes 50% of pain referred to ear in elderly
Cervical arthritis	Pain behind ear, worse with turning head	Pain reproduced by testing range of motion of neck; may be tender on palpation of posterior neck	Common
Temporomandibular joint dysfunction	Intermittent, sometimes sharp pain localized just anterior to tragus, which is worse on awakening, after talking, chewing, pipe smoking; may be history of recent dental work; history of bruxism (clenching the teeth)	Tenderness, crepitus on palpation of temporomandibular joints while patient opens, closes mouth, moves jaw side to side; may have strong masseter, malocclusion, absent molars, limitation of jaw opening	Common; radiographs usually normal; sometimes affected in rheumatoid arthritis

Table continues on following page

Table 160-1 (*Continued*)

Lesion	Subjective findings	Objective findings	Comments
Elongation of styloid process (Eagle's syndrome)	1. Post-tonsillectomy type: Pain extending from throat to ear, compulsion to swallow, pain on swallowing 2. Carotid artery type: Sharp pain in periauricular region caused by turning head	Both types demonstrate pain, sensation of bony resistance on palpation of tonsillar fossa with gloved finger; in carotid type, the temporal pulse decreases on contralateral head rotation	1. Thought to be caused by calcified stylohyoid ligament rubbing against tonsillectomy scar tissue 2. Thought to be caused by stylohyoid ligament compressing external carotid; panoramic jaw radiograph shows elongated styloid
Tonsillitis, peritonsillar abscess (quinsy)	Throat pain referred to ear, difficulty swallowing, drooling, fever, chills (peritonsillar abscess)	Inflamed pharynx with swollen tonsil(s) with exudate in crypts; unilateral swelling of soft palate and anterior pillar above tonsil denotes peritonsillar abscess	Peritonsillar abscess is infrequent complication of untreated streptococcal sore throat
Angina pectoris	Left neck, jaw, or teeth may occasionally be the sole location of anginal pain; brought on by exercise, relieved by rest; dyspnea, nausea, diaphoresis often present; positive cardiac risk factors	May have tachycardia, increased blood pressure, S_3 gallop, paradoxical split of S_2 during pain	History, electrocardiogram during pain, and exercise tolerance test are keys to diagnosis
Carotidynia	Unilateral, sometimes bilateral, persistent pain extending from just below the angle of the the jaw to the ear	Tender carotid bulb, no other adjacent tender structures	Responds to aspirin or prednisone; should be considered a diagnosis of exclusion
Spontaneous dissection of carotid artery	Unilateral neck, ear, face, head pain; pulsatile tinnitus	Tender over carotid; audible bruit; Horner's syndrome sometimes present; transient ischemic attacks or major stroke may occur	Rare; caused by degeneration of media; angiography verifies diagnosis
Prodrome of Bell's palsy, herpes zoster oticus, or herpes zoster of C2 or C3	Pain, sometimes severe, in or behind ear	Normal physical exam; vesicles occur 4–5 days after onset of pain, providing the diagnosis in zoster; facial weakness provides clue to diagnosis of Bell's palsy	Diagnosed only in retrospect
Glossopharyngeal neuralgia	Severe pain lasting a few seconds that radiates from posterior pharynx to ear; recurs frequently, sometimes for hours; triggered by swallowing cold liquids	Normal physical exam	Rare; history is key to diagnosis, but negative exam of the pharynx and larynx required to rule out lesions in these areas as cause of pain; should be considered a diagnosis of exclusion
Subacute thyroiditis	Neck, ear pain, dysphagia, malaise, chills, fever; may have symptoms of hyperthyroidism	Tender, enlarged, boggy thyroid gland; often fever, tachycardia	Elevated sedimentation rate; T_4 often elevated; diagnosis confirmed by very low radioactive iodine uptake
Cancer of external auditory canal	Ear pain, which may be severe	No visible lesion; localized pain on palpation of external canal with a tightly wound cotton-tipped wire applicator	Rare presentation; requires referral and biopsy

location of the lesion. If at this point there are still questions about the etiology of the pain, referred otalgia from a laryngeal or pharyngeal lesion must be considered. Examples are carcinoma of the pyriform fossa, base of the tongue, vallecula, or larynx; contact ulcer of the larynx; and arthritis of the cricoarytenoid joint. The patient should be referred to an otolaryngologist for careful examination and possible biopsy of these structures.

References

Birt D. Headaches and head pains associated with diseases of the ear, nose and throat. Med Clin North Am 1978; 62:523.

Bluestone CD, Klein JO. Otitis media in infants and children. Philadelphia: WB Saunders, 1988.

DeWeese DD, et al, eds. Textbook of otolaryngology. 7th ed. St. Louis: CV Mosby, 1988.

Gilman S, Winans SS. Essentials of clinical neuroanatomy and neurophysiology. 6th ed. Philadelphia: FA Davis, 1982:81.

Halstead C, et al. Otitis media. Am J Dis Child 1968; 115:542.

Paparella MM. Otalgia. In: Paparella MM, Shumrick DA, eds. Otolaryngology. 2nd ed. Philadelphia: WB Saunders, 1980:1354.

Price J. Otitis externa in children. J R Coll Gen Pract 1976; 26:610.

Williams PL, Warwick R. Fundamental neuroanatomy of man. Philadelphia: WB Saunders, 1975:1001.

Hearing Problems in the Elderly

Janice C. Hitzhusen, MD

161

Definition

Any process that impedes an individual's perception of sound manifests itself as a hearing problem of which the individual may or may not be aware. Hearing loss is expressed in decibels in low, middle, or high frequencies described as mild, moderate, severe, or profound. Most individuals with hearing loss have residual hearing, even when hearing loss is profound. Total deafness is rare. Hearing loss may be classified by side of involvement (unilateral or bilateral) or by onset (sudden or progressive). Tinnitus is a frequent but nonspecific complaint. A person recognizes a hearing loss when there is deterioration of social contacts or of the ability to cope with work responsibilities. The individual may complain of changes in the quality of the sound, so-called dysacusis.

Impaired hearing joins arthritis and cardiovascular disease as one of the most prevalent chronic conditions that affect the physical health of older people. Presbycusis, hearing loss common to older individuals, afflicts approximately 60 percent of individuals over age 65. An estimated 30 percent of people over age 65 and 50 percent of people over age 75 in the community experience overt disability. It is estimated that 90 percent of people living in nursing homes have a hearing loss that interferes with communication. Hearing loss is conductive, sensorineural, or a combination of the two. Conductive hearing problems are due to disorders of the external or middle ear. Sensorineural hearing problems occur when there is a disturbance of the cochlea, eighth cranial nerve, or central auditory channels, which together are referred to as hearing loss of peripheral origin. Sensorineural loss is further subdivided into sensory loss due to changes in the end organ, the cochlea, and neural loss due to changes in the first-order neurons in the eighth cranial nerve. Lesions of the second-order neurons (cochlear nuclei) and more central connections can produce difficulty in perception of speech, referred to as hearing loss of central origin. Mixed or combined hearing loss involves disturbances of both conductive and sensorineural mechanisms.

Diagnostic Approach

History

The first step in the assessment of hearing problems in the older patient is also the most difficult, and that is the simple recognition by the patient, the physician, and the patient's family that hearing impairment is present. There are several reasons why hearing loss may go unrecognized.

Hearing problems, like problems of other body functions, may become accepted by older people and their close associates as a "normal" aspect of aging. Also, hearing loss may develop so gradually that behavioral changes resulting from the hearing loss may be noted before the loss itself. Finally, other medical problems may be present that draw attention away from this impairment. Therefore, a hearing problem may be present for a long time without being brought to the physician's attention.

Identifying the problem requires alertness on the part of the physician. Suspicion of a hearing problem should be raised when the interviewer becomes aware of shouting at or being unable to converse easily with the patient. Family members may complain that the patient "never listens," "has a terrible memory," "is getting peculiar," or "seems to be depressed all the time" and "doesn't want to do anything anymore." Because hearing loss alters sensory experience, it may lead to isolation, detachment, and loss of motivation and independence. The patient's family may tell the physician that the patient is senile. Not infrequently, hard-of-hearing patients become convinced that people are talking about them behind their backs and may become angry and aggressive. The first visit to the physician may, in fact, be the required medical evaluation prior to placement of the individual in a nursing home because the family cannot continue to provide care.

Patients may be aware of a hearing loss but may be reluctant to admit it. They may criticize family members because they "don't speak up," while minimizing their own difficulty in hearing. Persistence on the physician's part is important in obtaining an accurate and full history.

History taking should characterize the hearing loss by side (unilateral or bilateral), type of onset, duration, course, and associated symptoms. Questions regarding occupation, avocation, family history of hearing loss, previous medical or surgical problems of the ear, and drugs taken in the past or at present should be included. The onset and location of the hearing loss may help to establish a differential diagnosis (Table 161-1).

Progressive, bilateral hearing loss is the most common presentation of hearing problems in older people and is often the result of presbycusis, a symmetric, progressive, high-frequency hearing loss. Occupational noise exposure of long duration may be a factor in the development of presbycusis. Certain chemicals and drugs (Table 161-2) may produce a hearing loss. The hearing loss is often bilateral and greatest in the higher frequencies. Ototoxic reactions may be distinguished by their association with symptoms of tinnitus and vertigo (Table 161-3).

Elderly patients often have significantly decreased renal

Table 161-1 Common Causes of Hearing Problems in the Elderly Patient

Progressive Bilateral Hearing Loss	**Sudden Unilateral Hearing Loss**
Presbycusis	Ototoxicity
Occupational noise exposure	Otitis media
Ototoxicity	Meniere's disease
Otosclerosis	Labyrinthitis
Paget's disease	Vascular lesion
Depression	Head trauma
	Barotrauma
Progressive Unilateral Hearing Loss	**Fluctuating Hearing Loss**
Cerumen plug	Ototoxic medications
Cholesteatoma	Meniere's disease
Otosclerosis	Syphilis
Occupational or recreational noise exposure	**Congenital or Longstanding Hearing Loss**
Cerebellopontine angle tumor	
Eighth cranial nerve lesion	
Cortical involvement	
Hearing aid dysfunction	

Table 161-2 Ototoxic Drugs

Antibiotics	Diuretics
Chloramphenicol	Ethacrynic acid
Colistin (polymyxin E)	Furosemide
Dihydrostreptomycin	**Miscellaneous Drugs**
Gentamicin	Atropine
Kanamycin	Barbiturates
Tobramycin	Caffeine
Minocycline	Chlordiazepoxide
Neomycin	Ergot
Pharmacetin	Morphine
Polymyxin B	Nitrogen mustard
Ristocetin	Procaine (Novocain)
Vancomycin	Quinine
Viomycin	Salicylates

function and, like patients with renal failure, are more susceptible to ototoxicity. Although most commonly the history of otosclerosis is that of worsening of hearing in a woman during or after pregnancy, the bilateral, slowly progressive quality of impairment may result in initial recognition in the elderly patient. Occasionally, hearing may improve in a noisy environment and increased loudness may be enjoyed, in contrast to the unpleasant quality of loudness of presbycusis, so-called recruitment.

When Paget's disease of bone involves the skull, narrowing of the cranial nerve foramina, changes in the ossicular chain, or compression of the auditory, vestibular, and seventh nerves may occur. The resulting hearing loss may be conductive, mimicking mixed or cochlear otosclerosis. The physical characteristics and radiographic findings suggest the etiology. Unilateral hearing loss may result from a cerumen plug that is occluding the external auditory canal. Although removal may completely resolve the impairment, attention should be given to an underlying hearing loss that may also be present.

Physical Examination

The examination of the ear may give some clues to the etiology of the hearing loss. The postauricular region may be scarred from previous surgery or swollen from an infection. Direct pressure over the mastoid may produce pain and suggest acute suppurative otitis media. As the pinna is pulled up and back to visualize the ear canal, pain, erythema, and edema may be evidence of external otitis. Cerumen may occlude the canal and may be removed with a curette under direct visualization. Perforation of the tympanic membrane may indicate suppurative or nonsuppurative otitis media (acute or chronic), ear trauma, or cholesteatoma, a tumor of the middle ear. A normal tympanic membrane is gray in color, and its anatomic landmarks can be identified, i.e., the handle and the short process of the malleus, the anterior and posterior malleolar folds, the pars flaccida and pars tensa, and occasionally the chorda tympani.

During routine inspection of a patient's hearing aid, remove wax from the earmold canal, look for cracks in the tubing, clear the microphone of debris, and check the battery for proper insertion in the battery case and for proper voltage (Fig. 161-1). The patient may complain of squeaking of the hearing aid, which may indicate that the mold does not fit properly or that wax in the earmold canal is adding acoustic feedback. Loss of amplification may be secondary to battery failure.

Tuning fork tests (the Weber and Rinné tests) aid in the differential diagnosis of conductive or sensorineural hearing loss. See Chapter 154, "Hearing Loss," and Figure 154-3 for a description of these tests. The tuning fork tests are not fully diagnostic alone. The audiometric examination provides a more accurate measure of the patient's hearing.

The audiologic assessment provides necessary diagnostic information about the hearing loss that is required for appropriate treatment, such as a hearing aid. The test should be ordered with this possible outcome in mind.

Before the audiologic examination, discuss with the patient the practical considerations of obtaining a hearing aid. Does the individual view the hearing loss as a social handicap? Is the individual motivated to wear a hearing aid? Would the individual require supervision in the care and use of a hearing aid? Would hand deformity or inadequate fine motor coordination make manipulation of small switches difficult? Does the individual require financial assistance? Will the individual wear two aids if hearing loss is bilateral? Prior discussion of these questions with patients will prepare them for the possible outcome of the audiologic assessment and may provide the encouragement necessary to overcome the fear or anxiety of wearing a hearing aid.

Audiometric Assessment

When the physicial examination and appropriate laboratory tests have been completed, the audiologist may proceed with the audiometric assessment of hearing.

Table 161-3 Characteristics of Ototoxic Drugs

	Characteristic Action				
Agent	*Cochleotoxic*	*Vestibulotoxic*	*Transient*	*Permanent*	*Delayed onset*
Dihydrostreptomycin	++	+	No	Yes	Yes
Streptomycin	+	++	No	Yes	No
Neomycin	++++	+	No	Yes	Yes
Kanamycin	+++	+	No	Yes	No
Gentamicin	+	+++	No	Yes	No
Viomycin	++	+++	No	Yes	No
Vancomycin	++	+			Yes
Minocycline		+			
Ethacrynic acid	+	+	Usually	Occasionally	No
Furosemide	+	±	Usually	Occasionally	No
Quinine	+	−	Usually	Rarely	Occasionally
Salicylates	+	+	Always	No	No
Nitrogen mustard	++	++	No	Yes	No

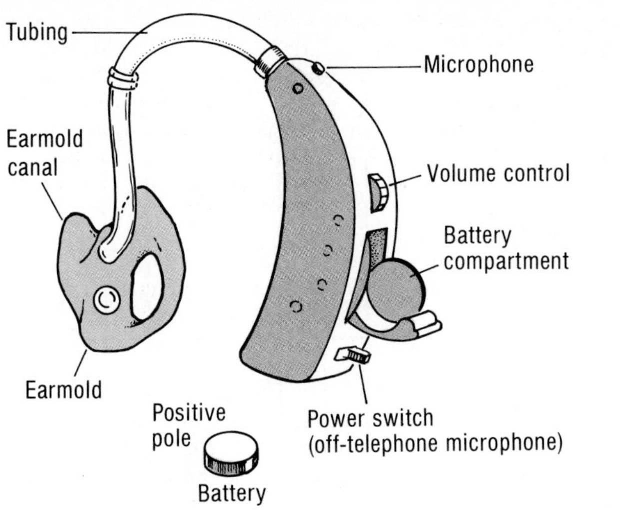

Figure 161-1 A behind-the-ear hearing aid.

The basic hearing test battery includes (1) pure tone testing of thresholds by air conduction and bone conduction, (2) speech reception threshold, (3) speech discrimination score, and (4) acoustic impedance evaluation.

Pure tone audiometry testing utilizes a sound-generating instrument that delivers auditory stimuli to either ear by earphones, an air-conduction pure tone test, or by a vibrator placed on the mastoid process behind the ear, a bone-conduction pure tone test. Specific frequencies (250, 500, 1,000, 2,000, 4,000, and 8,000 Hz) are presented at various intensities (0 to 110 dB) to determine the lowest intensity at which the patient can hear (the threshold). Threshold values measured for each ear are plotted on an audiogram as shown in Figure 161-2A, a normal audiogram. The thresholds for air-conduction and bone-conduction pure tone testing can be compared to determine the site of the hearing problem in the auditory system. A sensorineural hearing loss, a problem in the inner ear or eighth cranial nerve, is illustrated in Figure 161-2B. The air- and bone-conduction thresholds are the same, depressed from normal. A conductive hearing loss, a problem within the outer or middle ear, is represented by Figure 161-2C. Bone-conduction thresholds are in the normal range, whereas air-conduction thresholds are depressed. In hearing loss that is a combination of conductive and sensorineural problems, the air-conduction threshold demonstrates a greater threshold drop than does bone conduction (Fig. 161-2D).

Speech reception audiometry measures the effect of hearing loss on an individual's ability to understand speech. In speech reception threshold (SRT) tests, two-syllable (spondee) words are presented to the patient at decreasing levels of intensity through the earphones, and the patient repeats aloud what has been heard. The SRT is the intensity at which the patient can repeat correctly 50 percent of the words presented.

In speech discrimination testing, 50 single-syllable words are presented to the listener at a comfortable intensity through earphones; the listener's score is determined by the percentage of words that he or she can repeat correctly. Normal hearing is suggested by a score of 90 percent or higher. With a conductive hearing loss, speech discrimination is often normal. Discrimination scores tend to be lower with sensorineural hearing loss. Speech discrimination testing can predict the potential benefit of amplification.

Impedance audiometry testing consists of measurements of the intensity of sound reflected off the eardrum, an assessment of impedance, which is a measure of middle ear function. When sound is absorbed and little is reflected back, low impedance is suggested.

Other audiometric tests can be performed when appropriate. All of these tests require concentration and cooperation for reliable results.

Common Causes of Hearing Impairment in Elderly Patients

Presbycusis

Presbycusis is characterized by a symmetric, slowly progressive, high-frequency, sensorineural hearing loss, and it is common to all populations of people over the age of 40. It is generally noted around the age of 60, although the age of onset and rate of progression vary widely, possibly influenced by genetic and environmental factors. The predominant pathologic change is degeneration of the hair cells of the organ of Corti and the cochlear nerve fibers. Four types of presbycusis can be identified: sensory, neural, strial, and cochlear. *Sensory presbycusis* is characterized by degeneration in the organ of Corti. An abrupt high-tone hearing loss is noted on the audiogram. Speech discrimination is good. *Neural presbycusis* results from degeneration of cochlear neurons. The patient experiences loss of speech discrimination that is more severe than the hearing loss for pure tones noted on the audiogram. Elderly people with rapidly progressive neural presbycusis may also exhibit motor weakness, lack of coordination, tremors, irritability, loss of memory, and intellectual deterioration. *Strial presbycusis* is vascular in origin and manifests atrophy of the stria vascularis. Speech discrimination is excellent. The audiogram threshold line is flat. *Mechanical cochlear presbycusis* may result from stiffness of the basilar membrane, and is characterized by a descending pure tone audiometric pattern for tone conduction. Speech discrimination is inversely related to the steepness of the threshold line.

Typically, a family member complains to the physician about the need to shout to be heard by the patient, the patient's not "paying attention," and the patient's turning up the volume of the radio or television. The patient may deny any problem. High voices and background noise cause the most difficulty. As impairment develops gradually, patients may subconsciously begin to use visual cues such as watching facial expression and lip motion more closely. Recruitment, the patient's subjective experience of an abnormal loudness when sound volume increases, makes the problem worse. Loud sounds become irritating. Tinnitus often accompanies the hearing impairments of presbycusis and varies in quality and quantity. It is often the presenting complaint.

Ototoxicity

Hearing loss and tinnitus can result from the detrimental effects of drugs and chemicals on the inner ear, so-called ototoxic drugs. The common ones are (1) antibiotics (aminoglycoside group, including streptomycin and gentamicin, which cause primarily vestibular damage, and kanamycin, dihydrostreptomycin, and neomycin, which cause primarily cochlear damage); and (2) other drugs, including quinine, salicylates, and diuretics (ethacrynic acid and furosemide), which cause cochlear damage. With some drugs, damage is arrested after discontinuation of the drug, whereas with others, progressive loss may continue. There is individual variation in susceptibility, and toxicity may occur within so-called safe blood levels. Elderly patients are more susceptible to ototoxic damage because renal function decreases with increasing age, previous ear disease is more likely, and the general health status is usually more fragile than that of younger people. The onset of symptoms is related temporally to the administration of ototoxic drugs. Hearing loss is

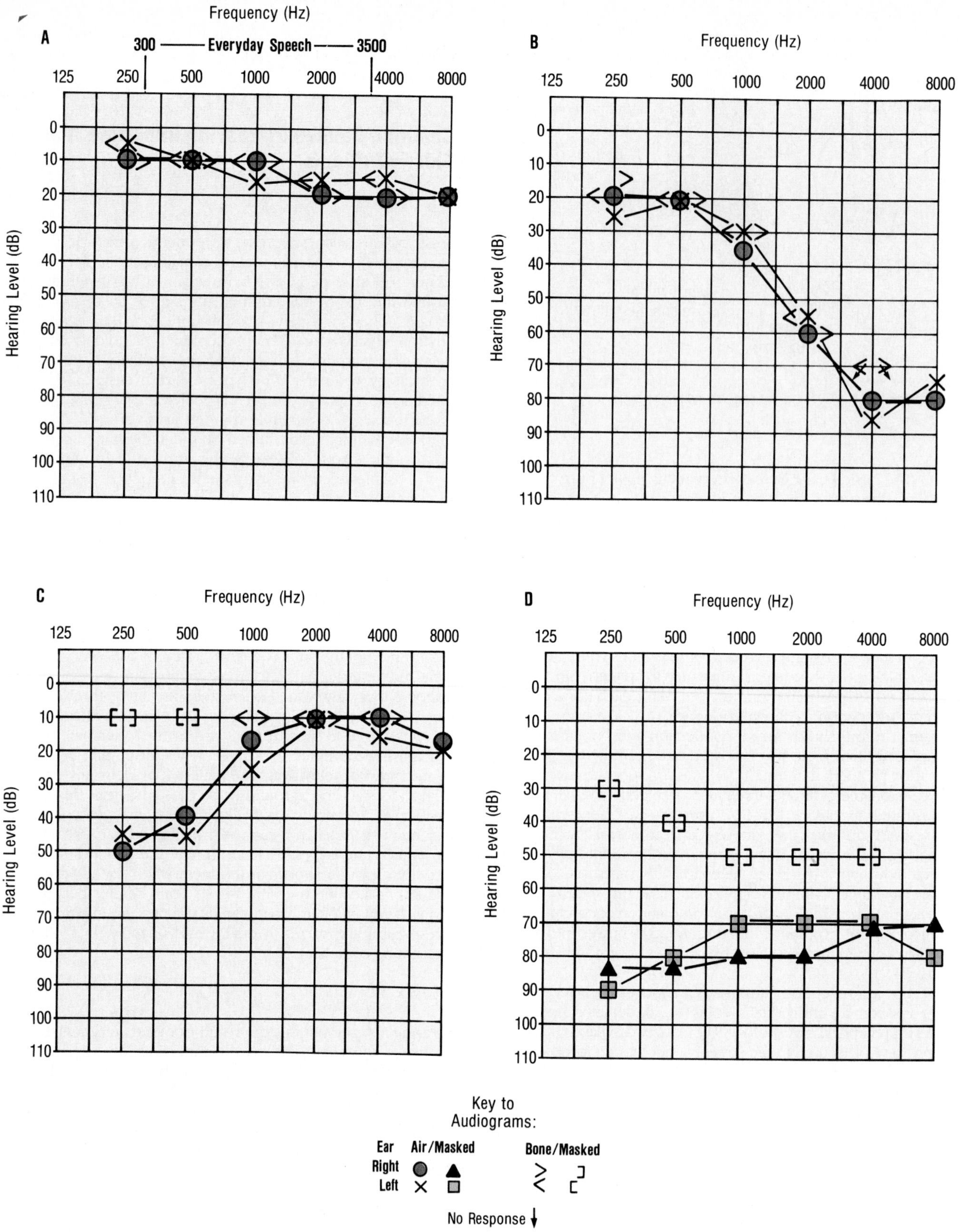

Figure 161-2 Audiograms. (**A**) Normal hearing. (**B**) Sensorineural hearing loss of presbycusis. (**C**) Conductive hearing loss. (**D**) Mixed hearing loss.

sensorineural, bilateral, symmetric, and abrupt, although gradual vestibular dysfunction (dizziness, loss of balance, or ataxia) may be noted for the first time when the patient has recovered from an illness and attempts to ambulate. Ataxia is more severe in darkness. Caloric responses are decreased or absent. The ear examination is normal. Discontinuation of the drug (e.g., salicylates) may reverse the undesirable effect, but more often the effect is irreversible.

Trauma

A variety of forces may injure middle and inner ear structures. Acoustic trauma—explosive pressure waves close to the ear—may disrupt middle and inner ear structures or perforate the tympanic membrane. Noise—unorganized sound waves or frequencies—may induce hearing impairment following chronic exposure to less intense sound pressure waves. Exposure to occupational noises causes more hearing loss than any other noise source. Hair cells become distorted, and vascular changes may result in anoxia. The basal cochlear turn is most susceptible, and initial impairment involves the 4,000-Hz range. Initially, impairment is temporary and reversible in a quiet environment; however, impairment becomes permanent as the time of exposure increases. The magnitude of hearing loss depends on noise intensity, frequency and duration of exposure, an individual's susceptibility, and pre-existing ear disease. High-frequency hearing loss occurs initially, and the individual may not notice the impairment. When the frequency widens to involve 500 to 2,000 cps (the speaking range), communication becomes difficult. Background noise becomes distracting, and women's voices (usually a higher frequency than men's voices) become difficult to hear.

Practical Considerations of the Hearing-Impaired Elderly Patient

Costs of Hearing Aids

Costs of obtaining a hearing aid are as follows: audiologic assessment, \$45.00 to \$75.00; hearing aid mold, \$15.00 to \$40.00; hearing aid fitting, \$80.00 to \$100.00; hearing aid (behind the ear, body aid, in the ear, glasses aid), \$350.00 to \$550.00.

Financial Assistance

All individuals who are on Medicaid may apply for assistance in purchasing an aid or aids. Medicaid will pay for a hearing aid only if a physician has examined the individual and the audiometric evaluation has been done by an audiologist certified by the American Speech-Language-Hearing Association.

Special Devices for the Hearing Impaired

Special devices for the hearing impaired include the following:

1. Captioned television (\$250.00 to \$500.00), Sears and Roebuck Co., Tele-Caption. The major television networks offer programs in which subtitles have been added beneath the picture. A special television set receives the captions (\$500.00). A caption adapter (\$250.00) can be attached to any set and may be used with cable television. For available programming, write to the Caption Center, WGBH-TV, 125 Western Avenue, Boston, MA 02134.
2. Vibravact (\$60.00). An acoustic signal activates vibration of an alarm clock, telephone, or fire alarm.
3. Television phone (\$395.00), Phonics Corporation. A television prerecords conversations for playback on a keyboard-controlled alphanumeric display screen (similar to airline terminals). A light signals that the telephone is ringing.
4. Doorbell and telephone signaler (\$98.95), Nationwide Flashing Signals System. A transmitter system activates a flashing light when the telephone or doorbell rings.
5. Telephone amplifier (no charge), AT&T. A two-button device, 100-A coupler, that adapts to the Trimline phone and amplifies the telephone signal by 10 to 20 dB.
6. Television earphone extension.

References

Meyeroff WL. Diagnosis and management of hearing loss. Philadelphia: WB Saunders, 1984.

Mulrow CD, et al. Quality of life changes and hearing impairment. Ann Intern Med 1990; 113:188.

Gynecology

Vaginitis

Nelson M. Gantz, MD
Susan Connor, RN
Todd W. Hunter, MD

Definition

Vaginitis is an inflammation of the vagina that frequently extends to the vulva. The primary symptoms are unusual vaginal discharge or genital pruritus. This inflammation may be caused by infectious agents, chemical agents, mechanical agents, or neoplasms.

Etiology

Physiologic changes in vaginal discharge are common in the newborn, in pregnancy and in the postpartum period, in puberty and menopause, premenstrually and at ovulation, with sexual excitement, and with the use of oral contraceptives. These are normal variations and should not be confused with symptoms of vaginitis. Physiologic vaginal discharge should be differentiated from nonphysiologic vaginal discharge (Table 162-1).

There are multiple causes for an abnormal vaginal discharge. The three most common types of vaginal infections are caused by *Gardnerella vaginalis, Trichomonas vaginalis,* and *Candida albicans. Gardnerella* (formerly *Haemophilus vaginalis*) is responsible for approximately 50 to 60 percent of vaginal infections. *Trichomonas* and *Candida* each cause about 15 to 20 percent of vaginal infections. A small percentage of vaginal infections are caused by herpesvirus. *Neisseria gonorrhoeae* rarely infects the adult vagina. The discharge associated with this organism originates in the endocervix and passes through the introitus and is perceived as vaginal discharge by the patient. Similarly, *Chlamydia* can cause an excessive cervical discharge. Symptoms of vaginitis are also noted by patients with cervicitis in whom no particular causative organism is identified.

Mechanical agents are also implicated in vaginal symptoms. Examples of these mechanical irritants are a retained tampon, an intrauterine device, or other foreign bodies in the vagina.

Table 162-1 Characteristics of Vaginal Discharge

Characteristics	Physiologic discharge	Nonphysiologic discharge
Odor	Not offensive	Offensive
Vulvar discomfort	Absent	Present
Polymorphonuclear leukocytes	Few	Many
Bacteriology	Predominantly gram-positive bacillus	Altered (see text)
Etiologies	Ovulation Premenses Use of birth control pills Sexual excitement	Dermatologic: allergic, chemical irritation Anatomic: fistula, proctitis, foreign body Infectious Neoplastic

Chemical agents, such as douches, vaginal sprays or perfumes, and contraceptive creams, jellies, foams, and suppositories, are known to produce symptoms of vaginitis in some individuals.

Gynecologic neoplasms may also cause symptoms of unusual vaginal discharge or genital pruritus. The neoplasm may be cervical, vaginal, vulval, or in rare cases, in the fallopian tube.

Diagnostic Approach

An approach to the evaluation of a patient with vaginal discharge is presented in Figure 162-1.

History

Important data to be collected during the patient history include a good menstrual history, including the first day of the last menstrual period. In developing the chief complaint, such information as chronology, type of onset (gradual or acute), history of similar problems in the past, previous therapies or home remedies, recent medication use, and relationship to the menstrual cycle should be explored. A sexual history, especially regarding changes in practices and the presence of symptoms in the partner, is helpful. A contraceptive history is essential, as are hygienic practices, such as the use of feminine hygiene products, douching and wiping practices, changes in soaps or detergents, as well as the wearing of nonporous undergarments or tight-fitting clothing. A medical history of diabetes or family history of diabetes is important information.

Symptoms

The most common symptoms reported by patients with vaginal complaints are a change in the amount or color of their vaginal discharge, a vaginal odor, and itching, discomfort, or burning of the vulvovaginal tissue. Some other frequently reported symptoms include local burning with urination, vulvovaginal redness and swelling, and pain with intercourse. Less frequent complaints include postcoital and intermenstrual bleeding.

Physical Examination

The physical examination includes inspection of the vulvovaginal and cervical tissue, as well as notation of the appearance of the discharge. The inguinal nodes are also checked for enlargement and tenderness.

Laboratory Tests

The most useful and least costly differential diagnostic aid in the evaluation of vaginal complaints is a microscopic examination of the vaginal discharge, using both a saline and a potassium hydroxide (KOH) preparation technique. Determination of vaginal pH is also a simple, cost-effective, and helpful aid.

A saline or wet prep is prepared by taking a sample of the vaginal discharge using a cotton swab. A small amount of discharge is placed on a clean, dry slide. A drop of normal saline is

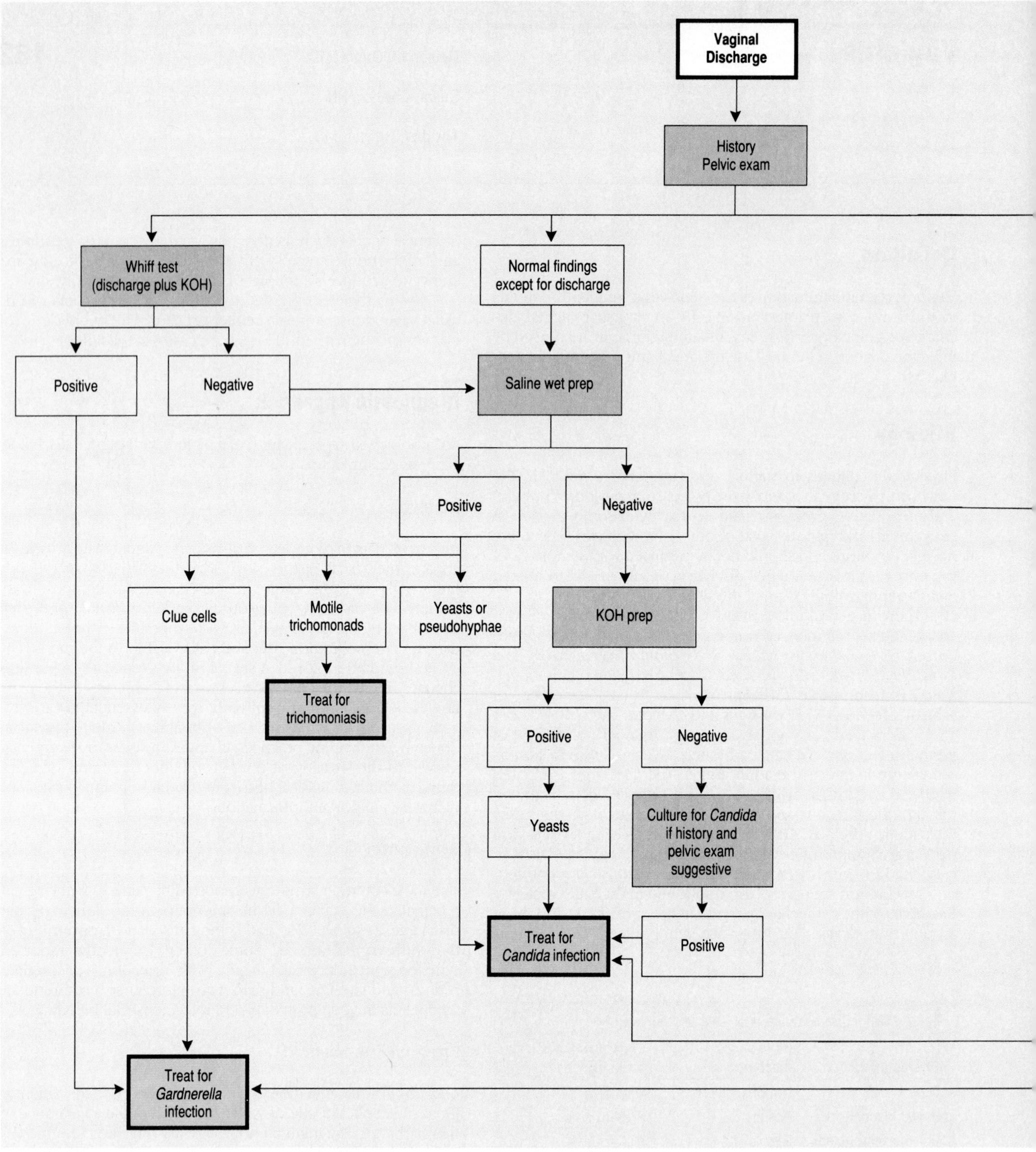

Figure 162-1 Algorithm for the diagnostic evaluation of vaginal discharge. KOH = potassium hydroxide, PMNs = polymorphonuclear leukocytes.

added and covered with a coverslip. This is then analyzed microscopically under 10× power.

A KOH prep is prepared in exactly the same manner, omitting the normal saline and adding a drop of 10 percent potassium hydroxide to the discharge. The combined mixture is then stirred and covered with a coverslip.

To determine the vaginal pH, a small strip of pHydrion tape is introduced into the vagina with a Kelly clamp or sponge forcep to allow the lateral vaginal wall to be touched without touching the speculum.

Other diagnostic tests, which are often unnecessary and can be costly, may be helpful in the differential diagnosis. These

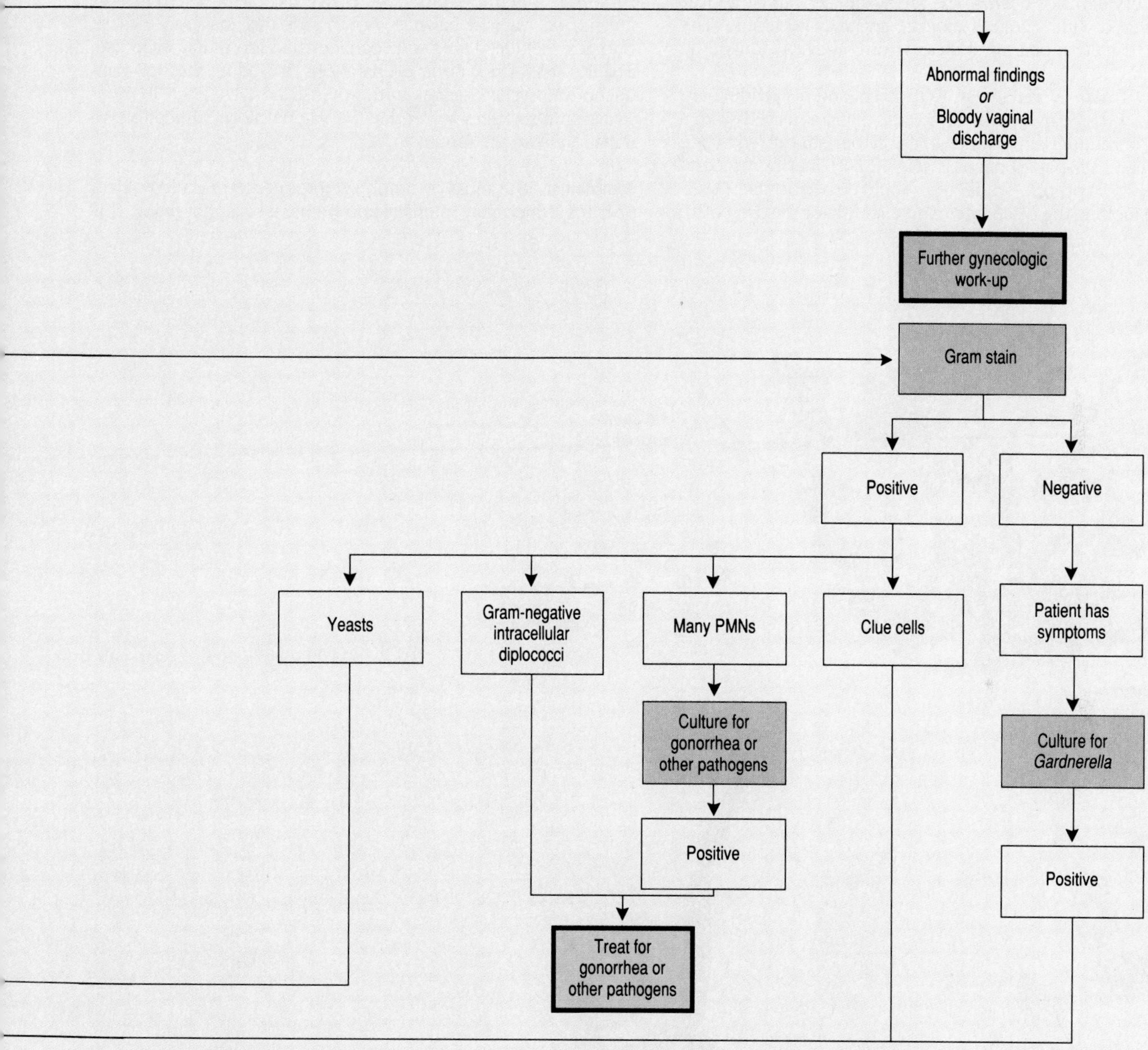

include a Gram stain, bacterial culture, viral culture, fungal culture, and a Papanicolaou (Pap) smear.

Common Vaginal Infections

The three most common vaginal infections are bacterial vaginosis, or *Gardnerella* vaginitis, moniliasis or candidiasis, and trichomoniasis. A more detailed explanation of these conditions may aid in the differential diagnosis of vaginal complaints.

Gardnerella Vaginitis (*Haemophilus vaginalis* Vaginitis)

Etiology. Bacterial vaginosis (formerly nonspecific vaginitis) is thought to account for 50 to 60 percent of vaginal infections. The most common pathogen thought to be implicated in "nonspecific" vaginitis is *Gardnerella vaginalis.* Gardner states that "probably more than 90 percent of vaginitides previously classified as 'nonspecific vaginitis' are caused by *H. vaginalis.*"

Symptoms. These patients generally present with the chief complaints of increased vaginal discharge and vaginal odor. The vaginal discharge is usually described as increased in amount, watery in consistency, and grayish in color. Some patients also complain of a bloody tinge to the discharge. The odor is usually noted to be foul, and many patients report the odor to be worse postcoitally. Some patients report vulval irritation; however, this is usually slight or nonexistent.

Physical Examination. The vulval exam usually reveals little or no vulval erythema or edema. The vagina and cervix may appear to be covered with a grayish exudate and may be friable. The discharge usually appears grayish and frothy and has a foul odor.

Laboratory Tests. A wet smear, KOH prep, and pH reading are done. The wet smear reveals "clue cells," squamous cells with a stippled or granular appearance to the cytoplasm caused by the intracellular rod-shaped bacteria (Fig. 162-2). During preparation of the KOH prep, a "whiff" test should be performed. This is done by smelling the discharge immediately after the drop of 10 percent potassium hydroxide is added. If *Gardnerella* is present, a "fishy" unpleasant odor is usually emitted.

Moniliasis (Candidiasis)

Etiology. *Candida albicans* is a fungus that causes most monilial vaginal infections. Approximately 20 percent of all vaginal infections are monilial vaginitis.

History. Although moniliasis can be sexually transmitted, it occurs more often in women who have experienced changes in the normal vaginal balance. Conditions that may cause these changes include diabetes, pregnancy, lactation, antibiotic use, and the use of hormone preparations, including the oral contraceptive. Cyclic changes in the menstrual cycle prior to menstruation also seem to render the vagina more susceptible to irritation from the fungus.

Symptoms. The most common symptom noted is vulvovaginal pruritus, which may intensify and be most severe at night. This

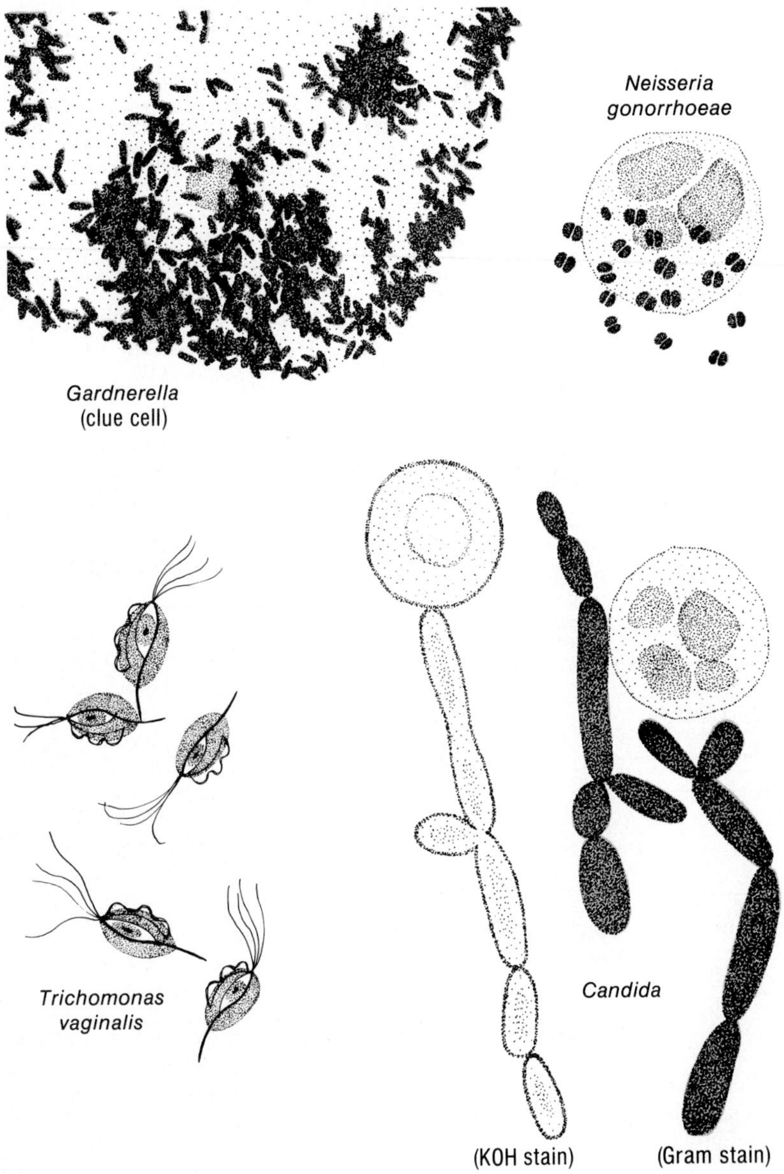

Figure 162-2 Microscopic appearance of common organisms that cause vaginal discharge.

may be accompanied by varying degrees of swelling and redness. Often there is a change in the character of the vaginal discharge, which is described as thick, whitish yellow in color, frequently increased in amount, and bland in odor. Many patients describe the discharge as curdy—like "cottage cheese." The vulvovaginal irritation often causes painful intercourse and local burning with urination.

Physical Examination. The vulva generally is edematous and erythematous and may be excoriated. Curdy, white discharge may be present in the labial folds. The vaginal tissue appears edematous and erythematous. Grayish white thrush-like patches may be present on the vaginal tissue. The vaginal discharge appears thick and whitish yellow in color. The cervix may also appear erythematous and be covered with grayish white, thrush-like patches.

Laboratory Tests. Microscopic analysis of the KOH preparation is the most helpful tool in the immediate diagnosis of candidiasis. The organism appears as budding hyphae and is easily identifiable (see Fig. 162-2). *Candida albicans* rarely survives in a vaginal pH greater than 5. Gram stain or specific fungal cultures may be indicated when there is a high suspicion of moniliasis and the KOH preparation appears negative.

Trichomoniasis

The trichomonad is the causative microorganism of trichomoniasis. It is a parasitic protozoan possessing motile flagella. This form of vaginitis is usually sexually transmitted; infrequently, however, it can be transmitted by close contact with contaminated articles.

History. In this form of vaginitis, prior history of trichomoniasis is useful information in determining the possibility of reinfection. Recent changes in sexual partners as well as the onset of symptoms in relation to the onset of menses are important data. The symptoms of trichomoniasis are generally more severe immediately after the menstrual period.

Symptoms. The most common complaint is that of an abnormal vaginal discharge. The discharge is usually described as thin, watery, bubbly, generally profuse, yellowish green, and foul in odor. Many patients compare the odor to a "fishy" smell. Most patients report some degree of vulvovaginal irritation; however, the severity varies, and it is usually less than in moniliasis. Some patients may note lower abdominal discomfort, other urinary tract complaints, and painful intercourse.

Physical Examination. A slight to moderate amount of abdominal discomfort may be present on palpation of the lower abdomen. The vulval examination may reveal varying amounts of erythema, and a yellowish green, frothy, thin discharge may be noted at the introitus. Increased amounts of this discharge are

Gynecology

Table 162-2 Infectious Vaginal Discharges

Trichomoniasis (*Trichomonas vaginalis*)	60–70% of consorts of infected women positive Usually sexually transmitted	25% asymptomatic, 25% vulvar pruritus, 50% pruritus and discharge Onset often at menses or immediately after; creamy, profuse, frothy discharge; offensive odor Erythematous, excoriated vulva, punctate hemorrhages of cervix	Wet mount of vaginal secretions Pap smear unreliable Culture
Candidiasis and monilial vaginitis (*Candida albicans*)	Sexual transmission plays a minor role Vaginal colonization in 25–50% of asymptomatic, sexually active women Increased prevalence with oral contraceptive use, diabetes, late pregnancy, steroids, and antibiotics	Premenstrual onset of marked vulvar pruritus Discharge odorous, scanty; at times thick, white Vulva erythematous, edematous, excoriated	KOH preparation or Gram stain Culture in symptomatic women with negative KOH preparation
Gonorrhea (*Neisseria gonorrhoeae*)	Sexually transmitted Increase in positive cultures and dissemination during menses	Asymptomatic infection common Vaginal discharge creamy, thick Presence of pelvic inflammatory disease	Gram stain detects 46%; 3% false positive Endocervical culture detects 80–90%, rectal culture an additional 5%
Bacterial vaginosis (anaerobes plus *Gardnerella*)	Sexually active women	Mild to moderate grayish white discharge, mild pruritus	Positive whiff test; few PMNs and sheets of small gram-negative rods; vaginal epithelial cells covered with coccobacilli—clue cells Culture
Purulent vaginitis (unclear etiology)		Vaginal discharge	Gram stain shows sheets of PMNs Culture

Abbreviation: PMNs = polymorphonuclear leukocytes

noted vaginally, and there may be small hemorrhagic petechiae, commonly termed "strawberry spots," noted on the vaginal mucosa. The cervix may appear inflamed and also contain these "strawberry spots." Slight discomfort may be noted on bimanual and rectovaginal examination (Table 162-2).

Laboratory Tests. The most helpful diagnostic aid in the immediate diagnosis of trichomoniasis is the saline wet preparation. Microscopically, trichomonads are smaller than vaginal squamous epithelial cells and larger than white blood cells. They are motile, and on higher power the flagella can be identified (see Fig. 162-1). Trichomonads are rarely found in a vaginal pH lower than 5.

References

Kaufman RH. Benign diseases of the vulva and vagina. Chicago: Year Book Medical Publishers, 1989.

McCue JD. Evaluation and management of vaginitis. Arch Intern Med 1989; 149:565.

Monif G. Infectious diseases in obstetrics and gynecology. 2nd ed. Philadelphia: Harper & Row, 1982.

Paevonen J, Stamm WE. Lower genital tract infections in women. Infect Dis Clin North Am 1987; 1:179.

Phillips RS, et al. Should tests for *Chlamydia trachomatis* cervical infections be done during routine gynecologic visits? An analysis of the costs of alternative strategies. Ann Intern Med 1987; 107:188.

Abnormal Vaginal Bleeding

Don P. Deprez, MD

163

Definition

In order to assess whether vaginal bleeding is abnormal, it is necessary to ascertain the chronologic phase of development of the individual's reproductive system. Five periods of time can be defined: (1) the premenarchal years (prior to menstruation), (2) the menarche (the establishment of a menstrual pattern during puberty), (3) the reproductive years (characterized by usually regular menses), (4) the perimenopausal years (the period of waning ovarian function), and (5) the postmenopausal years (after menses have ceased).

Any bleeding per vaginum during period 1 or 5 is abnormal and must be investigated. On the other hand, quite irregular and occasionally heavy bleeding is frequently seen and may be "physiologic" (i.e., "normal") during periods 2 and 4, and occasionally in period 3. In general, however, bleeding may be considered abnormal if it recurs more frequently than every 20 days (polymenorrhea) or less often than every 42 days (oligomenorrhea), if it lasts longer than 8 days (menorrhagia), if the blood loss during an episode is greater than 150 ml (hypermenorrhea), or if bleeding occurs between menstrual periods (metrorrhagia).

Pathophysiology

Normal menstruation results from a complex series of interactions involving numerous hormones and organs, including the uterus, ovaries, pituitary gland, central nervous system, and thyroid and adrenal glands. In conceptualizing the causes of abnormal bleeding, it is helpful to distinguish four categories: (1) bleeding during periods of no ovarian function, (2) bleeding related to ovulatory cycles, (3) anovulatory bleeding, and (4) bleeding related to pregnancy. Pregnancy disorders are not discussed here.

Clinically, one may distinguish ovulatory bleeding from anovulatory bleeding in that ovulatory bleeding is usually *regular* in periodicity and is associated with crampy lower abdominal pain (dysmenorrhea) and some degree of premenstrual symptoms (nausea, sensation of bloating, emotional lability). Anovulatory bleeding, conversely, occurs *irregularly,* without prodrome, and is usually painless. It is helpful to make the distinction because in abnormal ovulatory bleeding, (1) the bleeding is usually due to pelvic pathology, (2) the pelvic examination may suggest an abnormality, and (3) dilation and curettage or hysteroscopy is often diagnostically helpful and occasionally therapeutic. Anovulatory bleeding, however, is usually endocrine in origin and not associated with pelvic pathology; the pelvic examination is usually normal; and dilation and curettage are usually not indicated.

Anovulatory bleeding occurs physiologically during the menarche and the perimenopause. During menarche, a few months or years may elapse after the first episode of menstrual bleeding before the completion of the maturational process involving the central nervous system, hypothalamus, pituitary, ovaries, and uterus that leads to ovulation. The key milestone is the occurrence of regular ovulation. This event requires cyclic and interdependent fluctuations in circulating levels of hypothalamic releasing factors, pituitary gonadotropins, ovarian steroids, and perhaps uterine factors. Without ovulation, there is no formation of the corpus luteum, which is the source of progesterone. Without a periodic rise, and then fall, in serum progesterone, there is no maturation and subsequent sloughing of the estrogen-primed endometrium. Under unopposed estrogen stimulation, the endometrium continues to proliferate until it can no longer be maintained by the current (perhaps now waning) circulating level of estrogen, resulting in irregular, incomplete, and perhaps quite heavy endometrial sloughing. Prolonged unopposed estrogen stimulation (over a period of years) can lead to endometrial hyperplasia and carcinoma.

Once regular ovulatory cycles have been established, menstruation occurs with a set frequency, duration, and intensity; occasionally, however, ovulation may fail to occur, usually because of a minor, transient imbalance in the several circulating hormones. This frequently is caused by physical or emotional stress.

The menopausal years are characterized by a gradual depletion of ovarian follicles and, thus, a cessation of ovulation initially and eventually cessation of estrogen production, resulting in a complete disappearance of menstrual bleeding. Thus, anovulatory bleeding is common at both ends of that phase of a woman's life during which reproduction is possible.

Etiology

In discussing the etiology of abnormal vaginal bleeding, it is helpful to integrate the five stages of development of the reproductive system with the four conceptual categories outlined previously.

Initially, it is necessary to confirm that the bleeding is coming from the reproductive tract, and not from intestinal or urinary sources. Next, it is important to distinguish bleeding from the lower genital tract (vulva, vagina, and cervix) from the upper tract (uterus). Causes of the former include infection, trauma, neoplasm, foreign body, and atrophy (due to estrogen deficiency in the postmenopausal years).

Abnormal uterine bleeding related to ovulatory cycles is usually due to a demonstrable pelvic lesion such as an endometrial polyp, acute or chronic endometritis, uterine leiomyomas (fibroids), adenomyosis, an intrauterine contraceptive device, uterine neoplasm, chronic pelvic inflammatory disease, or ovarian tumor. Occasionally, however, it may be secondary to a bleeding tendency due to a blood disorder such as von Willebrand's disease, leukemia, or idiopathic thrombocytopenic purpura.

Abnormal uterine bleeding related to anovulation ("dysfunctional uterine bleeding") is usually endocrine in origin and not due to pelvic pathology, except in the case of a hormone-producing ovarian tumor. However, very heavy bleeding during menarche may be due to a bleeding diathesis in about 20 percent of cases. Anovulation implies lack of the mid-cycle luteinizing hormone surge. The hypothalamic-pituitary axis may be disturbed by either anatomic distortions (tumors, infiltrative processes, vascular lesions) or neuroendocrine perturbations. The latter include (1) the hyperprolactinemia syndromes (due to prolactinoma, medications, or afferent neural lesions, (2) the hyperandrogen syndromes (including ovarian and adrenal sources), (3) thyroid disorders, and most commonly (4) conditions of chronic stress, either psychological or physical. Common examples of the latter include extremes or fluctuations of body weight and strenuous physical conditioning. (See also Chapter 37, "Amenorrhea.")

Diagnostic Approach

An initial phase of the diagnostic (and therapeutic) process is to distinguish intense, acute bleeding requiring immediate hospitalization from those situations that may be investigated and managed without hospital admission. The history, physical examination, vital signs, and complete blood count will usually indicate how urgent the condition is and point to the two or three leading possibilities in the great majority of cases.

Specimens for cervical cytology and culture should be obtained routinely during pelvic examination. Aids that may be helpful in selected cases include pelvic ultrasound examination and sensitive and specific assays for hormones such as human chorionic gonadotropin (hCG), follicle-stimulating hormone, luteinizing hormone, prolactin, estrogens, androgens, or thyroid hormones. Finally, biopsies of the cervix or uterus may be obtained, the pituitary region may be investigated with specialized imaging techniques such as computed tomography, or the upper genital tract may be examined by laparoscopy and cervical dilation and uterine curettage, or hysteroscopy. With this armamentarium of diagnostic aids, and knowing the relative probabilities of the various etiologies depending upon the age of the patient, a rational approach may be followed.

In the premenarchal girl, any bleeding is abnormal. The source is usually the lower genital tract, and the cause is usually trauma (accidental straddle injury or molestation), a foreign body, occasionally infection, and rarely neoplasm (e.g., sarcoma botryoides). If the history and physical examination fail to yield an explanation, bleeding may rarely be from the uterus, usually resulting from a hormonally active ovarian tumor ("precocious pseudopuberty") or central nervous system lesion (causing true precocious puberty). Pelvic ultrasound examination, hormone assays, and pituitary imaging would then be helpful.

During menarche, the cause of abnormal bleeding in the majority of cases is physiologic anovulatory bleeding, but blood disorders, pregnancy-related disorders, and pelvic infection should also be considered. In addition to the history and physical examination, the appropriate clotting studies, hCG assay, complete blood count, sedimentation rate, and cervical cultures would be helpful.

In the adult menstruating woman, all categories of abnormal bleeding must be considered. Uterine leiomyomas and adenomyosis are common causes, as are pregnancy disorders, pelvic infections, and anovulatory bleeding. Cancer becomes increasingly important to exclude, as its incidence rises with age. Dilation and curettage or hysteroscopy assumes a larger role as a diagnostic measure.

During the menopausal years, anovulatory bleeding is common, but cervical and uterine cancer must be excluded by tissue sampling.

Any bleeding in the postmenopausal woman (more than 1 year since her last episode of vaginal bleeding) is abnormal, and cancer must be excluded. A more common cause of (usually light) bleeding, however, is vulvovaginal epithelial atrophic change.

It is obvious that unusual situations occasionally occur and that one must remain vigilant in the diagnostic process, but it is unnecessary and unwise to adopt a "shotgun" approach and request a large battery of laboratory tests and imaging studies at the initial patient encounter. By following a rational diagnostic approach, one may ensure the welfare of both the individual and society.

Gynecology

References

Glass RH. Office gynecology. 3rd ed. Baltimore: Williams & Wilkins, 1987.

Speroff, L, Kase NG, Glass RH. Clinical gynecologic endocrinology and infertility. 4th ed. Baltimore: Williams & Wilkins, 1988.

Female Sexual Dysfunction

Mai-Lan Rogoff, MD

164

Although human sexual function and dysfunction have presumably existed as long as there have been humans, the study of the physiology of sexuality really began with the work of Masters and Johnson. Since their publication of *Human Sexual Response,* the field has expanded considerably, with reports of various aspects of both male and female sexuality.

Definition

Masters and Johnson divided the sexual response cycle into four stages: excitement, plateau, orgasm, and resolution, each with genital and extragenital components. Helen Singer Kaplan later added a fifth stage to the scheme: desire (Fig. 164-1). It remains to be demonstrated that earlier stages are necessary for later ones, that everyone experiences all aspects of the cycle, or even that one of the stages (plateau) should be considered a separate "stage," as it has no clear beginning differentiating it from excitement. Despite these problems, Masters and Johnson's concept of the sexual response cycle remains widely accepted, probably because it ties together and organizes a great deal of data.

Desire

Desire is characterized by interest in sexuality, active seeking of opportunities for sexual engagement (proceptivity), and passive reception of advances (receptivity). The most common dysfunction of this phase of the cycle is hypoactive sexual desire, also often called lack of libido. Hormonally, the degree of sex drive appears to be androgen-dependent in both men and women (Waxenburg et al, 1960). For example, it is a common clinical observation that women receiving androgens for control of malignant breast tumors often report increased libido. It has also been reported that women who had a higher level of androgen at the midpoint of their menstrual cycle tended to have more intercourse throughout the cycle than did women with a lower level (Persky et al, 1982).

The relationship of the stage of the menstrual cycle to sexual desire is unclear. A peak of sexual interest has been shown, as measured by number of coital episodes, before or just after the initiation of menses, at a point where estradiol and progesterone are at their lowest. Because number of coital episodes in the woman can be determined by proceptivity or receptivity, each of which may be determined by different hormones, a more accurate way to examine the question would be to look only at female-initiated episodes (Adams et al, 1978). When this has been done, the peak of female desire was found to be at the midpoint of the cycle, with desire subsiding just before menses.

Psychological factors also determine degree of desire and may in fact be more significant (Bancroft et al, 1980). The levels of testosterone and estradiol in women taking oral contraceptives correlate with reported libido only in the group of women not reporting sexual difficulties. In those women who had difficulty, typically loss of libido while taking pills with return of libido during the days off pill, there was no correlation of hormone level with degree of sexual interest, suggesting that factors such as feelings about taking oral contraceptives may be more important than hormone levels.

Hypoactive sexual desire may be caused by physical factors, psychological factors, or a combination of factors. A less common disorder of this phase, sexual aversion disorder, in which there is persistent extreme aversion to and avoidance of genital sexual contact with a male or female partner, is psychologically caused.

Arousal is facilitated by the woman's confidence that she can be aroused as well as by aspects of sight, smell, and sound that have particular connotations for her. Learned behavior about sex roles or "proper" responsiveness may have facilitating or inhibiting effects. Physiologic arousal without subjective perception of arousal has been reported to cause a feeling of "disgust," suggesting a strong learned component to the subjective experience of sexual arousal as such. Most important, libido is affected by the woman's feelings about herself as a sexual being and her feelings of trust in her current relationship. Relationship issues, events and their meanings, are generally very important to women. Some investigators have suggested that relationship may be more of a primary motivating factor in women's psychology than in men's.

Hypoactive Sexual Desire Disorder (Decreased Libido)

Hypoactive sexual desire is both very common and often difficult to treat. Biologic causes are probably similar to those in men but have been less well studied in women. These include alcohol abuse and abuse of central nervous system depressants (barbiturates, narcotics), liver or other endocrine diseases that shift the estrogen-androgen ratio in favor of estrogens, and use of anticholinergic medication such as the psychotropics and some antihypertensives. Sexual interest is frequently diminished during the first and last trimesters of pregnancy and the first few months post partum, through a combination of hormonal and psychological factors. In addition, individuals vary in their usual levels of libido, probably on a constitutional basis.

Psychological factors leading to loss of libido include depression with vegetative signs, unconscious conflicts about sexuality or intimacy, sexual phobias, learned familial or societal messages about sexuality that have negative connotations about being aroused, and conflicted feelings about the partner. Many couples with sexual dysfunctions develop partnership styles that tend to maintain the dysfunction. Stopping affectionate behavior (avoidance of sensual behavior, scheduling other activities that preclude sex ["too tired" or "headaches"]) is a common example. Fear of failure and performance pressure, both of which diminish sexuality, also are common. Generally, despite the close association of aggression and sexuality in the limbic system and in many men, anxiety, guilt, embarrassment, and anger tend to diminish sexual responsiveness in women.

Disorders of later phases of sexual function tend eventually to develop into hypoactive sexual desire because of the anticipation of failure or of unpleasant experience. The multiplicity of possible causes of hypoactive sexual desire, together with the frequent finding that women experiencing this dysfunction often have a greater degree of psychosexual conflict than those

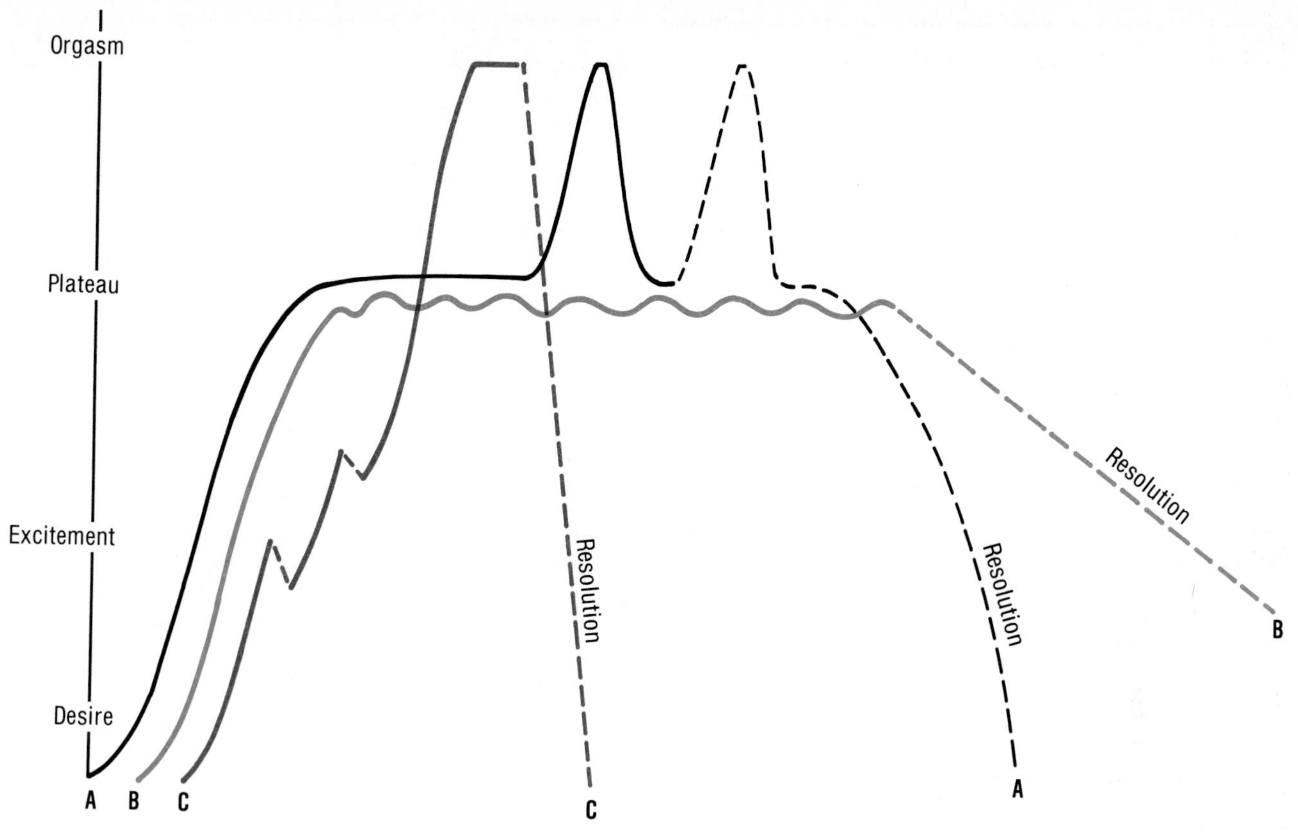

Figure 164-1 The female sexual response cycle.

experiencing disorders of later phases of the cycle such as anorgasmia, combine to make hypoactive sexual desire the most difficult of the sexual dysfunctions to treat. It is, unfortunately, also one of the most common.

Excitement

Excitement is characterized by a sex flush, nipple erection, increase in breast size, lubrication, elevation of labia majora, engorgement of labia minora, and elongation and increase in diameter of the clitoris. Lubrication is a transudate that appears on the walls of the vagina in a "sweating" response. Masters and Johnson also reported vaginal lubrication in women with vaginal reconstructions made from skin. Erectile tissue is present in the glans, body, and crura of the clitoris and the vestibular bulbs of the vagina. Engorgement is thought to take place by mechanisms similar to those in the man.

The clitoris is innervated by the dorsal nerve of the clitoris, via the pudendal nerve, analogous to the dorsal nerve of the penis. The dorsal nerve of the clitoris is smaller in diameter than the dorsal nerve of the penis, probably because of the different sizes of the two organs. The number of nerve endings per square millimeter in both the glans of the penis and of the clitoris is similar. The vagina and its counterpart in the male, the scrotum, are more poorly innervated. Members of both sexes get the most intense sexual stimulation by manipulation of the glans of the clitoris or penis, rather than by inserting objects into the vagina or manipulation of the scrotum.

One group has described finding another area of intense sexual stimulation in the vagina, the Grafenberg or "G" spot. This area is felt only in the excited woman, through the anterior vaginal wall 1 to 2 cm deeper than the pelvic bone with the woman in a supine position. Stimulation of the spot requires steady massage with upward pressure and is said to cause an initial urge to urinate followed by intense sexual pleasure. The existence of this spot is controversial, the innervation unclear, and the method of stimulation unlikely in penis-in-vagina intercourse.

Disorders of the Excitement Phase

The disorder of the excitement phase is female sexual arousal disorder. The two sexual pain disorders, vaginismus (involuntary contraction of the muscles underlying the outer third of the vagina) and dyspareunia (pain on intercourse), also often occur during this phase of the cycle. Dyspareunia, particularly due to organic cause, may also occur later in the response cycle.

Physical causes of disorders of the excitement phase include irritation of the vagina or pudendal area through infection or chemical irritation, central nervous system disorders that cause dysfunction of the autonomic nervous system or interruption of the pelvic nerves, and cardiovascular diseases causing difficulty sustaining the increased pulse and blood pressure or interruption of pelvic blood flow. In addition, postpartum women and postmenopausal women often report vaginal tightness and difficulty lubricating despite subjective feelings of excitement.

Treatment of the latter two conditions is most easily accomplished with artificial lubricants such as K-Y jelly (available without prescription) and reassurance. Treatment of other organic causes of excitement disorders depends on the underlying cause. The use of oral or vaginal estrogens in postmenopausal women is controversial, although these will relieve pain due to thinning mucosa and repromote lubrication. Use of local steroid creams does not solve the problem of side effects, as vaginal steroid preparations are even more effectively absorbed systemically than oral ones.

Plateau

Plateau is defined by Masters and Johnson as the phase of orgasmic inevitability. It has no clear events separating it from excitement and probably represents simply the late stage of excitement. During this time the clitoris retracts back under the clitoral hood. The vaginal barrel, which starts to relax and increase in diameter during excitement, reaches full expansion. There are no disorders specifically of this phase in the woman.

Orgasm

Orgasm is characterized by increased heart rate, respiratory rate, and blood pressure extragenitally. Genitally, there are rhythmic contractions of the muscles underlying the outer third of the vagina and uncoordinated contractions of the uterus. These uterine contractions increase in coordination in the pregnant woman. A few seconds before the orgasmic contractions start, there is a short "tonic" contraction of the outer third of the vagina. The subjective feeling of orgasm is one of intense pleasure and loss of control of voluntary muscles. Many women have reported achieving orgasm 80 to 90 percent of the time when masturbating but only 40 percent of the time through intercourse. This may correspond to the more effective clitoral stimulation during masturbation. On the other hand, unlike most men, many women report intercourse as deeply satisfying even without orgasm, depending on feelings toward the partner.

Inhibited Female Orgasm

The disorder of the orgasm phase is inhibited female orgasm, which may be primary, in a woman who has never had an orgasm, or secondary, in one who has had but has subsequently lost this ability. Primary inhibited orgasm is often found in women who have never masturbated, do not know how to stimulate themselves effectively, and therefore cannot teach their partners. Secondary inhibited orgasm is generally more difficult to treat and suggests physical or psychological (usually interpersonal) pathology. Interestingly, there is no female equivalent of premature ejaculation in the man.

Organic causes of inhibited orgasm include interruption of autonomic nervous system function by drugs or surgery and interruption of pelvic nerves. Conditions causing desire or excitement phase disorders will often cause inhibited orgasm because the phase will not be reached. When this problem is due to lack of lubrication, the use of artificial lubricants such as K-Y jelly may allow the sexual response cycle to proceed. Although antidepressants generally increase sexuality by relieving the loss of libido associated with depression, complaints of delayed orgasm and lack of orgasm have been documented in individual case reports of women taking neuroleptics, monoamine oxidase inhibitors, and tricyclic antidepressants (Gross, 1982). One report by Gross documented successful treatment of inhibited orgasm induced by antidepressants through the use of a cholinergic drug, suggesting that the mechanism of orgasmic dysfunction is through interference with autonomic nervous system function in at least some cases.

The picture in diabetes, a well-described source of sexual dysfunction in men, is more complicated in women. The incidence of dysfunction secondary to diabetes is lower in women than in men. The mechanism of sexual dysfunction in the male diabetic patient appears to involve autonomic pelvic neuropathy. Because the physiology of male and female sexual function is remarkably similar, one would expect similar reports of inhibited orgasm and arousal difficulties in diabetic women. Both dysfunction (Kolodny, 1971) and absence of dysfunction (Ellenberg, 1980) have been described in women with diabetes. (Both of these studies were conducted by questionnaire.) Male and female differences may be partially explained by the ability of the woman to feel sexually fulfilled and "satisfied" without orgasm, even in the absence of diabetes, whereas men are more likely to monitor closely any difficulties in achieving ejaculation.

The same psychological factors that may cause difficulty with desire or excitement (unconscious conflict, aversive learning, poor relationship with partner) may also cause dysfunctions of orgasm. Generally, women with orgasm-phase dysfunction are more likely to have difficulty with the sense of loss of control than the problems with intimacy often seen in women with hypoactive sexual desire.

"Faking It"

A problem related to difficulty in reaching orgasm is pretending to have one. At some point in their lives, most women "fake" an orgasm. Brunswick (1943) went so far as to suggest that this pretending is so common, it is at the root of the perception of women as "tricky." What seems more likely is that women feel compelled to live up to their own ego ideal of universal orgasm with intercourse or to placate what they perceive as a partner's "fragile male ego" with pretense. Faking orgasm as a response to perceived failure has obvious implications for self-esteem and self-perception as a sexual being. Faking it in deference to the perceived needs of the partner may reflect on the relationship. In either case, open communication is not fostered. Management of the woman who has been "pretending during most orgasms" in the relationship may be facilitated by suggesting that she discuss "intensity" of orgasm with the partner, as it is very difficult to reveal the absolute truth.

Treatment

A relatively high number of otherwise functional individuals and couples will experience a sexual dysfunction at some time in their lives (Fig. 164-2). Treatment of the individual with a sexual dysfunction can be thought of as proceeding in three stages. The first is that of education, listening, and permission giving. Most patients will not need more than this. Educating the patient about when it is safe to resume intercourse after procedures or illnesses, giving permission to talk about such things with their partners or to be concerned, and listening to fears of reactions of partners to procedures such as mastectomy are all tremendously helpful. Patients may have mild dysfunctions due to lack of knowledge of the possibilities or of specific techniques. Suggestions as simple as moving the bed away from the wall adjoining the children's room or trying a different sexual position may have a surprisingly beneficial effect.

Some patients will require more than this and may respond to structured interventions in sexual dysfunction therapy. Sexual dysfunction therapy, pioneered by Masters and Johnson, is focused, symptom-oriented, has limited goals, and is more structured than insight-oriented psychotherapy. Much of the focus is on improving physical aspects of nonverbal communication, and the therapy uses exercises that are done at home (*not* in front of the therapist) and are then discussed during the sessions. The underlying assumptions of sexual dysfunction therapy are based on those of behavioral psychology and learning theory. The success of this type of therapy is dependent on patient selection and absence of any other psychological problems.

A few patients will require intensive individual or couples psychotherapy and will not respond to the relatively brief interventions of sexual dysfunction therapy. These include patients whose dysfunction is based on unconscious conflict, patients whose psychological distress extends beyond the realm of sexual function, those whose marital problems are more extensive

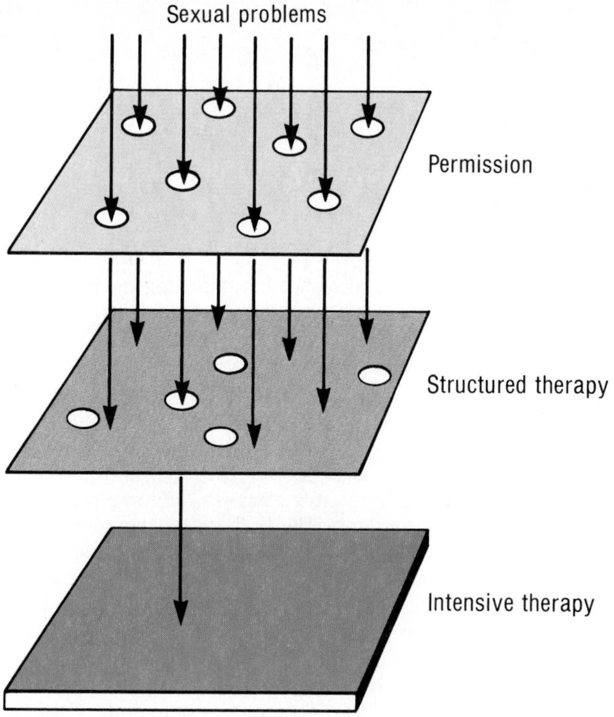

Figure 164-2 The sexual dysfunction filter.

than sexual dysfunctions, and most patients with hypoactive sexual desire, although short-term cognitive approaches have even been reported as successful in this disorder.

Significant marital problems beyond sexuality also suggest a need for more than structured sexual dysfunction therapy. Partner rejection was given by Masters and Johnson as the most common reason for treatment failure in their series (Lansky and Davenport, 1975). In Lansky's work, couples who avoided the exercises had interactions characterized by blame, projection, and depression. Therapy only aggravated their marital difficulties, probably by offering a concrete focus for repetition of the dysfunctional pattern.

One study (Derogatis et al, 1981) reported an increased incidence of psychiatric disorders as measured on a symptom checklist for women with sexual dysfunctions as compared with controls. Although half of the women with inhibited orgasm did not have other associated disorders, only 13 percent of the women with dyspareunia or vaginismus were symptom-free. Women with sexual dysfunctions, particularly vaginismus or dyspareunia, often have difficulty adjusting in other areas of psychological life.

Most physicians would agree that the first stage of therapy—permission giving, listening, and education—can and should be done by the primary physician. Most would also agree that the third stage, intensive psychotherapy, should be done by someone trained in intensive psychotherapy. Physicians and primary health care providers such as nurse-practitioners vary in their interest and willingness to take on structured behavioral interventions with patients, the second stage of therapy (see Fig. 164-2).

A detailed description of the methods of behavioral intervention is beyond the scope of this chapter. The interested reader is referred to one of the excellent texts available (Kaplan, 1974). Generally, sexual dysfunction therapy interrupts current nonfunctional patterns (such as lack of communication between the partners as to what feels good, or constant striving for orgasm) by placing a temporary ban on the anxiety-provoking behavior and setting up structured exercises, gradually leading to increasingly threatening situations. Goal-oriented behavior and the bedroom "self-observer" are discouraged. Sensuality and communication, both verbal and nonverbal, are encouraged. Specific interventions are also used, such as progressive dilators for vaginismus or masturbation training for primary anorgasmia.

Treatment is most likely to be successful if both partners are committed to the relationship and if there is no severe psychopathology in the individuals or in the couple. Couples are usually seen conjointly with one or two therapists. Prognosis is best for disorders later in the cycle (i.e., inhibited orgasm) than earlier (i.e., hypoactive sexual desire). Although vaginismus will respond well to treatment with dilators, the underlying hypoactive sexual desire often then becomes apparent. Prognosis is poorest when projection, blame, hidden contempt for the spouse, or fear of intimacy is a major factor.

Summary

Human sexual response and behavior is determined through a complex mixture of biology, psychological experience and understanding, relationship, and technical expertise. The physician is not infrequently called upon to act as a sexual counselor. Both physical and some psychological therapies are well within the province of the primary physician. Although some patients will require more structured therapy or even intensive psychotherapy, many can be managed by the primary physician using a combination of education, listening, and permission giving. The primary physician is a significant resource in helping women feel comfortable with themselves in this important aspect of human existence.

References

Adams DB, Gold AR, Burt AD. Rise in female initiated sexual activity at ovulation and its suppression by oral contraceptives. N Engl J Med 1978; 299:1145.

Bancroft J, et al. Androgens and sexual behavior in women using oral contraceptives. Clin Endocrinol 1980; 12:327.

Brunswick RM. The accepted lie. Psychoanal Q 1943; 12:458.

Derogatis LR, Meyer JK, King KM. Psychopathology in individuals with sexual dysfunction. Am J Psychiatry 1981; 138:757.

Ellenberg M. Sexual function in diabetic patients. Ann Intern Med 1980; 92(part 2):331.

Gross D. Reversal by bethanechol of sexual dysfunction caused by anticholinergic antidepressants. Am J Psychiatry 1982; 139:1393.

Hite S. The Hite report. New York: Macmillan, 1976.

Kaplan HS. The new sex therapy. New York: Brunner/Mazel, 1974.

Kolodny RC. Sexual dysfunction in diabetic females. Diabetes 1971; 20(B):557.

Kolodny RC, Masters WH, Johnson VE. Textbook of sexual medicine. Boston: Little, Brown, 1979.

Lansky MR, Davenport AE. Difficulties in brief conjoint treatment of sexual dysfunction. Am J Psychiatry 1975; 132:177.

Morley JE, Kaiser FE. Sexual function with advancing age. Med Clin North Am 1989; 73:1483.

Persky H, et al. The relation of plasma androgen levels to sexual behaviors and attitudes of women. Psychosom Med 1982; 44:305.

Sheahan SL. Identifying female sexual dysfunction. Nurse Pract 1989; 14(2):25.

Breast Pain

Michael D. Wertheimer, MD

165

Definition

Breast pain, or mastodynia, results from pain in one of the anatomic structures of the breast. The physician's first task in approaching the patient who complains of breast pain is to distinguish mammary and extramammary causes. Although the patient can generally distinguish between chest discomfort and breast pain, the physician must clearly distinguish musculoskeletal, cardiac, and gastrointestinal causes of breast pain from true mastodynia. Once it is clear that the pain is truly in the breast, the critical issue to be faced by the physician is whether the pain represents an exaggeration of normal physiology or whether it is a truly abnormal and pathologically significant problem.

Anatomy

The breast is composed of ducts, ligaments, lobules, fat, and skin, as illustrated in Figure 165-1. The ducts are lined by epithelium in much the same way that branching alveoli make up the structure of the lung. The ducts are subdivided and grouped together in lobules that are surrounded by ligaments. These (Cooper's) ligaments ramify through the breast and eventually connect to the skin of the breast, the chest wall, and rectus fascia, and encompass the mammary gland in between. Adipose tissue surrounds and is interspersed among the lobules. All pathologic entities in the breast can be related to one of the major anatomic structures mentioned: the ducts, ligaments, lobules, fat, and skin. Because Cooper's ligaments traverse all of these anatomic boundaries, they generally become involved in, or affected by, any pathologic process in the breast, whether benign or malignant. This may be manifest on physical examination by dimpling or tethering of the skin or by nipple retraction. Abnormal ductal epithelium (ductal hyperplasia, dysplasia, and neoplasia) is the most common and most important cause of the symptoms of breast disease—namely, pain, lump, and nipple discharge.

Differential Diagnosis

The mammary gland is a dynamic organ that shows profound responses to the normal and sometimes abnormal ebb and flow of endogenous hormones in the menstruating woman. The commonest type of breast pain results from the normal premenstrual engorgement of the mammary "gland," caused by the estrogen tide. The patient describes a pronounced cycle of swelling, pain, and tenderness that begins in the premenstrual period and occasionally continues with the menses. This corresponds histologically to a pattern of proliferation, edema, fibrosis, and regression that can be appreciated with light microscopy in patients with this clinical syndrome. The discomfort recedes with the onset of menses and may repeat itself regularly in a monthly cycle. Although it is generally bilateral, it may be unilateral. The intensity of the breast pain frequently fluctuates from cycle to cycle, but it usually disappears or is markedly diminished with menopause. Depending on the degree of premenstrual breast swelling, the patient's pain threshold, and the degree of fibrocystic change, this "physiologic" basis of breast pain and tenderness may be mild or severe. Most women experience some degree of this change in the breasts normally, and for most women it is mild, transitory, and does not require treatment. A detailed history will usually reveal the cyclic and bilateral nature of the problem, even when some asymmetry is initially described.

Fibrocystic "change" of the breast, the most common cause of breast discomfort, is frequently seen in women aged 25 to 60. Multiple, well-delineated, movable nodules feel somewhat firm in consistency. The pain and nodules are typically most prominent in the upper outer quadrant, but can be anywhere within the breast tissue. The discomfort is often, but not always, bilateral and symmetric; it is usually cyclic and most severe in the premenstrual phase. Palpation reveals multiple nodules that change throughout the menstrual cycle, are not consistent in all positions during examination, and are present in multiple breast quadrants.

Reassurance or mild symptomatic therapy should be all that is required. In rare instances, this seemingly physiologic aberration is the source of intense pain and anxiety, in which case further investigation and treatment are warranted. Xanthine (e.g., caffeine) restriction, vitamin E administration, hormone manipulation (danazol or antiestrogens), potent analgesics, and excisional surgery have all been advocated for intractable cases. Any or all of these may be tried once serious underlying pathology has been ruled out by careful physical examination and mammography.

Noncyclic breast pain in the premenopausal woman, or any breast pain in the postmenopausal woman, is generally not physiologic. The differential diagnosis in noncyclic breast pain includes mastitis, cysts, trauma, and malignancy.

Mastitis and fibrocystic disease are imprecise terms when referring to the common clinical syndrome of painful lumps or "nodularity" in otherwise normal women. Histologically, this is usually seen as proliferation of normal ductal lobular or connective tissue elements that can be extreme in some patients. This may still be a normal variant in some patients and should not be construed as pathologic unless a specific pathologic diagnosis, such as sclerosing adenosis or papillomatosis, can be made on biopsy. All of these are pathologic entities under the rubric of "fibrocystic disease," and whenever possible a specific histopathologic diagnosis should be made. Painful nodularity can therefore be a normal occurrence based on the known anatomy and physiology of the breast. It may be an exaggeration of the norm, may or may not represent fibrocystic change, and may prove very difficult to differentiate from more serious pathology on examination. This represents one of the major pitfalls in arriving at an accurate differential diagnosis in the patient with "painful nodularity"; it requires diligence on the part of the clinician, repeat examination, and often surgical consultation.

Benign cysts as well as some malignant tumors of the breast may cause pain in spite of the common assumption that malignant tumors generally present as painless lumps. Unfortunately, physicians and the public are frequently misled by this oversimplification, and it should be ignored. Rapidly enlarging cysts as well as small cancers may cause pain, which can be the primary presenting complaint.

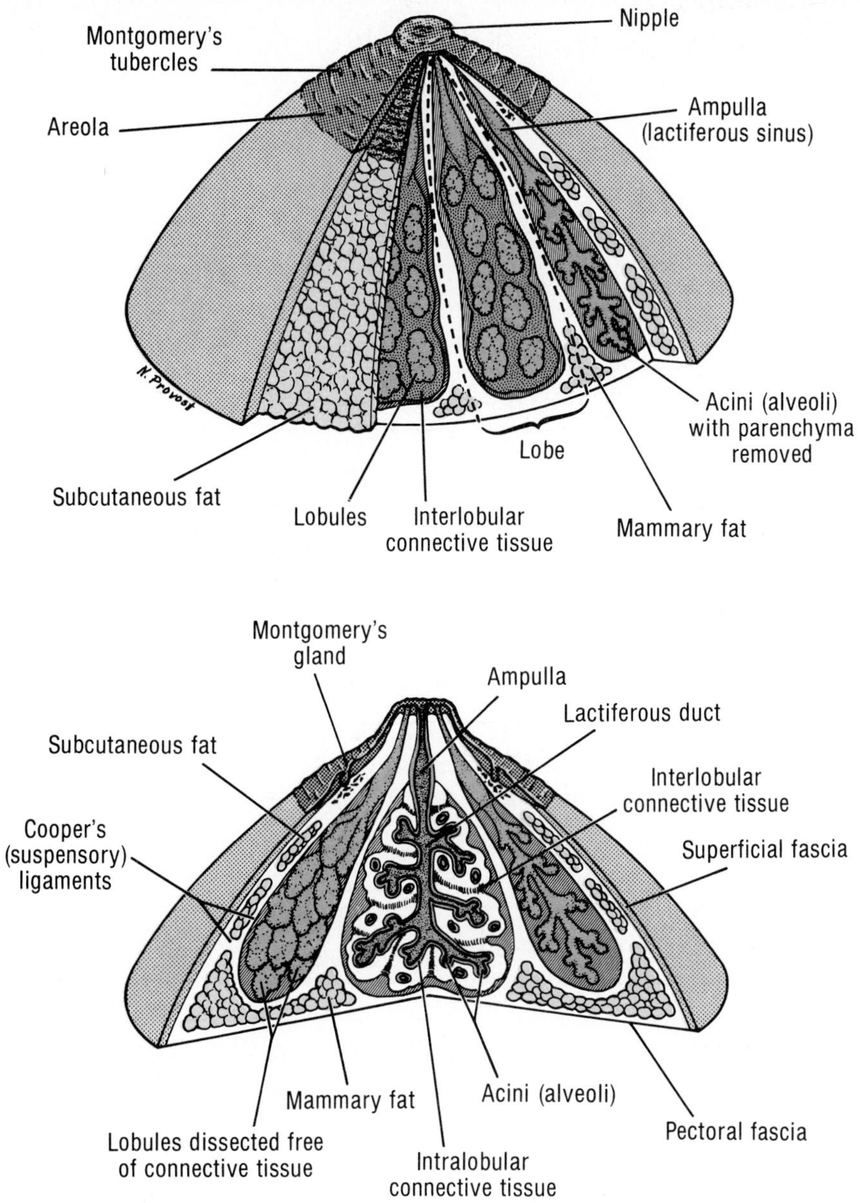

Figure 165-1 Anatomy of the breast.

Patients may describe breast pain and fail to mention an accompanying mass for fear of a diagnosis of cancer. Occasionally, carcinomas have pain as their first presenting symptom.

The breast is not an uncommon site of trauma resulting from accidents, sexual play, or self-abuse. Any clues by history or physical examination regarding abuse should be followed with appropriate counseling. Unusual extramammary causes of mastodynia include cervical radiculitis, costochondritis (Tietze's syndrome), and herpes zoster.

Diagnostic Approach

When the patient complains of breast pain, the physician's history is directed at obtaining information about endocrine, structural, or traumatic causes (Fig. 165-2). Symmetric, cyclic breast pain suggests an estrogen effect. Asymmetric but cyclic pain suggests fibrocystic change. Unilateral, noncyclic pain raises the suspicion of mastitis, trauma, or a mass lesion (benign or malignant).

The physical examination should include a careful search for lymphadenopathy in all regional node basins of the breast (axillary, supraclavicular, cervical). Skin and nipple abnormalities should be sought. Erythema might indicate mastitis or the early signs of inflammatory breast carcinoma. Ecchymosis, inflammation, or irritation could be secondary to trauma, infection, dermatologic disease, or carcinoma. Unexplained skin lesions in the breast should be biopsied to determine whether malignancy is present. Breast palpation is aimed specifically at a search for a mass that the patient did not detect or report.

If breast pain is noncyclic and persistent, a mammogram may be helpful even in the absence of a mass. Ambiguous or uncertain physical findings should be documented in the medical record, preferably diagrammed, and repeat examination should be requested in no more than 1 month. Close surveillance and diligent re-examination will usually clarify unclear

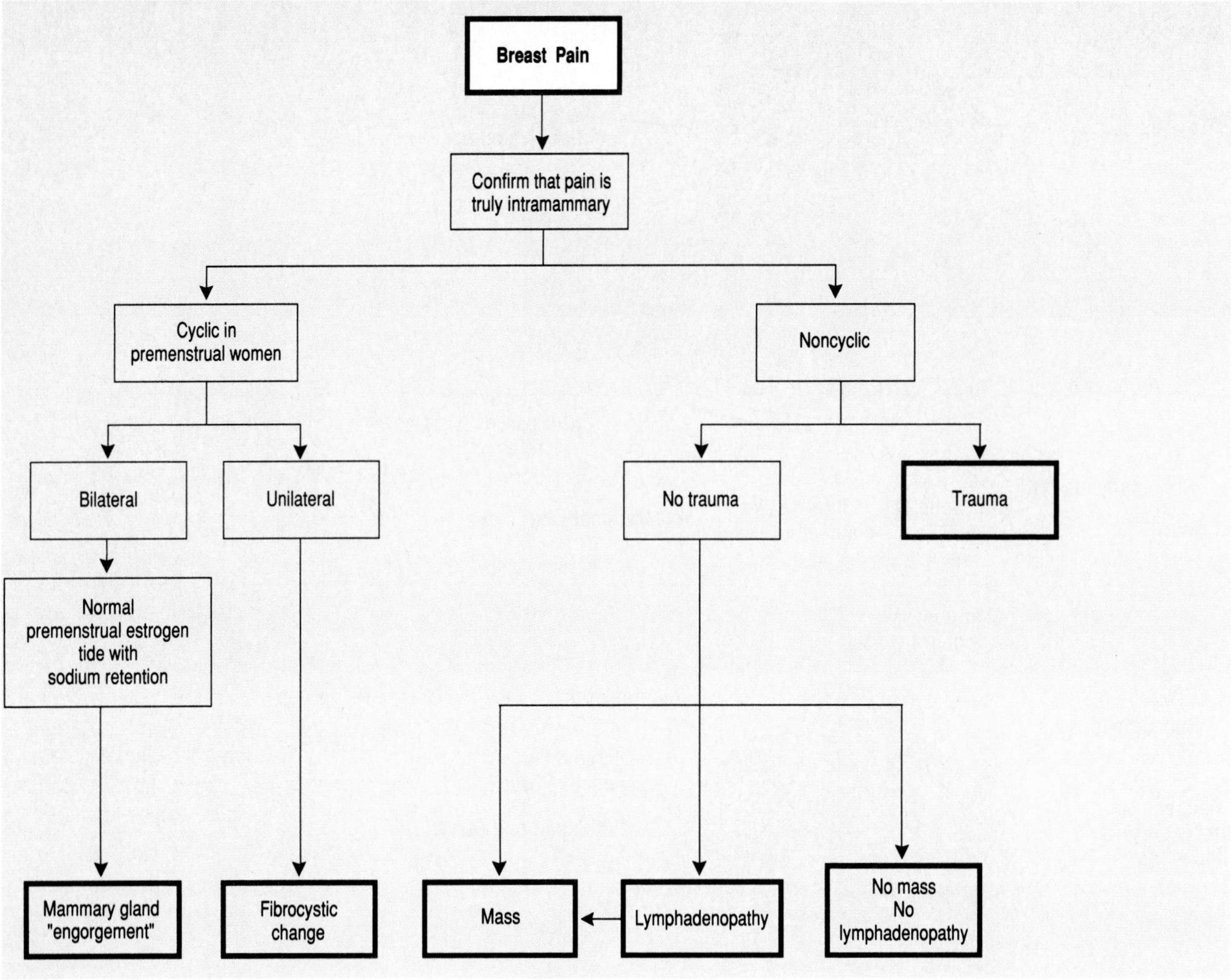

Figure 165-2 Algorithm for the diagnostic approach to the patient with breast pain.

physical findings and help establish the patient's unique pattern of cyclic nodularity so that pathologically significant findings are not overlooked. Frequent collaboration with the mammographer and surgical consultant are important parts of the armamentarium for the primary care physician to be successful in breast diagnosis.

References

Haagensen CD. Diseases of the breast. 3rd ed. Philadelphia: WB Saunders, 1987.
Townsend CM. Breast lumps. Clin Symp 1980; 32(2):405.

Nipple Discharge

Michael D. Wertheimer, MD

166

Definition

Discharge from the nipple is a very common office complaint, second only to a lump as a symptom in patients seen in the office for breast symptoms. The most common form of nipple discharge results from a physiologic aberration or benign duct ectasia; it may reflect significant endocrine pathology or, more commonly, be of no pathologic consequence. Other kinds of nipple discharge result from dermatologic conditions affecting the skin of the nipple or from diseases of the breast's ductal epithelium.

Differential Diagnosis

Discharge resulting from innocuous physiologic aberrations (including hormonal influences) may occur when a woman's

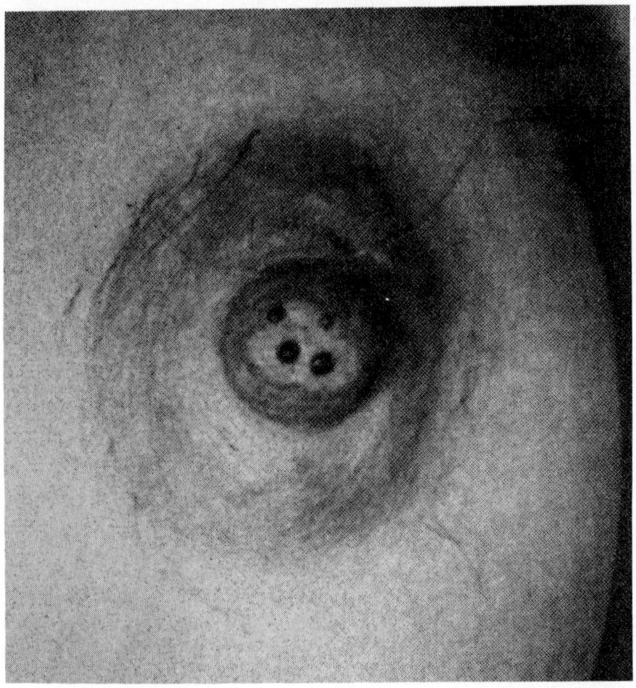

Figure 166-1 Bloody discharge from multiple ducts.

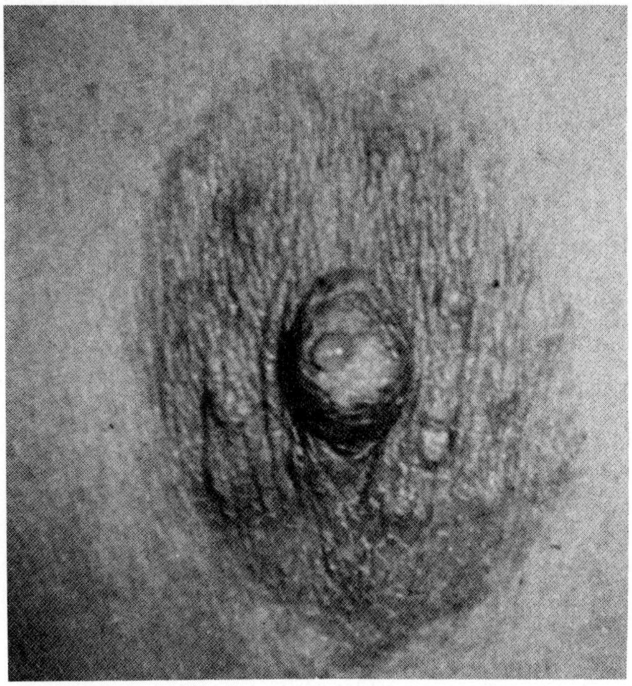

Figure 166-3 Serous discharge from a single duct.

breast is manipulated, particularly if she uses the birth control pill, tranquilizers, or rauwolfia alkaloids, or has recently become menopausal or undergone a surgical incision of the chest or abdomen. Pregnancy, prolonged lactation, and nonlactational galactorrhea also result in this kind of discharge. These systemic influences usually affect both breasts (the end organ) and lead to bilateral stimulation of breast ductal epithelium, which generates milky discharge. Occasionally, elevated serum prolactin levels can be identified in these patients; very rarely, a prolactinoma is present (see Chapter 38, "Galactorrhea").

Nipple discharge is called "true" when the effluent (discharge) is derived from an abnormality of the ductal epithelium. Benign causes of true nipple discharge include cystic mastitis, ductal epithelial hyperplasia, and some forms of extensive fibrocystic change, such as intraductal papilloma, papillomatosis, and sclerosing adenosis. Malignant causes of true nipple discharge are not uncommon and usually represent a sentinel of early disease. Approximately 7 percent of patients with nipple discharge have carcinoma. Dermatologic conditions causing nipple discharge may be benign (e.g., eczema) or malignant (Paget's

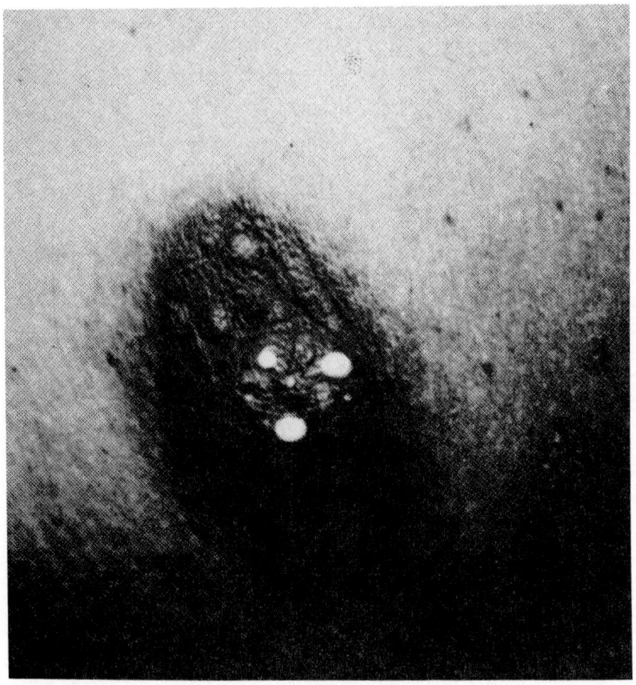

Figure 166-2 Milky discharge from multiple ducts.

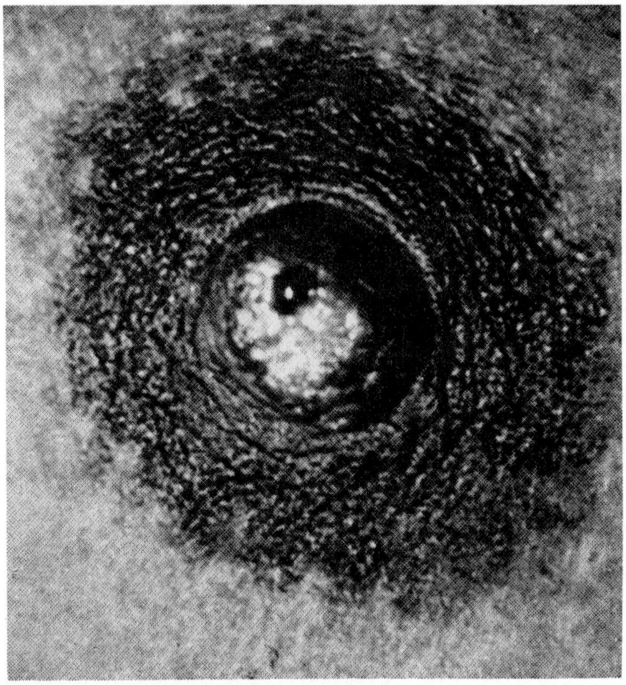

Figure 166-4 Bloody discharge from a single duct.

Table 166-1 Incidence of Malignancy in Patients with Nipple Discharge

Nipple discharge	No. of patients	Benign	Malignant
Without mass	103	92	11 (11%)
With mass	51	34	17 (33%)

disease of the breast—intradermal infiltration by underlying ductal carcinoma—or Bowen's disease, squamous carcinoma of the nipple). Cystic mastitis, ductal hyperplasia, and other forms of extensive fibrocystic disease (e.g., intraductal papilloma, papillomatosis, and sclerosing adenosis) may also cause bilateral serous or bloody nipple discharge.

Diagnostic Approach

The following discussion is offered to help the reader identify the likely etiology and character of the patient's nipple discharge. Attention should be directed toward distinguishing the exceedingly small subgroup of patients with nipple discharge who have serious underlying pathology.

The history, physical examination, cytology, and mammogram are paramount in the investigation of nipple discharge.

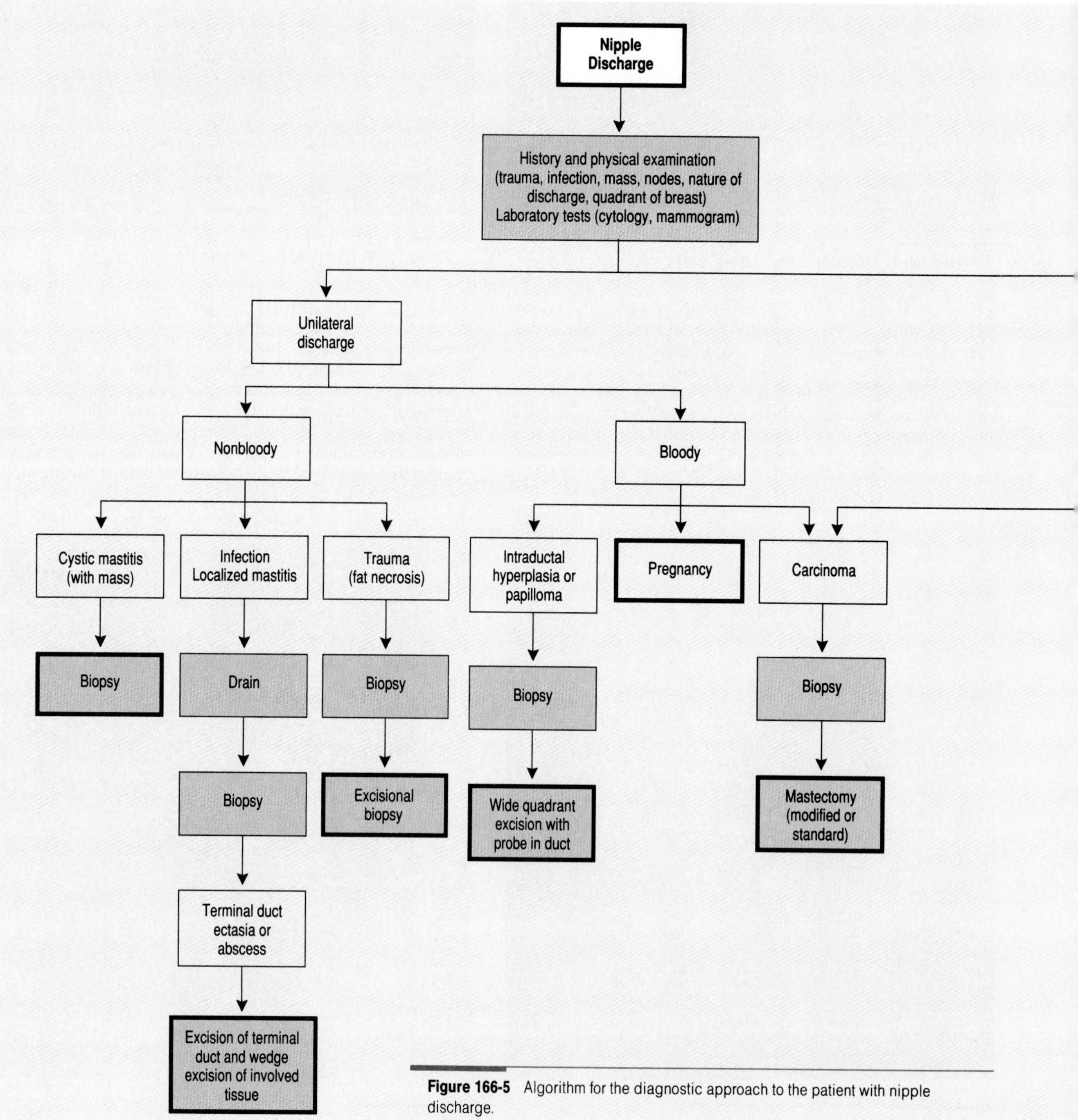

Figure 166-5 Algorithm for the diagnostic approach to the patient with nipple discharge.

The important points in the history concern whether the nipple discharge is unilateral or bilateral, spontaneous or elicited, persistent, or nonlactational. It is important to document whether the discharge results only when elicited by breast or nipple compression, and whether the discharge emanates from multiple ducts (Figs. 166-1 and 166-2) or a single duct (Figs. 166-3 and 166-4) in a given nipple. The color, character, and frequency of discharge are important, as are antecedent trauma, infection, pain, or mass. Past history of breast disease or cancer, lactation, associated medical history, and use of medications are important parts of the history. Family history for breast cancer is also important.

The physical examination should include the examination of the breast, nipple, and the regional lymph nodes. The nipple itself should be inspected for skin or other lesions. If no discharge is apparent on initial inspection, the nipple should be gently but firmly pressed between the first two fingers of the patient's or examiner's hands. If nipple discharge is neither clear nor milky, it is often helpful to touch the nipple's secretions with a white gauze. The discharge will spread by capillary action and allow a better view of its consistency and color. This is often helpful when the examiner is uncertain whether a dark nipple discharge is actually bloody. Hematesting of the discharge is often helpful if occult bloody discharge is suspected.

Bilateral nipple discharge that only occurs with active breast or nipple compression, never occurs spontaneously, and is serous, greenish, or milky rarely represents significant underlying pathology. This is the most common circumstance in the

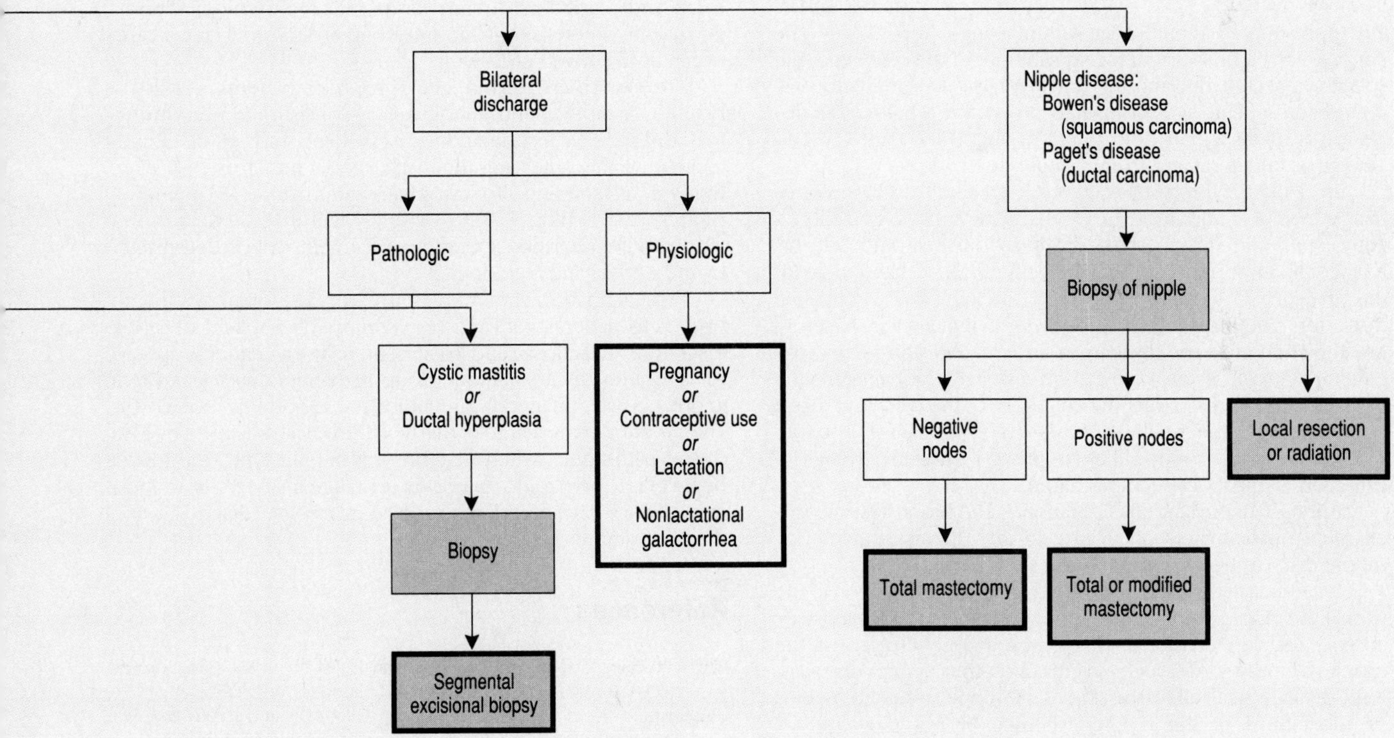

Figure 166-5 *Continued*

Table 166-2 Character and Etiology of Nipple Discharge

Character of nipple discharge	No. of patients	Diagnosis: *Galactorrhea*	*Ectasia*	*Infection*	*Papilloma*	*Fibrocystic disease*	*Cancer*
Bloody	40	—	2	—	22	10	6
Serosanguineous	39	—	2	—	21	9	7
Serous	42	—	1	—	19	18	4
Grumous	21	—	21	—	—	—	—
Purulent	5	—	—	5	—	—	—
Milky	2	2	—	—	—	—	—
Watery	3	—	—	5	—	—	—
Total	152	2	26	10	62	37	17

Figures based on 1,868 patients undergoing breast surgery. *Adapted from* Leis HP Jr. Diagnosis and treatment of breast lesions. New York: Medical Examination Publishing Co., 1970.

woman presenting with a complaint of nipple discharge. These patients usually have bilateral nipple discharge emanating from multiple ducts in both nipples and generally have an underlying systemic or organ-wide cause for the discharge. After endocrine pathology is ruled out (see Chapter 38, "Galactorrhea"), these patients generally require only reassurance and close follow-up to assure that no change occurs. This is in contrast to the patient who has *spontaneous, unilateral, bloody,* or *serous discharge* from a *single duct* of *one nipple.* The latter circumstance generally represents local pathology within a single duct system. The patient may be unaware of the specific site of the discharge, but specific directed questioning and a physical examination directed at a specific site can usually determine whether the discharge is bilateral and from multiple ducts (see Figs. 166-1 to 166-4), or unilateral and from a single duct.

In patients with a spontaneous, unilateral discharge emanating from a single duct, the discharge should be considered pathologic, and further work-up and biopsy should be performed. An important caveat to this generalization has to do with the presence or absence of a mass coincident with the nipple discharge. The incidence of underlying malignancy is threefold greater when mass and discharge coexist (Table 166-1). In those patients who ultimately come to surgery in order to determine the cause of the discharge, the character of the discharge has a relationship to the final diagnosis (Table 166-2). Serous or bloody discharge is more likely to prove pathologically significant than is milky or green discharge.

Another important consideration is the bloody nipple discharge. Approximately one-fourth of all patients with bloody nipple discharge have carcinoma as the cause.

A careful physical examination must include attention to the skin of the nipple-areolar complex to determine the presence or absence of skin erosions, ulcers, eczematous change of the nipple, or masses. Although eczema and other benign dermatologic disorders can affect the skin of the nipple, all skin erosions or ulcerations of the nipple, whether or not they are accompanied by a palpable mass, must be considered carcinoma until proved otherwise. Paget's disease and Bowen's disease frequently masquerade as eczema and are treated incorrectly, with disastrous consequences. All skin erosions of the nipple require immediate evaluation and mandatory biopsy.

Once all of the preceding criteria for diagnosis have been examined and satisfied, a very small subgroup of patients with potentially dangerous and pathologically significant discharge remains. To reiterate, this high-risk group is characterized by persistent, spontaneous, unilateral, uniductal, and bloody or serous nipple discharge. All patients with this complex of symptoms need a work-up to determine a definite diagnosis. In spite of the fact that pregnancy, intraductal hyperplasia or papilloma, and occasionally trauma or mastitis can mimic carcinoma, all patients in this subgroup must be considered to have carcinoma until proved otherwise.

The work-up in this latter group of patients should be prompt, complete, and definitive and consist of (1) careful history and physical examination, (2) cytologic study of the effluent (performed by smearing the discharge on a microscopic slide, fixing it, and sending it for cytologic examination), (3) mammography, and (4) biopsy. Biopsy usually will include duct cannulation and exploration. Definitive treatment will be determined by the underlying pathology.

The algorithm shown in Figure 166-5 summarizes the approach to patients with the very common complaint of nipple discharge. Diagnosis and treatment of these patients involve identification of a small subgroup of patients with persistent, spontaneous, unilateral, and uniductal bloody or serous discharge. Nipple discharge of this type is invariably caused by local ductal pathology, which may be of a benign type (intraductal hyperplasia or papilloma) or of a malignant type (intraductal carcinoma). These patients require aggressive diagnostic and therapeutic intervention.

References

Earley T. Nipple discharge. In: Eiseman B, Wotkyns RS, eds. Surgical decision making. Philadelphia: WB Saunders, 1978:254.

Fischermann K, et al. Nipple discharge: Diagnosis and treatment. Acta Chir Scand 1969; 135.

Haagensen CD. Diseases of the breast. 3rd ed. Philadelphia: WB Saunders, 1987.

Pilnik S, Leis HP. Nipple discharge. In: Gallage HS, et al, eds. The breast. St. Louis: CV Mosby, 1978:524.

Townsend CM. Breast lumps. Clin Symp 1980; 32(1):405.

Asymptomatic Pelvic Mass

William J. McLaughlin, MD

167

Definition

The asymptomatic pelvic mass can often prove to be an enigma to the student or physician. Must one be aggressive in the work-up and management of this problem, or should it simply be followed without intervention? Actually, either approach may be appropriate. By definition, we are most commonly describing a problem that the physician uncovers. The patient does not offer symptoms. The asymptomatic pelvic mass, therefore, is usually found on routine pelvic examination or by a diagnostic modality such as ultrasound or radiography used in the evaluation of another problem.

Etiology

Asymptomatic pelvic masses may be categorized according to type. The functional mass is of no pathologic importance. It is usually physiologic and often regresses or disappears. Examples include a corpus luteum cyst of the ovary, a pregnant uterus, and a dilated cecum. The inflammatory mass usually represents enlargement of a normal structure. Most inflammatory masses are symptomatic, although this is not always true, particularly in the case of chronic infection. Chronic inflammation may also involve adjacent anatomic structures, making characterization of the mass difficult. The neoplastic mass may be benign or malignant. Diagnosis and work-up may depend greatly on the patient's age. Effort is usually concentrated to exclude malignancy. The miscellaneous category includes other masses of gynecologic origin, i.e., embryonic remnants, as well as masses from other organ systems, particularly the urinary and gastrointestinal systems.

Several points in the present illness and past history are important. Very different diagnoses may be suggested, depending on the age of the patient, i.e., premenarchal, reproductive years, or postmenopausal. In the reproductive years, an ovarian mass must be greater than 5 cm in diameter to be pathologic, whereas a palpable ovary in a postmenopausal woman is distinctly abnormal. Questioning concerning gravidity and parity may reveal involuntary infertility. This could suggest the diagnosis of endometriosis or ovarian carcinoma. The date of the last menstrual period may suggest intrauterine or ectopic pregnancy or a functional ovarian cyst. Precise date of bleeding and the amount and character of the bleeding must be elicited. For example, did menses occur when expected? Did menses last the usual number of days? Was the amount of bleeding normal? A complaint involving an anatomically adjacent organ system may result in the discovery of an "asymptomatic" pelvic mass. For instance, the complaint of bladder pressure or urinary frequency may result from the "asymptomatic" pelvic enlargement of the uterus from a leiomyoma. It is of utmost importance that a complete past history be obtained. Has the mass been present previously? If so, what was the diagnosis? A woman previously "cured" of a pelvic tumor by hysterectomy may demonstrate recurrent disease by presenting with an asymptomatic mass on routine examination.

Meticulous abdominal and pelvic exams are necessary to characterize the asymptomatic mass. Auscultation, percussion, and palpation of the abdomen will help to characterize the mass as well as to determine its relations to abdominal viscera. Pelvic exam will further define the size, shape, and consistency of the mass. As always, normal pelvic structures should be identified. Location of the mass should be noted as well as any attachment or fixation to adjacent structures. Examination may cause the mass to become symptomatic, i.e., pressure discomfort or even frank pain. Pap smear, cultures, and biopsies should be performed, if necessary.

At this point in the work-up, the student and physician should realize that the diagnosis may remain very much in doubt. The reproductive, urinary, and gastrointestinal systems are in close anatomic relation. A precise diagnosis of an asymptomatic pelvic mass based on history and physical examination alone is often not possible. It is best at this time to continue to entertain a number of diagnostic possibilities.

Differential Diagnosis

Possible causes of an asymptomatic pelvic mass are listed in Table 167-1.

Reproductive Tract

Uterus. The normal retroflexed uterus may, at first, be construed as a pelvic mass. With experience this mistake will be avoided. The most common functional midline mass in the woman of reproductive age is a pregnant uterus. The uterus remains a pelvic organ until approximately 12 weeks of gestation. It is globular, symmetric, and soft. Uterine neoplasms may first be discovered as an asymptomatic mass. The most common is a benign leiomyoma, or fibroid. This is a smooth-muscle tumor originating in the myometrium. These tumors are of variable size, usually irregular to palpation, and quite firm. They may be embedded within the wall of the uterus or become pedunculated such that they feel separate from the uterus. Malignant neoplasms of the uterus, e.g., leiomyosarcoma, rarely present as a pelvic mass. Carcinoma of the uterine cervix can, on occasion, present as an asymptomatic pelvic mass. Obstruction of the uterine outflow tract, which can be congenital or secondary to tumor or surgery, results in hematometra, or pyometra if infection is involved. This could present as a symmetric enlargement of the uterus.

Ovary. A functional cyst (follicular or corpus luteum) is the most common asymptomatic ovarian mass. In women of reproductive age, a functional cyst will resorb physiologically at the onset of menses. Inflammatory processes such as salpingitis or abscess can cause a pelvic mass; however, unless chronic, these are usually symptomatic. Inflammatory processes usually involve the pelvis bilaterally so that the mass may be diffuse and difficult to define on examination. The most common benign ovarian neoplasm is a benign cystic teratoma or "dermoid cyst." Also common is an endometrioma or "chocolate cyst." This is a benign cystic mass of the ovary containing various amounts of old blood secondary to abnormal bleeding from the ovary at the time of menses. There may be scarring and adhesion formation in the area of endometriosis that "enlarges" the pelvic mass. The

Table 167-1 Possible Causes of an Asymptomatic Pelvic Mass

Reproductive System
Uterus:
Normal retroflexed
Pregnancy
Benign neoplasm (leiomyoma)
Malignant neoplasm (leiomyosarcoma)
Hematometra, pyometra
Ovary:
Functional cyst (follicular, corpus luteum cysts)
Infection (salpingitis, abscess)
Benign neoplasm (benign cystic teratoma, endometrioma)
Malignant neoplasm (cystadenocarcinoma)
Tube:
Pyosalpinx, hydrosalpinx, salpingitis (usually symptomatic)
Abscess
Embryonic remnant (paratubal cyst)
Ectopic pregnancy (usually symptomatic)
Gastrointestinal System
Fecal material
Inflammatory
Neoplasm (benign, malignant)
Urinary System
Distended bladder
Pelvic kidney
Urachal cyst
Miscellaneous
Hematoma
Abscess
Foreign body
Neoplasm

pelvis may even feel "frozen" on examination. Cystadenomas, serous or mucinous, should also be considered. Brenner tumors and ovarian fibromas are examples of benign solid neoplasms. Malignant neoplasms are most commonly of epithelial origin, such as serous, mucinous, and endometroid cystadenocarcinoma. These can be of various sizes and often present as asymptomatic masses in the postmenopausal woman.

Fallopian Tube. A paratubal cyst, often a wolffian remnant, may present as an asymptomatic pelvic mass. Pyosalpinx, salpingitis, hydrosalpinx, and ectopic pregnancy are other possibilities, but they are usually associated with pelvic symptomatology.

Gastrointestinal System

The gastrointestinal tract may be the source of a pelvic mass. Fecal material in the lower bowel is often interpreted as a pelvic mass. A pre-examination enema and careful rectovaginal examination should eliminate this problem. Inflammatory processes of the bowel, e.g., Crohn's disease, ulcerative colitis, diverticulitis, may have caused scarring and adhesions that may be interpreted as an ill-defined pelvic mass. Appendiceal or pericolic abscesses may have the same effect. Benign or malignant neoplasms of the bowel must also be considered.

Urinary System

A distended bladder or pelvic kidney may occasionally present as an asymptomatic pelvic mass. A urachal cyst may be present because of incomplete obliteration of the urachus during embryonic life. This would be palpated in the anterior abdominal wall and is actually extrapelvic in location.

Miscellaneous

Occasionally, rare problems may present as asymptomatic pelvic masses. Examples include hematoma formation secondary to previous trauma or surgery, a misplaced sponge or instrument from a previous surgical procedure, or other foreign body. Retroperitoneal hematoma or abscess as well as benign or malignant tumors of bone, nerve, or lymphatics of the retroperitoneum may, very rarely, present as pelvic masses.

Diagnostic Approach

The diagnostic evaluation of a woman presenting with an asymptomatic pelvic mass is variable. As suggested earlier, a great deal depends on the history despite the lack of symptoms. The age of the patient may dictate observation or surgery. The most common cause of an asymptomatic pelvic mass in a woman of reproductive age is a functional cyst. In this case, serial pelvic examinations after intervening menses would be appropriate. An asymptomatic pelvic mass in a postmenopausal woman, however, must be considered a malignancy until proved otherwise. Papanicolaou (Pap) smear and cervical culture are in order for the evaluation of most patients. Pelvic ultrasound examination, intravenous pyelography, or barium enema study may be helpful in further delineating a pelvic mass in terms of its location, composition, and association or effect on other anatomic structures. In some cases, the ureters should be demonstrated radiographically if an eventual surgical approach is contemplated. These diagnostic modalities should be undertaken only at the suggestion of an experienced examiner, who would be responsible for any surgical intervention. Colposcopy (microscopic visualization of the cervix) and directed biopsy may be helpful in the case of an abnormal Pap smear or a mass thought to be originating from the uterine cervix. Perhaps the most effective and efficient tool in the diagnosis of the asymptomatic pelvic mass is laparoscopy. Under general anesthesia, visualization of the pelvis is possible. Biopsies and intraperitoneal cultures may be performed. The need for further surgical exploration can be assessed by laparoscopy. Exploratory laparotomy, however, may become the ultimate diagnostic procedure. The individual circumstances will dictate the appropriateness and extent of such a procedure.

Although not appropriate or cost-effective as a screening measure, determination of CA125 levels may play a role in the work-up of some pelvic masses. CA125 is an antigen present in derivatives of coelomic epithelium. It may be elevated in cases of significant derangements of this epithelium, such as ovarian carcinoma, salpingitis, and endometriosis. An elevated CA125 (>35 U/ml) in the presence of a pelvic mass may indicate an extent of disease that might require the services of a tertiary referral center and an oncologic gynecologist. The CA125 analysis is just one of a number of immunologic tests being developed that may prove fruitful in the delineation of pelvic masses in the future. It is important to remember that the finding of a normal CA125 level still requires that the cause of the pelvic mass be elucidated.

References

Athey PA, Hadlock FP. Ultrasound in obstetrics and gynecology. 2nd ed. St. Louis: CV Mosby, 1985.

Cibils LA. Diagnostic and operative gynecologic laparoscopy. Philadelphia: Lea & Febiger, 1975.

Novak ER. Novak's textbook of gynecology. 11th ed. Baltimore: Williams & Wilkins, 1988.

Wynn RM. The clinical core. In: Obstetrics and gynecology. Philadelphia: Lea & Febiger, 1988.

Palliation, Medical-Legal Issues, Social Services

V

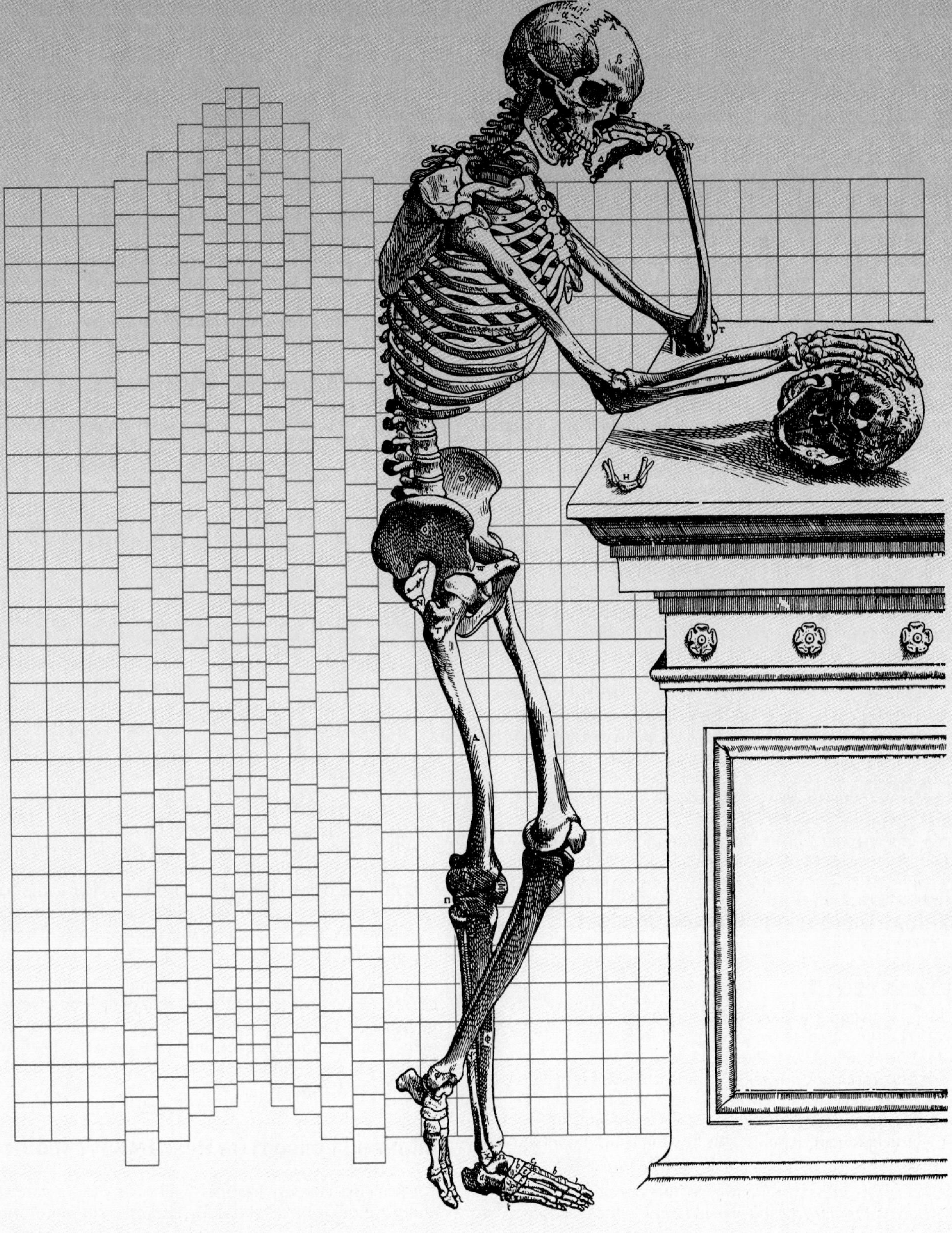

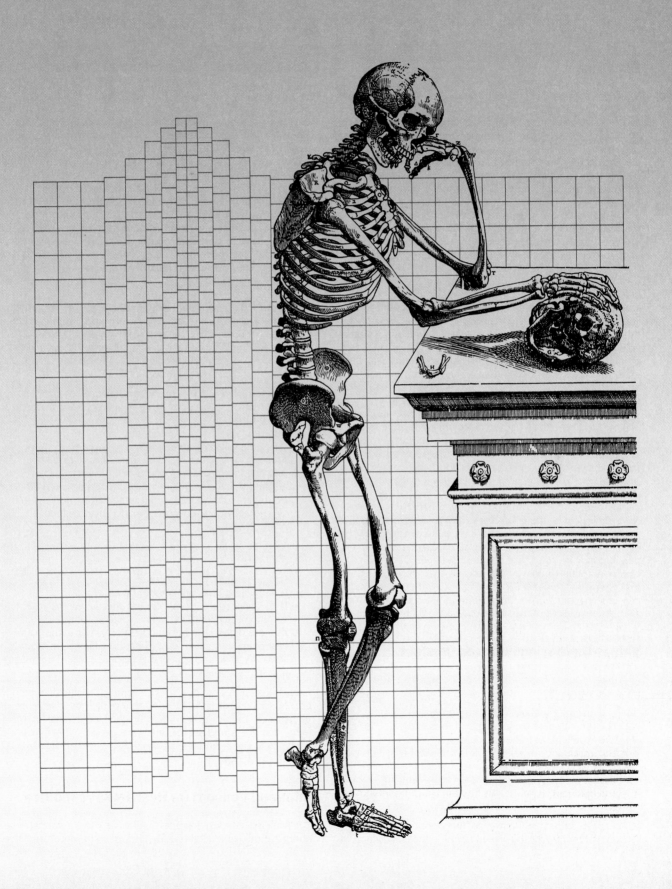

Informed Consent in Medical Practice and Research

Marcia K. Liepman, MD

168

Definition

Informed consent consists of two elements—information and consent. The principle was first well summarized in a 1914 legal case by Justice Cardozo: "Every human being of adult years and sound mind has a right to determine what shall be done with his own body." The nature of the doctor-patient relationship is a contractual one, with the doctor's special "fiduciary" duty to the patient to act in good faith with due regard for the patient's interests as a special feature. The doctrine of informed consent exemplifies this fiduciary relationship. Exact requirements for informed consent vary from state to state. In general, however, this doctrine simply states that a physician may not treat a patient until he or she has explained to the patient the risks and material facts concerning the treatments and all alternatives (including the option not to treat). The standards for informed consent in medical practice have been derived from the case law beginning with the principle as stated by Justice Cardozo; those for research have been derived from many sources, including ethical codes (Nuremburg Code, Declaration of Helsinki, and others). The physician must secure the patient's competent, voluntary, and understanding agreement in order to proceed with treatment. The more elective or experimental a procedure, the more important informed consent is, and the more detailed the information given should be.

The traditional arguments given by physicians against full disclosure and the patient's having a major role in decision making have been that (1) the patient will not be able to understand the information that the physician wishes to convey, and (2) the information will unduly scare the patient, leading the patient to withhold consent for a procedure that actually carries only minimal risk. There has been no hard evidence that full disclosure of the nature, risks, and benefits of a procedure, either routine or experimental, has been harmful to a person. Nevertheless, it is the physician's duty to inform the patient about a procedure or a study so that the patient may make up his or her own mind. The physician who believes that this task is not possible may be conveying another message: either the physician is not able to convey the risks of and alternatives to the procedures to the patient (perhaps because the physician does not understand the procedure), or the physician believes that if such disclosures were made, the patient would not consent.

Values Underlying Informed Consent

Alexander Capron has outlined several important functions of informed consent:

1. The promotion of individual autonomy
2. The protection of patients and subjects
3. The avoidance of fraud and duress
4. The importance of self-scrutiny by medical professionals
5. The promotion of rational decision making
6. The involvement of the public (in promoting autonomy as a general social value and in controlling biomedical research)

Most experts stress that the primary functions of informed consent are the *protection* and *promotion* of individual *autonomy*.

Consent Form Versus Informed Consent

It is generally accepted that for most significant therapeutic and research procedures, some documentation of the subject's consent must be obtained by the treating physician or investigator. This has come to take the form of a document called an *informed consent document*. In a recent survey of patients' attitudes toward these documents, more than three-quarters of the patients held the opinion that the consent form itself was a legal document with the purpose of protecting the interests of the physicians or hospital. Neither the doctrine of informed consent, nor the informed consent document itself, is a protection for the physician or the hospital involved in the procedures. Rather, the form is meant to provide written verification of the process of disclosure by the physician and consent by the patient. The written consent document, regardless of how complete or detailed, is not a substitute for the *processes* of disclosure and consent.

Informed consent laws vary from state to state and in general do not specify rigid guidelines for which specific routine diagnostic or therapeutic procedures require written documentation of consent. The consent document for routine procedures (e.g., elective surgery, thoracentesis) should contain certain elements that, in the broadest terms, include the following:

1. A description of the proposed procedure
2. A description of alternatives to the proposed treatment or procedure
3. Inherent risks of serious bodily injury in the proposed treatment or procedure
4. Problems related to recovery that are anticipated from the proposed treatment or procedure
5. Any additional information other physicians would disclose in similar circumstances or, in some states, information that a *reasonable person* would consider material in making his or her decision

Annas (1978) points out the following exceptions to these requirements:

1. In an emergency
2. If the patient does not want to be informed
3. If the procedure is simple and the danger remote, and commonly accepted and appreciated as remote
4. If in the physician's best judgment it is not in the patient's best interest to know, e.g., when the information would so seriously upset the patient that he or she would not make a decision rationally

Exceptions 3 and 4 can be particularly difficult. Little documentation of serious harm being done to a person by disclosure of information regarding a routine hospital procedure or treatment may be found in the literature. In fact, there is good evidence to the contrary (Annas, 1978; Levine, 1981; Lidz et al, 1983; Taub, 1982).

Informed Consent for Research Procedures

The principles underlying informed consent for research procedures are the same as those for informed consent in practice.

There are, however, some additional features relating to consent for research that should be emphasized. Medical research procedures are, for the most part, elective. Many are innovative or invasive, and it may not seem obvious to the lay subject why such procedures are being undertaken. The United States Department of Health and Human Services and the Food and Drug Administration have established regulations describing the elements of information that must be communicated with any subject of research on humans. These regulations include the following (Levine, 1981):

1. Invitation to the individual to become a research subject (the fact that the subject is being invited to participate in *research* should be clear)
2. Statement of purpose, which should include a clear indication that the study is a research study
3. Statement of basis for subject selection
4. Explanation of the procedures involved in doing research, including the specific identification of any *experimental procedures* and an estimate of the expected duration of the research subject's participation
5. A description of discomforts and risks
6. A statement of the availability of medical treatment and compensation in the event that disability is incurred as a result of the research
7. A description of any benefits to the subjects or to others that may reasonably be expected from the research
8. A statement that describes any appropriate alternative procedures or courses of treatment to the proposed research that might be advantageous to the research subject
9. A statement that describes the extent to which the records identifying the research subject will remain confidential

In addition, the Food and Drug Administration requires the following:

1. A statement of the financial costs that might result from the subject's participation in the research. Although not mentioned in the regulations, any payment or material inducements offered for participation by a research subject should also be detailed.
2. An offer to answer questions that the subject might have
3. A statement offering consultation in the event that the subject desires another opinion regarding participation in the research project
4. A statement that participation is voluntary and that refusal to participate will in no way penalize the research subject
5. Occasionally, because such disclosure might leave the study's results open to question, a research subject may be informed that some information (usually disclosure of purpose) is being deliberately withheld. In such a case, all other pertinent elements of information described here that might be of importance in the subject's decision must be disclosed.

There also may be statutes further regulating consent to research in particular states. Federal regulations also require the establishment of local review committees (Institutional Review Boards [IRBs]) located in institutions where research involving humans is conducted. IRBs are generally composed of individuals from science, medicine, and the lay public (including clergy) whose purpose is primarily to assure that the rights and welfare of research subjects are protected.

The detailed regulations outlined for the process of informed consent for research projects are not nearly so clearly defined (nor are they regulated) for consent to procedures in routine practice. Nevertheless, the *principles* underlying informed consent in either setting are *identical*: the patient's or subject's comprehension and autonomy should be assured whenever consent is sought.

Summary

The doctrine of informed consent has the primary function of protection and promotion of individual autonomy whether the individual is undergoing procedures in clinical practice or in experimental research. To some extent, this notion of consent is an ideal to which daily practice can only aspire. It may be difficult to assure any individual patient's or subject's understanding when consent is sought. The consent form is not a substitute for this process but only documentation of the dialogue that should have occurred between investigator or treating physician and subject or patient. Special problems exist when an attempt is made to secure full, free, informed, and knowing consent from particularly vulnerable groups such as mentally incompetent individuals, prisoners, terminally ill patients, and children. Informed consent in these cases has not been discussed here; it is reviewed elsewhere (Levine, 1981).

The securing of informed consent in practice or in research has become routine. It is much more than a mere formality in the relationship between doctor and patient. The doctrine of informed consent is bolstered by law in many states and by the universal ethical concern for individual autonomy.

References

Annas GJ. The rights of hospital patients. New York: Avon Books, 1975.

Annas GJ. Informed consent. Ann Rev Med 1978; 29:9.

Fitten LJ, Waite MS. Impact of medical hospitalization on treatment decision-making capacity in the elderly. Arch Intern Med 1990; 150:1717.

Lidz CW, et al. Barriers to informed consent. Ann Intern Med 1983; 99:539.

Levine RJ. Ethics and regulation of clinical research. 2nd ed. Baltimore: Urban and Schwarzenberg, 1986.

Schloendoff v. Society of New York Hospital. 105 N.E.92,93, New York, 1914.

Taub S. Cancer and the law of informed consent. Law Med Health Care 1982; 10:61.

Patients Wishing to Leave Against Medical Advice

Barry Ginsberg, MD

Barbara F. Katz, JD

Jonathan S. Rothman, MD

169

A physician whose patient threatens to sign out of the hospital against medical advice (AMA) may be justifiably concerned about the extent of the patient's legal rights and his or her psychiatric state. Nonetheless, the physician's initial task is to examine the patient's relationships to the staff and to the physician so that, where possible, he or she might reverse the process that culminates in discharge contrary to the patient's best interest.

Studies of patients signing out of general hospitals AMA have indicated a correlation with the presence of alcoholism and drug abuse. Perhaps twice as many men as women sign out AMA. These patients tend to be younger and lower on the socioeconomic ladder. The authors of one study speculated that AMA discharges had not resulted in serious disruptions of care, citing later return visits by these patients and vigorous efforts to prevent critically ill patients from leaving. However, another study at a Veterans Administration hospital found that, compared with controls, an unexpectedly high percentage of patients discharged AMA died within 6 months, suggesting that very ill patients were included in this group.

The wish to sign out AMA does not by itself mean that the patient is psychiatrically ill, and there is no single psychiatric illness that correlates with AMA discharge. Organic brain syndrome, psychosis, depression, and personality disorder each has sometimes been diagnosed. The emotion underlying the threat to sign out is often overwhelming fear or anger. Signs of emotional distress and difficulty in the treatment relationship tend to have been present before the actual threat to sign out. These signs include complaints of poor sleep, restlessness, displays of anger or fearfulness, and struggles over medication.

Ideally, efforts to rectify the problem should begin before the threat to sign out is made. Any of the aforementioned signs of emotional distress should alert the physician. The physician must then investigate how the patient's emotional turmoil came about. This is made more difficult by the possibility that the physician will have been perceived as a source of distress. Under the stress of hospitalization, patients may misinterpret their caregivers' behavior and motives; such misperceptions can usually be corrected. For this to take place, the physician must undertake a concerted effort to elicit and understand the patient's point of view. The emotional needs of some patients may necessitate flexibility in their management (e.g., a patient with a strong need to control might be allowed to participate more actively than usual in treatment decisions). Some patients may regularly, if unintentionally, engender frustration in their caregivers; when efforts at re-establishing a good working relationship are unsuccessful, and the signals of emotional distress continue to increase, psychiatric consultation may be helpful. Patients whose fear or anger reflects paranoid or other psychotic thinking may benefit from antipsychotic medication as well.

If these efforts fail and the patient maintains the wish to sign out, certain legal regulations apply. Efforts to restrict the ability of a competent adult patient to leave the hospital may be considered "false imprisonment," which is the intentional confinement of an individual against his or her will by the use of threats or physical barriers. In a lawsuit for false imprisonment, it is not necessary for the patient to prove that he or she was actually harmed by the conduct of the physician or hospital, because the law will assume harm to the patient. Although there have been relatively few cases of this type, they appear to be growing in number in recent years.

However, if a physician reasonably believes that an adult patient is incompetent, i.e., of unsound mind to the extent that he or she does not understand or appreciate the nature and consequences of his or her actions, the physician may prevent the patient from leaving the hospital, pending determination of guardianship by the court. The basis for the physician's conclusion should be well documented in the patient's record. In such circumstances, it is prudent to obtain a psychiatric consultation, which should also be included in the patient's record. It may also be determined, apart from the issue of competence, that the patient is mentally ill and dangerous to self or others. In that case, the patient may be committable under the involuntary commitment statute of that particular state, and be retained accordingly.

When dealing with minor patients, it is generally the decision of the parents or legal guardians as to when the patient will be discharged. Courts have found hospitals liable for interfering with the parent's right to custody of the child when attempts have been made to detain the child in the facility. If the actions of the parent place the life of the child in serious jeopardy, however, the health care provider may take whatever reasonable actions are necessary to protect the child, including preventing the parents from removing the child from the hospital. The hospital social services department should be helpful in these circumstances regarding necessary steps to take, including possible court action.

The hospital or physician may request that the departing patient sign a "Discharge Against Medical Advice" form. A sample form is provided in Figure 169-1. If signed, such a form should become part of the patient's medical record. However, the patient has no obligation to sign such a form as a precondition of release. Upon such a refusal, the health care provider should fully document in the patient's record the circumstances of the situation, indicating the patient's condition, his or her stated reasons for leaving, any noncoercive attempts made to persuade the patient to stay, and any instructions given to the patient regarding continued care outside the facility. Although not legally required to do so, the physician may make referrals to other health care providers or may make follow-up telephone calls to the patient after his or her departure.

In rare situations, such as those involving contagious disease, the state public health authorities may have the power to restrain a patient from leaving a hospital. This authority is explained in fuller detail in the state's public health laws, or you can find out more by contacting the state's public health agency.

Neither the author nor the publisher is engaged in rendering legal advice through this publication. Readers requiring or desiring such advice should consult a competent attorney of their own choosing.

UNIVERSITY OF MASSACHUSETTS HOSPITAL	NAME ADDRESS BIRTHDATE/AGE	MEDICAL RECORD NO. SEX

LEAVING HOSPITAL AGAINST ADVICE

DATE ____________________

This is to certify that ____________________ a patient in the above-named hospital, is leaving the hospital against the advice of the attending physician and the hospital administration. I acknowledge that I have been informed of the risk involved and hereby release the attending physician, and the hospital, from all responsibility and any ill effects which may result from this action.

____
(PATIENT)

____
(OTHER PERSON RESPONSIBLE)

Witness ____________________

____
(RELATIONSHIP)

Witness ____________________

Figure 169-1 A sample form documenting discharge against medical advice.

References

Adler v. Beverly Hills Hospital, 594 S.W. 2d 153 (Tex. Civ. App. 1980).

Albert HD, Kornfeld DS. The threat to sign out against medical advice. Ann Intern Med 1973; 79:888.

Corley MC, Link K. Men patients who leave a general hospital against medical advice; mortality rate within six months. J Studies Alcohol 1981; 42:1058.

Gawreys v. D.C. General Hospital, 480 F. Supp. 853 (D.D.C. 1979).

Health Law Center. Admitting and discharge. In: Hospital law manual. Germantown, MD: Aspen Systems Corp., 1980:46.

Holder AR. Legal issues in pediatrics and adolescent medicine. 2nd ed. New Haven: Yale University Press, 1985.

Horty J. Patient discharge, departure or transfer. In: Hospital law. Pittsburgh: Action-Kit for Hospital Law, 1981:1.

Jankowski, Drum. Diagnostic correlates of discharge against medical advice. Arch Gen Psychiatry 1977; 34:153.

Johnson v. Greer, 477 F 2d 101 (5th Cir. 1973).

Long Island Home, Ltd. v. Rotondi, 324 N.Y.S. 2d 834 (Sup. Ct. 1971).

Montague v. George J. London Memorial Hospital, j396 N.E. 2d 1289 (Ill. App. 1979).

Schlauch RW, Reich P, Kelly MJ. Leaving the hospital against medical advice. N Engl J Med 1979; 300:22.

Risk Management

170

Ardath Quinlan, BS

Harry L. Greene, MD

Technology and the public demand shape the delivery of health care. However, the greatest challenge for the practitioner in the 1990s may well be the issue of delivering quality health care in an era of increasingly restricted resources. There are financial restrictions imposed by the government's Medicare program, Medicaid, commercial insurers, and health maintenance organizations. All seek ways to curtail their payments for health care. And yet the public still believes it is their right to have any and all means of technology available for their individual health needs.

There are other restrictions that may be less obvious. When one realizes that approximately two-thirds of all malpractice claims are brought by the unhappy patient—one who has had an unexpected outcome, not necessarily one whose care fell below the medical standard—the additional burden imposed by potential liability is apparent.

The costs are many. There is the real cost in terms of insurance premiums, claims litigation, and settlements. There are also the indirect costs in the guise of defensive medicine, the physician's practice of ordering additional tests for self-protection. Finally, there is the very real cost in time and anguish for the practitioner involved in a malpractice suit. How will this challenge be met?

Background

Prior to 1970, hospitals and physicians paid little attention to the issue of malpractice or attendant costs. Most hospitals enjoyed some form of charitable immunity, and malpractice claims were infrequent. Many theories about why the malpractice claims picture changed in the 1970s have been espoused. Some suggestions include the following:

1. Rise in consumerism and an awareness of individual (including patient) rights
2. Increased belief in the "miracle" of technology
3. Rise in specialization and tertiary care, with the resultant depersonalization of health care delivery
4. An increase in the number of lawyers
5. A change in the practice of law from treating injuries under contract law to tort law
6. Awareness of availability of suit through advertisements in papers and television and motion picture promotions
7. Lack of adequate time for care
8. More proprietary and less charitable care

What is known is that over 90 percent of all suits have been filed since 1964. The average premium paid by physicians and hospitals quadrupled from 1960 to 1970. And between 1983 and 1985, premiums rose an additional 53 percent to an estimated annual cost of $14.7 billion. Since that time, the trend has not abated. Claims continue to increase in both frequency and severity in terms of dollars awarded. The total amount of claims paid by insurers rose 264 percent from 1980 to 1987. In the same period, the total amount of medical malpractice premiums paid by physicians and hospitals grew 235 percent.

Faced with the prospect of spiraling costs, hospitals and physicians have reacted with three responses. The first response was development of some form of self-insurance program. Many hospitals and physician groups have formed captive insurance companies. The goal of these groups is to provide coverage at the lowest possible cost. The second response was to develop a risk management program. In more recent years, the third response has been to combine the elements of a risk management program with those of a quality assurance program.

Prior to the mid-1970s, risk management programs in hospitals followed the industrial model and focused primarily on safety programs with emphasis on property insurance. Risk management, by definition, is a systematic and scientific approach to the identification, evaluation, reduction, or elimination of the possibility of an unfavorable deviation from expectations. The goal is to prevent the loss of financial assets of the individual practitioner or institution as a result of injuries to patients, visitors, employees, or independent medical staff. Further, the risk manager will attempt to control or transfer these risks at the lowest possible cost to the involved parties. In the hospital, the risks that cause the greatest financial loss are professional liability, including medical malpractice and worker's compensation. With the escalating cost of malpractice, risk managers changed their focus to the area where the institution and physicians find their greatest exposure, i.e., loss of assets as a result of malpractice claims. Patient safety programs were developed with the focus directed to those areas with the greatest likelihood of claims. Resources such as the National Association of Insurance Commissioners (NAIC) and the California Medical Insurance Feasibility (CMIF) study were the data sources for the early efforts. Risk managers began to focus on deficiencies within the delivery of medical care that resulted in patient injuries.

At the same time, the Joint Commission on Accreditation of Hospitals (JCAH) was rethinking its required quality assurance standards. Up until this time, the focus of the JCAH was primarily on quality control—again, an industrial model like the safety programs followed by traditional risk managers. The quality control requirements were supplemented by audits of identified or suspected problem areas. Since the mid-1980s, the JCAH requirements, having gone through a series of evolutions, have mandated consistent, ongoing monitoring of all important aspects of care being delivered within the hospital. The focus is on patient outcomes and the delivery of effective and efficient care. Change is to occur as a result of the findings.

The overlap and similarities between the monitoring functions of risk management and quality assurance are now evident.

Risk Management and Quality Assurance

The risk management process consists of the following five steps:

1. Identification of risk (injury), real or potential
2. Measurement of potential financial impact of each risk, identifying potential frequency and severity
3. Formulation of a policy of control for each risk
4. Implementation of the chosen technique
5. Periodic evaluation of the entire program to assess needed change

Because the first step in the process is identification, it is important to create a single, coherent system for risk detection. Until recently, the most widely used tool for detection has been the incident report. Incident reports exist in some form in almost every hospital. There may be a general policy and procedure with respect to filling out an incident report for all "unusual" occurrences, or there may be separate policies and procedures that deal with specific events for which an incident report must be filed. Although incident reports are used to identify events with potential for liability, they are not frequently used to report injuries. More often, they cumulatively represent a pattern of events. The problem with incident reports is that they are usually filled out by nurses and viewed as nursing documents.

Traditionally, physicians have been reluctant to use incident reports. Therefore, as risk management programs have become sophisticated, a series of tools have been developed to identify potential compensable events (PCEs).

A California physician, Dr. Joyce Craddick, developed a system to detect and prevent medically related patient injuries. The program is called the Medical Management Analysis (MMA) system and is usually referred to as generic or occurrence screening. It is designed to be both comprehensive and concurrent. Craddick used the study of claims in the CMIF study to develop a profile of most frequent claims allegations. From that, she developed a monitoring system that focuses on those variances in cases in which claims are most likely to develop. Medical records of patients who meet certain criteria are always reviewed and a determination made with respect to the reason for the problem. For example, any patient who incurs an adverse reaction to a medication, transfusion, or anesthetic will be reviewed, as will any patient who has an operation for perforation, laceration, tear, or injury received during intubations, catheterizations, incision, radiographic procedures, endoscopies, percutaneous aspirations, and percutaneous biopsies. Also reviewed are all unplanned removals of organs or parts of organs during an invasive procedure, all hospital-incurred trauma (patient accidents, procedural errors, shocks and burns), and other complications or unexplained major diagnostic and therapeutic maneuvers.

The program allows an objective examination of all events likely to lead to litigation. Patterns and trends relating to a particular department or practitioner become apparent, and remedial action may be possible before any claims have actually been initiated.

The quality assurance process incorporates the following five elements, which are similar to those found in the risk management process:

1. Identification of suspected deviations from the standard of care
2. Evaluation of these data to measure their validity and potential impact on patient's outcome
3. Formulation of a policy to address each identified variance
4. Implementation of the recommended change
5. Periodic assessment of the change to be sure of its continued effectiveness

Although the data sources for identification of risk or adverse patient outcomes and the assessment process for both programs are essentially the same, in most hospitals the programs exist independent of each other. Recognizing the value of having a single shared experience for both assuring patient outcomes and limiting the exposure of an institution and its physicians to liability, JCAH implemented a Risk Management Standard in 1989. This standard requires the two disciplines to share information that will be of mutual benefit to their common goals.

The result will be database programs that will not only spot patterns and trends of past and potential liability but will allow examination of both individual physician practice patterns and hospital practices relative to patient care. Such information will allow early intervention when there are lapses in quality care. The incentives for such a program are twofold: the escalating costs of malpractice awards, and the need for hospitals to become more efficient because of federal programs for prospective payment to hospitals.

Since the passage of the Tax Equity and Fiscal Responsibility Act (TEFRA) in 1982, hospitals have been paid for Medicare patients on a prospective basis, rather than a cost-reimbursed basis. Simply stated, this program requires that for each diagnosis there be a set payment. There are some exceptions, and certain considerations are given for regions of the country and patient mix. The intent, however, is to curtail the cost of health care by setting a fee paid per diagnosis. If the hospital spends less, it shares the reward. If it spends more, as in the case of a severely ill patient, it bears the cost. The result is an ever-increasing focus on reducing the length of stay, doing more outpatient procedures, and ordering fewer tests. Hospitals that are not aggressive in their cost-cutting will go out of business.

How does this relate to risk management? The first and most critical step in the risk management process remains identification. A systems approach allows a coordinated program of detection with all identification monitors, incident reports, generic quality screens, and maloccurrence reports channeled through a single location, the risk manager.

In addition to occurrence screens and incident reports, information is gathered from patient satisfaction and patient complaint forms. Quality assurance activity reports from individual services, infection control surveillance, and reports from outside monitors, such as JCAH and the Peer Review Organization (PRO), which oversees the federal Diagnosis Related Group (DRG) program, will be evaluated.

Each incident, pattern, or trend is evaluated in terms of frequency and severity. For example, falls (either patient falls or falls of others on hospital property) are high in frequency but low in severity in terms of losses paid. Surgical mishaps are low in frequency but high in severity. The identification indicators are used to spot new and emerging trends in PCEs to determine the formulation of a specific policy to control each risk. These loss control measures may be education, change in protocol and procedures, limitations of privilege, counseling, disciplinary action, claims management, and legal defense.

Physician Involvement

To this point, the discussion has focused on the identification process and tracking those findings. However, the next and most difficult step in the process is usually implementation. Risk management is by its nature a multidisciplinary function. Every health care provider and every hospital employee becomes a risk manager. To be effective, territorial prerogatives must be eliminated, and the goal of safe quality care must be the primary objective.

Just as it is no longer feasible for the physician to be concerned solely with his or her own liability exposure, it is also no longer possible for the physician to deny his or her collective responsibility for assuring quality patient outcomes. Given an awareness of the extent of the problem, and the institutional response to the problem, what is the responsibility of the individual practitioner and what can he or she do to minimize his or her own and the institution's exposure to liability?

The first step is to recognize the problem and approach it constructively. At least for the short term, everyone going into practice will have to deal with the realities of a litigious environment.

Quality care without "defensive" medicine must be the rule. In 1990, defensive medical care cost the health care industry $20 billion. With prospective payment, these costs must be eliminated.

Peer review as part of the medical staff function must no longer be regarded as a regulatory imposed requirement;

rather, it must be viewed as a desirable tool in the ongoing challenge to deliver safe patient care in a changing environment. Standards of care must be met to assure satisfactory patient outcomes and to preclude litigation. Therefore, every practitioner has a personal interest in assuring that an organized, systematic approach is in place to obtain that result.

Given that the quality assurance process ensures that professional standards of care are being met, what other resources does the physician have to protect himself or herself from litigation? The five best defenses are described in the following sections.

Good Rapport with Your Patient. Although patients who have longstanding relationships with their physicians do sometimes bring suit against them, it is usually the angry patient or family who brings a claim. The patient who feels rejected or "depersonalized," who has a sense of embarrassment, or who is humiliated or shamed in some way is likely to bring a claim if he or she incurs an injury. As a medical student you have only a short time to establish this rapport, so it must be worked at.

Good Documentation. It is probable that more claims have been won or lost over issues of documentation than any other. There is an axiom that states, "If it's not in the record, it didn't happen." The medical record is either your best friend or your worst enemy in a legal action. Careful consideration must be given to the implication of what is written in the chart. It is not the arena for argument. It is neither the place for philosophy nor the place to make a diagnosis or suggest procedures with which you are inexperienced or unfamiliar.

Prompt Reporting. If an incident does occur, there must be prompt reporting to the patient's physician of record and to the authority in the institution who handles the risk management function or to your insurance company's claim manager. Prompt interaction can often make the difference in terms of the potential financial loss.

Patient Confidentiality. Respect for your patient's confidentiality is critical. Avoid casual conversation about patients and their management or complications. The law is becoming increasingly restrictive regarding patient's rights and confidentiality. Be familiar with your state's laws and, when in doubt, contact your attending physician, risk manager, or legal consultant.

Informed Consent. The informed consent process is still frequently viewed as a legalistic requirement demanding that a form be filled out before permission is given for a certain event to occur. In *Informed Consent: Legal Theory and Clinical Practice,* Dr. Paul Applebaum suggests a more positive approach. The legel requirements for informed consent can be used as an opportunity to develop a therapeutic alliance with the patient. Such an alliance would significantly reduce unexpected outcomes, which, data suggest, constitute a significant portion of claims that are made.

Although many claims are made, negligence must be proved in order for a claim to be a viable malpractice action. This means that (1) there was a duty owed, (2) the duty was breached, (3) an injury occurred, and (4) the breach caused the injury.

Not every injury is negligence. The determination of who is negligent is usually decided by an evaluation of the standard of care. A medical student will be compared with other medical students, a second-year resident with other second-year residents, and so on. In the past, the standard was usually what was accepted practice in a given community or locality. Today, the trend is moving to a wider regional standard and, in some cases, to a national standard.

Medical Student Exposure

For the medical student, the greatest threat of claims occurs in two areas: fraud and improper supervision.

Fraud

The patient is usually unaware of whether the health care provider is a doctor or a medical student. In fact, medical students are often introduced as "doctors" or "young doctors." In this situation, the health care provider and the student have conspired to commit fraud. This fraud can lead to liability if the patient is injured as a result of the medical student's actions. Because fraud is an intentional tort, unlike medical malpractice, the patient may recover not only for any physical injuries but also for certain emotional injuries that resulted from intimate disclosures that would not have been made to a nonphysician. The court is also free to award punitive damages in cases of intentional torts. Punitive damages are not dependent on the amount of actual damages; rather, they are determined by the outrageous nature of the fraud. Even a minor injury may result in substantial punitive damages.

Although punitive damages may only be awarded for intentional fraud, unintentional or implicit fraud also has legal risks. This usually occurs when a patient is led to assume that the medical student is a doctor, as when the patient refers to the student as "doctor" and is not corrected. Confusion often results when a student has a doctorate-level degree. In a patient care setting, a patient expects "doctor" to mean physician. The best way to deal with this issue is to wear a name tag that identifies you as a medical student and identify yourself appropriately.

From the risk management perspective, the usual argument is that a patient may not consent if the student is not introduced as "doctor." That is precisely the issue. If a patient is tricked into treatment by a medical student, with the assumption that the student is a physician, the legal consequences may be serious. Most health care providers have found that patients are happy to be attended by medical students. Those patients who would not agree present the greatest threat of legal action.

Improper Supervision

The second major class of risk for the student involves injuries resulting from improper supervision. This can occur in two ways: because of improper delegation by the staff physicians or because of unauthorized care initiated and rendered by the medical student. In the first situation, the student would be liable if it could be shown that the student knew or should have known the acts would be improper, and the staff would be liable because they authorized the student's overreaching behavior. In the second situation, the staff would be liable for failing to supervise the student properly, and the student would be liable for taking unauthorized initiative. The implication of this finding is that you must seek supervision for procedures you have not done before. You should avoid functioning in situations in which you receive little, if any, supervision. Taking initiative may fulfill an ego need and a desire for autonomy, but it can have severe litigation consequences.

The problem with unauthorized actions may be twofold; they may result in either the issuance of unauthorized orders to other health care personnel or direct action by the student. The student who gives an order poses a problem only if the order is carried out without the authorization of the supervising physician. The problem of students acting on their own is more difficult, but it also has significant legal consequences.

Although traditionally medical students have not been named in lawsuits, the trend is changing. Hospitals and supervising physicians are usually the named defendants, but students need to be aware that plaintiffs' attorneys are beginning to be more specific in whom they name in claims. The trend is to name the individual(s) whose unauthorized or improper act resulted in the injury. This means that it is important to clear decisions and procedures with the attending physician before they are performed if there is any risk attendant to this performance.

Summary

In conclusion, the health care provider in the 1990s is faced with continued pressure to reduce costs associated with care while maintaining high quality. Insurance companies and federal and state agencies will be monitoring care given to patients and, at the same time, restricting payments made to hospitals for the care given. It is reasonable to expect that there will be similar restrictions on fees charged by physicians for unnecessary care.

Concurrently, the climate continues to favor increased numbers of malpractice claims and higher awards. The courts are becoming less restrictive with respect to expectations of care, and ever-increasing pressures are being placed on hospitals and physicians to provide incident-free care.

The challenge for the new physician will be to practice quality medicine within a cost-conscious environment given an awareness of the legal climate. It will be your responsibility to participate in self-policing through peer review and to join other physicians, health care providers, and lawmakers to see that the laws are changed. The current defensive and inequitable system must be restructured to protect the best of medical practice and provide reasonable compensation for those who are inadvertently injured during the course of medical practice.

When a Patient Leaves the Hospital

171

Judith P. Stone, MSW, LICSW

Judith Freiman Olson, MSW, LICSW

Assessing and planning for a patient's posthospital needs are a critical part of patient care. Shortened length of stay and technologic advances have an important impact on the discharge planning process. Nevertheless, one must consider the patient in the context of family and community. Although the hospitalization will focus upon specific symptoms, diagnoses, and interventions, this is but a time-limited, isolated experience for the patient. In other words, family and community are the constant themes. These themes will, to a large measure, frame continuity of care and, to a great extent, influence the outcome of hospital intervention.

The multidisciplinary health care team, working with and for the patient, includes the patient's family and community agencies. An example is the stroke patient who requires a full range of therapies in the acute care setting and requires the support of family and community agencies and services when discharged from the hospital.

Gains made during hospitalization are sustained through effective discharge planning. Concerns for quality care should continue beyond the acute care stay. Because the treatment team is complex, a comprehensive care plan emerges as an amalgam of many disciplines. In order to assure coordination and accountability of this intricate process, one discipline or department must assume responsibility. Although many disciplines (e.g., physical therapy, nutrition, occupational therapy, and physicians) make major contributions, traditionally social workers and nurses have taken leadership roles in case management for discharge planning purposes. Nurses have an overall understanding of patient care needs and community health nursing. Social work offers understanding of family systems and psychological issues, community resources, and how to use them.

There is an intimate relationship among discharge planning and family systems, societal changes, and the culture and resources of a given community. The increasing geriatric population and changing roles of women are two significant factors. Marked increases, especially in the over-80 population, are currently more rapid than the development of services to meet their needs. Their adult children (and presumed caretakers) may themselves be senior citizens. Employment of women outside the home has reduced the probability of caretaker availability for the disabled or frail elder. Finally, communities vary significantly insofar as available resources are concerned. In the provision of social service and economic support, one cannot assume that an affluent community will provide more social support than the inner city. Each community has its own traditions, networks, cultural attitudes, and resources. Effective discharge planning recognizes these variations and knows how to maximize use of community resources and adapt environments for optimal patient care.

Clinical Issues

Discharge planning raises a myriad of psychological stresses and pressures for patients and their families that are often framed by cultural and social realities. Serious illness is a crisis that provokes fears of change, the unknown, disability, and death. Although the patient is the focus, the entire family is affected. In a relatively short period of time, patients and families are expected to accept and adjust to consequences of illness that may be far reaching. Within a few days, families are asked to consider discharge planning options while they are still trying to adjust to the crisis of sudden illness. These families are fearful, anxious, and vulnerable as they are faced with significant changes and losses. An example is the coma patient who is medically stable and ready for a rehabilitation program, or the stroke patient ready for discharge who can never return home.

The hospitalized patient may be disabled, acutely or chronically ill, and experiencing multiple simultaneous losses. Although some of these losses may be transient (such as loss of privacy and independence), the irreversible losses require careful, sensitive consideration. Unresolved losses (such as death of a spouse) may even have contributed to the illness or accident. It is worth noting that gender differences may affect adjustment to loss. For example, widowers have a higher mortality rate during their first year of bereavement than widows.

Family adjustment relates to pre-existing family structure and relationships. Adult children may feel guilty about not caring for an ill parent, especially if raised in a culture in which elders were cared for at home. This may also be true if the patient blames his or her children for necessary placement or if relationships were conflicted prior to illness. It is helpful to involve a social worker in these situations because family dynamics need to be understood in order to resolve family conflicts. The resistant or demanding family can often be helped by empathic assessment and understanding. It is not unusual for discharge planning efforts to be frustrated by untreated family resistance (e.g., projections of blame onto caretakers).

Evaluation of Patients for Discharge Planning

In order to individualize a patient's discharge plan, a full spectrum of medical and psychosocial issues should be considered. This information comprises four interrelated and overlapping categories: history, current situation, needs, and preferences.

An evaluation of history and current situation involves the following elements:

1. Was the patient receiving home- or community-based services prior to hospitalization? If so, what were they and were they adequate?

2. How have the patient and family functioned in the past during periods of illness and dependency? What is their experience and attitude toward services or long-term care? Is their ability to cope now the same, enhanced, or compromised? What has the patient's home situation been (e.g., living alone or with whom, adequacy of housing, availability of caretakers, quality of relationships, and sources and adequacy of income)? Barriers to home care need to be evaluated, such as transportation, handicap accessibility, and safety factors.

3. Are there cultural, social, or religious affiliations to consider? For example, does the patient require kosher food or caretakers who speak a foreign language? Is this patient eligible for financial support from welfare, worker's compensation, veterans' programs, the American Cancer Society, Social Security, Commission for the Blind, or other agencies?

4. Is this situation adequate and appropriate without services, adequate and appropriate if services are provided, or inadequate or inappropriate?

Examples of questions related to the preceding outline would be as follows: Has anyone in this family had a history of institutionalization or a negative experience with a long-term care facility? If a patient is returning home with durable medical equipment, have architectural barriers and adequacy of wiring been assessed? Is the home situation comfortable, taking into account the patient's current limitations?

The needs of the patient and family are illness-related and psychosocial. Many disciplines provide clinical information essential for the plan. Areas of clinical needs to be assessed for appropriate planning include the following:

1. Medical (diagnoses, treatment, prognosis)
2. Nursing (skill-required treatments and monitoring; level of independence in activities of daily living; education [patient and family]; "high-tech" needs [intravenous lines, total parenteral nutrition, ventilators])
3. Restorative care (occupational therapy, physical therapy, speech therapy, respiratory therapy, rehabilitation potential)
4. Nutrition (special diets)
5. Psychosocial factors

Psychosocial factors often determine whether the patient can return home and whether the plan will be effective. Mental status and history of substance abuse are important. Attitude toward illness affects compliance and treatment goals. Cultural and religious values may affect behavior. Unrelated stresses in the home situation may influence current adjustment and cooperation. To what extent will lifestyle be altered (e.g., employment, income, living situation)? Has the patient been a caretaker for others?

Examples of psychosocial factors requiring attention include a Chinese-speaking patient who needs a nursing home, which raises cultural issues as well as communication problems; an 80-year-old frail widow who has been the sole caretaker of a retarded adult child; and a head-injured attorney who has been the sole financial support of a young family.

Patients and families may have strong opinions about the amount and type of service they want. An important consideration is who has the decision-making responsibility, be it patient, next of kin, or legal guardian.

Patient and family preference should always be respected and honored to the extent possible. Patient safety, availability of resources, and financial situation influence access and extent of choice. Third-party payments and government regulations also affect choice and timing.

No evaluation would be complete without consideration of legal issues that bear upon safety, liability of caretakers, and competence of patient and family to make decisions regarding care.

Timeliness of evaluation is vitally important for the patient, family, and institution. Shortened lengths of stay and termination of insurance coverage when the patient is no longer acute have streamlined the discharge-planning process as never before. It appears that this trend will continue.

Services Provided to Persons Living at Home

Home Health Care

Home health agencies fall into two broad categories: "certified" home health agencies (either nonprofit or proprietary), which are eligible for third-party reimbursement, and "noncertified" agencies, which are usually proprietary and depend upon private funding sources.

Services focus on the health care needs of the patient. Although there may be variations in the scope of services provided by a specific agency or in a particular community, these services may include high-tech needs; skilled nursing; physical, occupational, or speech therapy; social work and mental health; home health aides; and hospice care.

Payment by a third party is generally contingent upon whether the services are "skilled," as defined by the regulations of a health maintenance organization (HMO) or an insurance contract. In general, this means that services should be provided by professionals and be limited in duration. For example, a new diabetic patient may qualify for short-term teaching at home, but ongoing diabetic care (e.g., insulin shots) may not be covered. A new stroke patient returning home may qualify for Medicare-funded physical therapy, occupational therapy, and social work, but ongoing custodial care would not be funded by third-party payments.

These issues are significant, as ongoing services need an alternative source of funding (Medicaid or private funds). Medicaid (public welfare medical assistance) can vary from state to state in its coverage. It is important to be sensitive to the fact that patients and families find it difficult to understand that requiring considerable care may not qualify one for "skilled" reimbursable care.

In recent years, sophisticated services have been developed that allow such technologic care as intravenous lines and total parenteral nutrition to be delivered at home. The feasibility of sophisticated home health care may depend upon the support of reliable family or friends, the resources of a given community, and whether funding is available.

Medical equipment such as walkers, hospital beds, and oxygen may be available and reimbursable for certain conditions.

Other Support Services

Many communities offer support services that enable disabled and frail elderly to remain in their homes. These services may include homemakers, chore services, home-delivered meals, and transportation. There may be services at community sites, such as hot meals and social activities, that enhance the quality of life for many older persons. Adult day care is an expanding concept, offering social support and often medical and nursing care. These programs can prevent or delay institutionalization, and they can provide significant assistance to families caring for elderly relatives.

The availability of support in one's housing situation can affect the timing of the discharge plan. Many communities have special housing, often subsidized, for elderly, disabled, retarded, or chronic psychiatric patients. Supports often include supervision, nutrition, health monitoring, and transportation. In increasing numbers, people are living in congregate housing and continuing-care retirement communities. Their availability may be restricted by short supply or financial cost.

Having outlined an array of options, it is important to note that many social and economic trends affect availability and access. The individual who is "over income" for Medicaid but living on a fixed income may find it hard to finance needed services. Some states sponsor and underwrite the cost of home care services for persons meeting income guidelines.

Many regional and individual issues bear upon access. Only an individualized approach by knowledgeable discharge planners can responsibly discern and develop an appropriate plan. The depth and scope of individualized planning requires maximal lead time during the patient's hospital stay. The importance of early referral to the social worker cannot be overstated.

Services Provided to Persons Requiring Institutional Care

When ready for hospital discharge, many patients have needs that are met only in an institutional setting. This may be a short-term need, such as a rehabilitation program, or a permanent need, such as a long-term care facility.

Rehabilitation is provided both in specialized hospitals or hospital units and in some nursing homes (extended-care facilities or skilled nursing homes). Specific criteria and regulations determine whether someone is eligible and whether insurance will pay. For example, a patient with a non–weight-bearing fractured hip will not qualify until he or she can participate in active physical therapy. Alternative plans, if available, may be necessary for this interim period. The situation of a markedly confused patient with a fractured hip is likewise problematic. If the patient's confusion is transient, the plan is as above; if confusion is permanent, a rehabilitation program is an unlikely alternative.

Some states have chronic-care hospitals. These facilities provide custodial care with medical management for patients who may have significant nursing or rehabilitative needs. Examples include certain Veterans Administration hospitals, former tuberculosis hospitals, and the chronic hospitals, both public and voluntary, in states such as Massachusetts. There are also chronic-care hospitals specializing in the care of particular populations, such as disabled children and chronic psychiatric patients.

Nursing homes, rest homes, and homes for the aged vary significantly in the extent of services they offer. Skilled nursing facilities offer around-the-clock professional nursing and rehabilitative services, and they may offer high-tech care (feeding tubes, intravenous lines, ventilators). They may be certified for Medicare, but this benefit is quite limited. Many patients and families believe that Medicare covers long-term care for custodial needs; this is not the case.

Intermediate or Custodial Care

Nursing homes are for patients who require less care than provided in the facilities described previously. There is support for activities of daily living, and nursing supervision is provided. Most of the care is provided by paraprofessionals.

Nursing home care, with the exception of limited insurance benefits, is financed by Medicaid, private funds, or a combination thereof. Increasingly, both the insurance industry and the United States Congress are working on developing long-term care insurance.

There is tremendous variation in the scope of care in nursing homes, often defined by state regulations or reimbursement rates. There are local and regional variations in availability of beds, staffing, reimbursement, and regulations. The hardest patients to plan for are those with behavioral or addiction problems, those with heavy nursing care needs, and those dependent upon public financial support. These issues may delay timing of transfer of patients from the acute care setting. Again, this underscores the value of professional discharge planning, in order to maximize the benefits of acute care and treatment, to find resources able to meet a given patient's needs, and to minimize risk of readmission.

References

Kulys R. Future crisis and the very old: Implications for discharge planning. Health Social Work 1980; 1:450.

Lurie A. The social work advocacy role in discharge planning. Social Work Health Care 1982; 8(2):75.

Schrager J, et al. Impediment to the course and effectiveness in discharge planning. Social Work Health Care 1978; 4(1):65.

Shaughnessy PW, Kramer AM. The increased needs of patients in nursing homes and patients receiving home health care. N Engl J Med 1990; 322:21.

Legal Issues Surrounding a Patient's Death

Barbara F. Katz, JD

172

The Right to Refuse Treatment

In general, a competent adult patient (18 years of age or older) has the right to refuse treatment, including life-saving treatment. This includes "do not resuscitate" (DNR) orders. The Joint Commission on the Accreditation of Healthcare Organizations requires hospitals to have formal policies on DNR orders, and physicians should be familiar with the one in their particular institution. It is important in a competent patient's exercise of this right that the patient be fully informed of all information relevant to his or her decision making. Any refusal of treatment by the patient should be fully documented in the patient's medical record. This should include the patient's physical and mental condition, the information that was provided to the patient, the fact of and reasons for the patient's refusal, and the level of knowledge and reaction of any family. A form may be developed and used for these purposes that the patient signs and that is placed in the record. If no form is used, it may be wise to have the patient read and sign the medical record entry.

Incompetent Patients

Because the trend in the law is to give incompetent individuals the same rights as those who are competent, courts in many states have held that incompetent patients also have the right to refuse life-saving treatment. In the context of medical care, an adult is deemed to be competent if the patient can understand the nature and consequences of the illness or condition, the nature and consequences of the proposed medical procedure, and the likely result if the procedure is not performed. It should be remembered that an individual who is mentally ill, mentally retarded, or voluntarily or involuntarily institutionalized is *not* automatically legally incompetent for the purpose of refusing life-saving treatment. In addition, the mere fact that a patient's decision is contrary to that which his or her physician or family recommends, or contrary to that which a majority of people in a similar situation would make, does not by itself indicate incompetence.

In decision making for incompetent patients, the standard applied in many states is "substituted judgment," i.e., attempting to determine as closely as possible what the incompetent patient would do if able to indicate his or her own desires, taking into account his or her personal preferences and beliefs. This usually involves reviewing any written statement previously prepared by the patient (see discussion of living will); ascertaining whether the patient, although incompetent, is nevertheless capable of making some present expression of his or her desires; discussing with family and other available individuals close to the patient whether, through word or action, the patient had expressed a preference; and discussing with health care providers whether a patient who was competent for some portion of his or her hospital stay had given an indication of his or her wishes. In some situations involving minors (generally individuals under the age of 18) and patients who have never been competent, the standard used has been the "best interests" test, i.e., determining that which is in the patient's best interests.

In many states, there is no requirement for obtaining a court order before stopping treatment. Next of kin, guardians, and other patient proxies often make these decisions on behalf of incompetent patients. Courts are available for instances in which there is reason for uncertainty regarding the incompetent patient's wishes or other doubt about the appropriate course to take. However, it is important in this area to consult the law in your particular state, as there is a certain amount of variation among the states regarding treatment decision making for incompetent patients.

Living Wills

In making treatment decisions for terminally ill incompetent patients, a "living will" can be extremely helpful. A living will is a written declaration made by a person when competent, indicating his or her wishes regarding treatment if he or she should become incompetent or otherwise incapable of expressing his or her own desires. Thus, it permits individuals to refuse in advance to consent to certain procedures under certain circumstances.

At least 40 states have statutes dealing with living wills, and physicians practicing in those states should become familiar with their provisions. However, even in states without such a statute, it certainly is very good evidence of the patient's desires, and can help form the basis for a determination of the patient's "substituted judgment," as discussed previously. In cases involving living wills, a copy of the document should be placed in the medical record. Of course, if the living will was signed a long time prior to the present illness, and close family members or others provide plausible evidence, including verbal, that the patient in fact had changed his or her mind, this information should be documented and seriously considered in the analysis as well.

Determination of Death

In the determination of when a patient has died, some questions have been raised about the legality of the concept of brain death. As long as the definition and criteria used are accepted by the medical profession as an appropriate and medically valid means for determining death, the law will accept it as well. This is so even in those states that do not have "brain death" statutes. Again, in those states that do have specific statutes on the subject, physicians should be familiar with their content.

When a patient is determined to be brain dead, the time of and reasons for this decision should be documented in the medical record. Any machines sustaining the patient's bodily functions should be removed, unless there are independent reasons, such as organ donation, for continuing them. The family should be informed that the patient is dead. It is not necessary or advisable to ask family permission for discontinuing care, because the patient is already dead and there are no longer any treatment decisions that need to be made. When speaking to the

Neither the author nor the publisher is engaged in rendering legal advice through this publication. Readers requiring or desiring such advice should consult a competent attorney of their own choosing.

family, one should also avoid using terms such as "brain dead" or "clinically dead," because this is often confusing to a layperson and may be taken to imply the patient is not yet in fact "dead."

Organ Donation

The Uniform Anatomical Gift Act, with some minor variations, is law in all states. It provides that any individual 18 years of age or older and of sound mind may make a gift of all or any specific part of his or her body to the following parties for the following purposes:

1. To any hospital, surgeon, or physician, for medical or dental science, therapy, or transplantation
2. To any accredited medical or dental school, college, or university for education, research, advancement of medical or dental science, or therapy
3. To any bank or storage facility, for medical or dental education, research, advancement of medical or dental science, therapy, or transplantation
4. To any specified individual for therapy or transplantation needed by him or her.

The gift can be made by a provision in a will or by signing a donation card in the presence of two witnesses. The gift can be revoked in most states by destruction of the card or an oral declaration in the presence of two witnesses.

Following a patient's death, the next of kin may consent to organ donation. The line of kinship is the surviving spouse, if there is one, then other survivors in order of family relationship—usually adult children, parents, adult siblings. The statute provides that if there is actual notice of opposition to the gift by a member of the same or a prior class of kinship, then the gift may not be accepted.

Required Request

A growing trend in many states is to have what are termed "required request" laws, which obligate physicians responsible for the care of a patient to request organ donation from the patient's next of kin on or immediately before the patient's death. There are often certain exceptions to this requirement, such as if the request would not yield an organ suitable for transplant purposes, if the request would cause undue emotional stress to the next of kin, if the decedent had expressed a contrary wish while alive, or if the donation would be contrary to the decedent's religious or moral beliefs.

Autopsy

Under the laws of most states, the next of kin has the right to consent to an autopsy. The line of kinship and the treatment of situations in which there is opposition to the decision is essentially as discussed under organ donation. This right of the next of kin to determine the disposition of the dead body generally may be overridden only by an official coroner or medical examiner autopsy. Some states have specific statutes dealing with autopsies, and physicians should be aware of any such provisions. (The autopsy is discussed in greater detail in Chapter 174.)

References

Annas G, Glantz L, Katz B. The rights of doctors, nurses, and allied health professionals. New York: Avon Books, 1981:214.

Bartling v. Superior Court, 163 Cal. App. 3d 186, 209 Cal. Rptr. 220 (1984).

Bouvia v. Superior Court, 179 Cal. App. 3d 1127, 225 Cal. Rptr. 297 (1986).

Brophy v. New England Sinai Hospital, Inc., 398 Mass. 417, 497 N.E. 2d 626 (1986).

In re Conroy, 98 N.J. 321, 486 A.2d 1209 (1985).

Cruzan v. Director, Missouri Dep't of Health, 58 U.S.L.W. 4916 (June 26, 1990).

In re Dinnerstein, 6 Mass. App. 466, 380 N.E.2d 134 (1978).

In re Farrell, 108 N.J. 335, 529 A.2d 404 (1987).

Gray v. Romeo, 697 F. Supp. 580 (D.R.I. 1988).

In re Jobes, 108 N.J. 394, 529 A.2d 434 (1987).

John F. Kennedy Mem. Hosp., Inc. v. Bludworth, 452 So. 2d 921 (Fla. 1984).

In re Peter, 108 N. J. 365, 529 A.2d 419 (1987).

President's Commission for the Study of Ethical Problems in Medicine and Biomedical and Behavioral Research. Defining death: Medical, legal and ethical issues in the determination of death. Washington, DC: US Government Printing Office, 1981.

In re Quinlan, 70 N.J. 10, 355 A.2d 647 (1976).

In re Requena, 213 N.J. Super. 475, 517 A.2d 886 (N.J. Super. Ch. Div.), aff'd 213 N.J. Super. 443, 517 A.2d 869 (N.J. Super. App. Div. 1986).

Robertson J. The rights of the critically ill. New York: Bantam Books, 1983.

Satz v. Perlmutter, 362 So. 2d 160 (Fla. Dist. Ct. App. 1978).

In re Spring, 380 Mass. 629, 405 N.E.2d 115 (1980).

Matter of Storar and Eichner v. Dillon, 52 N.Y.2d 363, 438 N.Y.S.2d 266, 420 N.E.2d 64 (1981).

Superintendent of Belchertown State School v. Saikewicz, 373 Mass. 728, 370 N.E.2d 417 (1977).

In re Westchester County Medical Center on behalf of O'Connor, 531 N.E.2d 607 (N.Y. 1988).

When a Patient Dies: Pronouncement of Death

173

Allen D. Ward, MD

Brian D. Blackbourne, MD

Arthur R. Russo, MD

The major thrust of medical school training and residency programs is toward the treatment and cure of ill patients. A patient presents to a physician with an illness or disease that the physician diagnoses, treats, and, it is hoped, cures. We learn that our reward is the successful diagnosis and treatment and the patient's gratitude for this. Unfortunately, a successful outcome is not always the case, and the patient dies. When poorly handled, the death of a patient can leave many hard feelings among the patient's family, physicians, and the health care team. On the other hand, if well handled, a patient's death can be reasonably satisfactory; it can even lead to a life-long friendship and, if need be, a continuing medical relationship with the patient's survivors.

An expected death, as with cancer, heart disease, renal

failure, or chronic lung disease, presents one set of problems; the unexpected death presents another.

Definition

Although there is no uniform definition of death, it can be divided into two broad categories: determination of death by clinical means and determination of brain death. Death on a clinical basis can be most simply defined as irreversible cessation of circulatory and respiratory functions with no obvious neurologic activity. The definition of brain death, on the other hand, has been a source for great debate, primarily in legislative arenas, and the definition varies from state to state. Most definitions of brain death include irreversible cessation of entire brain function, including death of the brain stem. This is also accompanied by irreversible cessation of cardiopulmonary function. This latter event would make it difficult to obtain organs for transplantation; thus, criteria have been established to help guide the clinician. These issues are discussed later in this chapter.

The Expected Death

When a patient appears to be terminally ill with a known disease, it is important for the physician to review all aspects of the patient's case to make certain that he or she is dying of a known cause; e.g., a patient with cancer of the colon who presents with bowel obstruction should be evaluated to make certain that the obstruction is due to the cancer and not due to simple adhesions that could be corrected surgically, thus allowing the patient further good-quality survival. Another example is the patient with breast cancer who presents with confusion. The physician must rule out hypercalcemia as the cause of confusion before assuming the problem is due to brain metastases. Hypercalcemia is readily treatable with medications, and the patient can return to a reasonably productive life in this instance, whereas brain metastases may be part of the cause of the patient's death.

It is important that the physician communicate with the patient and his or her family and be certain that they understand what is going on. By understanding the disease and the goals of therapy, the family becomes part of the therapeutic team. In these days of increasing lawsuits, good rapport with a patient and the family prevents such problems. The most useful approach is the family conference; although it involves an investment of time, it is time well spent. It allows the family to know exactly what is going on, and it allows the patient and the family to express their feelings about the patient's illness.

Throughout the patient's terminal illness, it is important that the physician be available to the patient and the family. It is very easy for the physician to become suddenly unavailable or to avoid the terminally ill patient. Often on rounds the physician notes that the patient is sleeping and avoids a visit because the patient "needs his rest." Because the patient is likely to realize that he or she has been skipped that day and may feel abandoned, the physician should either wake the patient or return at a later time. The physician on rounds may be accosted by family members, and it is important to make time for them even when time is short.

When a terminally ill patient dies, the physician will be called upon to pronounce the patient dead.

Pronouncement

The physician may be called from the office, from home, or from another part of the hospital to pronounce a patient dead, or the physician may have been in attendance with a terminally ill patient at the time of death. In general, when pronouncing a patient dead clinically, the physician first observes for signs of any spontaneous activity, be it movement or respiratory effort. The physician should then provide the patient with a verbal stimulus; if there is no response to the verbal stimulus, the physician may inflict an uncomfortable stimulus. If there still is no response, the physician should then assess the patient's vital signs; the physician should palpate the carotid artery for sign of a pulse and then place a stethoscope on the chest and auscultate for either respiratory effort or cardiac function. If these signs are absent, the physician should do a brief neurologic assessment, including examination of the pupils for reaction to light. If there is absence of spontaneous movement, absence of spontaneous respiration, absence of cardiac function, and absence of neurologic function clinically, the patient may be assumed to be dead and pronounced as such.

When pronouncing the patient dead, the physician should write a note in the patient's chart clearly documenting the events leading to the determination of death, i.e., either the notification by the nursing staff that the patient expired or the physician's presence during the terminal event, the pertinent physical examination as just outlined, the associated medical problems that may have contributed to the patient's death, and finally, the time at which the patient was pronounced dead. Furthermore, the pronouncement note should include information concerning whether or not the next of kin was notified, whether or not a postmortem examination is desired by the family or is indicated on the basis of legal requirements, and what the disposition of the body will be.

Notifying the Family

When notifying the family of the patient's death, the physician should not be surprised by the family reaction, even if the death was totally expected. There may be a great deal of agonizing and anger, which at times may be directed toward the physician. In this situation, patience and courtesy will win out; sometimes the angriest confrontations at the death of a patient will be followed by expressions of gratitude. If at all possible, the doctor should make every effort to be with the family, even briefly, and comfort them. At this time, it is important to emphasize the positive aspects of the family's involvement in the patient's death. It is very important to commend the family, when reasonable, on their efforts at helping with the patient's terminal illness and to allay any fears that they did not do enough for the patient.

The Autopsy

In most instances, it is desirable to request permission for an autopsy. The autopsy is an important part of the total care of the patient. It helps us understand a specific disease process as well as the dynamics of the disease in a particular patient. Sometimes, when rapport with a family has been very good prior to death, it is possible to approach this subject while the patient is still alive. More often, the subject does not come up until the patient has expired. It is very important not to be demanding when requesting postmortem permission but to be matter of fact and explain that physicians are required to ask for autopsy permission, adding that such permission may clarify some points for the doctors and even benefit others in the future. If autopsy permission is refused by any members of the family, it is important not to be aggressive about it. There have been instances in which ill will developed when an autopsy was performed against the wishes of one or more family members.

Although the majority may rule in voting, this doesn't necessarily hold with autopsy permission (see Chapter 172, "Legal Issues Surrounding a Patient's Death," and Chapter 174, "The Autopsy"). It is necessary that the autopsy permission be obtained from the patient's next of kin, and not from a well-meaning relative or friend. When the next of kin cannot be contacted, an autopsy must not be performed, even when several family members agree to it. The following is the priority order of legal next of kin:

1. Spouse, if present, is always legal next of kin.
2. An adult son or daughter is next in line with authority for autopsy and should be contacted if there is no spouse.
3. Either parent.
4. Adult brother or sister.
5. Guardian of decedent at the time of his or her death.
6. Any other person authorized or under legal obligation to dispose of the remains.

Once permission has been obtained, and the appropriate forms are completed, it is important that the physician caring for the deceased patient notify the pathologist of the desire to perform an autopsy. The patient's clinical course, the presumed clinical cause of death, and any specific questions that the autopsy may clarify are discussed with the pathologist. It is important that information concerning possible infectious diseases or other rare conditions be communicated to the pathologist prior to the autopsy so that appropriate precautions can be taken and appropriate specimens obtained. Furthermore, if a postmortem examination is to be performed, all invasive lines (e.g., endotracheal tubes, Swan-Ganz catheters, and central venous lines) should be left in place so that any iatrogenic complication can be more easily diagnosed.

Finally, once the results of the autopsy are known, it is very important that the physician discuss these results with the family members. This may help them to understand more clearly the cause of death of their family member, to be aware of potential inheritable disease(s) within a family, and most important, to be reassured that the patient was properly cared for. (For more information, see Chapter 174, "The Autopsy"). This contact also provides the family the opportunity to discuss any unresolved issues surrounding the patient's death.

The Unexpected Death

A more difficult problem is the unexpected death, or the unexpected rapid decline in the patient's condition. This brings us to the issue of brain death.

With the advent of intensive care medicine and the ability of the physician to keep a patient alive, i.e., in terms of respiratory and circulatory support, it has become increasingly apparent that such maintained patients often have suffered irreversible brain damage leading to presumed brain death. For several years now, physicians, lawyers, legislators, and theologians have wrestled with the definition of brain death. This has become even more important in the era of organ transplantation; patients who are "most likely" brain dead can have their vital functions maintained by artificial means for a finite period before their organs are no longer suitable for transplantation.

To date, there is no uniform definition of brain death in the United States, despite the work of the President's Commission for the Study of Ethical Problems in Medicine and Biomedical and Behavioral Research on such guidelines. Many states do have specific criteria for the determination of brain death, with much state-to-state variation. In general terms, brain death has been defined as irreversible cessation of brain function, including cerebral function as well as brain-stem function. Furthermore, the criteria and the studies required to prove that a patient is brain dead are even more varied than the general definition of brain death. It is not the intent of this chapter to discuss these controversies in great detail but rather to make the physician aware of the increasing need for determination of brain death and the legal issues involved.

In 1968 a committee of the Harvard Medical School faculty confronted the problem of brain death and published a set of criteria they believed would represent "irreversible coma" in a patient presumed to be brain dead. The criteria as outlined are (1) unreceptivity and unresponsivity, (2) absence of movement and spontaneous respirations, (3) absence of reflexes, and (4) flat electroencephalogram in the absence of any factors that would or might depress the central nervous system activity. These tests should be repeated at least 24 hours later with no change.

The last criterion presented by the Harvard faculty is very important, because many conditions may mimic irreversible coma or brain death, especially the presence of pharmacologic agents (such as high levels of benzodiazepines or barbiturates), hypothermia, and shock. Also, it is known that the brains of infants and young children are much more resistant to damage and have potential for recovery even after prolonged insult.

This process of determination of brain death can be agonizing for the family, especially in the case of the unexpected death. Anger may be directed at the physician and other staff. For example, the patient with a brain tumor who has been doing well but suddenly deteriorates in a matter of hours and dies may leave the family wondering what the doctor has missed, when in fact recurrent tumor may be very hard to detect before a catastrophe happens. This requires patient listening on the part of the physician, and as much time as necessary should be spent explaining to the family what happened. Again, a family conference is most helpful here, although sometimes it is anxiety producing for the doctor. Often, questions raised may seem "silly," but it is time well spent, especially in terms of the well-being of those left behind.

There are certain situations in which the physician is required to notify the medical examiner of a patient's death. The circumstances vary from state to state; specific information is available from the office of the state medical examiner in the state where the physician practices. In general, the following instances warrant notification:

1. Violent deaths, including those due to sexual abuse
2. Death due to chemical, thermal, or electrical agents, including death of a child determined to be physically dependent upon addictive drugs at birth
3. Death following abortion
4. Death resulting from disease, injury, or an infection resulting from occupation
5. Sudden deaths in the absence of recognizable disease or malnutrition
6. Persons found dead

In central Massachusetts, for example, deaths that must be reported by order of the medical examiner include the following:

1. Any hospital death within 24 hours of admission
2. Any hospital death in which the person was unconscious on admission and remained so
3. Any death due to therapeutic misadventure
4. Deaths pronounced by a physician other than the attending doctor
5. Unexpected death in the course of pregnancy, obstetrical deliveries, anesthesia, or surgery
6. Any death occurring under suspicious circumstances
7. Any deaths of people in police custody
8. Any deaths of employees while at work
9. All deaths due to cirrhosis

The Death Certificate

Finally, there is the formality of filling out the death certificate. Note that the death certificate changes in format from time to time, but instructions are usually provided. A black pen must be used for copying purposes. Exactly what should be stated as the cause of death on the certificate remains somewhat controversial. Often the cause of death will be stated to be cardiopulmonary arrest, and the underlying cause may be stated as the disease that caused the cardiopulmonary arrest. It has been our experience that this has created some legal problems subsequently. For example, in some cities any firefighter who dies of cardiopulmonary arrest is entitled to a large pension for his family, and if a cardiac cause is implied in the death certificate, the pension will take effect even if the patient's cause of death was really carcinoma of the prostate. We prefer to use the major diagnosis as a cause of the patient's death, such as "carcinoma of the prostate with widespread metastases."

Summary

The death of a patient is one of the more unsettling aspects of the practice of medicine, primarily because much of a physician's training is focused on curing the patient. Often it is helpful to share your own feelings about the process with a trusted colleague. If it is a patient you were close to, you may grieve as well. This period of grief seems to shorten with experience, but it never goes away, and it is one factor that helps maintain our sensitivity as physicians. Finally, if properly handled, the events surrounding the patient's death can create goodwill toward the medical profession and satisfaction on the part of the physician. More important, they can ameliorate some of the family's suffering.

References

Bernat JL, et al. Defining death in theory and practice. The Hastings Center Report. February 1982.

Black PM. Brain death (first of two parts). N Engl J Med 1978; 299(7).

Black PM. Brain death (second of two parts). N Engl J Med 1978; 299(8).

Chianchiano DR. Legislative arena: Definition of death. Am J Kidney Dis 1982; 1(6).

Dornette WHL. How does your state define death? Legal Aspects of Medical Practice, May 1980.

Report of the Ad Hoc Committee of the Harvard Medical School to examine the definition of brain death: A definition of irreversible coma. JAMA 1978; 205(6).

Report of the Medical Consultant in the Diagnosis of Death to the President's Commission for the Study of Ethical Problems in Medicine and Biomedical and Behavioral Research: Guidelines for the determination of death. Crit Care Med 1982; 10(1).

The Autopsy

Carolyn C. Compton, MD, PhD

174

The autopsy is the most important quality control in the practice of medicine. Its acquisition is also a measure of the intellectual honesty of the physician. The declining autopsy rate is a threat to the medical profession and to the public health. Our knowledge of the natural history of disease, of our own accuracy in diagnosis, and of the efficacy and complications of treatment come largely from autopsy studies.

The sophisticated technology of modern medicine has insidiously engendered a misguided sense of security about diagnosis. Why bother to get an autopsy when the disease process and cause of death are already known? Hence the declining autopsy rate. It is clear from several recent studies, however, that the premortem diagnosis is accurate in only slightly more than half of cases. The rate at which autopsies detect major unexpected findings whose premortem diagnosis would actually improve survival is more than 10 percent. Obviously, then, even in this age of cost containment, the autopsy is one corner that medicine cannot afford to cut. What precedent could be more dangerous for medical professionals than learning to accept burying our mistakes? The physician's responsibility to the patient does not end at the moment of death.

Obtaining Autopsy Permission

As with many of the primary duties of patient care in teaching institutions, the responsibility of obtaining autopsy permission from the next of kin belongs to the house officer. Enlisting the cooperation of the family in any mode of medical care requires that the physician be both sensitive to the concerns of the family and willing to spend the time to inform them about the nature of and need for the procedure.

For help in determining who is the next of kin and what defines a medical-legal autopsy (no permission required from next of kin), see Chapter 172, "Legal Issues Surrounding a Patient's Death," and Chapter 173, "When a Patient Dies: Pronouncement of Death."

The following are some points to remember about autopsies:

1. The autopsy is just like a surgical procedure. It is performed by a physician with the same care, skill, and respectful attitude. Families understand this analogy. Imagined connotations of an autopsy are often more frightening and unnecessarily emotionally disturbing.

2. The routine complete autopsy is *not* cosmetically deforming in any way. Complete autopsies refer to examination of thoracic and abdominal viscera (usually removed from the body "en bloc") and the brain.

3. "Limited" autopsies are often agreeable to family members who may object to a full dissection. *This is very important.* Autopsy examination can be tailored to the patient's major disease process and the most important questions to be answered. You can be a gentle guide to the next of kin by indicating what examination would be most likely to yield the information you would like to have. Frequently, even family members who would be otherwise disinclined to have an autopsy done grant autopsy permission as a compensation to the physician for the care of their loved one.

Although a limited autopsy is better than no postmortem examination at all, be sure that the compromise is reasonable. Severe limitations (e.g., percutaneous needle biopsy of the heart in a patient with suspected myocardial infarction) may reduce the probability of obtaining useful information to almost zero.

It is very important to remember that negative emotional

responses to examination of the brain (such as would occur in a "complete" autopsy) are extremely common. Do not neglect to suggest an autopsy with a restriction on examination of the brain ("no head"). This is often a perfectly acceptable compromise.

4. Although most pathology departments usually perform autopsies only within specified hours during the week and on weekends, special arrangements can almost always be made to complete the autopsy outside those hours, should religious codes, personal dilemmas, or unusual circumstances dictate. It may be important to reassure family members that their wishes regarding any special considerations of the deceased will be honored by the pathologist to the fullest extent possible.

Informing the Pathologist

All autopsies are not equal. The pathologist tailors dissection technique and use of ancillary procedures to the case at hand. The more the pathologist knows about the patient, the more information will be derived from the autopsy, and the fewer points of interest to the physician will be inadvertently overlooked. *Be sure* to fill out the clinical summary that accompanies the autopsy permission form, and be explicit about your major concerns and unanswered questions. Direct communication with the pathologist before the autopsy is best.

It is also of utmost importance that the pathologist be informed of any communicable diseases, either diagnosed or suspected, that the patient might have. This is vital to the safety of the pathologist, who is at maximum risk of contracting such diseases if the proper autopsy precautions are not taken.

Try to attend at least part of the autopsy yourself or arrange to meet the pathologist in the autopsy suite later to review and discuss the findings. In teaching institutions, pathology autopsy conferences are held for pathologists to review their cases. These conferences provide a rich opportunity for clinicopathologic correlations. When the patient's autopsy is to be presented, it is important that physicians and students involved in the patient's care attend.

The Autopsy Report

Within a day or two after completion of the autopsy, a preliminary anatomic diagnosis is issued based on the gross findings in the case. If particularly critical to the diagnosis, a limited number of histologic specimens may be processed prior to issuing the preliminary anatomic diagnosis, but the complete histologic examination usually requires at least a week or two. The final anatomic diagnosis will be based upon the histologic and gross findings. The pathologist's analysis of the case is included in the diagnosis.

Conclusion

The autopsy is the only opportunity in medical practice to know *all* about your patient's illness. Understandably, diagnostic approaches to the living patient are limited by either technical or ethical parameters. Ironically, the autopsy is the only medical service that benefits others rather than the patient, but the benefits are great. The physician learns about the accuracy of his or her judgment, the patient's family members benefit from exact knowledge of their own family history (often with potential implications about their own health), and society benefits from validated vital statistics and public trust in a medical profession willing to discover the truth in its practices.

References

Gobbato J, et al. Inaccuracy of death certificate diagnoses in malignancy: An analysis of 1,405 autopsy cases. Hum Pathol 1982; 13:1036.

Goldman L, et al. The value of the autopsy in three medical areas. N Engl J Med 1983; 308:1000.

Landefeld CS. Diagnostic yield of the autopsy in a university hospital and a community hospital. N Engl J Med 1988; 313:1249.

Lundberg GD. Medical students, truth, and the autopsy. JAMA 1983; 250:1199.

Lundberg GD, Voigt GE. Reliability of a presumptive diagnosis in sudden unexpected death in adults: The case for autopsy. JAMA 1979; 242:2328.

Mortality statistics without autopsies: Wonderland revisited [editorial]. Hum Pathol 1987; 18:875.

Prutting J. The autopsy. JAMA 1972; 222:1556.

Rubenstone AI, et al. Autopsies in hospitals of the Chicago area. Proc Inst Med Chicago 1983; 36:39.

Bereavement and Grief

175

Sandra L. Bertman, PhD

Helen K. Sumpter, BA

Harry L. Greene, MD

Definitions

Grief is an adaptational response to loss through the death of or separation from an object of love, be it a person, a body part, or a body function. Even less tangible "losses," such as a change in status, retirement, a move to a new home or job, or the loss of an activity or an ideal, can trigger a grief reaction. Normal grief is self-limiting and resolved by reality. Interference with it is regarded as useless, even harmful. Grieving, then, is a healing process necessary to diminish and resolve the pain of the loss.

Phyllis Silverman, a social worker at Harvard University, has noted that with the death of a parent, one loses the past; of a spouse, one's present; and of a child, the future. The profound changes brought about by death can be regarded as a temporary disintegration of the life process. The healing that must take place may be considered a gradual reintegration of one's daily functions, physical as well as psychological, in the light of these changes.

Pathologic mourning is unresolved grief characterized by lifelong mourning that is never concluded. Its etiology has been hypothesized to be an inability to express the grief feelings.

Complications of inhibited, delayed, or morbid grief reactions include severe depressions, persistent self-disparagement, suicidal preoccupations, and even medical disease in which there is tissue change or damage (see also Chapter 142, "Depression").

Anticipatory grief is the working through of grief before a loss or death actually occurs. The process can be helpful in leading to a greater calm and acceptance of the ensuing death unless, having grieved so well, family members give up the patient long before he or she dies and at a time when family support, comfort, and reassurance are critically needed.

Manifestations of Grief

Acute grief has been identified as a definite syndrome with the following psychological and somatic symptoms:

1. Sensations of somatic distress that occur in waves lasting for 20 minutes to an hour, characterized by tightness in the throat, choking, shortness of breath, sighing, an empty feeling in the stomach, lack of muscular strength, and an intense subjective distress described as tension or pain
2. Intense preoccupation with the image of the deceased, as in waking dreams, accompanied by feelings of vagueness and unreality
3. Guilt feelings; the survivor reviews behaviors prior to the death for evidence of negligence and failure
4. Emotional distancing in relationships with others, accompanied by erratic responses of irritability, hostility, and anger
5. Disoriented behavior such as restlessness, insomnia, absentmindedness, and an inability to concentrate or to initiate and maintain normal daily activities

Grief Process

Although the grief process is gradual, it has a beginning, a middle, and an end, at which point the bereaved should be recovering. The process is phasic, approximating the stage theory developed by Elisabeth Kubler-Ross in her work with dying patients.

Phase 1: Shock, Denial, and Protest

Feelings of numbness, or being stunned, alternate with angry protest and yearning or pining in an attempt to regain or reunite with the lost object. This emotional paralysis or semianesthetized state serves as a buffer against overwhelming anxiety, and it allows one to function with therapeutic protocols (if terminally ill) or the details of funeral arrangements (if bereaved). The connection with the deceased is maintained by intense preoccupation with the departed, even to the point of adopting the symptoms of the illness. Preoccupied with searching for a lost perfection, the mourner tends to idealize the dead. (Kubler-Ross's first three stages of *shock* ["Not me!"]; *anger* ["Why me?"]; and a maneuver to postpone or put a condition on acceptance, i.e., *bargaining* ["I'll stop smoking if . . ." or "If only I can live to see my son's wedding . . ."], ward off the full impact of the loss for the terminally ill.)

Phase 2: Disorganization and Despair

The feelings of disbelief give way to the realization that there will be no reprieve and that the reality is neither a horrible hoax nor a bad dream. Confronting the sadness of the reality may involve considerable weeping, rage, and resentment at times toward the physician, God, fate, or even toward the dead person, whose "abandonment" is the cause for such pain and unhappiness. The bereft person is overwhelmed with guilt and confusion at these and previous hostile or negative feelings toward the deceased. As the survivor reviews the history of the attachment, he or she may be immobilized by feelings of self-recrimination or deprecation, helplessness, and hopelessness. Despair and suicide are common preoccupations at this time, as are withdrawn, brooding, and uncommunicative behaviors (Kubler-Ross's stage four, *depression*).

Phase 3: Reintegration, Recovery, or Transformation

Ties with the lost object or person are loosened. Memories have faded or are a source of solace and the presence of the departed is preserved in a positive way. The motions of living no longer seem meaningless; grief is no longer heavy. The survivor has come to terms with the loss, is energized, and gradually becomes free to seek new attachments. (Kubler-Ross's final stage of *acceptance* is viewed as a peaceful time reached after anticipated and actual losses are mourned and decathection from the world of the living has occurred.) (The American Psychiatric Association defines the word *decathect* as the opposite of *cathesis*, which is attachment, conscious or unconscious, of emotional feeling and significance to an idea or object, most commonly a person.) Table 175-1 presents a breakdown of the three phases of grief discussed in the preceding sections.

These phases or stages may be regarded as normal reactions to any loss. They overlap, may be of varying and unpredictable duration, occur in any order, may be present simultaneously, and may disappear or reappear at random. Anniversary reactions, reminders of the deceased, or new losses reactivate this original grief, although the intensity and duration of the feelings and behaviors are less severe.

Unresolved Grief

The physician is in a good position to detect pathologic mourning or unresolved grief and, upon suspecting a severe problem, will want to enlist psychotherapeutic help. Severe depression, hypochondriasis, psychophysiologic reactions, alcoholism, drug dependency, psychotic states, and inhibited or absent grieving are warning signals.

Dr. Aaron Lazare has compiled the following listing of symptoms and behaviors of unresolved grief:

1. A depressive syndrome of varying degrees of severity
2. A history of delayed or prolonged grief
3. Symptoms of guilt, self-reproach, panic attacks, and somatic expressions of fear such as choking sensations and hyperventilation
4. Somatic symptoms representing identification with the deceased, those of the terminal illness
5. Physical distress under the upper half of the sternum accompanied by expressions such as "There is something stuck" or "I feel there is a demon inside me"
6. Searching behavior (trying to locate the deceased symbolically or actually)
7. Recurrence of depressive symptoms and searching behavior on holidays or anniversaries
8. A feeling that the death occurred yesterday, even though the loss took place months or years ago
9. Unwillingness to move the material possessions of the deceased
10. Change in relationships (e.g., replacement of deceased with someone else)
11. Diminished participation in religious and ritualistic activities
12. The inability to discuss the deceased without crying or the voice cracking, particularly when the death occurred over a year ago
13. Recounting themes of loss

Table 175-1 Trajectory of Grief

	Phase 1 (shock, denial, and protest)	Phase 2 (disorganization)*	Phase 3 (reintegration)
Attitude toward deceased	Idealized preoccupation, pangs, pining/searching, sense of continued presence	Conflicting: anger, sadness	Spiritualized/memorialized
Physical manifestations	Numbness, shock, abnormal calm	Restlessness, muscular aches, insomnia, weeping, loss of appetite, lack of sexual interest, weakened immune system	Active
Energy level	Immobilized, going through the motions	Devoid of energy	Re-energized
Attitude toward world	Anger, bewilderment, sense of unreality	Apathetic, overwhelmed	Interested, manageable
Feelings	Lack of emotion, shock, disbelief	Conflicting and ambivalent mood swings: sadness, despair, depression, heaviness, emptiness, helplessness, withdrawal, uncommunicativeness, fear, brooding, anxiety, irritability, hopelessness, shame, guilt, anger, sense of going crazy, intense mental suffering	Shedding of grief, itself
Outlook	Focus on deceased	Focus on self	Looking outward
Tasks of grief	Acknowledge the loss, review history of attachment	Ventilate repertoire of emotion	Increase capacity to function

* Adaptive, i.e., attempts to manage the loss.

Grief Work or Mourning

The weaning of investment in a body part or attachment to a loved one and readjustment to a new reality is not an automatic or passive venture. Grief work is active. It requires remembering repetitively, over an extended period, experiences shared with the dead person, and talking about and manifesting the mixed emotional ties to the absent love object until the devastating potency of the loss is neutralized. To facilitate the grieving process, one must help the bereaved see the process as tasks that can, indeed, be completed.

The physician can offer presence and concern. Oftentimes not much needs to be said. The bereaved need to be listened to, encouraged to relive unpleasant as well as pleasant memories, assured that they are not going insane and especially that the pain they experience *is* the grief work and that it will not last forever.

Table 175-2 Frequent Topics of Discussion in Bereavement Meetings

Is time to have appropriate closure beneficial to bereavement?	Loneliness, emptiness, and lack of activity	Fear of cancer
Do we want to know how long a patient has to live?	Loved one is never lost to you	Hallucinations
Needing to tell one's own story	Life is pain and joy	Cemetery visits
Affirmation of feelings	Acknowledgment of dissension between the deceased and family, not always accord	Role change from grieving to supporting
Concern about appropriate length of bereavement	It takes time to feel normal again	Loss of physical contact
Frustrations about closures with the dying	Harder for men than women?	No longer being needed (volunteering?)
Myth about death bringing families closer	Last-minute "heroics"	Selfishness about the dying
Mental state related to amount of crying	Repression sometimes antidote for suffering?	Distractions and problems of bills, insurances
Crying and releasing as beneficial	Problems with establishment of new identification	Helping children understand
Crying not a sign of weakness	Help of religion	Remarriage
Guilt, sadness, and anger as components of healthy grief	Help of bereavement group	Inertia
Almost as many different ways of handling grief as people experiencing it	Alcohol use during bereavement period	Vulnerability of clergy and professionals as well as laymen
The dying themselves, facilitators for healthy bereavement	Desire to return the favor of the best possible care (volunteering)	Misplaced angers
Reflection of positive memories important	Possessions, and how and under what conditions to dispose of them	The hospital unit (where the patient died), a place closest to the lost one (like cemetery?)
Anniversaries and holidays as painful	Fear of one's own death and mortality	Satisfaction with last days (gratitude for good care)
Replacement versus no replacement of the lost one	Support systems	Setbacks after "controlled" periods
		Unhelpful responses from friends and family

Encourage the saying of goodbyes at the bedside, before death, whenever possible. A palliative care service or hospital staff may be particularly helpful in aiding family members to complete unfinished business and express their concerns and love. Such "anticipatory grieving" or predeath bereavement is a balm or antidote for the guilts that plague both the dying and the soon-to-be survivors.

Encourage active participation in care of the dying, in being present at the moment of death, and even in preparing the body for burial. There is great solace in being able to say "I was there, and I did all that I could."

Encourage involvement with the mourning rituals of funeral, eulogy, and memorial services. Such rites provide outlets for expression of sorrow and stage the grieving process. Viewing the dead body helps one accept the fact of death.

Listen, nonjudgmentally, realizing that part of the catharsis of grief is the need to tell and retell one's story. Encourage reminiscences, the painful as well as the positive, and expression of the hostile, angry, and *negative feelings* that seem to the bereaved so incompatible with their genuine love for the deceased.

Monitor your own feelings. The physician is not immune to sadness, anxiety, or the need to express personal concern. Your reactions are conditioned by your own experiences with earlier losses and by your ability to weather hostile reactions from patients. Build your own support systems, and don't be afraid to share your feelings with your colleagues and friends.

Apprise patients and family members of self-help support groups such as Candlelighters, Living with Cancer, and Widow-to-Widow and bereavement programs sponsored by YWCAs, churches, and hospitals. A bereavement group serves many functions. The group can assist in answering questions, in understanding feelings, and in providing a network through which the vulnerable can gradually become stronger within the community. It can enable these family members to reach out to others as they gain enlightenment about their own personal experiences. The group process stresses the importance of the individual. It helps each person realize that his or her journey is unique and that the tasks involved in his or her own healing may differ considerably from those of other group members. Expressions of sadness and anger are not prohibited. Any expression of grief, within reason, is encouraged, provided it gives relief. Sharing is cathartic, and the group, through its acceptance of thoughts and feelings, affirms the importance of each member. Table 175-2 outlines frequently recurring topics of discussion in bereavement meetings.

Grief has been likened to a disease or a physical injury, i.e., a "blow" in which the "wound" gradually heals. As is the case with "illness," the malady increases one's physical and emotional vulnerability. Although it is disabling, grief, when worked through, brings strength. As Parkes has said,

> Just as broken bones may end up stronger than unbroken bones, so the experience of grieving can strengthen and bring maturity to those who have previously been protected from misfortune. The pain of grief is just as much a part of life as the joy of love; it is, perhaps, the price we pay for love, the cost of commitment. To ignore this fact, or to pretend that it is not so, is to put on emotional blinders which leave us unprepared for the losses that will inevitably occur in our own lives and unprepared to help others to cope with the losses in theirs.

References

Bertman S. The language of grief: Social-science theories and literary practice. Mosaic 1982; XV(1):153.

Bowlby J. Process of mourning. Int J Psychoanalysis 1961; 42:317.

Freud S. Mourning and melancholia (1919). In: Collected Papers, vol 4. New York: Basic Books, 1959.

Fulton R, Gottesman D. Anticipatory grief: A psychosocial concept reconsidered. Br J Psychiatry 1980; 137:45.

Kubler-Ross E. On death and dying. New York: Macmillan, 1969.

Lazare A. Unresolved grief. In: Outpatient psychiatry, diagnosis and treatment. 2nd ed. Baltimore: Williams & Wilkins, 1988.

Lindemann E. The symptomatology and management of acute grief. Am J Psychiatry 1944; 101:141.

Parkes C. Bereavement. New York: International Universities Press, 1972.

Silverman P. In: Litzer N, ed. Understanding bereavement and grief. Hoboken, NJ: Yeshiva University, Ktav Publishing House, 1977:10.

Appendix I

Normal Laboratory Values

Table of Normal Laboratory Values—Chemistry

Test	Specimen requirement	Reference range	Your laboratory normal	Comments
Acetoacetate	Red top	Negative <3 mg/dl		
Acetone (ketone) screening	Red top Random urine	Negative Negative		Semiquantitative report with dilutions
Acid phosphatase	Red top (fresh)	0.1–0.6 IU/L (men)		
Alanine aminotransferase (ALT [SGPT])	Red top	7–40.U/L		
Albumin	Red top	3.5–5.0 g/dl		Usually a part of a chemistry profile
Alcohol, ethyl	Red top	Negative		
Aldolase	Red top	1.5–8.1 U/L		Varies with temperature and activity
Aldosterone	2 red tops 24-hr urine	10 ng/dl 2–26 μg/24 hr		Patient should be fasting
Alkaline phosphatase	Red top	30–115 U/L		Usually a part of a chemistry profile
Alkaline phosphatase fractionation (heat labile)	Red top	25–35% of total alk. phos.		<25% bone predominant >35% liver predominant
Ammonia	Arterial blood, green top (fresh on ice)	15–32 μmol/L		Send immediately
Amylase	Red top 2-hr urine specimen	25–85 U/L 4–37 U/2 hr		
Aspartate aminotransferase (AST [SGOT])	Red top	7–40 U/L		Usually a part of a chemistry profile
Bilirubin, total	Red top Urine	0.5–1.2 mg/dl Negative		Usually a part of a chemistry profile Specimen should be protected from light
Bilirubin, direct	Red top	0–0.2 mg/dl Negative		
Blood urea nitrogen (BUN)	Red top	7–26 mg/dl		Usually a part of a chemistry profile
Calcitonin	Call lab	Varies from lab to lab		
Calcium	Red top	8.5–10.5 mg/dl		Decreased when serum albumin is decreased
Carotene	Red top	40–200 μg/dl		Protect from light
Catecholamines	Green top (on ice) 24-hr urine (HCl preservative)	Call lab		Check drugs and foods that interfere with assay
Carbon dioxide (CO_2)	Red top	24–32 mmol/L		One of the electrolytes
Ceruloplasmin	Red top	23–50 mg/dl		
Chloride	Red top Random urine or 24-hr urine	97–110 mmol/L 110–250 mmol/L		One of the electrolytes
Cholesterol, total	Red top	150–720 mg/dl (recommended desirable 140–220)		Patient fasting 10 hr
Cholesterol fractionation	Red top	See individual analytes		Includes cholesterol, triglyceride, HDL, LDL, and VLDL
Copper	Large red top 24-hr urine (HCl preservative)	Serum—male: 70–140 μg/dl Serum—female: 80–155 μg/dl 0–50 mg 24 hours		
Cortisol	Red top	8 AM–10 AM 5–23 μg/dl 4 PM–6 PM 3–13 μg/dl		
CPK (creatine phosphokinase)	Red top	45–110 U/L		Fractions may include MM Muscle, MB Cardiac, BB Brain
CPK isoenzyme (MB)	Red top	MB >5% indicates possible myocardial damage		MM and BB fractions not normally present
Creatinine	Red top 24-hr urine (refrigerated)	0.6–1.2 mg/dl 1.0–1.8 g/24 hr 1.0–1.8 g/24 hr		Clearance Male 107–139 ml/min Female 85–110 ml/min

Table of Normal Laboratory Values—Chemistry *(Continued)*

Test	Specimen requirement	Reference range	Your laboratory normal	Comments
Creatinine clearance	24-hr urine (refrigerate) and blood for serum creatinine	80–130 ml/min		A serum creatinine must be ordered during the clearance time period
Erythroprotoporphyrin	Purple top	15–50 μg/dl		
Ferritin	Red top	Male: 15–200 ng/ml Female: 12–150 ng/ml		<12 ng/ml = iron deficiency anemia
Follicle-stimulating hormone	Serum	Male: 4–25; female: midcycle 10–90, with pregnancy low		
	Urine 24 hour	Adult: 6–50 mouse uterine units (muu)/24 hr Postmenopausal: <50 muu/24 hr		
GGTP (gamma-glutamyl transpeptidase)	Red top	5–50 IU/L		
Glucose	Red top Random urine CSF	65–105 mg/dl, 2 hr PC <120 mg/dl Negative 40–70 mg/dl		Fasting preferred Usually a part of a chemistry profile
Glycohemoglobins Hgb A_1C	Green or purple top	4–7%		Elevated suggests poor diabetes control
High-density lipoprotein (HDL) cholesterol	Red top	35–65 mg/dl		Patient should fast 10 hr
17-Hydroxycorticosteroids	Red top	0.2–1.8 ng/ml (0.04–0.5 ng/ml postmenopausal)		
	24-hr urine with boric acid or HCl preservative	Male: 3–10 mg/24 hr Female: 2–8 mg/24 hr		
5-Hydroxyindoleacetic acid (5-HIAA)	24-hr urine; refrigerate with 10 ml HCl preservative	2–8 mg/24 hr		
Hydroxyproline	24-hr urine; refrigerate with 10 ml HCl preservative			
Insulin	Red top (fresh)	R.A.I. 4–24 μIU/ml		
Iron (Fe)	Red top	Male: 50–160 μg/dl Female: 40–150 μg/dl		
Iron-binding capacity (IBC)	Red top	280–400 μg/dl		
17-Ketosteroids	24-hr urine with boric acid or HCl preservative	Male: 8–20 mg/24 hr Female: 4–15 mg/24 hr		Decreases in males >70 yr old
Lactate	Gray or green (on ice) CSF (on ice)	0.5–1.3 mmol/L (arterial) 0.6–2.2 mmol/L		Specimen must be fresh and on ice
Lactate dehydrogenase (LDH)	Red top	100–225 IU/L		Usually part of a chemistry profile
LDH isoenzymes	Red top	LD_1: 24–34% LD_2: 35–45% LD_3: 15–25% LD_4: 4–10% LD_5: 1–9%		
Lead		0–50 μg/dl		Toxic at ≥100 μg/dl
Lipase	Red top	0–1.5 U/ml		
Lipoprotein electrophoresis	Red top			Patient must be fasting
Lithium	Red top	Therapeutic 0.6–1.2 mEq/L		Toxic >2 mEq/L
Magnesium	Red top	1.8–2.4 mmol/dl		
Metanephrine	24-hr urine	0.3–1.20 mg/24 hr		
Osmolarity	Red top (serum) Urine	280–295 mOsm/kg 500–800 mOsm/kg		Depends on state of hydration
Parathormone (PTH)	Red top (fresh on ice)	210–310 pg/ml—intact PTH 230–630 pg/ml—N-terminal Lab dependent—C-terminal		Deliver immediately to lab
pH	Fluids or random urine	7.35–7.45		Fluids may need to be anticoagulated; check with your lab
Phosphorus	Red top 24 hr (refrigerate)	2.5–4.5 mg/dl 0.4–1.3 g/24 hr		Serum is usually part of a chemistry profile No preservative for excretion test
Potassium	Red top Random urine 24-hr urine (refrigerate)	3.5–5.3 mmol/L — 40–80 mmol/24 hr		One of the electrolytes No preservative for excretion test

Table of Normal Laboratory Values—Chemistry (*Continued*)

Test	Specimen requirement	Reference range	Your laboratory normal	Comments
Prolactin	Serum	Female: 1–25 ng/ml, follicular <23, luteal 5–40, pregnancy increases each trimester Male: 1–20 ng/ml		
Protein (total)	Red top CSF 24-hr urine (refrigerate)	6.0–8.0 g/dl 15–45 mg/dl 10–100 mg/24 hr		Serum is usually a part of a chemistry profile Urine needs no preservative
Sodium	Red top Random urine 24-hr urine (refrigerate)	136–142 mmol/L 80–180 mmol/L		 Urine needs no preservative Depends on diet
Specific gravity	Fluids or random urine	Urine 1.002–1.030		Should go above 1.025 after 12 hr of fluid restriction
Stool electrolytes	72-hr specimen			
Stool for occult blood	Random specimen	Negative		
Stool for pH and reducing substances	Random specimen			
Stool for fat	Random			
Testosterone, total	Red top	Male: 300–1,200 ng/dl Female: 30–95 ng/dl		
Thyroid studies:				
Free thyroxine	Red top	0.8–2.4 ng/dl		
Total T_4	Red top	4.3–9.5 μg/dl		
Resin uptake	Red top	24–33%		
TSH	Red top	0–5 μU/ml		
Triglycerides	Red top	Male: 44–248 mg/dl Female: 40–247 mg/dl		Should be fasting Reference range is age dependent
Urinalysis	Random urine			Fresh specimen
Urine occult blood	Random urine	Negative		
Urine porphobilinogen	24-hr urine (refrigerate) Random urine	Up to 2.0 mg/24 hr		No preservative and protect from light
Uric acid	Red top 24-hr urine (refrigerate)	3.5–8.0 mg/dl 0.25–0.75 g/24 hr (average diet)		Serum is usually part chemistry profile No preservative for urine
Urobilinogen	Random urine 2 hr	0.1–0.8 EU/2 hr		
Vanillylmandelic acid (VMA)	24-hr urine, 10 ml HCl preservative	2–8 mg/24 hr		Refrigerate
D-Xylose tolerance	24-hr blood in gray top and 5-hr urine collection	>25 mg/dl (with 25 g dose)		
Zinc	Trace element tube 24-hr urine (acid-washed container)			

Table of Normal Laboratory Values—Hematology

Test	Specimen requirement	Reference range	Your laboratory normal	Comments
Acid phosphatase stain	Blood or bone marrow smears	Interpreted		<3.0 ng/ml normal
Acid phos-tartaric acid	Blood or bone marrow smears	Interpreted		
Antithrombin III	Blue-top tube 2.7 or 4.5 ml	17–30 mg/dl		
Buffy coat smear	Purple-top tube 4 or 7 ml			To look for bacteria
Bleeding time	Performed on patient's forearm	4–6 min		
Blood smear prep	Purple-top tube 4 or 7 ml			
Clot retraction		>50%		
Cryofibrinogen	Blue-top tube 4.5 ml	Interpreted		

Table of Normal Laboratory Values—Hematology *(Continued)*

Test	Specimen requirement	Reference range	Your laboratory normal	Comments
Cerebrospinal fluid, cell count	Clean test tube	0 red blood cells, 0–8 lymphocytes		
Differential	Purple-top tube 4 or 7 ml			
Eosinophil count	Purple-top tube 4 or 7 ml	0–450/mm^3		
Erythropoietin	Red-top tube 10 ml	15–59 IU/ml		
Erythrocyte sedimentation rate (ESR)	Purple-top tube 4 or 7 ml	40–51%		Must be done within hours of drawing
Factor assays	Blue-top tube 4.5 ml	>70%		
Factor VIII or IX antigen	Blue-top tube 2.7 or 4.5 ml	>70%		
Fibrinogen	Blue-top tube 2.7 or 4.5 ml	150–400 mg/dl		
Fibrin split products (FSP)	Special tube 2-ml draw	<20 μg/dl		
Ham's test	Purple-top tube 7 ml	No hemolysis		
Haptoglobin	Red-top tube 4 or 10 ml	100–300 mg/dl		
Heinz body prep	Purple-top tube 4 or 7 ml	Negative		
Hematocrit	Purple-top tube 4 or 7 ml or microcontainer	Male: 47 ± 5 ml/dl Female: 42 ± 5 ml/dl		
Hemoglobin (Hgb)	Purple-top tube 4 or 7 ml or microcontainer	Male: 16.0 ± 2 g/dl Female: 14.0 ± 2 g/dl		
Hgb A_1C (see page 686)				
Hgb A_2	Purple-top tube 4 or 7 ml	1.5–3.5%		
Hgb electrophoresis	Purple-top tube 4 or 7 ml			
Hgb F stain	Heparin 4 or 10 ml			
Hemosiderin-urine	Specimen container	Negative		
Heparin assay	Blue-top tube 2.7 or 4.5 ml			
Inhibitor screen/1 : 1 mix	Blue-top tube 2.7 or 4.5 ml	Correction to normal range		
Iron stain	Bone marrow smear	(Present) increased or decreased		Look for ringed sideroblasts
Leukocyte alkaline phosphatase	Green-top tube 4 or 10	11–95		
Myoglobin, urine	Specimen container	Negative		
Nonspecific esterase	Blood or bone marrow smears			
Osmotic fragility	Green-top tube 4 or 10 ml			
Periodic acid–Schiff stain	Blood or bone marrow smears			
Peroxidase stain	Blood or bone marrow smears			
Platelet count	Purple-top tube 4 or 7 ml or microcontainer	130,000–400,000		
Platelet adhesiveness		>25%		
Platelet aggregation		>50%		
Platelet factor 3				
Plasminogen	Blue-top tube 2.7 or 4.5 ml			
Prothrombin time (PT)	Blue-top tube 2.7 or 4.5 ml	<13 sec		
Partial thromboplastin time (PTT)	Blue-top tube 2.7 or 5 ml	27–38 sec		
Reptilase	Blue-top tube 2.7 or 5 ml	18–22 sec		Should be done if TT >20 sec
Red blood cell count	Purple-top tube 4 or 7 ml or microcontainer	Male: 5.4 ± 0.7 million/mm^3 Female: 4.8 ± 0.6 million/mm^3		
Reticulocyte count	Purple-top tube 4 or 7 ml or microcontainer	0.8–2.5%		
Ristocetin aggregation	Blue-top tube 2.7 or 5 ml	70%		
Sickle cell prep	Purple-top tube 4 or 7 ml	Negative		
Sudan black stain	Blood or bone marrow smears	Interpreted		
Sugar water test sucrose lysis	Purple-top tube	<5% hemolysis		
Thrombin time (TT)	Blue-top tube 2.7 or 5 ml	<20 sec		
White blood cell count	Purple-top tube 4 or 7 ml or microcontainer	7,800 ± 3,000/mm^3		
Westergren sedimentation rate (ESR)	Purple top	1–3 mm/hr (adult male) 4–7 mm/hr (adult female)		

Table of Normal Laboratory Values—Hematology (*Continued*)

Test	Specimen requirement	Reference range	Your laboratory normal	Comments
Wintrobe ESR	Purple-top tube 4 or 7 ml	Male: 0–10 mm/hr Female: 0–20 mm/hr		Must be done within hours of drawing
Zeta sedimentation ratio	Lavender top tube 4 or 7 ml	40–51%		Must be done within hours of drawing

Table of Normal Laboratory Values—Immunology/Rheumatology

Test	Specimen requirement	Reference range	Your laboratory normal	Comments
Alpha-1-antitrypsin	Red top	85–213 mg/dl (adult)		
Alpha-2-macroglobulin	Red top	150–350 mg/dl (adult male) 175–420 mg/dl (adult female)		
Antiadrenal antibody (fluorescent antibody)	Red top	Negative		
Antimitochondrial antibody (fluorescent antibody)	Red top	Negative or <1:20		
Antinuclear antibody (fluorescent antibody)	Red top	Negative		
Anti–glomerular basement membrane antibody (fluorescent antibody)	Red top	Negative		
Antiheart antibody (fluorescent antibody)	Red top	Negative		
Anti–smooth muscle antibody (fluorescent antibody)	Red top	Negative or <1:20		
Bence-Jones protein (by immunoelectrophoresis)	Urine	Negative		Random or 24-hr specimen can be used No preservatives for 24-hr specimen
C1 esterase inactivator (qualitative screen)	Red top	Present		
Complement C3	Red top	83–177 mg/dl (adult)		
C3 activator	Red top	10–45 mg/dl (adult)		
Complement C4	Red top	15–45 mg/dl (adult)		
C-reactive protein (CRP) (qualitative)	Red top	Negative		
C-reactive protein (CRP) (quantitative)	Red top	0–0.8 mg/dl		
Cryoglobulin, cryocrit	Red top	Negative		Keep tube at temperature (37°C) and deliver *immediately*
DNA antibody (double-stranded DNA) (radioimmunoassay)	Red top	0–15 U/ml = normal >25 U/ml = systemic lupus erythematosus 15–25 U/ml = other diseases		
Extractable nuclear antibody (ENA) (counterimmunoelectrophoresis)	Red top	Negative		
Gastric parietal cell antibody (fluorescent antibody)	Red top	Negative		
LE cell prep	Green top	Negative		
Quantitative IgA, serum	Red top	70–312 mg/dl (adult)		
Quantitative IgE, serum (radioimmunoassay)	Red top	<20 U/ml—atopic genesis not probable >100 U/ml—atopic genesis highly probable		
Quantitative IgG, serum	Red top	639–1,349 mg/dl (adult)		
Quantitative IgM, serum	Red top	56–352 mg/dl (adult)		

Table of Normal Laboratory Values—Immunology/Rheumatology *(Continued)*

Test	Specimen requirement	Reference range	Your laboratory normal	Comments
Quantitative IgA, CSF	Clean, dry container	0–0.6 mg/dl (adult)		
Quantitative IgG, CSF	Clean, dry container	0.5–6.1 mg/dl		
Quantitative IgM, CSF	Clean, dry container	0–1.3 mg/dl		
RA latex (rheumatoid factor) (latex fixation)	Red top	Negative or <1:20		
Serum viscosity	Red top	1.4–1.8 (relative to water)		Minimum 10.0 ml blood
Synovial fluid analysis	Red top (1) Purple top (1)	See Chapter 96, page 407		
Total hemolytic complement	Red top	200–260 CH_{50} U/ml		Place tube *on ice* and deliver to lab immediately
Transferrin	Red top	204–360 mg/dl		

Appendix II

Commonly Prescribed Drugs

Scott R. Allen, MD

Harry L. Greene, MD

This appendix provides essential information on more than 200 commonly used medications. Important aspects of each drug are listed, and medication dosages conform to the recommendations outlined by the texts listed in the bibliography. Information on each drug is not comprehensive, and it is imperative that the reader be completely familiar with the manufacturer's product information before prescribing any medication.

Each drug is organized into nine sections: (1) generic name and up to two common brand names, (2) preparations, (3) adult dose, (4) indications, (5) action, (6) metabolism, (7) excretion, (8) contraindications and precautions, and (9) drug interactions. Brand names are cross-indexed to the generic name. Not all brand names appear, and those included do not necessarily come in all the preparation forms listed. Consult a *Physicians' Desk Reference* or pharmacy for further information on dosage forms. Only dosages for approved indications are provided; however, other common usage is included under the indications section. Dosages listed in this chapter are for adults; consult other texts for pediatric dosages. Many of the medications require a dosage adjustment for geriatric patients or for hepatic or renal function impairment; specific notation is made in these situations.

Adverse reactions are not listed. Hypersensitivity or allergic reaction to a drug or any of its components is a contraindication to its use. The use of a drug in a woman who is or anticipates being pregnant or who is currently breastfeeding requires an assessment of risk and benefit. Please note that pregnancy and breastfeeding are not listed as precautions in this chapter. The manufacturer's product information must be consulted before any medication is prescribed in these two situations.

Acetaminophen (Anacin-3, Tylenol, others)

Preparations: Tablets 160, 325, 650 mg; capsules, 325, 500 mg; elixir, 120 mg/5 ml, 160 mg/5 ml, 325 mg/5 ml; liquid, 160 mg/5 ml, 500 mg/15 ml; solutions, 100 mg/ml, 120 mg/2.5 ml; suppositories, 120, 325, 600 mg

Adult dosage: PO: 325–650 mg q4–6h prn or 1,000 mg q6–8h prn. PR: 650 mg q4–6h prn.

Note: Decrease dosage in hepatic impairment.

Indications: Relief of fever and pain

Action: Antipyretic and non-narcotic analgesic

Metabolism: Hepatic

Excretion: Renal

Contraindications and precautions

1. Use with caution in G6PD deficiency, alcoholism, hepatitis, hepatic disease.
2. May be hepatotoxic with chronic use or with large single doses.

Drug interactions

1. Diflunisal leads to elevated acetaminophen plasma level.
2. Chronic excessive alcohol intake leads to elevated acetaminophen toxicity.
3. Acute alcohol intoxication leads to decreased acetaminophen overdose toxicity.
4. Acetaminophen leads to elevated serum levels of chloramphenicol and zidovudine (AZT).

Acetazolamide (Diamox, others)

Preparations: Tablets, 125, 250 mg; ER capsules, 500 mg; injection (IM, IV), 500 mg/vial

Adult dosage

Antiglaucoma: *Open angle*—PO: Initially, 250 mg qd–bid. Titrate maintenance dosage to patient response. ER preparations administered bid. *Angle-closure, secondary*—PO: 250 mg bid up to 250 mg q4h. If acute, may administer 500 mg followed by 125–250 mg q4h. IM, IV (preferred): 500 mg for acute glaucoma.

Anticonvulsant—PO: 8–30 mg/kg/day in up to 4 divided doses. Usual dosage range is 375–100 mg/day. When used in combination with other anticonvulsants, initiate with 250 mg/day.

Indications: Treatment of open-angle, angle-closure, and secondary glaucoma and treatment of centrencephalic epilepsies (petit mal, unlocalized seizures)

Action: Carbonic anhydrase inhibitor

Metabolism: None

Excretion: Renal

Contraindications and precautions

1. Contraindicated in hyponatremia, hypokalemia, severe hepatic or renal function impairment, hyperchloremic acidosis, and adrenocortical insufficiency.
2. Use with caution in impaired alveolar ventilation, diabetes mellitus, and electrolyte imbalance.
3. Cross-sensitivity to antibacterial sulfonamides has been reported.

Drug interactions

1. Diuretics, amphotericin B, and glucocorticoids may increase risk of hypokalemia.
2. Acetazolamide may increase effects of quinidine, pseudoephedrine, and flecainide.
3. Acetazolamide may decrease effect of lithium.

Acyclovir (Zovirax)

Preparations: Ointment 5% (50 mg/g), 15-g tube; capsule, 200 mg; injection (IV), 500 mg/10 ml

Adult dosage

Topical: *Herpes genitalis and simplex*—apply with rubber glove/finger cot to skin and mucous membranes (excluding eyes) q3h while awake for 7 days

Systemic: *Herpes genitalis:* Initial therapy —PO 200 mg q4h while awake (5 capsules/day) for 10 days; if severe, IV 5 mg/kg infused over 1 h q8h for 5 days. Intermittent therapy—PO 200 mg q4h while awake (5 capsules/day) for 5 days. Chronic suppressive therapy—PO 200 mg q8h for up to 6 mo. *Mucocutaneous herpes simplex (HSV-1 and HSV-2) infections in immunocompromised patients:* IV 15 mg/kg q8h for 7 days *Herpes zoster, disseminated herpes simplex:* IV 5–10 mg/kg q8h for 7–10 days.

Note: Recommended dose adjustment in renal impairment is as follows:

Creatinine clearance (ml/min/1.73 m²)	Dose (mg/kg)	Dosing interval (hr)
>50	5	8
25–50	5	12
10–25	5	24
0–10	2.5	24

Indications: Treatment of initial episodes and management of recurrent episodes of herpes genitalis and simplex; treatment of herpes zoster (shingles) and varicella (chickenpox)

Action: Converted to acyclovir triphosphate, which interferes with viral DNA polymerase and inhibits viral DNA replication

Metabolism: Hepatic

Excretion: Renal

Contraindications and precautions (systemic therapy): Use with caution in dehydration, pre-existing renal function impairment, or underlying neurologic abnormalities.

Drug interactions (systemic therapy)

1. Intrathecal methotrexate or interferon may lead to neurologic abnormalities.
2. Probenecid leads to increased serum concentration and increased half-life.

Albuterol (Proventil, Ventolin)

Preparations: Tablets, 2, 4 mg; ER tablets, 4 mg; syrup, 2 mg/5 ml; aerosol, 0.09 mg per metered spray; solution for inhalation, 0.083, 0.5%

Adult dosage

Bronchodilator—PO: 2–4 mg tid–qid up to a maximum 32 mg/day. ER preparations may be administered bid

Aerosol: 0.18 mg (2 inhalations) q4–6h prn

Solution for inhalation via nebulization or intermittent positive-pressure breathing: 1.25–5 mg in 2–5 ml or more of sterile normal saline or water q4–6h prn

For prophylaxis of exercise-induced bronchospasm: 0.18 mg (2 inhalations) of aerosol 15 min before exercise.

Indications: Treatment of bronchospasm in patients with reversible obstructive airway disease and prophylaxis of exercise-induced bronchospasm

Action: Sympathomimetic bronchodilator (β_2)

Metabolism: Hepatic

Excretion: Renal

Contraindications and precautions: Use with caution in cardiac arrhythmias, coronary insufficiency, ischemic heart disease, hypertension, diabetes mellitus, hyperthyroidism and pheochromocytoma.

Drug interactions

1. Hydrocarbon inhalation anesthetics, digoxin, and levodopa may increase risk of arrhythmias.
2. Tricyclic antidepressants and MAO inhibitors may increase vascular system effects.
3. Sympathomimetics and xanthine-derivatives may increase risk of CNS stimulation.
4. Albuterol may decrease effect of antihypertensives, β-adrenergic blockers.
5. Albuterol may increase effect of thyroid hormones and vice versa.

Allopurinol (Zyloprim, others)

Preparations: Tablets, 100, 300 mg

Adult Dosage

Antihyperuricemic: *Gout*—PO: Initially, 100 mg qd and increase by 100 mg/day every week until desired serum uric acid concentration (usually ≤6 mg/dl) attained. Maintenance doses for mild gout are usually 200–300 mg/day and 400–600 mg/day for severe gout. Maximum total daily dosage is 800 mg. *Neoplastic disease*—PO: 600–800 mg/day starting 2–3 days before initiation of chemotherapy or radiation therapy.

Antiurolithic: *Uric acid calculi*—PO: 100–200 mg qd–qid. *Calcium oxalate calculi*—PO: 200–300 mg qd.

Note

1. Recommended dosage reduction in renal function impairment:

Creatinine clearance (ml/min)	Dose
10–20	200 mg qd
3–10	≤100 mg qd
<3	100 mg q24h or more

2. The total daily dose may be given as a single dose or in divided doses. Individual doses should not exceed 300 mg.

Indications: Treatment of chronic gouty arthritis; treatment and prophylaxis of uric acid nephropathy and hyperuricemia due to neoplastic disease; prophylaxis of recurrent uric acid and calcium oxalate renal calculi

Action: Xanthine oxidase inhibitor, resulting in decreased uric acid production

Metabolism: Hepatic

Excretion: Renal

Contraindications and Precautions

1. Not effective in the treatment of acute gouty attacks; may exacerbate an acute attack.
2. May increase the frequency of acute gouty attacks following the initiation of therapy; concurrent prophylactic doses of colchicine have been recommended during the first 3–6 mo of allopurinol therapy.
3. Use with caution in renal function impairment.

Drug interactions

1. Thiazide diuretics may increase risk of allopurinol toxicity.
2. Allopurinol may increase chlorpropamide, aminophylline, and theophylline blood levels.
3. Allopurinol may increase toxicity of mercaptopurine or azathioprine.
4. Allopurinol may increase anticoagulant effect of warfarin.

Aluminum hydroxide (ALternaGEL, Amphojel, others)

Preparations: Tablets, 300, 600, 608 mg; capsules, 475, 500 mg; suspension, 320, 600 mg/5 ml; liquid, 600 mg/5 ml

Adult dosage

Hyperacidity—PO: 500–1,800 mg 1 and 3 hr pc and qhs

Hyperphosphatemia—PO: 1,800–4,800 mg tid–qid

Indications: Relief of symptoms of hyperacidity

Action: Neutralizes gastric acid and binds phosphate in the intestine to form insoluble $AlPO_4$, which is excreted in the feces

Metabolism: None

Excretion: Fecal and renal

Contraindications and precautions

1. Chronic use may aggravate metabolic bone disease.
2. May exacerbate constipation.

Drug interactions: Aluminum hydroxide may decrease absorption of coumadin, digoxin, iron preparations, isoniazid, ketoconazole, phenothiazines, phosphates, tetracyclines, fat-soluble vitamins, and H_2-blockers.

Amiloride (Midamor, others)

Preparations: Tablets, 5 mg

Adult dosage: Diuretic or antihypertensive—PO: 5–10 mg qd

Indications: Treatment of edema and hypertension

Action: Antikaliuretic-diuretic agent

Metabolism: None

Excretion: Renal = fecal

Contraindications and precautions

1. Contraindicated in hyperkalemia.
2. Use with caution in anuria, renal insufficiency, hyperuricemia, gout, and diabetes mellitus.

Drug interactions

1. Blood transfusions, captopril, enalapril, lisinopril, cyclosporine, other potassium-sparing diuretics, potassium supplements, and salt substitutes may increase risk of hyperkalemia.
2. Amiloride leads to increased risk of lithium toxicity.

Amiloride and hydrochlorothiazide (Moduretic)

Preparations: Amiloride/hydrochlorothiazide tablets, 5 mg/50 mg

Adult dosage: Diuretic or antihypertensive—PO: 1–2 tablets qd

Indications: Treatment of edema and hypertension; not indicated for initial therapy; determine optimum maintenance dose of each drug separately, and use the combination preparation if it corresponds to the ratio of the separate drugs

Action, metabolism, excretion, contraindications and precautions, and drug interactions: See under *Amiloride* and *Hydrochlorothiazide*

Aminophylline (see *Xanthine derivatives*)

Amitriptyline (Elavil, Endep, others)

Preparations: Tablets, 10, 25, 50, 75, 100, 150 mg; injection (IM), 10 mg/ml

Adult dosage: PO: Initially, 25 mg bid–qid. Increase up to 150 mg/day in outpatients or 300 mg/day in in-patients. Maximum antidepressant effect may take ≥2 wk. Start with lower doses of 10 mg tid and 20 mg qhs in geriatric patients. IM: 20–30 mg qid. After control of symptoms, taper to lowest effective dose.

Indications: Treatment of depression. Unlabeled use includes treatment of neurogenic pain.

Action: Tricyclic antidepressant; increases CNS synaptic concentration of norepinephrine and/or serotonin, presumably by blocking presynaptic re-uptake; has sedative, anticholinergic, peripheral vasodilator, and direct quinidine-like myocardial effects

Metabolism: Hepatic

Excretion: Renal

Contraindications and precautions

1. Contraindicated during recovery from myocardial infarction and possibly concurrent MAO inhibitor use.
2. Use with caution in alcoholism, asthma, bipolar disorder, schizophrenia, cardiovascular disorders, blood disorders, gastrointestinal disorders, narrow-angle glaucoma, hepatic or renal function impairment, hyperthyroidism, prostatic hypertrophy or urinary retention, and seizure disorders.

3. Use caution while driving or performing other tasks requiring alertness.
4. Abrupt cessation following prolonged administration may cause withdrawal symptoms.
5. Prescribe the smallest quantity for patients considered at risk for suicide.

Drug interactions

1. Alcohol or CNS depressants lead to increased CNS depression.
2. Drugs with antimuscarinic activity lead to increased anticholinergic side effects.
3. Direct-acting sympathomimetics lead to increased cardiac effects.
4. MAO inhibitors lead to increased risk of hyperpyretic episodes, convulsions, hypertensive crises, and death.
5. Antithyroid agents lead to increased risk of agranulocytosis.
6. Barbiturates and carbamazepine may decrease plasma concentration of amitriptyline.
7. Cimetidine, methylphenidate, phenothiazines, estrogens, and possibly ranitidine may increase plasma concentration of amitriptyline.
8. Metrizamide leads to increased risk of seizures.
9. Thyroid hormone leads to increased therapeutic and toxic effects of both medications.
10. Amitriptyline leads to decreased hypotensive effect of guanethidine and clonidine.
11. Amitriptyline may increase plasma concentration of coumadin.

Amoxapine (Asendin)

Preparations: Tablets, 25, 50, 100, 150 mg

Adult dosage: PO: Initially, 50 mg bid–tid. Increase to 100 mg bid–tid by end of first week. Dosage may be increased to 400 mg/day (600 mg/day in hospitalized patients) after at least 2 wk at 300 mg/day. Single doses should not exceed 300 mg. Antidepressant effect usually apparent in <2 wk. Start with lower doses of 25 mg bid–tid in geriatric patients; can increase to 150 mg/day by end of first week, and then up to 300 mg/day after ≥2 wk. After control of symptoms, taper to lowest effective dose.

Indications: Treatment of depression

Action: Tricyclic antidepressant; increases CNS synaptic concentration of norepinephrine and/or serotonin, presumably by blocking presynaptic re-uptake; has sedative, anticholinergic, peripheral vasodilator, and direct quinidine-like myocardial effects

Metabolism: Hepatic

Excretion: Renal

Contraindications and precautions

1. Contraindicated during recovery from myocardial infarction and possibly concurrent MAO inhibitor use.
2. Use with caution in alcoholism, asthma, bipolar disorder, schizophrenia, cardiovascular disorders, blood disorders, gastrointestinal disorders, narrow-angle glaucoma, hepatic or renal function impairment, hyperthyroidism, prostatic hypertrophy or urinary retention, and seizure disorders.
3. Use caution while driving or performing other tasks requiring alertness.
4. Abrupt cessation following prolonged administration may cause withdrawal symptoms.
5. Prescribe the smallest quantity for patients considered at risk for suicide.

Drug interactions

1. Alcohol or CNS depressants lead to increased CNS depression.
2. Drugs with antimuscarinic activity lead to increased anticholinergic side effects.
3. Direct-acting sympathomimetics lead to increased cardiac effects.
4. MAO inhibitors lead to increased risk of hyperpyretic episodes, convulsions, hypertensive crises and death.
5. Antithyroid agents lead to increased risk of agranulocytosis.
6. Barbiturates and carbamazepine may decrease plasma concentration of amoxapine.
7. Cimetidine, methylphenidate, phenothiazines, estrogens, and possibly ranitidine may increase plasma concentration of amoxapine.
8. Metrizamide leads to increased risk of seizures.
9. Thyroid hormone leads to increased therapeutic and toxic effects of both medications.
10. Amoxapine leads to decreased hypotensive effect of guanethidine and clonidine.
11. Amoxapine may increase plasma concentration of coumadin.

Amphotericin B (Fungizone)

Preparations: Cream, 30 mg/g, 20-g tube; lotion, 30 mg/ml, 30-ml bottle; ointment, 30 mg/g, 20-g tube; injection (IV), 50 mg/vial (5 mg/ml after reconstitution)

Adult dosage

Topical: Apply to lesions bid–qid

Bladder irrigation: 50 mg/L D/W continuous irrigation at 1 L/day for 3–5 days or 5–15 mg in D/W instilled into bladder with retention for 20–30 min q6–8h for 3–5 days

Intravenous: Suspended at a concentration of 0.1 mg/ml or less. Each dose should be infused in D/W over 4–6 hr. Initial test dose of 1 mg in 50–150 ml D/W over 20–30 min. If tolerated, 0.2 mg/kg the next day, and increase daily dose by 0.1–0.2 mg/kg/day until 0.5–0.6 mg/kg/day up to 1 mg/kg/day for severe infection. May give twice the usual dose qod. Maximum daily dose 1.5 mg/kg.

Intrathecal and intraventricular: 0.1 mg initially, then gradually increase to a maximum of 0.5 mg q48–72h

Indications: Cutaneous or mucocutaneous fungal infection caused by *Candida* sp.; fungal cystitis, and progressive and potentially fatal fungal infections

Action: Fungistatic/fungicidal by binding to fungal cytoplasmic membrane sterols, increasing membrane permeability

Metabolism: Unknown

Excretion: Renal

Contraindications and precautions

1. Renal toxicity: reversible related to daily dose; permanent related to cumulative dose >4 g. Monitor BUN, creatinine, and serum electrolytes.
2. May cause transient acute reaction involving fever, rigors, nausea, vomiting and headache 1–3 hr after starting infusion; patient usually becomes tolerant with continued doses. May be attenuated by antipyretic, antihistamine, hydrocortisone, or IV meperidine.
3. May cause local thrombophlebitis. May be attenuated by adding heparin.
4. May cause bone marrow depression. Monitor complete blood count.

Drug interactions

1. Avoid concurrent use of nephrotoxic agents.
2. May increase effects of digoxin or skeletal muscle relaxants due to decreased K^+.
3. Corticosteroids may lead to decreased K^+.

Aspirin—Acetylsalicylic acid (Ecotrin, others)

Preparations: Tablets, 65, 81, 325, 500, 650 mg; EC tablets, 325, 500, 650, 975 mg; ER tablets, 650, 800 mg; EC capsules, 325, 500 mg; suppositories, 60, 120, 125, 130, 195, 200, 300, 325, 600, 650, 1,200 mg

Adult dosage

Analgesic, antipyretic—PO, PR: 325–650 mg q4h prn. For ER preparations, 650–1,300 mg q8h or 1,600 mg bid.

Antirheumatic—PO: 3.6–5.4 g/day in divided doses

Platelet aggregation inhibitor—PO: Optimal dose not established; most studies have used doses of 300–1,500 mg/day. Many clinicians recommend as little as 80–150 mg/day.

Note

1. Use lower doses in geriatric patients.
2. Therapeutic plasma concentration: analgesic—25–50 μg/ml; antirheumatic—150–300 μg/ml.

Indications: Treatment of minor pains, fever, rheumatoid and osteoarthritis, and rheumatic fever; prophylaxis of TIAs in men, myocardial infarction or reinfarction, and thrombosis or reocclusion of aortocoronary bypass grafts

Action: Acetylated salicylate with analgesic, antipyretic, and anti-inflammatory effects; antiplatelet effect and inhibition of prostaglandin synthesis due to irreversible inhibition of cyclo-oxygenase enzyme

Metabolism: Hepatic

Excretion: Renal

Contraindications and precautions

1. Patients intolerant of NSAIDs may be intolerant of aspirin.
2. Contraindicated in bleeding ulcers, other hemorrhagic states, hemophilia, and thrombocytopenia.
3. Use with caution in asthma, allergies, nasal polyps, gastritis, peptic ulcer disease, G6PD deficiency, hepatic and renal function impairment, and thyrotoxicosis.

Drug interactions

1. NSAIDs or alcohol may increase risk of GI side effects.
2. NSAIDs, oral anticoagulants, heparin, thrombolytic agents, platelet aggregation inhibitors, and other antiplatelet agents may increase risk of hemorrhage.

3. Carbonic anhydrase inhibitors lead to increased renal excretion.
4. Ototoxic medications may increase risk of ototoxicity.
5. Corticosteroids may decrease serum salicylate concentration.
6. Aspirin may increase plasma methotrexate concentration.
7. Aspirin may decrease uricosuric effect of probenecid and sulfinpyrazone.
8. High doses of aspirin may increase hypoglycemic effect of sulfonylureas and insulin.
9. Aspirin may increase toxicity of sulfonylureas, sulfonamides, methotrexate, nifedipine, verapamil, coumadin, and phenytoin, and vice versa.

Atenolol (Tenormin)

Preparations: Tablets, 50, 100 mg
Adult dosage
Antianginal—PO: Initially, 50 mg qd; increase to 100 mg in 1 week prn; may administer up to 200 mg
Antihypertensive—PO: Initially, 25–50 mg qd; increase to 50–100 mg in 2 wk prn
Note: Dosage adjustment in renal impairment as follows:

Creatinine clearance ($ml/min/1.73\ m^2$)	Maximum dose
15–35	50 mg qd
>15	50 mg qod

Indications: Treatment of chronic angina and hypertension
Action: Selective β-adrenergic blocking agent
Metabolism: Hepatic (minimal)
Excretion: Renal
Contraindications and precautions
1. Contraindicated in overt cardiac failure, cardiogenic shock, 2nd- or 3rd-degree AV block, sinus bradycardia, or hypotension associated with MI.
2. Use with caution in asthma, emphysema, CHF, diabetes mellitus, mental depression, or peripheral vascular disease.
3. Abrupt withdrawal after chronic administration can precipitate angina, MI and ventricular dysrhythmias. Dosage should be tapered over 2 wk.

Drug interactions
1. Hydrocarbon inhalation anesthetics may increase myocardial depression.
2. Insulin or antidiabetic agents may increase hypoglycemia.
3. Calcium channel blocking agents may increase conduction disturbance or CHF in patients with abnormal AV conduction or depressed left ventricular function.
4. Atenolol may increase or decrease cardiostimulating effect of sympathomimetics.
5. Atenolol leads to decreased bronchodilating effect of sympathomimetics and theophylline.
6. Atenolol may elevate BP with use of MAO inhibitor.

Atropine sulfate

Preparations: Injection (IM, IV, SC), 0.05, 0.1, 0.3, 0.4, 0.5, 0.8, 1, 1.2 mg/ml
Adult dosage
Bradyarrhythmias—IV: 0.4–1 mg q1–2h prn up to a maximum of 2 mg for bradycardia during CPR, the usual dose is 0.5 mg q5min not to exceed 2 mg until desired rate is achieved. The same dose may be administered via an endotracheal tube during CPR if IV access is not available.
Preoperative prophylaxis of excessive respiratory tract secretions—IM, SC: 0.4 mg (range: 0.2–0.6 mg) 30–60 min before surgery
Indications: Multiple uses, including treatment of sinus bradycardia and prophylaxis of excessive secretions of the respiratory tract during surgery.
Action: Antimuscarinic agent
Metabolism: Hepatic
Excretion: Renal
Contraindications and precautions
1. Contraindicated in angle-closure glaucoma, obstructive uropathy, myasthenia gravis, and tachycardia secondary to cardiac insufficiency or thyrotoxicosis.
2. Use with caution in cardiac disease, reflux esophagitis, ulcerative colitis, GI infection, GI obstruction, intestinal atony, paralytic ileus, acute hemorrhage with an unstable cardiac status, nonobstructive prostatic hypertrophy or urinary retention, hypertension, and hepatic or renal function impairment.

Drug interactions
1. Anticholinergic agents and other medications with antimuscarinic effects (e.g., tricyclic antidepressants) may increase antimuscarinic effect.
2. Antacids may decrease oral atropine absorption.
3. Oral atropine may increase GI lesions associated with wax-matrix potassium chloride preparations.

Azathioprine (Imuran)

Preparations: Tablets, 50 mg; Injection (IV), 100 mg/20-ml vial
Adult dosage
Immunosuppressant: Transplant rejection prophylaxis—PO, IV: 3–5 mg/kg 1–3 days prior to or on the day of surgery. Maintenance therapy is 1–3 mg/kg/day.
Antirheumatic—PO: Initially, 1 mg/kg/day. Can increase by 0.5 mg/kg/day after 6–8 wk if needed and tolerated. Daily dosage may then be increased by 0.5 mg/kg q4wk prn up to a maximum 2.5 mg/kg/day. For maintenance therapy, reduce by decrements of 0.5 mg/kg/day q4–6wk to the minimum effective dose. Consider drug failure if no response after 12 wk.
Note: Reserve IV administration for those patients unable to tolerate PO.
Indications: Adjunctive therapy for prevention of rejection of renal homotransplantation; also for management of severe, active rheumatoid arthritis unresponsive to conventional therapy
Action: Immunosuppressant of unclear mechanism of action; may be a purine metabolism antagonist
Metabolism: Hepatic
Excretion: Biliary, renal
Contraindications and precautions
1. Contraindicated in current or recent exposure to chickenpox and in herpes zoster.
2. Use with caution in gout, infection, hepatic or renal function impairment, and previous cytotoxic or radiation therapy.
3. Monitor periodic CBC and platelet count. Dosage should be reduced or stopped if a large or persistent decrease in WBC or platelet count occurs.

Drug Interactions
1. Allopurinol may increase toxicity.
2. Other immunosuppressants may increase risk of infection or neoplasm.
3. Bone marrow depressants or radiation therapy may increase risk of bone marrow depression.
4. Azathioprine may decrease antibody response to or potentiate the replication of live virus vaccines.

Azidothymidine (see *Zidovudine*)

AZT (see *Zidovudine*)

Beclomethasone dipropionate (Beconase, Vancenase)

Preparations: Aerosol, 42 μg/inhalation, 16.8-g inhaler canister; spray, 42 μg/inhalation (0.042%), 20-g bottle
Adult dosage: Intranasal inhalation: 42 μg (1 metered spray) in each nostril bid–qid. For rhinitis, do not continue beyond 3 wk if there is no symptomatic improvement. For polyps, several weeks may be required for a therapeutic effect.
Indications: Treatment of seasonal or perennial rhinitis when effectiveness of or tolerance to conventional therapy is unsatisfactory; treatment of postsurgical prophylaxis of nasal polyps
Action: Anti-inflammatory steroid
Metabolism: Hepatic
Excretion: Fecal > renal
Contraindications and precautions: Use with caution in fungal or systemic viral infections, ocular herpes simplex, and latent or active respiratory tract tuberculosis.

Beclomethasone dipropionate—Inhalation (Beclovent, Vanceril)

Preparations: Aerosol, 42 μg inhalation, 16.8-g inhaler canister
Adult dosage: PO inhalation: 84 μg (2 metered sprays) tid–qid. If severe asthma, start with 12–16 sprays/day and decrease according to patient response. Maximum dose is 20 sprays/day.
Note: If transferring from systemic to inhalation adrenocorticoids, the patient's asthma should be relatively stable. Full maintenance dosage of systemic adrenocorticoids should be continued for at least 1 wk when inhalation therapy is started. Systemic dosage may then be reduced very slowly at 1- to 2-wk intervals. Monitor for adrenal insufficiency.
Indications: Treatment of chronic asthma requiring corticosteroids in conjunction with other therapy
Action: Anti-inflammatory steroid
Metabolism: Hepatic > renal, pulmonary
Excretion: Fecal > renal
Contraindications and precautions
1. Not for treatment of status asthmaticus or acute episodes of asthma.
2. Adrenal suppression may occur if above dosages are exceeded, but it has been reported with usual inhalation doses.

3. Use with caution in diabetes, peptic ulcer disease. CHF, hypertension, systemic fungal infection, and ocular herpes simplex.

Benzoyl peroxide (Clearasil, Desquam-X, others)

Preparations: Bar, 5, 10%; cream, 5, 10%; lotion, 5,5.5, 10%; liquid, 5, 10%; gel, 2.5, 5, 10%
Adult dosage
Cleansers (bar, liquid)—TOP: Apply qd–bid.
Other dose forms—TOP: Initially, 2.5 or 5% cream, lotion, or gel, and change to 10% after 3–4 wk or sooner if tolerated. Apply once daily for several days, and increase to BID if tolerated.
Indications: Treatment of acne vulgaris
Action: Antibacterial via release of active oxygen; has some keratolytic, drying, and desquamative effects
Metabolism: Metabolized in skin to benzoic acid
Excretion: Renal
Contraindications and precautions
1. Concurrent use of other acne preparations, alcohol-containing preparations, abrasive or medicated soaps or cleansers may increase irritant or drying effect.
2. Use with caution on acutely inflamed or denuded skin.
3. May bleach hair or clothes.
4. Avoid mucous membranes.

Benztropine (Cogentin, others)

Preparations: Tablets, 0.5, 1,2 mg; injection (IM, IV), 1 mg/ml
Adult Dosage
Parkinsonism—PO: 1–2 mg/day; increase dose in 0.5-mg increments q5–6 days. Usual maintenance dose is 0.5–6 mg/day qhs or in divided doses. In idiopathic parkinsonism, start with 0.5–1 mg qhs. In postencephalitic parkinsonism, start with 2 mg qd in one or more doses; IM, IV: 1–2 mg/day; adjust as tolerated prn.
Drug-induced extrapyramidal reactions—PO: 1–4 mg qd–bid. If extrapyramidal reaction develops soon after initiating treatment with neuroleptic drugs, administer 1–2 mg bid–tid and attempt to withdraw benztropine in 1–2 wk to determine continued need. IM, IV: 1–2 mg usually relieves reaction. Follow with PO 1–2 mg bid to prevent recurrence.
Indications: Treatment of parkinsonism and drug-induced extrapyramidal reactions except tardive dyskinesia
Action: Synthetic anticholinergic agent with more selective CNS activity
Metabolism: Unknown
Excretion: Unknown
Contraindications and precautions
1. Use with caution in cardiovascular disease, tardive dyskinesia, glaucoma, intestinal obstruction, myasthenia gravis, prostatic hypertrophy, or urinary retention.
2. Geriatric patients may develop mental confusion, disorientation, agitation, hallucinations, and psychotic-like symptoms even with usual doses.
3. Hyperthermia is possible in geriatric, chronically ill, or alcoholic patients.

Drug interactions
1. Drugs with anticholinergic properties lead to increased antimuscarinic effects.
2. Antacids lead to decreased benztropine absorption.

Bisacodyl (Dulcolax, others)

Preparations: EC tablets, 5 mg; suppositories, 10 mg; enema suspension, 10 mg
Adult Dosage: PO: 5–15 mg qd (AM or hs) up to 30 mg/day for preparation of lower GI tract for special procedures. Onset of action in 6–8 h. PR: 10 mg. Onset of action in 15 min–1hr.
Indications: Treatment of constipation; bowel evacuation in preparation for surgery, radiography, and sigmoidoscopy
Action: Stimulant laxative; probably increases peristalsis by a direct effect on intestinal smooth muscle by stimulation of intramural nerve plexi
Metabolism: None (minimal absorption)
Excretion: Renal (of absorbed dose)
Contraindications and precautions
1. Contraindicated in nausea, vomiting, or other symptoms of appendicitis, acute surgical abdomen, undiagnosed rectal bleeding, intestinal obstruction, or fecal impactions.
2. May cause significant electrolyte loss with repeated use.
Drug interactions: Milk or antacids dissolve enteric coating.

Bumetanide (Bumex)

Preparations: Tablets, 0.5, 1,2 mg; injection (IM, IV), 0.25 mg/ml
Adult Dosage: PO: 0.5–2 mg/day as a single dose. Dose may be increased by adding a second or third daily dose at 4- to 5-hr intervals up to a maximum of 10 mg/day. Can use alternate-day schedule. IM, IV (IV preferred): 0.5–1.0 mg. Can repeat q2–3h up to 10 mg/day.
Note:
1. Forty times more potent than furosemide over the usual dosage range.
2. Onset of action: PO—30–60 min; IV—<5 min
3. Time to peak effect: PO—1–2 hr; IV—15–30 min
4. Duration of action: PO—4–6 hr; IV—4 hr
Indications: Treatment of edema associated with CHF, cirrhosis, and renal disease; adjunctive therapy in pulmonary edema and hypercalcemia
Action: Loop diuretic
Metabolism: Hepatic
Excretion: Renal
Contraindications and precautions
1. Contraindicated in anuria.
2. Use with caution in severe renal function impairment, hepatic impairment, and those at increased risk if hypokalemia occurs.
3. Patients with known sulfonamide sensitivity may show allergic reaction.
4. May exacerbate gout or diabetes mellitus.
Drug interactions
1. Adrenocorticoids may decrease natriuretic or diuretic effect.
2. NSAIDs, especially indomethacin, may decrease diuretic effect.
3. Bumetanide may increase toxicity of lithium, amphotericin B, and aminoglycoside antibiotics.
4. Bumetanide may increase toxicity of digoxin and nondepolarizing neuromuscular blocking agents by elevating K^+.
5. Bumetanide may decrease anticoagulant effects of coumadin.

Buspirone (BuSpar)

Preparations: Tablets, 5, 10 mg
Adult dosage: PO: Initially, 5 mg tid; increase by 5 mg/day q2–3 days prn up to 60 mg/day
Indications: Treatment of anxiety disorders (short-term)
Action: Unknown; unrelated to benzodiazepines or barbiturates
Metabolism: Hepatic
Excretion: Renal > fecal
Contraindications and precautions: May cause sedation, especially at higher doses.
Drug interactions
1. Buspirone leads to elevated BP with use of MAO inhibitors.
2. Buspirone may increase serum digoxin level.

Butorphanol tartrate (Stadol)

Preparations: Injection (IM, IV), 1,2 mg/ml
Adult dosage: Analgesic—IM: 1–4 mg (usually 2 mg) q3–4h prn; IV: 0.5–2 mg (usually 1 mg) q3–4h prn
Note
1. Use lower doses in geriatric patients.
2. Administer smallest effective dose and as infrequently as possible to minimize tolerance and physical dependence.
Indications: Pain relief
Action: Mixed agonist/antagonist narcotic analgesic; consult other texts for effect profile compared to agonist narcotics
Metabolism: Hepatic
Excretion: Renal >> biliary
Contraindications and precautions
1. Contraindicated in diarrhea associated with pseudomembranous colitis, diarrhea caused by poisoning until the toxic material has been eliminated, and acute respiratory depression.
2. Psychological and physical dependence and tolerance to many of the effects of butorphanol may develop with chronic administration.
3. Use with caution in patients with opioid agonist analgesic dependence (butorphanol may not suppress withdrawal symptoms).
4. Use with caution in acute myocardial infarction, acute abdominal conditions, acute asthma or chronic respiratory impairment, head injury, increased intracranial pressure, intracranial lesions, hepatic or renal function impairment, hypothyroidism, gallbladder disease, inflammatory bowel disease, recent GI tract surgery, prostatic hypertrophy or obstruction, urethral stricture, acute alcoholism, Addison's disease, epilepsy, suicidal ideation, emotional instability, or history of drug abuse.
5. Use with caution in patients performing tasks requiring mental alertness or physical coordination.

Drug interactions
1. Alcohol or other CNS depressants may increase CNS depression.
2. Antidiarrheals or antimuscarinics may increase risk of constipation.
3. Naltrexone, naloxone, and buprenorphine may block certain opioid actions. Consult other texts for further information.

Calcitonin—Human (Cibacalcin)

Preparations: Injection (SC), 0.5 mg/vial in double-chamber vials
Adult dosage: SC: Initially, 0.5 mg qd. Maintenance dose varies from 0.25 mg qd to 0.5 mg 2–3 times/week. If severe, may require up to 0.5 mg bid. Continue for 6 mo and then stop if symptoms improved.
Indications: Treatment of moderate to severe symptomatic Paget's disease; has been used (not approved) for postmenopausal osteoporosis and hypercalcemia
Action: Reduces the rate of bone turnover by blocking bone resorption; inhibits renal tubular reabsorption of Na^+, Ca^{++}, and phosphate
Metabolism: Renal > blood, peripheral tissues
Excretion: Renal
Contraindications and precautions
1. Possibility of systemic allergic reaction exists because calcitonin is a protein.
2. Antibodies to calcitonin develop but less frequently than to calcitonin-salmon and may diminish efficacy.

Drug interactions: No clinically significant interactions

Calcitonin—Salmon (Calcimar, Miacalcin)

Preparations: Injection (SC, IM), 100 IU/ml, 200 IU/ml
Adult dosage
Paget's disease—SC, IM: Initially, 100 IU qd. Monitor serum alkaline phosphatase and symptoms. If there is improvement, maintenance dose is 50 IU qd–qod.
Postmenopausal osteoporosis—SC, IM: 100 IU qd–qod.
Hypercalcemia—SC, IM: Initially, 4 IU/kg q12h. If response is unsatisfactory after 1–2 days, increase to 8 IU/kg q12h. If response remains unsatisfactory, increase to 8 IU/kg q6h.
Indications: Treatment of moderate to severe symptomatic Paget's disease and hypercalcemic emergencies; treatment adjunct for postmenopausal osteoporosis
Action: Reduces the rate of bone turnover by blocking bone resorption; inhibits renal tubular reabsorption of Na^+, Ca^{++}, and phosphate
Metabolism: Renal > blood, peripheral tissues
Excretion: Renal
Contraindications and precautions
1. Possibility of systemic allergic reaction exists because calcitonin is a protein.
2. Antibodies to calcitonin develop in >50% of patients on long-term treatment and may diminish efficacy.

Drug interactions: No clinically significant interactions

Calcium carbonate (Os-Cal, Tums, others)

Preparations: Tablets, 650, 667, 750, 1,250, 1,500 mg; chewable tablets, 350, 420, 500, 625, 750, 850, 1,250 mg; capsules, 1,512 mg; suspension, 1,250 mg/5 ml. Calcium carbonate = 40% elemental calcium (750 mg of calcium carbonate = 300 mg elemental calcium)
Adult dosage: PO: 500–2,000 mg bid–qid
Indications: Treatment of chronic hypocalcemia and prophylaxis of calcium deficiency
Action: Multiple physiologic functions, primarily for bone growth.
Excretion: Fecal > renal
Contraindications and precautions
1. Contraindicated in hypercalcemia, hypercalciuria, calcium renal calculi, or sarcoidosis.
2. Use with precaution in renal function impairment or electrolyte imbalance.

Drug interactions
1. Thiazide diuretics lead to increased calcium excretion.
2. Calcium carbonate leads to decreased absorption of tetracycline, phenytoin, iron salts, and etidronate.

Captopril (Capoten)

Preparations: Tablets, 12.5, 25, 50, 100 mg
Adult dosage
Antihypertensive—PO: Initially, 12.5 mg bid–tid. Increase in 1–2 wk prn to 25 mg bid–tid. Doses up to 100 mg tid can be used.
Vasodilator—PO: Initially, 12.5 mg bid–tid. Increase daily prn up to 50 mg tid. Doses up to 100 mg tid can be used.
Note: An initial dose of 6.25 mg should be used in patients who are salt-volume depleted, are on diuretics, or have renal function impairment.
Indications: Treatment of hypertension and CHF; unlabeled uses include hypertensive crisis and hypertension related to scleroderma renal crisis
Action: Angiotensin converting enzyme inhibitor with antihypertensive and vasodilator effects
Metabolism: Hepatic
Excretion: Renal
Contraindications and precautions
1. May cause profound hypotension after the first dose, especially if patient is salt-volume depleted.
2. Use with caution in hyperkalemia, bilateral renal artery stenosis, solitary kidney, renal function impairment, and salt-volume depletion.

Drug interactions
1. Potassium-sparing diuretics, potassium supplements, and salt substitutes lead to increased risk of hyperkalemia.
2. Diuretics and other renin-releasing antihypertensive agents lead to increased antihypertensive effect.

Carbamazepine (Epitol, Tegretol, others)

Preparations: Tablets, 100, 200 mg; suspension, 100 mg/5 ml
Adult dosage
Anticonvulsant—PO: Initially, 200 mg bid on the first day. Increase by 200 mg/day every week prn until best response obtained. Usual maintenance is 600 mg/day. Can give up to 1,200 mg/day.
Antineuralgic—PO: Initially, 100 mg bid on the first day. Increase by 200 mg qod in increments of 100 mg q12h. Usual maintenance is 400–800 mg/day.
Indications: Treatment of partial seizures with simple or complex symptomatology (psychomotor, temporal lobe), generalized tonic-clonic seizures, mixed seizure patterns, and other partial or generalized seizures; treatment of pain associated with trigeminal neuralgia; unlabeled uses include other neurogenic pain disorders, central diabetes insipidus, certain psychiatric disorders, and alcohol withdrawal
Action: Unknown anticonvulsant and antineuralgic effect; stimulates ADH release
Metabolism: Hepatic
Excretion: Renal > fecal
Contraindications and precautions
1. Contraindicated in absence, atonic, or myoclonic seizures; history of bone marrow depression or other blood disorders with low blood counts; and concurrent use of MAO inhibitors.
2. Use with precaution in patients who are intolerant of tricyclic antidepressants, those who have cardiac impairment, glaucoma, SIADH, hepatic impairment, urinary retention, or history of adverse hematologic reactions to other medications.

Drug interactions
1. Cimetidine, erythromycin, isoniazid, propoxyphene, diltiazem, and verapamil may increase carbamazepine toxicity.
2. Tricyclic antidepressants lead to increased CNS depressant effects and decreased anticonvulsant effects.
3. MAO inhibitors may cause hyperpyretic crises, hypertensive crises, convulsions, and death.
4. Carbamazepine may decrease effect of coumadin, phenytoin, phenobarbital, benzodiazepines, primidone, valproic acid, estrogens, and quinidine.

Carbidopa (see *Levodopa*)

Charcoal—Activated

Preparations: Powder for suspension, 15, 30, 40, 120, 240 g; suspension, 12.5, 15, 25, 30, 40, 50 g/5 ml; charcoal and sorbitol suspension, 25, 30, 50 g with various amounts of sorbitol
Adult dosage: PO: 30–100 g as a single dose (or 5–10× weight of ingested poison). For multiple-dose therapy, 25–50 g q4–6h. Do not use activated charcoal and sorbitol preparation for multiple-dose therapy because of excessive catharsis.
Indications: Treatment of poisoning by most drugs and chemicals
Action: Adsorbs ingested toxic substances; sorbitol (if used), a hyperosmotic laxative, reduces intestinal transit time
Metabolism: Not absorbed; sorbitol poorly absorbed
Excretion: Fecal
Contraindications and precautions: Not effective in adsorbing cyanide and relatively ineffective for ethanol, methanol, ferrous sulfate, caustic alkalis, and mineral acids.
Drug interactions: Adsorbs and inactivates syrup of ipecac.

Chloral hydrate (Aquachloral, Noctec, others)
Preparations: Capsules, 250, 500 mg; syrup, 250, 500 mg/5 ml;
suppositories, 324, 500, 648 mg
Adult dosage
Sedative—PO: 250 mg tid. PR: 324 mg tid.
Hypnotic—PO: 500–1,000 mg qhs or 30 min before surgery. PR: 324 mg qhs.
Indications: Adjunctive therapy for preoperative sedation and postoperative care and control of pain; short-term treatment of insomnia
Action: Unknown
Metabolism: Hepatic > renal
Excretion: Renal
Contraindications and precautions
1. Use caution while performing tasks requiring mental alertness.
2. Use with caution in severe cardiac disease, marked hepatic or renal impairment, and gastritis.
3. Prolonged use may result in psychic and physical dependence.

Drug interactions
1. Alcohol, CNS depressants, and coumadin lead to increased effect.
2. IV furosemide following chloral hydrate may cause a hypermetabolic state owing to displacement of bound thyroxine.

Chlordiazepoxide (Librium, others)
Preparations: Tablets, 5, 10, 25 mg; capsules 5, 10, 25 mg; powder for injection (IM, IV), 100 mg
Adult dosage
Antianxiety—PO: 5–25 mg tid–qid. IM, IV: Initially, 50–100 mg; then 25–50 mg tid–qid
Preoperative—IM: 50–100 mg 1 hr prior to surgery
Sedative-hypnotic for alcohol withdrawal—PO: Initially, 50–100 mg; repeat as needed up to 300 mg/day. IM, IV: Initially, 50–100 mg repeated in 2–4 hr.
Note: Use lower doses for anxiety in elderly or debilitated patients.
Indications: Treatment of anxiety disorders, acute alcohol withdrawal, and preoperative anxiety
Action: Anxiolytic sedative-hypnotic benzodiazepine; may potentiate CNS gamma-aminobutyric acid effects
Metabolism: Hepatic (oxidation)
Excretion: Renal
Contraindications and precautions
1. Contraindicated in acute alcohol intoxication with depressed vital signs, depressive neuroses, or psychoses without prominent anxiety.
2. Use with caution in acute narrow-angle glaucoma, myasthenia gravis, shock, severe chronic obstructive pulmonary disease, hepatic or renal impairment, patients with depressed respirations, or those receiving concurrent respiratory depressants.
3. Long-term therapy may result in psychic or physical dependence.
4. Use caution while performing tasks requiring alertness and coordination.

Drug interactions
1. Cimetidine, disulfiram, erythromycin, isoniazid, ketoconazole, and oral contraceptives may increase effects.
2. Alcohol or other CNS depressants lead to increased CNS depression.

Chlorothiazide (Diuril, others)
Preparations: Tablets, 250, 500 mg; suspension, 250 mg/5 ml; injection (IV), 500 mg/20-ml vial
Adult dosage
Diuretic—PO, IV: Initially, 500–2,000 mg/day in single or bid doses or 250 mg bid–qid. Reduce to lowest effective maintenance dose.
Antihypertensive—PO, IV: Initially, 500–1,000 mg/day in single or bid doses. Maintenance dose determined by BP response. If adding to another antihypertensive agent, start with 250 mg qd and adjust according to BP response.
Indications: Treatment of hypertension and edema
Action: Thiazide diuretic that inhibits renal tubular reabsorption of sodium and water in the distal tubule. It also increases urinary excretion of potassium and decreases urinary excretion of calcium and uric acid. Antihypertensive mechanism is unknown.
Metabolism: Minimal
Excretion: Renal
Contraindications and precautions
1. Contraindicated in anuria and hypersensitivity to thiazides or other sulfonamide derivatives.
2. Use with caution in diabetes mellitus, history of gout, hyperuricemia, hepatic function impairment, hypercalcemia, systemic lupus erythematosus, sympathectomy, or electrolyte disturbances.
3. Electrolyte disturbances may occur; monitor serum electrolytes.

Drug interactions
1. Cholestyramine and colestipol lead to decreased absorption.
2. Glucocorticoids and amphotericin B lead to increased risk of hypokalemia.
3. Chlorothiazide leads to increased risk of lithium toxicity.
4. Chlorothiazide leads to increased risk of toxicity of digoxin, amiodarone, and nondepolarizing neuromuscular blocking agents owing to hypokalemia.

Chlorpromazine (Thorazine, others)
Preparations: Tablets, 10, 25, 50, 100, 200 mg; SR capsules, 30, 75, 150, 200, 300 mg; syrup, 10 mg/5 ml; solution, 30 mg/ml, 100 mg/ml; suppositories, 25, 100 mg; injection (IM, IV), 25 mg/ml
Adult dosage
Antipsychotic: *Nonhospitalized or mild symptoms*—PO: Initially, 30–75 mg/day in 2–4 divided doses. Increase by 20–50 mg q3–4d until symptoms controlled. When optimum dosage achieved, continue for 2 wk, then taper to lowest effective dose (usually 200 mg up to 800 mg/day). *Hospitalized and severe symptoms*—IM: Initially, 25 mg. If necessary, administer an additional dose of 25–50 mg in 1 hr. Increase gradually over days to a maximum of 400 mg q4–6h until the patient is controlled and then transfer to oral therapy.
Nausea and vomiting—PO: 10–25 mg q4–6h prn. Increase dose if necessary. PR: 50–100 mg q6–8h prn. IM: Initially, 25 mg. If no hypotension, 25–50 mg q3–4h until PO tolerated.
Intraoperative acute nausea and vomiting—IM: 12.5 mg repeated in 30 min if no hypotension. IV: Dilute with normal saline to 1 mg/ml, and administer 2 mg/fractional injection q2min up to a total of 25 mg.
Presurgical anxiety—PO: 25–50 mg 2–3 hr prior to surgery. IM: 12.5–25 mg 1–2 hr prior to surgery.
Hiccups—PO: 25–50 mg tid–qid. IM: 25–50 mg tid–qid; IV: Dilute with normal saline to 1 mg/ml, and administer at a rate of 1 mg/min.
Porphyria—PO: 25–50 mg tid–qid. IM: 25 mg tid–qid until PO tolerated.
Tetanus—IM: 25–50 mg tid–qid usually with barbiturates. IV: 25–50 mg diluted with normal saline to 1 mg/ml and administered at a rate of 1 mg/ml.
Note: Use lower doses with geriatric or debilitated patients.
Indications: Treatment of psychotic disorders, preoperative anxiety, nausea and vomiting, intractable hiccups, and acute intermittent porphyria; treatment adjunct for tetanus
Action: Antipsychotic effect due to inhibition of CNS dopaminergic receptors; antiemetic effect from inhibition of medullary chemoreceptor trigger-zone dopaminergic receptors; has strong anticholinergic and sedative effects; peripheral α-adrenergic blocking effect causes vasodilation
Metabolism: Hepatic
Excretion: Renal > biliary
Contraindications and precautions
1. Contraindicated in comatose states, severe CNS depression, subcortical brain damage, bone marrow depression, and severe cardiovascular disease.
2. Use with caution in cardiovascular disease, seizure disorders, hepatic function impairment, glaucoma, urinary retention, prostatic hypertrophy, chronic respiratory disorders, blood dyscrasias, and active alcoholism.
3. Tartrazine in some products may cause allergic reactions.

Drug interactions
1. CNS depressants lead to increased sedative effect.
2. Anticholinergic agents lead to increased antimuscarinic effects
3. Aluminum- or magnesium-containing antacids or lithium may decrease oral absorption.
4. Epinephrine leads to severe hypotension and tachycardia.
5. Propranolol and possibly other β-blockers lead to increased levels and vice versa.
6. Opioids lead to increased risk of constipation.
7. Chlorpromazine may increase phenytoin or tricyclic antidepressant levels.
8. Chlorpromazine may increase risk of metrizamide-induced seizures.
9. Chlorpromazine may decrease effect of levodopa.

Chlorpropamide (Diabinese, Glucamide)
Preparations: Tablets, 100, 200 mg
Adult dosage
Antidiabetic—PO: Initially, 100–250 mg qd. Start with 100 mg in geriatric or debilitated patients. Increase by 50–125 mg q5–7d

until optimal control or a maximum dose of 750 mg. Patients previously on insulin doses of <40 units/day should start chlorpropamide and have the insulin stopped abruptly. Patients previously on ≥40 units/day should start oral therapy with a concurrent 50% reduction in insulin dose. Taper insulin and increase chlorpropamide according to clinical response.
Antidiuretic—PO: 100–250 mg qd; adjust q2–3d as needed up to 500 mg/day
Indications: Treatment of non–insulin-dependent diabetes mellitus and partial central diabetes insipidus
Action: Sulfonylurea that promotes insulin release from beta cells, decreases hepatic gluconeogenesis, and increases insulin sensitivity; potentiates the effect of antidiuretic hormone
Metabolism: Hepatic
Excretion: Renal
Contraindications and precautions
1. Contraindicated in significant acidosis, severe burns, diabetic coma, severe infection, significant ketosis, ketoacidosis, major surgery, or severe trauma.
2. Cross-sensitivity to other sulfonamide-type medications can occur.
3. Use with caution in adrenal or pituitary insufficiency, thyroid function impairment, renal, hepatic or cardiac function impairment, malnourishment, debilitated physical condition, or nausea and vomiting.
4. SIADH has occurred with chlorpropamide therapy.

Drug interactions
1. Chronic alcohol use, phenobarbital, and rifampin lead to decreased hypoglycemic effect.
2. Chloramphenicol, cimetidine, clofibrate, coumadin, ketoconazole, sulfonamides, and sulfinpyrazone lead to increased hypoglycemic effect.
3. Ethanol may lead to disulfiram-like reaction.

Chlorthalidone (Hygroton, others)
Preparations: Tablets, 25, 50, 100 mg
Adult dosage
Diuretic–PO: Initially, 50–100 mg qd or 100 mg qod or 100 mg 3 times per week. May require up to 150–200 mg/day.
Antihypertensive—PO: Initially, 25 mg qd. Increase to 50 mg qd up to a maximum daily dose of 100 mg.
Indications: Treatment of hypertension and edema
Action: Thiazide diuretic that inhibits renal tubular reabsorption of sodium and water in the distal tubule. It also increases urinary excretion of potassium and decreases urinary excretion of calcium and uric acid. Antihypertensive mechanism is unknown.
Metabolism: Minimal
Excretion: Renal
Contraindications and precautions
1. Contraindicated in anuria and hypersensitivity to thiazides or other sulfonamide derivatives.
2. Use with caution in diabetes mellitus, history of gout, hyperuricemia, hepatic function impairment, hypercalcemia, systemic lupus erythematosus, sympathectomy, or electrolyte disturbances.
3. Electrolyte disturbances may occur; monitor serum electrolytes.

Drug interactions
1. Cholestyramine and colestipol lead to decreased absorption.
2. Glucocorticoids and amphotericin B lead to increased risk of hypokalemia.
3. Chlorthalidone leads to increased risk of lithium toxicity.
4. Chlorthalidone leads to increased risk of toxicity of digoxin, amiodarone, and nondepolarizing neuromuscular blocking agents owing to hypokalemia.

Cholestyramine (Cholybar, Questran)
Preparations: Powder for suspension, 4 mg of dried resin/9 g of powder; chewable bar, 4 g of dried resin/bar
Adult dosage
Antihyperlipidemic or antipruritic—PO: 4 g of dried resin tid before meals. Increase up to 24 g/day in 2–5 divided doses. For the powder, mix in 60–180 ml of noncarbonated beverage. One level scoop or 1 packet = 4 g.
Indications: Treatment of hyperlipidemia and pruritus associated with partial biliary obstruction (cholestasis). Unlabeled uses include treatment of diarrhea due to bile acids.
Action: Binds with bile acids in the intestine, producing an insoluble complex that is excreted in the feces; results in a reduction of serum LDL (cholesterol) with minimal change in triglyceride or HDL levels
Metabolism: Not absorbed
Excretion: Not absorbed
Contraindications and precautions
1. Contraindicated in complete biliary obstruction.
2. Use with caution in bleeding disorders, gastrointestinal dysfunction, especially constipation or malabsorption states, peptic ulcer, and hemorrhoids.

Drug interactions
1. Cholestyramine may decrease absorption of many drugs. It is recommended that other drugs be administered 1 hr before or 4–6 hr after cholestyramine.
2. Cholestyramine is known to decrease absorption of coumadin, digoxin, thiazide diuretics, penicillin G, tetracycline, phenylbutazone, phenobarbital, thyroid hormones, and fat-soluble vitamins.

Cimetidine (Tagamet)
Preparations: Tablets, 200, 300, 400, 800 mg; liquid, 300 mg/5 ml; injection (IM, IV), 300 mg/2 ml; aqueous solution, 300 mg/50 ml normal saline
Adult dosage
Duodenal ulcer treatment–PO: 300 mg qid (with meals and qhs) or 400 mg bid or 800 mg qhs (considered by some to be first choice); 1,600 mg qhs may produce more rapid healing in patients with an endoscopically proven ulcer >1 cm and who abuse tobacco. IM, IV: 300 mg q6–8h.
Duodenal ulcer prophylaxis—PO: 400 mg qhs
Gastric ulcer treatment—PO: 300 mg qid (with meals and qhs) or 800 mg qhs. IM, IV: 300 mg q6–8h.
Gastric hypersecretory states—PO: 300 mg qid (with meals and qhs); may give up to 2.4 g/day. IM, IV: 300 mg q6–8h.
Note
1. If higher total daily parenteral doses are used, increase the frequency of 300-mg doses.
2. Dosage reduction in renal function impairment: 300 mg PO/IM/IV q12h up to q8h if necessary. Further reduction may be required if there is concurrent hepatic function impairment.

Indications: Treatment of active, benign gastric, or duodenal ulcers and gastric hypersecretory conditions (Zollinger-Ellison syndrome, systemic mastocytosis, multiple endocrine adenomas); prophylaxis of duodenal ulcer; unlabeled uses include treatment of gastroesophageal reflux, upper gastrointestinal bleeding, and stress-related mucosal damage
Action: H_2-receptor blocker; inhibits gastric secretion; inhibits cytochrome P-450 mixed function oxidase, and antagonizes dihydrotestosterone (antiandrogenic effect)
Metabolism: Hepatic
Excretion: Renal
Contraindications and precautions: Use with caution in hepatic or renal function impairment.
Drug interactions
1. Antacids lead to decreased absorption.
2. Cimetidine leads to increased effects/toxicity of benzodiazepines, calcium channel blockers, carbamazepine, coumadin, ethanol, labetalol, metoprolol, propanolol, lidocaine, metronidazole, mexiletine, phenytoin, quinidine, sulfonylureas, triamterene, tricyclic antidepressants, and xanthines.
3. Cimetidine leads to decreased absorption of ketoconazole
4. Cimetidine leads to decreased renal excretion of procainamide.
5. Alkylating agents lead to increased risk of neutropenia.
6. Tobacco abuse leads to decreased cimetidine-induced inhibition of nocturnal gastric secretion.

Clemastine fumarate (Tavist)
Preparations: Tablets, 1.34, 2.68 mg; syrup, 0.67 mg/5 ml
Adult dosage: Antihistaminic—PO: 1.34 mg bid for rhinitis; for urticaria and angioedema, up to 2.68 mg tid
Indications: Treatment of allergic rhinitis and allergic urticaria or angioedema
Action: H_1-receptor blocker
Metabolism: Hepatic
Excretion: Renal
Contraindications and precautions: Use with caution in prostatic hypertrophy, bladder neck obstruction, angle-closure glaucoma, asthma, and COPD.
Drug interactions
1. Alcohol or other CNS depressants may increase CNS depression.
2. Anticholinergics may increase antimuscarinic effects.
3. MAO inhibitors may increase antimuscarinic and CNS depressant effects.

Clonazepam (Klonopin)
Preparations: Tablets, 0.5, 1, 2 mg
Adult dosage: PO: Initially, 0.5 mg tid. Increase by 0.5–1 mg q3d until seizures are controlled or side effects preclude further increase. Maximum dose is 20 mg/day.
Indications: Treatment of Lennox-Gastaut syndrome (petit mal variant epilepsy), akinetic and myoclonic seizures; treatment of absence (petit mal) seizures refractory to succinimides or valproic acid
Action: Unknown; suppresses spread of seizure activity
Metabolism: Hepatic (oxidation)
Excretion: Renal
Contraindications and precautions: Use with caution in acute narrow-angle glaucoma, severe chronic obstructive pulmonary disease, patients with depressed respirations or concurrent respiratory depressants, or renal impairment.
Drug interactions
1. Cimetidine, disulfiram, erythromycin, isoniazid, ketoconazole and oral contraceptives may increase effects.
2. Phenytoin, phenobarbital, or carbamazepine may decrease clonazepam serum levels.

Clonidine (Catapres, others)
Preparations: Tablets, 0.1, 0.2, 0.3 mg; transdermal Catapres-TTS-1, -2, -3, supply 0.1, 0.2, 0.3 mg/24 hr
Adult dosage
Antihypertensive—PO: Initially, 0.1 mg bid; increase by 0.1–0.2 mg/day q2–4d until desired BP control or a maximum daily dose of 2.4 mg/day. Topical: Initially, 0.1 mg/day system applied to hairless skin once q7d: increase to next larger dose system q1–2wk until desired BP response or 0.6 mg/24 hr using two systems. The hypotensive effect of transdermal clonidine may not begin for 2–3 days.
Indications: Treatment of hypertension. Unlabeled uses include prophylaxis of migraine headache and treatment of vasomotor symptoms of menopause, opioid withdrawal, Gilles de la Tourette syndrome, and nicotine withdrawal.
Action: Central α_2-adrenergic stimulant that results in decreased sympathetic outflow
Metabolism: Hepatic
Excretion: Renal > biliary/fecal
Contraindications and precautions
1. Rebound hypertension may follow abrupt withdrawal; a 2- to 4-day taper is advised.
2. Use with caution in severe coronary insufficiency, recent MI, cerebrovascular disease, chronic renal function impairment, history of mental depression, Raynaud's syndrome, or thromboangiitis obliterans.
3. Avoid placing transdermal patches on irritated skin.

Drug interactions
1. Tricyclic antidepressants lead to decreased hypotensive effects.
2. Discontinuation of concurrent β-adrenergic blockers may increase risk of clonidine-withdrawal rebound hypertension.
3. Clonidine may increase CNS depressant effects of other sedatives.

Clorazepate (Tranxene, others)
Preparations: Tablets, 3.75, 7.5, 15 mg; single-dose tablets, 11.25, 22.5 mg; capsules, 3.75, 7.5, 15 mg
Adult dosage
Antianxiety—PO: Initially, 7.5–15 mg bid–tid or 15 mg qhs. Adjust dose to 15–60 mg/day in divided doses. Single-dose tablets are for maintenance therapy only.
Sedative-hypnotic for alcohol withdrawal—PO: Initially, 30 mg followed by 15 mg bid–qid on day 1; 15 mg tid to 6 times/day on day 2; 7.5–15 mg tid on day 3; 7.5 mg bid–qid on day 4. Thereafter, gradually reduce the dose to 7.5–15 mg qd. Avoid excessive reduction in daily dose.
Anticonvulsant—PO: Initially, 7.5 mg tid. Increase by no more than 7.5 mg every week up to 90 mg/day.
Note: Use lower doses for anxiety in elderly or debilitated patients.
Indications: Treatment of anxiety disorders and acute alcohol withdrawal; adjunctive therapy in partial seizures
Action: Anxiolytic sedative-hypnotic benzodiazepine may potentiate CNS gamma-aminobutyric acid effects; suppresses spread of seizure activity possibly by augmenting presynaptic inhibition
Metabolism: Hepatic (oxidation)
Excretion: Renal
Contraindications and precautions
1. Contraindicated in acute alcohol intoxication with depressed vital signs, depressive neuroses, or psychoses without prominent anxiety.
2. Use with caution in acute narrow-angle glaucoma, myasthenia gravis, shock, severe chronic obstructive pulmonary disease, hepatic or renal function impairment, patients with depressed respirations, or those receiving concurrent respiratory depressants.
3. Long-term therapy may result in psychic or physical dependence.
4. Use caution in performing tasks requiring alertness and coordination.

Drug interactions
1. Cimetidine, disulfiram, erythromycin, isoniazid, ketoconazole, and oral contraceptives may increase effects.
2. Alcohol or other CNS depressants lead to increased CNS depression

Codeine—Schedule II
Preparations Codeine phosphate: tablets, 30, 60 mg; solution, 15 mg/5 ml; injection (IM, IV, SC), 15, 30, 60 mg/ml Codeine sulfate: tablets, 15, 30, 60 mg
Adult dosage
Analgesic—PO, IM, IV, SC: 15–60 mg (usually 30 mg) q4–6h prn
Antitussive—PO: 10–20 mg q4–6h up to a maximum of 120 mg/day
Note
1. Use lower doses in geriatric patients.
2. Give smallest effective dose and as infrequently as possible to minimize tolerance and physical dependence.

Indications: Relief of pain and treatment of cough. Unlabeled use includes treatment of diarrhea.
Action: Narcotic analgesic with antitussive and antidiarrheal effects
Metabolism: Hepatic
Excretion: Renal
Contraindications and precautions
1. Contraindicated in diarrhea associated with pseudomembranous colitis, diarrhea caused by poisoning until the toxic material has been eliminated, and acute respiratory depression.
2. Psychological and physical dependence and tolerance to many of the effects of codeine may develop with chronic administration.
3. Use with caution in acute abdominal conditions, acute asthma or chronic respiratory impairment, head injury, increased intracranial pressure, intracranial lesions, hepatic or renal function impairment, hypothyroidism, gallbladder disease, inflammatory bowel disease, recent GI tract surgery, prostatic hypertrophy or obstruction, urethral stricture, acute alcoholism, Addison's disease, epilepsy, suicidal ideation, emotional instability, or history of drug abuse.
4. Use with caution in patients performing tasks requiring mental alertness or physical coordination.
5. Use with caution in patients being administered MAO inhibitors.

Drug interactions
1. Alcohol, other opioid agonist analgesics, and other CNS depressants (including antihistamines, phenothiazines, tricyclic antidepressants, benzodiazepines, sedative-hypnotics, barbiturates) may increase risk of CNS depression.
2. Antidiarrheals and anticholinergics lead to increased risk of constipation.
3. Antihypertensives and diuretics lead to increased risk of hypotension.
4. Naltrexone, naloxone, and buprenorphine may block certain opioid actions. Consult other texts for further information.

Codeine and acetaminophen (Tylenol with codeine) (see individual drugs)—Schedule III
Preparations
No. 1: 7.5 mg codeine phosphate and 300 mg acetaminophen (Schedule III)
No. 2: 15 mg codeine phosphate and 300 mg acetaminophen (Schedule III)
No. 3: 30 mg codeine phosphate and 300 mg acetaminophen (Schedule III)
No. 4: 60 mg codeine phosphate and 300 mg acetaminophen (Schedule III)

Colchicine
Preparations: Tablets, 0.5, 0.6, 0.65 mg; injection (IV), 1 mg/2 ml
Adult dosage
Antigout (acute gouty arthritis)—PO: Initially, 0.5–1.3 mg, then 0.5–0.65 mg q1–2h or 1–1.3 mg q2h until pain is relieved or until nausea, vomiting, or diarrhea occurs. IV: Initially, 2 mg followed by 0.5 mg q6h until relief. Some recommend 1 mg initially followed by 0.5 mg qd–bid or a single dose of 3 mg. Generally, do not exceed 4 mg/day or 4 mg for one course of treatment.
Prophylaxis—PO (preferred): 0.5–0.65 mg qd for 3–4 days/wk if ≤1 attack/year or 0.5–0.65 mg qd if >1 attack/year. For patients with gout undergoing surgery, administer 0.5–0.65 mg qd for 3 days

before and after surgery. IV: 0.5–1.0 mg qd–bid.
Indications: Treatment or prophylaxis of gouty arthritis. Unlabeled uses include treatment of familial Mediterranean fever and hepatic cirrhosis.
Action: Unknown; decreases leukocyte motility, phagocytosis, and lactic acid production, leading to decreased deposition of urate crystals
Metabolism: Hepatic
Excretion: Biliary > renal
Contraindications and precautions
1. Use with caution in severe cardiac or gastrointestinal disorders, severe hepatic or renal impairment, geriatric or debilitated patients.
2. Alcoholics are at greater risk of gastrointestinal toxicity, especially with oral therapy.
3. Severe local irritation occurs with extravasation during IV therapy.

Drug interactions
1. Drugs that impair blood clotting (e.g., coumadin, NSAIDs) lead to increased risk of hemorrhage.
2. Alcohol leads to increased risk of GI toxicity.
3. Colchicine leads to increased sensitivity to CNS depressants, sympathomimetics, and bone marrow suppressants.
4. Colchicine leads to increased reversible malabsorption of vitamin B_{12}.

Colestipol (Colestid)
Preparations: Granules for suspension, 5 g/packet or level scoop.
Adult dosage: Antihyperlipidemic—PO: 15–30 g/day before meals bid–qid. Prepare by mixing in liquids, soups, or pulpy fruit.
Indications: Treatment of hyperlipidemia
Action: Binds with bile acids in the intestine, producing an amino-soluble complex that is excreted in the feces; results in a reduction of serum LDL (cholesterol) with minimal change in triglyceride or HDL levels
Metabolism: Not absorbed
Excretion: Not absorbed
Contraindications and precautions
1. Contraindicated in complete biliary obstruction.
2. Use with caution in bleeding disorders, gastrointestinal dysfunction, especially constipation or malabsorption state, peptic ulcer and hemorrhoids.

Drug interactions
1. Colestipol may decrease absorption of many drugs. It is recommended that other drugs be administered 1 hr before or 4–6 hr after colestipol.
2. Colestipol is known to decrease absorption of coumadin, digoxin, thiazide diuretics, penicillin G, tetracycline, phenylbutazone, phenobarbital, thyroid hormones, and fat-soluble vitamins.

Cortisone acetate
Preparations: Tablets, 5, 10, 25 mg; injections (IM), 25, 50 mg/ml
Adult dosage: PO, IM: 25–30 mg/day as a single dose or in divided doses depending on the indication
Indications: Replacement therapy in the treatment of adrenal insufficiency states; used for anti-inflammatory and immunosuppressant effects in the treatment of many disorders. Consult further texts for specific therapeutic regimens in selected disorders.
Action: Adrenocorticoid with anti-inflammatory, immunosuppressant, and moderate mineralocorticoid effects. Other effects include suppression of the hypothalamic-pituitary-adrenal (HPA) axis, increased protein catabolism, increased blood glucose concentrations, insulin resistance, reduced intestinal absorption and increased renal excretion of calcium, and neutrophilia. See also table, page 708.
Metabolism: Primarily hepatic
Excretion: Renal
Contraindications and precautions
1. Use with caution in cardiac disease, CHF, hypertension, hepatic or renal function impairment, AIDS or other immunodeficiency states, uncontrolled bacterial or viral infection, systemic-fungal infection, tuberculosis (active, latent or positive skin test), ocular herpes simplex, diabetes mellitus, nonspecific ulcerative colitis, diverticulitis, esophagitis, gastritis, history of peptic ulcer, recent intestinal anastamosis, open-angle glaucoma, hyperthyroidism, hypoalbuminuria, myasthenia gravis, osteoporosis, or seizure disorder.
2. Administer daily dose in the morning to reduce HPA-axis suppressive effects. Alternate-day dosing may reduce the risk of adrenal suppression.
3. Withdrawal following long-term therapy with pharmacologic doses requires a gradual taper until the HPA-axis recovers.

Drug interactions
1. Alcohol, aspirin, and NSAIDs may increase risk of GI ulceration.
2. Amphotericin B and diuretics may increase risk of hypokalemia.
3. Estrogens may increase effects.
4. Ephedrine, phenytoin, phenobarbital, and rifampin may decrease effects.
5. Immunosuppressants lead to increased risk of infection.
6. Cortisone acetate may decrease effects of coumadin, oral antidiabetic agents, and insulin.
7. Cortisone acetate may decrease effect of isoniazid.
8. Pharmacologic doses of cortisone acetate may potentiate replication of live virus in vaccines or decrease antibody response to the vaccine.

Cromolyn sodium—Nasal (Nasalcrom)
Preparations: Nasal solution, 5.2 mg/metered spray in 13-ml canister
Adult dosage: Intranasal: 5.2 mg in each nostril tid–qid up to 6 times per day; in perennial rhinitis, symptomatic relief may require 2–4 wk of therapy
Indications: Treatment and prophylaxis of allergic rhinitis
Action: Inhibits degranulation of mast cells
Metabolism: None (<7% absorbed)
Excretion: Renal = biliary
Contraindications and precautions: Use with caution in severe hepatic or renal function impairment.

Cromolyn sodium—Inhalation (Intal)
Preparations: Aerosol, 0.8 mg/metered spray in 8.1- and 14.2-mg canister; capsule for inhalation, 20 mg; solution for inhalation, 20 mg/2-ml ampule.
Adult dosage
Asthma—aerosol: 2 metered sprays qid; nebulizer solution and capsules: 20 mg qid.
Bronchospasm—aerosol: 2 metered sprays as a single dose 15 min before exposure to the precipitating factor; nebulizer solution and capsules: 20 mg as a single dose just prior to exposure to the precipitating factor; for chronic prophylaxis, use the same doses but administer qid
Indications: Prophylaxis of bronchial asthma and bronchospasm due to inhaled precipitating factor or exercise; cromolyn has no role in the treatment of acute asthma
Action: Inhibits degranulation of mast cells
Metabolism: None (7–8% absorbed)
Excretion: Renal = biliary
Contraindications and precautions
1. Use aerosol preparation with caution in coronary artery disease or cardiac arrhythmias.
2. Use with caution in severe hepatic or renal function impairment.

Cyclosporine (Sandimmune)
Preparations: solution, 100 mg/ml; injection (IV), 50 mg/ml
Adult dosage: PO: Initially, 12–15 mg/kg/day as a single dose 4–12 hr prior to surgery and continue postoperatively for 1–2 wk. Taper dose by 5%/wk to a maintenance dose of 5–10 mg/kg/day. IV: Initially, 5–6 mg/kg/day as a single dose 4–12 hr before surgery (slow IV infusion over 2–6 hr), and continue postoperatively until PO tolerated.
Note
1. Corticosteroids should be used concurrently for allograft rejection prophylaxis. Consult further texts for dosing.
2. Cyclosporine blood levels as well as BUN and creatinine should be monitored.

Indications: Treatment of prophylaxis of organ rejection in renal, hepatic, and cardiac transplants
Action: Mechanism unknown; inhibits immunocompetent T lymphocytes, in part owing to inhibition of interleukin-2
Metabolism: Hepatic
Excretion: Biliary >> renal
Contraindications and precautions
1. Contraindicated in active varicella (chickenpox) or herpes zoster infection.
2. Use with caution in hepatic or renal function impairment, hyperkalemia, and infection.
3. Use live virus vaccines with caution.

Drug interactions
1. Cimetidine, corticosteroids, danazol, diltiazem, erythromycin, and estrogens may increase cyclosporine levels.
2. Carbamazepine, isoniazid, phenobarbital, phenytoin, and rifampin may decrease cyclosporin levels.
3. Concurrent immunosuppressants may increase risk of infection.
4. Aminoglycosides, amphotericin B, and NSAIDs may increase risk of nephrotoxicity.

Desipramine (Norpramin, Pertofrane)
Preparations: Tablets, 10, 25, 50, 75, 100, 150 mg; capsules, 25, 50 mg
Adult dosage: PO: 75–200 mg/day, in single or divided doses. Increase up to 300 mg. Maximum antidepressant effect may take ≥2 wk. Start with lower doses of 25–50 mg/day in geriatric patients, and increase up to 150 mg/day. After control of symptoms, taper to lowest effective dose.
Indications: Treatment of depression; unlabeled uses include treatment of anxiety, neurogenic pain, narcolepsy/cataplexy, and cocaine withdrawal
Action: Tricyclic antidepressant; increases CNS synaptic concentration of norepinephrine or serotonin presumably by blocking presynaptic re-uptake; has sedative, anticholinergic, peripheral vasodilator, and direct quinidine-like myocardial effects
Metabolism: Hepatic
Excretion: Renal
Contraindications and precautions

1. Contraindicated during recovery from myocardial infarction and possibly concurrent MAO inhibitor use.
2. Use with caution in alcoholism, asthma, bipolar disorder, schizophrenia, cardiovascular disorders, blood disorders, GI disorders, narrow-angle glaucoma, hepatic or renal function impairment, hyperthyroidism, prostatic hypertrophy, or urinary retention and seizure disorders.
3. Use caution while driving or performing other tasks requiring alertness.
4. Abrupt cessation after prolonged administration may cause withdrawal symptoms.
5. Prescribe the smallest quantity feasible to patients considered at risk for suicide.

Drug interactions

1. Alcohol or CNS depressants lead to increased CNS depression.
2. Drugs with antimuscarinic activity lead to increased anticholinergic side effects.
3. Direct-acting sympathomimetics lead to increased cardiac effects.
4. MAO inhibitors lead to increased risk of hyperpyretic episodes, convulsions, hypertensive crises, and death.
5. Antithyroid agents lead to increased risk of agranulocytosis.
6. Barbiturates and carbamazepine may decrease plasma concentration of desipramine.
7. Cimetidine, methylphenidate, phenothiazines, estrogens, and possibly ranitidine may increase plasma concentration of desipramine.
8. Metrizamide leads to increased risk of seizures.
9. Thyroid hormone leads to increased therapeutic and toxic effects of both medications.
10. Desipramine leads to decreased hypotensive effect of guanethidine and clonidine.
11. Desipramine may increase plasma concentration of coumadin.

Dexamethasone (Decadron, others)
Preparations: Tablets, 0.25, 0.5, 0.75, 1, 1.5, 2, 4, 6 mg; elixir, 0.5 mg/5 ml; solution, 0.5 mg/5 ml, 0.5 mg/0.5 ml; dexamethasone acetate injection (IM, intra-articular, intralesional), 8, 16 mg/ml; dexamethasone sodium phosphate injection (IM, IV, intra-articular, intralesional), 4, 10, 20, 24 mg/ml (24 mg/ml for IV only)
Adult dosage: PO, IV: 0.5–9 mg/day as a single dose or in divided doses depending on the indication. IM, intra-articular, intralesional: Consult other texts.
Dexamethasone suppression test: *For Cushing's syndrome*—PO: 1 mg as a single dose at 11 PM, and draw plasma cortisol at 8 AM the following day. Or 0.5 mg q6h for 48 hr, and collect 24-hr urine for 17-OHCS during the second 24 hr of dexamethasone administration. *To distinguish Cushing's syndrome due to pituitary ACTH excess from Cushing's syndrome due to other causes*—PO: 2 mg q6h for 48 hr, and collect 24-hr urine for 17-OHCS.
Cerebral edema: Initially, 10 mg (dexamethasone phosphate) IV followed by 4 mg IM q6h. Reduce dosage after 2–4 days, and discontinue over 5–7 days. If maintenance therapy is required, use 2 mg IM bid–tid or 2 mg PO bid–tid.
Indications: Use for anti-inflammatory and immunosuppressant effects in the treatment of many disorders. Consult other texts for specific therapeutic regimens in selected disorders.
Action: Adrenocorticoid with anti-inflammatory, immunosuppressant and minimal mineralocorticoid effects. Other effects include suppression of the hypothalamic-pituitary-adrenal (HPA) axis, increased protein catabolism, increased blood glucose concentrations, insulin resistance, reduced intestinal absorption and increased renal excretion of calcium, and neutrophilia. See also table, page 708.
Metabolism: Primarily hepatic
Excretion: Renal
Contraindications and precautions

1. Use with caution in cardiac disease, CHF, hypertension, hepatic or renal function impairment, AIDS or other immunodeficiency states, uncontrolled bacterial or viral infection, systemic fungal infection, tuberculosis (active, latent or positive skin test), ocular herpes simplex, diabetes mellitus, nonspecific ulcerative colitis, diverticulitis, esophagitis, gastritis, history of peptic ulcer, recent intestinal anastomosis, open-angle glaucoma, hyperthyroidism, hypoalbuminuria, myasthenia gravis, osteoporosis or seizure disorder.
2. Administer daily dose in the morning to reduce HPA-axis suppressive effects. Alternate-day dosing may reduce the risk of adrenal suppression.
3. Withdrawal following long-term therapy with pharmacologic doses requires a gradual taper until the HPA-axis recovers.

Drug interactions

1. Alcohol, aspirin, and NSAIDs may increase risk of GI ulceration.
2. Amphotericin B and diuretics may increase risk of hypokalemia.
3. Estrogens may increase effects.
4. Ephedrine, phenytoin, phenobarbital and rifampin may decrease effects.
5. Immunosuppressants lead to increased risk of infection.
6. Antacids may decrease absorption.
7. Dexamethasone may decrease effects of coumadin, oral antidiabetic agents, and insulin.
8. Dexamethasone may decrease effect of isoniazid.
9. Pharmacologic doses of dexamethasone may potentiate replication of live virus in vaccines or decrease antibody response to the vaccine.

Dextran
Preparations
Dextran 40—injection (IV): 10% in normal saline or D5W
Dextran 70 or 75—injection (IV): 6% in normal saline or D5W
Adult dosage
Shock—IV infusion: For dextran 40, total dosage during the first 24 hr should not exceed 20 ml/kg with the first 10 ml/kg infused rapidly. After 24 hr, total daily dosage should not exceed 10 ml/kg; therapy should not continue beyond 5 days. For dextran 70 or 75, total dosage during the first 24 hr should not exceed 20 ml/kg. The usual dosage is 500–1,000 ml, which may be infused at a rate of 20–40 ml/min. In nearly normovolemic patients, do not exceed rate of 4 ml/min. After 24 hr, total daily dosage should not exceed 10 ml/kg.
Prophylaxis of venous thrombosis—IV infusion of dextran 40 only: Start therapy during surgery with a dose of 500–1,000 ml. Continue therapy with 500 ml qd for 2–3 days. Thereafter, according to the risk of thromboembolism, 500 ml may be given q2–3d for up to 2 wk.
Indications: Emergent adjunctive treatment of shock due to hemorrhage, burns, surgery, or trauma; dextran 40 also used for prophylaxis of deep vein thrombosis in patients undergoing surgical procedures associated with a high risk of thromboembolic complications
Action: Branched polysaccharide plasma-volume expanders with an average molecular weight of 40,000 (dextran 40), 70,000 (dextran 70), or 75,000 (dextran 75) that increase blood volume and inhibit vascular stasis and platelet adhesiveness
Excretion: Renal
Contraindications and precautions

1. Dextran 40 can cause anaphylactoid reactions; monitor during first few minutes of infusion.
2. Contraindicated in renal disease with oliguria or anuria, severe dehydration, pulmonary edema, thrombocytopenia hypofibrinogenemia, or concurrent therapy with heparin or oral anticoagulants.
3. Use with caution in CHF or active hemorrhage.
4. Monitor urine output and hematocrit during therapy. If oliguria or a decrease in hematocrit <30 occurs during infusion, consider discontinuing dextran.

Drug interactions: No clinically significant interactions.

Diazepam (Valium, others)
Preparations: Tablets, 2, 5, 10 mg; SR capsules, 15 mg; solution, 5 mg/ml; injection (IM, IV), 5 mg/ml

Commonly Prescribed Drugs

Adult dosage
Antianxiety—PO: 2–10 mg bid–qid. IM, IV: 2–10 mg repeated in 3–4 hr. Preoperatively, usually 10 mg IM or IV 1–2 hr before surgery.
Sedative-hypnotic for alcohol withdrawal —PO: 10 mg tid–qid. Reduce to 5 mg tid–qid prn. IM, IV: Initially, 10 mg, then 5–10 mg q3–4h as necessary.
Anticonvulsant—PO: 2–10 mg bid–qid. For status epilepticus and severe recurrent convulsive seizures: IM, IV (preferred): Initially, 5–10 mg; repeat if necessary q10–15min up to a maximum dose of 30 mg. If necessary, repeat in 2–4 hr.
Skeletal muscle relaxant—PO: 2–10 mg tid–qid. IM, IV: Initially, 5–10 mg, then 5–10 mg in 3–4 hr if necessary. Larger doses may be needed in tetanus.
Amnestic: *Cardioversion*—IV: 5–15 mg for 5–10 min before the procedure.
Endoscopic procedure—IV (preferred): Usually up to 10 mg administered slowly just before procedure. Titrate to desired sedative response. IM: 5–10 mg 30 min before procedure.
Note
1. Use lower doses for elderly or debilitated patients.
2. Sustained-release forms given once qd can be used for anxiety, alcohol withdrawal, or muscle spasm when the total daily dosage is determined.

Indications: Treatment of anxiety disorders and acute alcohol withdrawal and adjunctive therapy for skeletal muscle spasm; parenterally for treatment of status epilepticus and severe recurrent seizures; adjunctive therapy before surgery, endoscopic procedures, and cardioversion for anxiolytic and amnestic effects
Action: Anxiolytic sedative-hypnotic benzodiazepine; may potentiate CNS gamma-aminobutyric acid effects; amnestic, anticonvulsant, and skeletal muscle relaxant effects of unclear mechanism
Metabolism: Hepatic (oxidation)
Excretion: Renal
Contraindications and precautions
1. Contraindicated in acute alcohol intoxication with depressed vital signs, depressive neuroses, or psychoses without prominent anxiety.
2. Use with caution in acute narrow-angle glaucoma, myasthenia gravis, shock, severe chronic obstructive pulmonary disease, hepatic or renal function impairment, patients with depressed respirations, or those receiving concurrent respiratory depressants.
3. Long-term therapy may result in psychic or physical dependence.
4. Use caution in performing tasks requiring alertness and coordination.

Drug interactions
1. Cimetidine, disulfiram, erythromycin, isoniazid, ketoconazole, and oral contraceptives may increase effects.
2. Alcohol or other CNS depressants lead to increased CNS depression.

Diclofenac (Voltaren)
Preparations: EC tablets, 25, 50, 75 mg
Adult dosage
Antirheumatic—PO: *Rheumatoid arthritis*—150–200 mg/day in 2–4 divided doses.
Osteoarthritis—100–150 mg/day in 2–3 divided doses.
Ankylosing spondylitis—100–125 mg/day in 4–5 divided doses.
Indications: Treatment of rheumatic disease; unlabeled uses include treatment of nonrheumatic inflammatory disorders
Note: Use lower doses in geriatric patients.
Action: Nonsteroidal anti-inflammatory drug that inhibits cyclo-oxygenase, resulting in decreased formation of prostaglandins; effects include antirheumatic, analgesic, antipyretic, and inhibition of platelet aggregation
Metabolism: Hepatic
Excretion: Renal > biliary
Contraindications and precautions
1. Contraindicated in a history of severe allergic reaction to aspirin or other NSAIDs.
2. Use with caution in patient with a history of peptic ulcer, upper GI disease or ulcerative colitis, renal or hepatic function impairment, bleeding disorders, asthma, CHF, diabetes mellitus, hypertension, and pre-existing edema.

Drug interactions
1. Acetaminophen, gold compounds, or nephrotoxic medications may increase risk of renal toxicity.
2. Glucocorticoids, alcohol, potassium supplements, other NSAID, or aspirin may increase risk of GI side effects.
3. Anticoagulants, thrombolytic agents, aspirin, platelet aggregation inhibitors, or colchicine may increase risk of hemorrhage.
4. Probenecid may increase diclofenac serum level.
5. Diclofenac may increase methotrexate toxicity.
6. Diclofenac may decrease antihypertensive effects of diuretics and antihypertensives.
7. Diclofenac may decrease diuretic effect of diuretics.
8. Diclofenac may increase hypoglycemic effect of sulfonylureas.
9. Diclofenac may increase digoxin, lithium, nifedipine, and verapamil blood levels.

Diflunisal (Dolobid)
Preparations: Tablets, 250, 500 mg
Adult dosage
Antirheumatic—PO: 250–500 mg bid
Analgesic—PO: 1 g followed by 250–500 mg q8–12h prn
Note: Use lower doses in geriatric patients.
Indications: Treatment of rheumatic and nonrheumatic inflammatory disorders and headache
Action: Nonsteroidal anti-inflammatory drug that inhibits cyclo-oxygenase, resulting in decreased formation of prostaglandins; effects include antirheumatic, analgesic, antipyretic, and inhibition of platelet aggregation
Metabolism: Hepatic
Excretion: Renal
Contraindications and precautions
1. Contraindicated in patient with history of severe allergic reaction to aspirin or other NSAIDs.
2. Use with caution in patient with history of peptic ulcer, upper GI disease or ulcerative colitis, renal or hepatic function impairment, bleeding disorders, asthma, CHF, diabetes mellitus, hypertension, and pre-existing edema.

Drug interactions
1. Acetaminophen, gold compounds, or nephrotoxic medications may increase risk of renal toxicity.
2. Glucocorticoids, alcohol, potassium supplements, other NSAID, or aspirin may increase risk of GI side effects.
3. Anticoagulants, thrombolytic agents, aspirin, platelet aggregation inhibitors, or colchicine may increase risk of hemorrhage.
4. Probenecid may increase diflunisal serum level.
5. Diflunisal may increase methotrexate toxicity.
6. Diflunisal may decrease antihypertensive effects of diuretics and antihypertensives.
7. Diflunisal may decrease diuretic effect of diuretics.
8. Diflunisal may increase hypoglycemic effect of sulfonylureas.

Digoxin (Lanoxin, others)
Preparations: Tablets, 0.125, 0.25, 0.5 mg; capsules, 0.05, 0.1, 0.2 mg; elixir, 0.05 mg/ml; injection (IV), 0.1 mg/ml, 0.25 mg/ml
Adult dosage
Antiarrhythmic, cardiotonic—PO: *Rapid digitalization:* Initially, 0.4–0.6 mg, then 0.1–0.3 mg q6–8h as tolerated until desired effect. Generally, a loading dose of 8–12 μg/kg should provide therapeutic effect for CHF and normal sinus rhythm. Up to 10–15 μg/kg is required for control of ventricular rate in atrial flutter or fibrillation. Loading doses in renal insufficiency are usually 6–10 μg/kg. Administer 50% of the loading dose at the first dose followed by additional fractions (25–35%) of the loading dose q6–8h PO or q4–8h IV until a therapeutic response, toxicity, or total loading dose is given. *Slow digitalization, maintenance*—PO: Tablets or elixir, 0.125–0.5 mg qd; capsules, 0.05–0.35 mg qd–bid. IV: 0.125–0.5 mg as a single dose or in divided doses per day.
Note
1. When changing from tablets or elixir to either capsule or IV therapy, reduce dosage by about 20–25%.
2. Dosage should be reduced in patients with hypokalemia, hypothyroidism, conduction disorders, renal function impairment, and in geriatric patients.
3. Daily maintenance dosage can be estimated by the following formula:

$$\text{Maintenance dose} = \text{Loading dose} \times \frac{14 + \text{Creatinine clearance}/5}{100}$$

4. Serum digoxin levels: therapeutic, 0.5–2.0 ng/ml; toxic, >2.5 ng/ml

Indications: Treatment of CHF and possibly cardiogenic shock; treatment and prophylaxis of atrial fibrillation, atrial flutter, and paroxysmal atrial tachycardia
Action: Positive inotrope; decreases conduction rate and increases effective refractory period of the AV node
Metabolism: Hepatic (slight)
Excretion: Renal >> fecal
Contraindications and precautions
1. Contraindicated in ventricular fibrillation and the presence of digitalis toxicity.

2. Use with caution in ischemic heart disease, acute myocardial infarction, acute myocarditis, incomplete AV block, sick sinus syndrome, Wolff-Parkinson-White syndrome, frequent premature ventricular contractions, carotid sinus hypersensitivity, hypercalcemia, hypokalemia, hypomagnesemia, severe pulmonary disease, myxedema, and renal function impairment

Drug interactions

1. Cholestyramine, colestipol, aluminum hydroxide, magnesium hydroxide, kaolin-pectin, and sulfasalazine lead to decreased absorption.
2. Glucocorticoids, mineralocorticoids, amphotericin B, diuretics, and laxatives may increase digoxin toxicity due to decreased K^+.
3. Amiodarone, quinidine, and verapamil lead to increased serum digoxin level.
4. β-Blockers, verapamil, and diltiazem may increase AV block.
5. Antiarrhythmics, parenteral calcium salts, succinylcholine, adrenergic agents, and sympathomimetics may increase the risk of cardiac arrhythmias.

Diltiazem (Cardizem)

Preparations: Tablets, 30, 60, 90, 120 mg; SR tablets, 60, 90, 120 mg

Adult dosage

Antianginal—PO: Initially, 30 mg qid. Increase q1–2d up to 180–360 mg/day in divided doses 3–4 times daily. SR preparation is not approved for angina.

Antihypertensive—PO: Initially, 30 mg qid. Increase q1–2d up to 180–360 mg/day in divided doses 3–4 times daily. For SR preparation, initially, 60–120 mg bid, increased q14d up to 360 mg/day.

Indications: Treatment of chronic stable angina pectoris, vasospastic angina, unstable angina, and hypertension

Action: Calcium-ion influx inhibitor (slow channel blocker), resulting in peripheral and coronary vasodilation, some depression of SA and AV nodal conduction, and minimal negative inotropic effects

Metabolism: Hepatic

Excretion: Renal

Contraindications and precautions

1. Contraindicated in 2nd- or 3rd-degree AV block and SA nodal function impairment, except in patients with a functioning artificial ventricular pacemaker, Wolff-Parkinson-White syndrome with atrial flutter or fibrillation, and severe hypotension.
2. Use with caution in hepatic or renal function impairment, bradycardia, mild or moderate hypotension, and CHF.

Drug interactions

1. β-Adrenergic blockers may elevate SA and AV nodal conduction delay and may increase risk of CHF.
2. Cimetidine may increase effects and toxicity.
3. Diltiazem may increase drug levels of carbamazepine, cyclosporine, digoxin, quinidine, or theophylline.

Diphenhydramine (Benadryl, others)

Preparations: Tablets, 25, 50 mg; capsules, 25, 50 mg; elixir, 12.5 mg/5 ml; syrup, 12.5 mg/5 ml; injection (IM, IV), 10 mg/ml, 50 mg/ml

Adult dosage

Antihistaminic, antivertigo agent, antiemetic—PO: 25–50 mg q4–6h prn, not to exceed 300 mg/24 hr. IM, IV: 10–50 mg; for vertigo, 10 mg initially and increase to 20-50 mg q2–3h if needed.

Antitussive—PO: (syrup only) 25 mg q4–6h prn

Sedative-hypnotic—PO: 50 mg qhs

Antidyskinetic—PO: Initially, 25 mg tid; increase up to 50 mg qid. IM, IV: 10–50 mg tid up to 400 mg/day.

Indications: Antihistaminic treatment for the symptoms associated with perennial and seasonal allergic rhinitis, vasomotor rhinitis, allergic conjunctivitis, mild, uncomplicated urticaria and angioedema, allergic reactions to blood or plasma, and dermatographism; treatment of vertigo, cough, insomnia, and parkinsonism or drug-induced extrapyramidal reactions; prophylaxis and treatment of motion sickness and nausea; used as a sedative-hypnotic; adjunctive therapy for anaphylactic reactions.

Action: Antihistamine (H_1-receptor blocker); blocks CNS muscarinic receptors, diminishes vestibular stimulation, suppresses the cough reflex at the level of the medullary cough center, and acts as a sedative-hypnotic

Metabolism: Hepatic

Excretion: Renal

Contraindications and precautions

1. Use with caution in angle-closure glaucoma, bladder neck obstruction, prostatic hypertrophy, predisposition to urinary retention, stenosing peptic ulcer, pyloroduodenal obstruction, and acute asthma.
2. Contraindicated with concurrent MAO inhibitor use.

Drug interactions

1. MAO inhibitors lead to increased antimuscarinic and CNS depressant effects.
2. Alcohol and CNS depressants lead to increased CNS depression.

Diphenoxylate with atropine (Lomotil, others)

Preparations: Tablets, 2.5 mg diphenoxylate and 0.025 mg atropine sulfate; liquid, 2.5 mg diphenoxylate and 0.025 mg atropine sulfate/5 ml

Adult dosage: PO: Initially, 2.5–5 mg of diphenoxylate qid. Continue until symptoms are controlled, and then taper to maintenance dose (may be as low as ¼ of initial daily dose). If no response within 48 hr, it is unlikely to be effective.

Indications: Treatment of diarrhea

Action: Diphenoxylate is an opiate agonist with little or no analgesic activity that inhibits gastrointestinal motility. Atropine has antimuscarinic activity (included to discourage deliberate overdosage).

Metabolism: Diphenoxylate—hepatic

Excretion: Diphenoxylate—biliary/fecal > renal

Contraindications and precautions

1. Contraindicated in pseudomembranous colitis.
2. Use with caution in acute ulcerative colitis, infectious diarrhea, hepatic function impairment, diarrhea due to poisoning, history of drug abuse, gallbladder disease, or respiratory impairment.
3. Because of atropine content, use with caution in angle-closure glaucoma, hypertension, intestinal atony, myasthenia gravis, prostatic hypertrophy, or urinary retention.

Drug interactions

1. MAO inhibitors lead to increased risk of hypertensive crisis.
2. Alcohol and CNS depressants lead to increased CNS depression.

Dipyridamole (Persantine, others)

Preparations: Tablets, 25, 50, 75 mg

Adult dosage: PO: 75–100 mg qid in combination with coumadin

Indications: Adjunct to coumadin anticoagulants in prophylaxis of platelet aggregation to prevent postoperative thromboembolic complications associated with heart valves. Unlabeled uses include prophylactic adjunct for myocardial infarction and transient ischemic attacks.

Action: Platelet aggregation inhibitor; decreases coronary and peripheral vascular resistance

Metabolism: Hepatic

Excretion: Biliary/fecal >> renal

Contraindications and precautions: Use with caution in hypotension.

Drug interactions: Heparin, salicylates, aspirin, thrombolytic agents, and possibly coumadin lead to increased risk of hemorrhage.

Dobutamine (Dobutrex)

Preparations: Injection (IV), 250 mg/20-ml vial

Adult dosage: IV: Infusion at a rate of 2.5–10 μg/kg/min. Titrate to patient's response determined by heart rate, BP, urine flow, cardiac output, and central venous or pulmonary wedge pressures.

Note: Correct hypovolemia prior to starting dobutamine.

Indications: Treatment of cardiogenic shock

Action: Inotropic agent via direct stimulation of cardiac β_1-adrenergic receptors; it results in mildly decreased systemic vascular resistance via β_2 stimulation (afterload reduction), reduces elevated ventricular filling pressure (preload reduction), and has positive chronotropic effects at higher doses.

Metabolism: Hepatic

Excretion: Renal

Contraindications and precautions

1. Contraindicated in idiopathic hypertrophic subaortic stenosis.
2. Use with caution in atrial fibrillation, hypovolemia, myocardial infarction, and ventricular ectopic activity.

Drug interactions

1. Halogenated hydrocarbon anesthetics lead to increased risk of arrhythmia.
2. β-Adrenergic blockers may decrease β_1 effect.

Docusate—Dioctyl sodium sulfosuccinate (Colace, others)

Preparations: Tablets, 50, 100 mg; capsules, 60, 100, 240, 250, 300 mg; liquid, 150 mg/15 ml; syrup, 50 mg/15 ml, 60 mg/15 ml

Adult dosage: PO: 50–200 mg qd up to 500 mg/day in single or divided doses

Indications: Treatment and prophylaxis of constipation; prophylactic use in patients with hard stools and in those who should not strain during defecation (post-MI, anorectal conditions)
Action: Stool softener; surface-active agent promoting permeation of liquid into stool
Metabolism: Unknown
Excretion: Fecal
Contraindications and precautions: Contraindicated in nausea, vomiting, or other symptoms of appendicitis, acute surgical abdomen, or intestinal obstruction.
Drug interactions: Docusate leads to increased absorption of mineral oil or phenolphthalein.

Dopamine (Dopastat, Intropin, others)

Preparations: Injection (IV), 40 mg/ml, 80 mg/ml, 160 mg/ml; in dextrose, 0.8 mg/ml, 1.6 mg/ml, 3.2 mg/ml
Adult dosage: IV: Infusion initially at a rate of 1–5 μg/kg/min; increased by 1–4 μg/kg/min q10–30min. For chronic refractory CHF, start at 0.5–2 μg/kg/min. If occlusive vascular disease is present, start at 1 μg/kg/min. Titrate to patient's response determined by heart rate, BP, urine flow, peripheral perfusion, presence of ventricular ectopic activity, and cardiac output.
Note
1. If urine output decreases in the absence of hypotension, consider reducing dosage.
2. Dopamine should be administered through a large vein. Extravasation may cause local necrosis.
3. Correct hypovolemia before starting dopamine.

Indications: Treatment of acute hypotension, cardiogenic shock, low cardiac output, or congestive heart failure
Action: Stimulates β_1-adrenergic receptors directly and indirectly via release of norepinephrine from storage sites; vasodilates the renal and mesenteric vascular beds via stimulation of dopaminergic receptors. Effects are dose-dependent. In low doses (0.5–2 μg/kg/min), there is predominantly dopaminergic stimulation, causing renal and mesenteric vasodilation. In moderate doses (2–10 μg/kg/min), dopaminergic and β_1 stimulation cause renal vasodilation and increased cardiac output. In high doses (>10 μg/kg/min), β_1- and α-adrenergic stimulation cause increased cardiac output and increased peripheral vascular resistance, including renal vasoconstriction.
Metabolism: Hepatic, renal, plasma
Excretion: Renal
Contraindications and precautions
1. Contraindicated in pheochromocytoma, tachyarrhythmias, or ventricular fibrillation.
2. Use with caution in occlusive vascular disease, ischemic heart disease, acidosis, hypercapnia, or hypoxia.

Drug interactions
1. Drugs with α-adrenergic blocking action lead to decreased vasoconstriction.
2. β-Adrenergic blockers lead to decreased cardiac effects.
3. Hydrocarbon inhalation anesthetics or digoxin may increase risk of arrhythmias.
4. MAO inhibitors lead to increased effects.
5. Tricyclic antidepressants may increase effects.
6. Phenytoin may decrease BP as well as heart rate.

Doxepin (Adapin, Sinequan, others)

Preparations: Capsules, 10, 25, 50, 75, 100, 150 mg; solution, 10 mg/ml
Adult dosage: PO: 30–150 mg/day, in single or divided doses depending on the severity of symptoms. Increase up to 150 mg for outpatients or 300 mg/day for in-patients. Maximum antidepressant effects may take ≥2 wk. Start with lower doses in geriatric patients. After control of symptoms, taper to lowest effective dose.
Indications: Treatment of depression and depression in manic-depressive illness. Unlabeled uses include treatment of anxiety and neurogenic pain.
Action: Tricyclic antidepressant; increases CNS synaptic concentration of norepinephrine or serotonin, presumably by blocking presynaptic reuptake; has sedative, anticholinergic, peripheral vasodilator, and direct quinidine-like myocardial effects
Metabolism: Hepatic
Excretion: Renal
Contraindications and precautions
1. Contraindicated during recovery from myocardial infarction and possibly concurrent MAO inhibitor use.
2. Use with caution in alcoholism, asthma, bipolar disorder, schizophrenia, cardiovascular disorders, blood disorders, gastrointestinal disorders, narrow-angle glaucoma, hepatic or renal function impairment, hyperthyroidism, prostatic hypertrophy or urinary retention, and seizure disorders.
3. Use caution while driving or performing other tasks requiring alertness.
4. Abrupt cessation following prolonged administration may cause withdrawal symptoms.
5. Prescribe the smallest quantity feasible to patients considered at risk for suicide.

Drug interactions
1. Alcohol or CNS depressants may increase CNS depression.
2. Drugs with antimuscarinic activity lead to increased anticholinergic side effects.
3. Direct-acting sympathomimetics lead to increased cardiac effects.
4. MAO inhibitors lead to increased risk of hyperpyretic episodes, convulsions, hypertensive crises, and death.
5. Antithyroid agents lead to increased risk of agranulocytosis.
6. Barbiturates and carbamazepine may decrease plasma concentration of doxepin.
7. Cimetidine, methylphenidate, phenothiazines, estrogens, and possibly ranitidine may increase plasma concentration of doxepin.
8. Metrizamide leads to increased risk of seizures.
9. Thyroid hormone leads to increased therapeutic and toxic effects of both medications.
10. Doxepin leads to decreased hypotensive effect of guanethidine and clonidine.
11. Doxepin may increase plasma concentration of coumadin.

Enalapril (Vasotec)

Preparations: Tablets, 5, 10, 20, 40 mg; injection (IV), 1.25 mg of enalaprilat/ml
Adult dosage:
Antihypertensive—PO: Initially, 5 mg qd. Increase in 1–2 wk prn up to 40 mg/day as a single or divided dose. Use initial dose of 2.5 mg in patients who are salt-volume depleted, are on diuretics, or have renal failure (creatinine clearance <30 ml/min). IV: 1.25 mg over 5 min q6h. Use initial dose of 0.625 mg in patients previously described under PO. If BP response is inadequate after 1 hr, repeat 0.625 mg dose and continue at 1.25 mg q6h.
Vasodilator—PO: 2.5 mg qd. Increase in 1–2 wk prn up to 20 mg/day as a single or divided dose.
Indications: Treatment of hypertension or CHF.
Action: Angiotensin coverting enzyme inhibitor with antihypertensive and vasodilator effects
Metabolism: Hepatic (to enalaprilat, which has no metabolism)
Excretion: Enalapril—renal > fecal; enalaprilat—renal
Contraindications and precautions
1. May cause profound hypotension after first-dose, especially if patient is salt-volume depleted.
2. Use with caution in hyperkalemia, bilateral renal artery stenosis, solitary kidney, renal function impairment, and salt-volume depletion.

Drug interactions
1. Potassium-sparing diuretics, potassium supplements, and salt substitutes lead to increased risk of hyperkalemia.
2. Diuretics and other renin-releasing antihypertensive agents lead to increased antihypertensive effect.

Encainide (Enkaid)

Preparations: Capsules, 25, 35, 50, mg
Adult dosage: Antiarrhythmic—PO: Initially, 25 mg q8h. Increase to 35 mg q8h in 3–5 days if needed. Increase to 50 mg q8h after 3–5 days if necessary. Higher doses such as 50–75 mg q6h have been used in selected cases. In severe renal function impairment (serum creatinine >3.5 mg/dl or creatinine clearance <20 ml/min), initiate therapy with 25 mg qd and increase to 25 mg q12h in 7 days if needed, followed by 25 mg q8h after an additional 7 days (up to a maximum 150 mg/day).
Indications: Treatment of symptomatic and life-threatening ventricular arrhythmias
Action: Class IC antiarrhythmic
Metabolism: Hepatic
Excretion: Renal/fecal
Contraindications and precautions
1. Contraindicated in either 2nd- or 3rd-degree AV block or bifascicular block without pacemaker and cardiogenic shock.
2. Use with caution in cardiomyopathy, CHF, hypo- or hyperkalemia, hepatic or renal function impairment, sick sinus syndrome, and in patients with pacemakers.
3. Encainide may be proarrhythmic.
4. Encainide has a negative inotropic effect.

5. Encainide may increase the P-R interval and prolong the QRS duration.

Drug interactions
1. β-Adrenergic blocking agents may increase negative inotropic effect.
2. Cimetidine may increase encainide plasma concentration.

Epinephrine

Preparations: Aerosol, 300 μg epinephrine bitartrate (= 160 μg epinephrine)/metered spray; 200, 250 μg epinephrine/metered spray; solution for nebulization, epinephrine hydrochloride 1%, racemic epinephrine hydrochloride equivalent to 1.25, 2.25% epinephrine base; injection (SC), 0.5 mg/ml; injection (IM, SC): 1 mg/ml (1 : 1,000). Injection (IV): 0.1 mg/ml (1 : 10,000).

Adult dosage:
Bronchodilator—aerosol: 160–250 μg (1 inhalation) repeated in 1–2 min if needed. Subsequent doses should not be administered for 3–4 hr. Solution for nebulization: all dose forms, 1–2 inhalations repeated up to q3–4h prn; may also be administered via a respirator. Injection (IM, SC): 0.2–0.5 ml of 1 : 1,000 solution q20min prn for up to 4 hr.
Anaphylactic reactions—Injection (IM, SC): 0.2–0.5 mg (0.2–0.5 ml of 1 : 1,000 solution) q10–15min prn. May increase dose up to 1 mg if needed. For anaphylactic shock, IM or SC injection of 0.5 mg followed by IV injection of 0.025–0.05 mg (0.25–0.5 ml of 1 : 10,000 solution) q15min prn. Alternatively, slow IV injection (over 5–10 min) of 0.1–0.25 mg (1–2.5 ml of 1 : 10,000 solution) repeated q5–15min prn or followed by a continuous IV infusion at an initial rate of 1 μg/min and increased up to 4 μg/min if needed.
Cardiac arrest—injection (IV): 0.1–1 mg (5–10 ml of 1 : 10,000 solution) repeated q5min prn. In extreme emergency, it may be given via an endotracheal tube, usually at a dose of 1 mg or as an intracardiac injection at a dose of 0.1–1 mg.

Note: SC administration preferred over IM.

Indications: Multiple uses, including treatment of reversible bronchospasm, anaphylaxis, and as adjunctive treatment in cardiac arrest

Action: Both α- and β-adrenergic agonist with peripheral vasodilatory, bronchial smooth muscle relaxant, and positive inotropic and chronotropic effects

Metabolism: Hepatic, neuronal

Excretion: Renal

Contraindications and precautions
1. Contraindicated in shock other than anaphylactic shock, most patients with arrhythmias, organic heart disease, coronary insufficiency, organic brain damage, cerebral arteriosclerosis, and during general anesthesia with halogenated hydrocarbons; parenteral epinephrine contraindicated in angle-closure glaucoma
2. Use with caution in angina pectoris, arrhythmias, cardiac dilatation, CHF, hypertension, diabetes mellitus, hyperthyroidism, pheochromocytoma, and psychoneurotic disorders.

Drug interactions
1. α-Adrenergic blockers may lead to severe hypotension and tachycardia.
2. β-Adrenergic blockers may lead to hypertension and bradycardia.
3. Hydrocarbon inhalation anesthetics, digoxin, and levodopa lead to increased risk of arrhythmias.
4. Tricyclic antidepressants and thyroid hormone may increase cardiovascular effects.
5. CNS stimulants, sympathomimetics, and xanthine derivatives may increase CNS stimulation.
6. Ergotamine and methyldopa may lead to hypertension.

Estrogens, conjugated (Premarin, others)

Preparations: Tablets, 0.3, 0.625, 0.9, 1.25, 2.5 mg; injection (IM, IV), 25 mg/vial; vaginal cream, 0.625 mg/g (0.0625%)

Adult dosage:
Vulvar atrophic dystrophy, atrophic vaginitis—PO: 0.3–1.25 mg or more qd depending on the tissue response of the patient. Administer for 21 days followed by 7 days without the drug repeated cyclically. Vaginal cream: 2–4 g intravaginally or topically qd for 21 days followed by 7 days without drug therapy repeated cyclically.
Female hypogonadism—PO: 2.5–7.5 mg qd in divided doses for 20 days with no drug therapy for 10 days. Dosage is repeated cyclically until menstruation occurs. If bleeding occurs before the end of the 10-day drug-free period, use a similar 20-day estrogen cycle and combine an oral progestin during the last 5 days of therapy. If bleeding occurs before this regimen is concluded, consult further texts.
Menopausal vasomotor symptoms—PO: 0.625–1.25 mg qd for 21 days followed by 7 days of no drug therapy. If the woman has not menstruated for >2 mo, begin arbitrarily. If menstruating, begin on day 5 of menstrual bleeding.
Primary ovarian failure, ovariectomy—PO: 1.25 mg qd for 21 days followed by 7 days of no drug therapy. Dose is adjusted (increased or decreased) according to severity of symptoms.
Breast carcinoma—PO: 10 mg PO qd for at least 3 mo
Prostate carcinoma—PO: 1.25–2.5 mg tid
Osteoporosis prophylaxis—PO: 0.625 mg qd cyclically for 21 days followed by 7 days of no drug therapy
Abnormal uterine bleeding—IM, IV (preferred): 25 mg repeated in 6–12 hr if necessary.

Note
1. Use the lowest effective dose for the shortest possible time.
2. Except for cancer treatment and possibly posthysterectomy, estrogens are administered on a 21-day-on and 7-day-off cycle. A progestin is usually given during the last 10–13 days of the cycle to decrease the risk of endometrial hyperplasia and, possibly, carcinoma.

Indications: Treatment of estrogen deficiency, atrophic vaginitis, female hypogonadism, vulvar atrophic dystrophy, primary ovarian failure, vasomotor symptoms of menopause, uterine bleeding due to hormonal imbalance, palliative treatment of carcinoma of the breast or prostate, and prophylaxis of postmenopausal osteoporosis

Action: Same effects as endogenous estrogens; increases cellular synthesis of DNA, RNA, and certain proteins in responsive tissue, and reduces the release of gonadotropin-releasing hormone from the hypothalamus

Metabolism: Primarily hepatic

Excretion: Primarily renal

Contraindications and precautions
1. Contraindicated in pregnancy; undiagnosed vaginal bleeding; estrogen-dependent neoplasia; breast cancer, except in selected patients treated for metastatic disease; and thromboembolic disorders or thrombophlebitis.
2. Use with caution in asthma, epilepsy, migraine headaches, and cardiac or renal function impairment.
3. Use with caution in metabolic bone disease associated with hypercalcemia, gallbladder disease, hepatic dysfunction, hypertension, endometriosis, uterine fibroids (leiomyomas), and acute intermittent porphyria.

Drug interactions
1. Barbiturates, carbamazepine, phenylbutazone, phenytoin, primidone, and rifampin lead to decreased effect.
2. Tobacco abuse leads to increased risk of cardiovascular side effects.
3. Estrogens lead to decreased effect of coumadin.
4. Estrogens lead to increased effect and toxicity of glucocorticoids.
5. Estrogens may increase cyclosporine levels.

Ethinyl estradiol (Estrogen, see *Oral contraceptives*)

Etidronate (Didronel)

Preparations: Tablets, 200, 400 mg; injection (IV), 300 mg/6 ml

Adult dosage
Paget's disease of bone—PO: Initially, 5–10 mg/kg/day as a single dose or in 2 divided doses for a period not to exceed 6 mo.; may use 10–20 mg/kg/day for a period not to exceed 3 mo. Doses >10 mg/kg/day are recommended when lower doses are ineffective or an overriding requirement for suppression for increased bone turnover exists. Retreatment regimens are the same as for initial therapy and should be separated by drug-free periods of at least 3 mo.
Hypercalcemia of malignancy—IV: Initially, an infusion of 7.5 mg/kg/day administered over at least 2 hr for 3 days. Treatment for >3 days increases the risk of hypocalcemia. Retreatment dosage after at least a 7-day drug-free period is the same as for initial therapy.
For maintenance therapy—PO: 20 mg/kg/day starting the day following the last IV dose for 30 days up to a maximum of 90 days

Indications: Treatment of symptomatic Paget's disease of bone and adjunctive therapy for hypercalcemia associated with malignancy

Action: A diphosphonate that reduces bone resorption and secondarily reduces bone formation by unclear mechanisms

Metabolism: None

Excretion: Renal

Contraindications and precautions
1. Contraindicated in severe renal function impairment (serum creatinine >5 mg/dl)
2. Use with caution in bone fractures, known lytic lesions of long bones, enterocolitis, and renal function impairment.

Drug interactions: Medications containing aluminum, calcium, iron, or magnesium may decrease absorption.

Famotidine (Pepcid)
Preparations: Tablets, 20 mg; powder for oral suspension, 40 mg/5 ml after reconstitution; injection (IV), 10 mg/ml
Adult dosage
Duodenal ulcer treatment—PO: 20 mg bid or 40 mg qhs. IV: 20 mg q12h.
Duodenal ulcer prophylaxis—PO: 20 mg qhs
Gastric hypersecretory conditions—PO: 20 mg q6h; doses up to 160 mg q6h reported
Note: Dosage reduction in renal function impairment. For creatinine clearance <10 ml/min, use 20 mg qhs or prolonged to q36–48 h.
Indications: Treatment of active, benign duodenal ulcers and gastric hypersecretory states (Zollinger-Ellison syndrome, systemic mastocytosis, multiple endocrine adenomas), and prophylaxis of duodenal ulcer. Unlabeled uses include treatment of gastric ulcer, gastroesophageal reflux, upper GI bleeding, and stress-related mucosal damage.
Action: Histamine H_2 blocker; inhibits gastric acid secretion
Metabolism: Hepatic
Excretion: Renal
Contraindications and precautions: Use with caution in hepatic or renal function impairment.
Drug interactions
1. Antacids lead to decreased absorption.
2. Famotidine leads to decreased absorption of ketoconazole.

Ferrous fumarate (see *Iron*)

Ferrous gluconate (*see Iron*)

Ferrous sulfate (see *Iron*)

Flecainide (Tambocor)
Preparations: Tablets, 100 mg
Adult dosage (Antiarrhythmic)
Sustained ventricular tachycardia—PO: Initially, 100 mg q12h. Increase in increments of 50 mg bid q4d until an effective response or until a maximum of 400 mg/day. Usual maintenance dose is 150 mg q12h.
Symptomatic nonsustained ventricular tachycardia—PO: Initially, same as above. Can increase up to 400 mg/day. If patient still symptomatic and a trough level is <0.6 μg/ml, dose can increase to a maximum of 600 mg/day.
Note
1. In CHF or myocardial dysfunction, initiate dosage at 50–100 mg q12h, not to exceed 200 mg q12h.
2. In renal function impairment, initiate dose at 100 mg q12h but increase dosage at intervals >4 days.
3. Therapeutic trough plasma levels are reportedly 0.2–1 μg/ml.

Indications: Treatment of symptomatic and life-threatening ventricular arrhythmias and frequent premature ventricular complexes
Action: Class IC antiarrhythmic
Metabolism: Hepatic
Excretion: Renal > fecal
Contraindications and precautions
1. Contraindicated in either 2nd- or 3rd-degree AV block or bifascicular block without pacemaker and cardiogenic shock.
2. Use with caution in cardiomyopathy, CHF, hypo- or hyperkalemia, hepatic or renal function impairment, sick sinus syndrome, and in patients with pacemakers.
3. Flecainide may be proarrhythmic.
4. Flecainide has a negative inotropic effect.
5. Flecainide may increase the P-R and Q-T intervals and prolong the QRS duration.

Drug interactions
1. β-Adrenergic blocking agents may increase negative inotropic effect.
2. Flecainide may increase plasma digoxin concentration.

Flunisolide—Nasal (Nasalide)
Preparations: Spray, 25 mg/inhalation, 25-ml bottle
Adult dosage: Intranasal inhalation: Initially, 50 μg (2 metered sprays) in each nostril bid; can increase to tid. For maintenance, reduce to lowest effective dose.
Indications: Treatment of seasonal or perennial rhinitis when effectiveness of or tolerance to conventional therapy is unsatisfactory; treatment of postsurgical prophylaxis of nasal polyps
Action: Anti-inflammatory steroid
Metabolism: Hepatic
Excretion: Fecal > renal
Contraindications and precautions: Use with caution in fungal or systemic viral infections, ocular herpes simplex, and latent or active respiratory tract tuberculosis.

Fluoxetine (Prozac)
Preparations: Capsules, 20 mg
Adult dosage: PO: Initially, 20 mg qd. Increase to 40 mg after several weeks if needed; maximum daily dose = 80 mg. Use bid dosing for doses >20 mg/day.
Note: Because of the long elimination half-life of fluoxetine (2–3 days) and its metabolite (7–9 days), dosing changes are not reflected in plasma levels for several weeks.
Indications: Treatment of major depressive disorder
Action: A nontricyclic antidepressant that inhibits CNS neuronal uptake of serotonin
Metabolism: Hepatic
Excretion: Renal >> biliary
Contraindications and precautions
1. Use with caution in hepatic or renal function impairment or a history of seizures.
2. There is limited clinical information on side effects and drug interactions.
3. Prescribe the smallest quantity feasible to patients considered at risk for suicide.

Drug interactions
1. Concurrent MAO inhibitors may cause severe side effects. When stopping fluoxetine, at least 5 wk should elapse before starting an MAO inhibitor.
2. Alcohol or CNS depressants lead to increased CNS depression.
3. Fluoxetine leads to increased drug levels of highly protein-bound medications (e.g., digoxin, coumadin).

Fluphenazine (Permitil, Prolixin)
Preparations: Tablets, 1, 2.5, 5, 10 mg; solution, 5 mg/ml; elixir, 2.5 mg/5 ml; injection (IM), 2.5 mg/ml
Adult dosage: PO: Initially, 0.5–10 mg/day in 3–4 divided doses. Increase gradually until symptoms are controlled (usually <20 mg/day), then taper to a daily maintenance dose of 1–5 mg/day, usually given as a single dose. IM: Initially, 2.5–10 mg/day in 3–4 divided doses; average initial dose is 1.25 mg. In general, IM dose is ½ to ⅓ of PO dose. Use >10 mg/day with caution. As with PO, increase gradually until symptoms are controlled and then transfer to oral therapy.
Note: Use lower doses with geriatric or debilitated patients.
Indications: Treatment of psychotic disorders
Action: Antipsychotic effect due to inhibition of CNS dopaminergic receptors; has weak anticholinergic and sedative effects; peripheral α-adrenergic blocking effect causes vasodilation
Metabolism: Hepatic
Excretion: Renal
Contraindications and precautions
1. Contraindicated in comatose states, severe CNS depression, subcortical brain damage, bone marrow depression, and severe cardiovascular disease.
2. Use with caution in cardiovascular disease, seizure disorders, hepatic function impairment, glaucoma, urinary retention, prostatic hypertrophy, chronic respiratory disorders, blood dyscrasias, and active alcoholism.
3. Tartrazine in some products may cause allergic reactions.

Drug interactions
1. CNS depressants lead to increased CNS depression.
2. Anticholinergic agents lead to increased antimuscarinic effects.
3. Aluminum- or magnesium-containing antacids or lithium may decrease oral absorption.
4. Epinephrine leads to severe hypotension and tachycardia.
5. Propranolol and possibly other β-blockers lead to increased levels and vice versa.
6. Opioids lead to increased risk of consupation.
7. Fluphenazine may increase phenytoin or tricyclic antidepressant levels.
8. Fluphenazine may increase risk of metrizamide-induced seizures.
9. Fluphenazine may decrease effect of levodopa.

Flurazepam (Dalmane, others)
Preparations: Capsules, 15, 30 mg
Adult dosage: Sedative-hypnotic—PO: 15–30 mg qhs. Initiate therapy with 15 mg in elderly or debilitated patients.
Indications: Treatment of insomnia
Action: Sedative-hypnotic benzodiazepine may potentiate CNS gamma-aminobutyric acid effects.
Metabolism: Hepatic (oxidation)

Excretion: Renal
Contraindications and precautions
1. Contraindicated in acute alcohol intoxication with depressed vital signs, depressive neuroses, or psychoses without prominent anxiety.
2. Use with caution in acute narrow-angle glaucoma, myasthenia gravis, shock, severe chronic obstructive pulmonary disease, hepatic or renal function impairment, patients with depressed respirations, or those receiving concurrent respiratory depressants.
3. Long-term therapy may result in psychic or physical dependence.
4. Exercise caution in performing tasks requiring alertness and coordination.

Drug interactions
1. Cimetidine, disulfiram, erythromycin, isoniazid, ketoconazole, and oral contraceptives may increase effect.
2. Alcohol or other CNS depressants lead to increased CNS depression.

Folic acid
Preparations: Tablets, 0.1, 0.4, 0.8, 1 mg; injection (IM, IV, SC), 5 mg/ml, 10 mg/ml
Adult dosage
Dietary supplement—PO: 0.1 mg qd; increase to 0.5–1 mg qd depending on conditions causing increased requirements. For pregnancy, 1 mg qd. For tropical sprue, 3–15 mg qd.
Folate deficiency—PO, IM, IV, SC: Initially, 0.25–1 mg qd until a hematologic response occurs; then give 0.4 mg (0.8 mg in pregnancy or lactation) qd as maintenance.
Indications: Treatment and prophylaxis of folic acid deficiency states
Action: Vitamin B_9; necessary for normal erythropoiesis and nucleoprotein synthesis
Metabolism: Hepatic
Excretion: Renal
Contraindications and precautions: Pernicious anemia must be ruled out before starting folic acid therapy (corrects anemia but not neurologic damage).
Drug interactions:
1. Phenytoin and primidone may decrease serum folate levels.
2. Folic acid may decrease phenytoin serum level.
3. Folic acid may interfere with antimicrobial effects of pyrimethamine.

Furosemide (Lasix, others)
Preparations: Tablets, 20, 40, 80 mg; solution, 10 mg/ml, 40 mg/5 ml; injection (IM, IV), 10 mg/ml
Adult dosage
Diuretic—PO: Initially, 20–80 mg/day as a single dose; can increase by 20–40 mg q6–8h until adequate diuresis. When total daily dose is determined, give daily as a single dose or divided bid. Can use alternate-day schedule. IM, IV (IV preferred): Initially, 20–40 mg; can increase by 20 mg in 2 hr. Give maintenance dose as a single dose or divided bid. For acute pulmonary edema, initially 40 mg; increase in 1 hr if diuresis inadequate.
Antihypertensive—PO: Initially, 40 mg bid and titrate to BP response.
Note
1. Administration of high-dose parenteral therapy should be by controlled IV infusion at ≤4 mg/min.
2. Onset of action: PO—30–60 min, IV—5 min
3. Time to peak effect: PO—1–2 hr, IV—20–60 min
4. Duration of action: PO—6–8 hr, IV—2 hr.
5. Person with renal function impairment may require higher doses.

Indications: Treatment of hypertension and edema associated with CHF, cirrhosis, and renal disease; adjunctive therapy in pulmonary edema and hypercalcemia
Action: Loop diuretic; also inhibits NaCl reabsorption in the distal tubule
Metabolism: Hepatic
Excretion: Renal > biliary
Contraindications and precautions
1. Contraindicated in anuria.
2. Use with caution in severe renal function impairment, hepatic impairment, and those at increased risk if hypokalemia occurs.
3. Patients with known sulfonamide sensitivity may show allergic reaction.
4. May exacerbate gout or diabetes mellitus.

Drug interactions
1. Adrenocorticoids may decrease natriuretic/diuretic effect.
2. NSAIDs, especially indomethacin, may decrease diuretic effect.
3. Furosemide may increase toxicity of lithium, amphotericin B, salicylates, and aminoglycoside antibiotics.
4. Furosemide may increase toxicity of digoxin and nondepolarizing neuromuscular blocking agents by decreasing K^+
5. Furosemide may decrease anticoagulant effect of coumadin.

Gemfibrozil (Lopid)
Preparations: Capsules, 300 mg
Adult dosage: PO: 1,200 mg/day (range, 900–1,500 mg/day) in 2 divided doses 30 min before morning and evening meals
Indications: Treatment of hyperlipidemia
Action: Reduces plasma VLDL (decreases triglyceride), slightly reduces LDL and increases HDL
Metabolism: Hepatic
Excretion: Renal >> fecal
Contraindications and precautions: Contraindicated in pre-existing gallbladder disease and hepatic (including primary biliary cirrhosis) or severe renal function impairment.
Drug interactions: Gemfibrozil leads to increased anticoagulant effects of coumadin.

Glipizide (Glucotrol)
Preparations: Tablets, 5, 10 mg
Adult dosage: PO: Initially, 5 mg qd. Start with 2.5 mg in geriatric, debilitated, or malnourished patients and in those with renal or hepatic function impairment. Increase by 2.5–5 mg every week until optimal control or a maximum daily dose of 40 mg. Use bid dosing for daily doses >15 mg. Patients being transferred from chlorpropamide should be monitored closely for hypoglycemia the first 2 wk. Transfer from other sulfonylureas does not require a conversion period. Patients previously on insulin doses <20 units/day should start glipizide and have the insulin stopped abruptly. Patients previously on ≥20 units/day should start oral therapy with a concurrent 50% reduction in insulin dose. Taper insulin, and increase glipizide according to clinical response.
Indications: Treatment of non–insulin-dependent diabetes mellitus
Action: Sulfonylurea that promotes insulin release from pancreatic beta cells, decreases hepatic gluconeogenesis, and increases insulin sensitivity
Metabolism: Hepatic
Excretion: Renal
Contraindications and precautions
1. Contraindicated in significant acidosis, severe burns, diabetic coma, severe infection, significant ketosis, ketoacidosis, major surgery, or severe trauma.
2. Cross-sensitivity to other sulfonamide-type medications is possible.
3. Use with caution in adrenal or pituitary insufficiency; thyroid function impairment; renal, hepatic, or cardiac impairment; malnourishment; debilitated physical condition; or nausea and vomiting.

Drug interactions
1. Chronic ethanol use, phenobarbital, and rifampin lead to decreased hypoglycemic effects.
2. Chloramphenicol, cimetidine, clofibrate, coumadin, ketoconazole, MAO inhibitors, methyldopa, NSAIDs, phenylbutazone, probenecid, salicylates, sulfonamides, and sulfinpyrazone lead to increased hypoglycemic effect.
3. Ethanol may lead to disulfiram-like reaction.

Glucocorticoids (see table "Glucocorticoid Pharmacology," page 708)

Glyburide (DiaBeta, Micronase)
Preparations: Tablets, 1.25, 2.5, 5 mg
Adult dosage: PO: Initially, 2.5–5 mg qd. Start with 1.25 mg in geriatric, debilitated, or malnourished patients and in those with renal or hepatic function impairment. Increase by no more than 2.5 mg every week until optimal control or a maximum daily dose of 20 mg. Use bid dosing for daily doses >10 mg. Patients being transferred from chlorpropamide should be monitored closely for hypoglycemia the first 2 wk. Transfer from other sulfonylureas does not require a conversion period. Patients previously on insulin doses of <40 units/day should start glyburide and have the insulin stopped abruptly. Patients previously on ≥40 units/day should start oral therapy, with a concurrent 50% reduction in insulin dose. Taper insulin, and increase glyburide according to clinical response.
Indications: Treatment of non–insulin-dependent diabetes mellitus
Action: Sulfonylurea that promotes insulin release from pancreatic beta cells, decreases hepatic gluconeogenesis, and increases insulin sensitivity
Metabolism: Hepatic
Excretion: Renal = biliary
Contraindications and precautions
1. Contraindicated in significant acidosis, severe burns, diabetic coma, severe infection, significant ketosis,

Glucocorticoid Pharmacology

Glucocorticoid	Equivalent dose (mg)	Relative glucocorticoid activity	Relative mineralocorticoid activity
Short-acting			
Cortisone	25	0.8	2+
Hydrocortisone	20	1	2+
Intermediate-acting			
Prednisone	5	4	1+
Prednisolone	5	4	1+
Methylprednisolone	4	5	0
Triamcinolone	4	5	0
Long-acting			
Paramethasone	2	10	0
Dexamethasone	0.75	20–30	0
Betamethasone	0.6	20–30	0

ketoacidosis, major surgery, or severe trauma.
2. Cross-sensitivity to other sulfonamide-type medications is possible.
3. Use with caution in adrenal or pituitary insufficiency; thyroid function impairment; renal, hepatic or cardiac impairment; malnourishment; debilitated physical condition; or nausea and vomiting.

Drug interactions
1. Chronic ethanol use, phenobarbital, and rifampin lead to decreased hypoglycemic effects.
2. Chloramphenicol, cimetidine, clofibrate, coumadin, ketoconazole, MAO inhibitors, methyldopa, NSAIDs, phenylbutazone, probenecid, salicylates, sulfonamides, and sulfinpyrazone lead to increased hypoglycemic effect.
3. Ethanol may lead to disulfiram-like reaction.

Haloperidol (Haldol, others)

Preparations: Tablets, 0.5, 1, 2, 5, 10, 20 mg; solution, 2 mg/ml; injection (IM), 5 mg/ml, 50 mg (of decanoate)/ml
Adult dosage: Antipsychotic—PO: Initially, 0.5–2 mg bid–tid in patients with moderate symptoms, geriatric, or debilitated patients. For severe symptoms, start with 3–5 mg bid–tid. Increase prn up to 100 mg/day. After symptoms are controlled, reduce to the lowest effective daily dose. IM: For acute psychosis, initially 2–5 mg; repeat q4–8h or as frequent as q1h if symptoms not controlled. For chronic psychosis, use IM haloperidol decanoate. Patients should be stable on PO haloperidol. Initially, 10–15 times previous daily PO dose, not to exceed 100 mg. Adjust dose q4wk.
Indications: Treatment of psychotic disorders and Gilles de la Tourette syndrome; unlabeled use includes treatment of severe nausea and vomiting.
Action: Similar to piperazine phenothiazines; blocks CNS postsynaptic dopamine receptors; also has mild α-adrenergic blocking effect
Metabolism: Hepatic
Excretion: Renal > biliary
Contraindications and precautions
1. Contraindicated in coma, severe CNS depression, and parkinsonism.
2. Use with caution in active alcoholism, history of allergies or other drug allergies, severe cardiovascular disorders, seizure disorders, thyrotoxicosis, and urinary retention.
3. Exercise caution while driving or performing activities requiring alertness.

Drug interactions
1. Alcohol or other CNS depressants lead to increased CNS depression.
2. Tricyclic antidepressants, MAO inhibitors, or trazodone may increase sedative and anticholinergic effects.
3. Lithium may increase risk of adverse CNS effects.
4. Haloperidol may block α-adrenergic effects of epinephrine.
5. Haloperidol may decrease effects of levodopa.

Heparin

Preparations: Injection (SC, IV): Heparin sodium injection, 1,000, 2,500, 5,000, 7,500, 10,000, 15,000, 20,000, 40,000 units/ml; heparin sodium in dextrose injection, 20, 40, 50, 100 units/ml; heparin sodium in NaCL injection, 2, 50, 100 units/ml; heparin sodium lock flush solution, 10, 100 units/ml; heparin calcium injection, 25,000 units/ml
Adult dosage
Full-dose regimen (therapeutic): *Continuous IV infusion (preferred):* Initially, a loading dose of 5,000 units IV is usually administered followed by 20,000–40,000 units in 1,000 ml normal saline or D/W as a continuous infusion. The initial infusion is usually, 1,000 units/hr, but adjust dosage according to results of coagulation tests. *Intermittent IV injection:* Initially, 10,000 units IV, followed by 5,000–10,000 units IV q6–24h as determined by coagulation test results. *Intermittent SC injection:* Initially a loading dose of 5,000 units IV is usually administered concurrently with 10,000–20,000 units SC, followed by 8,000–10,000 units SC q8h or 15,000–20,000 units SC q12h.
Low-dose regimen (prophylactic)—SC: 5,000 units 2 hr before surgery and then 8–12 hr thereafter for 7 days or until the patient is ambulatory
Lock-flush regimen—IV: 10 or 100 ml/unit solution injected into the diaphragm of the device after each use, after designated intervals or prn
Disseminated intravascular coagulation (DIC), cardiovascular surgery: Consult other texts.

Note
1. Low-dose therapy usually does not require coagulation test monitoring.
2. With full-dose therapy, coagulation tests should be monitored. The activated partial thromboplastin time (aPTT) is the most commonly used. For continuous IV infusion, check 1.5–2 hr after start of infusion, q4h during the early stages of treatment and at least daily thereafter. For intermittent injection, check before each dose during the early stages of treatment and at least daily thereafter. The generally accepted therapeutic value for the aPTT is 1.5–2.5 times the control value in seconds.
3. Full-dose heparin therapy is generally continued for 7–10 days in acute venous thrombosis. Consult medical texts for optimal duration in specific disorders.
4. When oral anticoagulants are administered for follow-up treatment after full-dose therapy, both drugs are usually overlapped until an adequate response to the oral anticoagulant is obtained (as determined by the prothrombin time). The optimal duration of concurrent therapy is controversial.

Indications: Treatment and prophylaxis of deep venous thrombosis and thromboembolism (including pulmonary and arterial); treatment of DIC or adjunctive therapy in acute myocardial infarction with heparin is controversial; used for prophylaxis against blood clotting in procedures such as cardiac surgery and hemodialysis and as a lock-flush solution to maintain the potency of indwelling venipuncture devices; consult other texts for specific heparin therapeutic regimen used in each indication
Action: Potentiates the inhibitory action of antithrombin III on thrombin (factor IIa) and factors IXa, Xa, and XIIa; results in inhibition of the conversion of fibrinogen to fibrin
Metabolism: Reticuloendothelial system uptake hepatic
Excretion: Renal
Contraindications and precautions
1. Full-dose therapy is contraindicated if coagulation tests cannot be performed at required intervals.
2. Contraindicated in uncontrollable hemorrhage (unless due to DIC), severe thrombocytopenia, and cerebrovascular hemorrhage.
3. Use with caution in conditions with increased risk of hemorrhage, including subacute bacterial endocarditis, arterial sclerosis, dissecting aneurysm, severe hypertension, pericarditis or pericardial effusion, spinal puncture, spinal anesthesia, recent or contemplated ocular or neurosurgery, hemorrhagic blood dyscrasias, gastrointestinal ulcerative lesions, continuous gastric or intestinal tube drainage, menstruation, threatened abortion, recent childbirth, severe hepatic or renal disease, major surgery, severe trauma, and indwelling catheters.
4. Patients with a history of allergies or asthma have a greater risk of allergic reaction to heparin.
5. Heparin may cause hyperkalemia due to

hypoaldosteronism; use with caution in renal function impairment.
6. Heparin may cause thrombocytopenia; monitor platelet count.

Drug interactions
1. Coumadin, NSAIDs, aspirin, dipyridamole, dextran, and thrombolytic agents lead to increased risk of hemorrhage.
2. High-dose penicillin, chloroquine, hydroxychloroquine, methimazole, propylthiouracil, and probenecid may increase risk of hemorrhage.
3. IV nitroglycerin leads to decreased anticoagulant effects.

Hycodan (Hydrocodone bitartrate and Homatropine methylbromide)—Schedule III

Preparations: Per tablet or 5 ml of syrup, 5 mg hydrocodone bitartrate and 1.5 mg homatropine methylbromide
Adult dosage: Antitussive—PO: 5 mg of hydrocodone bitartrate q4–6h prn
Indications: Treatment of cough
Action: Opioid agonist (hydrocodone) with antitussive effects
Metabolism: Hepatic (hydrocodone)
Excretion: Renal (hydrocodone)
Contraindications and precautions
1. Contraindicated in diarrhea associated with pseudomembranous colitis, diarrhea caused by poisoning until the toxic material has been eliminated, and acute respiratory depression.
2. Psychological and physical dependence and tolerance to many of the effects of hydrocodone may develop with chronic administration.
3. Use with caution in post-thoracotomy or postlaparotomy patients, acute abdominal conditions, acute asthma or chronic respiratory impairment, head injury, increased intracranial pressure, intracranial lesions, hepatic or renal function impairment, hypothyroidism, gallbladder disease, inflammatory bowel disease, recent GI tract surgery, prostatic hypertrophy or obstruction, urethral stricture, acute alcoholism, Addison's disease, epilepsy, suicidal ideation, emotional instability or history of drug abuse.
4. Use with caution in patients performing tasks requiring mental alertness or physical coordination.
5. Use with caution in patients being given MAO inhibitors.

Drug interactions
1. Alcohol, other opioid agonist analgesics, and other CNS depressants (including antihistamines, phenothiazines, tricyclic antidepressants, benzodiazepines, sedative-hypnotics, barbiturates) may increase risk of CNS depression.
2. Antidiarrheals and anticholinergics lead to increased risk of constipation.
3. Antihypertensives and diuretics lead to increased risk of hypotension.
4. Naltrexone, naloxone, and buprenorphine may block certain opioid actions. Consult other texts for further information.

Hydralazine (Alazine, Apresoline, others)

Preparations: Tablets, 10, 25, 50, 100 mg; injection, (IM, IV) 20 mg/ml
Adult dosage: PO: Initially, 10 mg qid for 2–4 days. Increase to 25 mg qid for the balance of the first week. Increase to 50 mg qid starting the second week, if needed, up to a daily dose of 300 mg; bid maintenance dosing may be adequate. IM, IV: 10–40 mg repeated prn.
Indications: Treatment of hypertension; unlabeled use includes treatment of CHF.
Action: Direct peripheral vasodilator resulting in decreased BP, decreased peripheral vascular resistance, and increased cardiac output
Metabolism: Hepatic (slow vs. fast acetylation)
Excretion: Renal
Contraindications and precautions
1. Hydralazine may cause drug-induced lupus; monitor ANA and CBC during therapy even if asymptomatic.
2. Contraindicated in mitral valvular rheumatic heart disease.
3. Use with caution in cerebrovascular disease, coronary artery disease, and severe renal function impairment.

Drug interactions: Diuretics, MAO inhibitors, or other hypotensive agents lead to increased risk of excessively decreased BP.

Hydrochlorothiazide (HydroDIURIL, others)

Preparations: Tablets, 25, 50, 100 mg; solutions, 50 mg/5 ml
Adult dosage
Diuretic—PO: Initially, 25–200 mg/day in single or bid doses. Usual maintenance doses are 25–100 mg qd given daily or intermittently.
Antihypertensive—PO: Initially, 50–100 mg qd. If adding to another antihypertensive agent, start with 25 mg qd and adjust according to blood pressure response.
Indications: Treatment of hypertension and edema
Action: Thiazide diuretic that inhibits renal tubular reabsorption of sodium and water in the distal tubule; increases urinary excretion of potassium and decreases urinary excretion of calcium and uric acid; antihypertensive mechanism unknown
Metabolism: Minimal
Excretion: Renal
Contraindications and precautions
1. Contraindicated in anuria and hypersensitivity to thiazides or other sulfonamide derivatives.
2. Use with caution in diabetes mellitus, history of gout, hyperuricemia, hepatic function impairment, hypercalcemia, systemic lupus erythematosus, sympathectomy, or electrolyte disturbances.
3. Electrolyte disturbances may occur; monitor serum electrolytes.

Drug interactions
1. Cholestyramine and colestipol lead to decreased absorption.
2. Glucocorticoids and amphotericin B lead to increased risk of hypokalemia.
3. Hydrochlorothiazide leads to increased risk of lithium toxicity.
4. Hydrochlorothiazide leads to increased risk of toxicity of digoxin, amiodarone, and nondepolarizing neuromuscular blocking agents owing to hypokalemia.

Hydrocortisone—Systemic

Preparations: Tablets, 5, 10, 20 mg; cypionate suspension, 10 mg/5 ml; acetate injection (intra-articular, intralesional, soft-tissue), 25, 50 mg/ml; sodium phosphate injection (IM, IV, SC), 50 mg/ml; sodium succinate injection (IM, IV), 100, 250, 500, 1,000 mg/vial
Adult dosage: PO: 20–240 mg/day as a single dose or in divided doses depending on the indication. IM, IV, SC: 100–500 mg (sodium succinate) repeated q2–6h prn depending on patient response or 15–240 mg/day (sodium phosphate) depending on the indication. Higher doses of either form may be required in life-threatening situations. Intra-articular, intralesional, soft-tissue: Consult other texts.
Indications: Replacement therapy in the treatment of adrenal insufficiency states; used for anti-inflammatory and immunosuppressant effects in the treatment of many disorders; consult further texts for specific therapeutic regimens in selected disorders
Action: Adrenocorticoid with anti-inflammatory, immunosuppressant, and mineralocorticoid effects; other effects include suppression of the hypothalamic-pituitary-adrenal (HPA) axis, increased protein catabolism, increased blood glucose concentrations, insulin resistance, reduced intestinal absorption and increased renal excretion of calcium, and neutrophilia. See also table, page 708.
Metabolism: Primarily hepatic
Excretion: Renal
Contraindications and precautions
1. Use with caution in cardiac disease, CHF, hypertension, hepatic or renal function impairment, AIDS or other immunodeficiency states, uncontrolled bacterial or viral infection, systemic-fungal infection, tuberculosis (active, latent or positive skin test), ocular herpes simplex, diabetes mellitus, nonspecific ulcerative colitis, diverticulitis, esophagitis, gastritis, history of peptic ulcer, recent intestinal anastomosis, open-angle glaucoma, hyperthyroidism, hypoalbuminuria, myasthenia gravis, osteoporosis, or seizure disorder.
2. Give daily dose in the morning to reduce HPA-axis suppressive effects. Alternate-day dosing may reduce the risk of adrenal suppression.
3. Withdrawal following long-term therapy with pharmacologic doses requires a gradual taper until the HPA axis recovers.

Drug interactions
1. Alcohol, aspirin, and NSAIDs may increase risk of GI ulceration.
2. Amphotericin B and diuretics may increase risk of hypokalemia.
3. Estrogens may increase effects.
4. Ephedrine, phenytoin, phenobarbital, and rifampin may decrease effects.
5. Immunosuppressants lead to increased risk of infection.
6. Hydrocortisone may decrease effect of coumadin, oral antidiabetic agents, and insulin.
7. Hydrocortisone may decrease effect of isoniazid.
8. Pharmacologic doses of hydrocortisone

may potentiate replication of live virus in vaccines or decrease antibody response to the vaccine.

Hydrocortisone retention enema (Cortenema)
Preparations: Retention enema, 100 mg/60 ml
Adult dosage: PR: 100 mg qhs for 21 days or until clinical improvement. Patient should lie on left side. The enema should be retained for at least 1 hr and preferably all night. Discontinue if no improvement is seen within 2–3 wk. If therapy exceeds 21 days, taper gradually.
Indications: Adjunctive therapy for ulcerative colitis
Action: Adrenocorticoid with anti-inflammatory
Metabolism: Hepatic (of absorbed dose)
Excretion: Renal
Contraindications and precautions: Contraindicated in intestinal obstruction, intestinal perforation, abdominal infection, extensive sinus tracts or fistulae, or soon after ileocolostomy
Drug interactions
1. Alcohol, aspirin, and NSAIDs may increase risk of GI ulceration
2. Amphotericin B and diuretics may increase risk of hypokalemia.
3. Immunosuppressants may increase risk of infection.
4. Hydrocortisone may decrease effect of coumadin, oral antidiabetic agents, and insulin.

Hydromorphone hydrochloride (Dilaudid, others)—Schedule II
Preparations: Tablets, 1, 2, 3, 4 mg; suppositories, 3 mg; injection (IM, SC), 1, 2, 3, 4, 10 mg/ml
Adult dosage
Analgesic—PO: 2 mg q4–6h prn; for severe pain, 4 mg q4–6h prn. PR: 3 mg q6–8h prn. IM, SC: 2 mg q4–6h prn; for severe pain, 3–4 mg q4–6h prn.
Antitussive—PO: 1 mg q3–4h
Note
1. Use lower doses in geriatric patients.
2. IM preferred over SC administration.
3. Give smallest effective dose and as infrequently as possible to minimize tolerance and physical dependence.

Indications: Treatment of pain and cough
Action: Narcotic analgesic with antitussive and antidiarrheal effects
Metabolism: Hepatic
Excretion: Renal
Contraindications and precautions
1. Contraindicated in diarrhea associated with pseudomembranous colitis, diarrhea caused by poisoning until the toxic material has been eliminated, and acute respiratory depression.
2. Psychological and physical dependence and tolerance to many of the effects of hydromorphone may develop with chronic administration.
3. Use with caution in acute abdominal conditions, acute asthma or chronic respiratory impairment, head injury, increased intracranial pressure, intracranial lesions, hepatic or renal function impairment, hypothyroidism, gallbladder disease, inflammatory bowel disease, recent GI tract surgery, prostatic hypertrophy or obstruction, urethral stricture, acute alcoholism, Addison's disease, epilepsy, suicidal ideation, emotional instability, or history of drug abuse.
4. Use with caution in patients performing tasks requiring mental alertness or physical coordination.
5. Use with caution in patients being administered MAO inhibitors.

Drug interactions
1. Alcohol, other opioid agonist analgesics, and other CNS depressants (including antihistamines, phenothiazines, tricyclic antidepressants, benzodiazepines, sedative-hypnotics, barbiturates) may increase risk of CNS depression.
2. Antidiarrheals and anticholinergics lead to increased risk of constipation.
3. Antihypertensives and diuretics lead to increased risk of hypotension.
4. Naltrexone, naloxone, and buprenorphine may block certain opioid actions. Consult other texts for further information.

Hydroxyzine (Atarax, Vistaril, others)
Preparations: Tablets, 10, 25, 50, 100 mg; capsules, 25, 50, 100 mg; syrup, 10 mg/5 ml; suspension, 25 mg/5 ml; injection (IM), 25, 50 mg/ml
Adult dosage
Antianxiety, sedative-hypnotic—PO: 50–100 mg qid. *For prompt control of hysterical patients or agitation caused by alcohol withdrawal*—IM: Initially, 50–100 mg; repeat q4–6h prn. *For preoperative sedation*—PO: 50–100 mg. IM: 25–100 mg.
Antihistaminic, antipruritic—PO: 25 mg tid–qid
Antiemetic—IM: 25–100 mg. Adjust dose to individual response.
Indications: Treatment of anxiety and psychosis-related anxiety or tension, alcohol withdrawal symptoms, pruritus due to allergic conditions, histamine-mediated pruritus, and nausea and vomiting; also used as adjunctive sedation pre- and postoperatively
Action: H_1-receptor blocker; has CNS subcortical suppressive, antiemetic, and anticholinergic effects
Metabolism: Hepatic
Excretion: Biliary/fecal
Contraindications and precautions
1. Use with caution in angle-closure glaucoma, prostatic hypertrophy, stenosing peptic ulcer, urinary retention, asthma, chronic obstructive pulmonary disease, hyperthyroidism, cardiovascular disease, or hypertension.
2. Exercise caution while driving or performing activities requiring mental alertness.

Drug interactions
1. Alcohol or CNS depressants lead to increased CNS depression.
2. Anticholinergic agents lead to increased antimuscarinic effects.

Ibuprofen (Advil, Motrin, others)
Preparations: Tablets, 200, 300, 400, 600, 800 mg
Adult dosage
Antirheumatic—PO: 1.2–3.2 g/day in 3–4 divided doses
Analgesic, antipyretic, antidysmenorrheal—PO: 200–400 mg q4–6h prn
Note: Use lower doses in geriatric patients.
Indications: Treatment of rheumatic and nonrheumatic inflammatory disorders, dysmenorrhea pain, headache, and fever; unlabeled uses include acute gouty arthritis, calcium pyrophosphate deposition disease, and chronic prophylaxis of headaches.
Action: Nonsteroidal anti-inflammatory drug that inhibits cyclo-oxygenase, resulting in decreased formation of prostaglandins. Effects include antirheumatic, analgesic, antipyretic, and inhibition of platelet aggregation.
Metabolism: Hepatic
Excretion: Renal
Contraindications and precautions
1. Contraindicated in patient with a history of severe allergic reaction to aspirin or other NSAID
2. Use with caution in patient with a history of peptic ulcer, upper GI disease, ulcerative colitis, renal or hepatic function impairment, bleeding disorders, asthma, CHF, diabetes mellitus, hypertension, and pre-existing edema.

Drug interactions
1. Acetaminophen, gold compounds, or nephrotoxic medications may increase risk of renal toxicity.
2. Glucocorticoids, alcohol, potassium supplements, other NSAID, or aspirin may increase risk of GI side effects.
3. Anticoagulants, thrombolytic agents, aspirin, platelet aggregation inhibitors, or colchicine may increase risk of hemorrhage.
4. Probenecid may increase ibuprofen serum level.
5. Ibuprofen may increase methotrexate toxicity.
6. Ibuprofen may decrease antihypertensive effects of diuretics and antihypertensives.
7. Ibuprofen may decrease diuretic effect of diuretics.
8. Ibuprofen may increase hypoglycemic effect of sulfonylureas.
9. Ibuprofen may increase digoxin, lithium, nifedipine, and verapamil blood levels.

Imipramine (Tofranil, others)
Preparations: Tablets, 10, 25, 50 mg; injection (IM) 25 mg/2 ml
Adult dosage: PO: Initially, 75–100 mg qd. Increase up to 200 mg/day for outpatients or 300 mg/day for in-patients. Maximum antidepressant effects may take ≥2 wk. Start with lower doses of 30–40 mg/day in geriatric patients. IM: Up to 100 mg/day in divided doses. After control of symptoms, taper to lowest effective dose.
Indications: Treatment of depression; unlabeled uses include treatment of anxiety, neurogenic pain, narcolepsy, cataplexy, and cocaine withdrawal.
Action: Tricyclic antidepressant; increases CNS synaptic concentration of norepinephrine or serotonin, presumably by blocking presynaptic reuptake; has sedative, anticholinergic, peripheral vasodilator, and direct quinidine-like myocardial effects
Metabolism: Hepatic

Excretion: Renal
Contraindications and precautions
1. Contraindicated during recovery from myocardial infarction and possibly concurrent MAO inhibitor use.
2. Use with caution in alcoholism, asthma, bipolar disorder, schizophrenia, cardiovascular disorders, blood disorders, gastrointestinal disorders, narrow-angle glaucoma, hepatic or renal function impairment, hyperthyroidism, prostatic hypertrophy or urinary retention, and seizure disorders.
3. Use caution while driving or performing other tasks requiring alertness.
4. Abrupt cessation following prolonged administration may cause withdrawal symptoms.
5. Prescribe the smallest quantity feasible to patients considered at risk for suicide.

Drug interactions
1. Alcohol or CNS depressants lead to increased CNS depression.
2. Drugs with antimuscarinic activity lead to increased anticholinergic side effects.
3. Direct-acting sympathomimetics lead to increased cardiac effects.
4. MAO inhibitors lead to increased risk of hyperpyretic episodes, convulsions, hypertensive crises, and death.
5. Antithyroid agents lead to increased risk of agranulocytosis.
6. Barbiturates and carbamazepine may decrease plasma concentration of imipramine.
7. Cimetidine methylphenidate, phenothiazines, estrogens, and possibly ranitidine may increase plasma concentration of imipramine.
8. Metrizamide leads to increased risk of seizures.
9. Thyroid hormone leads to increased therapeutic and toxic effects of both medications.
10. Imipramine leads to decreased hypotensive effect of guanethidine and clonidine.
11. Imipramine may increase plasma concentration of coumadin.

Indapamide (Lozol)

Preparations: Tablets, 2.5 mg
Adult dosage: Diuretic, antihypertensive—PO: Initially, 2.5 mg qd. If inadequate response, increase to 5 mg qd after 1 wk for edema for 4 wk for hypertension.
Indications: Treatment of hypertension and edema
Action: Thiazide-like diuretic that inhibits renal tubular reabsorption of sodium and water in the distal tubule. It also increases urinary excretion of potassium and decreases urinary excretion of uric acid. Although reported to decrease urinary calcium excretion, it does not appear to change serum calcium concentrations. Antihypertensive mechanism unknown.
Metabolism: Hepatic
Excretion: Renal biliary
Contraindications and precautions
1. Contraindicated in anuria and hypersensitivity to sulfonamide derivatives.
2. Use with caution in diabetes mellitus, history of gout, hyperuricemia, hepatic function impairment, sympathectomy, or electrolyte disturbances.
3. Electrolyte disturbances may occur; monitor serum electrolytes.

Drug interactions:
1. Glucocorticoids and amphotericin B lead to increased risk of hypokalemia.
2. Indapamide leads to increased risk of lithium toxicity
3. Indapamide leads to increased risk of toxicity of digoxin, amiodarone, and nondepolarizing neuromuscular blocking agents owing to hypokalemia.

Indomethacin (Indocin, others)

Preparations: Capsules, 25, 50, 75 mg; SR capsules, 75 mg; suspension, 25 mg/5 ml; suppositories, 50 mg
Adult dosage
Antirheumatic—PO: Initially, 25 mg bid–tid. Increase by 25–50 mg/day every week prn. For acute exacerbations of rheumatoid arthritis, increase dose by 25–50 mg daily prn. Dosage may be increased until a satisfactory response or a maximum daily dosage of 150–200 mg. SR capsules may be substituted for capsules when the effective and tolerated dose of indomethacin has been established. PR: 50 mg up to qid.
Antigout—PO, PR: 50 mg tid until pain is relieved. Rapidly reduce dose to cessation. Do not use SR capsule preparation.
Nonrheumatic anti-inflammatory—PO: 75–150 mg/day in 3–4 divided doses. PR: 50 mg up to TID. Discontinue several days after control of inflammation.
Note: Use lower doses in geriatric patients.
Indications: Treatment of rheumatic and nonrheumatic inflammatory disorders, acute gouty arthritis, and headache. Unlabeled uses include treatment of dysmenorrhea, acute calcium pyrophosphate deposition disease, and chronic prophylaxis of headache.
Action: Nonsteroidal anti-inflammatory drug that inhibits cyclo-oxygenase, resulting in decreased formation of prostaglandins. Effects include antirheumatic, analgesic, antipyretic, and inhibition of platelet aggregation.
Metabolism: Hepatic
Excretion: Renal > biliary
Contraindications and precautions
1. Contraindicated in patient with history of severe allergic reaction to aspirin or other NSAID.
2. Rectal dosage form contraindicated in recent anorectal bleeding, proctitis, or hemorrhoids.
3. Use with caution in patient with history of peptic ulcer, upper GI disease or ulcerative colitis, renal or hepatic function impairment, bleeding disorders, asthma, CHF, diabetes mellitus, hypertension, and pre-existing edema.

Drug interactions
1. Acetaminophen, gold compounds, or nephrotoxic medications may increase risk of renal toxicity.
2. Glucocorticoids, alcohol, potassium supplements, other NSAID, or aspirin may increase risk of GI side effects.
3. Anticoagulants, thrombolytic agents, aspirin, platelet aggregation inhibitors, or colchicine may increase risk of hemorrhage.
4. Probenecid may increase indomethacin serum level.
5. Indomethacin may increase methotrexate toxicity.
6. Indomethacin may decrease antihypertensive effects of diuretics and antihypertensives.
7. Indomethacin may decrease diuretic effect of diuretics.
8. Indomethacin may increase hypoglycemic effect of sulfonylureas.

Insulin (Humulin, Lente, others)

Preparations: See table, page 737.
Adult dosage: Dosage must be individualized. Selection of a particular treatment program depends on the clinical situation and the experience and judgment of the clinician. Therapy with regular insulin is generally 5–10 units SC 15–45 min before meals and qhs. Intermediate-acting insulins may be given as a single daily dose 30–60 min before breakfast.
Indications: Replacement therapy in diabetes mellitus. Insulin injection (regular) has been added to IV glucose solutions to shift potassium intracellularly in the treatment of severe hyperkalemia.
Action: Hormone that controls storage and metabolism of carbohydrate, fat, and protein. It facilitates transport of glucose into cells, hepatic glycogenesis, lipogenesis, and protein synthesis.
Metabolism: Hepatic > renal, muscle
Excretion: Renal
Contraindications and precautions
1. Insulin requirements may change in patients who become ill.
2. Hypoglycemia may result from excessive insulin dose.

Drug interactions
1. Alcohol, guanethidine, MAO inhibitors, salicylates, NSAIDs, and sulfonylureas may increase hypoglycemic effect.
2. Drugs that increase serum glucose (e.g., glucocorticoids; consult other texts for complete list) may decrease hypoglycemic effect.
3. β-Adrenergic blocking agents may mask symptoms of hypoglycemia.

Iron supplements

Preparations
Ferrous fumarate—tablets, 63, 100, 195, 200, 324, 325; ER capsules, 325; suspension, 100 mg/5 ml; drops, 45 mg/0.6 ml
Ferrous gluconate—tablets 300, 320, 325 mg; capsules, 86, 325, 435 mg; elixir, 300 mg/5 ml
Ferrous sulfate—tablets, 195, 300, 325 mg; ER capsules, 150, 250, 525 mg; elixir, 220 mg/5ml; syrup, 90 mg/5 ml; drops, 75 mg/0.6 ml, 125 mg/ml
Ferrous sulfate, dried—tablets, 200 mg; ER tablets, 160 mg; capsules, 200 mg; ER capsules, 159 mg
Adult dosage
Therapeutic—PO: The equivalent of 100–200 mg of elemental iron tid
Prophylactic—PO: The equivalent of 30–60 mg of elemental iron qd
Indications: Treatment and prophylaxis of iron deficiency anemia
Action: Iron is an essential component of hemoglobin, myoglobin, and other cellular enzymes.

Elemental Iron Content of Iron Salts

Iron salt	Percent elemental iron	Elemental iron (mg/g)
Ferrous fumarate	33	330
Ferrous gluconate	11.6	120
Ferrous sulfate	20	200
Ferrous sulfate, dried	~30	300

Metabolism: None
Excretion: None; small amounts lost in urine, feces, hair, etc.
Contraindications and precautions

1. Contraindicated in hemochromatosis, hemosiderosis, and hemolytic anemias. It is generally contraindicated in peptic ulcer, regional enteritis, or ulcerative colitis.
2. Use with caution in patients receiving repeat blood transfusions.

Drug interactions

1. Antacids, calcium supplements, coffee, eggs, milk products, tea, whole-grain breads or cereals, and tetracyclines lead to decreased absorption.
2. Vitamin C may increase absorption.
3. Iron leads to decreased absorption of penicillamine.

Isoetharine (Bronkometer, Bronkosol, others)

Preparations: Isoetharine mesylate inhalation aerosol (Bronkometer), 0.34 mg/metered spray (0.61%) in 10-, 15-ml vials with oral nebulizer; isoetharine hydrochloride inhalation solution for nebulization (Bronkosol, others), 0.062, 0.08, 0.1, 0.125, 0.14, 0.167, 0.17, 0.2, 0.25, 0.5, 1%
Adult dosage: Hand nebulizer: *Isoetharine mesylate*—1–2 inhalations q4h prn. *Isoetharine HCl*—4 inhalations (range 3–7) q4h prn. Oxygen aerosolization, intermittent positive-pressure breathing: *Isoetharine HCl*—0.5–1 ml in 0.5% or 0.25–0.5 ml of a 1% solution diluted 1:3 q4h prn. For undiluted doses, consult other texts.
Indications: Treatment of bronchospasm in patients with reversible obstructive airway disease
Action: Sympathomimetic bronchodilator (β_2)
Metabolism: Hepatic > pulmonary
Excretion: Renal
Contraindications and precautions: Use with caution in cardiovascular disease, especially coronary artery disease, hypertension, limited cardiac reserve, hyperthyroidism, and pheochromocytoma.
Drug interactions

1. Digoxin and levodopa may increase cardiac arrhythmias.
2. Tricyclic antidepressants and MAO inhibitors may increase effects on vascular system.
3. Thyroid hormone may increase effect of isoetharine and vice versa.
4. Isoetharine may increase CNS stimulation of other sympathomimetics and xanthines.

Isoproterenol—Parenteral (Isuprel, others)

Preparations: Injection (IM, IV, SC), 0.2 mg/ml (1 : 5,000 solution)
Adult dosage: Cardiac stimulant: *Shock*—IV: IV infusion of 1 mg in 500 ml D5W at a rate of 0.5–5 μg/min adjusted to clinical response (BP, heart rate urine output, etc). Infusion rates >30 μg/min have been reported. *Cardiac arrest, arrhythmias:* For emergency treatment, administer by IV injection or infusion. The table below summarizes recommended dosage regimens for cardiac arrest and cardiac arrhythmias.
Indications: Adjunctive treatment of shock and cardiac standstill or arrest; treatment of Adams-Stokes syndrome, symptomatic heart block, carotid sinus hypersensitivity, and ventricular arrhythmias that require increased inotropic cardiac activity
Action: β_1- and β_2-receptor agonist resulting in positive inotropic and chronotropic effects
Metabolism: Hepatic
Excretion: Renal
Contraindications and precautions

1. Contraindicated in tachycardia or AV block caused by digitalis intoxication and cardiac arrhythmias (primarily ventricular) other than those requiring increased inotropic cardiac activity. Generally contraindicated in cardiac arrhythmias associated with tachycardia.
2. Use with caution in hypertension, coronary artery disease, coronary insufficiency, angina pectoris, hyperthyroidism, diabetes mellitus, and pheochromocytoma.

Drug interactions

1. Inhalation hydrocarbon anesthetics, digoxin, and levodopa may increase risk of arrhythmias.
2. Tricyclic antidepressants and MAO inhibitors may increase cardiovascular effects.
3. β-Adrenergic blockers may decrease cardiovascular effects of isoproterenol and vice versa.
4. Xanthine derivatives and other CNS stimulants may increase CNS stimulation.
5. Isoproterenol may increase cardiovascular effects of sympathomimetics.

Isosorbide dinitrate—Oral (Isordil, others)

Preparations: Tablets, 5, 10, 20, 30, 40 mg; SR tablets, 40 mg; capsules, 40 mg; SR capsules, 40 mg.
Adult dosage: PO: Initially, 5–20 mg q6h. Usual dosage range is 20–40 mg qid. For SR tablets or capsules: Initially, 40–80 mg q8–12h.
Note: Tolerance to nitrates has been reported and may result in increased requirements. Tolerance may be reversed with short periods (8–24 hr) of nitrate withdrawal.
Indications: Treatment and prophylaxis of chronic angina pectoris; unlabeled use includes treatment of CHF
Action: Relaxes vascular smooth muscle, reduces myocardial oxygen demand due to reduction in left ventricular preload and afterload as a result of venous > arterial dilation.
Metabolism: Hepatic
Excretion: Renal
Contraindications and precautions: Use with caution in severe anemia, cerebral hemorrhage or head trauma, glaucoma, hyperthyroidism, hypertrophic cardiomyopathy, hypotension, recent myocardial infarction, or severe hepatic or renal function impairment.
Drug interactions

1. Alcohol, antihypertensives, phenothiazines, narcotic analgesics, β-blockers, calcium channel blockers, and other hypotension-producing medications lead to increased hypotension.
2. Isosorbide leads to decreased effect of norepinephrine.

Ketoprofen (Orudis)

Preparations: Capsules, 25, 50, 75 mg
Adult dosage:
Antirheumatic—PO: Initially, 50 mg qid or 75 mg tid. Maintenance doses are 150–300 mg/day in 3–4 divided doses.

Dosage Regimens for Treatment of Cardiac Arrest and Cardiac Arrhythmias

Route	Dilution	Initial dose	Subsequent dose range
IV infusion	2 mg (10 ml) in 500 ml D5W (injection = 1:250,000)	5 μg/min (1.25ml/min)	2–20 μg/min (0.5–5 ml/min)
IV injection	0.2 mg (1 ml) in 10 ml D5W (injection = 1:50,000)	20–60 μg/min (1–3 ml/min)	10–200 μg/min (0.5–10 ml/min)
IM	undiluted = 1:5,000	200 μg (1 ml)	20 μm–1 mg prn (0.1–5 ml)
SC	undiluted = 1:5,000	200 μg (1 ml)	150–200 μg prn (0.75–1 ml)
Intracardiac	undiluted = 1:5,000	20 μg (0.1 ml)	—

* *Adapted from* Drugs used in shock. In: Olin BR. Drug facts and comparisons. Philadelphia: JB Lippincott, 1990:570.

Analgesic, antidysmenorrheal—PO: 25–50 mg q6–8h prn
Indications: Treatment of rheumatic (and nonrheumatic inflammatory) disorders, dysmenorrhea, pain, and headache. Unlabeled uses include treatment of acute gouty arthritis and calcium pyrophosphate deposition disease.
Action: Nonsteroidal anti-inflammatory drug that inhibits cyclo-oxygenase, resulting in decreased formation of prostaglandins. Effects include antirheumatic, analgesic, antipyretic, and inhibition of platelet aggregation.
Metabolism: Hepatic
Excretion: Renal (? biliary)
Contraindications and precautions
1. Contraindicated in a history of severe allergic reaction to aspirin or other NSAID.
2. Use with caution in a history of peptic ulcer, upper gastrointestinal disease or ulcerative colitis, renal or hepatic function impairment, bleeding disorders, asthma, CHF, diabetes mellitus, hypertension, and pre-existing edema.

Drug interactions
1. Acetaminophen, gold compounds, or nephrotoxic medications may increase risk of renal toxicity.
2. Glucocorticoids, alcohol, potassium supplements, other NSAID, or aspirin may increase risk of GI side effects.
3. Anticoagulants, thrombolytic agents, aspirin, platelet aggregation inhibitors, or colchicine may increase risk of hemorrhage.
4. Probenecid may increase ketoprofen serum level.
5. Ketoprofen may increase methotrexate toxicity.
6. Ketoprofen may decrease antihypertensive effects of diuretics and antihypertensives.
7. Ketoprofen may decrease diuretic effect of diuretics.
8. Ketoprofen may increase hypoglycemic effect of sulfonylureas.
9. Ketoprofen may increase digoxin, lithium, nifedipine, and verapamil blood levels.

Labetalol (Normodyne, Trandate)
Preparations: Tablets, 100, 200, 300 mg; injection (IV), 5 mg/ml
Adult dosage: PO: Initially, 100 mg bid; increase dose by 100 mg q2–3d prn. Maintenance dose is usually 200–400 mg bid. IV: Repeated IV injection—20 mg (0.25 mg/kg for 80-kg patient) over 2 min. Additional injections of 40–80 mg q10min until desired BP achieved or a total of 300 mg given. Maximum effect is 5 min after injection. IV infusion—rate of 2 mg/min, and adjust according to response. Dose range is 50–300 mg. Discontinue IV infusion when desired response obtained and start PO.
Indications: Treatment of hypertension
Action: Nonselective β-adrenergic blocking agent and selective α_1-adrenergic blocking agent
Metabolism: Hepatic
Excretion: Renal > biliary/fecal
Contraindications and precautions
1. Contraindicated in overt cardiac failure, cardiogenic shock, 2nd- or 3rd-degree AV block, sinus bradycardia, or hypotension associated with MI.
2. Use with caution in asthma, emphysema, CHF, diabetes mellitus, or mental depression.
3. Abrupt withdrawal after chronic administration can precipitate angina, MI and ventricular dysrhythmias. Dosage should be tapered over 2 wk.

Drug interactions
1. Hydrocarbon inhalation anesthetics may increase myocardial depression.
2. Insulin and antidiabetic agents may increase hypoglycemia.
3. Calcium channel blocking agents may potentiate conduction disturbance or CHF in patients with abnormal AV conduction or depressed left ventricular function.
4. Labetalol may decrease or increase cardiostimulating effect of sympathomimetics.
5. Labetalol leads to decreased bronchodilatory effect of sympathomimetics and theophylline.
6. Labetalol may significantly increase BP with MAO inhibitor use.

Lactulose (Cephulac, Cholac, others)
Preparations: Syrup, 10 g/15 ml
Adult dosage:
Constipation—PO: 15–30 ml (10-20 g) qd up to 60 ml/day; onset of action in 24–48 hr
Portosystemic encephalopathy—PO: 30–45 ml (20–30 g) q1h for initial therapy. When laxative effect is achieved, reduce to 30–45 ml tid–qid titrated to produce about 3 soft stools per day. PR: Mix 300 ml with 700 ml water or normal saline as a retention enema for 30–60 min; repeat q4–6h prn. Use when oral therapy is not possible.
Indications: Treatment of constipation; treatment and prevention of portosystemic encephalopathy
Action: Synthetic disaccharide metabolized to acids in the colon, that facilitate conversion of ammonia to ammonium ion; laxative effect from osmotic effect promotes expulsion of ammonium
Metabolism: Unknown (<3% absorbed)
Excretion: Renal (of absorbed dose)
Contraindications and precautions
1. Oral preparation contraindicated in nausea, vomiting, or other symptoms of appendicitis, acute surgical abdomen, or intestinal obstruction.
2. Use with caution in diabetes or patients requiring low galactose diet, colostomy, or ileostomy.

Levodopa (Dopar, Laradopa), **Carbidopa** (Lodosyn), **Carbidopa and Levodopa** (Sinemet)
Preparations:
Levodopa: Tablets, 100, 250, 500 mg; capsules, 100, 250, 500 mg
Carbidopa: tablets, 25 mg
Carbidopa/levodopa: Tablets, 10 mg/100 mg, 25 mg/100 mg, 25 mg/250 mg
Adult dosage
Levodopa—PO: Initially, 250 mg bid–qid. Increase by 100–750 mg q3–7d until desired response, a maximum of 8 g/day, or intolerable side effects. Usual optimal dose is 3–6 g/day. Some sources recommend 6 or 7 divided doses/day.
Carbidopa/levodopa: *Patients not currently receiving levodopa*—PO: initially, 10/100 mg tid–qid or 25/100 mg tid. Increase dose by 1 tablet q1–2d until maximum of 8 tablets of 10/100 mg or 6 tablets of 25/100 mg/day. If higher doses of levodopa are required, use 25/250 mg tid–qid and increase by ½–1 tablet q1–2d until a maximum of 8 tablets/day. *Patients currently receiving levodopa:* Levodopa must be discontinued at least 8h before initiating therapy. The initial dose should provide no more than 25% of the previous levodopa dosage. *Patients who require <1.5 g of levodopa/day*—PO: Initially, 25/100 mg tid–qid and increase q1–2d prn. *Patients who require >1.5 g of levodopa/day*—PO: Initially, 25/250 mg tid–qid, and increase q1–2d prn.
Note
1. Peripheral carboxylase is fully inhibited at carbidopa doses of 70–100 mg/day. Additional carbidopa may be given to those requiring low doses of levodopa and utilizing the 10/100 preparation.
2. Geriatric and postencephalitic patients may be more sensitive to usual doses.

Indications: Treatment of parkinsonism
Action: Levodopa crosses the blood-brain barrier and is decarboxylated into dopamine in the basal ganglia. Carbidopa inhibits peripheral decarboxylation of levodopa, increasing availability of levodopa for transport to the central nervous system.
Metabolism: Carbidopa—minimal; levodopa—bowel, hepatic
Excretion: Carbidopa—renal; levodopa—renal
Contraindications and precautions
1. Contraindicated in concurrent MAO inhibitor use.
2. Use with caution in severe pulmonary disease, severe cardiovascular disease, or history of MI with residual dysrhythmias, angle-closure glaucoma, history of or suspected melanoma, history of peptic ulcer disease, psychoses, renal function impairment, urinary retention, hypothalamic/pituitary function disorders, or diabetes mellitus.

Drug interactions
1. MAO inhibitors lead to hypertensive crises.
2. Phenytoin, phenothiazines, butyrophenones, thioxanthines, and possibly benzodiazepines lead to decreased effect.
3. Cocaine and inhalation hydrocarbon anesthetics lead to increased risk of arrhythmia.
4. Pyridoxine (vitamin B_6) reverses toxic and therapeutic effects of levodopa. Antagonistic effect lost with administration of carbidopa.
5. Anticholinergics lead to mild increased effect; higher doses lead to decreased GI absorption of levodopa.
6. Hypotension-producing agents lead to additive decreased BP effect.

Levorphanol tartrate (Levo-Dromoran)—Schedule II
Preparations: Tablets, 2 mg; injection (SC), 2 mg/ml

Adult dosage: Analgesic —PO: 2 mg or 3–4 mg if pain is severe. SC: 2 mg or 3 mg if pain is severe; frequency of administration not well defined

Note

1. Use lower doses in geriatric patients.
2. Administer smallest effective dose and as infrequently as possible to minimize tolerance and physical dependence.

Indications: Treatment of pain as an adjunct to anesthesia

Action: Narcotic analgesic

Metabolism: Hepatic

Excretion: Renal

Contraindications and precautions

1. Contraindicated in diarrhea associated with pseudomembranous colitis, diarrhea caused by poisoning until the toxic material has been eliminated, and acute respiratory depression.
2. Psychological and physical dependence and tolerance to many of the effects of levorphanol tartrate may develop with chronic administration.
3. Use with caution in acute abdominal conditions, acute asthma or chronic respiratory impairment, head injury, increased intracranial pressure, intracranial lesions, hepatic or renal function impairment, hypothyroidism, gallbladder disease, inflammatory bowel disease, recent GI tract surgery, prostatic hypertrophy or obstruction, urethral stricture, acute alcoholism, Addison's disease, epilepsy, suicidal ideation, emotional instability, or history of drug abuse.
4. Use with caution in patients performing tasks requiring mental alertness or physical coordination.
5. Use with caution in patients being administered MAO inhibitors.

Drug interactions

1. Alcohol, other opioid agonist analgesics, and other CNS depressants (including antihistamines, phenothiazines, tricyclic antidepressants, benzodiazepines, sedative-hypnotics, barbiturates) may increase risk of CNS depression.
2. Antidiarrheals and anticholinergics lead to increased risk of constipation.
3. Antihypertensives and diuretics lead to increased risk of hypotension.
4. Naltrexone, naloxone, and buprenorphine may block certain opioid actions. Consult other texts for further information.

Levothyroxine sodium—L-Thyroxine, T$_4$ (Synthroid, others)

Preparations: Tablets, 25, 50, 75, 100, 112, 125, 150, 175, 200, 300 μg; injection (IV), 200, 500 μg/vial

Adult dosage

Mild hypothyroidism—PO: Initially, 50 μg qd; increase by 25–50 μg/day q2–4wk until desired response

Severe hypothyroidism—PO: Initially, 12.5–25 μg qd; increase by 25 μg/day q2–3wk until desired response

Hypothyroidism maintenance—PO: Usual dose range is 75–200 μg/day as a single dose. IV: Usual dose approximately ½ previously established PO dose

Myxedema coma or stupor—IV: Initially, 200–500 μg as a single dose; if no improvement after 24 hr, may administer additional 100–300 μg. Give daily parenteral maintenance dose of 50–200 μg qd until stabilized and PO can be taken.

Note: In the elderly and in patients with longstanding hypothyroidism or cardiovascular disease, initial replacement doses should be lower (12.5–25 μg qd) and increased q3–4wk. Maintenance doses are also usually lower.

Indications: Treatment of hypothyroidism; treatment and prophylaxis of various types of euthyroid goiters, thyrotropin-dependent thyroid gland carcinoma, and, in conjunction with antithyroid agents, treatment of thyrotoxicosis

Action: Unclear mechanism of action; results in increased metabolic rate of body tissues. Effects include increased protein synthesis, decreased serum cholesterol concentration, and increased gluconeogenesis; necessary for growth and development.

Metabolism: Hepatic

Excretion: Biliary/fecal

Contraindications and precautions

1. Contraindicated in thyrotoxicosis, acute myocardial infarction uncomplicated by hypothyroidism, and uncorrected adrenal insufficiency.
2. Use with caution in cardiovascular disease, history of hyperthyroidism, thyrotoxicosis being treated with antithyroid medication, diabetes mellitus, and pituitary insufficiency.
3. Patients with longstanding hypothyroidism or myxedema may be more sensitive to the effects levothyroxine; start replacement therapy with low doses.

Drug interactions

1. Cholestyramine and colestipol lead to decreased absorption.
2. Tricyclic antidepressants lead to increased effect.
3. β-Adrenergic blockers lead to decreased peripheral conversion of thyroxine (T$_4$) to triiodothyronine (T$_3$).
4. Estrogens may increase requirements of levothyroxine.
5. Ketamine leads to hypertension and tachycardia.
6. Levothyroxine may decrease effect of digoxin.
7. Levothyroxine leads to increased antidepressant effect of tricyclic antidepressants.
8. Levothyroxine leads to increased adrenergic effect of catecholamines and sympathomimetics.
9. Levothyroxine leads to increased effect of coumadin.

Lidocaine—Systemic (Xylocaine, others)

Preparations: Injection (IM), 100 mg/ml; (IV) for direct IV injection, 10 mg/ml, 20 mg/ml; (IV) for infusion and admixtures, 40 mg/ml, 100 mg/ml, 200 mg/ml; (IV) with 5% dextrose for IV infusion, 2 mg/ml, 4 mg/ml, 8 mg/ml

Adult dosage: IV: An IV bolus is used to establish rapid therapeutic levels. The usual bolus dose is 50–100 mg (1 mg/kg) given at a rate of 25–50 mg/min. If the desired response is not obtained, a second bolus of ⅓ to ½ of the first dose may be given in 5 min. Maintenance infusion to maintain antiarrhythmic effect is administered at a rate of 20–50 μg/kg/min (1–4 mg/min). Use lower rates for geriatric patients or those with CHF or hepatic function impairment. If arrhythmias reappear during continuous IV infusion, administer a small bolus and increase the infusion rate unless signs or symptoms of toxicity are present. IM (not preferred route): 300 mg (4.3 mg/kg) repeated in 60–90 min if necessary.

Indications: Treatment of ventricular arrhythmias

Action: A class IB antiarrhythmic; decreases phase 4 diastolic depolarization, automaticity, and excitability ventricles

Metabolism: Hepatic

Excretion: Renal

Contraindications and precautions

1. Contraindicated in known hypersensitivity to amide type anesthetics, Adams-Stokes syndrome, Wolff-Parkinson-White syndrome, and severe heart block (sinoatrial, atrioventricular, or intraventricular)
2. Use with caution in CHF, hepatic and renal function impairment, reduced hepatic blood flow, hypovolemia, shock, sinus bradycardia, incomplete heart block, and atrial fibrillation or flutter.
3. Continuous ECG monitoring is required. Stop lidocaine if there is prolongation of the P-R interval, widening of the QRS complex, or if aggravation of arrythmias occurs.

Drug interactions

1. Phenytoin lead to additive cardiac depressant effects.
2. Cimetidine and β-adrenergic blockers lead to increased serum lidocaine concentration.
3. Lidocaine leads to increased neuromuscular blocking effect of succinylcholine.

Lindane—Gamma benzene hexachloride (Kwell, others)

Preparations: Cream, 1%; lotion, 1%; shampoo, 1%

Adult dosage

Scabicide—cream or lotion: Apply to all skin surfaces from neck to soles of feet. After 8–12 hr, remove by washing. One application of 20–30 g is usually curative.

Pediculosis—cream or lotion: Apply to affected hairy areas and adjacent areas. After 8–12 hr, remove by washing. Reapply only if living lice are demonstrable after 7 days. Shampoo: Apply 15–60 ml (short or long-hair) and lather for 4–5 min. Rinse thoroughly and dry. Comb with fine-tooth comb to remove remaining nit shells. Reapply if living lice are demonstrable after 7 days.

Indications: Treatment of scabies and pediculosis captitis (head lice) or pubis (crab lice)

Action: Ectoparasiticide

Metabolism: Hepatic (slow topical absorption)

Excretion: Renal, fecal

Contraindications and precautions

1. Use with caution in seizure disorder.
2. Avoid mucous membranes and acutely inflamed skin.
3. Sexual partners and household contacts should receive prophylactic treatment for scabies.

Drug interactions: No clinically significant interactions

Lisinopril (Prinivil, Zestril)

Preparations: Tablets, 5, 10, 20, 40 mg
Adult dosage: Antihypertensive—PO: Initially, 10 mg qd. Increase prn up to 40 mg/day as a single daily dose. An initial dose of 5 mg should be used in patients who are salt/volume depleted, on diuretics, or have renal function impairment (creatinine clearance ≥10, ≤30 ml/min). Use 2.5 mg if creatinine clearance <10.
Indications: Treatment of hypertension
Action: Angiotensin converting enzyme inhibitor with antihypertensive and vasodilator effects
Metabolism: None
Excretion: Renal
Contraindications and precautions
1. May cause profound hypotension following the first dose, especially if patient is salt-volume depleted.
2. Use with caution in hyperkalemia, bilateral renal artery stenosis, solitary kidney, renal function impairment, or salt-volume depletion.

Drug interactions
1. Potassium-sparing diuretics, potassium supplements, and salt substitutes lead to increased risk of hyperkalemia.
2. Diuretics and other renin-releasing antihypertensive agents lead to increased antihypertensive effect.

Lithium carbonate (Eskalith, Lithobid, others)

Preparations: Tablets, 300 mg; SR tablets, 300, 450 mg; capsules, 150, 300 mg
Adult dosage
Acute mania—PO: Initially, 300–600 mg tid or 600–900 mg bid for SR tablets. An effective serum level is usually 1–1.5 mEq/L. Titrate dose to clinical response and patient tolerance. Monitor serum level q3–4d.
Bipolar disorder—PO: Usually 300 mg tid–qid. An effective serum level is usually 0.6–1.2 mEq/L. Maximum daily dosage is 2.4 g. Monitor serum levels q2–3m.
Note
1. Use lower doses in geriatric or debilitated patients.
2. Lithium toxicity may occur at or near therapeutic serum lithium levels (0.8–1.2 mEq/L for acute mania; 0.5–1.0 mEq/L for maintenance).
3. During episodes of acute mania, the patient may have a greater ability to tolerate lithium. This tolerance decreases with resolution of the mania and may require a corresponding adjustment.

Indications: Treatment of acute mania, and treatment and prophylaxis of bipolar disorder. Unlabeled uses include treatment of neutropenia and prophylaxis of vascular headache.
Action: Unknown mechanism of action
Metabolism: None
Excretion: Renal
Contraindications and precautions
1. Relatively contraindicated in history of leukemia, severe cardiovascular or renal disease, severe debilitation, dehydration, or sodium depletion.
2. Use with caution in cardiovascular disease, renal function impairment, CNS disorders, dehydration, concurrent diuretics, sodium depletion, hypothyroidism, and psoriasis.
3. Lithium has caused an acquired nephrogenic diabetes insipidus.
4. Use with caution while performing tasks requiring mental alertness.

Drug interactions
1. Diuretics lead to increased risk of lithium toxicity.
2. NSAIDs, haloperidol, phenothiazines, methyldopa, metronidazole, and molindone may increase effects of lithium.
3. Iodide salts lead to increased risk of hypothyroidism.
4. Sympathomimetic amines may decrease effects of lithium.
5. Lithium may increase effects of depolarizing and nondepolarizing neuromuscular blocking agents.

Loperamide (Imodium)

Preparations: Capsules, 2 mg; solution, 1 mg/5 ml
Adult dosage
Acute diarrhea—PO: Initially, 4 mg followed by 2 mg after each unformed stool. Maximum daily dosage is 16 mg. Discontinue if no improvement after 48 hr of therapy.
Chronic diarrhea—PO: Initially, 4 mg followed by 2 mg after each unformed stool until symptoms are controlled. Taper to maintenance dose, usually 4–8 mg/day as a single dose or in divided doses.
Indications: Treatment of diarrhea
Action: Slows intestinal motility by inhibiting peristalsis via a direct effect on intestinal wall muscles
Metabolism: Hepatic
Excretion: Fecal >> renal
Contraindications and precautions
1. Contraindicated in diarrhea associated with organisms that penetrate the intestinal mucosa or in pseudomembranous colitis associated with broad-spectrum antibiotics.
2. Use with caution in acute ulcerative colitis, infectious diarrhea, or hepatic function impairment.

Lorazepam (Ativan, others)

Preparations: Tablets, 0.5, 1, 2 mg; injection (IM, IV), 2 mg/ml, 4 mg/ml
Adult dosage
Antianxiety—PO: 2–3 mg/day in divided doses. IM: 0.05 mg/kg up to 4 mg. IV: 0.044 mg/kg up to 2 mg, or whichever is less.
Sedative-hypnotic—PO: 2–4 mg qhs. IM, IV: As for antianxiety.
Amnestic—IM: As for antianxiety; administer at least 2 hr before surgery. IV: As for antianxiety; administer 15–20 min before surgery. For greater amnestic effect, may use up to 0.05 mg/kg, not to exceed a maximum of 4 mg.
Note: Use lower doses in elderly or debilitated patients.
Indications: Treatment of anxiety disorders or anxiety associated with depression; parenterally, adjunctive therapy prior to surgery, endoscopic procedures, or cardioversion for anxiety and to diminish patient's recall
Action: Anxiolytic sedative-hypnotic benzodiazepine may potentiate CNS gamma-aminobutyric acid effects; amnestic effect of unclear mechanism
Metabolism: Hepatic (glucuronidation)
Excretion: Renal
Contraindications and precautions
1. Contraindicated in acute alcohol intoxication with depressed vital signs, depressive neuroses, or psychoses without prominent anxiety.
2. Use with caution in acute narrow-angle glaucoma, myasthenia gravis, shock, severe chronic obstructive pulmonary disease, hepatic or renal impairment, patients with depressed respirations, or those receiving concurrent respiratory depressants.
3. Long-term therapy may result in psychic or physical dependence.
4. Exercise caution in performing tasks requiring alertness and coordination.

Drug interactions
1. Lorazepam may increase zidovudine (AZT) toxicity
2. Alcohol or other CNS depressants lead to increased CNS depression.

Lovastatin (Mevacor)

Preparations: Tablets, 20, 40 mg
Adult dosage: PO: Initially, 20 mg with the evening meal; increase by 20 mg q4wk up to 80 mg/day as single or bid doses
Indications: Treatment of hyperlipidemia (primary hypercholesterolemia due to elevated LDL)
Action: Inhibits HMG-CoA reductase, causing decreased hepatic cholesterol synthesis and increased LDL catabolism; results in a reduction of serum LDL (cholesterol), VLDL, and triglyceride levels, and slightly increases HDL levels
Metabolism: Hepatic
Excretion: Fecal > renal
Contraindications and precautions
1. Contraindicated in active hepatic disease.
2. Use with caution in patient with alcoholism, past history of hepatic disease, or any risk factor predisposing to the development of rhabdomyolysis.
3. Slit-lamp ophthalmic examination for lenticular opacities should be done before therapy and yearly thereafter.
4. Stop therapy if serum transaminases increase three times or more the upper limit of normal or if myopathy or markedly elevated creatine kinase levels occur.
5. Contraindicated in pregnancy and in women who may become pregnant.

Drug interactions: Cyclosporine, gemfibrozil, or high doses of niacin may increase risk of myositis.

Magnesium sulfate

Preparations: Injection (IM, IV), 10, 12.5, 25, 50%; contains 1, 1.25, 2.5, 5 g/10 ml and 8, 10, 20, 40 mEq of magnesium/10 ml, respectively
Adult dosage
Anticonvulsant—IM: 1–5 g as a 25–50% solution up to 6 times/day into alternate buttocks. IV: 1–4 g as a 10–20% solution at a rate not to exceed 150 mg/min (equivalent of 1.5 ml of a 10% solution). For continuous IV infusion: 4 g in 250 ml

of D/W or normal saline at a rate not to exceed 3–4 ml/min.
Hypomagnesemia: Mild–IM: 1 g q6h for 4 doses. Severe—IM: 250 mg (2mEq/kg) over a 4-hr period. IV infusion: 5 g in 1 L D/W or normal saline administered over 3 hr
Total parenteral nutrition—IV: Usually 8–24 mEq/day
Indications: Treatment of seizures in eclampsia, pre-eclampsia, or other conditions in which hypomagnesemia may be a contributing cause; treatment and prophylaxis of hypomagnesemia
Note: Use lower doses in geriatric patients and those with renal function impairment.
Action: Depresses the CNS and blocks peripheral neuromuscular transmission
Metabolism: None
Excretion: Renal
Contraindications and precautions
1. Contraindicated in renal failure, heart block, or myocardial damage.
2. Use with caution in renal function impairment.
3. An IV calcium salt preparation should be readily available. IV calcium gluconate, 5–10 mEq or 10–20 ml of a 10% solution, will usually reverse heart block or respiratory depression.

Drug interactions
1. CNS depressants may increase CNS depression.
2. Neuromuscular blocking agents may increase risk of excessive blockade.
3. Digoxin may increase risk of cardiac conduction changes such as heart block.

Meclizine (Antivert, others)
Preparations: Tablets, 12.5, 25, 50 mg
Adult dosage
Antivertigo—PO: 25–100 mg/day in divided doses
Antimotion sickness—PO: 25–50 mg 1 hr before travel, repeated q24h prn
Indications: Prophylaxis and treatment of vertigo associated with diseases affecting the vestibular system and motion sickness
Action: Antiemetic, antivertigo, and antimotion sickness effect of unclear mechanism; has antihistaminic and anticholinergic activity
Metabolism: Unknown
Excretion: Renal, fecal
Contraindications and precautions
1. Use with caution in bladder neck obstruction, prostatic hypertrophy, or angle-closure glaucoma.
2. Use with caution in activities requiring mental alertness or physical coordination.

Drug interactions: Alcohol or other CNS depressants lead to increased CNS depression.

Medroxyprogesterone acetate (Provera, others)
Preparations: Tablets, 2.5, 5, 10 mg; injection (IM), 25 mg/ml, 100 mg/ml, 400 mg/ml
Adult dosage
Secondary amenorrhea, dysfunctional uterine bleeding—PO: 5–10 mg qd for 5–10 days. For amenorrhea, start any time but preferably during the assumed latter half (e.g., 16th–21st day) of the menstrual cycle. For dysfunctional uterine bleeding, start on the calculated day 16 or 21 of the menstrual cycle. To induce optimum secretory transformation of an endometrium that has been adequately primed with endogenous or exogenous estrogen, give 10 mg for 10 days starting on day 16 of the cycle. Withdrawal bleeding usually occurs within 3–7 days after stopping therapy.
Endometrial or renal carcinoma—IM: Initially, 400–1,000 mg every week. If improvement is noted, it may be possible to maintain improvement with as little as 400 mg every month.
Indications: Treatment of secondary amenorrhea and abnormal uterine bleeding due to hormonal imbalance; adjunctive and palliative treatment of advanced and inoperable endometrial or renal carcinoma, hypoventilation syndromes
Action: A progestin; transforms proliferative into secretory endometrium, and with high doses, inhibits release of luteinizing hormone from the anterior pituitary; mechanism of antineoplastic activity unknown
Metabolism: Hepatic
Excretion: Fecal > renal
Contraindications and precautions
1. Contraindicated in carcinoma of the breast or reproductive organs, hepatic dysfunction, thrombophlebitis or thromboembolic disorder, undiagnosed vaginal bleeding, missed abortion, or suspected pregnancy.
2. Use with caution in asthma, epilepsy, migraine headaches, and cardiac or renal function impairment.
3. Use with caution in hyperlipidemia or mental depression.

Drug interactions: Progestins interfere with effects of bromocriptine.

Menadiol sodium diphosphate (see *Vitamin K*)

Meperidine hydrochloride (Demerol, others)—Schedule II
Preparations: Tablets, 50, 100 mg; solution, 50 mg/5 ml; injection (IM, IV, SC), 25, 50, 75, 100 mg/ml
Adult dosage
Analgesic—PO, injection, IM, SC: 50–150 mg q3–4h prn; IV: continuous infusion at 15–35 mg/hr
Anesthesia adjunct—*Preoperatively*—Injection (IM, SC): 50–100 mg, 30–90 min prior to anesthesia. *Intraoperatively*—Injection (IV): Repeated slow IV injections of a solution diluted to 10 mg/ml or continuous infusion of a solution diluted to 1 mg/ml; individualize dosage
Note
1. IM preferred over SC administration.
2. Administer smallest effective dose and as infrequently as possible to minimize tolerance and physical dependence.

Indications: Treatment of pain and as an adjunct to anesthesia
Action: Narcotic analgesic
Metabolism: Hepatic
Excretion: Renal
Contraindications and precautions
1. Contraindicated in MAO inhibitor use, diarrhea associated with pseudomembranous colitis, diarrhea caused by poisoning until the toxic material has been eliminated, and acute respiratory depression.
2. Psychological and physical dependence and tolerance to many of the effects of meperidine hydrochloride may develop with chronic administration.
3. Use with caution in acute abdominal conditions, acute asthma or chronic respiratory impairment, head injury, increased intracranial pressure, intracranial lesions, hepatic or renal function impairment, atrial flutter or supraventricular tachycardias, hypothyroidism, gallbladder disease, inflammatory bowel disease, recent GI tract surgery, prostatic hypertrophy or obstruction, urethral stricture, acute alcoholism, Addison's disease, epilepsy, suicidal ideation, emotional instability, or history of drug abuse.
4. Use with caution in patients performing tasks requiring mental alertness or physical coordination.
5. Use with caution in patients being administered MAO inhibitors.

Drug interactions
1. MAO inhibitors may cause severe unpredictable and possibly fatal reactions.
2. Alcohol, other opioid agonist analgesics, and other CNS depressants (including antihistamines, phenothiazines, tricyclic antidepressants, benzodiazepines, sedative-hypnotics, barbiturates) may increase risk of CNS depression.
3. Antidiarrheals and anticholinergics lead to increased risk of constipation.
4. Antihypertensives and diuretics lead to increased risk of hypotension.
5. Naltrexone, naloxone, and buprenorphine may block certain opioid actions. Consult other texts for further information.

Mestranol—Estrogen (see *Oral contraceptives*)

Metaproterenol (Alupent, Metaprel)
Preparations: Tablets, 10, 20 mg; syrup, 10 mg/5 ml; aerosol, 650 μg (0.65 mg) per metered spray in 225 mg/canister; solution for inhalation, 0.4, 0.6% in unit-dose vials, 5% in 225 mg/canister
Adult dosage: PO: 20 mg tid–qid; aerosol: 1.3–1.95 mg (2–3 inhalations) q3–4h not to exceed 12 inhalations/day; solution for inhalation: Usually not more than q4h for acute bronchospasm and tid–qid for chronic bronchospastic disease. For 0.4 or 0.6% unit-dose vial, use one vial per nebulization treatment or 0.2–0.3 ml of 5% solution diluted to 2.5 ml administered through nebulizer or intermittent positive-pressure breathing (each vial of 0.4% = 0.2 ml of 5% solution diluted to 2.5 ml with normal saline; each vial of 0.6% = 0.3 ml of 5% solution diluted to 2.5 ml with normal saline).
Indications: Treatment of bronchospasm in patients with reversible obstructive airway disease
Action: Sympathomimetic bronchodilator (β_2)
Metabolism: Hepatic
Excretion: Renal

Contraindications and precautions: Use with caution in diabetes, hyperthyroidism, pheochromocytoma, and cardiovascular disease, especially arrhythmias, CHF, coronary artery disease, and hypertension

Drug interactions

1. Inhalation anesthetics lead to increased cardiovascular toxicity.
2. Digoxin and levodopa lead to increased cardiac arrhythmias.
3. β-Adrenergic blocking agents lead to decreased bronchodilating effect
4. Metaproterenol lead to increased CNS stimulation with use of other sympathomimetics or xanthines.
5. Metaproterenol leads to increased effect of thyroid hormone and vice versa.

Methadone hydrochloride (Dolophine hydrochloride, others)—Schedule II

Preparations: Tablets, 5, 10 mg; solution 5 mg/5 ml, 10 mg/5 ml; injection (IM, SC), 10 mg/ml

Adult dosage

Analgesic—PO, IM, SC: 2.5–10 mg q3–4h. Individualize dosage, especially in severe pain or if tolerance develops.

Detoxification—PO, IM, SC: 15–40 mg qd depending on opiate tolerance of patient. Consult other texts for further details.

Maintenance—PO: Dosage must be individualized. Consult other texts for further details.

Note

1. Use lower doses in geriatric patients.
2. Administer smallest effective dose and as infrequently as possible to minimize tolerance and physical dependence.
3. The oral concentrate containing 10 mg/ml is used only for methadone detoxification and maintenance.
4. IM preferred over SC administration.

Indications: Treatment of pain and treatment and prophylaxis of opioid narcotic abstinence syndrome; used for detoxification from illicit narcotic drug use

Action: Narcotic analgesic

Metabolism: Hepatic

Excretion: Renal >> biliary

Contraindications and precautions

1. Contraindicated in diarrhea associated with pseudomembranous colitis, diarrhea caused by poisoning until the toxic material has been eliminated, and acute respiratory depression.
2. Psychological and physical dependence and tolerance to many of the effects of methadone hydrochloride may develop with chronic administration.
3. Use with caution in acute abdominal conditions, acute asthma or chronic respiratory impairment, head injury, increased intracranial pressure, intracranial lesions, hepatic or renal function impairment, hypothyroidism, gallbladder disease, inflammatory bowel disease, recent GI tract surgery, prostatic hypertrophy or obstruction, urethral stricture, acute alcoholism, Addison's disease, epilepsy, suicidal ideation, emotional instability or history of drug abuse.
4. Use with caution in patients performing tasks requiring mental alertness or physical coordination.
5. Use with caution in patients being administered MAO inhibitors.

Drug interactions

1. Alcohol, other opioid agonist analgesics, and other CNS depressants (including antihistamines, phenothiazines, tricyclic antidepressants, benzodiazepines, sedative-hypnotics, barbiturates) may increase risk of CNS depression.
2. Antidiarrheals and anticholinergics lead to increased risk of constipation.
3. Antihypertensives and diuretics lead to increased risk of hypotension.
4. Naltrexone, naloxone, and buprenorphine may block certain opioid actions. Consult other texts for further information.

Methimazole (Tapazole)

Preparations: Tablets, 5, 10 mg

Adult dosage

Hyperthyroidism—PO: Initially, 15, 30–40, or 60 mg/day in 1–2 divided doses for mild, moderate, or severe hyperthyroidism, respectively. When patient is euthyroid, continue for additional 2 mo and then reduce to maintenance dosage, usually 5–30 mg/day in 1–2 divided doses.

Thyrotoxic crisis—PO: As adjunct to other measures, 15–20 mg q4h on the first day and then reduced as symptoms are controlled.

Indications: Treatment of hyperthyroidism

Action: Inhibits synthesis of thyroid hormone

Metabolism: Hepatic

Excretion: Renal

Contraindications and precautions

1. Monitor for signs or symptoms of illness, particularly infection; perform CBC in patients who develop fever or illness.
2. Use with caution in bone marrow depression, infection, or hepatic function impairment.

Drug interactions: Lithium, potassium iodide, or iodinated glycerol may increase risk of hypothyroidism and goiter.

Methylprednisolone (Medrol, others)

Preparations: Tablets, 2, 4, 8, 16, 24, 32 mg; acetate injection (IM, intra-articular, intralesional, soft-tissue), 20, 40, 80 mg/ml; sodium succinate injection (IM, IV), 40, 125, 500, 1,000, 20,000 mg/vial

Adult dosage: PO: 4–48 mg/day as a single dose or in divided doses depending on indication; IM (acetate): Usually 40–120 mg at intervals of qd to q2wk depending on indication; intra-articular, intralesional, soft tissue: Consult other texts; IM, IV (sodium succinate): Usually 10–40 mg repeated up to q4h with higher doses for life-threatening situations. Direct IV injection is given over 1 min. For high-dose "pulse" therapy, administer 30 mg/kg IV infusion over 30 min q4–6h prn up to 48–72 hr.

Indications: Replacement therapy in the treatment of adrenal insufficiency states, and for anti-inflammatory and immunosuppressant effects in the treatment of many disorders, consult further texts for specific therapeutic regimens in selected disorders

Action: Adrenocorticoid with anti-inflammatory, immunosuppressant, and minimal mineralocorticoid effects. Other effects include suppression of the hypothalamic-pituitary-adrenal (HPA) axis, increased protein catabolism, increased blood glucose concentrations, insulin resistance, reduced intestinal absorption and increased renal excretion of calcium, and neutrophilia. See also table, page 708.

Metabolism: Primarily hepatic

Excretion: Renal

Contraindications and precautions

1. Use with caution in cardiac disease, CHF, hypertension, hepatic or renal function impairment, AIDS or other immunodeficiency states, uncontrolled bacterial or viral infection, systemic-fungal infection, tuberculosis (active, latent or positive skin test), ocular herpes simplex, diabetes mellitus, nonspecific ulcerative colitis, diverticulitis, esophagitis, gastritis, history of peptic ulcer, recent intestinal anastamosis, open-angle glaucoma, hyperthyroidism, hypoalbuminuria, myasthenia gravis, osteoporosis, or seizure disorder.
2. Administer daily dose in the morning to reduce HPA-axis suppressive effects. Alternate-day dosing may reduce the risk of adrenal suppression.
3. Withdrawal following long-term therapy with pharmacologic doses requires a gradual taper until the HPA axis recovers.

Drug interactions

1. Alcohol, aspirin, and NSAIDs may increase risk of GI ulceration.
2. Amphotericin B and diuretics may increase risk of hypokalemia.
3. Estrogens may increase effects.
4. Ephedrine, phenytoin, phenobarbital, and rifampin may decrease effects.
5. Immunosuppressants lead to decreased risk of infection.
6. Erythromycin may increase effects.
7. Methylprednisolone may decrease effect of coumadin, oral antidiabetic agents, and insulin.
8. Methylprednisolone may decrease effect of isoniazid.
9. Pharmacologic doses of methylprednisolone may potentiate replication of live virus in vaccines or decrease antibody response to the vaccine.

Metolazone (Diulo, Mykrox, Zaroxolyn)

Preparations: Prompt metolazone—Mykrox: Tablets, 0.5 mg; extended metolazone—Diulo and Zaroxolyn: tablets, 2.5, 5, 10 mg

Note: Prompt preparation is more rapidly and extensively absorbed than extended form. Do not substitute one for another.

Adult dosage

Diuretic—PO: *Extended preparations*—Initially, 5–10 mg qd for edema of CHF and 5–20 mg qd for edema of renal disease

Antihypertensive—PO: *Extended preparation*—Initially, 2.5–5 mg qd; adjust according to BP response. If adding to another antihypertensive agent, start with 2.5 mg qd. *Prompt preparation*—Initially, 0.5 mg qd. If inadequate BP response, the dose can be increased to a maximum 1 mg qd.

Indications: Treatment of hypertension and edema

Action: Thiazide diuretic that inhibits renal tubular reabsorption of sodium and water in the distal tubule. Unlike the thiazides, it may produce diuresis in patients with a GFR <20 ml/min. It also increases urinary excretion of potassium and decreases urinary excretion of calcium and uric acid. Antihypertensive mechanism unknown.
Metabolism: Minimal
Excretion: Renal
Contraindications and precautions
1. Contraindicated in anuria, hepatic coma or pre-coma, and hypersensitivity to thiazides or other sulfonamide derivatives.
2. Use with caution in diabetes mellitus, history of gout, hyperuricemia, hepatic function impairment, hypercalcemia, systemic lupus erythematosus, sympathectomy, or electrolyte disturbances.
3. Electrolyte disturbances may occur; monitor serum electrolytes.

Drug interactions
1. Cholestyramine and colestipol lead to decreased absorption.
2. Glucocorticoids and amphotericin B lead to increased risk of hypokalemia.
3. Metolazone leads to increased risk of lithium toxicity.
4. Metolazone leads to increased risk of toxicity of digoxin, amiodarone, and nondepolarizing neuromuscular blocking agents due to hypokalemia.

Metoprolol tartrate (Lopressor)

Preparations: Tablets, 50, 100 mg; injection (IV), 1 mg/ml
Adult dosage
Antianginal—PO: Initially, 100 mg/day in 2 divided doses; increase q7d up to 400 mg/day
Antihypertensive—PO: Initially, 100 mg/day in single or divided doses; increase q7d up to 450 mg/day
Myocardial infarction prophylaxis: *Early treatment:* Initiate as soon as possible if definite or suspected acute MI. Administer 3 IV bolus injections of 5 mg q2min for 3 doses. If full IV dose (15 mg) tolerated, start 50 mg PO q6h 15 min after last IV dose for 48 hr. If full IV dose not tolerated, start 25–50 mg PO q6h 15 min after last IV dose for 48 hr. *Late treatment:* In patients with contraindications to early treatment, in those whose therapy was delayed, or in those who complete early treatment, start 100 mg PO bid for 3 or more months.
Indications: Treatment of chronic angina and hypertension and prophylaxis of myocardial infarction
Action: Selective β_1-adrenergic blocking agent
Metabolism: Hepatic
Excretion: Renal
Contraindications and precautions
1. Contraindicated in overt cardiac failure, cardiogenic shock, 2nd- or 3rd-degree AV block, sinus bradycardia, and hypotension associated with MI.
2. Use with caution in asthma, emphysema, CHF, diabetes mellitus, mental depression, or peripheral vascular disease.
3. Abrupt withdrawal after chronic administration can precipitate angina, MI, and ventricular dysrhythmias. Dosage should be tapered over 2 wk.

Drug interactions
1. Hydrocarbon inhalation anesthetics may increase myocardial depression.
2. Insulin or antidiabetic agents may increase hypoglycemia.
3. Calcium channel blocking agents may increase conduction disturbance or CHF in patients with abnormal AV conduction or depressed left ventricular function.
4. Metoprolol may increase or decrease cardiostimulating effects of sympathomimetics.
5. Metoprolol leads to decreased bronchodilatory effect of sympathomimetics and theophylline.
6. Metoprolol may significantly increase BP with MAO inhibitor use.

Midazolam (Versed)

Preparations: Injection (IM, IV), 1 mg/ml, 5 mg/ml
Adult dosage
Preoperative sedation and amnesia: IM, 0.07–0.08 mg/kg, 30–60 min before surgery
Preprocedure conscious sedation: *Healthy and <60 yr old:* Individualize dose and titrate slowly. Unpremedicated—IV: Initially, no more than 2.5 mg given over 2 min immediately prior to the procedure. Evaluate sedative effect after at least 2 min; may titrate further in small increments with intervals of ≥2 min for each increment. Premedicated with narcotics or concurrent CNS depressants—IV: As above, but reduce dose by 30%. *Debilitated, chronically ill, or >60 yr old:* Unpremedicated—IV: As for <60 yr old except initially no more than 1.5 mg and further doses given at a rate of no more than 1 mg over 2 min. Premedicated with narcotics or concurrent CNS depressant—IV: As above, but reduce dose by 50%.
Maintenance for conscious sedation: Give dose in increments of 25% of the dose used to first reach sedation.
Induction of general anesthesia: Consult other texts.
Adjunct to anesthesia for short surgical procedures: Consult other texts.
Indications: Preoperative sedation and amnesia, conscious sedation for procedures, and as an adjunct to both local and general anesthesia
Action: Short-acting benzodiazepine CNS depressant
Metabolism: Hepatic
Excretion: Renal
Contraindications and precautions
1. Because of potential for cardiorespiratory depression, resuscitative equipment and personnel must be available.
2. Contraindicated in shock, coma, or acute alcohol intoxication with depressed vital signs.
3. Use with caution in acute narrow-angle glaucoma, myasthenia gravis, shock, severe chronic obstructive pulmonary disease, patients with depressed respirations, or receiving concurrent respiratory depressants.
4. Careful individual dosage and titration in renal impairment or CHF.

Drug interactions: Alcohol or other CNS depressants lead to increased CNS depression.

Morphine sulfate (MS Contin, others)—Schedule II

Preparations: Tablets, 10, 30 mg; soluble tablets, 10, 15, 30 mg; ER tablets, 30, 60 mg; solution, 10 mg/5 ml, 20 mg/5 ml, 20 mg/ml, 100 mg/5 ml; suppositories, 5, 10, 20, 30 mg; injection (IM, IV, SC), 1, 2, 4, 5, 8, 10, 15 mg/ml
Adult dosage: Analgesic—PO: Individualize dosage for chronic pain; usually 10–30 mg q4h. For ER tablets, 30 mg q8–12h; patients being transferred from immediate-release to extended-release preparations should receive the same total daily dose given in 2 divided doses bid. PR: Usually 10–20 mg q4h. IM, SC: 5–20 mg q4h, usually 10 mg. IV: 2.5–15 mg diluted in 4–5 ml sterile water injected slowly over 4–5 min. For continuous IV infusion, initiate at 0.8–1.0 mg/hr and increase to effective dose prn.
Note
1. Use lower doses in geriatric patients.
2. Administer smallest effective dose and as infrequently as possible to minimize tolerance and physical dependence.

Indications: Treatment of pain, pain associated with myocardial infarction, and as an adjunct in anesthesia and acute pulmonary edema due to left ventricular failure
Note: Do not administer IV unless a narcotic antagonist is immediately available.
Action: Narcotic analgesic; may cause preload reduction
Metabolism: Hepatic
Excretion: Renal >> biliary
Contraindications and precautions
1. Contraindicated in diarrhea associated with pseudomembranous colitis, diarrhea caused by poisoning until the toxic material has been eliminated and acute respiratory depression.
2. Psychological and physical dependence and tolerance to many of the effects of morphine sulfate may develop with chronic administration.
3. Use with caution in acute abdominal conditions, acute asthma or chronic respiratory impairment, head injury, increased intracranial pressure, intracranial lesions, hepatic or renal function impairment, hypothyroidism, gallbladder disease, inflammatory bowel disease, recent GI tract surgery, prostatic hypertrophy or obstruction, urethral stricture, acute alcoholism, Addison's disease, epilepsy, suicidal ideation, emotional instability, or history of drug abuse.
4. Use with caution in patients performing tasks requiring mental alertness or physical coordination.
5. Use with caution in patients being administered MAO inhibitors.

Drug interactions
1. Alcohol, other opioid agonist analgesics, and other CNS depressants (including antihistamines, phenothiazines, tricyclic antidepressants, benzodiazepines, sedative-hypnotics, barbiturates) may increase risk of CNS depression.
2. Antidiarrheals and anticholinergics lead to increased risk of constipation.

3. Antihypertensives and diuretics lead to increased risk of hypotension.
4. Naltrexone, naloxone, and buprenorphine may block certain opioid actions. Consult other texts for further information.

Nadolol (Corgard)

Preparations: Tablets, 20, 40, 80, 120, 160 mg
Adult dosage
Antianginal—PO: Initially, 40 mg qd; increase by 40–80 mg q3–7d up to a total of 240 mg/day
Antihypertensive—PO: Initially, 40 mg qd; increase by 40–80 mg q7d up to a total of 320 mg/day
Note: Dosage adjustment in renal impairment as follows:

Creatinine clearance (ml/min/1.73 m²)	Dosage interval (hr)
>50	24
31–50	24–36
10–30	24–48
<10	40–60

Indications: Treatment of chronic angina and hypertension
Action: Nonselective β-adrenergic blocking agent (β_1, β_2)
Metabolism: None
Excretion: Renal
Contraindications and precautions
1. Contraindicated in overt cardiac failure, cardiogenic shock, 2nd- or 3rd-degree AV block, sinus bradycardia, and hypotension associated with MI.
2. Use with caution in asthma, emphysema, CHF, diabetes mellitus, mental depression, or peripheral vascular disease.
3. Abrupt withdrawal after chronic administration can precipitate angina, MI and ventricular dysrhythmias. Dosage should be tapered over 2 wk.

Drug interactions
1. Hydrocarbon inhalation anesthetics may increase myocardial depression.
2. Insulin or antidiabetic agents may increase hypoglycemia.
3. Calcium channel blocking agents may increase conduction disturbance or CHF in patients with abnormal AV conduction or depressed left ventricular function.
4. Nadolol may increase or decrease cardiostimulating effect of sympathomimetics.
5. Nadolol leads to decreased bronchodilating effect of sympathomimetics and theophylline.
6. Nadolol may significantly increase BP with MAO inhibitor use.

Naloxone hydrochloride (Narcan, others)

Preparations: Injection (IM, IV, SC), 0.4, 1 mg/ml
Adult dosage
Narcotic overdosage known or suspected—IM, IV (preferred), SC: 0.4–2 mg q2–3min prn. Question the diagnosis if no response after a total dose of 10 mg; may use smaller initial doses if the patient is physically dependent on narcotics. For continuous IV infusion, add 2 mg to 500 ml normal saline or D/W to prepare a 0.004 mg/ml solution. Some clinicians recommend an initial IV loading dose of 0.005 mg/kg or 0.4 mg/kg followed by initial infusion rates of 0.4 mg/hr or 0.0025 mg/hr, respectively. Titrate infusion rate to clinical response.
Postoperative narcotic depression—IV: Initially, 0.1–0.2 mg q2–3 min until there is adequate ventilation and alertness without significant pain. May repeat q1–2hr prn.
Indications: Treatment of narcotic toxicity, including respiratory depression and diagnosis of suspected acute narcotic overdosage
Action: Opiate narcotic antagonist
Metabolism: Hepatic
Excretion: Renal
Contraindications and precautions
1. Use with caution in opioid-dependent patients; naloxone may precipitate withdrawal.
2. Monitor patients who respond to naloxone because the duration of action of some opiates may exceed that of naloxone. Patients may require additional single doses or continuous IV infusion.
3. Use with caution in cardiovascular disease.

Naproxen (Anaprox, Naprosyn)

Preparations: Tablets, 275, 550 mg naproxen sodium (Anaprox), equivalent to 250, 500 mg naproxen; tablets, 250, 375, 500 mg naproxen (Naprosyn)
Adult dosage
Antirheumatic—PO: 250, 375, or 500 mg naproxen or 275 mg naproxen sodium bid, or 275 mg naproxen sodium every morning and 550 mg every evening
Analgesic, antidysmenorrheal, nonrheumatic anti-inflammatory—PO: Initially, 500 mg naproxen or 550 mg naproxen sodium, then 250 mg naproxen or 275 mg naproxen sodium q6–8h prn
Antigout—PO: Initially, 750 mg naproxen or 825 mg naproxen sodium, then 250 mg naproxen or 275 mg naproxen sodium q8h until attack subsides
Indications: Treatment of rheumatic and nonrheumatic inflammatory disorders, acute gouty arthritis, pain, dysmenorrhea, and headache; unlabeled uses include treatment of calcium pyrophosphate deposition disease and chronic prophylaxis of headache
Action: Nonsteroidal anti-inflammatory drug that inhibits cyclo-oxygenase, resulting in decreased formation of prostaglandins. Effects include antirheumatic, analgesic, antipyretic, and inhibition of platelet aggregation.
Metabolism: Hepatic
Excretion: Renal
Contraindications and precautions
1. Contraindicated in a history of severe allergic reaction to aspirin or other NSAIDs.
2. Use with caution in patient with history of peptic ulcer, upper gastrointestinal disease or ulcerative colitis, renal or hepatic function impairment, bleeding disorders, asthma, CHF, diabetes mellitus, hypertension, and pre-existing edema.

Drug interactions
1. Acetaminophen, gold compounds, or nephrotoxic medications may increase risk of renal toxicity.
2. Glucocorticoids, alcohol, potassium supplements, other NSAIDs, or aspirin may increase risk of GI side effects.
3. Anticoagulants, thrombolytic agents, aspirin, platelet aggregation inhibitors, or colchicine may increase risk of hemorrhage.
4. Probenecid may increase naproxen serum level.
5. Naproxen may increase methotrexate toxicity.
6. Naproxen may decrease antihypertensive effects of diuretics and antihypertensives.
7. Naproxen may decrease diuretic effect of diuretics.
8. Naproxen may increase hypoglycemic effect of sulfonylureas.

Niacin (Nicobid, Nicolar, others)

Preparations: Tablets, 25, 50, 100, 250, 400, 500 mg; SR tablets, 150, 250, 500, 750 mg; SR capsules, 125, 250, 300, 400, 500 mg; elixir, 50 mg/ml
Adult dosage: Antihyperlipidemic—PO: Initially, 100 mg tid and increase by 300 mg/day q4–7d until a maintenance dose of 1–2 g tid. For SR tablets or capsules, start with 125–150 mg bid. To ameliorate flushing, administer with meals or 30 min after aspirin. Maximum daily dose is 8 g/day.
Indications: Treatment of hyperlipidemia and treatment and prophylaxis of niacin (vitamin B_2) deficiency
Action: Unknown antihyperlipidemic action; results in a reduction of serum LDL (cholesterol) and VLDL levels, and increases HDL levels
Metabolism: Hepatic
Excretion: Renal
Contraindications and precautions
1. Contraindicated in arterial hemorrhage, severe hypotension, active peptic ulcer, and hepatic disease.
2. Use with caution in diabetes mellitus or gout.
3. Flushing may occur.

Drug interactions
1. Lovostatin may increase risk of myositis.
2. Niacin may increase hypotension due to ganglionic blocking drugs.
3. Aspirin administered 30 min before niacin may reduce flushing.

Nifedipine (Adalat, Procardia)

Preparations: Capsules, 10, 20 mg; SR tablets, 30, 60, 90 mg
Adult dosage
Antianginal—PO: Initially, 10 mg tid. Increase q7–14d prn up to 20–30 mg tid–qid. If symptoms warrant and the patient is assessed frequently, dosage may be increased up to 90 mg/day in increments of 30 mg/day over 3 days. For hospitalized and closely monitored patients, dosage may be increased by 10 mg q4–6 hr. For EC preparation, initiate with 30 or 60 mg. Limited clinical information is available on doses >90 mg/day.
Antihypertensive—PO: Only the EC preparation is indicated; initially, 30–60 mg qd. May increase q7–14d up to 120 mg qd.
Indications: Treatment of chronic stable angina pectoris, vasospastic angina, and hypertension; unlabeled uses include hypertensive emergencies
Action: Calcium-ion influx inhibitor (slow

channel blocker), resulting in peripheral and coronary artery vasodilation
Metabolism: Hepatic
Excretion: Renal
Contraindications and precautions
1. Contraindicated in severe hypotension.
2. Use with caution in hepatic or renal function impairment, mild or moderate hypotension, CHF, and aortic stenosis.

Drug interactions
1. Cimetidine may increase effects and toxicity.
2. β-Adrenergic blockers may increase risk of hypotension, exacerbation of angina, or arrhythmias.
3. Nifedipine may increase drug levels of digoxin.

Nitroglycerin—Sublingual (Nitrostat, others), Ointment (Nitro-Bid, Nitrol, others), Transdermal system (Nitro-Dur, Transderm-Nitro, others)

Preparations: Tablets, 0.15 mg (1/400), 0.3 mg (1/200), 0.4 mg (1/150), 0.6 mg (1/100 gr); ointment, 2%; transdermal system, 2.5, 5, 7.5, 10, 15 mg/24 hr; injection (IV), 0.5, 0.8, 5, 10 mg/ml
Adult dosage
Sublingual—PO: 0.15–0.6 mg repeated q5min prn for relief of anginal attack. If relief is not obtained after a total of 3 tablets over 15 min, have patient call a physician or go to the nearest emergency room. May be used prophylactically 5–10 min before activities known to precipitate an acute attack.
Topical ointment: Initially, 0.5 in. q8h. Titrate dose upward until angina is controlled or side effects preclude further increase. If angina occurs after the ointment has been in place for several hours, increase frequency to q6h. Apply in a thin, even layer on nonhairy skin. Cover with plastic wrap to spread ointment over 3.5 × 2.25 inch area or greater. Keep dose/area ratio constant, and rotate application site. One inch is the equivalent of approximately 15 mg nitroglycerin.
Topical transdermal systems: Apply pad qd to nonhairy skin not subject to excessive movement. Initially, use 5 mg/24-hr system qd. Titrate to higher-dose system as needed. Rotate application site.
Parenteral—IV: Initially, 5 μg/min through infusion pump. Increase by 5 μg/min q3–5min until desired reduction in BP or a rate of 20 μg/min. If no BP response or desired change in clinical status, increase by 10 μg/min q3–5min and later, if necessary, by 20 μg/min. When a partial BP effect is observed, reduce increments of dosage increase and lengthen interval between dosage increases. Titrate to BP and heart rate; continuous monitoring of BP and heart rate required.
Note
1. For oral and topical preparations, tolerance to nitroglycerin has been reported and may result in increased requirements. Tolerance may be reversed with short periods (8–24 hr) of nitrate withdrawal.
2. For parenteral preparations, polyvinyl chloride (PVC) IV infusion sets may absorb up to 40–80% of the nitroglycerin in diluted infusion solutions.

Indications: Treatment of acute angina pectoris (sublingual), chronic angina pectoris (sublingual, topical, parenteral), perioperative hypertension (parenteral), and CHF associated with MI (parenteral), and prophylaxis of acute angina pectoris (sublingual) and chronic angina pectoris (sublingual, topical). Unlabeled use of sublingual/topical preparations is CHF whether or not it is associated with MI.
Action: Relaxes vascular smooth muscle; reduced myocardial oxygen demand due to reduction in left ventricular preload and afterload as a result of venous > arterial dilatation.
Metabolism: Hepatic
Excretion: Renal
Contraindications and precautions
1. Parenteral preparations are contraindicated in hypotension, uncorrected hypovolemia, constrictive pericarditis, pericardial tamponade, increased intracranial pressure, or inadequate cerebral circulation.
2. All preparations should be used with caution in severe anemia, cerebral hemorrhage or head trauma, glaucoma, hyperthyroidism, hypertrophic cardiomyopathy, hypotension, recent MI, or severe hepatic or renal function impairment.
3. With sublingual tablets, loss of potency occurs 3–6 mo after opening bottle; discard unused tablets.

Drug interactions
1. Alcohol, antihypertensives, phenothiazines, narcotic analgesics, β-blockers, calcium channel blockers, and other hypotension-producing medications lead to increased hypotension.
2. Nitroglycerin leads to decreased effect of norepinephrine.
3. Substitute sublingual nitroglycerin for isosorbide.

Nitroprusside sodium (Nipride, others)

Preparations: Injection (IV), 50 mg/vial for reconstitution
Adult dosage: Antihypertensive—IV (continuous infusion): Initially, 0.5 μg/kg/min and increase by 0.5 μg titrated to BP response; Average dose is 3 μg/kg/min (range 0.5–10 μg/kg/min)
Note: Discontinue if administration of 10 μg/kg/min for 10 min does not produce adequate reduction of BP.
Indications: Treatment of hypertensive crisis; unlabeled uses include adjunctive treatment of severe CHF, MI, and severe mitral regurgitation.
Action: Direct vasodilation of arterial and venous vessels
Metabolism: Erythrocytic, then hepatic
Excretion: Renal
Contraindications and precautions
1. Contraindicated in compensatory hypertension such as arteriovenous shunt or coarctation of the aorta.
2. Use with caution in cerebrovascular or coronary artery insufficiency, hepatic or renal function impairment, hypothyroidism, hypovolemia, and vitamin B_{12} deficiency.
3. Cyanide toxicity can result from excessive amounts of nitroprusside. Monitor plasma thiocyanate concentrations daily if nitroprusside is administered for more than 48 hr, especially in patients with hepatic or renal function impairment.
4. If tolerance to the pharmacologic effects occurs, consider cyanide toxicity. Development of metabolic acidosis may be an early sign of cyanide toxicity.

Drug interactions: Ganglionic blocking agent and other hypotension-producing medications lead to increased hypotension.

Norethindrone—Progestin (see *Oral contraceptives*)

Norgestrel—Progestin (see *Oral contraceptives*)

Nortriptyline (Aventyl, Pamelor)

Preparations: Capsules, 10, 25, 50, 75 mg; solution, 10 mg/5 ml
Adult dosage: PO: Initially, 25 mg tid–qid. Increase up to 150 mg/day. Maximum antidepressant effects may take ≥2 wk. Start with lower doses of 30–50 mg/day in geriatric patients. After control of symptoms, taper to lowest effective dose. Some recommend monitoring plasma concentration (therapeutic = 50–150 ng/ml), especially at doses >100 mg/day.
Indications: Treatment of depression; unlabeled use includes treatment of neurogenic pain
Action: Tricyclic antidepressant; increases CNS synaptic concentration of norepinephrine and/or serotonin, presumably by blocking presynaptic reuptake, has sedative, anticholinergic, peripheral vasodilator, and direct quinidine-like myocardial effects
Metabolism: Hepatic
Excretion: Renal
Contraindications and precautions
1. Contraindicated during recovery from MI and possibly concurrent MAO inhibitor use.
2. Use with caution in alcoholism, asthma, bipolar disorder, schizophrenia, cardiovascular disorders, blood disorders, GI disorders, narrow angle glaucoma, hepatic or renal function impairment, hyperthyroidism, prostatic hypertrophy, or urinary retention and seizure disorders.
3. Exercise caution while driving or performing other tasks requiring alertness.
4. Abrupt cessation after prolonged administration may cause withdrawal symptoms.
5. Prescribe the smallest quantity feasible to patients considered at risk for suicide.

Drug interactions
1. Alcohol or CNS depressants lead to increased CNS depression.
2. Drugs with antimuscarinic activity lead to increased anticholinergic side effects.
3. Direct-acting sympathomimetics lead to increased cardiac effects.
4. MAO inhibitors lead to increased risk of hyperpyretic episodes, convulsions, hypertensive crises, and death.
5. Antithyroid agents lead to increased risk of agranulocytosis.
6. Barbiturates and carbamazepine may decrease plasma concentration of nortriptyline.

7. Cimetidine methylphenidate, phenothiazines, estrogens, and possibly ranitidine may increase plasma concentration of nortriptyline.
8. Metrizamide leads to increased risk of seizures.
9. Thyroid hormone leads to increased therapeutic and toxic effects of both medications.
10. Nortriptyline leads to decreased hypotensive effect of guanethidine and clonidine.
11. Nortriptyline may increase plasma concentration of coumadin.

Oral Contraceptives (Lo/Ovral, Ortho-Novum, others)

Preparations: Combination of an estrogen (ethinyl estradiol or mestranol) and a progestin (norethindrone or norgestrel). Products differ in the potency of the components and in the relative predominance of progestational or estrogenic activity. Consult further texts for specific product contents. Monophasic preparations provide a fixed dosage of estrogen to progestin throughout the cycle. Biphasic preparations provide a constant dosage of estrogen with a decreased progestin/estrogen ratio in the first half of the cycle, followed by an increased ratio in the second half. A triphasic preparation provides a constant dosage of estrogen with a progressively increased progestin dosage. Examples of such preparations include the following:

Monophasic—Ortho-Novum: 1/50 21, 1/50 28, 1/35 21, 1/35 28; Ovral, Ovral-28, Lo/Ovral-21, Lo/Ovral-28

Biphasic—Ortho-Novum: 10/11 21, 10/11 28

Triphasic—Ortho-Novum: 7/7/7

Adult dosage

Monophasic: *21-day cycle*—PO: 1 tablet qd for 21 days starting on day 5 of the cycle (day 1 = first day of menstrual bleeding) followed by no tablets for 7 days. Withdrawal bleeding usually occurs 2–3 days after the last tablet. Repeat the dosage cycle beginning on day 5 of the menstrual cycle or on the eighth day after taking the last tablet of the previous cycle, whichever occurs first. *28-day cycle*—PO: 1 tablet qd for 28 days starting on day 5 of the cycle. Repeat the dosage cycle on day 5 of the menstrual cycle or on the day after taking the last tablet of the previous cycle, whichever occurs first.

Biphasic and triphasic: *21- and 28-day cycles*—PO: 1 tablet qd for 21 or 28 days starting on the first Sunday after or on which menstrual bleeding has started. No tablets are then taken for 7 days for the 21-day cycle. Repeat the dosage cycle beginning on the eighth day after taking the last hormonally active tablet.

Note

1. The last 7 tablets in the 28-day cycle preparations are inert (contain no hormone).
2. Use the product with the least estrogenic activity that is compatible with an acceptable pregnancy rate.
3. First time users should generally be started on preparations containing <50 μg estrogen.
4. Do not rely on contraceptive effect until after 7 consecutive days of administration.
5. For missed doses or menstrual periods during contraceptive use, consult other texts.

Indications: Prevention of pregnancy

Action: Inhibits ovulation by suppressing secretion of FSH and LH; also inhibits implantation and alters cervical mucus

Metabolism: Hepatic

Excretion: Renal > fecal

Contraindications and precautions

1. Contraindicated in thrombophlebitis, thromboembolic disorders, history of deep vein thrombosis, cerebrovascular disease, coronary artery disease, known or suspected breast carcinoma or estrogen-dependent neoplasia, cholestatic jaundice, hepatic tumors, known or suspected pregnancy, breastfeeding, and undiagnosed abnormal vaginal bleeding.
2. Cigarette smoking increases the risk of cardiovascular side effects, especially in heavy smokers and women >35 years of age.
3. Use with caution in asthma, cardiac insufficiency, epilepsy, migraine headaches, endometriosis, gallbladder disease, renal or hepatic function impairment, hypercalcemia, hyperlipidemia, hypertension, history of jaundice during pregnancy, immobilization, history of mental depression, acute intermittent hepatic porphyria, or uterine fibroids.
4. When possible, discontinue oral contraceptives 4–6 wk before surgery.

Drug Interactions

1. Ampicillin, penicillin V, chloramphenicol, dihydroergotamine, hepatic enzyme inducers (e.g., rifampin, barbiturates, phenytoin, and others), sulfonamides, tetracyclines, or tranquilizers may decrease contraceptive efficacy.
2. Tobacco use leads to increased risk of cardiovascular side effects.
3. Oral contraceptives may decrease effectiveness of tricyclic antidepressants, oral anticoagulants, anticonvulsants, antihypertensives, and oral hypoglycemic agents.
4. Oral contraceptives may decrease metabolism of diazepam, chlordiazepoxide, and metoprolol.
5. Oral contraceptives may increase metabolism of lorezepam and oxazepam.

Oxazepam (Serax, others)

Preparations: Tablets, 15 mg; capsules, 10, 15, 30 mg

Adult dosage

Antianxiety—PO: 15–30 mg tid–qid

Sedative-hypnotic and for alcohol withdrawal—PO: 15–30 mg tid–qid

Indications: Treatment of anxiety disorders, anxiety associated with mental depression, and alcohol withdrawal

Action: Anxiolytic sedative-hypnotic benzodiazepine; may potentiate CNS gamma-aminobutyric acid effects

Metabolism: Hepatic (glucuronidation)

Excretion: Renal

Contraindications and precautions

1. Contraindicated in acute alcohol intoxication with depressed vital signs, depressive neuroses, or psychoses without prominent anxiety.
2. Use with caution in acute narrow-angle glaucoma, myasthenia gravis, shock, severe COPD, hepatic or renal impairment, patients with depressed respirations, or those receiving concurrent respiratory depressants.
3. Long-term therapy may result in psychological or physical dependence.
4. Exercise caution in performing tasks requiring alertness and coordination.

Drug interactions

1. Oxazepam may increase zidovudine (AZT) toxicity.
2. Alcohol or other CNS depressants lead to increased CNS depression.

Oxycodone (Roxicodone)—Schedule 2

Preparations: Tablets, 5 mg; solution, 5 mg/5 ml

Adult dosage: Analgesic—

PO: 5 mg q6h prn

Indications: Treatment of pain

Note

1. Use lower doses in geriatric patients.
2. Administer smallest effective dose and as infrequently as possible to minimize tolerance and physical dependence.

Action: Narcotic analgesic

Metabolism: Hepatic

Excretion: Renal

Contraindications and precautions

1. Contraindicated in diarrhea associated with pseudomembranous colitis, diarrhea caused by poisoning until the toxic material has been eliminated, and acute respiratory depression.
2. Psychological and physical dependence and tolerance to many of the effects of oxycodone may develop with chronic administration.
3. Use with caution in acute abdominal conditions, acute asthma or chronic respiratory impairment, head injury, increased intracranial pressure, intracranial lesions, hepatic or renal function impairment, hypothyroidism, gallbladder disease, inflammatory bowel disease, recent GI tract surgery, prostatic hypertrophy or obstruction, urethral stricture, acute alcoholism, Addison's disease, epilepsy, suicidal ideation, emotional instability, or history of drug abuse.
4. Use with caution in patients performing tasks requiring mental alertness or physical coordination.
5. Use with caution in patients being administered MAO inhibitors.

Drug interactions

1. Alcohol, other opioid agonist analgesics, and other CNS depressants (including antihistamines, phenothiazines, tricyclic antidepressants, benzodiazepines, sedative-hypnotics, barbiturates) may increase risk of CNS depression.
2. Antidiarrheals and anticholinergics lead to increased risk of constipation.
3. Antihypertensives and diuretics lead to increased risk of hypotension.
4. Naltrexone, naloxone, and buprenorphine may block certain opioid

actions. Consult other texts for further information.

Oxycodone and Acetaminophen (Percocet, Tylox)—Schedule II (see individual drugs)

Oxycodone hydrochloride, oxycodone terephthalate, and acetaminophen (Percodan)—Schedule II (see individual drugs)
Preparations: 4.5 mg oxycodone HCl and 0.38 mg oxycodone terephthalate and 325 mg acetaminophen (see individual drugs)

Pentazocine hydrochloride (Talwin)—Schedule IV
Preparations: Tablets, 50 mg with 0.5 naloxone hydrochloride (Talwin Nx); injection (IM, IV, SC), 30 mg/ml (Talwin)
Adult dosage: Analgesic—PO: 50 mg of pentazocine (base) q3–4h prn; may increase to 100 mg q3–4h, not to exceed 600 mg/day. IM, IV, SC: 30 mg q3–4h prn, not to exceed 30 mg IV or 60 mg IM or SC per dose and not to exceed 360 mg/day.
Note
1. Use lower doses in geriatric patients.
2. IM preferred over SC administration.
3. Administer smallest effective dose and as infrequently as possible to minimize tolerance and physical dependence.

Indications: Treatment of pain and as an adjunct to anesthesia
Action: Mixed agonist/antagonist narcotic analgesic; consult other texts for effect profile compared to agonist narcotics
Metabolism: Hepatic
Excretion: Renal
Contraindications and precautions
1. Contraindicated in diarrhea associated with pseudomembranous colitis, diarrhea caused by poisoning until the toxic material has been eliminated, and acute respiratory depression.
2. Psychological and physical dependence and tolerance to many of the effects of pentazocine may develop with chronic administration.
3. Use with caution in patients with opioid agonist analgesic dependence (pentazocine may not suppress withdrawal symptoms).
4. Use with caution in acute MI, acute abdominal conditions, acute asthma or chronic respiratory impairment, head injury, increased intracranial pressure, intracranial lesions, hepatic or renal function impairment, hypothyroidism, gallbladder disease, inflammatory bowel disease, recent GI tract surgery, prostatic hypertrophy or obstruction, urethral stricture, acute alcoholism, Addison's disease, epilepsy, suicidal ideation, emotional instability, or history of drug abuse.
5. Use with caution in patients performing tasks requiring mental alertness or physical coordination.

Drug interactions
1. Alcohol or other CNS depressants may increase CNS depression.
2. Antidiarrheals or antimuscarinics may increase risk of constipation.
3. Naltrexone, naloxone, and buprenorphine may block certain opioid actions. Consult other texts for further information.

Pentobarbital (Nembutal, others)
Preparations: Capsules, 50, 100 mg; elixir, 18.2 mg/5 ml; suppositories, 30, 60, 120, 200 mg; injection (IM, IV), 50 mg/ml
Adult dosage
Hypnotic—PO: 100 mg qhs. PR: 120–200 mg qhs. IM: 150–200 mg QHS. IV: Initially, 100 mg. After 1 min, additional small doses may be given q/min up to a total of 200–500 mg.
Sedative—PO: 20 mg tid–qid. PR: 30 mg bid–qid. *Preoperative sedation*—IM: 150–200 mg.
Anticonvulsant—IV: Initially, 100 mg. After 1 min, additional small dose may be given q1min up to a total of 500 mg.
Indications: Used for short-term treatment of insomnia, preoperative sedation, and acute convulsive episodes such as status epilepticus
Action: CNS depressant with sedative-hypnotic, anticonvulsant, and respiratory depressant effects
Metabolism: Hepatic
Excretion: Renal
Contraindications and precautions
1. Contraindicated in porphyria. Large doses contraindicated in respiratory insufficiency and nephritis.
2. Use with caution in history of drug abuse or dependence, hepatic or renal function impairment, hyperthyroidism, diabetes mellitus, severe anemia, acute or chronic pain, and a history of mental depression or suicidal tendencies.
3. Use with caution in performing activities requiring mental alertness or physical coordination.
4. Prolonged administration may result in psychological or physical dependence and tolerance.
5. Withdraw pentobarbital gradually to avoid withdrawal symptoms.

Drug interactions
1. Alcohol or other CNS depressants may increase CNS depression.
2. Valproic acid or MAO inhibitors may increase pentobarbital serum concentration.
3. Rifampin and other hepatic microsomal enzyme inducers may decrease pentobarbital serum concentration.
4. Pentobarbital may decrease effect of acetaminophen, glucocorticoids, cyclosporine, quinidine, oral anticoagulants, doxycycline, levothyroxine, oral contraceptives, estrogens, theophylline, and mexilitine.
5. Pentobarbital may increase or decrease phenytoin blood levels.

Perphenazine (Trilafon, others)
Preparations: Tablets, 2, 4, 8, 16 mg; repeat-action tablets, 8 mg; solution, 16 mg/5 ml; injection (IM, IV), 5 mg/ml
Adult dosage
Antipsychotic: *Nonhospitalized, moderate symptoms*—PO: Initially, 8–16 mg bid–qid, or repeat-action tablets, 8–32 mg bid. *For rapid control of symptoms*—IM: Initially, 5 mg q6h prn, not to exceed 15 mg/day in nonhospitalized and 30 mg/day in hospitalized patients. IM onset of action is 10 min.
Nausea and vomiting—PO: Initially, 8–16 mg/day in divided doses up to 24 mg if needed. IM: Initially, 5 mg; increase to 10 mg in hospitalized patients if needed. IV: 5 mg diluted to 0.5 mg/ml with normal saline as an infusion at a rate of 1 mg/min or less or as fractional injections of 1 mg or less, not less than q1–2min.
Note: Use lower doses in geriatric or debilitated patients.
Indications: Treatment of psychotic disorders and severe nausea and vomiting
Action: Antipsychotic effect due to inhibition of CNS dopaminergic receptors; antiemetic effect from inhibition of medullary chemoreceptor trigger-zone dopaminergic receptors; has moderate anticholinergic and weak to moderate sedative effects; peripheral α-adrenergic blocking effect causes vasodilation
Metabolism: Hepatic
Excretion: Renal
Contraindications and precautions
1. Contraindicated in comatose states, severe CNS depression, subcortical brain damage, bone marrow depression, and severe cardiovascular disease.
2. Use with caution in cardiovascular disease, seizure disorders, hepatic function impairment, glaucoma, urinary retention, prostatic hypertrophy, chronic respiratory disorders, blood dyscrasias, and active alcoholism.
3. Tartrazine in some products may cause allergic reactions.

Drug interactions:
1. CNS depressants lead to increased effect.
2. Anticholinergic agents lead to increased antimuscarinic effects.
3. Aluminum- or magnesium-containing antacids or lithium may decrease oral absorption.
4. Epinephrine leads to severe hypotension and tachycardia.
5. Propranolol and possibly other β-blockers lead to increased levels and vice versa.
6. Opioids lead to increased risk of constipation.
7. Perphenazine may increase phenytoin or tricyclic antidepressants levels.
8. Perphenazine may increase risk of metrizamide-induced seizures.
9. Perphenazine may decrease effect of levodopa.

Phenobarbital
Preparations: Tablets, 8, 15, 16, 30, 32, 100 mg; capsules, 16 mg; elixir, 15, 20 mg/5 ml; injection (IM, IV), 30, 60, 65, 130 mg/ml
Adult dosage
Hypnotic—PO: 100–320 mg qhs. IM, IV: 100–325 mg qhs. Not recommended for >2 wk of administration.
Sedative—PO: 30–120 mg/day in 2–3 divided doses. IM, IV: 30–130 mg in 2–3 divided doses. *For preoperative sedation*—IM: 130–200 mg 60–90 min before surgery.
Anticonvulsant—PO: 100–300 mg/day usually given as a single dose qhs. IM, IV: 100–320 mg repeated, if necessary, up to a total dose of 600 mg during a 24-hr period. *For acute seizure states*—IV: Recommended regimens vary from 200–600 mg repeated, if necessary, to initially

300–800 mg, then 120–240 mg q20min prn up to a maximum of 1–2 g/24 hr.

Note

1. Use lower doses in elderly and in hepatic function impairment.
2. IV administration should not exceed a rate of 60 mg/min.

Indications: Treatment of tonic-clonic and simple partial (cortical focal) seizures; used for acute seizure states, including status epilepticus, but is not first-line therapy; also used for short-term treatment of insomnia

Action: CNS depressant with sedative-hypnotic, anticonvulsant, and respiratory depressant effects

Metabolism: Hepatic

Excretion: Renal

Contraindications and precautions

1. Contraindicated in porphyria. Large doses contraindicated in respiratory insufficiency and nephritis.
2. Use with caution in history of drug abuse or dependence, hepatic or renal function impairment, hyperthyroidism, diabetes mellitus, severe anemia, acute or chronic pain, and a history of mental depression or suicidal tendencies.
3. Use with caution when performing activities requiring mental alertness or physical coordination.
4. Prolonged administration may result in psychological or physical dependence and tolerance.
5. Withdraw phenobarbital gradually to avoid withdrawal symptoms.

Drug interactions

1. Alcohol or other CNS depressants may increase CNS depression.
2. Valproic acid or MAO inhibitors may increase phenobarbital serum concentration.
3. Rifampin and other hepatic microsomal enzyme inducers may decrease phenobarbital serum concentration.
4. Phenobarbital may decrease effect of acetaminophen, glucocorticoids, cyclosporine, quinidine, oral anticoagulants, doxycycline, levothyroxine, oral contraceptives, estrogens, theophylline, and mexilitine.
5. Phenobarbital may increase or decrease phenytoin blood levels.

Phenytoin (Dilantin, others)

Preparations

Phenytoin: Tablets, 50 mg, suspension, 30, 125 mg/5 ml

Phenytoin sodium: Capsules, 30, 100 mg; ER capsules, 30, 100 mg; injection (IM, IV), 50 mg/ml

Adult dosage: Anticonvulsant—PO: Initially, 125 mg of phenytoin or 100 mg of phenytoin sodium tid. If higher doses are needed, increase by the equivalent of 100 mg of phenytoin sodium q7–14d. Optimal daily dosage is usually 6–7 mg phenytoin sodium/kg. Patients stabilized on 100 mg tid of the ER preparation may be switched to once-daily dosing with 300 mg. Loading doses may be used in a closely supervised setting and in patients without a history of renal or hepatic disease. Consult other texts for published protocols. One recommended regimen is initially 1 g phenytoin sodium administered in doses of 400, 300, and 300 mg q2h, followed by maintenance dosage 24 hr after the loading dose. IV: Status epilepticus—IV injection of 150–250 mg phenytoin sodium at a rate ≥50 mg/min. May give 100–150 mg 30 min after the first dose if needed. Some clinicians recommend a single initial dose of 15–18 mg/kg. Infusion rate should be ≤25 mg/min in geriatric or debilitated patients or in those with hepatic function impairment. If administration does not terminate the seizure, consider alternative therapies. For parenteral maintenance dosing, IV injection of 100 mg q6–8h at a rate ≤50 mg/min.

Note

1. Therapeutic serum level is 10–20 μg/ml.
2. Each 100 mg of phenytoin sodium contains 92 mg of phenytoin.
3. Only the ER preparation can be used for once-daily dosing.
4. For parenteral administration, IV infusions are not recommended. The IM route is not recommended unless PO and IV routes are unavailable. Consult other texts for IM dosage.
5. Reduce dosage in geriatric or debilitated patients or those with impaired hepatic function.

Indications: Treatment of tonic-clonic (grand-mal) and simple or complex partial seizures and status epilepticus; unlabeled use includes treatment of digitalis-induced arrhythmias

Action: Hydantoin anticonvulsant that stabilizes neuronal membranes and inhibits the spread of seizure activity. Cardiac effects include negative inotropy and facilitated AV conduction.

Metabolism: Hepatic

Excretion: Renal

Contraindications and precautions

1. IV administration is contraindicated in sinus bradycardia, sinoatrial block, 2nd- or 3rd-degree AV block, or Adams-Stokes syndrome.
2. Use with caution in active alcoholism, blood dyscrasias, diabetes mellitus, and hepatic or renal function impairment.
3. Lymph node hyperplasia has been associated with phenytoin.
4. Use caution in activities requiring mental alertness or physical coordination.
5. Abrupt withdrawal in patients with seizure disorders may precipitate seizures or status epilepticus.

Drug interactions

1. Phenytoin has many drug-drug interactions. Consult other texts for complete listings.
2. Drugs that may increase effect of phenytoin include the following: acute alcohol ingestion, allopurinol, amiodarone, chloramphenicol, cimetidine, diazepam, isoniazid, phenylbutazone, sulfonamides, valproic acid.
3. Drugs that may decrease effect of phenytoin include the following: antacids, barbiturates, calcium (dietary), chronic alcohol ingestion, enteral feedings, folic acid (dietary), carbamazepine.
4. Phenytoin may increase the effects of the following drugs: carbamazepine, cyclosporine, disopyramide, doxycycline, estrogens, glucocorticoids, haloperidol, levodopa, methadone, oral contraceptives, quinidine, and xanthine derivatives.
5. Alcohol or other CNS depressants may increase CNS depression.
6. Lidocaine may increase cardiac depressant effects.

Phosphorus (as monobasic and dibasic phosphates) (K-Phos, Neutra-Phos, others)

Preparations: See table below.

Adult dosage: Hypophosphatemia—PO: The equivalent of 228–250 mg (7.4–8 mM) of phosphorus qid. IV: Slow infusion of approximately 10–15 mM of phosphorus/day.

Indications: Treatment and prophylaxis of hypophosphatemia

Action: Phosphorus is essential for normal cellular function. Supplemental phosphates promote hydrogen secretion in the distal renal tubule, resulting in urine acidification.

Metabolism: None

Excretion: Renal

Contraindications and precautions

1. Contraindicated in hyperphosphatemia, severe renal function impairment, and

Phosphorus-Containing Preparations

Preparations	Potassium (mEq)	Sodium (mEq)	Total equivalent dose of phosphorus in mg (mM)
K-Phos Original tablets	3.7	0	114 (3.7)
K-Phos Neutral tablets	1.15	12.9	250 (8)
Neutra-Phos capsules or solution*	7.125	7.125	250 (8)
Neutra-Phos K capsules or solution†	14.25	0	250 (8)
Potassium phosphate (IV)/ml	4.4	0	93 (3)
Sodium phosphate (IV)/ml	0	4.0	93 (3)

* Neutra-Phos solution: 1 cap dissolved in 75 ml of liquefied (2.5 fluid oz) = 75 ml of a solution made from 1 bottle (64 g) of powder reconstituted in 1 gallon of solution

† Neutra-Phos K solution: 1 capsule dissolved in 75 ml of liquid (2.5 oz) = 75 ml of a solution made from 1 bottle (71 g) of powder reconstituted in 1 gallon of solution

magnesium ammonium phosphate (struvite) urolithiasis.
2. Use all phosphate with caution in hypoparathyroidism, chronic renal disease, osteomalacia, acute pancreatitis, and rickets.
3. Use potassium-containing phosphates with caution in Addison's disease, acute dehydration, extensive tissue breakdown, myotonia congenita, digitalized patients, and in patients on a potassium-restricted diet.
4. Use sodium-containing phosphates with caution in cardiac failure, severe hepatic disease or cirrhosis, peripheral or pulmonary edema, hypernatremia, toxemia of pregnancy, and in patients on a sodium-restricted diet.

Drug interactions
1. Aluminum-, calcium- or magnesium-containing antacids may decrease PO absorption.
2. Glucocorticoids or mineralocorticoids may increase risk of hypernatremia with sodium phosphates.
3. Captopril, enalapril, potassium-sparing diuretics, or potassium-containing medications may increase risk of hyperkalemia with potassium phosphates.
4. Calcium-containing medications may increase risk of deposition of calcium in soft tissues.

Phytonadione (see *Vitamin K*)

Piroxicam (Feldene)
Preparations: Capsules, 10, 20 mg
Adult dosage: Antirheumatic—PO: 20 mg qd
Indications: Treatment of rheumatic disease; unlabeled uses include treatment of acute gouty arthritis and calcium pyrophosphate deposition disease
Action: Nonsteroidal anti-inflammatory drug that inhibits cyclo-oxygenase, resulting in decreased formation of prostaglandins; effects include antirheumatic, analgesic, antipyretic, and inhibition of platelet aggregation
Metabolism: Hepatic
Excretion: Renal > biliary
Contraindications and precautions
1. Contraindicated in a history of severe allergic reaction to aspirin or other NSAIDs.
2. Use with caution in a history of peptic ulcer, upper GI disease or ulcerative colitis, renal or hepatic function impairment, bleeding disorders, asthma, CHF, diabetes mellitus, hypertension, and pre-existing edema.

Drug interactions
1. Acetaminophen, gold compounds, or nephrotoxic medications may increase risk of renal toxicity.
2. Glucocorticoids, alcohol, potassium supplements, other NSAIDs, or aspirin may increase risk of GI side effects.
3. Anticoagulants, thrombolytic agents, aspirin, platelet aggregation inhibitors, or colchicine may increase risk of hemorrhage.
4. Probenecid may increase piroxicam serum level.
5. Piroxicam may increase methotrexate toxicity.
6. Piroxicam may decrease antihypertensive effects of diuretics and antihypertensives.
7. Piroxicam may decrease diuretic effect of diuretics.
8. Piroxicam may increase hypoglycemic effect of sulfonylureas.

Potassium chloride
Preparations: Tablets, 1.33, 8, 10 mEq; EC tablets, 4, 13.4 mEq; ER tablets, 6.7, 8, 10 mEq; ER tablets (microcrystalloids), 10, 20 mEq, ER capsules, 8, 10 mEq; powder for solution, 15, 20, 25 mEq per packet or dose; solution, 5, 7.5, 10, 15, 20% containing 10, 15, 20, 30, 40 mEq K^+Cl^-/15 ml, respectively; injection (IV), various volumes containing the equivalent of 1, 1.5, 2, 2.4, 3 mEq/ml; injection (IV), KCl in D5/W 0.075, 0.15, 0.224, 0.3% containing 10, 20, 30, 40 mEq K^+/L, respectively
Adult dosage
Hypokalemia: Dosage must be individualized for each patient depending on clinical condition, EKG, and plasma K^+ level. *For K+ depletion*—PO: usually, 40–100 mEq/day in divided doses not to exceed 150 mEq/day; IV: general guidelines are the following:

K^+ serum level (mEq/L)	Dosage (mEq/hr)
>2.5	10–20
<2.0	40

Prophylaxis of hypokalemia—PO: Usually 16–24 mEq/day in 2–3 divided doses
Note
1. EC tablet preparations are not preferred owing to ulcerogenic tendency.
2. For IV administration, K^+ concentrations in IV fluids should not exceed 40–60 mEq/L unless infused via a central line. Consult individual hospital policies regarding rates of infusion.

Indications: Treatment and prophylaxis of hypokalemia
Action: Potassium is the major cation of intracellular fluid and essential for cellular function.
Metabolism: None
Excretion: Renal >> fecal
Contraindications and precautions
1. Contraindicated in hyperkalemia.
2. Use with caution in renal function impairment, oliguria, chronic renal insufficiency, untreated Addison's disease, heat cramps, acute dehydration, familial periodic paralysis, heart block, severe burns, crush injuries, or other conditions with extensive tissue breakdown.
3. Solid dosage forms are contraindicated in gastrointestinal obstruction or ulceration.
4. Use with caution in patients being administered digoxin.

Drug interactions
1. Glucocorticoids, mineralocorticoids, NSAIDs, blood, potassium-sparing diuretics, potassium-containing medications, salt substitutes, captopril, enalapril, lisinopril, heparin, and cyclosporine may increase risk of hyperkalemia.
2. Antimuscarinics may increase risk of GI lesions.
3. Potassium chloride should be used with caution in patients being administered digoxin.

Prazocin (Minipress)
Preparations: Capsules, 1, 2, 5 mg
Adult dosage: Antihypertensive—PO: Initially, 1 mg bid–tid. Dosage may be increased gradually up to a total daily dose of 20 mg. Usual maintenance dose is 6–15 mg/day in divided doses.
Note: First dose should be 1 mg given when patient will be recumbent for several hours. Lower dosage may be required in renal function impairment. Initial dosage in renal failure is 1 mg bid.
Indications: Treatment of hypertension. Unlabeled uses include adjunctive treatment of severe CHF, pheochromocytoma, and Raynaud's phenomenon.
Action: Postsynaptic α-adrenergic blocking agent producing both venous and arterial vasodilation
Metabolism: Hepatic
Excretion: Biliary, fecal >> renal
Contraindications and precautions
1. Use with caution in severe cardiac disease and renal function impairment.
2. Prazocin can cause marked hypotension with the first few doses.

Drug interactions: Diuretics and antihypertensives lead to increased hypotension.

Prednisone
Preparations: Tablets, 1, 2.5, 5, 10, 20, 25, 50 mg; solution, 1 mg/5 ml, 5 mg/ml; syrup, 5 mg/ml
Adult dosage: PO: 5–60 mg/day as a single dose or in divided doses depending on the indication
Indications: Replacement therapy in the treatment of adrenal insufficiency states; used for anti-inflammatory and immunosuppressant effects in the treatment of many disorders; consult further texts for specific therapeutic regimens in selected disorders
Action: Adrenocorticoid with anti-inflammatory, immunosuppressant, and minimal to moderate mineralocorticoid effects. Other effects include suppression of the hypothalamic-pituitary-adrenal (HPA) axis, increased protein catabolism, increased blood glucose concentrations, insulin resistance, reduced intestinal absorption and increased renal excretion of calcium, and neutrophilia. See also table, page 708.
Metabolism: Primarily hepatic
Excretion: Renal
Contraindications and precautions
1. Use with caution in cardiac disease, CHF, hypertension, hepatic or renal function impairment, HIV+, AIDS or other immunodeficiency states, uncontrolled bacterial or viral infection, systemic-fungal infection, tuberculosis (active, latent or positive skin test), ocular herpes simplex, diabetes mellitus, nonspecific ulcerative colitis, diverticulitis, esophagitis, gastritis, history of peptic ulcer, recent intestinal anastomosis, open-angle glaucoma, hyperthyroidism, hypoalbuminuria, myasthenia gravis, osteoporosis, or seizure disorder.
2. Administer daily dose in the morning to reduce HPA-axis suppressive effects.

Alternate-day dosing may reduce the risk of adrenal suppression.
3. Withdrawal following long-term therapy with pharmacologic doses requires a gradual taper until the HPA-axis recovers.

Drug interactions
1. Alcohol, aspirin, and NSAIDs may increase risk of GI ulceration.
2. Amphotericin B and diuretics may increase risk of hypokalemia.
3. Estrogens may increase effects.
4. Ephedrine, phenytoin, phenobarbital, and rifampin may decrease effects.
5. Immunosuppressants lead to increased risk of infection.
6. Antacids may decrease absorption.
7. Prednisone may decrease effects of coumadin, oral antidiabetic agents, and insulin.
8. Prednisone may decrease effect of isoniazid.
9. Pharmacologic doses of prednisone may potentiate replication of live virus in vaccines or decrease antibody response to the vaccine.

Procainamide (Procan SR, Pronestyl, others)

Preparations: Tablets, 250, 375, 500 mg; SR tablets, 250, 500, 750, 1,000 mg; capsules, 250, 375, 500 mg; injection (IM, IV), 100, 500 mg/ml

Adult dosage: Antiarrhythmic: *Atrial arrhythmias*—PO: Initially, 125 g followed by 750 mg in 1 hr if necessary, then 500–1,000 mg q2–3h until normal sinus rhythm or toxicity. Maintenance dosage is usually 500–1,000 mg q4–6 h. For SR preparations, administer ¼ of total daily dose q6h. *Ventricular tachycardia*—PO: Initially, 1 g followed by 50 mg/kg/day in 8 divided doses (q3h). *Ventricular premature contractions*—PO: 50 mg/kg/day in divided doses q3h. For SR preparations, administer ¼ of total daily dose q6h. Suggested guidelines for maintenance dosing are as follows:

Weight (kg)	Dose (mg) q3h	SR dose (mg) q6h
<55	250	500
55–91	375	750
>91	500	1,000

Parenteral administration—IM: 500–1,000 mg q4–8 hr. IV injection: 100 mg diluted in D5W q5min at a rate not exceeding 50 mg/min until arrhythmia is controlled or a maximum dose of 1 g. IV infusion: 500–600 mg diluted in D5W at a rate not exceeding 25–50 mg/min. May administer up to 1,000 g. Monitor BP and EKG continuously. Maintenance dosage following injection or infusion is a continuous infusion at a rate of 2–6 mg/min.

Note
1. Dosage reduction in CHF, renal functional impairment, and critical illness.
2. Therapeutic serum concentration for procainamide is 4–8 μg/ml.

Indications: Treatment and prophylaxis of atrial fibrillation, paroxysmal supraventricular tachycardia, premature ventricular contractions, and ventricular tachycardia

Action: Class 1A antiarrhythmic

Metabolism: Hepatic

Excretion: Renal

Contraindications and precautions
1. Contraindicated in complete AV block, 2nd- and 3rd-degree AV block unless controlled by electrical pacemaker and Torsade des Pointes. Generally contraindicated in myasthenia gravis.
2. Use with caution in AV block, bundle branch block, severe digitalis intoxication, CHF, hepatic or renal function impairment, history of SLE, and ventricular tachycardia during coronary occlusion.
3. Prolonged administration often leads to the development of a positive ANA test with or without symptoms of SLE. A positive ANA dictates reassessment of the relative benefits and risks.
4. Procainamide is partially metabolized to N-acetyl procainamide (NAPA) by acetylation. Fast acetylators convert a greater percentage of procainamide to NAPA with subsequent greater NAPA blood levels.

Drug interactions
1. Other antiarrhythmics may produce additive cardiac effects.
2. Cimetidine may increase plasma levels of procainamide and NAPA.
3. Anticholinergics may increase antimuscarinic effects.
4. Antihypertensives may increase hypotensive effect.
5. Procainamide may increase effect of neuromuscular blocking agents.

Prochlorperazine (Compazine, others)

Preparations: Tablets, 5, 10, 25 mg; SR capsules, 10, 15, 30 mg; suppositories, 2.5, 5, 25 mg; injection (IM) 5 mg/ml

Adult dosage

Antipsychotic: *Nonhospitalized or mild symptoms*—PO: Initially, 5–10 mg tid–qid. *Hospitalized or well-supervised patients with moderate to severe symptoms*—PO: 10 mg tid–qid. Increase q2–3d until control of symptoms or limiting side effects. Usual dose is 50–75 mg/day up to 100–150 mg/day. PR: Initially, 10 mg tid–qid and increase by 5–10 mg q2–3d prn. *For rapid control of symptoms*—IM: Initially, 10–20 mg repeated q2–4h if needed up to 3–4 additional doses. If prolonged IM therapy indicated, administer 10–20 mg q4–6h.

Antianxiety—PO: 5–10 mg tid–qid or SR capsule, 15 mg every morning, or SR capsule, 10 mg bid, for not longer than 12 wk. IM: 5–10 mg repeated q3–4h prn up to 40 mg/day.

Nausea and vomiting—PO: 5–10 mg tid–qid or SR capsule 15 mg every morning or SR capsule 10 mg bid. PR: 25 mg bid. IM: 5–10 mg repeated q3–4h prn up to 40 mg/day. *For intraoperative control*—IM: 5–10 mg 1–2 hr before induction of anesthesia or for acute symptoms during surgery; repeat once in 30 min if needed. IV: 5–10 mg as an injection at a rate ≤5 mg/min 15 min before induction of anesthesia or, for acute symptoms during surgery, repeat once if needed. Alternatively, for an IV infusion, consult further texts.

Note: Use lower doses for geriatric or debilitated patients.

Indications: Treatment of psychotic disorders, nausea and vomiting, and nonpsychotic anxiety (short-term; not first-line)

Action: Antipsychotic effect due to inhibition of CNS dopaminergic receptors; antiemetic effect from inhibition of medullary chemoreceptor trigger-zone dopaminergic receptors; has weak anticholinergic and moderate sedative effects; peripheral α-adrenergic blocking effect causes vasodilation

Metabolism: Hepatic

Excretion: Renal

Contraindications and precautions
1. Contraindicated in comatose states, severe CNS depression, subcortical brain damage, bone marrow depression, and severe cardiovascular disease.
2. Use with caution in cardiovascular disease, seizure disorders, hepatic function impairment, glaucoma, urinary retention, prostatic hypertrophy, chronic respiratory disorders, blood dyscrasias, and active alcoholism.
3. Tartrazine in some products may cause allergic reactions.

Drug interactions
1. CNS depressants lead to increased effects.
2. Anticholinergic agents lead to increased antimuscarinic effects.
3. Aluminum- or magnesium-containing antacids or lithium may decrease oral absorption.
4. Epinephrine leads to severe hypotension and tachycardia.
5. Propranolol and possibly other β blockers lead to increased levels and vice versa.
6. Opioids lead to increased risk of constipation.
7. Prochlorperazine may increase phenytoin or tricyclic antidepressant levels.
8. Prochlorperazine may increase risk of metrizamide-induced seizures.
9. Prochlorperazine may decrease effect of levodopa.

Promethazine (Phenergan, others)

Preparations: Tablets, 12.5, 25, 50 mg; syrup, 6.25, 25 mg/5 ml; suppositories, 12.5, 25, 50 mg; injection (IM, IV), 25 mg/ml; injection (IM only), 50 mg/ml

Adult dosage

Antihistaminic—PO: 12.5 mg qid or 25 mg qhs as needed. PR, IM, IV: 25 mg repeated in 2 hr if needed.

Antiemetic—PO, PR: Initially, 25 mg, then 12.5–25 mg q4–6h prn. IM, IV: Initially, 12.5–25 mg, then 12.5–25 mg q4–6h prn.

For motion sickness—PO, PR: 25 mg 30–60 min before travel, repeated in 8–12 hr prn; it may be given bid thereafter. IM, IV: 12.5–25 mg 30–60 min before travel, repeated in 4–6 hr prn.

Sedative-hypnotic—PO, PR, IM, IV: 25–50 mg

Note: Preferred parenteral route is deep IM injection. For IV administration, use a concentration ≤25 mg/ml and infuse at a rate ≤25 mg/min.

Indications: Treatment of symptoms associated with perennial and seasonal allergic rhinitis, vasomotor rhinitis, allergic conjunctivitis, pruritus, urticaria, angioedema, and dermatographism; treatment and prophylaxis of motion sickness and nausea and vomiting; adjunctive treatment for anaphylactoid reactions; used for pre- and postoperative sedation

Action: Histamine (H_1)-receptor blocker

Metabolism: Hepatic

Excretion: Renal, fecal

Contraindications and precautions

1. Contraindicated in comatose patients, in those who have received large doses of CNS depressants, or in those with a previous history of phenothiazine-induced jaundice or bone marrow suppression.
2. Use with caution in asthma or other respiratory disorders, bladder neck obstruction, prostatic hypertrophy, predisposition to urinary retention, angle-closure glaucoma, hepatic function impairment, stenosing peptic ulcer or pyloroduodenal obstruction, bone marrow depression, cardiovascular disease, hypertension, or seizure disorder.
3. Use with caution in activities requiring mental alertness or physical coordination.

Drug interactions

1. Alcohol or other CNS depressants may increase CNS depression.
2. Amantadine, antihistamines, and other anticholinergic agents may increase antimuscarinic effect.
3. Adsorbent antidiarrheal agents or aluminum- or magnesium-containing antacids may decrease absorption.
4. Antithyroid agents may increase risk of agranulocytosis.
5. Promethazine may block α-adrenergic effects of dopamine and epinephrine.
6. Promethazine may decrease antiparkinsonian effects of levodopa.
7. Promethazine may increase cardiac effects of quinidine.
8. Promethazine may decrease the seizure threshold of intrathecal metrizamide.

Propoxyphene (Darvon, others)—Schedule IV

Preparations

Propoxyphene hydrochloride, capsules, 32, 65 mg; propoxyphene napsylate, tablets, 100 mg; solution, 50 mg/ml

Adult dosage: Analgesic—PO: 65 mg propoxyphene hydrochloride q4h prn, not to exceed 390 mg/day, or 100 mg propoxyphene napsylate q4h prn, not to exceed 600 mg/day

Note

1. Propoxyphene hydrochloride 65 mg is equipotent to propoxyphene napsylate 100 mg.
2. Use lower doses in geriatric patients.
3. Administer smallest effective dose and as infrequently as possible to minimize tolerance and physical dependence.

Indications: Treatment of pain

Action: Narcotic analgesic

Metabolism: Hepatic

Excretion: Renal

Contraindications and precautions

1. Contraindicated in diarrhea associated with pseudomembranous colitis, diarrhea caused by poisoning until the toxic material has been eliminated, and acute respiratory depression.
2. Psychological and physical dependence and tolerance to many of the effects of propoxyphene may develop with chronic administration.
3. Use with caution in acute abdominal conditions, acute asthma or chronic respiratory impairment, head injury, increased intracranial pressure, intracranial lesions, hepatic or renal function impairment, hypothyroidism, gallbladder disease, inflammatory bowel disease, recent GI tract surgery, prostatic hypertrophy or obstruction, urethral stricture, acute alcoholism, Addison's disease, epilepsy, suicidal ideation, emotional instability, or history of drug abuse.
4. Use with caution in patients performing tasks requiring mental alertness or physical coordination.
5. Use with caution in patients being administered MAO inhibitors.

Drug interactions

1. Alcohol, other opioid agonist analgesics, and other CNS depressants (including antihistamines, phenothiazines, tricyclic antidepressants, benzodiazepines, sedative-hypnotics, barbiturates) may increase risk of CNS depression.
2. Antidiarrheals and anticholinergics lead to increased risk of constipation.
3. Antihypertensives and diuretics lead to increased risk of hypotension.
4. Naltrexone, naloxone, and buprenorphine may block certain opioid actions. Consult other texts for further information.
5. Propoxyphene may increase carbamazepine blood levels.

Propoxyphene and acetaminophen (Darvocet-N)—Schedule IV (see individual drugs)

Preparations: Darvocet-N 50, 50 mg propoxyphene and 325 mg acetaminophen; Darvocet-N 100, 100 mg propoxyphene and 650 mg acetaminophen

Propoxyphene hydrochloride and acetaminophen (Wygesic)—Schedule IV (see individual drugs)

Preparations: 65 mg propoxyphene hydrochloride and 650 mg acetaminophen

Propranolol (Inderal)

Preparations: Tablets, 10, 20, 40, 60, 80, 90 mg; SR capsules, 60, 80, 120, 160 mg; solution, 20 mg/5 ml, 80 mg/ml; injection (IV), 1 mg/ml

Adult dosage

Antianginal—PO: 10–20 mg tid–qid or 80 mg SR qd; increase dose q3–7d up to 320 mg/day

Antiarrhythmic—PO: 10–30 mg tid–qid; increase prn. IV: 1–3 mg at a rate ≤1 mg/min; repeat after 2 min and again after 4 hr if necessary.

Antihypertensive—PO: 40 mg bid or 80 mg SR qd; increase dose prn up to 640 mg/day

Hypertrophic subaortic stenosis—PO: 20–40 mg tid–qid or 80–160 mg SR qd

Myocardial infarction prophylaxis—PO: 180–240 mg/day in divided doses

Pheochromocytoma—PO: 20 mg tid to 40 mg tid–qid as necessary for β-blockade for 3 days before surgery. Do not administer until α-adrenergic blocking agent established. If inoperable, 30–160 mg/day in divided doses.

Vascular headache prophylaxis—PO: 20 mg qid up to 240 mg/day *in divided dose*

Thyrotoxicosis—PO: 10–40 mg tid–qid

Indications: Treatment of chronic angina, supraventricular arrhythmias, ventricular tachycardias, digitalis-induced tachyarrhythmias, hypertension, hypertrophic subaortic stenosis, mitral valve prolapse syndrome, and tremors; adjunctive treatment of pheochromocytoma and thyrotoxicosis; prophylaxis of myocardial infarction and vascular headache

Action: Nonselective β-adrenergic blocking agent (β_1, β_2)

Metabolism: Hepatic

Excretion: Renal

Contraindications and precautions

1. Contraindicated in asthma, overt cardiac failure, cardiogenic shock, 2nd- or 3rd-degree AV block, sinus bradycardia, and hypotension associated with MI.
2. Use with caution in emphysema, CHF, diabetes mellitus, mental depression, or peripheral vascular disease.
3. Abrupt withdrawal after chronic administration can precipitate angina, MI, and ventricular dysrhythmias. Dosage should be tapered over 2 wk.

Drug interactions

1. Hydrocarbon inhalation anesthetics may lead to increased myocardial depression.
2. Insulin or antidiabetic agents may increase hypoglycemia
3. Calcium channel blocking agents may increase conduction disturbance or CHF in patients with abnormal AV conduction or depressed left ventricular function.
4. Propranolol may increase or decrease cardiostimulating effect of sympathomimetics.
5. Propranolol leads to decreased bronchodilating effect of sympathomimetics and theophylline.
6. Propranolol may significantly increase BP with MAO inhibitor use.

Propylthiouracil (PTU)

Preparations: Tablets, 50 mg

Adult dosage

Hyperthyroidism—PO: Initially, 300–450 mg/day in 3 divided doses up to 1,200 mg/day for severe hyperthyroidism. When euthyroid, continue for additional 2 mo and then reduce to maintenance dosage, usually ⅓ to ⅔ of initial dosage.

Thyrotoxic crisis—PO: As an adjunct to other measures, 200–400 mg q4–6h on the first day and then decreased as symptoms are controlled

Indications: Treatment of hyperthyroidism

Action: Inhibits synthesis of thyroid hormone and peripheral conversion of thyroxine (T_4) to triiodothyronine (T_3)

Metabolism: Hepatic

Excretion: Renal

Contraindications and precautions

1. Monitor for signs or symptoms of leukopenia, particularly infection; perform CBC in patients who develop fever or illness.
2. Use with caution in bone marrow depression, infection, or hepatic function impairment.

Drug interactions

1. Propylthiouracil may increase risk of hemorrhage due to anticoagulants.
2. Lithium, potassium iodide, or iodinated glycerol may increase risk of hypothyroidism and goiter.

Protriptyline (Vivactyl)
Preparations: Tablets, 5, 10 mg
Adult dosage: PO: Initially, 5–10 mg qid. Increase up to 60 mg/day. Maximum antidepressant effects may take ≥2 wk. Start with lower doses in geriatric patients. After control of symptoms, taper to lowest effective dose.
Indications: Treatment of depression; unlabeled uses include treatment of obstructive sleep apnea and narcolepsy/cataplexy syndrome
Action: Tricyclic antidepressant; increases CNS synaptic concentration of norepinephrine or serotonin, presumably by blocking presynaptic reuptake; has sedative, anticholinergic, peripheral vasodilator, and direct quinidine-like myocardial effects
Metabolism: Hepatic
Excretion: Renal
Contraindications and precautions
1. Contraindicated during recovery from MI and possibly concurrent MAO inhibitor use.
2. Use with caution in alcoholism, asthma, bipolar disorder, schizophrenia, cardiovascular disorders, blood disorders, GI disorders, narrow-angle glaucoma, hepatic or renal function impairment, hyperthyroidism, prostatic hypertrophy or urinary retention, and seizure disorders
3. Exercise caution while driving or performing other tasks requiring alertness.
4. Abrupt cessation after prolonged administration may cause withdrawal symptoms.
5. Prescribe the smallest quantity feasible for patients considered at risk for suicide.

Drug interactions
1. Alcohol or CNS depressants lead to increased CNS depression.
2. Drugs with antimuscarinic activity lead to increased anticholinergic side effects.
3. Direct-acting sympathomimetics lead to increased cardiac effects.
4. MAO inhibitors lead to increased risk of hyperpyretic episodes, convulsions, hypertensive crises, and death.
5. Antithyroid agents lead to increased risk of agranulocytosis.
6. Barbiturates and carbamazepine may decrease plasma concentration of protriptyline.
7. Cimetidine methylphenidate, phenothiazines, estrogens, and possibly ranitidine may increase plasma concentration of protriptyline.
8. Metrizamide leads to increased risk of seizures.
9. Thyroid hormone leads to increased therapeutic and toxic effects of both medications.
10. Protriptyline leads to decreased hypotensive effect of guanethidine and clonidine.
11. Protriptyline may increase plasma concentration of coumadin.

Pseudoephedrine hydrochloride (Sudafed, others)
Preparations: Tablets, 30, 60 mg; ER capsules, 120 mg; liquid, 15, 30 mg/5 ml
Adult dosage: Decongestant—PO: 60 mg q4–6h or 120 mg bid of the ER preparation up to a maximum 240 mg/day
Indications: Treatment of nasal, sinus, and eustachian tube congestion
Action: α-Adrenergic agonist that results in vasoconstriction of the respiratory tract mucosa; has minimal β-adrenergic agonist activity
Metabolism: Hepatic
Excretion: Renal
Contraindications and precautions
1. Contraindicated in severe hypertension or coronary artery disease and in concurrent MAO inhibitor use.
2. Use with caution in cardiovascular disease, coronary artery disease, hypertension, diabetes mellitus, prostatic hypertrophy, and hyperthyroidism.

Drug interactions
1. MAO inhibitors may cause intense cardiac stimulant or vasopressor effects; concurrent use is contraindicated.
2. Pseudoephedrine may decrease effect of β-adrenergic blockers.
3. Pseudoephedrine may increase cardiovascular effects of sympathomimetics or digoxin.

Psyllium (Metamucil, others)
Preparations: Powder, 3.3, 3.4, 3.5, 4.94 g/dose; effervescent powder, 3.0, 3.4 g/dose; granules, 2.5, 4.03 g/dose; chewable pieces, 3.4 g/2 pieces; wafers, 3.4 g/wafer (consult other sources for full contents of above preparations that contain sugars and salts)
Adult dosage: PO: *Powder*—1 tsp; *effervescent powder*—1 packet; or *granules*—1 rounded tsp mixed in liquid qd–tid or 2 pieces taken with liquid qd–tid or 1 wafer taken with liquid qd–tid
Indications: Treatment and prophylaxis of constipation; treatment of irritable bowel syndrome
Action: Bulk-forming laxative
Metabolism: Not absorbed
Excretion: Fecal
Contraindications and precautions:
1. Contraindicated in nausea, vomiting, or other symptoms of appendicitis, acute surgical abdomen, intestinal obstruction, or fecal impaction.
2. Use with caution in dysphagia, CHF, hypertension, and diabetes.

Drug interactions: Psyllium may decrease absorption of coumadin, digoxin, and salicylates.

Quinidine
Preparations
Quinidine sulfate: Tablets, 100, 200, 300 mg; SR tablets, 300 mg; capsules, 200, 300 mg; injection (IM, IV), 200 mg/ml
Quinidine gluconate: SR tablets, 324, 330 mg; injection (IM, IV), 80 mg/ml. On a molar basis, 267 mg quinidine gluconate = 200 mg quinidine sulfate. Quinidine gluconate used for maintenance dosing only.
Adult dosage: Antiarrhythmic: *Premature atrial and ventricular contractions*—PO: 200–300 mg tid–qid. *Paroxysmal supraventricular tachycardia*—PO: 400–600 mg q2–3h until paroxysm is terminated. Higher doses (up to 600 mg q1h × 10 hr) have been reported for paroxysmal ventricular tachycardia. *Atrial flutter*—PO: Individual titration after digitalization. *Conversion of atrial fibrillation*—PO: 200 mg q2–3h for 5–8 doses. Increase daily dosage until normal sinus rhythm or toxicity. Alternatively, 300–400 mg q6h until conversion. *Parenteral administration for acute arrhythmias*—Quinidine gluconate (IM): Initially, 600 mg, then 400 mg q2h prn adjusted by the effect of the previous dose. Quinidine gluconate (IV): Dilute 800 mg (10 ml) in 40 ml D5W administered at an infusion rate of 1 ml/min with EKG and BP monitoring. Discontinue if normal sinus rhythm restored or toxicity develops. Usually <300 mg is required for conversion of ventricular arrhythmias. Quinidine sulfate (IV): Dilute 600 mg in 40 ml D5W, and follow guidelines for IV quinidine gluconate. *Maintenance*—PO: Quinidine gluconate—324–660 mg q8–12 h; quinidine sulfate—200–300 mg tid–qid or 300–600 mg of SR preparation q8–12h.
Note
1. Therapeutic serum concentration is 2–6 μg/ml.
2. A test dose of 200 mg may be given to check for intolerance.

Indications: Treatment and prophylaxis of cardiac arrhythmias: paroxysmal and chronic atrial fibrillation, atrial flutter, paroxysmal supraventricular tachycardia, paroxysmal AV junctional rhythm, paroxysmal ventricular tachycardia not associated with complete heart block, and premature atrial and ventricular contractions
Action: Class 1A antiarrhythmic
Metabolism: Hepatic
Excretion: Renal
Contraindications and precautions
1. Contraindicated in complete AV block, severe intraventricular conduction defects, ectopic impulses and rhythms due to escape mechanisms, and digitalis toxicity with AV conduction disorder.
2. Generally contraindicated in myasthenia gravis.
3. Use with caution in asthma, muscle weakness, and infection with fever because hypersensitivity reactions may be masked.
4. Use with caution in incomplete AV block, digitalis intoxication, and hepatic or renal function impairment.
5. Monitor serum quinidine levels with daily doses >2 g. Widening of the QRS complex signifies possible quinidine toxicity.

Drug interactions
1. Hepatic enzyme inducers (e.g., phenobarbital, phenytoin, rifampin) may decrease serum quinidine level.
2. Amiodarone, cimetidine, acetazolamide, and thiazides may increase serum quinidine level.
3. Phenothiazines or other antiarrhythmics may have additive cardiac effects.
4. Anticholinergics may increase antimuscarinic effects.
5. Quinidine may increase effect of neuromuscular blocking agents and oral anticoagulants.
6. Quinidine leads to increased serum level of digoxin.

Quinine sulfate (Quinamm, others)
Preparations: Tablets, 260, 325 mg; capsules, 64.8, 130, 195, 200, 300, 325 mg
Adult dosage: Nocturnal leg cramps—PO: 260–300 qhs. An additional dosage may be taken after the evening meal.
Indications: Treatment and prophylaxis of nocturnal recumbency leg muscle cramps; treatment of malaria
Action: Quinine has skeletal muscle relaxant effects.
Metabolism: Hepatic
Excretion: Renal
Contraindications and precautions
1. Contraindicated in G6PD deficiency, history of thrombocytopenic purpura associated with previous quinine administration, tinnitus, or optic neuritis.
2. Use with caution in myasthenia gravis and atrial fibrillation.

Drug interactions
1. Aluminum-containing antacids may decrease absorption.
2. Quinine may increase risk of hemorrhage associated with oral anticoagulants.
3. Quinine may increase serum concentrations of digoxin.
4. Quinine may increase effects of neuromuscular blocking agents.

Ranitidine (Zantac)
Preparations: Tablets, 150, 300 mg; injection (IM, IV), 25 mg/ml
Adult dosage
Duodenal ulcer treatment—PO: 150 mg bid or 300 mg qhs; IM, IV: 50 mg q6–8h
Duodenal ulcer prophylaxis—PO: 150 mg hs
Gastric ulcer treatment—PO: 150 mg bid; IM, IV: 50 mg q6–8h
Gastric hypersecretory conditions—PO: 150 mg bid; doses up to 6 g/day reported; IM, IV: 50 mg q6–8h
Gastroesophageal reflux—PO: 150 mg bid
Note: Dosage reduction in renal function impairment: For creatinine clearance <50 mg/ml—PO: 150 mg q24h. IM, IV: 50 mg q18–24h. Further reduction may be required if there is concurrent hepatic function impairment.
Indications: Treatment of active benign gastric and duodenal ulcers, gastroesophageal reflux, and gastric hypersecretory conditions (Zollinger-Ellison syndrome, systemic mastocytosis, multiple endocrine adenomas), and prophylaxis of duodenal ulcer. Unlabeled uses include upper gastrointestinal bleeding and stress-related mucosal damage.
Action: Histamine H_2 blocker; inhibits gastric acid secretion; weak inhibitor of cytochrome P-450 mixed function oxidase
Metabolism: Hepatic
Excretion: Renal
Contraindications and precautions: Use with caution in hepatic or renal function impairment.
Drug interactions
1. Antacids lead to decreased absorption.
2. Ranitidine may increase effects and toxicity of benzodiazepines, calcium channel blockers, carbamazepine, coumadin, ethanol, labetolol, metoprolol, propanolol, lidocaine, quinidine, metronidazole, phenytoin, sulfonylureas, tricyclic antidepressants, and xanthines (much less effect than cimetidine).
3. Ranitidine leads to decreased absorption of ketoconazole.
4. Ranitidine leads to decreased renal excretion of procainamide.

Salsalate (Disalcid, others)
Preparations: Tablets, 500, 750 mg; capsules, 500 mg
Adult dosage: Antirheumatic—PO: Usual initial dose is 3 g/day in 2–3 divided doses. Maintenance dosage is usually 2–4 g/day in divided doses.
Indications: Treatment of rheumatoid and osteoarthritis; unlabeled use includes treatment of nonrheumatic inflammatory disorders
Action: Nonacetylated salicylate with anti-inflammatory effects; no clinically significant antiplatelet effects
Metabolism: Hepatic
Excretion: Renal
Contraindications and precautions
1. Contraindicated in bleeding ulcers, other hemorrhagic states, and hemophilia.
2. Use with caution in erosive gastritis, peptic ulcer disease, hepatic and renal function impairment, and thyrotoxicosis.

Drug interactions
1. Alcohol or NSAIDs may increase risk of GI side effects.
2. Oral anticoagulants, NSAIDs, heparin, thrombolytic agents, and other antiplatelet agents may increase risk of hemorrhage.
3. Carbonic anhydrase inhibitors lead to increased renal excretion.
4. Ototoxic medications may increase risk of ototoxicity.
5. Corticosteroids may decrease serum salicylate concentration.
6. Salsalate may increase plasma methotrexate concentration.
7. Salsalate may decrease uricosuric effect of probenecid.
8. High doses of salsalate may increase hypoglycemic effect of sulfonylureas and insulin.

Senna (Senokot, others)
Preparations: Standardized senna concentrate: Tablets, 187, 217 mg; syrup, 218 mg/5 ml; granules, 326 mg/tsp; suppositories, 625 mg
Adult dosage: PO: 1–2 tablets or 1 tsp of granules or 10–15 ml of syrup qd up to bid. PR: 1 suppository qhs.
Indications: Treatment of constipation; bowel evacuation in preparation for surgery, radiography, and sigmoidoscopy
Action: Stimulant laxative; probably increases peristalsis by a direct effect on intestinal smooth muscle by stimulation of intramural nerve plexi
Metabolism: None (minimal absorption)
Excretion: Unknown
Contraindications and precautions
1. Contraindicated in nausea, vomiting, or other symptoms of appendicitis, acute surgical abdomen, undiagnosed rectal bleeding, intestinal obstruction, or fecal impaction.
2. May cause significant electrolyte loss with repeated use.

Spironolactone (Aldactone, others)
Preparations: Tablets, 25, 50, 100 mg
Adult dosage
Diuretic—PO: Initially, 25–200 mg/day in 2–4 divided doses for at least 5 days. Titrate to maintenance doses. If there is inadequate diuresis after 5 days, consider adding a second diuretic that acts more proximally in the renal tubule.
Antihypertensive—PO: Initially, 50–100 mg/day in a single dose or 2–4 divided doses. After 2 wk, titrate up to 200 mg/day if needed.
Aldosterone antagonist—PO: *Diagnostic aid for primary hyperaldosteronism*—consult other texts. *Treatment of primary hyperaldosteronism*—100–400 mg/day in divided doses prior to surgery; if patient is not a candidate for surgery, use lowest possible dose for long-term maintenance.
Antihypokalemic—PO: 25–100 mg/day
Indications: Treatment of edema, hypertension, primary hyperaldosteronism, and hypokalemia
Action: Blocks sodium exchange for potassium in distal renal tubule, resulting in increased excretion of water and sodium and retention of potassium; competitive inhibitor of aldosterone
Metabolism: Hepatic
Excretion: Renal > biliary
Contraindications and precautions
1. Contraindicated in hyperkalemia.
2. Use with caution in anuria, renal insufficiency, hyperuricemia, gout, breast enlargement, and diabetes mellitus.

Drug interactions:
1. Blood transfusions, captopril, enalapril, lisinopril, cyclosporine, other potassium-sparing diuretics, potassium supplements, and salt substitutes may increase risk of hyperkalemia.
2. Spironolactone leads to increased risk of lithium toxicity.

Spironolactone with hydrochlorothiazide (Aldactazide, others)
Preparations: Spironolactone/hydrochlorothiazide tablets, 25/25, 25/50 mg
Adult dosage
Diuretic—PO: 25–200 mg/day of each component
Antihypertensive—PO: 50–100 mg/day of each component
Indications: Treatment of edema and hypertension. This combination is not indicated for initial therapy. Determine the optimum maintenance dose of each drug separately, and use the combination preparation if it corresponds to the ratio of the separate drugs.
Action: Hydrochlorothiazide inhibits sodium reabsorption in the distal renal tubule, and spironolactone blocks sodium exchange for potassium in the distal renal tubule. The combination has additive diuretic and antihypertensive effects.
Metabolism: Spironolactone—hepatic; hydrochlorothiazide—minimal
Excretion: Spironolactone—renal > biliary; hydrochlorothiazide—renal

Spironolactone
Contraindications and precautions
1. Contraindicated in hyperkalemia.
2. Use with caution in anuria, renal

insufficiency, hyperuricemia, gout, breast enlargement, and diabetes mellitus.

Drug interactions

1. Blood transfusions, captopril, enalapril, lisinopril, cyclosporine, other potassium-sparing diuretics, potassium supplements, and salt substitutes may increase risk of hyperkalemia.
2. Spironolactone leads to increased risk of lithium toxicity.

Hydrochlorothiazide

Contraindications and precautions

1. Contraindicated in anuria and hypersensitivity to thiazides or other sulfonamide derivatives.
2. Use with caution in diabetes mellitus, history of gout, hyperuricemia, hepatic function impairment, hypercalcemia, systemic lupus erythematosus, sympathectomy, or electrolyte disturbance.

Drug interactions

1. Cholestyramine and colestipol lead to decreased absorption.
2. Glucocorticoids and amphotericin B lead to increased risk of hypokalemia.
3. Hydrochlorothiazide leads to increased risk of lithium toxicity.
4. Hydrochlorothiazide leads to increased risk of toxicity of digoxin, amiodarone, and nondepolarizing neuromuscular blocking agents due to hypokalemia.

Sucralfate (Carafate)

Preparations: Tablets, 1 g
Adult dosage: PO: 1 g 1 hr ac and qhs on an empty stomach
Indications: Treatment of duodenal ulcer. Unlabeled use includes treatment of gastric ulcer.
Action: Sucralfate forms an ulcer-adherent complex that protects the ulcer site from acid, pepsin, and bile salts.
Metabolism: <5% absorption
Excretion: Renal (of absorbed dose)
Contraindications and precautions: No clinically significant precautions

Drug interactions

1. Sucralfate may decrease absorption of cimetidine, digoxin, phenytoin, or tetracycline.
2. Antacids may decrease effectiveness of sucralfate.

Sulfasalazine (Azulfidine, others)

Preparations: Tablets, 500 mg; EC tablets, 500 mg; suspension, 250 mg/5 ml
Adult dosage: Inflammatory bowel disease—PO: Initially, 1–2 g q6–8h. After clinical and endoscopic improvement, reduce to maintenance dose, usually 500 mg qid. Take doses with or after meals and do not exceed 8 hr between doses.

Note

1. May require dosage reduction in renal function impairment.
2. Adverse reactions tend to increase when total daily doses exceed 4 g.

Indications: Treatment and prophylaxis of inflammatory bowel disease
Action: Mechanism unknown; cleaved in the colon by bacteria to sulfapyridine and 5-aminosalicylic acid, which may act locally
Metabolism: Hepatic
Excretion: Renal (sulfapyridine); fecal > renal (5-aminosalicylic acid)

Contraindications and precautions

1. Patients intolerant of any sulfonamide, furosemide, thiazides, sulfonylureas, acetazolamide, or salicylates may be intolerant of sulfasalazine.
2. Use with caution in blood dyscrasias, G6PD deficiency, intestinal or urinary tract obstruction, hepatic or renal function impairment, or porphyria.

Drug interactions

1. Probenecid may increase toxicity of sulfasalazine.
2. Methenamine may increase risk of crystalluria.
3. Sulfasalazine may decrease absorption of iron preparations, folic acid, and digoxin.
4. Sulfasalazine may increase toxicity of coumadin, phenytoin, sulfonylureas, methotrexate, hemolytic agents, other hepatotoxic medications, or bone marrow depressants.

Sulindac (Clinoril)

Preparations: Tablets, 150, 200 mg
Adult dosage:
Antirheumatic—PO: 150 mg bid
Nonrheumatic anti-inflammatory, antigout—PO: Initially, 200 mg bid, then reduce according to patient response
Indications: Treatment of rheumatic and nonrheumatic inflammatory disorders and acute gouty arthritis; unlabeled use includes treatment of calcium pyrophosphate deposition disease
Action: Nonsteroidal anti-inflammatory drug that inhibits cyclo-oxygenase, resulting in decreased formation of prostaglandins; effects include antirheumatic, analgesic, antipyretic, and inhibition of platelet aggregation
Metabolism: Hepatic
Excretion: Renal > biliary

Contraindications and precautions

1. Contraindicated in a history of severe allergic reaction to aspirin or other NSAIDs.
2. Use with caution in a history of peptic ulcer, upper gastrointestinal disease or ulcerative colitis, renal or hepatic function impairment, bleeding disorders, asthma, CHF, diabetes mellitus, hypertension, and pre-existing edema.

Drug interactions

1. Acetaminophen, gold compounds, or nephrotoxic medications may increase risk of renal toxicity.
2. Glucocorticoids, alcohol, potassium supplements, other NSAIDs, or aspirin may increase risk of GI side effects.
3. Anticoagulants, thrombolytic agents, aspirin, platelet aggregation inhibitors, or colchicine may increase risk of hemorrhage.
4. Probenecid may increase sulindac serum level.
5. Sulindac may increase methotrexate toxicity.
6. Sulindac may decrease antihypertensive effects of diuretics and antihypertensives.
7. Sulindac may decrease diuretic effect of diuretics.
8. Sulindac may increase hypoglycemic effect of sulfonylureas.

Tamoxifen citrate (Nolvadex)

Preparations: Tablets, 10 mg
Adult dosage: Breast carcinoma—PO: 10–20 mg bid
Indications: Treatment of metastatic breast carcinoma in postmenopausal women; adjuvant therapy for breast carcinoma following surgery in postmenopausal women or women ≥50 yr of age with positive axillary nodes
Action: Nonsteroidal antiestrogen
Metabolism: Hepatic
Excretion: Fecal > renal
Contraindications and precautions: Use with caution in leukopenia or thrombocytopenia.
Drug interactions: No clinically significant interactions.

Temazepam (Restoril, others)

Preparations: Capsules, 15, 30 mg
Adult dosage: Sedative-hypnotic—PO: 15–30 mg qhs. Initiate therapy with 15 mg in elderly or debilitated patients.
Indications: Treatment of insomnia
Action: Sedative-hypnotic benzodiazepine; may potentiate CNS gamma-aminobutyric acid effects
Metabolism: Hepatic (glucuronidation)
Excretion: Renal

Contraindications and precautions

1. Contraindicated in acute alcohol intoxication with depressed vital signs, depressive neuroses, or psychoses without prominent anxiety.
2. Use with caution in acute narrow-angle glaucoma, myasthenia gravis, shock, severe COPD, hepatic or renal function impairment, patients with depressed respirations, or those receiving concurrent respiratory depressants.
3. Long-term therapy may result in psychological or physical dependence.
4. Exercise caution in performing tasks requiring alertness and coordination.

Drug interactions

1. Temazepam may increase zidovudine (AZT) toxicity.
2. Alcohol or other CNS depressants lead to increased CNS depression.

Terbutaline (Brethine, others)

Preparations: Tablets, 5 mg; aerosol, 0.20 mg per metered spray in 7.5-ml canister; injection (SC), 1 mg/ml
Adult dosage: Bronchodilator—PO: 2.5–5 mg tid. Aerosol: 0.4 mg (2 inhalations) separated by 60 sec q4–6h. SC: 0.25 mg repeated in 15–30 min if necessary up to a dose not to exceed 0.5 mg within a 4-hr period.
Indications: Treatment of bronchospasm in patients with reversible obstructive airway disease. Unlabeled use includes inhibition of premature labor.
Action: Sympathomimetic bronchodilator (β_2)
Metabolism: Hepatic
Excretion: Renal
Contraindications and precautions: Use with caution in cardiovascular disease, especially arrhythmias and hypertension, diabetes, hyperthyroidism, pheochromocytoma, and history of seizures.

Drug interactions

1. Digoxin and levodopa may increase cardiac arrhythmias.

2. Tricyclic antidepressants and MAO inhibitors may increase effects on vascular system.
3. Thyroid hormone may increase effect of terbutaline and vice versa.
4. Terbutaline may increase CNS stimulation of other sympathomimetics and xanthines.

Terfenadine (Seldane)

Preparations: Tablets, 60 mg
Adult dosage: Antihistaminic—PO: 60 mg bid
Indications: Treatment of allergic rhinitis
Action: H_1-receptor blocker. Terfenadine lacks the significant antimuscarinic effects of other antihistamines.
Metabolism: Hepatic
Excretion: Fecal > renal
Contraindications and precautions: Terfenadine lacks significant antimuscarinic effects but should still be used with caution in prostatic hypertrophy, bladder neck obstruction, angle-closure glaucoma, asthma, and COPD.
Drug interactions: No clinically significant interactions.

Theophylline (see *Xanthine derivatives*)

Thiamine hydrochloride

Preparations: Tablets, 5, 10, 25, 50, 100, 250, 500 mg; injection (IM, IV), 100, 200 mg/ml
Adult dosage
Thiamine deficiency: *In critically ill*—injection (IM, IV): Initially, 5–10 mg tid. *Following improvement in critically ill or initially in noncritically ill*—PO: 5–30 mg/day as a single dose or in 3 divided doses.
Nutritional supplement—PO: 1–2 mg qd
Indications: Treatment and prophylaxis of thiamine deficiency
Action: Thiamine combines with ATP to form a coenzyme essential for carbohydrate metabolism.
Metabolism: Hepatic
Excretion: Renal
Contraindications and precautions: Wernicke's encephalopathy may be precipitated or worsened after IV glucose administration. Administer thiamine before glucose.
Drug interactions: No clinically significant interactions.

Thioridazine (Mellaril, others)

Preparations: Tablets, 10, 15, 25, 50, 100, 150, 200 mg; solution, 30 mg/ml, 100 mg/ml; suspension, 25 mg/5 ml, 100 mg/5 ml
Adult dosage
Antipsychotic—PO: Initially, 25–100 mg tid. Increase dose gradually up to 300 mg/day or 800 mg/day in 2–4 divided doses if patient is hospitalized or has severe symptoms. Once a response is obtained, taper to lowest effective dose, in 2–4 divided doses.
Depression with anxiety—PO: Initially, 25 mg tid. Adjust dose from 10 mg bid–qid to 50 mg tid–qid.
Note: Use lower doses in geriatric or debilitated patients.
Indications: Treatment of psychotic disorders and short-term treatment of major depression with variable degrees of anxiety
Action: Antipsychotic effect due to inhibition of CNS dopaminergic receptors; has strong anticholinergic and sedative effects; peripheral α-adrenergic blocking effect causes vasodilation
Metabolism: Hepatic
Excretion: Renal, biliary
Contraindications and precautions
1. Contraindicated in comatose states, severe CNS depression, subcortical brain damage, bone marrow depression, and severe cardiovascular disease.
2. Use with caution in cardiovascular disease, seizure disorders, hepatic function impairment, glaucoma, urinary retention, prostatic hypertrophy, chronic respiratory disorders, blood dyscrasias, and active alcoholism.
3. Tartrazine in some products may cause allergic reactions.

Drug interactions
1. CNS depressants lead to increased CNS depression.
2. Anticholinergic agents lead to increased antimuscarinic effects.
3. Aluminum- or magnesium-containing antacids and lithium may decrease oral absorption.
4. Epinephrine leads to severe hypotension and tachycardia.
5. Propranolol and possibly other β-blockers lead to increased levels and vice versa.
6. Opioids lead to increased risk of constipation.
7. Thioridazine may increase phenytoin and tricyclic antidepressant levels.
8. Thioridazine may increase risk of metrizamide-induced seizures.
9. Thioridazine may decrease effect of levodopa.

Timolol maleate—Ophthalmic (Timoptic)

Preparations: Solution, 0.25, 0.5%
Adult dosage: Topical, to the conjunctiva: 1 drop of 0.25 or 0.5% solution bid. Dosage may be reduced to 1 drop qd if satisfactory intraocular pressure is maintained.
Indications: Treatment of open-angle and secondary glaucoma, glaucoma in aphakic eyes, and ocular hypertension
Action: Nonselective β-adrenergic blocker; reduces intraocular pressure, presumably by decreasing aqueous humor production
Metabolism: Minimal absorption
Excretion: Minimal absorption
Contraindications and precautions
1. Contraindicated in history of bronchial asthma, severe chronic obstructive pulmonary disease, CHF, cardiogenic shock, sinus bradycardia, and 2nd, or 3rd-degree AV block.
2. Use with caution in bronchitis, emphysema, CHF, diabetes mellitus, severe cardiac disease, cerebrovascular disease, and hyperthyroidism.

Drug interactions
1. β-Adrenergic blockers (systemic) may have additive effects.
2. Digoxin and calcium channel blockers may produce AV conduction disturbances.

Tocainide (Tonocard)

Preparations: Tablets, 400, 600 mg
Adult dosage: Antiarrhythmic—PO: Initially, 400 mg q8h. Usual dosage rate is 1,200–1,800 mg/day in 3 divided doses up to a maximum 2,400 mg/day.
Note: May need to reduce dosage in hepatic or renal function impairment
Indications: Treatment and prophylaxis of ventricular arrhythmias
Action: Class IB antiarrhythmic
Metabolism: Hepatic
Excretion: Renal
Contraindications and precautions
1. Contraindicated in 2nd- or 3rd-degree AV block without pacemaker.
2. Use with caution in CHF, atrial fibrillation or flutter, bone marrow failure, or cytopenia.
3. Tocainide may be proarrhythmic.
4. Tocainide has a mild negative inotropic effect.

Drug interactions: β-Adrenergic blocking agents may increase negative inotropic effect.

Tolazamide (Ronase, Tolinase, others)

Preparations: Tablets, 100, 250, 500 mg
Adult dosage: PO: Initially, 100–250 mg qd. Start with lower doses in geriatric, debilitated, or malnourished patients, and in those with renal or hepatic function impairment. Increase gradually until there is optimal control or a maximum daily dose of 1 g. Use bid dosing for daily doses >500 mg. Patients being transferred from chlorpropamide should be monitored closely for hypoglycemia the first 2 wk. Transfer from other sulfonylureas does not require a conversion period. Patients previously on insulin doses <40 units/day can start tolazamide and have the insulin abruptly stopped. Patients previously on ≥40 units/day should start oral therapy with a concurrent 50% reduction in insulin dose. Taper insulin, and increase tolazamide according to clinical response.
Indications: Treatment of non–insulin-dependent diabetes mellitus
Action: Sulfonylurea that promotes insulin release from pancreatic β cells, decreases hepatic gluconeogenesis, and increases insulin sensitivity
Metabolism: Hepatic
Excretion: Renal
Contraindications and precautions
1. Contraindicated in significant acidosis, severe burns, diabetic coma, severe infection, significant ketosis, ketoacidosis, major surgery, or severe trauma.
2. Cross-sensitivity to other sulfonamide-type medications possible.
3. Use with caution in adrenal or pituitary insufficiency, thyroid function impairment, renal, hepatic or cardiac impairment, malnourishment, debilitated physical condition, or nausea and vomiting.

Drug interactions
1. Chronic ethanol use, phenobarbital, and rifampin lead to decreased hypoglycemic effects.
2. Chloramphenicol, cimetidine, clofibrate, coumadin, ketoconazole, MAO inhibitors, methyldopa, NSAIDs,

phenylbutazone, probenecid, salicylates, sulfonamides, and sulfinpyrazone lead to increased hypoglycemic effect.
3. Ethanol may lead to disulfiram-like reaction.

Tolbutamide (Oramide, Orinase, others)

Preparations: Tablets, 250, 500 mg

Adult dosage: PO: Initially, 500 mg–1 g qd. Start with lower doses in geriatric, debilitated, or malnourished patients, and in those with renal or hepatic function impairment. Increase gradually until optimal control or a maximum daily dose of 3 g. Divided doses may be better tolerated. Patients being transferred from chlorpropamide should be monitored closely for hypoglycemia the first 2 wk. Transfer from other sulfonylureas does not require a conversion period. Patients previously on insulin doses <20 units/day can start tolbutamide and have the insulin abruptly stopped. Patients previously on 20–40 units/day should start tolbutamide with a concurrent 30–50% reduction in insulin dose. Those on >40 units/day should start oral therapy with a concurrent 20% reduction in insulin dose. Taper insulin, and increase tolbutamide according to clinical response.

Indications: Treatment of non–insulin-dependent diabetes mellitus

Action: Sulfonylurea that promotes insulin release from pancreatic β cells, decreases hepatic gluconeogenesis, and increases insulin sensitivity

Metabolism: Hepatic

Excretion: Renal > biliary

Contraindications and precautions
1. Contraindicated in significant acidosis, severe burns, diabetic coma, severe infection, significant ketosis, ketoacidosis, major surgery, or severe trauma.
2. Cross-sensitivity to other sulfonamide-type medications is possible.
3. Use with caution in adrenal or pituitary insufficiency, thyroid function impairment, renal, hepatic or cardiac impairment, malnourishment, debilitated physical condition, or nausea and vomiting.

Drug interactions
1. Chronic ethanol use, phenobarbital, and rifampin lead to decreased hypoglycemic effects.
2. Chloramphenicol, cimetidine, clofibrate, coumadin, ketoconazole, MAO inhibitors, methyldopa, NSAIDs, phenylbutazone, probenecid, salicylates, sulfonamides, and sulfinpyrazone lead to increased hypoglycemic effect.
3. Ethanol may lead to disulfiram-like reaction.

Trazodone (Desyrel, others)

Preparations: Tablets, 50, 100, 150 mg

Adult dosage: PO: Initially, 150 mg in divided doses. Increase by 50 mg q3–4d prn up to 400 mg/day in outpatients and 600 mg/day in in-patients. Maximum antidepressant effect usually occurs within 2 wk. When symptoms are controlled, taper to lowest effective dose.

Indications: Treatment of major depressive episodes with or without anxiety

Action: A nontricyclic antidepressant; it presumably inhibits CNS neuronal uptake of serotonin

Metabolism: Hepatic

Excretion: Renal

Contraindications and precautions
1. Contraindicated during the acute recovery period of myocardial infarction.
2. Use with caution in cardiac disease (especially arrhythmias), active alcoholism, or hepatic or renal function impairment.
3. Trazodone should be discontinued if leukocyte or absolute neutrophil counts fall below normal.
4. Exercise caution while driving or performing tasks requiring alertness.
5. Prescribe the smallest quantity feasible to patients considered at risk for suicide.

Drug interactions
1. Alcohol or CNS depressants lead to increased CNS depression.
2. Antihypertensives lead to increased risk of hypotension.
3. Trazodone may increase plasma levels of digoxin and phenytoin.

Triamcinolone acetonide (Azmacort)

Preparations: Aerosol, 100 μg/inhalation, 20-g inhaler canister

Adult dosage: PO inhalation: 200 μg (2 metered sprays) tid–qid. If patient has severe asthma, start with 12–16 metered sprays/day and decrease according to patient response.

Note: If transferring from systemic to inhalation adrenocorticoids, the patient's asthma should be relatively stable. Full maintenance dosage of systemic adrenocorticoids should be continued for at least 1 wk when inhalation therapy is started. Systemic dosage may be reduced very slowly at 1 to 2 wk intervals, monitoring for adrenal insufficiency.

Indications: Treatment of seasonal or perennial rhinitis when effectiveness of or tolerance to conventional therapy is unsatisfactory; treatment of postsurgical prophylaxis of nasal polyps

Action: Anti-inflammatory steroid

Metabolism: Hepatic

Excretion: Fecal

Contraindications and precautions: Use with caution in fungal or systemic viral infections, ocular herpes simplex, and latent or active respiratory tract tuberculosis.

Triamterene (Dyrenium)

Preparations: Capsules, 50, 100 mg

Adult dosage: PO: 25–100 mg qd–bid up to 300 mg/day

Indications: Treatment of edema

Action: Blocks sodium exchange for potassium in distal renal tubule, resulting in increased excretion of water and sodium and retention of potassium

Metabolism: Hepatic

Excretion: Biliary > renal

Contraindications and precautions
1. Contraindicated in hyperkalemia.
2. Use with caution in anuria, renal insufficiency, hyperuricemia, gout, history of renal stones, and diabetes mellitus.

Drug interactions
1. Blood transfusions, captopril, enalapril, lisinopril, cyclosporine, other potassium-sparing diuretics, potassium supplements, and salt substitutes may increase risk of hyperkalemia.
2. Spironolactone leads to increased risk of lithium toxicity.

Triamterene and hydrochlorothiazide (Dyazide, Maxide, others)

Preparations: Triamterene/hydrochlorothiazide: Tablets, 37.5 mg/25 mg (Maxide, 25 mg), 75 mg/50 mg (Maxide); capsules, 50 mg/25 mg (Dyazide)

Adult dosage: Diuretic or antihypertensive—PO: *Dyazide*—1–2 capsules bid up to 4 capsules day. Some patients may be maintained on 1 cap qd or qod. *Maxide*—1 tablet qd.

Note: Although Dyazide and Maxide contain the same ingredients, they are not generic equivalents. They contain different amounts and ratios of the ingredients and have different oral bioavailability.

Indications: Treatment of edema and hypertension. This combination is not indicated for initial therapy. Determine the optimum maintenance dose of each drug separately, and use the combination preparation if it corresponds to the ratio of the separate drugs.

Action: Hydrochlorothiazide inhibits sodium reabsorption in the distal renal tubule, and spironolactone blocks sodium exchange for potassium in the distal renal tubule. The combination has additive diuretic and antihypertensive effects.

Metabolism: Spironolactone—hepatic; hydrochlorothiazide—minimal

Excretion: Spironolactone—renal > biliary; hydrochlorothiazide—renal

Triamterene

Contraindications and precautions
1. Contraindicated in hyperkalemia.
2. Use with caution in anuria, renal insufficiency, hyperuricemia, gout, breast enlargement, and diabetes mellitus.

Drug interactions
1. Blood transfusions, captopril, enalapril, lisinopril, cyclosporine, other potassium-sparing diuretics, potassium supplements, and salt substitutes may increase risk of hyperkalemia.
2. Spironolactone leads to increased risk of lithium toxicity.

Hydrochlorothiazide

Contraindications and precautions
1. Contraindicated in anuria and hypersensitivity to thiazides or other sulfonamide derivatives.
2. Use with caution in diabetes mellitus, history of gout, hyperuricemia, hepatic function impairment, hypercalcemia, systemic lupus erythematosus, sympathectomy, or electrolyte disturbance.

Drug interactions
1. Cholestyramine and colestipol lead to decreased absorption.
2. Glucocorticoids and amphotericin B lead to increased risk of hypokalemia.
3. Hydrochlorothiazide leads to increased risk of lithium toxicity.

4. Hydrochlorothiazide leads to increased risk of toxicity of digoxin, amiodarone, and nondepolarizing neuromuscular blocking agents due to hypokalemia.

Triazolam (Halcion)

Preparations: Tablets, 0.125, 0.25, 0.5 mg
Adult dosage: Sedative-hypnotic—PO: 0.25–0.5 mg qhs. Initiate therapy with 0.125 mg in elderly or debilitated patients.
Indications: Treatment of insomnia
Action: Sedative-hypnotic benzodiazepine; may potentiate gamma-aminobutyric acid effects
Metabolism: Hepatic (oxidation)
Excretion: Renal and fecal
Contraindications and precautions

1. Contraindicated in acute alcohol intoxication with depressed vital signs, depressive neuroses, or psychoses without prominent anxiety.
2. Use with caution in acute narrow-angle glaucoma, myasthenia gravis, shock, severe COPD, hepatic or renal function impairment, patients with depressed respirations, or those receiving concurrent respiratory depressants.
3. Long-term therapy may result in psychological or physical dependence.
4. Exercise caution in performing tasks requiring alertness and coordination.

Drug interactions

1. Cimetidine, disulfiram, erythromycin, isoniazid, ketoconazole, and oral contraceptives may increase effects.
2. Alcohol or other CNS depressants lead to increased CNS depression.

Trifluoperazine (Stelazine, others)

Preparations: Tablets, 1, 2, 5, 10 mg; solution, 10 mg/ml; injection (IM), 2 mg/ml
Adult dosage
Antipsychotic—PO: Initially, 2–5 mg bid. Increase gradually; optimum response usually occurs within 2–3 wk at 15–20 mg/day. IM: 1–2 mg q4–6h prn up to 6 mg/24 hr.
Antianxiety—PO: 1–2 mg bid up to 6 mg/day for not longer than 12 wk.
Note: Use lower doses in geriatric and debilitated patients.
Indications: Treatment of psychotic disorders and nonpsychotic anxiety (short-term; not first-line)
Action: Antipsychotic effect due to inhibition of CNS dopaminergic receptors; has weak anticholinergic and sedative effects; peripheral α-adrenergic blocking effect causes vasodilation
Metabolism: Hepatic
Excretion: Renal
Contraindications and precautions

1. Contraindicated in comatose states, severe CNS depression, subcortical brain damage, bone marrow depression, and severe cardiovascular disease.
2. Use with caution in cardiovascular disease, seizure disorders, hepatic function impairment, glaucoma, urinary retention, prostatic hypertrophy, chronic respiratory disorders, blood dyscrasias, and active alcoholism.
3. Tartrazine in some products may cause allergic reactions.

Drug interactions

1. Central nervous system depressants lead to increased effect.
2. Anticholinergic agents lead to increased antimuscarinic effects.
3. Aluminum- or magnesium-containing antacids or lithium may decrease oral absorption.
4. Epinephrine leads to severe hypotension and tachycardia.
5. Propranolol and possibly other β-blockers lead to increased levels and vice versa.
6. Opioids lead to increased risk of constipation.
7. Trifluoperazine may increase phenytoin or tricyclic antidepressant levels.
8. Trifluoperazine may increase risk of metrizamide-induced seizures.
9. Trifluoperazine may decrease effect of levodopa.

Trihexyphenidyl (Artane, others)

Preparations: Tablets, 2, 5 mg; SR capsules 5 mg; elixir, 2 mg/5 ml
Adult dosage
Parkinsonism—PO: Initially, 1–2 mg the first day; increase in 2 mg/day increments q3–5d until desired response or until the total daily dose is 6–10 mg/day (up to 15 mg/day). Usual maintenance dose is 6–10 mg/day in 3–4 divided doses. SR capsules are used when maintenance dose is determined.
Drug-induced extrapyramidal reactions—PO: Initially, single 1-mg dose. If reaction is not controlled in a few hours, progressively increase dose until control is achieved. Usual dose is 5–15 mg/day in 3–4 divided doses.
Indications: Treatment of parkinsonism and drug-induced extrapyramidal reactions, except tardive dyskinesia
Action: Synthetic anticholinergic agent with more selective CNS activity
Metabolism: Unknown
Excretion: Renal
Contraindications and precautions

1. Use with caution in cardiovascular disease, tardive dyskinesia, glaucoma, intestinal obstruction, myasthenia gravis, prostatic hypertrophy, or urinary retention.
2. Geriatric patients may develop mental confusion, disorientation, agitation, hallucinations, and psychotic-like symptoms, even with usual doses.
3. Hyperthermia is possible in geriatric, chronically ill or alcoholic patients.

Drug interactions

1. Drugs with anticholinergic properties lead to significantly increased antimuscarinic effects.
2. Antacids lead to decreased trihexyphenidyl absorption.

Valproic acid (Depakene, Depakote, others)

Preparations: Capsules, 250 mg (valproic acid); EC tablets, 125, 250, 500 mg (divalproex sodium); syrup, 250 mg/5 ml (valproate sodium)
Adult dosage: Anticonvulsant—PO: Initially, 5–15 mg/kg/day in a single dose. Increase by 5–10 mg/kg/day every week until seizures are controlled or side effects prevent further increase. Maximum daily dose is 60 mg/kg/day. Give in 2 or more divided doses if the total daily dosage exceeds 250 mg.
Note

1. Abrupt withdrawal may precipitate seizures; dosage should be reduced gradually.
2. A correlation between plasma valproic acid concentration and therapeutic effect has not been established.
3. Use lower doses in geriatric patients.

Indications: Treatment of simple and complex absence (petit mal) seizures; treatment adjunct in patients with multiple seizure types
Action: Anticonvulsant effect of unknown mechanism, but it may be due to increased GABA concentrations
Metabolism: Hepatic
Excretion: Renal
Contraindications and precautions

1. Contraindicated in hepatic disease or significant hepatic function impairment.
2. Use with caution in blood dyscrasias, history of hepatic disease, organic brain disease, or renal function impairment.
3. Use with caution in performing tasks that require mental alertness or physical coordination.
4. Valproic acid is associated with serious hepatotoxicity; monitor hepatic function tests.
5. Valproic acid is associated with thrombocytopenia and inhibition of platelet aggregation; monitor platelet count and bleeding time.

Drug interactions

1. Alcohol or other CNS depressants may increase CNS depression.
2. Oral anticoagulants, aspirin, heparin, platelet aggregation inhibitors, and thrombolytic agents may increase risk of hemorrhage.
3. Hepatotoxic agents may increase risk of hepatotoxicity.
4. Carbamazepine may decrease serum concentration of valproic acid.
5. Valproic acid may increase serum concentration of primidone or barbiturates.
6. Valproic acid may increase or decrease serum concentration of phenytoin.

Verapamil (Calan, Isoptin, others)

Preparations: Tablets, 40, 80, 120 mg; ER tablets, 240 mg; injection (IV), 2.5 mg/ml
Adult dosage
Antianginal—PO: Initially, 80–120 mg tid (40 mg in elderly or hepatic function impairment). Increase every day (unstable angina) every week up to 240–480 mg/day in 3–4 divided doses.
Antihypertensive—PO: Initially, 80 mg tid (40 mg in elderly or hepatic function impairment). Increase every week up to 360 mg/day. For extended-release, initially, 120–240 mg qd. Increase by 120 mg/day every week up to 480 mg/day in 2–4 divided doses.
Antiarrhythmic—PO: *For chronic atrial fibrillation in digitalized patients*—Initially, 80 mg tid, and increase to 240–320 mg/day in 3–4 divided doses. *For prophylaxis of paroxysmal supraventricular tachycardia in nondigitalized patients*—Initially, 80 mg tid, and increase to 240–480 mg/day in 3–4 divided doses. IV: Initially, 5–10 mg (0.075–0.15 mg/kg) injected via slow IV over 2 min. If response is not adequate,

administer 10 mg (0.15 mg/kg) 15–30 min after initial dose.
Indications: Treatment of chronic stable angina pectoris, vasospastic angina, unstable angina, hypertension, and supraventricular tachycardias
Action: Calcium-ion influx inhibitor (slow channel blocker), resulting in peripheral and coronary artery vasodilation, depression of SA and AV nodal conduction, and negative inotropic effects
Metabolism: Hepatic
Excretion: Renal
Contraindications and precautions
1. Contraindicated in 2nd- or 3rd-degree AV block, SA nodal function impairment, except in patients with a functioning artificial ventricular pacemaker, Wolff-Parkinson-White syndrome with atrial flutter or fibrillation, and severe hypotension.
2. Use with caution in hepatic or renal function impairment, bradycardia, mild-moderate hypotension, and CHF.

Drug interactions
1. β-Adrenergic blockers may increase SA and AV nodal conduction delay.
2. Cimetidine may increase effects and toxicity.
3. Calcium salts, vitamin D, and rifampin may decrease effects.
4. Disopyramide leads to increased negative inotropic effect.
5. Verapamil may decrease drug levels of lithium.
6. Verapamil may increase drug levels of carbamazepine, cyclosporine, digoxin, quinidine, or theophylline. It may increase levels of protein-bound drugs such as coumadin, phenytoin, NSAIDs, salicylates, and sulfonylureas.
7. Verapamil may potentiate effects of nondepolarizing muscle relaxants.

Vitamin K (Mephyton, Synkavite, others)
Preparations
Menadiol sodium diphosphate: Tablets, 5 mg (Synkavite); injection (IM, IV, SC), 5, 10, 37.5 mg/ml (Synkavite)
Phytonadione: Tablets, 5 mg (Mephyton); injection (IM, IV, SC), 2, 10 mg/ml (Aquamephyton); injection (aqueous dispersion for IM only), 2, 10 mg/ml (Konakion)
Adult dosage
Menadiol: *Nutritional supplement, hypoprothrombinemia secondary to obstructive jaundice and biliary fistulas*—PO: 5 mg qd. *Hypoprothrombinemia secondary to drugs (antibacterials, salicylates)*—PO: 5–10 mg qd. Injection (IM, IV, SC): 5–15 mg qd–bid.
Phytonadione: *Hypoprothrombinemia secondary to oral anticoagulants*—PO: 2.5–10 mg up to 25 mg, repeated in 12–48 hr prn. Injection (IM, IV, SC): 2.5–10 mg up to 25 mg, repeated in 6–8 hr prn. Determine subsequent doses by prothrombin time (PT) response. *Hypoprothrombinemia secondary to other causes*—Injection (IM, IV, SC): 2–25 mg, repeated if necessary.
Indications: Treatment and prophylaxis of coagulation disorders due to impaired formation of factors II, VII, IX, and X, resulting from vitamin K deficiency or interference with vitamin K activity

Note
1. Phytonadione has a more rapid and prolonged effect than menadiol and is generally more effective, especially for the treatment of oral anticoagulant–induced hypoprothrombinemia. Onset of action for parenteral menadiol is 8–24 hr; for PO phytonadione, 6–12 hr; and for parenteral phytonadione, 1–2 hr, with control of bleeding usually within 3–8 hr.
2. Use the smallest effective dose to counteract oral anticoagulant–induced hypoprothrombinemia to avoid temporary refractoriness to further anticoagulant therapy.
3. IV administration of phytonadione should not exceed 1 mg/min.

Action: Vitamin K promotes the hepatic synthesis of factors II (prothrombin), VII, IX, and X by an unknown mechanism. Menadiol sodium diphosphate (vitamin K_4) is a water-soluble derivative, and phytonadione (vitamin K_1) is a synthetic lipid-soluble form of vitamin K.
Metabolism: Hepatic
Excretion: Unknown
Contraindications and precautions
1. Severe reactions have occurred rarely during or immediately following IV administration of phytonadione. IV route not recommended unless other routes are not feasible.
2. Use menadiol with caution in G6PD deficiency.
3. Use vitamin K with caution in hepatic function impairment.

Drug interactions
1. Cholestyramine, colestipol, mineral oil, or sucralfate may decrease absorption.
2. Vitamin K leads to decreased effect of oral anticoagulants.

Warfarin sodium (Coumadin, others)
Preparations: Tablets, 2, 2.5, 5, 7.5, 10 mg
Adult dosage: Anticoagulant—PO: Initially, 10–15 mg qd for 2–4 days, then 2–10 mg qd as indicated by prothrombin-time determinations.
Indications: Treatment and prophylaxis of deep venous thrombosis and pulmonary embolism, and prophylaxis of thromboembolism associated with chronic atrial fibrillation and myocardial infarction. Unlabeled uses include treatment of TIAs and prophylaxis of recurrent cerebral thromboembolism, myocardial reinfarction, and thromboembolism associated with prosthetic heart valves and cardioversion of chronic atrial fibrillation.
Action: Inhibits hepatic synthesis of vitamin K–dependent clotting factors (II, VII, IX, X)
Metabolism: Hepatic
Excretion: Renal biliary
Contraindications and precautions
1. Contraindicated in hemorrhagic blood dyscrasias, hemophilia or other hemorrhagic tendency, recent or contemplated ophthalmic or neurologic surgery, major surgery, active bleeding, threatened abortion, cerebral or dissecting aortic aneurysm, cerebrovascular hemorrhage, severe uncontrolled hypertension, pericardial effusion, or pericarditis.
2. Use with caution in conditions associated with an increased risk of hemorrhage, such as severe diabetes mellitus, GI or respiratory or urinary tract ulceration, severe renal function impairment, and vasculitis.
3. Use with caution in conditions associated with an increased anticoagulant effect such as visceral carcinoma, CHF, severe hepatic function impairment or cirrhosis, or vitamin C or K deficiency.
4. Use with caution in subacute bacterial endocarditis, mild to moderate hypertension, polyarthritis, and protein C deficiency.
5. Use with caution in procedures associated with an increased risk of hemorrhage, such as lumbar block anesthesia or spinal puncture and indwelling catheters.
6. Use with caution in patients with alcoholism, emotional instability, psychosis, or senility, or who are uncooperative.

Drug interactions
1. Consult other texts for a complete listing.
2. Drugs associated with an increased anticoagulant effect include acetaminophen chloral hydrate, acute alcohol intoxication, allopurinol, aminosalicylic, amiodarone, androgens, cephalosporins, chloramphenicol, cimetidine, clofibrate, diflunisal, erythromycin, fenoprofen, gemfibrozil, ibuprofen, indomethacin, influenza, isoniazid, phenylbutazone, phenytoin, propylthiouracil, salicylates, sulfinpyrazone intoxication, sulfonamide, sulfonylureas, sulindac acid, thyroid hormones, tricyclic antidepressants, quinidine, quinine, and vaccines.
3. Drugs associated with a decreased anticoagulant effect include chronic alcohol abuse, barbiturates, carbamazepine, cholestyramine, colestipol, estrogens, griseofulvin, phenytoin, rifampin, sulfonylureas, and vitamin K.
4. Salicylates, platelet aggregation inhibitors, dextran, NSAIDs, heparin, and thrombolytic agents lead to increased risk of hemorrhage.

Xanthine derivatives—aminophylline, theophylline (Slo-Phyllin, Theodur, others)
Preparations: Aminophylline (hydrous): Tablets, 100, 200 mg; ER tablets, 225 mg; theophylline (anhydrous): Tablets, 100, 125, 200, 225, 250, 300 mg; ER tablets, 100, 200, 250, 300, 400, 450, 500 mg; capsules, 100, 200, 250 mg; ER capsules (q8, 12, and 24 hr), 50, 65, 75, 100, 125, 130, 200, 250, 260, 300 mg; elixir, 80, 150 mg/15 ml; solution, 80, 150 mg/15 ml; syrup, 80, 150 mg/15 ml; injection (IV), 0.4, 0.8, 1.6, 2, 3.2, 4 mg/ml D5W
Adult dosage: Bronchodilator: Acute attack (leading dose): *For patients not currently receiving theophylline preparations*—PO, IV: The equivalent of 5–6 mg theophylline/kg. *For patients currently receiving theophylline preparations*—PO, PR, IV: Obtain serum theophylline level immediately, if possible; each equivalent of

Recommended Dosages of Xanthine Derivatives

	Oral		IV	
Group	*Dosage for next 12–16 hr after loading dose**	*Maintenance dosage**	*Dosage for next 12–16 hr after loading dose**	*Maintenance dosage*
Young adult smoker	3 mg/kg q4h × 3 doses (3.8)	3 mg/kg q6h (3.8)	0.79 mg/kg/hr (1.0)	0.63 mg/kg/hr (0.8)
Healthy, nonsmoking	3 mg/kg q6h × 2 doses (3.8)	3 mg/kg q8h (3.8)	0.55 mg/kg/hr (0.7)	0.39 mg/kg/hr (0.5)
Older patients Patients with cor pulmonale	2 mg/kg q6h × 2 doses (2.5)	2 mg/kg q8h (2.5)	0.47 mg/kg/hr (0.6)	0.24 mg/kg/hr (0.3)
CHF, hepatic function impairment	2 mg/kg q8h × 2 doses (2.5)	1–2 mg/kg q12h (1.3–2.5)	0.39 mg/kg/hr (0.5)	0.08–0.16 mg/kg/hr (0.1–0.2)

* Expressed as theophylline. Aminophylline dosages are given in parentheses.

0.5 mg of theophylline/kg will result in a 1 (range 0.5–1.6) μg/ml increase in serum theophylline. If the level cannot be obtained rapidly, one can administer a single dose equivalent to 2.5 mg theophylline/kg if there are no symptoms of theophylline toxicity.

Chronic therapy—PO: For rapidly absorbed preparations, initially, 6–8 mg/kg up to a maximum of 400 mg/day in 3–4 divided doses q6–8h. For extended-release preparations, initially, 4 mg/kg q8–12h or 400 mg as a single dose q24h. Can increase the dose by 25% increments for rapidly absorbed preparations or by 2–3 mg/kg/day for extended-release preparations q3d up to a maximum of 13 mg/kg or 900 mg/day, whichever is less, without measurement of serum theophylline concentration.

Note

1. Except for EC and ER preparations, the immediate-release tablets, liquids, or injection can be used for acute attacks, with IV administration providing the most rapid effect.
2. The therapeutic theophylline concentration is as follows: bronchodilator (10–20 μg/ml); respiratory stimulant (5–10 μg/ml).
3. Dosage should be calculated from lean (ideal) body weight.
4. Monitor serum theophylline concentration with higher than usual dosage or prolonged use.
5. The equivalent dose of aminophylline (hydrous) is 79% theophylline (anhydrous).

Indications: Treatment of reversible airway obstruction associated with asthma, bronchitis, and COPD and prophylaxis of asthma. Unlabeled uses include adjunctive treatment of CHF and pulmonary edema.

Action: Direct relaxation of the smooth muscle of the bronchial airways and pulmonary blood vessels. Additional actions include diuresis and respiratory, cardiac, cerebral, and skeletal muscle stimulation.

Metabolism: Hepatic

Excretion: Renal

Contraindications and precautions: Use with caution in pre-existing arrhythmias, severe cardiac disease, severe hypoxemia, cor pulmonale, alcoholism, hepatic or renal function impairment, gastritis, peptic ulcer disease, or hyperthyroidism.

Drug interactions

1. Cigarette smoking, phenobarbital, carbamazepine, phenytoin, primidone, or rifampin may decrease serum theophylline level.
2. Cimetidine, erythromycin, or oral contraceptives may increase serum theophylline level.
3. Theophylline may decrease effect of phenytoin, lithium, and β-adrenergic blocking agents.
4. Theophylline may increase effect of digoxin and oral anticoagulants.

Zidovudine—Azidothymidine, AZT

(Retrovir)

Preparations: Capsules, 100 mg

Adult dosage: PO: 100 mg q4h around the clock

Indications: Treatment of symptomatic HIV infection (AIDS and advanced ARC) in adults with a history of *Pneumocystis carinii* pneumonia or an absolute CD4 (T4 helper/inducer) lymphocyte count of less than 200/mm^3

Action: Zidovudine is converted to zidovudine triphosphate, which interferes with viral RNA-dependent DNA polymerase (reverse transcriptase)

Metabolism: Hepatic

Excretion: Renal

Contraindications and precautions

1. Use with caution in bone marrow depression and hepatic or renal function impairment.
2. Zidovudine is associated with hematologic toxicity; monitor CBC.

Drug interactions

1. Acetaminophen, aspirin, benzodiazepines, cimetidine, indomethacin, morphine, probenecid, or sulfonamides may increase risk of toxicity.
2. Bone marrow depressants or radiation therapy may increase risk of bone marrow suppression.

Antidepressant Pharmacology

Drug	Anticholinergic effect	Sedative effect	Orthostatic hypotension	Arrhythmias
Amitriptyline	High	High	Moderate	High
Amoxapine	Low to moderate	Low to moderate	Low to moderate	Moderate
Clomipramine	Moderate	Low	Moderate	Moderate
Desipramine	Low	Low	Moderate	Moderate
Doxepin	Moderate	High	Moderate	Moderate
Fluoxetine	Low to none	None	None	Low to none
Imipramine	Moderate	Moderate	High	High
Maprotiline	Low	Moderate	Low	Low to moderate
Nortriptyline	Moderate	Low to moderate	Low	Low
Protriptyline	Moderate to high	Low	Low to moderate	High
Trazodone	Low	Moderate	Moderate	Low
Trimipramine	Moderate to high	High	Moderate to high	High

Schedules of Controlled Substances

Schedule I:	High abuse potential, no accepted medical use in the United States Narcotics: Heroin Hallucinogens: Mescaline, methaqualone, peyote, LSD, MDA, STP, DMT, DET Other: Marijuana
Schedule II:	High abuse potential, severe psychological or physical dependence, liability, therapeutic utility Narcotics: Morphine, codeine, fentanyl (Innovar, Sublimaze), hydromorphone (Dilaudid), levorphanol (Levo-Dromoran), meperidine (Demerol), methadone (Dolophine), oxycodone (Percodan, Percocet), oxymorphone (Numorphan), opium, anileridine (Levitine), alpha-prodine (Nisentil) Stimulants: Amphetamine (Dexedrine), methamphetamine (Desoxyn), methylphenidate (Ritalin), phenmetrazine (Preludin) Depressants: Amobarbital (Amytal), pentobarbital (Nembutal), secobarbital (Seconal), phencyclidine (PCP) Other: Dronabinol (THC), Marinol, nabilone (Cesamet)
Schedule III:	Abuse potential less than those in Schedules I and II Narcotics: Nalorphine (Nalline) and mixtures of limited specified quantities of codeine, dihydrocodeine, hydrocodone, morphine, or opium with noncontrolled active ingredients Stimulants: Benzphetamine (Didrex), phendimetrazine (Plegine) Depressants: Mixtures of Schedule II barbiturates (amobarbital, pentobarbital, secobarbital) with noncontrolled active ingredients, aprobarbital, butabarbital, butalbital, talbutal, thiopental, glutethimide (Doriden), methyprylone (Noludar) Other: Naltrexone (Trexane)
Schedule IV:	Abuse potential less than those listed in Schedule III Narcotics: Dosage forms of propoxyphene (Darvon) and pentazocine (Talwin) Stimulants: Phentermine (Ionamin), fenfluramine (Pendimin), mazindol (Sanorex), diethylpropion (Tenuate), pemoline (Cylert) Depressants: Benzodiazepines—alprazolam (Xanax), chlordiazepoxide (Librium), clonazepam (Klonopin), clorazepate (Tranxene), diazepam (Valium), flurazepam (Dalmane), halazepam (Daxipam), lorazepam (Ativan), midazolam (Versed), oxazepam (Serax), prazepam (Centrax), quazepam (Dormalin), temazepam (Restoril), triazolam (Halcion); barbiturates—barbital, mephobarbital, phenobarbital, methohexital (Brevital); chloral hydrate; ethchlorvynol (Placidyl), ethinamate (Valmid); meprobamate (Miltown); paraldehyde
Schedule V:	Abuse potential less than those listed in Schedule IV Narcotics: Limited specified quantities of buprenorphine, codeine, dihydrocodeine, diphenoxylate (Lomotil), ethylmorphine, opium

Weights and Measures

Metric Weight Equivalents

1 kilogram (kg)	= 1,000 grams
1 gram (g)	= 1,000 milligrams
1 milligram (mg)	= 0.001 gram
1 microgram (mcg, μg)	= 0.001 milligram

Metric Volume Equivalents

1 liter (L)	= 1,000 milliliters (ml)
1 deciliter (dl)	= 100 milliliters

Weight/Volume Equivalents

1 mg/dl	= 10 mcg/ml
1 mg/dl	= 1 mg%

Conversion Equivalents

1 gram (g)	= 15.43 grains
1 ounce (oz)	= 28.35 grams
1 pound (lb)	= 453.6 grams
1 kilogram (kg)	= 2.2 pounds
1 fluid ounce (fl)	= 29.57 ml
1 pint (pt)	= 473.2 ml

Conversion Equivalents

0.1mg	= 1/600 gr
0.12 mg	= 1/500 gr
0.15 mg	= 1/400 gr
0.2 mg	= 1/300 gr
0.3 mg	= 1/200 gr
0.4 mg	= 1/150 gr
0.5 mg	= 1/120 gr
0.6 mg	= 1/100 gr
0.8 mg	= 1/80 gr
1.0 mg	= 1/65 gr

Formula for Estimating Creatinine Clearance in Adults with Stable Renal Function (Aged 18 yr and older)

$$Cl_{cr}\,(\text{men}) = \frac{(140 - \text{age}) \times (\text{weight})}{Cr_s \times 72}$$

$$Cl_{cr}\,(\text{women}) = 0.85 \times \text{above value}$$

where Cl_{cr} = creatinine clearance in ml/min, and Cr_s = serum creatinine in mg/dl. Age is in years, and weight is in kilograms.

Narcotic-Type Analgesics Used for Pain

Generic name (trade name)	Route	Equianalgesic dose (mg)	Onset of action (min)	Peak effect (min)	Duration of action (hr)	Comments
Codeine	IM	120	10–30	30–60	4–6	
	PO	200	30–45	60–120	4–6	
Meperidine (Demerol)	IM	75	10–15	30–50	2–4	
	IV	—	1	5–7	2–4	
	PO	300	15	60–90	2–4	
Pentazocine (Talwin)	IM	60	15–20	30–60	2–3	Mixed agonist-antagonist
	PO	180	15–30	60–90	3	
Morphine	IM	10	10–30	30–60	4–5	Extended-release tablets available
	IV	—	—	20	4–5	
	SC	—	10–30	50–90	4–5	
	PO	60	—	60–120	4–5	
Oxycodone	PO	30	—	60	3–4	
Methadone (Dolophine)	IM	10	10–20	60–120	4–5	Increased duration of action with continued dosing
	PO	20	30–60	90–120	4–6	
Nalbuphine (Nubain)	IM	10	≤15	60	3–6	Mixed agonist-antagonist
Levorphanol (Levo-dromoran)	IM	2	—	60	4–5	
	SC	—	—	60–90	4–5	
	PO	4	10–60	90–120	4–5	
Hydromorphone (Dilaudid)	IM	1.5	15	30–60	4–5	
	IV	—	10–15	15–30	2–3	
	SC	—	15	30–90	4	
	PO	7.5	30	90–120	4	
Oxymorphone (Numorphan)	IM	1	10–15	30–90	3–6	
	IV	—	5–10	15–30	3–4	
	SC	—	10–20	—	3–6	

Relative Potency of Some Topical Steroid Products

Potency	Brand Name	Generic name	Dosage form	Strength (%)
Very high	Diprolene	Betamethasone dipropionate	Optimized vehicle cream or ointment	0.05
	Psorcon	Diflorasone diacetate	Optimized vehicle ointment	0.05
	Temovate	Clobetasol dipropionate	Cream, ointment	0.05
High	Aristocort	Triamcinolone acetonide	Cream, ointment	0.5
	Cyclocort	Amcinonide	Cream, lotion, ointment	0.1
	Diprolene	Betamethasone dipropionate	Cream, lotion	0.05
	Diprosone	Betamethasone dipropionate	Cream, lotion, ointment	0.05
	Florone	Diflorasone diacetate	Cream, ointment	0.05
	Halog	Halcinonide	Cream, ointment, solution	0.1
	Kenalog	Triamcinolone acetonide	Cream, ointment	0.5
	Lidex	Fluocinonide	Cream, gel, ointment, solution	0.05
	Maxiflor	Diflorasone diacetate	Cream, ointment	0.05
	Psorcon	Diflorasone diacetate	Ointment	0.05
	Synalar-HP	Fluocinolone acetonide	Cream	0.2
	Topicort	Desoximetasone	Cream, ointment	0.25

Relative Potency of Some Topical Steroid Products *(continued)*

Potency	Brand Name	Generic name	Dosage form	Strength (%)
Intermediate	Aristocort	Triamcinolone acetonide	Cream, ointment	0.1
	Benisone	Betamethasone benzoate	Cream, gel, lotion, ointment	0.025
	Cordran	Flurandrenolide	Lotion, ointment	0.05
	Cordran SP	Flurandrenolide	Cream	—
	Diprosone	Betamethasone dipropionate	Cream, lotion, ointment	0.05
	Elocon	Mometasone furoate	Cream, ointment	0.1
	Halog	Halcinonide	Cream	0.025
	Kenalog	Triamcinolone acetonide	Cream, ointment	0.1
	Locoid	Hydrocortisone butyrate	Cream, ointment	0.1
	Synalar	Fluocinolone acetonide	Cream, ointment	0.025
	Topicort	Desoximetasone	Gel	0.05
	Topicort LP	Desoximetasone	Cream	0.05
	Uticort	Betamethasone benzoate	Cream, gel, lotion	0.025
	Valisone	Betamethasone valerate	Cream, lotion, ointment	0.1
Low	Aclovate	Aclometasone dipropionate	Cream, ointment	0.05
	Aristocort	Triamcinolone acetonide	Cream	0.025
	Cloderm	Clocortolone pivalate	Cream	0.1
	Cordran	Flurandrenolide	Ointment	0.025
	Kenalog	Triamcinolone acetonide	Cream, ointment	0.025
	Synalar	Fluocinolone acetonide	Solution	0.01
	Tridesilon	Desonide	Cream, ointment	0.05
	Valisone	Betamethasone valerate	Cream	0.1
	Westcort	Hydrocortisone valerate	Cream, ointment	0.2
Very low	Decaderm	Dexamethasone	Gel	0.1
	Medrol acetate topical	Methylprednisolone acetate	Ointment	0.1, 0.25
	Various	Hydrocortisone acetate	Cream, lotion, ointment	Up to 2.5
	Various	Hydrocortisone base	Cream, gel, lotion, ointment, solution	Up to 2.5

Comparison of Common Insulin Preparations

Insulin preparations	Strength (units/ml)		Insulin effect after SC source injection (hr)			Insulin effect after IV bolus injection (min)		
			Onset	*Peak*	*Duration*	*Onset*	*Peak*	*Duration*
Rapid-Acting								
Insulin injection Regular insulin	U-40	Mixed	0.5–1	2–4	5–7	10–30	15–30	30–60
	U-100	Mixed, purified beef, pork, purified pork, semi-synthetic human, biosynthetic human						
	U-500	Purified pork						
Prompt insulin zinc suspension (Semilente insulin)	U-40	Mixed	1–3	2–8	12–16	Not for IV use		
	U-100	Mixed, beef, purified pork						
Intermediate-Acting								
Isophane insulin suspension (NPH insulin)	U-40	Mixed	3–4	6–12	18–28	Not for IV use		
	U-100	Mixed, beef, purified beef, purified pork, semisynthetic human, biosynthetic human						
Insulin zinc suspension (Lente insulin)	U-40	Mixed	1–3	8–12	18–28	Not for IV use		
	U-100	Mixed, beef, purified beef, purified pork, semisynthetic human, biosynthetic human						
Long-Acting								
Protamine zinc insulin suspension (PZI insulin)	U-40	Mixed	4–6	14–24	36	Not for IV use		
	U-100	Mixed, purified beef, purified pork						
Extended insulin zinc suspension (Ultralente insulin)	U-40	Mixed	4–6	18–24	36	Not for IV use		
	U-100	Mixed, beef, purified beef						
Insulin injection (30%) and isophane insulin suspension (70%)	U-100	Purified pork, semisynthetic human	0.5	4–8	24	Not for IV use		

Appendix III

Common Abbreviations

A	ampere
A_1	aortic first heart sound
A_2	aortic second heart sound
a	before
aa	of each
AA	Alcoholics Anonymous
AAA	abdominal aortic aneurysm
A-aDo$_2$	alveolar-arterial oxygen difference
AAL	anterior axillary line
AAO	amino acid oxidase
AARF	acute alveolar respiratory failure
AAROM	active assisted range of motion
ab	abortion
abd	abdomen
ABD	abduction
Abd Hyst	abdominal hysterectomy
ABE	acute bacterial endocarditis
ABG	arterial blood gases
ABI	atherosclerotic brain infarction
abnl	abnormal
ABP	arterial blood pressure
ABS	acute brain syndrome
abs	absent
AC	acromioclavicular
ac	before meals
ACB	antibody-coated bacteria
acc	accident
accom	accommodation
Acet	acetone
ACL	anterior cruciate ligament
ac phos	acid phosphatase
ACT	activated clotting time
ACTA	automatic computerized transverse axial
ACTH	adrenocorticotropic hormone
AD	right ear
ADA diet	American Diabetic Association diet
ADD	adduction
adenoca	adenocarcinoma
ADH	antidiuretic hormone
ADL	activities of daily living
ad lib	as desired
adm	admission
admin	administer
adol	adolescent
ADP	adenosine diphosphate
ADR	adverse drug reaction
ADT	adenosine triphosphate
AEG	air encephalogram
AFB	acid-fast bacillus
AFib	atrial fibrillation
Afl	atrial flutter
AFO	ankle, foot orthosis
AFP	alpha-fetoprotein
AGA	acute gonococcal arthritis
agglut	agglutination
agit	shake
AGL	acute granulocytic leukemia
AGN	acute glomerulonephritis
AgNO$_3$ sol	silver nitrate solution
A/G ratio	albumin/globulin ratio
AGS	adrenogenital syndrome
AHA	autoimmune hemolytic anemia
AHD	autoimmune hemolytic disease
AHF	antihemophilic factor
AHG	antihemophilic globulin
AHM	ambulatory Holter monitoring
AI	aortic insufficiency
AICD	autoimplantable cardioverter defibrillator
AID	acute infectious disease
AIDS	acquired immunodeficiency syndrome
AIH	artificial insemination—husband
AIP	acute intermittent porphyria
AJ	ankle jerk
AK	above knee
AKA	above-knee amputation
alb	albumin
ALD	alcoholic liver disease
ALG	antilymphocyte globulin
A-line	arterial line
alk	alkaline
ALL	anterior longitudinal ligament
ALRI	anterolateral rotary instability
ALS	amyotrophic lateral sclerosis
ALT	alanine aminotransferase
alt	alternate
alt day	alternate days, every other day
alv	alveolar
AM	before noon
AMA	against medical advice
amb	ambulate
AMI	acute myocardial infarction
AML	acute myelogenous leukemia
AMP	adenosine monophosphate
amp	ampule
AMRI	anteromedial rotary instability
amt	amount
ANA	antinuclear antibody
anes	anesthesia
ANF	antinuclear factor
ANLL	acute nonlymphocytic leukemia
ANS	autonomic nervous system
A & O	alert and oriented
ant	anterior
AOD	arterial occlusive disease
AODM	adult-onset diabetes mellitus
AOM	acute otitis media
AP	apical pulse
AP	anteroposterior
A & P	auscultation and percussion
APB	atrial premature beat
APCs	atrial premature contractions
appt	appointment
AP repair	anteroposterior repair
APTT	activated partial thromboplastin time
aq	aqueous
aq dist	distilled water
AR	aortic regurgitation
A/R	apical/radial (pulse)
ARE	active resistive exercise
ARD	acute respiratory disease
ARDS	adult respiratory distress syndrome
ARF	acute renal failure
AROM	active range of motion
AS	aortic stenosis
ASA	acetylsalicylic acid
ASAP	as soon as possible
A-S attack	Adams-Stokes attack
ASCVD	arteriosclerotic cardiovascular disease
ASD	atrial septal defect
ASHD	arteriosclerotic heart disease
ASMI	atrial septal myocardial infarction
ASO	arteriosclerosis obliterans
assn	association
ass't	assistance
AST	aspartate aminotransferase
as tol	as tolerated
ATG	antithymocyte globulin
ATN	acute tubular necrosis
ATP	adenosine triphosphate
AU	both ears
AV	atrioventricular
AV	arteriovenous
AVM	arteriovenous malformation
AVN	avascular necrosis
AVR	aortic valve replacement

AVS	arteriovenous shunt
A & W	alive and well
ax	axis
Ⓑ	both
B	bacillus
b	born
BA	brachial artery
Ba	barium
bact	bacteria
Ba E	barium enema
bands	banded neutrophilis
barb	barbiturate
baso	basophils
Ba swallow	barium swallow
BB	bundle branch
BBA	born before arrival
BBB	bundle branch block
BBBB	bilateral bundle branch block
BBT	basal body temperature
B Bx	breast biopsy
B & C	biopsy and curettage
BC	blood culture
BCC	basal cell carcinoma
BCE	barium contrast enema
BCN	bilateral cortical necrosis
BCP	birth control pills
BD	bile duct
BEI	butanol extractable iodine
bf	boyfriend
BFB	bifascicular block
BFP	biological false positive
BFR	blood flow rate
BG	blood glucose
BHS	beta-hemolytic streptococcus
bid	two times a day
BIH	benign intracranial hypertension
bil	bilateral
bili	bilirubin
bili D/I	bilirubin, direct & indirect
bili T	bilirubin, total
BJ protein	Bence-Jones protein
BK	below knee
BKA	below-knee amputation
bkfst	breakfast
bl	blood
BLE	bilateral lower extremity
Bl T	blood type
bl time	bleeding time
BM	bowel movement
BMAP	bone marrow acid phosphatase
BMR	basal metabolic rate
BNO	bladder neck obstruction
BOM	bilateral otitis media
BOS	base of support
BP	blood pressure
BPD	bronchopulmonary dysplasia
BPH	benign prostatic hypertrophy
BR	bed rest
bro	brother
BRP	bathroom privileges
br sounds	breath sounds
BS	blood sugar
B & S glands	Bartholin and Skene glands
BSD	bedside drainage
BSE	breast self-examination
BSI	bound serum iron
BSO	bilateral salpingo-oophorectomy
BSP	bromsulphalein
BT	brain tumor
BTB	breakthrough bleeding
BTL	bilateral tubal ligation
BTPD	body temperature and ambient pressure, dry
BTPS	body temperature and ambient pressure, saturated with water vapor
BTU	British thermal unit
BUE	bilateral upper extremity
BUN	blood urea nitrogen
BV	blood vessel
BVH	biventricular hypertrophy
BVL	bilateral vas ligation
bx	biopsy
C	centigrade
c	cubic
C1,C2	cervical vertebrae 1,2
c̄	with
CA	carcinoma
Ca	calcium
C & B	chair and bed (rest)
CABG	coronary artery bypass graft
CAD	coronary artery disease
Cal	calorie
cal	caliber
C alb	albumin clearance
CALD	chronic active liver disease
C am	amylase clearance
CAO	chronic airway obstruction
cap	capacity
caps	capsules
CAS	carotid artery system
CAT	computed axial tomography
cath	catheter
caut	cauterize
CBC	complete blood count
CBD	common bile duct
CBR	complete bed rest
CBT	computed body tomography
CC	chief complaint
cc	cubic centimeter
CCA	common carotid artery
CCE	clubbing, cyanosis, or edema
CCM	congestive cardiomyopathy
CCMSU	clean catch midstream urine
CCU	coronary care unit
CD	cardiovascular disease
C/d	cigarettes per day
C & D	cystoscopy and dilatation
CDH	congenital dislocation of hip
CE	cholesterol esters
CEA	carcinoembryonic antigen
ceph floc	cephalin flocculation
CF	cardiac failure
CFP	chronic false positive
CFT	complement fixation test
CG	chorionic gonadotropin
CGD	chronic granulomatous disease
CGL	chronic granulocytic leukemia
CGN	chronic glomerulonephritis
CGP	chorionic growth hormone prolactin
CGTT	cortisone glucose tolerance test
CHB	complete heart block
CHD	coronary heart disease
CHE	cholinesterase
CHF	congestive heart failure
chol	cholesterol
chol est	cholesterol esters
chr	chronic
CICU	coronary intensive care unit
circ	circulation
ck	check
Cl	chloride
CLD	chronic lung disease
cldy	cloudy
CLL	chronic lymphocytic leukemia
cm	centimeter
CK	creatine kinase
CM	costal margin
CMF	cyclophosphamide, methotrexate, 5-fluorouracil
CN	cranial nerve
CNE	chronic nervous exhaustion
CNS	central nervous system
CO	carbon monoxide
c/o	complains of
^{60}Co	radioactive cobalt
CO_2	carbon dioxide
COAD	chronic obstructive airway disease
coag	coagulation
coag time	coagulation time
COG	closed angle glaucoma
Cog	cognitive
COHB	carboxyhemoglobin
COLD	chronic obstructive lung disease
Comp	compound
conc	concentration
cond	condition
cont	continue
Coor	coordination
COP	capillary osmotic pressure
COPD	chronic obstructive pulmonary disease
COPE	chronic obstructive pulmonary emphysema
COTA	Certified Occupational Therapy Assistant
CP	cerebral palsy
C & P	cystoscopy and panendoscopy
CPB	cardiopulmonary bypass
CPD	cephalopelvic disporportion
Cpd E	cortisone (compound E)
Cpd F	hydrocortisone (compound F)
CPK	creatine phosphokinase
CPPB	continuous positive-pressure breathing
CPPV	continuous positive-pressure ventilation

CPR	cardiopulmonary resuscitation
CPT	chest physiotherapy
Cr	radioactive chromium
CR	cardiorespiratory
CRA	central retinal artery
CRBBB	complete right bundle branch block
creat	creatinine
CRF	chronic renal failure
CRIF	closed reduction internal fixation
CRV	central retinal vein
C & S	culture and sensitivity
CS	corticosteroid
CSF	cerebrospinal fluid
CSH	chronic subdural hematoma
CSP	carotid sinus pressure
CSR	corrected sedimentation rate
CT	computed tomography
ct	count
CTD	connective tissue disease
Cu	copper
CV	cardiovascular
CVA	cerebrovascular accident
CVD	cardiovascular disease
CVG	coronary vein graft
CVI	cerebrovascular insufficiency
CVP	central venous pressure
CVRD	cardiovascular renal disease
CVS	cardiovascular system
Cysto	cystoscopy

D	dorsal
d	day
D1, D2	dorsal vertebrae 1,2
DAPT	direct agglutination pregnancy test
DAT	diphtheria antitoxin
DOB	date of birth
db	decibel
DBM	diabetic management
DBP	diastolic blood pressure
D/C	discontinue
D & C	dilation and curettage
DCABG	double coronary artery bypass graft
DCG	dynamic electrocardiography
DDx	differential diagnosis
DDST	Denver Developmental Screening test
DDx	differential diagnosis
D & E	dilation and evacuation
decr	decrease
deform	deformity
deg	degeneration
depr	depression
DES	diethylstilbestrol
desc	descending
dev	deviation
dgm	decigram
DI	diabetes insipidus
diab	diabetic
diam	diameter
DIC	disseminated intravascular coagulation
diff	differential blood count
diff diag	differential diagnosis
dig	digitalis
Dil	dilantin
dil	dilute
dim	diminished
DIP	distal interphalangeal joint
dis	disease
disch	discharge
disloc	dislocation
disp	dispense
dissem	disseminated
dist	distance
DJD	degenerative joint disease
DJS	Dubin-Johnson syndrome
DKA	diabetic ketoacidosis
dl	deciliter
DLE	disseminated lupus erythematosus
DM	diabetes mellitus
DOA	dead on arrival
DOB	date of birth
DOD	date of death
DOE	dyspnea on exertion
DOI	date of injury
DOT	Doppler ophthalmic test
DPD	diffuse pulmonary disease
DPT	diphtheria, pertussis, tetanus
DQ	developmental quotient
dr	dram
DR	diabetic retinopathy
D/S	dextrose and saline
D5/S	dextrose (5%) in saline
DSA	digital subtraction angiography
DSD	dry sterile dressing
dsg	dressing
DTO	deodorized tincture of opium
DTP	diphtheria, tetanus, pertussis
DTR	deep tendon reflex
DTs	delirium tremens
DUB	dysfunctional uterine bleeding
DV	dilute volume
DVI	digital video imaging
DVISA	digital video imaging subtraction angiography
DVT	deep vein thrombosis
D5W	dextrose (5%) in water
Dx	diagnosis

EA	erythrocyte antibody
ea	each
EAC	erythrocyte antibody complement
EAM	external auditory meatus
EBL	estimated blood loss
EBV	Epstein-Barr virus
EC	enteric-coated
ECBV	effective circulating blood volume
ECCE	extracapsular cataract extraction
ECF	extended-care facility
ECFV	extracellular fluid volume
ECG	electrocardiogram
ECHO	echocardiogram
ECIB	extracorporeal irradiation of blood
E. coli	Escherichia coli
ECRB	extensor carpi radialis brevis
ECRL	extensor carpi radialis longus
ECS	electrocerebral silence
ECT	electroconvulsive therapy
ECU	extensor carpi ulnaris
ED	Emergency Department
EDC	extensor digitorum communis
EDD	expected date of delivery
EDL	extensor digitorum longus
EE	eye and ear
EDS	Ehlers-Danlos syndrome
EEE	Eastern equine encephalitis
EEF	extracellular fluid volume
EEG	electroencephalogram
EENT	eyes, ears, nose and throat
EF	ejection fraction
e.g.	for example
EGG	electrogastrogram
EHBF	estimated hepatic blood flow
EHO	extrahepatic obstruction
EHP	extra high potency
EI	enzyme inhibitor
EIB	exercise-induced bronchospasm
EIP	extensor indicis proprius
EKG	electrocardiogram
ELB	elbow
ELISA	enzyme-linked immunosorbent assay
elix	elixir
EM	electron microscope
EMC	encephalomyocarditis
EMG	electromyogram
EMHS	Emergency Mental Health Service
EMT	Emergency Medical Technician
emul	emulsion
ENG	electronystagmogram
ENT	ears, nose, and throat
EO	eyes open
eo	eosinophil
EOG	electro-oculogram
EOM	extraocular movements
EPA	eicosapentaenoic acid
EPB	extensor pollicis brevis
EPC	epilepsy
Epi	epinephrine
epith	epithelial
EPL	extensor pollicis longus
ER	extended release
EPS	electrophysiologic study
EPSX	extrapyramidal symptoms
eq	equivalent
ER	external rotation
ERA	evoked response audiometry
ERBF	effective renal blood flow
ERCP	endoscopic retrograde cholangiopancreatography
ERG	electroretinogram
ERP	effective refractory period
ERV	expiratory refractory volume
ES	electric stimulation
ESM	ejection systolic murmur

ESR erythrocyte sedimentation rate
ESRD end-stage renal disease
et al. and others
ETH elixir terpin hydrate
ETH/C elixir terpin hydrate with codeine
ETOH ethyl alcohol
ETT exercise tolerance test
EUA examination under anesthesia
eval evaluation
ex example
exam examination
expt expectorant
Ext extract

F Fahrenheit
Fa father
FA folic acid
FANA fluorescent antinuclear antibodies
FB finger breadth
FBS fasting blood sugar
FCR flexor carpi radialis
FCU flexor carpi ulnaris
FD fatal dose
FDA Food and Drug Administration
FDL flexor digitorum longus
FDP flexor digitorum profundus
FDR flexor digitorum radialis
FDS flexor digitorum sublimus
Fe iron
FECG fetal electrocardiogram
Fe def iron deficiency
fem female
FF fat-free (diet)
FFA free fatty acids
FFB flexible fiberoptic bronchoscope
FH family history
FHB flexor hallucis brevis
FHL flexor hallucis longus
FHR fetal heart rate
fib fibrillation
fibrin fibrinogen
fld fluid
fld ext fluid extract
fl dr fluid dram
Flex flexion
fl oz fluid ounce
fluor fluorescent
FMF familial Mediterranean fever
FOI flight of ideas
FP frozen plasma
FPB flexor pollicis brevis
FPL flexor pollicis longus
freq frequent
FRF follicle-stimulating hormone–releasing factor
FROM full range of motion
FSF fibrin stabilizing factor
FSH follicle-stimulating hormone
ft feet/foot
FT_4 free thyroxine
FTE free thyroxine equivalent
FTG full-thickness graft
FTI free thyroxine index
FTN finger to nose
FTND full-term normal delivery
FTT failure to thrive
5-FU 5-fluorouracil
f/u follow up
Func functional
FUO fever of unknown origin
FV fluid volume
FVU first voided urine
FWB full weight bearing
Fx fracture

G glucose
g gram
^{67}Ga radioactive gallium
GA general anesthesia
gal gallon
GB gallbladder
GB series gallbladder series
GC *Gonococcus*
g-cal gram-calorie
g-cm gram-centimeter
GDH gonadotropic hormone
G/E granulocyte/erythroid ratio
gen general
GERD gastroesophageal reflux disorder
GF glomerular filtration
GFD gluten-free diet
GG gamma globulin
GGT gamma glutamyl transpeptidase
GH growth hormone
GHD growth hormone deficiency
GHRF growth hormone–releasing factor
GI gastrointestinal
GI series gastrointestinal series
gl gland
glob globulin
gluc glucose
gm gram
Gm– Gram stain negative
Gm+ Gram stain positive
gm % grams per hundred milliliters
gm-m gram-meter
G/NS glucose in normal saline
G6PD glucose-6-phosphate dehydrogenase
gr grain
gran granular
GRF gonadotropin-releasing factor
G/S glucose and saline
GSD glycogen storage disease
GSW gunshot wound
GT glutamyl transferase
GTH gonadotropic hormone
GTI genital tract infection
GTT glucose tolerance test
gtts drops
GU genitourinary
GVHR graft versus host reaction
G/W glucose in water
GWE glycerin and water enema
Gyn gynecology

H/A headache
HA hemagglutination
HAA hepatitis associated antigen
HAI hemagglutination inhibition
HASCVD hypertensive arteriosclerotic cardiovascular disease
HASHD hypertensive arteriosclerotic heart disease
HAV hepatitis A virus
Hb hemoglobin
HBAg hepatitis B antigen
HBE His-bundle electrogram
HBIG hepatitis B immunoglobulin
HBP high blood pressure
HBV hepatitis B virus
hCG human chorionic gonadotropin
HCl hydrochloric acid
Hct hematocrit
HCVD hypertensive cardiovascular disease
HDL high-density lipoproteins
HDN hemolytic disease of the newborn
H & E hematoxylin & eosin
HEAT human erythrocyte agglutination test
HEENT head, eyes, ears, nose, throat
HEP home exercise program
HF Hageman factor
HFHL high-frequency hearing loss
HFI hereditary fructose intolerance
Hg mercury
Hgb hemoglobin
HGG human gamma globulin
HGH human growth hormone
H&H hemoglobin and hematocrit
HHA hereditary hemolytic anemia
HHD hypertensive heart disease
HI hemagglutination inhibition
HIA hemagglutination inhibition antibody
5-HIAA 5-hydroxyindoleacetic acid
H-K heel to knee
HKAFO hip, knee, ankle, foot orthosis
H&L heart and lungs
HLH human luteinizing hormone
HMD hyaline membrane disease
HNP herniated nucleus pulposus
HO House Officer
h/o history of
H_2O water
HOCM hypertrophic obstructive cardiomyopathy
HOH hard of hearing
HOR ABD horizontal abduction
HOR ADD horizontal adduction
hosp hospital
HP hot pack
H & P history and physical
HP diet high protein (diet)
HPE history and physical examination
HPG human pituitary gonadotropin
HPI history of present illness
HPS high-protein supplement
HPVD hypertensive pulmonary vascular disease
HR heart rate

hr	hour
HRS	hepatorenal syndrome
hs	at bedtime
HSM	hepatosplenomegaly
Ht	height
HTAT	human tetanus antitoxin
HTE	hypertensive encephalopathy
HTN	hypertension
HUS	hemolytic-uremic syndrome
HV	hyperventilation
HVG stim	high-voltage galvanic stimulation
Hx	history
hypo	hypodermic injection
Hz	Hertz
I	Independent
^{131}I	radioactive iodine
IABC	intra-aortic balloon counterpulsation
IAC	internal auditory canal
IADHS	inappropriate antidiuretic hormone syndrome
IAM	internal auditory meatus
IASD	intra-atrial septal defect
IBC	iron-binding capacity
IBS	irritable bowel syndrome
IC	intracutaneous (injection)
ICA	intracranial aneurysm
ICCE	intracapsular cataract extraction
ICCM	idiopathic congestive cardiomyopathy
ICD	idiopathic cerebral dysfunction
ICF	intracellular fluid
ICM	intercostal margin
ICP	intracranial pressure
ICS	intercostal space
ICSH	interstitial cell-stimulating hormone
ict	icterus
ICU	intensive care unit
id	the same
ID	intradermal (injection site)
I & D	incision and drainage
IDA	iron-deficiency anemia
IDD	insulin-dependent diabetes
IDS	immune deficiency state
I/E	inspiratory/expiratory ratio
IEMG	integrated electromyogram
IEP	immunoelectrophoresis
IF	intrinsic factor
IFC	intrinsic factor concentrate
IFR	inspiratory flow rate
IFV	intracellular fluid volume
Ig	immunoglobulin
IH	infectious hepatitis
IHA	indirect hemagglutination
IHBT	incompatible hemolytic blood transfusion
IHD	ischemic heart disease
IHO	idiopathic hypertrophic osteoarthropathy
IHSS	idiopathic hypertrophic subaortic stenosis
IICP	increased intracranial pressure
IM	intramuscular
IMA	internal mammary artery
IMBC	indirect maximum breathing capacity
IMI	inferior myocardial infarction
imp	impression
IMV	intermittent mandatory ventilation
In	insulin
in	inch
incl	include
incr	increase
Inf	inferior
info	information
ing	inguinal
inj	injection
inoc	inoculation
Inpt	in-patient
INPV	intermittent negative-pressure assisted ventilation
INS	idiopathic nephrotic syndrome
int	internal
int rot	internal rotation
I & O	intake and output
IO	intestinal obstruction
IOFB	intraocular foreign body
IOP	intraocular pressure
IP	interphalangeal
IPF	idiopathic pulmonary fibrosis
IPG	impedance plethysmography
IPH	idiopathic pulmonary hemosiderosis
IPPB	intermittent positive-pressure breathing
IPPO	intermittent positive-pressure inflation with oxygen
IPPV	intermittent positive-pressure ventilation
IQ	intelligence quotient
IR	internal rotation
IRBBB	incomplete right bundle branch block
IRDS	idiopathic respiratory distress syndrome
irrig	irrigation
IRV	inspiratory reserve volume
IS	intercostal space
ISF	interstitial fluid
ISG	immune serum globulin
IT	inhalation therapy
ITP	idiopathic thrombocytopenic purpura
ITT	insulin tolerance test
IUCD	intrauterine contraceptive device
IUD	intrauterine device
IV	intravenous
IVC	inferior vena cava
IVCD	intraventricular conduction defect
IVCV	inferior venacavography
IVD	intervertebral disk
IVGTT	intravenous glucose tolerance test
IVP	intravenous pyelography
IVSD	intraventricular septal defect
JDM	juvenile diabetes mellitus
jej	jejunum
JOD	juvenile onset diabetes
JPB	junctional premature beat
JPC	junctional premature contraction
JRA	juvenile rheumatoid arthritis
jt	joint
JV	jugular vein
JVD	jugular venous distention
JVPT	jugular venous pulse tracing
K	potassium
k	constant
17K	17-ketosteroid excretion
KAFO	knee, ankle, foot orthosis
KB	ketone bodies
kcal	kilocalorie
KCl	potassium chloride
kg	kilogram
kg/cal	kilogram-calorie
kilo	a thousand grams
KJ	knee jerk
KK	knee kick
Klebs	*Klebsiella*
KLS	kidney, liver, spleen
km	kilometer
KOH	potassium hydroxide
KS	ketosteroid
KUB	kidneys, ureters, bladder
L	liter
(L)	left
L & A	light and accommodation
LA	left atrium
lab	laboratory
lac	laceration
LAD	left anterior descending
LAH	left anterior hemiblock
LAIT	latex agglutination inhibition test
LAO	left anterior oblique
LAP	leukocyte alkaline phosphatase
lat	lateral
LATS	long-acting thyroid stimulator
lax	laxative
LB	low back
lb	pound
LBBB	left bundle branch block
LBP	low back pain
LCA	left coronary artery
LCL	lateral collateral ligament
LD	left deltoid
L & D	labor and delivery
LD_{50}	median lethal dose
LDD	light-dark discrimination
LDH	lactate dehydrogenase
LDL	low-density lipoproteins
L-dopa	levodopa
LED	lupus erythematosus disseminatus
LF	latex fixation
LFD	lactose-free diet
LFP	left frontoposterior
LFS	liver function series
LFT	latex flocculation test
LG	left gluteus
lg	large
LH	luteinizing hormone
LHF	left-heart failure
Li	lithium

LICSW licensed independent clinical social worker
lig ligament
LIH left inguinal hernia
LIMA left internal mammary artery
liq liquid
LL lower lobe
LLC long leg cast
LLE left lower extremity
LLL left lower lobe
LLQ left lower quadrant
LMCA left main coronary artery
L/min liters per minute
LMP last menstrual period
LOA leave of absence
LOB loss of balance
LOCc loss of consciousness
LOM left otitis media
LOQ lower outer quadrant
LOS length of stay
LP lumbar puncture
LPE lipoprotein electrophoresis
LPN Licensed Practical Nurse
LPO light perception only
LPV left pulmonary veins
L & R left and right
LS lumbosacral
LSB left sternal border
LSD lysergic acid diethylamide
LSO left salpingo-oophorectomy
LSV left subclavian vein
LTC long-term care
LTG long-term goal
LTH luteotrophic hormone
LU left upper
L & U lower and upper
LUE left upper extremity
LUL left upper lobe
LUQ left upper quadrant
LV left ventricle
LVDP left ventricular diastolic pressure
LVET left ventricular ejection time
LVF left ventricular failure
LVH left ventricular hypertrophy
L & W living and well
LWP large whirlpool
lymphs lymphocytes
lytes electrolytes

MAO-I monoamine oxidase inhibitor
M_1 mitral first heart sound
M_2 mitral second heart sound
MABP mean arterial blood pressure
MAL midaxillary line
malig malignant
manip manipulation
MAP mean arterial pressure
MAT multifocal atrial tachycardia
max maximum
MBC maximum breathing capacity
MBD minimal brain dysfunction
MBF married black female
MBM married black male
MBP mean blood pressure
MC metacarpal
MCA middle cerebral artery
MCCH mean corpuscular hemoglobin concentration
mcg microgram
MCL medial collateral ligament
MCP metacarpophalangeal (joint)
MCR metabolic clearance rate
mcU microunit
MCV mean corpuscular volume
MD Medical Doctor
MDI manic-depressive illness
MDM mid-diastolic murmur
MDUO myocardial disease of unknown origin
MDV multiple-dose vial
ME Medical Examiner
MEA multiple endocrine adenomatosis
meas measurement
MEC minimum effective concentration
meds medications
MEF maximal expiratory flow
memb membrane
mEq milliequivalent
MER mean ejection rate
met metastatic
metab metabolism
M & F mother and father
MG myasthenia gravis
Mg magnesium
mg milligram
mg% milligrams percent
MGN membranous glomerulonephritis
$MgSO_4$ magnesium sulfate
MH medical history
MHb methemoglobin
MHC Mental Health Counselor
M/hct microhematocrit
MHR maximum heart rate
MI myocardial infarction
MIC minimum inhibitory concentration
mid middle
millisec millisecond
min minute
MIP maximum inspiratory pressure
misc miscellaneous
mixt mixture
ml milliliter
ML middle lobe
MLAP mean left atrial pressure
MLD minimal lethal dose
MLNS mucocutaneous lymph node syndrome
M/L ratio monocyte/lymphocyte ratio
mm millimeter
mm^3 cubic millimeter
mm Hg millimeters of mercury
MMPI Minnesota Multiphasic Personality Inventory
MMT manual muscle test
Mn manganese
MO mineral oil
mo month
MGF maternal grandfather
MGM maternal grandmother
Mo mother
mod moderate
MOM milk of magnesia
Mono infectious mononucleosis
mono monocyte
MOPP nitrogen mustard, oncovin, procarbazine, and prednisone
MP metacarpophalangeal (joint)
MPA main pulmonary artery
MPI multiphasic personality inventory
MR mitral regurgitation
mr milliroentgen
MRAP mean right atrial pressure
MRF mitral regurgitant flow
MRVP mean right ventricular pressure
MS multiple sclerosis
MSAP mean systemic arterial pressure
MSER mean systolic ejection rate
MSL midsternal line
MSt mitral stenosis
MSW Master of Social Work
MT metatarsal (joint)
MTP metatarsophalangeal
MTT maximal treadmill test
MTU methylthiouracil
MTX methotrexate
mu (μ) micron
musc muscles
MV mitral valve
MVP mitral valve prolapse
MVR mitral valve replacement
MVV maximum voluntary ventilation
MWF married white female
MWM married white male
myelo myelocyte

NA Nurse Assistant
Na sodium
N/A not available
NaCl sodium chloride
NAD no appreciable disease
NAG narrow-angle glaucoma
NBTE nonbacterial thrombotic endocarditis
NBW normal birth weight
ND neurotic depression
NE norepinephrine
NEC necrotizing enterocolitis
NEFA nonesterified fatty acids
neg negative
Neuro neurology
neut neutrophil
NF National Formulary
NFTD normal full-term delivery
NG nasogastric
ng nanogram
NH_3 ammonia
NH_4Cl ammonium chloride
n/l normal limits
NM neuromuscular
NMA neurogenic muscular atrophy
NMR nuclear magnetic resonance
no number

noc	night
non rep	do not repeat
NOS	not otherwise specified
NP	nasopharyngeal
NPB	nodal premature beat
NPC	nodal premature contraction
NP cult	nasopharyngeal culture
NPD	Neimann-Pick disease
NPH	neutral protamine Hagedorn
NPI	no present illness
NPN	nonprotein nitrogen
NPO	nothing by mouth
NR	do not repeat
NREM	nonrapid eye movement
NRI	neutral regular insulin
NS	nervous system
NS	normal saline
NSFTD	normal spontaneous full-term delivery
NSR	normal sinus rhythm
NSS	normal saline solution
N/T	not tested
N & T	nose and throat
NTG	nitroglycerin
NTMI	nontransmural myocardial infarction
nucl	nucleus
NV	normal value
Nv	naked vision
N & V	nausea and vomiting
NVA	near visual acuity
NVD	nausea, vomiting, diarrhea
NVS	neurologic vital signs
NWB	non-weight-bearing
NYD	not yet diagnosed
O_2	oxygen
OA	osteoarthritis
O & A	observation and assessment
OAD	obstructive airway disease
OAG	open-angle glaucoma
OAP	ophthalmic artery pressure
obl	oblique
OC	oral contraceptive
O_2 cap	oxygen capacity
od	daily
OD	right eye
OFC	occipitofrontal circumference
OGTT	oral glucose tolerance test
17-OH	17-hydroxycorticosteroids
OHA	oral hypoglycemic agents
oint	ointment
oj	orange juice
OK	all right
OM	otitis media
om	every morning
OMVC	open mitral valve commissurotomy
OOB	out of bed
O & P	ova and parasites
OPD	Outpatient Department
OPG	ocular pneumoplethysmography
Ophth	ophthalmology
OR	operating room
ORIF	open reduction with internal fixation
ORTHO	orthopedics
OS	left eye
O_2 sat	oxygen saturation
OT	occupational therapy
Oto	otolaryngology
OTR	Registered Occupational Therapist
OU	both eyes
OURQ	outer upper right quadrant
OV	office visit
O/W	oil in water
oz	ounce
Ⓟ	passive
P	pulse
$\bar{P}$	after
P & A	percussion and auscultation
PA	pulmonary artery
PABA	para-aminobenzoic acid
PAL	posterior axillary line
PAN	polyarteritis nodosa
PAP	Papanicolaou smear
Para 1	having borne one child
PAS	pulmonary artery stenosis
PAT	paroxysmal atrial tachycardia
Path	pathology
Pb	lead
PBC	primary biliary cirrhosis
PBF	pulmonary blood flow
PBI	protein-bound iodine
PC	phosphocreatine
pc	after food
PCA	plasma catecholamines
PCD	polycystic disease
PCF	prothrombin conversion factor
PCG	phonocardiogram
PCL	posterior cruciate ligament
PCN	penicillin
Pco_2	partial pressure of carbon dioxide
PCP	phencyclidine HCl
PCS	portacaval shunt
PCV	packed cell volume
PD	Parkinson's disease
p/d	packs per day
PDA	patent ductus arteriosus
PDR	*Physicians' Desk Reference*
PE	physical examination
Pec	pectoralis
Ped	pediatrics
PEEP	positive end-expiratory pressure
PEF	peak expiratory flow
PEG	pneumoencephalogram
PEP	pre-ejection period
Perc	perception
PERLA	pupils equal and react to light and accommodation
PES	programmed electric study
PFR	peak flow rate
PFT	pulmonary function test
pg	picogram
PGF	paternal grandfather
PGM	paternal grandmother
PH	past history
pH	hydrogen ion concentration
PHA	phytohemagglutinin
phar	pharmacy
PHMD	pseudohypertrophic muscular dystrophy
PHP	pseudohypoparathyroidism
PHT	pulmonary hypertension
PI	present illness
PIA	plasma insulin activity
PID	pelvic inflammatory disease
PIFR	peak inspiratory flow rate
PIP	proximal interphalangeal
PIVD	protruded intervertebral disk
PJB	premature junctional beat
PKU	phenylketonuria
PLL	posterior longitudinal ligament
plt	platelet
PM	after noon
PMB	postmenopausal bleeding
PMH	past medical history
PMI	point of maximum impulse
PMNs	polymorphonuclear leukocytes
PMP	past menstrual period
PMR	polymyalgia rheumatica
PMS	premenstrual syndrome
PMV	prolapsed mitral valve
PN	peripheral nerve
PNC	premature nodal contraction
PND	paroxysmal nocturnal dyspnea
PNE	pneumoencephalography
PNS	peripheral nervous system
PO	by mouth
Po_2	partial pressure of oxygen
PO_4	phosphate
POAG	primary open-angle glaucoma
POD	postoperative day
polys	polymorphonuclear leukocytes
POMP	prednisone, oncovin, methotrexate, and 6-mercaptopurine
post	after
postop	postoperative
pp	near point of accommodation
PPA	palpitation, percussion, auscultation
PPBS	postprandial blood sugar
PPD	purified protein derivative
PPF	plasma protein fraction
ppm	parts per million
PPV	positive-pressure ventilation
PR	per rectum
PR	pulse rate
pr	pair
PRA	plasma renin activity
PRBC	packed red blood cells
PRC	plasma renin concentration
PRE	progressive resistive exercise
preop	preoperative
PRF	prolactin-releasing factor
prn	whenever necessary
Pro	pronation
proc	procedure
PROM	passive range of motion
pro time	prothrombin time
PS	pyloric stenosis

PSMA progressive spinal muscular atrophy
PSMF protein-sparing modified fast
PSP phenolsulfonphthalein
PSVT paroxysmal supraventricular tachycardia
Psych psychiatry
PT physical therapy
pt patient
PTA prior to admission
PTB patella tendon bearing
PTC plasma thromboplastin component
PTCA percutaneous transluminal coronary angioplasty
PTED pulmonary thromboembolic disease
PTH parathyroid hormone
PTSS post-traumatic stress syndrome
PTT partial thromboplastin time
PTU propylthiouracil
PUD peptic ulcer disease
PUO pyrexia of unknown origin
PV peripheral vascular
PVB premature ventricular beat
PVC premature ventricular contraction
PVD peripheral vascular disease
PVE prosthetic valve endocarditis
PVT paroxysmal ventricular tachycardia
PWB partial weight-bearing
PZI protamine zinc insulin

q every
qAM every morning
qd every day
q2d every second day
qh every hour
q2h every 2 hours
qhs at bedtime
qid four times a day
qns quantity not sufficient
qod every other day
qoh every other hour
qon every other night
qs as much as will suffice
qt quart
qv as much as you wish
quads quadriceps

Resp respirations
Ⓡ right
r roentgen
Ra radium
RA rheumatoid arthritis
RAD right axis deviation
RAE right atrial enlargement
RA factor rheumatoid factor
RAH right atrial hypertrophy
RAI radioactive iodine
RAIU radioactive iodine uptake
RAM rapid alternating movements
RAO right anterior oblique
RAP right atrial pressure
RB right bundle
RBBB right bundle branch block
RBC red blood cell count
rbc red blood cells
RBCV red blood cell volume
RBF renal blood flow
RCA right coronary artery
RCV red cell volume
RD respiratory disease
RDS respiratory distress syndrome
RECG radioelectrocardiology
ref phys referring physician
rehab rehabilitation
REM rapid eye movement
rep let it be repeated
retics reticulocytes
RF rheumatic fever
RFA right femoral artery
RFS renal function studies
Rh^+ Rhesus positive factor
Rh^- Rhesus negative factor
Rh agglut rheumatoid agglutinins
RHD rheumatic heart disease
RHF right-heart failure
Rh factor Rhesus factor
RHL right hepatic lobe
RIA radioimmunoassay
RIH right inguinal hernia
RISA radioactive iodine serum albumin
RIU radioactive iodine uptake
RLC residual lung capacity
RLE right lower extremity
RLF retrolental fibroplasia
RLL right lower lobe
RLQ right lower quadrant
RML right middle lobe
RMV respiratory minute volume
RN Registered Nurse
RNC Certified Nurse Practitioner
RND radical neck dissection
R/O rule out
ROM range of motion
ROS review of systems
rot rotate
rout routine
ROV return office visit
Rp pulmonary resistance
RPA right pulmonary artery
RPG retrograde pyelogram
RPR rapid plasma reagin
RPV right pulmonary artery
R & R rate and rhythm
RRE round, regular, equal
RROM resisted range of motion
RRP relative refractory period
RSIVP rapid sequence intravenous pyleogram
RSO right salpingo-oophorectomy
RSR regular sinus rhythm
RSV right subclavian vein
RT respiratory therapy
RTC return to clinic
RTN renal tubular necrosis
RUE right upper extremity
RUL right upper lobe
RUQ right upper quadrant
RUR resin-uptake ratio
RV right ventricle
RVH right ventricular hypertrophy
RVol residual volume
RVT renal vein thrombosis
Rx prescription

s sign
s̄ without
SA serum albumin
S&A sugar and acetone
SAC short arm cast
SAH subarachnoid hemorrhage
SAP serum alkaline phosphatase
SAQ short arc quad
sat saturate
sat sol saturated solution
SB side bend
SBA stand-by assist
SBE subacute bacterial endocarditis
SBF single black female
SBM single black male
SBP systolic blood pressure
SBQC small base quad cane
SBR strict bed rest
SC subcutaneous
S/C self care
SCABG single coronary artery bypass graft
SCD sudden cardiac death
SCFE slipped capital femoral epiphysis
sched schedule
SCID severe combined immunodeficiency disease
SCK serum creatine kinase
SCS shaken child syndrome
SDH subdural hematoma
SDS sensory deprivation syndrome
SE saline enema
sec second
sed rate sedimentation rate
segs segmented white cells
sens sensitivity
SEP systolic ejection period
serv service
SFA superficial femoral artery
SFP spinal fluid pressure
SFT skinfold thickness
SG skin graft
SGOT serum glutamic-oxaloacetic transaminase
SGPT serum glutamic-pyruvic transaminase
SH social history
SHO secondary hypertrophic osteoarthropathy
SI serum iron
SIADH syndrome of inappropriate antidiuretic hormone secretion
sib sibling
SICU surgical intensive care unit
SIDS sudden infant death syndrome
sig let it be labeled
sis sister
SIW self-inflicted wound

SK	streptokinase
SL	sublingual
SLC	short leg cast
SLDH	serum lactate dehydrogenase
SLE	systemic lupus erythematosus
SLR	straight-leg raising
sm	small
SMA-6	Sequential Multiple Analysis-6 tests
SMA-12	Sequential Multiple Analysis-12 tests
SMC	special mouth care
SMON	subacute myelo-optic neuropathy
SNB	scalene node biopsy
SND	sinus node disease
SNP	sodium nitroprusside
SNS	sympathetic nervous system
SNV	systemic necrotizing vasculitis
SO	salpingo-oophorectomy
SO_4	sulphate
SOB	short of breath
soln	solution
SOM	serous otitis media
SOP	standard operating procedure
sos	one dose if necessary
SP	systolic pressure
S/P	status post
SPA	salt-poor albumin
SPCA	serum prothrombin conversion accelerator
SPEP	serum protein electrophoresis
sp fl	spinal fluid
sp gr	specific gravity
spont	spontaneous
SPP	suprapubic prostatectomy
SQ	subcutaneous
sq	square
SR	sedimentation rate
SR	sustained-release
SRM	superior rectus muscle
S & S	signs and symptoms
ss	one-half
SSA	side-to-side anastomosis
SSE	soapsuds enema
SS enema	saline-solution enema
SSKI	saturated solution of potassium iodide
SSPE	subacute sclerosing panencephalitis
ST	speech therapy
STA	superficial temporal artery
staph	*Staphylococcus*
STAT	immediate
std	standard
STD	sexually transmitted disease
stet	let it stand
Stim	stimulation
STF	special tube feeding
STK	streptokinase
STP	standard temperature and pressure
strep	*Streptococcus*
STSG	split-thickness skin graft
SUA	serum uric acid
subcut	subcutaneous
subling	sublingual
SUN	serum urea nitrogen
Sup	supination
supp	suppository
Susp	suspension
SVCG	spatial vectorcardiogram
SVE	supraventricular ectopic
SVG	saphenous vein graft
SVT	supraventricular tachycardia
SW	Social Worker
S & W enema	soap-and-water enema
SWF	single white female
SWM	single white male
SWP	small whirlpool
sympt	symptom
synd	syndrome
syr	syrup
sys	system
T(A)	temperature, axillary
T & A	tonsillectomy and adenoidectomy
tab	tablet
TAH	total abdominal hysterectomy
talc	talcum powder
TAO	thromboangiitis obliterans
TAT	Thematic Apperception Test
tbc	tuberculosis
TBG	thyroxine-binding globulin
TBI	total body irradiation
TBM	tuberculous meningitis
tbsp	tablespoonful
TBV	total blood volume
TC	total capacity
TCA	tricyclic antidepressant
TCABG	triple coronary artery bypass graft
TDWB	touch-down weight-bearing
TED	thromboembolic disease
TET	treadmill exercise test
TFA	total fatty acids
TG	triglycerides
TGA	transient global amnesia
TGT	thromboplastin generation time
Thal	thalassemia
ther	therapy
TIA	transient ischemic attack
TIBC	total iron-binding capacity
tid	three times daily
tinct	tincture
TJ	triceps jerk
TKO	to keep open
TLV	total lung volume
TM	transmetarsal (joint)
TMA	transmetatarsal amputation
TMJ	temporomandibular joint
TNTC	too numerous to count
T(O)	temperature, oral
T/O	telephone order
TOA	tubo-ovarian abscess
TOF	tetralogy of Fallot
tol	tolerate
Top	topical
TPA	tissue protein activator
TPBF	total pulmonary blood flow
TPI	*Treponema pallidum*–immobilization
TPN	total parenteral nutrition
TPR	temperature, pulse, respirations
T(R)	temperature, rectal
trach	tracheostomy
tract	traction
TRBF	total renal blood flow
TRF	thyrotropin-releasing factor
TRIC	trachoma inclusive conjunctivitis
trig	triglycerides
TRP	tubular reabsorption of phosphate
TSD	Tay-Sachs disease
TSH	thyroid-stimulating hormone
tsp	teaspoonful
TSP	total serum protein
TT	thrombin time
TTP	thrombotic thrombocytopenic purpura
TTT	tolbutamide tolerance test
TU	tuberculin units
TUG	total urinary gonadotropin
T_3 uptake	triiodothyronine uptake
T_4 uptake	thyroxine uptake
TUR	transurethral resection
TURB	transurethral resection of bladder
TURP	transurethral resection of prostate
tuss	cough
TVH	total vaginal hysterectomy
TVU	total volume urine
TW	tap water
TWE	tap-water enema
typ	typical
U	unit
UA	urine analysis
UAO	upper airway obstruction
UCG	urinary chorionic gonadotropin
UCHD	usual childhood diseases
UE	upper extremity
UGI	upper gastrointestinal
UIBC	unsaturated iron-binding capacity
UIQ	upper inner quadrant
UL	upper lobe
U & L	upper and lower
ung	ointment
unilat	unilateral
unk	unknown
UOQ	upper outer quadrant
up ad lib	out of bed, as desired
UQ	upper quadrant
UR	utilization review
URI	upper respiratory infection
Urol	urology
URQ	upper right quadrant
US	ultrasonic
USN	ultrasonic nebulizer
UT	urinary tract
UTI	urinary tract infection
UU	urine urobilinogen

V	vein
vacc	vaccinate
vag hyst	vaginal hysterectomy
VAMP	vincristine, amethopterin, 6-mercaptopurine, and prednisone
VBI	vertebrobasilar insufficiency
VBL	vinblastine
VCG	vectorcardiogram
VCT	venous clotting time
VCU	voiding cystourethrogram
VD	venereal disease
VDA	visual discriminatory acuity
VDP	vincristine, daunorubicin, prednisone
VDRL	Venereal Disease Research Laboratory
VEA	ventricular ectopic activity
VEB	ventricular ectopic beat
VEP	visual evoked potentials
VER	visual evoked response
VF	ventricular fibrillation
VGM	ventriculogram
VHD	valvular heart disease
Vit	vitamin
vit cap	vital capacity
VLDL	very low density lipoproteins
V/O	verbal order
VOD	vision right eye
vol	volume
VOS	vision left eye
VPB	ventricular premature beat
VPC	ventricular premature contraction
V/S	vital signs
VSD	ventricular septal defect
VT	ventricular tachycardia
VV	varicose veins
WAIS	Wechsler Adult Intelligence Scale
WAIS-R	Wechsler Adult Intelligence Scale–Revised
Wass	Wassermann test
WBAT	weight bearing as tolerated
WBC	white blood cell count
W/C	wheelchair
WD/WN	well developed, well nourished
W/E	weekend
WF	white female
WFL	within functional limits
whpl	whirlpool
WISC-R	Wechsler Intelligence Scale for Children–Revised
wk	week
WM	white male
WNL	within normal limits
w/o	without
WPW	Wolff-Parkinson-White
wt	weight
w/u	work-up
X-match	cross-match
XX chromosome	normal female chromosome type
XY chromosome	normal male chromosome type
Y	yes
Y/O	year old
yr	year
ZE syndrome	Zollinger-Ellison syndrome
ZIG	zoster immune globulin
ZSR	zeta sedimentation rate

Symbols

+	positive
?	question
↑	up, increase
↓	below, decrease
>	greater than
<	less than
≤	less than or equal to
≥	greater than or equal to
=	equal
Δ	change
±	plus or minus
+	slight trace
++	trace
+++	moderate amount
++++	large amount
x	times
1x	one time
°	degree
1°	first degree
′	foot
″	inch
#	number
@	at
/	per
♂	male
♀	female
Λ	diastolic blood pressure
V	systolic blood pressure
μc	microcurie
μEq	microequivalent
μg	microgram
μμg	micromicrogram
μ	micron
μμ	micromicron
≠	is not equal to
%	percent
÷	divided by
↔	reversible reaction
:	is to (ratio)
−	negative
≅	approximately
~	approximate

Appendix IV

Defined Data Base Form

30315998PK

DEPARTMENT OF MEDICINE
EMORY UNIVERSITY SCHOOL OF MEDICINE
GRADY MEMORIAL HOSPITAL

DEFINED DATA BASE*

Date ______________________

Name ______________________ Initial Data Base ? ☐

Age ____________ Sex ____________ Interval Data Base? ☐

See Data Base of

Source ____________ Reliability ____________ ______ Month ______ Day ______ Year

Patient's Major Physician or Pre-Admission Clinic Area *(Enter "none" if none)* ______________

Nearest Relative ______________________ *Phone* ____________

THE HISTORY

1. Chief Complaint and Present Illness:

Continue on Reverse

* Courtesy of H. Kenneth Walker, M.D. Used with permission

Defined Data Base Form

Present Illness (cont'd):

Instructions: Check *no* or *yes* for the history; check *normal* or *abnormal* for the physical. Leave blank if not asked or not done. Write *NA* if not applicable. Write *NK* if unknown by the patient or examiner. Give narrative description in space on right for all *yes* answers.

	NO		YES
		General	
2	( )	Weight change	( )
3	( )	Fever/chills	( )
4	( )	Night sweats	( )
5	( )	Dizziness	( )
	( )	Other	( )
		Endocrine System	
6	( )	Heat/cold intolerance	( )
7	( )	Thyroid problems	( )
8	( )	Neck surgery/irradiation	( )
9	( )	Diabetes/diabetic indicators	( )
		Eye	
10	( )	Visual dysfunction	( )
	( )	Other	( )
		Ear, Nose, Throat	
11	( )	Difficulty hearing/deaf	( )
12	( )	Tinnitus	( )
13	( )	Epistaxis	( )
14	( )	Hoarseness	( )
15	( )	Sinusitis	( )
16	( )	Vertigo	( )
	( )	Other	( )
		Gastrointestinal System	
17	( )	Nausea/retching	( )
18	( )	Vomiting	( )
19	( )	Hematemesis	( )
20	( )	Melena	( )
21	( )	Dysphagia	( )
22	( )	Indigestion	( )
23	( )	Heartburn	( )
24	( )	Abdominal pain	( )
25	( )	Abdominal swelling	( )
26	( )	Jaundice	( )
27	( )	Hematochezia	( )
28	( )	Diarrhea	( )
29	( )	Constipation	( )
30	( )	Hernia	( )
31	( )	Hemorrhoids	( )
32	( )	Peptic ulcer disease	( )
33	( )	Gallbladder disease	( )

	NO		YES
34	( )	Pancreatitis	( )
35	( )	GI surgery	( )
36	( )	Alcohol intake	( )
	( )	Other	( )
		Pulmonary System	
37	( )	Dyspnea/breathlessness/shortness of breath	( )
38	( )	Cough/sputum production	( )
39	( )	Hemoptysis	( )
40	( )	Wheezing/asthma	( )
41	( )	Tuberculosis/tbc exposure	( )
42	( )	Past PPD	( )
43	( )	Previous chest	( )
44	( )	Respiratory infections/pneumonia	( )
45	( )	Smoking history	( )
46	( )	Environmental inhalation	( )
	( )	Other	( )
		Cardiovascular System	
47	( )	Inadequate exercise level	( )
48	( )	Orthopnea/paroxysmal nocturnal dyspnea	( )
49	( )	Chest discomfort/pain	( )
50	( )	Palpitations	( )
51	( )	Syncope	( )
52	( )	Edema	( )
53	( )	Phlebitis	( )
54	( )	Claudication	( )
55	( )	Hypertension	( )
56	( )	Rheumatic	( )
57	( )	Past heart disease	( )
58	( )	Family history heart disease	( )
	( )	Other	( )
		Genitourinary System	
59	( )	Urinary frequency/urgency/dysuria	( )
60	( )	Urinary tract infection	( )
61	( )	Flank pain	( )
62	( )	Nocturia	( )
63	( )	Hematuria	( )
64	( )	Past stones	( )
65	( )	Urinary stream flow abnormality	( )
66	( )	Urethral discharge	( )
67	( )	Syphilis/positive serology	( )
68	( )	Male genital lesions	( )
69	( )	Testicular mass/pain	( )
70	( )	Impotence	( )
71	( )	Family history renal disease	( )
		Other	( )

	NO		YES
		Birth Control	
72	( )	Birth control method	( )
		Gynecologic System	
73	( )	Pelvic pain	( )
74	( )	Vaginal discharge	( )
75	( )	Abnormal vaginal bleeding	( )
		A. Menarche: Age ________ yr.	
		B. Menopause: Age ________ yr.	
		C. Menstrual flow, interval: ________ days	
		D. Menstrual flow, duration: ________ days	
		E. Menstrual flow, amount: ________	
		F. Date last menstrual period: ________	
		G. Postcoital bleeding	
		H. Postmenopausal bleeding	
76	( )	Pelvic Mass	( )
	( )	Other	( )
		Sexual History	
77	( )	Sexual difficulties	( )
		Breast	
78	( )	Breast lump	( )
79	( )	Breast pain	( )
80	( )	Nipple discharge	( )
	( )	Other	( )
		Skin	
81	( )	Skin disorder	( )
82	( )	Itching	( )
83	( )	Mole(s)	( )
84	( )	Skin cancer	( )
	( )	Other	( )
		Neurological System	
85	( )	Headaches	( )
86	( )	Epileptic seizures	( )
87	( )	Episodic neurological symptoms	( )
88	( )	Pain/sensory perversions	( )
89	( )	Weakness	( )
90	( )	Head trauma	( )
91	( )	Muscle cramps	( )
92	( )	Stroke	( )
93	( )	Sleep disorder	( )
	( )	Other	( )
		Hematopoietic System	
94	( )	Excessive bleeding/bruising	( )
95	( )	Anemia	( )
96	( )	Pica	( )
97	( )	Family history sickle cell	( )
	( )	Other	( )

	NO		YES
		Musculoskeletal System	
98	( )	Joint stiffness	( )
99	( )	Joint pain	( )
100	( )	Joint swelling	( )
101	( )	Family history musculoskeletal disease	( )
	( )	Other	( )
		Psychiatric	
102	( )	Previous psychiatric problems or hospitalizations	( )
103	( )	Interpersonal relationship difficulties	( )
104	( )	Anxiety	( )
105	( )	Depression	( )
106	( )	Loss of control/violence potential	( )
107	( )	Disturbances of vegetative function	( )
108	( )	Substance abuse	( )
	( )	Other	( )
		Allergies	
109	( )	Drug allergies	( )
	( )	Other	( )
		Immunizations	
110	( )	Past immunizations	( )
		Family History	
111	( )	Heritable disease potential	( )
		Hospitalizations and Medications	
112	( )	Past hospitalizations	( )

Date	Location	Reason

113	( )	Current/recent medications	( )

	Drug (current)	Dose	Frequency		Drug (current)	Dose	Frequency
1.				6.			
2.				7.			
3.				8.			
4.				9.			
5.				10.			

( ) Other history data not included in Data Base Items 1 - 113 ( )

THE PATIENT PROFILE

114 Occupation ______________________________

115 Usual day's activities:

Morning ______________________________

Afternoon ______________________________

Evening ______________________________

116 Hobbies/interests

____

117 Nutritional history

____

____

118 Education:

____

119 Financial difficulties:

____

Other comments relevant to patient profile;

____

THE PHYSICAL EXAMINATION

	NORMAL *		ABNORMAL*
		General	
120	( )	General appearance	( )
121	( )	Temperature (oral ☐ rectal ☐), ______C°	( )
122	( )	Respiratory	( )
		a. Rate: ____/min.	
		b. Rhythm:__________	
123	( )	Pulse	( )
		a. Rate:_____/min.	
		b. Rhythm:___________	
124	( )	Blood pressure:_______/_____ mm Hg	
		If abnormal:	
		a. Leg: ______/_____ mm Hg	
		b. Standing: _______/______ mm Hg	
125a	( )	Height _________ (cm ☐ in ☐)	( )
125b	( )	Weight _________ (kg ☐ lb ☐)	( )
		a. Ideal body weight _____________	
		b. % of ideal body weight _______ %	
126	( )	Body habitus	( )
127	( )	Hair	( )
128	( )		( )
129	( )	Nails	( )
	( )	Other	( )
		Head, Ears, Nose	
130	( )	Cranial/orbital bruit	( )
131	( )	Pinnae/canals/drums	( )
132	( )	Nose	( )
	( )	Other	( )
		Eyes	
133	( )	External eye	( )
134	( )	Fundi	( )
135	( )	Pupil	( )
	( )	Other	( )

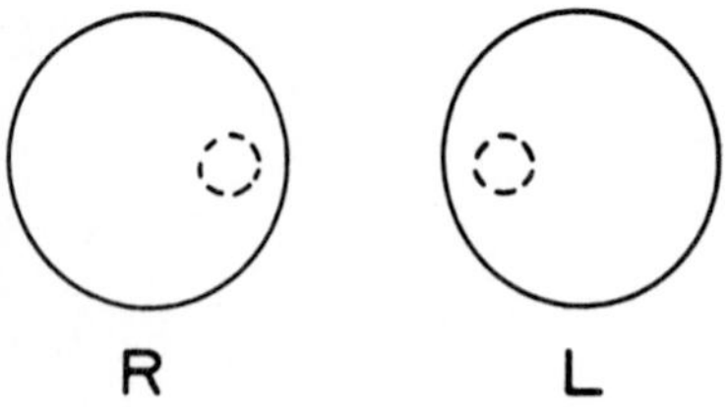

		Oral Cavity	
136	( )	Teeth/gums/oral mucosa	( )
137	( )	Tongue	( )
138	( )	Tonsils/pharynx	( )
139	( )	Parotid enlargement	( )
	( )	Other	( )

NORMAL ABNORMAL

Neck

140 ( ) Inspection ( )
141 ( ) Carotid bruit (R) (L) ( )
142 ( ) Venous hum ( )
143 ( ) Thyroid ( )
( ) Other ( )

Nodes

144 ( ) Lymphadenopathy ( )
If present indicate location:

	R	L
Cervical	a	b
Epitrochlear	c	d
Axillary	e	f
Inguinal	g	h
Other	i	j

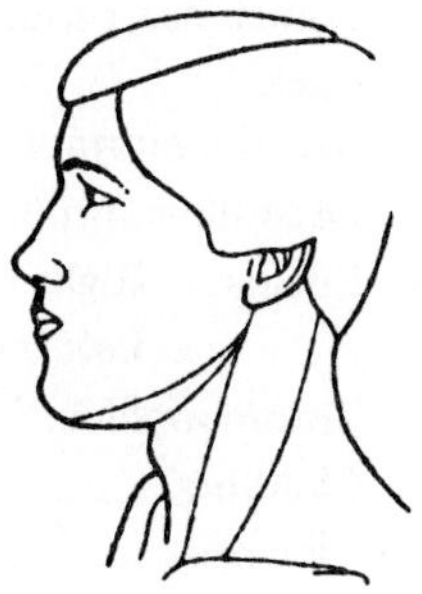

Chest

145 ( ) Chest structure ( )
146 ( ) Chest motion ( )
147 ( ) Chest auscultation ( )
148 ( ) Chest percussion ( )
( ) Other ( )

Breast

149 ( ) Mass ( )
150 ( ) Nipple/areola ( )
( ) Other ( )

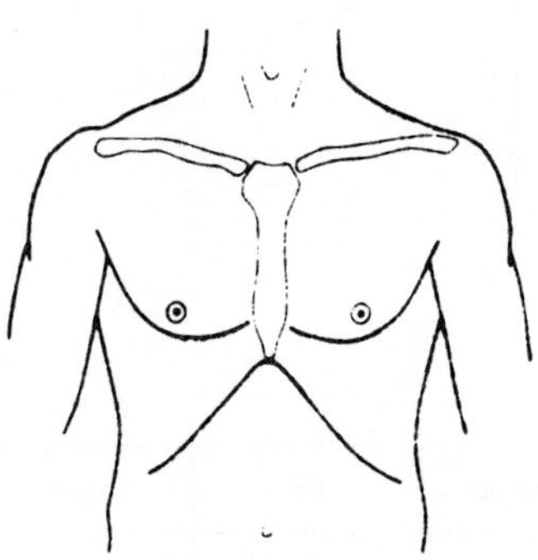

(Anterior)

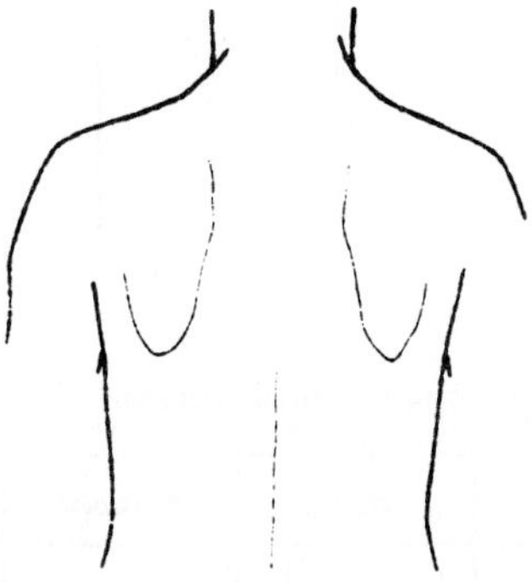

(Posterior)

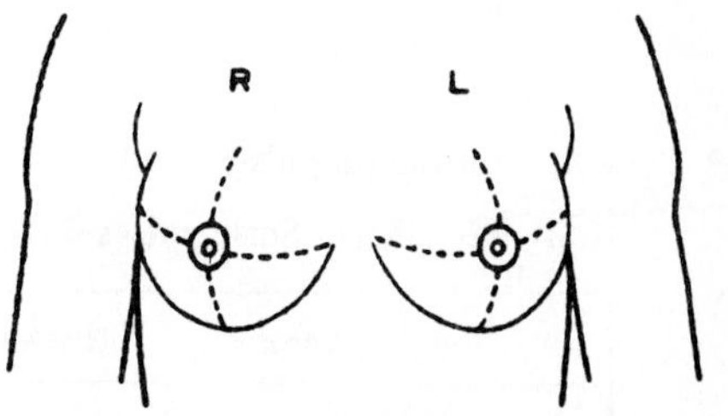

NORMAL — ABNORMAL

Cardiovascular System

151 ( ) Jugular venous pressure: ______cm at ______° ( )
152 ( ) Jugular venous pulsations ( )
153 ( ) Carotid pulse upstroke ( )
154 ( ) Apex impulse ( )
155 ( ) Parasternal impulse ( )
156 ( ) Pulmonary artery pulsation ( )
157 ( ) First heart sound ( )
158 ( ) Second heart sound ( )
159 ( ) Third heart sound ( )
160 ( ) Fourth heart sound ( )
161 ( ) Click ( )
162 ( ) Systolic murmur ( )
163 ( ) Diastolic murmur ( )
164 ( ) Edema: Right leg 1 2 3 4 ( )
Left leg 1 2 3 4
165 ( ) Thrombophlebitis ( )
166 ( ) Clubbing ( )
167 ( ) Cyanosis ( )
168 ( ) Pulsus alternans ( )
( ) ( )

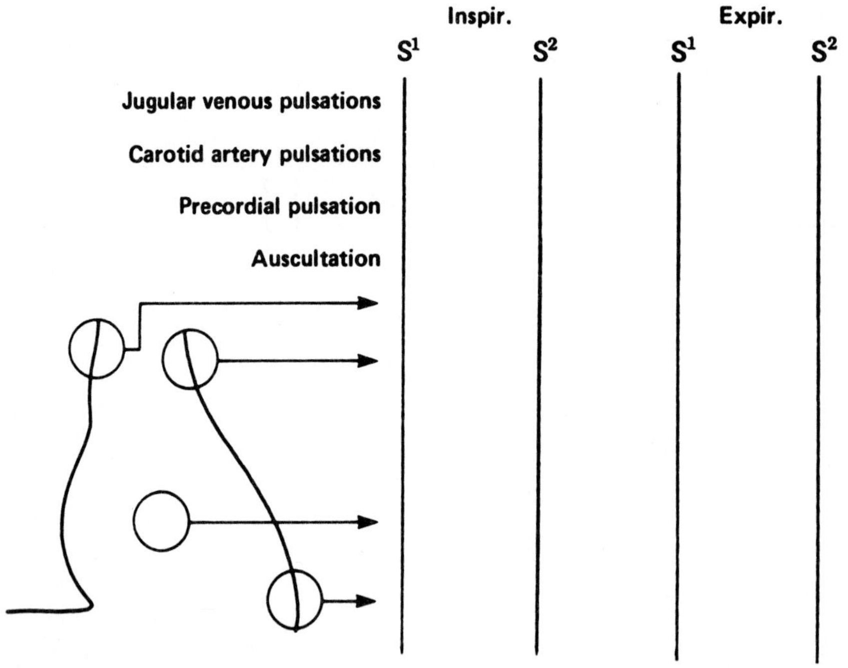

169 ( ) Peripheral pulses/bruits ( )

Complete chart. Scale pulses 0 - 4 (normal = 3) and circle if bruit present.

	Carotid	Brachial	Radial	Aorta	Femoral	Popliteal	PT	DP
Right	a	c	e		h	j	l	n
Left	b	d	f	g	i	k	m	o

	NORMAL		ABNORMAL
		Abdomen	
170	( )	Inspection	( )
171	( )	Auscultation: bowel sounds/bruits/rubs	( )
172	( )	Palpation: pain/tenderness	( )
173	( )	Ascites	( )
174	( )	Liver: auscultation	( )
175	( )	Liver: shape/size	( )
176	( )	Spleen	( )
177	( )	Inguinal canal	( )
	( )	Other	( )

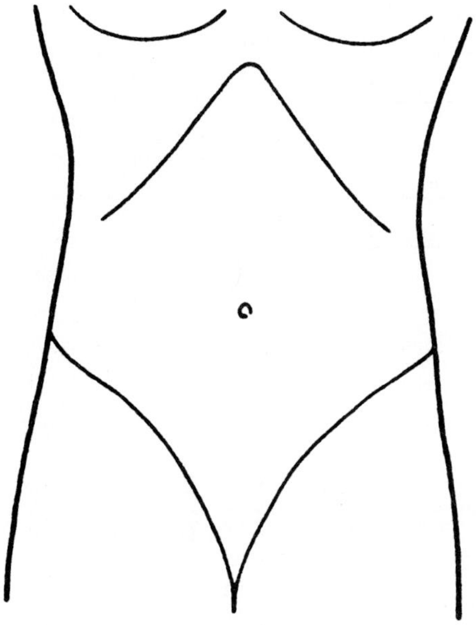

		Male Genitalia	
178	( )	External male genitalia	( )
		Female Genitalia	
179	( )	Pelvic exam:	( )
		Indicate site(s) of abnormality	
		a. External genitalia	
		b. Vagina	
		c. Cervix	
		d. Uterus	
		e. Adnexa	
		f. Pap test: done ☐ not done ☐	
	( )	Other	( )

	NORMAL		ABNORMAL
		Rectal Examination	
180	( )	Rectal: inspection/tone/hemorrhoids	( )
181	( )	Prostate	( )
182	( )	Stool occult blood: ________________	( )
		Musculoskeletal	
183	( )	Musculoskeletal exam:	( )

	R	L
Hands and wrists	a	b
Elbow	c	d
Shoulder	e	f
TMJ	g	h
Cervical spine	i	
Thoracic and lumbar spine	j	
Hip	k	l
Knee	m	n
Foot and ankle	o	p

	NORMAL		ABNORMAL
	( )	Other	( )
		Neurological and Psychiatric	
184	( )	Appearance/affect/motor behavior	( )
185	( )	General intellectual functions	( )
186	( )	Attention span	( )
187	( )	Judgment	( )
188	( )	Abstration	( )
189	( )	Delusions/hallucinations/illusions	( )
190	( )	Associations of thought	( )
191	( )	Orientation	( )
192	( )	Memory	( )
193	( )	Level of consciousness	( )
194	( )	Speech and other lateralizing cortical functions	( )
		Cranial Nerves:	
195	( )	I. Olfactory nerve	( )
196	( )	II. Optic nerve A. Visual acuity B. Visual fields	( )
197	( )	III, IV, VI. Oculomotor, Trochlear and Abducens nerves	( )
198	( )	V. Trigeminal nerve	( )
199	( )	VII. Facial nerve	( )
200	( )	VIII. Acoustic nerve Weber/Rinne tuning fork test	( )
201	( )	IX, X. Glossopharyngeal and Vagus nerves	( )
202	( )	XI. Spinal accessory nerve	( )
203	( )	XII. Hypoglossal nerve	( )

NORMAL ABNORMAL

207 ( ) Sensation: (specify modalities tested) ( )

Upper extremities:

Lower extremities:

208 ( ) Motor system (strength, atrophy, fasciculations, drift, fine movements) ( )

Upper extremities:

Lower extremities:

Gait:

209 ( ) Cerebellum ( )

210 ( ) Involuntary Movements ( )

a. Tremor

b. Chorea

c. Athetosis

d. Myoclonus

e. Asterixis

211 ( ) Suck/snout, grasp reflexes ( )

212 ( ) Deep tendon reflexes ( )

213 ( ) Plantar reflex

Grade 0 - 4 where 4 = repeating clonus; plantar reflex ↑, ↓ or →

	Biceps (C5–6)	Br-Rad (C5–6)	Triceps (C5–7)	FJ (C8T1)	Knee Jerk (L3–4)	Ankle Jerk (S1–2)	Plantar Reflex
Right	a	c	e	g	i	k	213a
Left	b	d	f	h	j	l	213b

Other

( ) Other physical examination data not included in Data Base Items 123 - 213 ( )

THE LABORATORY EXAMINATION

	NORMAL			ABNORMAL
		Hematology		
211	( )	Hematocrit ____________ vol %		( )
212	( )	White blood cell count __________/mm^3		( )
213	( )	Differential: ____ S, ____ L, ____ M, ____ E, ____ B		( )
214	( )	Platelets _____/hpf or _______/mm^3		( )
215	( )	RBC morphology		( )
		Urinalysis		
216	( )	Urine color/odor		( )
217	( )	Urine specific gravity 1.0 ________		( )
218	( )	Proteinuria	1 2 3 4	( )
219	( )	Glycosuria/Ketonuria	G: Neg Tr 1 2 3 4	( )
			K: Neg Tr 1 2 3 4	
220	( )	Urine sediment: ____ wbc/hpf; _____rbc/hpf		( )
		Other: ________________________________		
		Chemistries		
221	( )	BUN	_______mg/dl	( )
222	( )	Glucose: (serum □ plasma □)	_______mg/dl	( )
223	( )	Serum sodium (Na)	_______meq/L	( )
224	( )	Serum potassium (K)	_______meq/L	( )
225	( )	Serum chloride (Cl)	_______meq/L	( )
226	( )	Serum total CO_2 Content (CO_2)	_______meq/L	( )
227	( )	SGOT	_______mu/ml	( )
228	( )	LDH	_______mu/ml	( )
229	( )	Alkaline phosphatase	_______mIu/ml	( )
230	( )	Total bilirubin:		
			_______mg/dl	( )
231	( )	Uric acid	_______mg/dl	( )
232	( )	Creatinine	_______mg/dl	( )
233	( )	Calcium	_______mg/dl	( )
234	( )	Serum inorganic phosphorus	_______mg/dl	( )
235	( )	Cholesterol	_______mg/dl	( )
236	( )	Total protein:	_______gm/dl	( )
	( )	Albumin/globulin	_______/_______gm/dl	( )
		Miscellaneous		
237	( )	Intermediate PPD:_______mm induration		( )
238	( )	VDRL/RPR		( )

NORMAL ABNORMAL

Electrocardiogram

239 ( ) EKG ( )

a. Rate: ______/min. b. Rhythm: ________

Intervals: c. PQ ______; d. QRS ________;

e. QT ________;

f. Interpretation: ______________________________

____

____

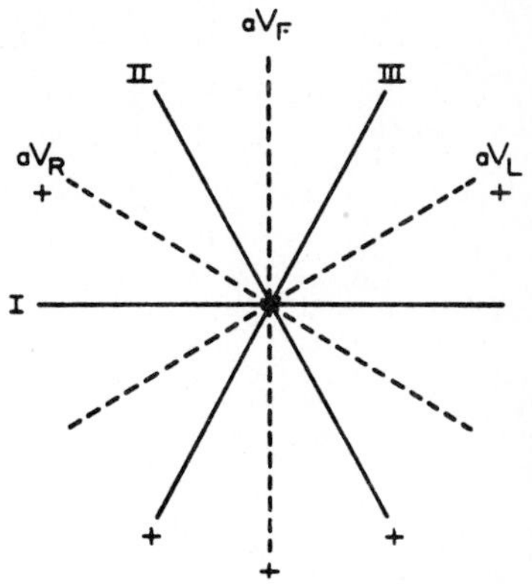

Chest X-Ray

240 ( ) Chest X-Ray ( )

Interpretation: ______________________________

____

____

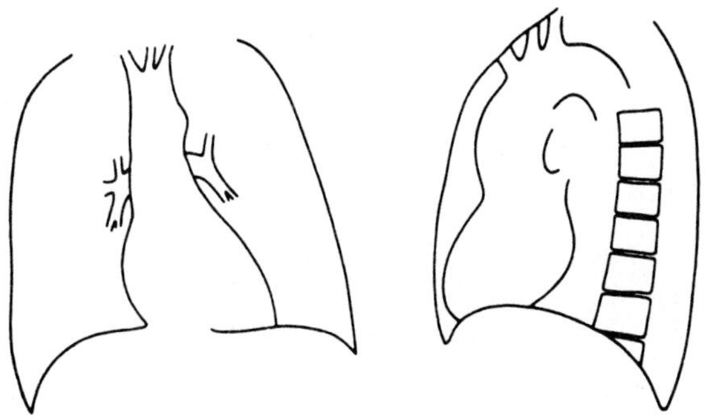

( ) Other laboratory data not included in Data Base Items 211-240. ( )

Signatures indicate agreement with Data Base content. Exceptions and additions should be noted, initialed, and dated on the Data Base.

Signed: ______________________________
Student

____
House Officer

____
Subspecialty Fellow

____
Attending Physician

Index

Page numbers in *italics* refer to illustrations; page numbers followed by the letter "t" refer to tables.

B

C

E

G

H

I

J

K

P

Q

R

S

U

V